Phacoemulsification

System requirement:
- **Windows XP or above**
- **Power DVD player (Software)**
- **Windows media player 11.0 version or above (Software)**

Accompanying Photo CD ROM is playable only in Computer and not in DVD player.

Kindly wait for few seconds for Photo CD to autorun. If it does not autorun then please do the following:
- Click on my computer
- Click the **CD/DVD drive** and after opening the drive, kindly double click the file **Jaypee**

DVD Contents

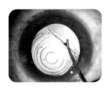
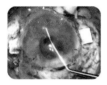
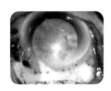
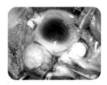
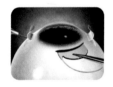
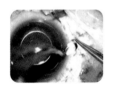
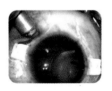
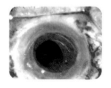

Phacoemulsification

FOURTH EDITION

Editors

Amar Agarwal MS FRCS FRCOphth

Athiya Agarwal MD DO FRSH

Soosan Jacob MS FRCS DNB MNAMS

All of Dr Agarwal's Group of Eye Hospitals & Eye Research Centre
19 Cathedral Road, Chennai, India

Foreword to the First Edition
John J Alpar

Foreword to the Second Edition
Spyros Georgaras

Foreword to the Third Edition
Robert H Osher

Foreword to the Fourth Edition
Thomas John

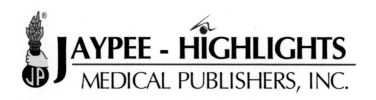

JAYPEE - HIGHLIGHTS
MEDICAL PUBLISHERS, INC.

Jaypee Brothers Medical Publishers (P) Ltd.

Headquarter

Jaypee Brothers Medical Publishers (P) Ltd
4838/24, Ansari Road, Daryaganj
New Delhi 110 002, India
Phone: +91-11-43574357
Fax: +91-11-43574314
Email: jaypee@jaypeebrothers.com

Overseas Offices

J.P. Medical Ltd.,
83 Victoria Street London
SW1H 0HW (UK)
Phone: +44-2031708910
Fax: +02-03-0086180
Email: info@jpmedpub.com

Jaypee-Highlights Medical Publishers Inc.
City of Knowledge, Bld. 237, Clayton
Panama City, Panama
Phone: 507-317-0160
Fax: +50-73-010499
Email: cservice@jphmedical.com

Website: www.jaypeebrothers.com
Website: www.jaypeedigital.com

Inquiries for bulk sales may be solicited at: jaypee@jaypeebrothers.com

This book has been published in good faith that the contents provided by the contributors contained herein are original, and is intended for educational purposes only. While every effort is made to ensure accuracy of information, the publisher and the contributors specifically disclaim any damage, liability, or loss incurred, directly or indirectly, from the use or application of any of the contents of this work. If not specifically stated, all figures and tables are courtesy of the author(s). Where appropriate, the readers should consult with a specialist or contact the manufacturer of the drug or device.

Publisher: Jitendar P Vij
Publishing Director: Tarun Duneja
Editor: Dr Richa Saxena
Cover Design: Seema Dogra

Phacoemulsification

First Edition :   1998
Second Edition :   2000
Third Edition :   2004
Fourth Edition: **2012**

ISBN-13: 978-93-5025-483-7

Printed in India

To

A True Visionary

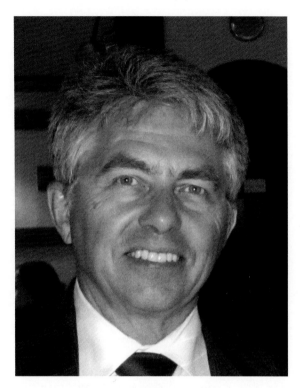

Steve Arshinoff

Contributors

A Beléndez MD
Spain

A Fimia MD
Universidad de Murcia
Murcia, Spain

Abhay R Vasavada MS FRCS
Iladevi Cataract &
IOL Research Centre
Raghudeep Eye Clinic
Gurukul Road, Memnagar
Ahmedabad, India

Alejandro Espaillat MD
ELK County Eye Clinic
765 Johnsonburg Road, St Marys
PA 15857, USA

Amar Agarwal MS FRCS FRCOphth
Dr Agarwal's Group of Eye Hospitals
& Eye Research Centre
19 Cathedral Road, Chennai, India

Ana Claudia Arenas MD
Calle 104 # 46 A 10
Casa 9, Santa Fe De Bogota 8
Colombia

Andrea M Izak MD
40 Bee St # 323
Charleston SC 29403
USA

Aritz Bidaguren
Department of Ophthalmology
Hospital Donostia
Basque Health Service-Osakidetza
Paseo Dr. Beguiristáin, 115
Donostia-San Sebastián, Spain

Ashok Garg MS PhD
Garg Eye Hospital
235, Model Town
Dabra Chowk
Hisar, Haryana, India

AT Gasch MD
Department of Health and
Human Services
Bethesda, USA

Athiya Agarwal MD FRSH DO
Dr Agarwal's Group of Eye Hospitals
& Eye Research Centre
19 Cathedral Road, Chennai, India

Barry S Seibel MD
1515 Vermon Avenue
7th Floor, Station C
Los Angeles, California, USA

Benjamin F Boyd MD FACS
Consultant Editor
Highlights of Ophthalmology
Panama, Rep. of Panama

Bonnie An Henderson MD
Ophthalmic Consultants of Boston
Boston, MA, USA

Brian Little
Moorfields Eye Hospital
London, UK

C González MD
Universidad de Murcia
Murcia, Spain

Carlos F Fernandez
Retina and Vitreous Service
Clinica Oftalmologica Oftalmolaser
Lima, Peru

Charles D Kelman MD
USA

Chi-Chao Chan MD
National Institute of Health
Building 10, Room 10N/206
Bethesda, MD 20892
USA

Christopher Khng MD
Cincinnati Eye Institute
10494 Montgomery Road
Cincinnati, OH 45242, USA

Clement K Chan MD FACS
Medical Director
Southern California Desert Retina
Consultants, M.C.
and Inland Retina Consultants
Palm Springs, California, USA
Associate Clinical Professor
Department of Ophthalmology
Loma Linda University
Loma Linda, California, USA

Cristela F Aleman MD
Director Cataract Department
Director, Clinica Boyd
Panama, Rep. of Panama

Cristina Irigoyen
Department of Ophthalmology
Hospital Donostia
Basque Health Service-Osakidetza
Paseo Dr. Beguiristáin, 115
Donostia-San Sebastián, Spain

David F Chang MD
762 Altos Oaks Drive, Suite 1
Los Altos, CA 94024, USA

David J Apple MD
John A. Moran Eye Center
Department of Ophthalmology and
Visual Sciences, Fifth Floor
University of Utah
50 North Medical Drive
Salt Lake City, Utah-84132, USA

David Meyer MD
Faculty of Medicine
Department of Ophthalmology
Cape Town
South Africa

Dhivya Ashok Kumar MD
Dr Agarwal's Group of
Eye Hospitals & Eye Research Centre
19 Cathedral Road, Chennai
India

Douglas D Koch MD
Department of Ophthalmology
Baylor College of Medicine
Houston, TX, USA

E Villegas MD
Universidad de Murcia
Murcia, Spain

Ellen Anderson Penno MD
Gimbel Eye Centre
Calgary, Alberta
Canada

Enrique Chipont MD
Instituto Oftalmologico De Alicante
Alicante, Spain

Esteban Pertejo-Fernández
Spain

F Mateos MD
Universidad Miguel Hernandez de
Elche, Alicante, Spain

Francisco Contreras-Campos MD
Clinica Ricardo Palma
Av. Javier Prado Este 1038
PISO 10 San Isidro Lima, Peru

Gabor B Scharioth
Germany

Gaurav Prakash
Dr Agarwal's Eye Hospital &
Eye Research Centre
19 Cathedral Road, Chennai
India

Glauco Reggiani Mello
Cole Eye Institute
Cleveland Clinic Foundation
Cleveland OH, USA

Guillermo L Simón-Castellvi
Chief Anterior Segment Surgeon
Refractive Surgery Unit
Simon Eye Clinic, Barcelona, Spain

Hampton Roy MD
Hampton Roy Eye Center
9800 Lile Drive, Suite 660
Little Rock, Arkansas, USA

Howard V Gimbel MD
Gimbel Eye Centre
Suite 450, 4935-40, Avenue N.W.
Calgary, Alberta
Canada T3A 2N1

I Howard Fine MD FACS
Oregon Eye Surgery Center
1550, Oak Street
#5, Eugene, USA

I Pascual MD
Departmet I De Optica
Universidad De Alicante
Apartado 99 E-03080 Alicante
Spain

Issac lipschitz
Israel

J Fernando Arevalo
Retina and Vitreous Service
Clínica Oftalmológica Centro Caracas,
Caracas, Venezuela

Javier Mendicute
Chairman
Department of Ophthalmology
Hospital Donostia
Basque Health Service-Osakidetza
Paseo Dr. Beguiristáin, 115
Donostia-San Sebastián Begitek Clínica
Oftalmológica Plaza Teresa de
Calcuta, 7
20012 Donostia-San Sebastián, Spain

JM Legeais MD PhD
Ophthalmology Department
Hotel Dieu
1 Place Du Parvis Notre Dame
Paris 775181, France

Jonathan H Talamo
Cole Eye Institute
Cleveland Clinic Foundation
Cleveland OH, USA

Jorge L Alio MD PhD
Instituto Oftalmologico De Alicante
Alicante, Spain

José Maria Simón-Castellvi
Chairman
Simon Eye Clinic, Barcelona
Spain

José Maria Simón-Tor
Barcelona, Spain

Kaladevi Satish
Dr Agarwal's Eye Hospital &
Eye Research Centre
19 Cathedral Road, Chennai
India

L Carretero MD
Univerisidad de Alicante
Alicante, Spain

L Samuel Boyd MD
Editor in Chief and Executive Vice
President, Highlights of Ophthalmology
Director
Laser Section, and Associate Director
Retina and Vitreous Department
Clinica Boyd - Ophthalmology Center
Panama, Rep. of Panama

Li Wang MD PhD
Department of Ophthalmology
Baylor College of Medicine
Houston, TX, USA

Liliana Werner MD PhD
John A. Moran Eye Center
Department of Ophthalmology and
Visual Sciences, Fifth Floor
University of Utah
50 North Medical Drive
Salt Lake City, Utah-84132
USA

Louis D "Skip" Nichamin
Nichamin Eye Centre
USA

Luis W Lu MD FACS
Eye Physician and Surgeon Director
Pennsylvania Eye Consultants
Pennsylvania, USA

M Edward Wilson MD
Miles Center for Pediatric
Ophthalmology
Charleston
USA

Mark Packer MD
Oregon Eye Surgery Center
1550, Oak Street, #5 Eugene
Or 97401, USA

Marta Ubeda
Department of Ophthalmology
Hospital Donostia
Basque Health Service-Osakidetza
Paseo Dr. Beguiristáin, 115
Donostia-San Sebastián, Spain

Nick Mamalis
Professor of Ophthalmology
Director, Intermountain Ocular
Research Center
Director, Ocular Pathology
John A. Moran Eye Center
University of Utah
Salt Lake City, Utah , USA

P Klonowski
Spain

Pandelis A Papadopoulos MD PhD FEBO
Director, Ophthalmology Department
Athens Metropolitan Hospital
Director, Diagnostic & Therapeutic Eye
Center Ophthalmo-Check Ltd
General Secretary, Hellenic Society of
Cataract and Refractive Surgery
42, Poseidon Avenue
Paleo Faliro 175 61
Athens, Hellas, Greece

Paul Liebenberg MD
Faculty of Medicine
Department of Ophthalmology
Cape Town
South Africa

R Fuentes MD
Universidad de Alicante
Alicante, Spain

Richard S Hoffman
Oregon, USA

Robert J Weinstock
USA

Roberto Bellucci MD
Camo-Cebtro Ambrosiano
Microchirurgia Oculare
Milano
Italy

Roger F Steinert MD
Professor of Ophthalmology
Professor of Biomedical Engineering
Vice Chair of Clinical Ophthalmology
Director of Cornea, Refractive and
Cataract Surgery, University of
California, Irvine, 118 Med Surge I
Irvine CA, USA

Ronald Kreuger MD
USA

Rupal H Trivedi
Miles Center for Pediatric
Ophthalmology, Storm Eye Institute
Department of Ophthalmology
Medical University of South Carolina
Charleston, SC
USA

Samuel Masket MD
2080, Century Park East
Suite 911, Los Angeles, CA 90067
USA

Sarabel Simón-Castellvi
Simon Eye Clinic
Barcelona, Spain

Shetal M. Raj MS
Iladevi Cataract & IOL Research Centre
Raghudeep Eye Clinic
Gurukul Road, Memnagar,
Ahmedabad, India

Smita Narasimhan
Dr Agarwal's Eye Hospital &
Eye Research Centre,
19 Cathedral Road, Chennai
India

Soosan Jacob MS FRCS DNB MNAMS
Dr Agarwal's Group of Eye Hospitals
& Eye Research Centre
19 Cathedral Road, Chennai
India

Stanley Fuller
Ophthalmic Pathology / Research Fellow
John A. Moran Eye Center
University of Utah
Salt Lake City, Utah, USA

Steve Charles MD
Charles Retina Institute
6401 Poplar Avenue, Suite 190
Memphis, Tennessee, USA

Sunil Thadani MD
Ophthalmic Consultants of Boston
Boston, MA, USA

Sunita Agarwal MS DO FSVH (Germany)
Dr. Agarwal's Eye Hospital
19 Cathedral Road
Chennai-600 086, India
15 Eagle Street, Langford Town
Bengaluru, India

Suresh K Pandey MD
Center for Research on Ocular
Therapeutics and Biodevices
Storm Eye Institute
Charleston, USA

Terence M Devine
Chief of Ophthalmology at the Guthrie
Clinic in Sayre, Pennsylvania
Associate Professor of Ophthalmology
at the State University of New York,
USA

Thomas A Oetting
USA

Tobias Neuhann MD
Founder and Medical Director
Aam Augenklinik AM Marienplatz
Marienplatz 18, Munich, Germany

Uday Devgan MD
Devgan Eye Surgery
11600 Wilshire Blvd, Suite 200
Los Angeles, CA 90025, USA

Vaishali Vasavada
Iladevi Cataract &
IOL Research Centre
Raghudeep Eye Clinic
Memnagar, Ahmedabad, India

Viraj A Vasavada
Iladevi Cataract &
IOL Research Centre
Raghudeep Eye Clinic
Memnagar, Ahmedabad
India

Warren E Hill MD
7525 E Broadway Road
#6 Mesa, AZ 85208-2057
USA

William J Fishkind MD
5599 N. Oracle Rd.
Tucson, Arizona, USA

Yolanda Gallego
Department of Ophthalmology
Hospital Donostia
Basque Health Service-Osakidetza
Paseo Dr. Beguiristáin, 115
Donostia-San Sebastián, Spain

Foreword to the Fourth Edition

Worldwide, seniors are the fastest growing population and this will contribute to continued increase in age-related eye diseases of which cataract is an important clinical entity that all ophthalmologists will be spending a significant segment of their clinical time in the surgical management and postoperative follow-up in the road to postcataract, visual rehabilitation of our patients. Such an age-related segmental increase in population towards the elderly group can be related to the incremental advances in the fields of medicine, science, and technology. According to the United Nation News Center, the world population is expected to surpass 9 billion by the year 2050 from the current 6.7 billion. This population growth is most concentrated in the 60-plus age group according to H Zlotnik, Director, UN Population Division. Due to the high prevalence of cataracts among the aging population worldwide, cataract surgery will continue to dominate the center stage as the most common ophthalmic surgery among general ophthalmologists. As such, cataract surgery will be one of the main surgical revenue sources for the ophthalmic surgeon. It is certainly very timely to introduce the fourth edition of Professor Amar Agarwal's book on *Phacoemulsification* published by Jaypee-Highlights Medical Publishers, a world leader in medical publishing.

Professor Amar Agarwal is a recognized world leader in ophthalmic surgery who has received prestigious awards from leading ophthalmic societies both in India and globally. He has edited numerous textbooks in both medical and surgical aspects of ophthalmology, a true attestation to his continued dedication to ophthalmic education. He is the pioneer of phakonit and microphakonit cataract surgery that focuses on cataract removal using a 0.7 mm phaco tip. He has also contributed to secondary intraocular lens (IOL) implantation using a glued IOL technique. His interests do expand beyond the anterior to posterior segment of the eye with his pioneering surgical

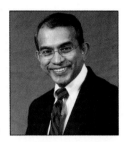

implantation of the new mirror telescopic IOL (LMI) for macular degeneration. He has improved epiretinal membrane visualization during retinal surgery by using intraoperative trypan blue staining technique. Truly, we are all fortunate to have Professor Agarwal bring this latest edition of his surgical textbook on phacoemulsification for us to rely upon to refer and learn both the well-established and the most-advanced techniques, and everything in between, and thus continue to raise our own skill set in the area of cataract surgery to the benefit of our patients.

Professor Amar Agarwal, Athiya Agarwal, and Soosan Jacob have channeled their energies to bring together a group of world leaders in cataract surgery whose cohesive input and countless hours of dedication has resulted in this excellent, current, state-of-the-art cataract surgery book on *Phacoemulsification* which covers all aspects of phacoemulsification from the historic perspective, to phaco-hardware (phaco machines and pumps) and phaco-software (fluidics, software-assisted torsional phaco), viscosurgical devices, surgical techniques, to premium IOLs, complication management, and much more, "all-in-one" comprehensive textbook on *Phacoemulsification*. It is a "one-stop-shopping" approach to learn all aspects of modern-day cataract surgery and hence I recommend this book as a must have surgical textbook for all those interested in cataract surgery from residents in training, to practicing ophthalmologists at all levels of surgical expertise in cataract and IOL surgery. The book should be incorporated in all medical libraries worldwide as an important source of comprehensive information on cataract surgery for all those who have an interest in age-related eye diseases especially, cataract.

Thomas John MD
Clinical Associate Professor
Loyola University at Chicago
Visiting Professor
Department of Defense, MMA, Belgrade
Private Practice in Oak Brook
Oak Lawn and Tinley Park, Illinois
USA

Foreword to the Third Edition

Authoring a medical textbook is a labor of love. For months and months, the act of writing, correcting, rewriting, editing, proofreading, corresponding, negotiating, etc. replaces hobbies and recreational pursuits. Yet when all is said and done, an immense sense of satisfaction embraces the author, who by this time has aged considerably.

The authors of the third edition are to be congratulated for bringing this collaborative work to fruition. The encyclopedic table of contents in combination with an erudite and highly experienced international faculty offer two volumes of information to the reader. Moreover the microphacoemulsification section reflects the leading contribution that Dr. Agarwal's group is making in the evolution toward even smaller incision surgery.

Being on the "cutting edge" can be a mixed blessing, but investing the time and effort necessary to share information is always a rewarding task for those surgeons who have contributed their work. I hope that the reader is also rewarded by becoming a more knowledgeable cataract surgeon after digesting the contents of the third edition of this textbook on phacoemulsification.

Robert H Osher MD
Professor of Ophthalmology
University of Cincinnati
College of Medicine
Medical Director Emeritus
Cincinnati Eye Institute

Foreword to the Second Edition

Dr Amar Agarwal's brilliant mind has captured the idea of presenting the most advanced techniques of Cataract Surgery, at the dawn of the new millennium in this splendid book, *Phacoemulsification, Laser Cataract Surgery and Foldable IOLs*.

The reader can enjoy not only a skilful description of classic cataract surgery, but also Dr Agarwal's great experience, opening new horizons in this field. I wholeheartedly recommend the book and am honored to Foreword this second edition which will almost certainly be as great a success as the first one. I am very proud to share the knowledge arising from Dr Agarwal's book who is one of the leaders in the field of cataract surgery and a great colleague and friend.

Spyros Georgaras MD
President of the
Hellenic Union of Specialized Ophthalmologists
Greek Intraocular Implant and Refractive Surgery Society
Research & Therapeutic Institute "Ophthalmos"
Ophthalmological Center "Hygeia-Ophthalmos"

Foreword to the First Edition

One of the great joys and honors in my life was my frequent visits to India and my meetings with great clinicians, surgeons, teachers and human beings of the Indian ophthalmological community... among them, the wonderful Agarwal family of Chennai. So I am very much honored by their request to write a Foreword to the new book edited and written by them and by other superb surgeons and teachers such as Keiki R Mehta, Mahipal Singh Sachdev, Kenneth J Hoffer, I Howard Fine and all the other internationally known and respected teachers and experts. The table of contents, both concerning the titles of the chapters and the authors, speaks for itself. Some of the world's greatest authorities on the subject, speaking from both scientific and clinical experience, are gracing this book. Every aspect of modern successful cataract surgery is covered, so the book will be extremely useful—not only for the beginners, but also for the accomplished surgeons who need to look at some different points of views and approaches to surgery or for information. The worldwide brotherhood of ophthalmic surgeons, researchers and teachers is deeply and greatly indebted to the editors of the book who assembled the panel and chose the topics and to the writers of the chapters who devoted their time and knowledge to this undertaking. I congratulate and thank the authors and wish them God's blessings.

John J Alpar MD FACS
Clinical Professor at Texas Tech University
Honorary Member of All India Ophthalmological Society

Preface to the Fourth Edition

When the concept of Phacoemulsification was developed by Charles Kelman, it revolutionized cataract surgery but it has today come a long way from where it started. From being essentially a therapeutic procedure for elderly people with cataracts, it has now also come to encompass people of all ages and expectations. With the baby boomer generation coming of age, there is a large population who not only want their cataracts removed but also want it to be done in a faster, better and smarter manner. In keeping with this, there have been huge developments in phacoemulsification in all aspects right from the techniques used to the instruments, machines and intraocular lenses.

Newer machines with enhanced software and hardware features, better power modulation and fluidics are being introduced in a regular manner by the industry. We, as surgeons, also tend to constantly evolve and improve our techniques be it in moving to smaller and smaller incisions utilizing biaxial phaco, microincisional coaxial phaco and so on or in incorporating newer techniques to manage complex situations such as small pupils or subluxated lenses. Add to all this, the desire to regain their youthful vision by the cataract patient – the need to see clearer and sharper for all distances without spectacles has meant a very demanding and aware patient. In response to this, a host of newer intraocular lenses with varying properties for distance, intermediate and near; dark and light have been introduced into the market and it becomes imperative for the surgeon desiring to perform refractive cataract surgery to be aware of the intricacies, potential advantages and disadvantages of all these lenses.

This onslaught of newer information which is required to be engrained into their practice by the cataract surgeon is a daunting task. In an effort to make this easier, we have brought out this fourth edition of *Phacoemulsification*. The entire gamut of cataract surgery right from the basics such as IOL power calculation in simple and complex cases, phaco machine, phaco steps, etc. to advanced phaco such as microincision phaco, challenging cases and premium IOLs to the very recent advances such as femtosecond laser-assisted cataract surgery and 3-dimensional viewing systems for cataract surgery have been covered in detail. We have also included a section on complications as every surgeon needs to know how to manage these undesirable scenarios. The chapters have been written by world renowned authors from an international faculty of cataract experts in an easy-to-understand format. We sincerely hope that this book will serve the reader as an excellent resource material and guide for enhancing his/her cataract practice.

Editors

Preface to the Third Edition

A lot of toil, blood, tears, and sweat has been poured through these pages from so many authors working in so many countries serving so many people. This two volume book on cataract surgery in its most advanced fashion, is an attempt to spread knowledge and letting you know that each one of us believes a much greater force has helped us compile this into fruition.

We may have claimed many a research project, however each one who has done any research knows fully well and can hear fully well that inner voice calling out. Every time we write whether it is for our own gratification or towards a more sublime learning and teaching once again whether we want to accept it or not we know that it is something else that makes us do these things. It is something far more powerful than we can ever imagine that guides our thinking,

our hands, our profession or whatever direction the guide wants us to. And yet there is a choice of free will given to all of us. And yet we choose to burn the midnight oil, we choose to forsake sensual pleasures in a quest of that something that gives us much more peace and understanding of the world, much more joy than owning all the gold in Fort Knox would ever give us.

Here my dear friends is where we are today to say Thank You to the world to the Cosmos to everyone of you who read this and to those who benefit through your reading because this may just be a small drop in the ocean of knowledge, yet it is a small drop in the right direction. In the spirit of serving the human race and all who come after us our attempt is to give them a springboard where they can take off where we have left off.

Editors

Preface to the Second Edition

Coming from a background where ophthalmology ordained the dining table conversation for over seven decades and three generations it is not surprising that the need for revised second edition was thought necessary and mandatory. Especially since our understanding of cataract surgery has been in a perpetually accelerating flux.

Sometimes revelations have been quite by accident however most often progress is steady and slow, depending on many factors like available resources and necessity. The more we read and more we try to assimilate information the more we realize how far we are from the understanding of the topic.

Of late it is difficult to understand progress in the coming years of the new millennium without the assistance and utilization of lasers, computers and advanced technology. More often than nought the space traveler it seems enjoys more information and technological advancements than does the mundane operation theater of medical personnel. However even this equation seems to be changing and much like a science fiction movie our operation theaters reel away progress only thought of to exist in future centuries.

Retaining the same concept of cataract surgery this edition throws much light on the why and wherefores with an insight into the modalities of treatment. Along comes research from the offices of Dr David Apple, a person who has brought glamor into ocular pathology and the understanding of different treatment types, along with Dr SK Pandey have explained the reasons why they have come to a conclusion where there seems to be no difference between intracameral anesthesia, topical anesthesia, and now venturing into new grounds—No anesthesia itself.

However good a surgery comes to nought when plagued with bacterial or microbial invasion, many ophthalmic surgeons have gone through sleepless nights in the pursuit of infection control and its management. This leads us to believe that it was essential to have detailed chapter written on the subject. Much to our chagrin there was hardly any material on the topic of Sterilization. It seems to be we all know about it, understand its importance in the surgical field, yet have never really written about it. The maximum one finds in known literature is something written as a chapter of a microbiology book. Still nothing much from a clinician's point of view, still nothing much in terms of explaining to us what works best, and still nothing more

telling us how to work it. Quoting a cop friend of mine, "An assassin has to be lucky just once, I have to be lucky every day, every instant." In the same light we as surgeons have to be on our guard every time, every instant, the bacteria need be lucky only once. Add to this is sometimes the diplomatic approach of instrument engineers who wave aside grave consequences to patient's wellbeing in the interest of their product image. Sometimes we overlook the obvious, just like we look for the source of light standing right under the sun, similarly the internal tubing of an ultrasound machine that gauges the pressure inside the eye, is actually the prime source of infection in phacoemulsification.

With the Mediterranean influence of L Burrato we have a new chapter on the adversities of a small pupil and still manage to perform phacoemulsification with the greatest of finesse, "Pushing an elephant through a keyhole". Giving importance to Incisions is S Pallin, small steps of the surgery which go a long way in its success. Posterior Polar Cataract has new light from A Vasavada whose immense knowledge on phacoemulsification makes him a leader in this field.

Coupled with this progress is the inroads made by Indian ophthalmology along with Indian engineering and scientific skill that have been displayed for all to see at the pinnacle body internationally as far as cataract and refractive surgery are concerned, the American Society for Cataract and Refractive Surgery (ASCRS) were witness to live surgery telecast from India to America at the 1999 ASCRS meeting. This instruction course made history with it being the first time such an event had occurred and displayed live—No Anesthesia Laser Phakonit (under 1 mm) Cataract Surgery. Thus all that we had written about came to pass when delegates were able to see the surgery in its full form. Such feats would be repeated more often at different meetings since seeing is believing!

As the volume of knowledge has expanded, so too the need for multiple contributors. To strengths of diversity and multiple forms of expertise, this trend has created a burden on the editorial. Thus consistency of writing form is difficult to maintain, however this also adds to the texts' value as a learning and teaching tool. The whole volume of the book has therefore extended and with more color plates and more reading material, we hope dear reader you enjoy reading this as much as we have in writing it!

Editors

Preface to the First Edition

Forewords rarely touch the reader's heart unless the writer sends them out from the same location. That gives us a fighting chance, because we have spent our entire life in the pursuit of ophthalmic sciences and still count this as one of our good friends that always reserves its gratitude and encourages our chances of discovering further and further in its wake.

To write a book today in the world of entertainment with video, movies and the whirlwind of computers seems gratuitous. Still the beauty and magic of reading will never fade and the history of writing that dates back more than 5000 years can never be surpassed. To the memory of the writers of yore and to encourage the many more writers to come, we have taken the task of bringing you the latest synopsis of the trends in cataract surgery through the nineties.

The scientists and researchers of today are full time clinicians who have placed their energy in the development of new ideas. In fact if you go back in time, most discoveries and inventions have been made by the person attempting to correct human malady, and while doing so perchance steps onto some discovery or invention.

It was in this same manner the father of Intraocular lenses while treating pilots from the Royal Airforce during the Second World War came to the conclusion that IOLs were a possibility. He noticed that pieces of windshield material lay immersed in ocular tissue producing no reaction and were transparent and could thus be implanted into the eye (in the place) of spectacles. Dr Harold Ridley thus brought about one of the greatest advancements in this century as far as ophthalmic sciences are concerned. To him and his batch of pioneers, ophthalmology down the ages will always have a place of honor. Salutations to such torchbearers and more to come.

When we look down at the achievements that the human mind has achieved in the realm of ophthalmology and its progress, we are baffled by its enormity especially when we know that there is still so much more to be discovered and so much more to be invented. The scientific progress that has occurred in the last 100 years has bypassed all that could have occurred in the last 5000 years from the Neanderthal cousin of ours, and that which will occur in the next decade itself will be a renaissance in ophthalmology. We still know only a drop in the ocean of the ophthalmic sciences and we realize that what we can dream, we can certainly achieve in the forthcoming years. This book aims at giving you dear Reader not only food

for thought but also in contributing to this Renaissance, thereby, achieving the dreams our forefathers had in this beautiful world of Vision.

Through the reading of this book you will find subjects divided into six basic structures to ease you in the understanding of what cataract and its management mean today. The contributing authors are themselves authorities on the topics of their choice. All stages of learning have been taken care of through these six stages from the learner through the advanced surgeon, bringing you to bear down on mayhap a forgotten episode, for we all know "Trifles make perfection, though perfection is no trifle."

The computer has brought into our world a dream of precision and this has come to become a part of every machinery developed in the modern world. In fact when we look into what "robotics" have done to this factor, we realize we are very close to making the blind man see. Many have been the times that patients have asked their eye surgeon, "Cannot you change my eye itself?" Yes, now we can reply them with the idea of repositioning a video camera and sending the signals into the brain directly. Unthought of till only yesterday, and today will soon be a reality.

A surgeon in the midst of surgery in his or her home town can now think of operating in orbit around the world with a little help from satellites and robotics. Now most distant of patients can get the precise expertise from the dexterous experience of the surgeon. Very soon no one will be bereft of resourceful opinion and/or surgery in this world and that beyond the stars.

Marching towards the next millennium we have accessed cataract surgery with an intraocular lens insertion under the 2 mm mark with the latest "laser cataract surgery," becoming a reality. Coupled with changes in ultrasound technology it will create many newer trends in the years "beyond 2000". Phakonit has brought the incision of cataract surgery to 0.9 mm. Computers and lasers have crossed many marks, and "intrastromal lasers" will soon see the light of the day. Spectacles will not be worn for the want of refractive errors with the latest modalities of the LASIK laser and its contemporaries.

This reading hopes to take you down the lane from humble beginnings of a retrobulbar to peribulbar anesthesia and now to the present exodus of topical anesthesia to the advanced "No anesthesia" ophthalmic surgery, taking its first few steps of infancy in India. After all, have we all not seen sudden injuries to the eye reflecting no pain to the patient? It hopes to give you food for thought and may be rethink the corneal reflex, rethink the anatomy and physiology of the eye itself and delve into the basic sciences of our specialty, "the eye".

It is said that the pen is mightier than the sword (here the surgical knife) and in this case both go hand in hand, and thus, whatever the knife has done the pen has put it down for you to read.

Contributing authors have already left footprints on the sands of time. Let us further your objective in strengthening the armor of ophthalmology.

Editors

Contents

Section 1: Introduction

Section 2: Instrumentation, Medication and Machines

Section 3: Phaco Steps

Section 4: MICS/Phakonit

Section 5: Premium IOLs

Section 6: Difficult Cases

Section 7: Complications

Section 8: IOL Implantation in Eyes Without a Capsule

Section 9: Miscellaneous

SECTION 1

Introduction

CHAPTER 1

Cataract Etiology

David Meyer, Paul Liebenberg

INTRODUCTION

The term cataract is derived from the Latin *cataracta* and from the Greek *katarraktes* which denotes a waterfall or a portcullis. Analogously a cataract is a complete or partial opacification of sufficient severity, on or in the human lens or capsule, to impair vision.

Vision is one of the most valued senses. Proper vision is achieved by a series of eye tissues working harmoniously in concert. Most eye debilities involve dysfunction in the lens or retina, and hence this chapter will focus on and elucidate etiological factors which may affect the proper function of the lens as target organ.

The lens is an elegantly simple tissue. It is made up of only two types of cells.

- *Epithelial cells*, which have not yet completely differentiated and not yet elaborated the major gene products, and
- *Fiber cells*, in which these processes have been initiated or even completed.

Cataract is one of the major causes of visual impairment leading eventually to blindness. In the USA alone 1.35 million cataract extractions are performed annually. In developing countries, the magnitude of the problem is overwhelming.

Management of this age-old impairment of vision requires one of the three following approaches, or a combination of these approaches.

1. Surgical, i.e. extracapsular lens extraction (either manually or by phacoemulsification) and intraocular lens (IOL) implantation;
2. Development and application of drug-related strategies to counteract the development of cataract;
3. Identification and elimination of risk factors.

It is now well-established that cataract formation is a multifactorial disease. Several of the etiological factors are constitutional and hence difficult to manipulate. Others are environmental in nature and a little easier to control whilst a significant number are behavioral in nature and fall well within the individuals' own ability to control or modify.

- This review will briefly touch on congenital and infantile cataract but will focus on etiological factors in adults **(Figure 1.1)** and especially those implicated as risk factors in age-related cataract.

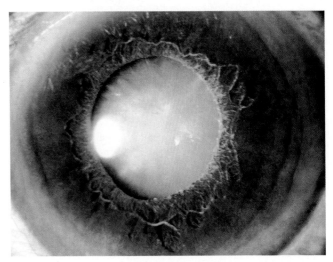

FIGURE 1.1: Mature senile cataract (*Courtesy:* Dr Agarwal's Eye Hospital, India)

CONGENITAL AND INFANTILE CATARACT

Congenital cataract is numerically the most important cause of remediable blindness in children, being far more common than, for example, retinoblastoma or congenital glaucoma.

The prevalence of infantile cataract has been reported to be between 1.2 and 6 cases per 10,000 births. Furthermore, it has been estimated that between 10% and 38.8% of all blindness in children is caused by congenital cataract **(Figures 1.2 to 1.4)** and that one out of

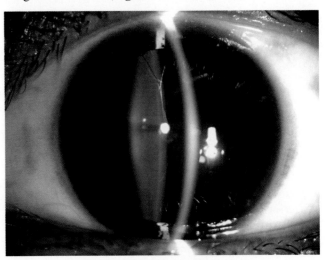

FIGURE 1.2: Anterior polar cataract (*Courtesy:* Dr Agarwal's Eye Hospital, India)

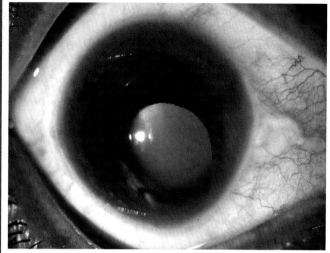

FIGURE 1.3: Brown cataract with iris coloboma (*Courtesy:* Dr Agarwal's Eye Hospital, India)

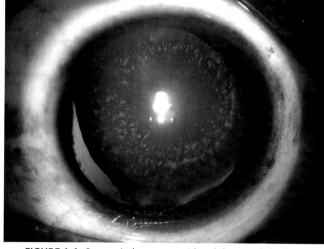

FIGURE 1.4: Congenital cataract with coloboma of the lens (*Courtesy:* Dr Agarwal's Eye Hospital, India)

every 250 newborns (0.4%) has some form of congenital cataract.

The etiology of infantile cataract **(Table 1.1)** can be established in up to one-half of children with bilateral cataract, but in a smaller proportion of infants with unilateral cataract. Infantile cataract most commonly occurs secondary to genetic or metabolic diseases, intrauterine infections or trauma. Less commonly they may occur as a side effect of treatment with certain medications or radiation therapy.

TABLE 1.1 Etiology of infantile cataract

A. Idiopathic	**K. Inherited with systemic abnormalities**
B. Intrauterine infection	• **Chromosomal abnormalities**
1. Rubella	1. Trisomy 21
2. Varicella	2. Turner syndrome
3. Toxoplasmosis	3. Trisomy 13
4. Herpes simplex	4. Trisomy 18
C. Drug induced	5. Translocation 3;4
Corticosteroids	6. Cri-du-chat syndrome
D. Metabolic disorders	7. Translocation 2;14
1. Galactosemia	• **Craniofacial syndromes**
2. Galactokinase deficiency	Cerebro-oculo-facio- skeletal syndrome (COFS)
3. Hypocalcemia	• **Mitochondrial abnormalities**
4. Hypoglycemia	Complex I deficiency
5. Mannosidosis	**L. Skeletal disease**
E. Trauma	1. Smith-Lemli-Opitz syndrome
1. Accidental	2. Conradi syndrome
2. Non-accidental	3. Weill-Marchesani syndrome
F. Miscellaneous	**M. Syndactyly, polydactyl or digital abnormalities**
1. Radiation	1. Bardet-Biedl syndrome
2. Laser photocoagulation	2. Rubinstein-Taybi syndrome
G. Other ocular diseases	**N. Central nervous system abnormalities**
1. Microphthalmia	1. Zellweger syndrome
2. Aniridia	2. Meckel-Gruber syndrome
3. Persistent hyperplastic primary vitreous (PHPV)	3. Marinesco-Sjögren syndrome
4. Prematurity	4. Infantile neuronal ceroid-lipofuscinosis
5. Peters' anomaly	(Batten's disease)
6. Corneal guttata	**O. Dermatological**
7. Endophthalmitis	1. Crystalline cataract and uncombable hair
H. Dental anomalies	2. Cockayne syndrome
1. Nance-Horan syndrome	3. Rothmund-Thomson syndrome
I. Cardiac disease	4. Atopic dermatitis
Hypertrophic cardiomyopathy	5. Incontinentia pigmenti
J. Renal disease	6. Progeria
1. Lowe syndrome	7. Ichthyosis
2. Hallermann-Streiff-Francois syndrome	8. Ectodermal dysplasia

GENETIC

Infantile cataract may be inherited as autosomal dominant, autosomal recessive or X-linked recessive traits. Autosomal dominant cataracts are most commonly bilateral nuclear opacities, but marked variability can be present even within the same pedigree. In an extended pedigree of 28 patients with autosomal dominant nuclear cataract, Scott et al reported that 19 of the affected family members had unilateral cataract while 9 had bilateral cataract. Less commonly, anterior polar, posterior polar, and posterior lentiglobus cataract can be autosomal dominantly inherited. In the United States, infantile cataracts are most commonly inherited as autosomal dominant traits, however, in countries where there is a high prevalence of parental consanguinity, infantile cataracts are more commonly inherited as autosomal recessive traits. In Egypt, where one-third of all marriages are consanguineous, Mostafa et al reported autosomal recessive inheritance for six of seven pedigrees with inherited infantile cataract. Linkage analysis has been used to determine the genetic loci of certain autosomal dominant cataract. Coppock-like cataract has been linked to the gamma E-crystalline gene on chromosome 2, Coppock cataract to chromosome 1q21-q25, Marner cataract to 16q22, and cerulean cataract to 17q24. The Cerulean cataract links closely to the galactokinase gene, but galactokinase levels in these patients are normal.

METABOLIC

The most common metabolic disturbance causing cataract during infancy is galactosemia. Galactosemia may be caused by a transferase, galactokinase or epimerase deficiency. Galactose-1-phosphate uridyl transferase (GALT) deficiency occurs in 1:40,000 newborns in the United States and 1:23,000 newborns in Ireland. A homozygous mutation of Q188R on exon 6 of the GALT gene on chromosome 9 is found in two-thirds of children with the transferase deficiency. This results in the accumulation of galactose 4-phosphate in the blood. Galactose is then converted to galactitol in the crystalline lens, resulting in an influx of water into the lens by osmosis. The hydration of the lens then disrupts the normal structure of the lens fibers, resulting in a loss of transparency. Early on, these lens changes have the appearance of an oil-droplet in the center of the lens. These changes are initially reversible with the elimination of galactose from the diet. If left untreated, a lamellar cataract develops which may then progress to a total cataract. In addition to cataract, these children have failure to thrive as infants, which may lead to death if milk and milk products are not eliminated from their diet. Later in childhood, these children may have delayed development, abnormal speech, growth delay, ovarian failure and ataxia. While eliminating galactose from the diet can prevent the life-threatening problems which occur during infancy, dietary compliance does not always correlate closely with the formation of cataract in later childhood or with the associated abnormalities of late childhood. The N314D

mutation of the GALT gene causes the milder Duarte form of galactosemia. Combinations of Q188R, N314D and unknown mutations may result in phenotypically different forms of galactosemia.

Galactokinase deficiency may cause cataract with few or no systemic abnormalities. The galactokinase gene is on chromosome 17 and has recently been cloned and found to harbor homozygous mutations in some patients with cataract. Heterozygotes for galactokinase deficiency have half normal values on blood tests. Conflicting results have been reported in the literature as to whether partial loss of enzyme activity leads to presenile cataract. Alpha manno-sidosis can also be associated with early onset cataract.

Lamellar cataract may also develop in children with neonatal hypoglycemia or hypocalcemia. Neonatal hypoglycemia is more common in low birth weight infants.

INFECTIOUS

The congenital rubella syndrome was one of the most common causes of congenital cataract in the United States until the widespread employment of the rubella vaccine. During the rubella epidemic in the United States during 1963-64, 16% of all children with the congenital rubella syndrome developed cataract. Infantile cataract also occurs occasionally in children after intrauterine varicella, toxoplasmosis and herpes simplex infections, or after bacterial or fungal endophthalmitis. Cataract may also develop after a varicella infection during early childhood.

PREMATURITY

Transient cataract occurs occasionally in premature infants. They are usually bilateral and begin as clear vacuoles along the apices of the posterior lens suture. They may progress to posterior subcapsular vacuoles. In most cases, they clear completely over the course of several months. All of the premature infants with transient cataract reported by Alden et al were septic and had been treated with Kanamycin, 80% of these infants also had an unexplained metabolic acidosis. These authors suggested that osmotic changes in the lens of these infants might have caused these cataract.

TRAUMA

While trauma is not a common cause of cataract during infancy it should be considered, particularly when a cataract is associated with other ocular signs suggestive of a traumatic injury. The trauma can be either blunt or penetrating. Nonaccidental causes for the trauma must always be considered. Eyes with suspected traumatic cataract should also be examined carefully for both retinal and optic nerve injuries.

LASER PHOTOCOAGULATION

Laser photocoagulation has been used in recent years to ablate the avascular retina of infants with threshold retinopathy of prematurity (ROP). Laser-induced cataracts are transient in some instances, but progress in some cases to total opacification of the lens. Drack et al reported cataract in six eyes following argon laser photoablation of the avascular retina in four infants with threshold retinopathy of prematurity.

RADIATION INDUCED

Radiation used to treat ocular and periocular tumors may induce cataract in children. A radiation dose of 15 Gy has been shown to be associated with a 50% risk of cataract formation. Radiation usually causes posterior subcapsular cataract, which typically have their onset 1 to 2 years after the completion of radiation therapy.

MEDICATIONS

Systemic corticosteroids cause cataract in up to 15% of children once a cumulative dose of 1000 mg of prednisone or the equivalent has been reached. This cataract usually begins as central posterior subcapsular opacities, but may progress to involve the entire lens.

IDIOPATHIC

In most series, at least 50% of bilateral infantile cataracts are idiopathic. The percentage of idiopathic unilateral infantile cataract is even higher.

AGE-RELATED CATARACT

PERSONAL FACTORS

Gender

It has often been observed that more females than males have cataract and undergo cataract surgery. This is partly explicable by the longer life span of women and therefore their over-representation in the age groups where cataract is most common. It does appear, however, that there is an additional effect—a true excess risk of cataract in females. In Nepal the prevalence of cataract was greater in females than in males at all ages. The overall risk ratio was 1.4, which would be detectable only in larger studies. In most case-control studies, the two groups were age- and sex-matched so that the effect of sex could not be explored. Hiller et al had to combine the results from three earlier studies in the United States and India to find a significant excess relative risk of 1.13 in females. This follow-up study of data from the National Health and Nutrition Examination Survey (NHANES) also suggested that such an excess risk for women is specific to cortical cataract. In a population-based prevalence survey in Beaver Dam, Wisconsin, women had more cortical opacities compared to men within similar age groups. The Beaver Dam Study reported a protective effect for nuclear opacities with current use of postmenopausal estrogens. Older age at menopause was associated with decreased risk of cortical opacities, suggesting hormonal influences in cataractogenesis. It was also suggested that hormone replacement therapy (HRT)

may protect against cortical cataract. The Epidemiology of Cataract in Australia study found that a protective relationship of HRT and cortical cataract exists at the univariate level, but that this relationship was not significant in multivariate analysis. Nuclear cataract cases were more likely to be female in the above study, even after age adjustment. They were, however, unable to support the hypothesis that HRT is protective against nuclear cataract.

Tavani et al studied 287 Italian women who had undergone cataract extraction and 1277 control subjects who were in the hospital for acute, nonneoplastic, nonophthalmologic, nonmetabolic, nongastroenterologic diseases in a case-control study in Northern Italy. The results of this study support the association in women between cataract extraction and diabetes, (OR 4.6 for those younger than 60 years and 1.7 for those age 60 and over) current overweight, (OR 2.2) history of clinically relevant obesity, (OR 1.5) hypertension(OR 1.5) and hyperlipidemia (OR 1.8). They suggest that these factors may have some biologically independent impact on the risk of cataract in women and therefore support the association in women between cataract extraction on the other hand and diabetes, current overweight, history of clinically relevant obesity, hypertension and hyperlipidemia on the other.

Body Mass Index

Body mass index (BMI) is computed as weight in kilograms divided by the square of the height in meters (kg/m²) and is frequently identified as a risk factor for cataract, but the nature of the association is unclear. Several mechanisms may play a role:
- BMI affects glucose levels, which are associated with increased risk of cataract
- Higher BMI also increases uric acid concentrations and the risk of gout, which were associated with cataract in some studies
- BMI is also an important determinant of hypertension which has a controversial relationship with cataract.

Experimental evidence also supports a possible protective effect of restriction of energy intake on the risk of cataract by protection against oxidative stress to the lens.

In developing countries, some studies have associated low BMI with cataract. A recent case control study in India, however, failed to confirm this association.

Hankinson et al in a prospective study examined the association of BMI with cataract extraction in a large cohort of women and found elevated rates of cataract in those with higher BMI. Women with BMI of 23 or above had significantly elevated rates of extraction, between 46% and 65% higher than those with BMI of less than 21. Glynn et al in a prospective cohort study of a total of 17,764 apparently healthy US male physicians aged 40 to 84 years who were free of cataract at baseline were followed for 5 years. In this group higher BMI was especially strongly related to risk of posterior subcapsular and nuclear sclerotic cataract and was also significantly related to risk of cataract extraction. Furthermore, BMI below 22 appeared especially protective against posterior subcapsular cataract, with reductions in risk of 50% or more relative to each of the groups with a higher BMI. They concluded that BMI appears to be a strong and independent risk factor for cataract in this well-nourished and socioeconomically homogeneous study population. Even modest elevations in weight were associated with increased risk.

In so far as BMI index is modifiable, cataract caused by overweight is therefore potentially preventable.

Social Economic Status

Less education and lower income are related to increased morbidity and mortality from a number of diseases, even after controlling the known risk factors. These relations have been attributed to underuse of health care resources, high-risk behaviors, exposure to noxious work or adverse home environment, and poor nutrition. In population studies, less education and lower income consistently have been associated with impaired vision and cataract. The relationship of education, income, marital status, employment status to age-related cataract and impaired vision was addressed in the population-based Beaver Dam Eye Study.

A private census of the population of Beaver Dam, Wisconsin, was performed from September 15, 1987 to May 4, 1988. Eligibility requirements for entry into the study included living in the city or township of Beaver Dam and being 43 to 84 years of age at the time of the census. A total of 5924 eligible people were identified. Of these, 4926 (83.1%) participated in the examination.

While controlling for age and sex in this study, less education was significantly (P< 0.05) related to higher frequency of nuclear sclerotic and cortical cataract. Lower reported total household income was significantly associated with higher frequen-cies of cortical and posterior subcapsular cataract. These relations between total household income and cataract were observed in both men and women.

Less education has been associated with higher frequencies of history of heavy drinking, cigarette smoking and less vitamin supplement intake, all of which have been found to be related to specific types of cataract. However, the association of education and income with cataract persisted, despite controlling these exposures in their population. It is possible that poorer nutrition occuring earlier in life, may be related to the development of age-related cataract. A second possible reason explaining the relation of education and income to cataract is that people with less education or lower income are less likely to see an ophthalmologist or have cataract surgery.

Marital status is a measure of social support which is postulated to be an important factor in developing and managing complications associated with disease. While controlling for age and sex, people who were never married had a higher frequency of impaired vision than those currently married. This may be due to the fact that married people may have more social pressure to seek health care and to maintain familial responsibilities, and they may have more transportation assistance than their unmarried/widowed counterparts.

In summary, less education and income are related to cataract and visual impairment, but not to age-related maculopathy. These data suggest that access to medical, surgical, and low vision care may be of benefit to people with low socioeconomic status.

SOCIAL FACTORS

Smoking

Tobacco is the leading preventable cause of disease, disability and premature death.

Tobacco smoking is considered a major risk factor for 6 of the 15 leading causes of death. An individual who smokes has about twice the risk of premature death as a non-smoker, and the heavier the cigarette consumption, the higher the risk.

Of the 4,000 active substances in tobacco smoke, most are hazardous to human health. More than 40 of these chemicals are carcinogens and many others are deleterious to the cardiovascular and the pulmonary systems. They include nicotine, tars, nitrosamines, polycyclic aromatic hydrocarbons, hydrogen cyanide, formaldehyde, and carbon monoxide. Cigarette smoking is also a substantial source of intake of heavy metals and toxic mineral elements, such as cadmium, aluminum, lead, and mercury, all known to be poisonous in high concentrations.

Tobacco smoke also contains numerous compounds with oxidative properties; their existence is linked to the pathogenesis of several of the most common eye disorders, such as cataract and age-related macular degeneration.

Epidemiological data link cigarette smoking to several ophthalmologic disorders like ocular irritation, ocular ischemia, age-related macular degeneration (AMD), cataract, thyroid ophthalmopathy, tobacco-alcohol amblyopia, primary open-angle glaucoma, conjunctival intra-epithelial neoplasia, uveal melanoma, Leber hereditary optic neuropathy, type II diabetes, ocular sarcoidosis and strabismus in the offspring of smoking mothers. The effects of smoking on ocular disorders show significant dose dependence; higher levels of smoking increase the risk of developing cataract. It is important to note, however, that the interpretation of results of different studies may be inherently biased, as smokers in these studies use cigarettes of different types, containing different concentrations of toxic substances. Moreover, some of the cigarettes have filters and others do not. Smoking habits may also be associated with other potentially noxious habits, such as excessive alcohol consumption, which may contribute a further bias to the results.

Table 1.2 summarizes five very thought-provoking studies all supporting the view that smoking is associated with the development of cataract.

Several authors have reported a significant link between tobacco smoking and an increased risk of cataract

TABLE 1.2	Smoking and the risk of cataract		
Study	**Relative risk (RR)**	**95% CI**	**Comments**
Leske *et al*, 1991	1.68	0.96-1.94	Association was found to nuclear cataract
Hankinson *et al*, 1992	1.63	1.8-2.26	Conducted on 50,828 women; RR for developing posterior subcapsular cataract is 2.59
Christen *et al*, 1992	2.16	1.46-3.20	N = 22,071 males; RR for nuclear cataract is 2.24 and for posterior subcapsular, 3.17
Klein *et al*,1993	1.09	1.04-1.16	Beaver Dam Eye Study; same RR for women and men
West *et al*,1995	2.40	1.00-6.00	Conducted on 442 watermen of the Chesapeake Bay

development. Nuclear sclerosis appears to be the type of cataract most commonly associated with smoking.

In the Beaver Dam Eye Study, the relationship between cigarette smoking and lens opacities was examined in 4926 adult subjects. A significant correlation was found between severe levels of nuclear sclerosis and the number of pack-years smoked. For both sexes, the odds ratio associated with 10 years was 1.09 (confidence interval, 1.04–1.16). The frequency of posterior subcapsular opacities was also increased (odds ratios, 1.05 [confidence interval, 1.00–1.11] for men and 1.06 [confidence interval, 0.98–1.14] for woman). Cortical opacities were not found to be linked to smoking. Leske et al studied, 1380 patients with cataract, aged 40 to 79 years, in an attempt to identify possible risk factors for the development of cataract, current smoking was correlated with the risk of developing nuclear cataract (odds ratio, 1.68; confidence interval, 0.96–1.94), but not other forms of cataract. The City Eye Study reported epidemiological data concerning 1029 volunteers, aged 54 to 65 years, from London, UK. The findings showed a significant relationship between nuclear lens opacities and moderate to heavy cigarette smoking. The relative risk for nuclear-type cataract ranged from 1.0 for past light smokers to 2.6 for past heavy smokers, and 2.9 for current heavy smokers.

Klein et al presented evidence that smoking has a detrimental effect on the development of cataract in the type II diabetic population.

Several prospective studies have investigated the relationship between cataract formation and cigarette smoking. In an 8-year prospective study, Hankinson et al examined the association between cigarette smoking and the risk of cataract extraction in 50,828 female nurses aged 45 to 67 years. The age-adjusted relative risk among female smokers of at least 65 pack-years was 1.63 (confidence interval, 1.18–2.26).

Smoking was also strongly associated with posterior subcapsular opacities for smokers of 65 or more pack-years (relative risk 2.59). In a 5-year prospective study of 22,071 men aged 40 to 84 years, current smokers of at least 20 cigarettes a day showed a significantly increased risk of developing cataract (relative risk 2.16; confidence interval, 1.46–3.20). When calculated for the different types, the relative risk was 2.24 for developing nuclear sclerosis and 3.17 for posterior subcapsular cataract. Past smokers were also at increased risk of developing posterior subcapsular opacities (relative risk 1.44), whereas current light smokers had the same chance of developing any type of cataract as subjects who had never smoked. In a study of 838 watermen from Chesapeake Bay, Maryland, West et al found a significantly increased risk of development of nuclear opacities associated with cigarette smoking (relative risk 2.40; confidence interval, 1.00–6.00).

A 5-year prospective study of this cohort of subjects reported an increase in the incidence and degree of nuclear opacities with increasing age. The risk of progression of nuclear opacities from less than grade 3 at baseline to grade 3 or worse was 2.4-fold higher among current smokers than among ex-smokers or non-smokers.

A significant increase (18%) in the risk of cataract progression was associated with each pack-year that a subject had smoked during the 5-year study period.

Mechanism The way in which smoking induces cataract formation is probably through its effect on the oxidant-antioxidant status of the lens. Oxidative damage plays a major role in cataractogenesis. Animal, laboratory, clinical, and epidemiological data support the relationship between cataract prevention and diets rich in nutritional factors with antioxidant properties, such as riboflavin, vitamins C and E, and the carotenoids.

Smoking appears to further impair lenticular function by imposing an additional oxidative challenge as well as by contributing to the depletion of endogenous anti-oxidant pools. Tobacco smoke also contains large amounts of heavy metals, such as cadmium, lead and copper, which appear to accumulate in the lens and exert further toxicity.

The above data strongly support an association between tobacco smoking and cataract formation. Given the magnitude and seriousness of the cataract problem, an important preventive measure in fighting this disorder is to quit smoking. It is important to note that smoking is on the increase in the developing world, where cataract surgery is not always readily available.

Alcohol

Excessive alcohol use is associated with numerous chronic health problems, such as liver disease, varicosities, blood dyscrasias, and elevated blood pressure. Some studies have reported a relationship between alcohol consumption and cataract, while other studies have found no relationship. One study reported that both abstainers and heavy drinkers were more likely to have cataract than moderate users, while another found that total abstainers were more likely to have cataract than alcohol users.

As far back as 1973 Sabiston clinically observed in 40 patients over a 5-year period a definite correlation between alcohol intake, Dupuytren's contracture, and cataract. He stated that the mechanism of cataract formation was uncertain, but that an element of chronic dehydration was possible. In New Zealand, where he did his observations, heavy drinking often commenced with the ingestion of large quantities of beer. The national average consumption of beer there is 100 liters per head annually, with manual laborers ingesting a daily total of 4 liters of beer per person per day on average. These persons were almost invariably heavy cigarette smokers as well. He further noted that the cataract commenced in a posterior subcapsular position, and could progress to almost full maturity in six months. There was almost universally a history of heavy cigarette smoking as well. Malnutrition was only sometimes seen.

Drews in 1970 also drew attention to the association of ethanol and cataract. Two decades later he writes: "A patient in his or her 40s or 50s who appears with a posterior subcapsular cataract should be investigated for alcoholism…In the author's practice, about 25% of patients younger than age 65 years who present with cataract are found to be alcoholic on careful investigation. It has been his experience that if the opacities are incipient and if the consumption of alcohol is stopped completely, the posterior subcapsular changes may reverse and even disappear."

Two decades later attention is once again drawn to the possible link between alcohol and cataract in the Archives of Ophthalmology by two different sets of authors. Munoz et al from the Wilmer Eye Institute, Baltimore, MD, USA conducted a follow-up study of surgical cases of posterior subcapsular cataract (PSC) and their controls to evaluate the possible association of alcohol intake and posterior subcapsular opacities. Two hundred thirty-eight cases and controls were interviewed. Current alcohol intake and usual and maximum weekly consumption ever were assessed. In this population, 57% of the cases and 56% of the controls were nondrinkers, 22% of the cases and 36% of the controls had an average of seven or fewer drinks per week, and 17% of the cases and 8% of the controls had more than seven drinks per week. Heavy drinkers were more likely to be cases than were nondrinkers (odds ratio, 4.6; $P<0.05$), and light drinkers were not at an increased risk. Light drinkers, defined as those who drink less than 91 g/wk (i.e. one drink or less per day), were at a lower risk than were nondrinkers, although this difference did not reach statistical significance. Moderate to heavy drinkers, that is, those drinking an average of more than one drink per day (more than 91 g/wk) were 2.7 times more likely to have PSC. This U-shaped relationship between alcohol and the risk of PSC was more pronounced in the logistic regression model when controlling for all the factors found to be related to PSC. Some studies have suggested that heavy drinking patterns are associated with lower socioeconomic status. In this study after adjustment for education level, the risk of PSC was still higher among drinkers. Smoking was also not related to PSC. Heavy alcohol use has been linked to poor nutritional status, so the presence of PSC may be related to poor nutrition rather than alcohol consumption *per se*. Dietary assessment however, was not performed in this study. In summary, this study concluded that moderate to heavy alcohol consumption is associated with a four-fold increase of PSC cataract whereas light drinkers, those consuming one drink per day or less, were not at an increased risk.

The second study reported in the same journal was on alcohol use and lens opacities in the Beaver Dam Eye Study group of patients. The relationship between alcohol use and lens opacities was examined in a large (N = 4926) population-based study of adults. Alcohol history was determined by a standardized questionnaire and the cataract severity was determined by masked grading of photographs obtained using a slit lamp camera and retroillumination. Several significant findings were made and conclusions drawn:

- In both sexes and every age group, a higher percentage of current heavy drinkers had late nuclear sclerotic changes. Similar results were seen for cortical and PSC changes.
- Past heavy drinkers were found to have increased odds of nuclear sclerosis (OR, 1.34; 95% confidence interval [CI], 1.12 to 1.59). There was an additional significant effect of past heavy drinking on the severity of cortical opacity (OR, 1.36; 95% CI, 1.04 to 1.77). The presence of posterior subcapsular opacity was also significantly associated with past heavy drinking (OR, 1.57; 95% CI, 1.10 to 2.25).

- Wine was associated with less severe nuclear sclerosis (OR, 0.84; 95% CI, 0.74 to 0.94) in general. Participants who drank liquor were less likely to have severe nuclear sclerosis than those who did not (OR, 0.81; 95% CI, 0.72 to 0.95). Liquor use was also associated with lower frequencies of any cataract (OR, 0.83; 95% CI, 0.72 to 0.94) and fewer past cataract surgeries (OR, 0.75; 95% CI, 0.57 to 0.98).

- A significant relationship was found between beer consumption and cortical cataract. Those who drank larger amounts of beer were more likely to have cortical cataract than those who drank smaller quantity of beer. An increased risk of cortical cataract was associated with increased beer consumption. An increased risk of cortical cataract was not associated with consumption of wine, hard liquor, or a combination of alcohol types when considered as continuous variables. These different relationships for the different types of alcohol (wine and hard-liquor consumption was generally associated with OR's or less than 1, while beer consumption was associated with OR's of more than 1) raises the possibility that other components of wine or hard liquor confer protective effects on cataract development. However, no such theoretical links have yet been established.

Alcohol has many metabolic effects, and modifies the absorption of drugs and dietary components. These effects may be important in the alcohol-cataract relationship. However, one cannot exclude the possibility that alcohol itself, especially when consumed in high volume, may be a direct toxin to the human phacos.

METABOLIC FACTORS

Diabetes Mellitus

Juvenile diabetic cataract classically known as the "snow flake cataract" is now uncommon with the advent of effective hypoglycemic therapy. It occurs in insulin-dependent diabetics whose onset was before the age of 30. The limited period over which snow flake cataract may occur (chiefly in the first two decades of life) contrasts with the extended period over which lenticular change occurs (from youth into the eighth decade). It is of interest that snow flake cataract occurs at a period of life when the lens is undergoing a major physiological shape change, with negligible sagittal and major equatorial expansion. It may very well be that the mechanisms for refractive change and cataract are the same but age-related factors such as the decreasing ability of the lens to swell may protect the older lens from this type of cataract formation. Other typical features of this type of cataract are subcapsular and cortical "snow flakes", and polychromatic opacities and vacuoles **(Figure 1.5)**. These may proceed to mature cataract within weeks or months and rarely, may be reversible after normalization of blood glucose over some weeks or even as rapidly as 24 hours.

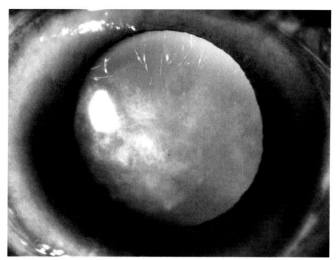

FIGURE 1.5: Diabetic mature cataract (*Courtesy:* Dr Agarwal's Eye Hospital, India)

The rat sugar cataract model is an attractive model for juvenile diabetic cataract in terms of its acute development and other features. It is also relevant to human galactosemic cataract, in which the lens is exposed to high levels of aqueous galactose. The first visible indication of galactosemic cataract is the "oil-droplet" change on retroillumination, due to a change in refractive index between the inner and outer parts of the lens.

It has been noted that there are difficulties in accepting a role of aldose reductase in human cataract. Even though sorbitol is found in increased amount in the human diabetic lens, the amounts detected have been quite low, and insufficient on a lens mass basis to account for osmotic damage.

Data on a cell-to-cell basis, which would be appropriate, are not available.

Although Vadot and Guibal considered that there was sufficient sorbitol in young diabetic lenses to induce cataract, Lerman and Moran could not demonstrate the accumulation of significant amounts in sugar-incubated lenses over the age of 20 years. There is no information about levels in juvenile diabetic cataract itself. Jedziniak et al found a higher aldose reductase activity in the young lens than in the adult lens and calculated that it was sufficient to generate a significant osmotic stress. However, these calculations referred to the lens epithelium and assumed that sorbitol was not removed. Since polyol dehydrogenase is more active than aldose reductase in the human lens, the calculated levels would be expected to be lower. Lin et al demonstrated accumulation of dulcitol and loss of myoinositol in 72-hour cultures of infantile human lens epithelium in a 30 mlQI galactose medium, associated with vacuolar changes at ultrastructural level. Sorbinil and AL1576 reversed these changes. Similar changes have been produced in dog epithelial culture within 6 hours. Lin et al suggest that damage in the human lens may reflect compartmentalization of aldose reductase activity, for instance in the epithelium. If sorbitol accumulation in the epithelium (and not the fibers) were the basis of juvenile cataract, then a failure of epithelial permeability or pumping functions would be a more likely cause of lens swelling and cataract than an osmotic mechanism. There is no information available as to whether an oxidative mechanism, dependent on the polyol pathway or not, is operative in juvenile diabetic cataract.

Cataract in diabetic adults Cataract has a greater pre- valence in diabetics with a greater risk for women, and is dependent on the duration of diabetics. The morphology is no different from that of age-related cataract, although the frequency of some subtypes is increased.

Klein et al in a population study found cataract to be more prevalent in early and late onset diabetes with significant association with age, severity of retinopathy and diuretic usage. Diabetes duration and the level of glycosyla- ted hemoglobin were also associations in early onset diabe- tics. In a second report, cataract was found to be the second most common cause of severe visual loss in adult onset diabetics. Various other reports have shown an association between cataract, and diabetes duration or retinopathy.

The frequency of cataract extraction is greater in diabe- tics than non-diabetics. The Framingham study showed a significant excess risk in the 50 to 64 years age group (relative risk 4.02), while the HANES study showed a relative risk of 2.97 in this age group and 1.63 in the 65 to 74 years age group. Both studies reported an excess prevalence of cataract in diabetics in 50 to 64 years age groups, which disappeared at an older age. This has been attributed to the higher mortality in diabetics with cataract. However, a case-control study in Oxford found an increased risk for cataract extraction in diabetics in the age group of 50 to 79 years, and a small increase in risk for women relative to men.

As has been noted, the morphology of cataract in the adult diabetic resembles that seen in age-related cataract in the absence of diabetes. Thus the major features are nuclear cataract (increased nuclear scattering and brunescence) and cortical spoke and posterior subcapsular cataract. In the Lens Opacity Case Control study, diabetes increased the risk of posterior subcapsular, cortical and mixed forms of cataract. Individual features may not have an identical etiology, but it is likely that those metabolic changes identified in experi- mental cataract are relevant for the human are in varying degrees. There is no relation between cataract type, and the level of either sorbitol or myoinositol in lens epithelium from patients with cataract and diabetes.

It has been suggested that the increased nuclear scattering and brunescence in diabetic lenses is likely to be the result of increased glycation and the formation of advanced glycation end products.

There is evidence for a fall in free lysine amino groups in the human diabetic lens. It is also possible to induce a change in tertiary structure in alpha-crystalline (bovine) incubated with glucose and glucose-6-phosphate.

A three-fold increase in glycation was measured in diabetics and controls by Vidal et al but there was no correlation with the degree of browning of the lenses measured spectrophotometrically, and they concluded that other chromophores were responsible for the browning at the relevant wavelengths.

Certainly a number of other factors have been proposed to contribute to nuclear brunescence of the non-diabetic lens, but since the diabetic state is not anticipated to increase their concentration, glycation products are still the most likely candidates responsible for diabetic cataract.

Cortical cataract can be caused experimentally by agents which interfere with membrane permeability, ion and water control. The non-diabetic, aging human lens, free of cataract, has an increased membrane permeability which parallels the increase in optical density which occurs from about the fifth decade. There is evidence of degradation of the lens protein MIP26 with age in non-diabetics, which could be responsible for a functional abnormality. This channel protein has until recently been regarded as the gap junctional protein, but may, in fact, serve as a volume regulating channel. Disturbance of either function could increase the risk of cataract. It would be of interest to examine these events in the diabetic lens. The greater thickness of the diabetic compared to the non-diabetic lens could be relevant to this point. The disturbance in Na' K'- ATPase kinetics reported by Garner and Spector during exposure to glucose-6-phosphate is similar to the change noted in diabetic human lenses. Hydrogen peroxide is present in normal human aqueous, and present at raised levels in the aqueous of patients with cataract. Higher levels are found in the aqueous of diabetic patients with cataract. Simonelli et al have also shown an increase in malon- dialdehyde in cataractous compared with non-cataractous lenses which is greater in the cataract of diabetic patients. Malondialdehyde is a product of lipid peroxidation of cell membranes, and is regarded as an indicator of oxidative membrane damage. These are important findings, although the methods of measurement are not entirely specific.

The potential role of the sorbitol (polyol) pathway in juvenile cataract was discussed earlier. Recent studies of cultured lens epithelium from cataract patients have shown negligible or absent levels of sorbitol in the epithelium of non-diabetics. In diabetic epithelium sorbitol levels are higher than blood glucose levels, while there is an inverse relationship between blood glucose and myoinositol.

It has been noted that oxidative stress may cause lens membrane damage experimentally. It may also cause damage to DNA. Subcapsular cataract may be regarded as due to an aberration of lens mitosis and lens fiber differentiation, and could be the result of oxidative damage. There are no data, which link this to human subcapsular cataract.

Other cataract-related events A higher rate of capsular rupture reported in diabetics undergoing intracapsular or extracapsular extraction could be related to structural and chemical changes which are known to occur in the capsule. There is an increased risk for death in patients with cataract and diabetes. Cohen et al found lens opacities to be a powerful predictor of death, independent of other factors and with an odd ratio of 2.4 (95% confidence interval 1.5-3.9).

Dyslipidemia

Lens opacification and cardiovascular disease are two of the main causes of morbidity worldwide. Lens opacity, manifesting as cataract, is responsible for an estimated 40% of the 42 million cases of blindness in the world. On the other hand, heart disease is the single greatest cause of death in developed countries. The relationship between cholesterol and cardiovascular heart disease is well documented. The relationship between cholesterol and lens opacity is, however, far less well-appreciated.

Issues relating to drug safety and inherited defects in enzymes mediating cholesterol metabolism have brought renewed attention to a possible inter-relationship between lipid metabolism and cataract induction in humans. The lens is unique in that it contains a relative abundance of cholesterol in the fiber cell plasma membrane, (the highest of any cell group in the body) and furnishes its needs for cholesterol by onsite biosynthesis. It has been shown that inhibition of cholesterol synthesis in the lens leads to cataract formation in man.

Smith-Limli-Opitz syndrome, mevalonic aciduria and cerebrotendinous xanthomatosis are inherited disorders of cholesterol metabolism and affected patients may present with lens opacities. Triparanol, a hypolipidemic agent that inhibits cholesterol biosynthesis was withdrawn from clinical use because of its propensity to induce cataract formation in humans. The very widely used vastatin class of hypolipidemic medicines is potent inhibitors of cholesterol biosynthesis and is able to lower serum lipid concentration effectively. Although high ocular safety in older patients over periods of up to 5 years, has been reported, it is still not clear whether these agents have the potential to be cataractogenic, particularly in younger patients and over longer periods.

In order to assess the prevalence of lenticular opacities in patients with dyslipidemia (raised serum cholesterol and triglycerides) a group of 80 dyslipidemic patients were subjected to a general physical examination and an ophthalmic examination of the fully dilated eye at the Tygerberg Academic Hospital, University of Stellenbosch, South Africa (unpublished data).

Patients (n = 80) of both genders and irrespective of age were enrolled in the trial if they met the inclusion criteria for dyslipidemia. Patients were included if their fasting serum cholesterol and triglyceride concentrations were > 5.2 mmol/l and > 2.3 mmol/l, respectively when measured on three separate occasions over a one-month period **(Figure 1.6)**. Patients were excluded if they suffered from any condition known to cause or predispose them to elevated lipid levels or lenticular opacification.

Results The study group was predominantly male Caucasian and smokers. Most patients—68.8% admitted regular alcohol consumption. The mean systolic and diastolic blood pressure data, 134 ± 18 and 84 ± 9 mm Hg, respectively, fell within the normal range for age. The BMI of the group was significantly greater than the norm (i.e. 28.89 ± 4.82 kg/m^2).

The prevalence of lenticular opacities divided the study group into two cohorts, i.e. those with normal lenses (62%) and those with opacities (39%) **(Figure 1.7)**.

The prevalence of lenticular opacity in dyslipidemic patients in the age group of 30 to 40 years was 33%. This age group was not studied in the Barbados Eye Study (BES) or in The Beaver Dam Eye Study (BDES) and consequently data for comparison are not available **(Table 1.3)**. In the 40 to 50 year age group, the prevalence of lenticular opacity in our patients was 50% compared to 4.7% in the BES and 8.3% in BDES. Differences in the older age groups were not prominent **(Figure 1.8)**.

Modern medicine today aspires to early detection of disease processes with the aim of early intervention in an attempt either to halt the progression or to reverse the process.

Although the classic systemic signs of dyslipidemia are well-appreciated, i.e. xanthomata, xanthelasma, thickening

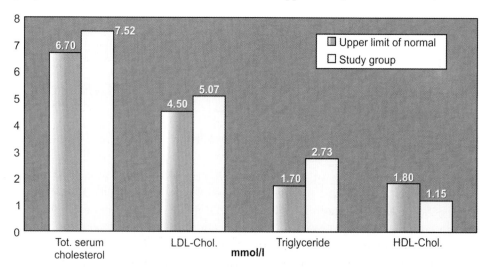

FIGURE 1.6: The lipid profile of the study group

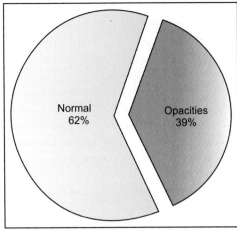

FIGURE 1.7 : The prevalence of lens opacities in the study group

TABLE 1.3	Age distribution of patients with lenticular opacities compared to other population based studies		
Age group Study group	Percentage of opacities	BES	BDES (years)
30–40	33.33	N/A	N/A
40–50	50.00	4.7	8.3
50–60	18.51	24.5	26.5
60–70	33.33	57.5	56.7
70–80	66.67	85.9	70.5
80+	33.33	98.3	N/A

BES: Barbados Eye Study
BDES: Beaver Dam Eye Study N/A: Not available.

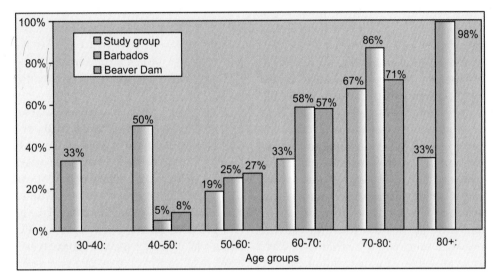

FIGURE 1.8: Prevalence of lenticular opacities in two population-based studies compared to the dyslipidemic study group

of the Achilles tendon and corneal arcus, in our study the prevalence of one or more of the ocular signs was far greater than that of the systemic signs, 23.8% for the former as opposed to 47.3% for the latter.

The distribution of dyslipidemia-related signs in this study was:
- Xanthelasma—7.5%
- Corneal arcus—8.8%
- Achilles tendon involvement—16.3%
- Cortical lenticular opacity—31.0%.

It is noteworthy that the most frequent ocular sign—cortical lenticular opacity—occurred twice as frequently as the most frequent systemic sign—Achilles tendon thickening **(Figure 1.9)**.
This work leads the investigators to conclude that:
- Dyslipidemic patients are more likely to develop cortical opacification than the normal population.
- Cortical lens opacification in dyslipidemics manifests at a younger age than does nuclear opacification.
- Cortical lens opacification in the patient younger than 50 years of age should alert the ophthalmologist to arrange for diagnostic serum lipid assessment.

- Cortical lenticular opacification should be regarded as one of the most common, and hence reliable, clinical signs of dyslipidemia.

Jahn et al attempted to determine the role of glucose and lipid metabolism in the formation of cataract in elderly people undergoing cataract extraction. They found that patients with posterior subcapsular cataract had higher concentrations of fasting serum triglycerides and were significantly younger than patients with nuclear or cortical cataract. Their results furthermore suggest that the association of hypertriglyceridemia, hyperglycemia and obesity favors the formation of a specific morphologic type of lens opacity, posterior subcapsular cataract, occuring at an early age. Because these factors are potentially modifiable by lifestyle changes, these observations may prove important as the modification of these parameters could constitute an effective mode of prevention or retardation in a subgroup of patients developing cataract at an early age.

Acetylator Status

The human acetylation polymorphism has been known for more than three decades since its discovery during the

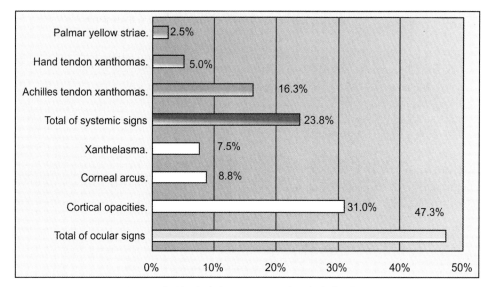

FIGURE 1.9: Physical signs associated with dyslipidemia

metabolic investigation of the antituberculous hydrazine drug, isoniazid. The trait was originally known as the "isoniazid acetylation polymorphism" but is now usually abbreviated as "acetylation polymorphism" because acetylation of numerous hydrazine and arylamine drugs and other chemicals are subject to this trait. Individuals phenotype as "slow" acetylators when homozygous for the slow acetylator gene, "rapid" when homozygous for the rapid acetylator gene or "intermediate" when heterozygous. The acetylator phenotype is a life-long, relatively stable characteristic of the individual that can phenotypically be determined by procedures using any of several test agents (e.g. caffeine, isoniazid, sulfamethazine, sulfapyridine). Certain disease states such as AIDS can change the phenotype expression in an individual. On the other hand, acetylator genotype can be determined by specialized polymerase chain reaction (PCR) methods.

Several diseases have been linked to acetylator pheno- and/or genotype. The best documented are bladder cancer (slow), colorectal adenomas (rapid), Gilbert's syndrome (slow), allergic diseases Type I diabetes mellitus (fast), Type II diabetes mellitus (slow) and familial Parkinson's disease (slow).

Recent work (PhD level, unpublished) at the departments of Ophthalmology and Pharmacology at the University of Stellenbosch, South Africa, have also established an association between age-related cataract and acetylation status as determined both phenotypically and genotypically. Sixty adult patients of both sexes with classic age-related lens opacities presenting for cataract surgery were enrolled in a prospective controlled study. Patients were included in the trial if they perceived themselves to be colored and if this was verified by at least one independent observer. The South African population of mixed ancestry (including Malay, Khoisan, Negroid and Caucasoid stock) is referred to as "colored" and all patients were selected from this well studied subgroup of the population. Care was taken to exclude all patients with well-known etiological factors for cataract formation such as diabetes mellitus, previous ocular trauma, other metabolic and/or inherited diseases. One

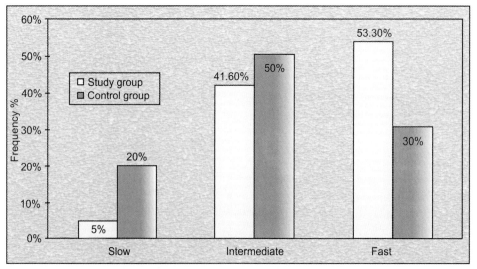

FIGURE 1.10: Acetylator status of cataract vs normal patients

hundred and twenty patients of the same race group served as controls.

Figure 1.10 demonstrates that in the control group (representing the population at large) the distribution of the phenotypic acetylation status was 20% "rapid", 50% "intermediate" and 30% "slow". In the cataract group the distribution was 5% "rapid", 42% "intermediate" and 53% "slow". This clearly seems to suggest that cataract possibly occurs more frequently in slow acetylators than in the rest of the population. Could this finding perhaps suggest a possible etiologic role for chemical substances possessing a primary aromatic amine or hydrazine group in human lenticular opacification?

Lipid Peroxidation, Free Radicals and Nutritional Influences on Cataract Formation

Oxygen and oxygen-derived free radicals and a failure of intracellular calcium homeostatic mechanisms are recurring themes in a wide variety of cell injuries.

The addition of electrons to molecular oxygen leads to the formation of toxic free oxygen radicals or reactive oxygen species (ROS), e.g.

O_2^- = superoxide (one electron)
H_2O_2 = hydrogen peroxide (two electrons)
OH^- = hydroxyl radical (three electrons)

Iron is very important in this process according to the Haber-Weiss reaction:

$$H_2O_2 + O_2^- \overset{Fe^{2+}}{\rightarrow} . OH + OH^- + O_2$$

These free radical species cause lipid peroxidation and other deleterious effects on cell structure. Recent studies have shown that lipid peroxidation, an event caused by imbalance between free radical production and antioxidant defense, may play a role in the genesis of cataract. Higher levels of malondialdehyde (MDA), a final product of the lipid peroxidation process, have been observed in diabetic and myopic cataract compared with senile cataract.

Protection of the cell against damage by these free radicals takes place indirectly (enzymatically) by antioxidant enzymes—superoxide dismutase (SOD), glutathione peroxidase (GPX) and catalase (CAT). Direct protection is offered by mainly dietary antioxidants—ascorbate (Vit C), tocopherol (Vit E), carotenoids(Vit A) and glutathione (GSH).

Light and oxygen as risk factors for cataract Various epidemiological studies demonstrate associations between elevated risk of various forms of cataract and exposure to higher intensities of incident and/or reflected ultraviolet light (**Table 1.4**).

Elevated levels of oxygen exposure perhaps show the clearest causal relationship between oxidative stress and cataract. Nuclear cataract was observed in patients treated with hyperbaric oxygen therapy, and markedly elevated levels of mature cataract were observed in mice that survived exposure to 100% oxygen twice weekly for 3 hours. A higher incidence of cataract was noted in lenses exposed to hyperbaric oxygen *in vitro*. Very early stages of cataract in guinea pigs exposed to hyperbaric oxygen was noted by Giblin.

Role of cellular antioxidants against lens damage Protection of the organism against photooxidative insult can be viewed as two interrelated processes. Primary defenses offer protection of proteins and other lens constituents by lens antioxidants and antioxidant enzymes whereas secondary defenses include proteolytic and repair processes. The primary defenses shall form the focus of our attention.

The major aqueous antioxidants in the lens are ascorbate and GSH.

Ascorbate is probably the most effective, least toxic antioxidant identified in mammalian systems. The following has been observed:

• The lens and aqueous concentrate ascorbate >10 times the level found in human plasma.

| TABLE 1.4 | Extent of light expoxure and the risk of cataract |

Study	Exposure		PR	95% CI
USA: NHANES survey	Daily hours of sunlight in area; ages 65–74	< 6.6 h	1.0	
		7.1–7.7 h	1.7	1.2–2.7
		>8.2 h	2.7	1.6–4.6
Australia	Daily hours of sunlight in area	<8 h	1.0	
		8.5–9 h	2.9	0.6–13.2
		>9.5 h	4.2	0.9–18.9
	Average mean erythemal dose of area	2000	1.0	
		2500	1.3	0.8–2.3
		3000	1.8	1.0–3.4
Nepal	Average hours of sunlight	7–9 h	1.0	
		10–11 h	1.2	0.9–1.4
		>12 h	2.5	2.1–3.0

PR = prevalence ratio   CI = confidence interval

- The concentration of ascorbate in the lens nucleus is only 25% that of the surrounding cortex.
- Ascorbate levels in normal lenses are higher than in cataractous lenses.
- Ascorbate levels are higher in the older guinea pig lens than in younger animals despite the same dietary intake of ascorbate.
- Increasing lens ascorbate concentrations by two-fold is associated with protection against cataract-like damage.

With this basic science knowledge, several epidemiological, clinical and even interventional studies have been undertaken. Vitamin C was considered in approximately 9 published studies and observed to be inversely associated with at least one type of cataract in eight of these studies.

In the Nutrition and Vision Project, age-adjusted analyses bases on 165 women with high vitamin C intake (mean = 294 mg/day) and 136 women with low vitamin C intake (mean = 77 mg/day) indicated that the women who took vitamin C supplements for $\geq$ 10 years had > 70% lower prevalence of early opacities (RR: 0.23; CI: 0.09-0.60) and > 80% lower risk of moderate opacities (RR: 0.17; CI: 0.03-0.87) at any site compared with women who did not use vitamin C supplements.

In comparison to the above data, Mares-Perlman et al report that past use of supplements containing vitamin C was associated with a reduced prevalence of nuclear cataract, but an increased prevalence of cortical cataract after controlling for age, sex, smoking, and history of heavy alcohol consumption.

Glutathione (GSH) levels in the lens are several fold the levels found in whole blood and plasma. GSH levels also diminish in the older and cataractous lenses. Pharmacological opportunities could be suggested by observations that incorporating the industrial 0.4% butylated hydroxytoluene in diets of galactose-fed (50% of diet) rats diminished prevalence of cataract. Clinical studies, however, have not yet been forthcoming.

Vitamin E, a natural lipid-soluble antioxidant, can inhibit lipid peroxidation and appears to stabilize lens cell membranes. Consumption of Vit E supplements was inversely correlated with cataract risk in two studies. Robertson et al found among age- and sex-matched cases and controls that the prevalence of advanced cataract was 56% lower (RR: 0.44; CI: 0.24–0.77) in persons who consumed vitamin E supplements (>400 IU/day) than in persons not consuming supplements. Jacques and Chylack (unpublished) observed a 67% (RR: 0.33; CI:0.12–0.96) reduction in prevalence of cataract for vitamin E supplement users after adjusting for age, sex, race and diabetes.

Two prospective studies demonstrated a reduced cataract progress among individuals with higher plasma vitamin E. Rouhianen et al found a 73% reduction in risk for cortical cataract progression (RR:027; CI: 0.08–0.83), whereas Leske et al reported a 42% reduction in risk for nuclear cataract progression (RR: 0.58; CI: 0.36–0.94). Vitamin E

supplementation was related to a lower risk for progress of nuclear opacity (RR:0.43; CI: 0.19–0.99).

The carotenoids, like vitamine E, are also natural lipid-soluble antioxidants. Beta-carotene is the best known carotenoid because of its importance as a vitamin A precursor. However, it is only one of the 400 naturally occuring carotenoids, and other carotenoids may have similar or greater antioxidant potential. In addition to β-carotene, α-carotene, lutein and lycopene are important carotenoid components of the human diet.

Jacques and Chylack were the first to observe that persons with carotene intakes above 18,700 IU/day had the same prevalence of cataract as those with intakes below 5,677 IU/day (RR:0.91; CI:0.23–3.78). Hankinson et al followed this report with a study that reported that the multivariate-adjusted rate of cataract surgery was about 30% lower (RR: 0.73; CI: 0.55–0.97) for women with high carotene intakes (median = 14,558 IU/day) compared with women with low intakes of this nutrient (median = 2,935 IU/day). However, while cataract surgery was inversely associated with total carotene intake, it was not strongly associated with consumption of carotene-rich foods, such as carrots. Rather, cataract surgery was associated with lower intakes of foods such as spinach that are rich in lutein and xanthin carotenoids, rather than β-carotene. This would appear to be consistent with the observation that the human lens contains lutein and zeaxanthin but no β-carotene.

This observation would appear to be consistent with the observation that lutein and zeaxanthin are the most prevalent carotenoids in lens. However, Mares-Perlman did not detect a significantly altered risk for cataract among consumers of these nutrients.

Intervention studies To date only one intervention trial designed to assess the effect of vitamin supplements on cataract risk has been completed. Sperduto et al took advantage of two ongoing, randomized, double-blinded vitamin and cancer trials to assess the impact of vitamin supplements on cataract prevalence. The trials were conducted among almost 4,000 participants aged 45 to 74 years from rural communities in Linxian, China. Participants in one trial received either a multisupplement or placebo. In the second trial, a more complex factorial design was used to evaluate the effects of four different vitamin/mineral combinations:

- Retinol (5000 IU) and zinc (22 mg)
- Riboflavin (3 mg) and niacin (40 mg)
- Vitamin C (120 mg) and molybdenum (30 mg)
- Vitamin E (30 mg), β-carotene (15 mg), and selenium (50 mg).

At the end of the five to six years follow-up, the investigators conducted eye examinations to determine the prevalence of cataract. In the first trial there was a significant 43% reduction in the prevalence of nuclear cataract for persons aged 65 to 74 years receiving the multisupplement (RR: 0.57; CI: 0.36–0.90). The second trial demonstrated a significantly reduced prevalence of nuclear cataract in persons receiving the riboflavin/niacin supplement relative to those persons not receiving the supplement (RR: 0.59; CI: 0.45–0.79). The effect was strongest in those aged 65 to 74 years (RR: 0.45; CI: 0.31–0.64). However, the riboflavin/niacin supplement appeared to increase the risk of posterior subcapsular cataract (RR:2.64; CI: 1.31–5.35). The results further suggested a protective effect of the retinol/zinc supplement (RR: 0.77; CI: 0.58–1.02) and the vitamin C/molybdenum supplement (RR:0.78; CI: 0.50–1.04) on prevalence of nuclear cataract.

Conclusion Although light and oxygen are necessary for physiological function, when present in excess they seem to be causally related to cataractogenesis. Aging might diminish the bodies primary antioxidant reserves, antioxidant enzyme abilities, and diminished secondary defenses such as proteases.

The literature creates the strong impression that antioxidant intake might diminish the risk for cataract formation.

Longitudinal studies and more intervention studies are essential in order to establish the value of dietary antioxidants and to determine the extent to which cataract progress is affected by nutritional supplements. This fact becomes significant when one appreciates that poor education and lower socioeconomic status are directly related to poor nutrition. It is, therefore, not irrational to contemplate the value of intervention for populations at risk. The work available, albeit preliminary, indicates that nutrition may provide the least costly and most practicable means to attempt the objectives of delaying cataract.

OCULAR DISEASE

Many ocular diseases have been associated with cataract formation either as direct cause and effect relationships or as common associations.

Myopia

Weale suggested that lenses of myopes are subject to excessive mechanical stress which could lead to cataract. This hypothesis was tested by several investigators and Harding et al during their Oxford case-control studies found that the risk of cataract after the age of 50 was doubled in myopes. Weale (1980) also suggested that there is a graded risk for increasing degrees of myopia. This was eloquently confirmed two decades later by Lim et al in the Blue Mountains Eye Study. Eyes with onset of myopia before age 20 had the greatest posterior subcapsular (PSC) cataract risk (odds ratio [OR] 3.9; confidence interval [CI] 2.0–7.9) Refraction-related increasing odds were found between PSC cataract and myopia: low myopia (OR 2.1; CI: 1.4–3.5), moderate myopia (OR 3.1; CI: 1.6–5.7), and high myopia (OR 5.5; CI: 2.8–10.9). High myopia was associated with PSC, cortical, and late nuclear cataract. Conversely PSC cataract was inversely associated with hyperopia (OR 0.6; CI: 0.4–0.9). They finally concluded that early-onset myopia (before 20 years of age) may be a strong and independent risk factor for PSC cataract, that

nuclear cataract was associated with presumed acquired myopia, whereas high myopia was associated with all three types of cataract.

Wensor et al demonstrated that a myopic shift is associated with nuclear cataract. In the population based study of 3,271 Australians an association between myopia of 1 Diopter or more and both nuclear and cortical cataract was observed. Between posterior subcapsular cataract and myopia such a relationship did not exist. It is not sure that a causal relationship exists between cortical cataract and myopia or rather that a myopic shift occurs after people develop cortical cataract. The temporality of this relationship should still be explored in future prospective analyses.

Glaucoma

Glaucoma has been shown to be strongly associated with the pathogenesis of cataract **(Figure 1.11)** in many studies undertaken in many countries. The relative risk (odds ratio [OR]) of cataract developing in a glaucoma patient can be as high as six times normal. This risk more than doubles to an OR of 14.3 after glaucoma filtration surgery. This rise in risk is most probably due to the trauma of surgery for glaucoma. Vesti in Helsinki, Finland investigated cataract progression after trabeculectomy in a study of 47 eyes with exfoliative glaucoma (EXG) and in 20 eyes with primary open-angle glaucoma (POAG). EXG, age, hypotony (IOP < or = 5 mm Hg) lasting > or = 5 days and early postoperative IOP rise > 30 mm Hg were observed to be risk factors for cataract progression.

Besides formal filtering procedures like full thickness procedures, laser procedures for the management of different types of glaucomas are frequently performed such as argon laser trabeculoplasty, argon laser iridoplasty and Nd-YAG peripheral iridotomy. Each of these procedures carries the risk of inducing a cataract especially of the focal type. Zadok et al has described a previously unreported complication of a posterior chamber intraocular lens (IOL)

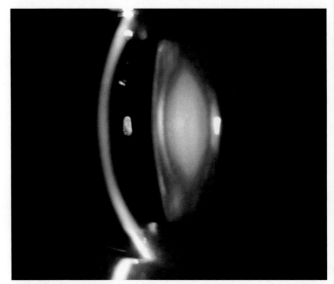

FIGURE 1.11: Immature cataract (*Courtesy:* Dr Agarwal's Eye Hospital, India)

implanted in a phakic eye. The left eye of a 25-year old patient with high myopia was treated prophylactically with Nd: YAG laser iridotomy prior to phakic IOL implantation. Slit lamp examination of the same eye disclosed an opacity of the anterior capsule of the crystalline lens under the iridotomy site.

Miotics, particularly long-acting cholinesterase inhibitors, if used for long term, may cause tiny anterior subcapsular vacuoles and, occasionally, more advanced opacities. Cessation of medication may stop, retard or occasionally reverse their progression.

Acute congestive angle-closure glaucoma is associated with the subsequent formation of glaukomflecken consisting of small, gray-white, anterior, subcapsular or capsular opacities in the pupillary zone.

Ophthalmic Surgical Procedures

Many different ophthalmic procedures carry the risk of inducing cataract. Among others are surgical iridectomy, filtration surgery, corneal transplants, retinal detachment surgery with and without intraocular silicone oil as well as pars plana vitrectomy especially in diabetics. Assessing the surgical outcome in a series of 63 consecutive patients treated for rhegmatogenous retinal detachment by primary vitrectomy Oshima reported the reattachment rate by final examination as 100%, but there was a high incidence (53.8%) of cataract progression in phakic eyes.

More recently with the advent of minus power phakic, IOL implantation surgery, several reports have appeared of cataract induction secondary to the implantation of these lenses into the ciliary sulcus. These cataracts have occurred both with silicone and collamer materials. Some have taken as short a time as 6 months, whilst others took 7 years to form. In another series of 38 consecutive eyes with high myopia implanted with a silicone posterior chamber plate-style intraocular lens (Chiron, Adatomed) over a period of 21 months and followed for between 3 and 24 months not a single cataract occurred. The lens style and design may play a significant role in the cataract pathogenesis, because in a recent study Brauweiler et al attempted to assess the effectiveness and safety of implantation of a silicone, posterior chamber IOL in the ciliary sulcus of phakic, highly myopic eyes in a noncomparative consecutive interventional series. Eighteen eyes of 10 patients underwent implantation of a Fyodorov 094M-1 IOL by the same surgeon and were evaluated for a 2-year postoperative period. Cataract formation of the anterior subcapsular (8 eyes) or nuclear (only 1 eye) type was observed in overall 9 (52.9%) of 17 eyes. When considering only the patients with a follow-up of 2 years, the incidence of cataract formation was 81.9% (9 of 11 eyes). Obviously this very high incidence of cataract formation should discourage the implantation of the type of IOL used in this study.

Ocular Trauma

The development of cataract (**Figure 1.12**) is a known complication following blunt or penetrating ocular trauma.

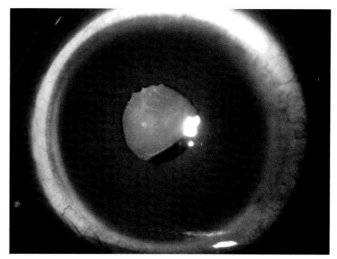

FIGURE 1.12: Traumatic subluxated cataract
(*Courtesy:* Dr Agarwal's Eye Hospital, India)

However traumatic cataract and zonular dehiscence is only one complication of the injured ocular tissues. Other complications include glaucoma, retinal detachment, optic nerve damage, extraocular muscle imbalance and injury to the bony orbit.

Ocular trauma is a major cause of monocular blindness in both the developed and developing world, but this is not seen as a significant cause of bilateral blindness. Trauma can, therefore, be considered as a major cause of blind eyes but not of blind people.

Crystalline lens subluxation, total dislocation, or localized cortical or diffuse opacities are often observed secondary to blunt ocular trauma. An unusual complication of blunt trauma is rupture of the posterior capsule with subsequent lens fiber hydration leading to rapidly progressive lens opacification. Posterior capsular breaks have been reported to develop thick, fibrous, opaque margins approximately 6 weeks after blunt trauma.

Secondary Cataract

Uveitis A secondary cataract develops as a result of some other primary ocular disease. The most common cause of secondary cataract is chronic anterior uveitis. The earliest finding is a polychromatic luster at the posterior pole of the lens. If the uveitis is controlled, the progression of cataract may be arrested. If the inflammation cannot be controlled, anterior and posterior subcapsular opacities develop and the lens may become completely opaque. The lens opacification seems to progress more rapidly in the presence of posterior synechiae.

Hereditary posterior segment disease Hereditary fundus dystrophies such as retinitis pigmentosa, Leber's congenital amaurosis, gyrate atrophy, Wagner's and Stickler's syndromes may be associated with posterior subcapsular lens opacities. In a study of 384 eyes of 192 patients with a mean age of 39.1 years who presented with typical retinitis pigmentosa, cataract was found in 46.4% of the eyes.

Among these, 93.6% showed posterior subcapsular opacification. The incidence of cataract increased with age.

Wagner's vitreoretinal degeneration is characteristically associated with high myopia, glaucoma, choroidal atrophy, retinal detachment and presenile cataract.

Persistent hyperplastic primary vitreous (PHPV) is a congenital disorder that manifests a range of ocular anomalies including leukoria, microphthalmia, a retrolental fibrovascular membrane and cataract. In general the prognosis for visual acuity with PHPV is poor.

Iris color McCarty et al in their Australian population study of 3,271 adults aged 40 years and older found an association between cortical cataract and brown or dark brown irides for all ages that was not explained by country of birth or language spoken. In all age categories, brown iris color was also associated with nuclear cataract. No such association was found for posterior subcapsular cataract.

In the Italian-American Cataract Study, there was an increased, although not significant, risk of cortical cataract in people with brown irides. Dark iris color was not associated with cortical cataract in the Lens Opacities Case-Control Study. In the National Health and Nutrition Examination Survey, blacks, who have dark brown irides, were found to have significantly increased risk of cortical cataract. In both the above mentioned studies, dark iris color was also found to be a significant risk factor for nuclear cataract.

The relationship of nuclear cataract and iris color could result from genetic susceptibility associated with iris color or other factors not yet determined. This finding may partially explain the variation in the prevalence of nuclear cataract observed in different countries with different racial groups.

SYSTEMIC DISEASES

Hypertension

The association between hypertension and cataract was first noted in the Framingham study where earlier detection of elevated blood pressure was more common in those later found to have cataract. It was also noted in the same study that consumption of diuretics which restores normal blood pressure in many patients does not protect against this risk. There may, however, be a variety of interactions in these patients in that hypertension may be associated with high blood glucose, diabetes and other conditions as well as with use of diuretics. Diuretics have different effects on plasma urea levels, with frusemide and acetazolamide associated with the highest levels, and parallel effects on cataract. Overall diuretic use was associated with an odds ratio of 1:6 but cyclopenthiazide (Navidrex), which had least effect on plasma urea, was reported by a greater proportion of controls than cases. Loop diuretics were reported by more than twice the proportion of cases than of controls. Hypertension and diuretic consumption did not appear as risk factors in Oxford but the graded properties of different diuretics did emerge and with a similar sequence to that found in Edinburgh. The only significant association of individual diuretics was an apparent protective effect by cyclopenthiazide and a risk associated with spironolactone which itself is a steroid. There was no significant association of particular sites of opacity with diuretic use.

Dehydrational Crisis

Harding has proposed that frequent episodes of diarrhea may be related to cataractogenesis and may account for the excess prevalence in some developing countries. Four intermediate events have been suggested to explain the role of diarrhea in the development of cataract
- Malnutrition secondary to malabsorption of nutrients
- Relative alkalosis from administration of rehydrating fluids with bicarbonate
- Dehydration induced osmotic disturbance between the lens and the aqueous humor, and
- Increased levels of urea and ammonium cyanate which may denature lens proteins by the process of carbamylation.

Six case-control studies have examined the relationship of severe diarrhea and increased risk of cataract, with discordant results. Two case-control, clinic-based studies done in Madhya Pradesh and Orissa, India have suggested a three- to four-fold increase in the risk for cataract for those with remembered episodes of life-threatening dehydration crises, severe enough to render the patient bedridden for at least three days. However, these findings were not replicated in two other epidemiologic investigations done in India. Using a less stringent definition of diarrhea (confinement to bed for one day), the India-US Case-Control Study found no associations with cataract. Also, a village-based case-control study in Southern India showed no association between severe diarrhea and risk of cataract. Furthermore, an observational study done in Matlab, Bangladesh, revealed that diarrhea from all causes was not significantly associated with cataract, although it was difficult to determine how cataract was defined in the study. The case-control study in Oxford found a marginally significant excess risk of cataract with reported severe diarrhea, but a significant risk in the subgroup aged 70 and older. Adjustments for the other possible confounding factors also found in the study were not done. Considering the potential public health importance of diarrhea as a risk factor, as well as the biologically plausible role of dehydration in cataractogenesis, further research to clarify this association is needed. Prospective studies involving closer follow-up of groups of patients who suffered from acute life-threatening diarrhea may provide more convincing evidence. Moreover, studies that examine the cumulative effect of milder, chronic dehydration episodes in cataractogenesis may also add to the current understanding of this issue.

Renal Failure

Cataract has been reported in many cases of renal failure. Sometimes cataract, often transient, was associated with hemodialysis and thought to be caused by the osmotic shock that dialysis causes, but Laqua (1972) noted lens opacities before dialysis and suggested they were caused by uremia. Increased blood urea could lead to cataract in a similar way to that postulated in severe diarrhea. After renal transplantation patients are treated with immunosuppressants usually including corticosteroids that may cause cataract. Posterior subcapsular lens opacities were observed in 19 out of 22 renal transplant recipients, aged 21 to 54 years in Hiroshima. Half of the patients suffered visual loss, attributed to steroid-induced cataract. In a study of diabetic patients receiving renal transplants in the USA, only one patient developed a visually-impairing cataract but lesser degrees of lens opacification were seen in 26% of eyes. Fourteen of 55 non-diabetic renal transplant patients were found to have cataract. The case-control study in Edinburgh did not report on renal failure as such but did find that the mean urea level was significantly higher in the plasma of cataract patients compared with controls. The level was not high enough to indicate renal failure. The raised urea levels are still present when subjects are subdivided by age and sex. Diuretics may raise urea levels and thus contribute to these differences but when all diabetics and individuals receiving diuretics were excluded, a relationship between high plasma urea and cataract remained.

ENVIRONMENTAL FACTORS: ULTRAVIOLET RADIATION

There is considerable international interest in the association **(Figures 1.13 and 1.14)** between solar ultraviolet B (UVB) radiation and cataract. Much of this interest has resulted from concern about the health effects of the increasing levels of UVB reaching the earth's surface as a consequence of depletion of the stratospheric ozone layer.

Young suggests that sunlight is the primary causal factor in cataractogenesis, and strongly advocates the widespread distribution of sunglasses to prevent cataract. Harding on

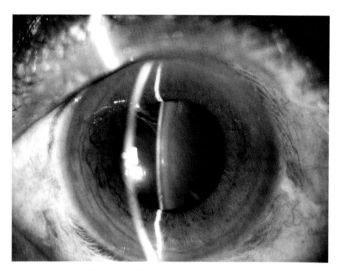

FIGURE 1.14: Black cataract (*Courtesy:* Dr Agarwal's Eye Hospital, India)

the other hand suggests that sunlight is not a major etiological factor in human cataract formation.

The lens is known to absorb UVB and UVA and change in lens clarity has been linked in animal experiments with short-term, high intensity exposure and chronic exposure to UVB.

Epidemiologic studies have demonstrated cataract to be more prevalent in sunny countries, such as Israel, than in cloudy countries, such as England. Moreover, in Romania and the United States, cataracts are more prevalent in dry hot areas with more sun exposure within each country than in areas with prolonged cloud cover. The Beaver Dam Eye Study found an association between ultraviolet B radiation exposure and cortical cataract in men only.

The Lens Opacity Case-Control Study did not find an association between sun exposure and any type of cataract development. However, this study investigated only urban populations, and this may explain why no association was found. In both the Italian-American Cataract Study and India-US Case-Control Study, sunlight exposure was associated with cataract formation. Taylor studied 797 watermen and went to great lengths to calculate an ultraviolet radiation exposure index on the basis of field variables such as outdoor hours worked, work location, and attenuation due to spectacle use and hat cover. He found a significant association between ultraviolet B radiation index and cortical cataract but found no association with other morphological cataract types.

Bochow et al studied the relationship between ultraviolet radiation exposure and posterior subcapsular cataract. He not only discovered a significant association but also a dose-response relationship.

Two unique studies, one prospective and one case-control, provide indirect evidence that ultraviolet light plays a role in cataract formation. Schein et al studied the distribution of cortical opacities by lens quadrant in a prospective study of Chesapeake Bay watermen. The prevalence of cortical lens opacities increased with age, with a high degree of concordance between eyes. The infero-

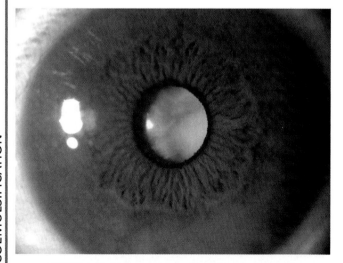

FIGURE 1.13: Mature cataract (*Courtesy:* Dr Agarwal's Eye Hospital, India)

nasal lens quadrant was the most common location involved both for new cataract development and for progression of preexisting cataract. Cataract formation in this quadrant was presumed to be the most consistent with ultraviolet radiation damage on the basis of greater exposure in this area of the lens. Resnikoff et al studied the association of lens opacities with two other presumed ultraviolet radiation-associated ocular diseases, climatic droplet keratopathy and exfoliation syndrome. There was a strong correlation between the diseases in this case-control study.

Based on the available epidemiological evidence, the following conclusions can be drawn:

- There is sufficient experimental evidence that exposure to artificial sources of UVB can cause lens opacities in laboratory animals.
- There is limited evidence suggesting that exposure to solar UVB causes cortical opacities in humans.
- There is also limited evidence suggesting that exposure to solar UVB causes posterior subcapsular cataract in humans.
- The epidemiological evidence is consistent in suggesting that nuclear cataracts are not causally associated with exposure to solar UVB.

DRUG-RELATED FACTORS

A number of well-known and widely used drugs have been implicated in cataract etiology with oral corticosteroids probably the widest recognized of all.

Corticosteroids

In 1930, Hench postulated that a naturally occuring substance might be responsible for the clinical improvement seen in women with rheumatoid arthritis when they became pregnant. He called this substance "compound E", but it was not until 1948 that this substance (soon to be called cortisone) was synthesized and became available for clinical use. In the 50 years since then, corticosteroids have had an enormous impact in medicine, however, it soon became clear that hydrocortisone has significant mineral corticoid as well as anti-inflammatory activity and that this could produce dose-related toxicity. It is now known that the principal naturally occurring corticosteroids secreted by the adrenal cortex are hydrocortisone (cortisol), a glucocorticoid involved in the regulation of carbohydrate, protein and lipid metabolism and aldosterone, a mineralocorticoid affecting fluid and electrolyte balance. Because hydrocortisone also exerts some mineralocorticoid (salt-retaining) effects, several structurally modified glucocorticoids with relatively greater anti-inflammatory and lower salt-retaining properties were synthesized once the therapeutic potential of their anti-inflammatory and immunosuppressive properties became apparent. Anti-inflammatory and immunosuppressive effects occur at doses above the normal physiological levels of daily glucocorticoid production, i.e. at pharmacological doses. However, since many physio-

logical and pharmacological actions are mediated by the same receptor, it is not surprising that prolonged use of pharmacological doses can lead to adverse physiological effects.

It is estimated that between 10 to 60% of patients using systemic corticosteroids develop cataract, especially of the posterior subcapsular (PSC) type. Glucocorticosteroids are lipophilic and therefore diffuse easily across the cell membrane after which they bind and activate a cytoplasmic glucocorticoid receptor. The resulting receptor steroid complex enters the cell nucleus, binds to the glucocorticoid response elements on the DNA and up- or downregulates the expression of corticosteroid-responsive genes with resultant effects on protein synthesis in target tissues.

Several ways have been identified in which corticosteroids may induce cataract formation including:

- Elevation of glucose level
- Inhibition of Na, K-ATPase
- Increased cation permeability
- Inhibition of glucose-6-dehydrogenase
- Inhibition of RNA-synthesis
- Loss of ATP
- Covalent bonding of steroids to lens proteins.

Posterior subcapsular cataract is the hallmark of steroid cataract. It starts as fine granular and vacuolated opacities at the posterior aspect of the lens. PSC opacities occur frequently with high doses (more than 15 mg prednisone or equivalent per day) and prolonged use (more than one year) of corticosteroids. Clinical trials have shown that PSC opacities secondary to oral corticosteroids may develop within as short a time as 4 months.

Recent studies have suggested that the use of inhaled corticosteroids may be a significant risk factor for the development of cataract, may be even more so than the use of oral corticosteroids. These studies have again pointed out the importance of the "first-order effect". A drug absorbed through the nasal mucosa or conjunctiva "drains" to the right atrium and ventricle. The drug is then pumped in part, to the head (i.e. the eye as a target organ) before returning to the left atrium and ventricle. The second passage is then to the liver and kidneys, where the drug is metabolized and detoxified. With oral medication—the first pass includes absorption from the gut via the liver where, depending on the drug, more than 90% of the drug is detoxified before going to the right atrium. Therefore, oral medications are metabolized even before the first pass, while ocular or nasally administered drugs are not metabolized until the second pass. This, in part, may be a reason why more potent steroid inhalants have greater ocular exposure and some ocular medications cause significant systemic adverse effects.

Considering the widespread use of corticosteroids and their association with PSC cataract, clinicians should be aware of a patient's medication history and recognize the distinguishing features of PSC cataract.

Allopurinol

Allopurinol is an antihyperuricemic drug widely used for the treatment of hyperuricemia and chronic gout. It inhibits the terminal step in uric acid synthesis, which results in a reduction of uric acid concentrations in both serum and urine. In about 85% of patients with gout, serum urate concentrations can be normalized by an allopurinol dose of 300 mg/d, and in some patients a dose of 100 to 200 mg/d is sufficient. Treatment with allopurinol is usually well tolerated, with hypersensitivity reactions constituting the most common adverse effects.

In 1982, Fraunfelder et al reported 30 cases of cortical and subcapsular cataract associated with long-term use of allopurinol reported to the National Registry of Drug-Induced Ocular Side Effects (Oregon Health Sciences University, Portland). The observed lens changes appeared to have the characteristics of early age-related cataract. At about the same time, Lerman et al used phosphorescence spectroscopy to demonstrate *in vitro* the probable presence of allopurinol in cataractous lenses that had been extracted from patients treated with allopurinol. The phosphorescence peaks characteristic of allopurinol could not be demonstrated in lenses from patients who had not ingested allopurinol. Evidence from epidemiologic studies on the possible cataractogenic effects of allopurinol is, however, inconclusive. Two separate epidemiologic studies did not show an increased risk. Another study reported an unusual morphologic thinning of the anterior clear zone of the lens in patients receiving long-term treatment with allopurinol. In the Lens Opacities Case Control Study, wherein gout medications were found to be associated with a 2.5-fold increased risk of mixed cataract, no distinction was made between allopurinol and other medications for gout. In a case control study conducted by Garbe et al using data from the Quebec universal health program for all elderly patients they established that a clear relationship exists between the long-term administration of allopurinol and an increased risk for cataract extraction.

Phenothiazines

In 1965, the occurrence of ocular pigmentation and lens opacity in patients on high dose phenothiazine drugs, particularly chlorpromazine, was reported in several papers. Phenothiazine has been thought to cause pigmentation by virtue of its ability to combine with melanin and form a photosensitive product. It is also postulated that this process might accelerate any predisposition to lens opacification from environmental insults such as solar radiation. A study involving schizophrenic patients showed an association between severity or grade of lenticular pigmentation and equivalent dose of phenothiazine intake. Epidemiologic research on the role of phenothiazines in cataractogenesis is limited. A case-control study done in North Carolina found a two-fold increased risk of cataract in those with history of tranquilizer use, although the types of tranquilizers and cataract were not characterized. A health maintenance organization based, non-concurrent prospective study that controlled for steroid use and diabetes documented at least three-fold increased risk for cataract extraction among current and past (two to five years prior to extraction) users of two groups of tranquilizers: "antipsychotic phenothiazine drugs" (chlorpromazine, thioridazine, trifluoperazine, perphenazine, fluphenazine) and "other phenothiazine drugs" (chlorperazine, prochlorperazine, promethazine, trimeprazine).

Given the paucity and limitations of available epidemiologic data, more studies, such as those characterizing the specific types of senile cataract and phenothiazines, are needed to verify any association.

Diuretics and Antihypertensives

Harding and van Heyningen reported that thiazide diuretics were used less frequently by patients who underwent cataract surgery than control subjects. More recently, the Beaver Dam Eye Study found that use of thiazides was associated with lower prevalence of nuclear cataract and increased prevalence of posterior subcapsular cataract. Several other studies have found that use of diuretics was associated with increased risk of cataract. The Beaver Dam Eye Study also found a raised overall risk (OR, 1.3) for potassium-sparing diuretics, but this was not statistically significant. A cataractogenic effect of potassium-sparing diuretics is biologically plausible, as these diuretics disturb sodium transport across the lens fiber membrane.

The calcium channel blocker nifedipine has been associated with increased risk of cataract extraction and angiotensin-converting enzyme inhibitors with decreased risk of nuclear cataract. Hypertension and other cardiovascular conditions is a potential confounding problem in studies of cataract and antihypertensive medications, including diuretics.

Antimalarial Drugs

Most drugs used in the treatment of malaria produce phototoxic side effects in both the skin and the eye. Cutaneous and ocular effects that may be caused by light include: cataract formation, changes in skin pigmentation, corneal opacity and other visual disturbances including irreversible retinal damage (retinopathy) leading to blindness. The mechanism for these reactions in humans is unknown. A number of studies have been published that suggest a strong relationship between chloroquine use and cataract formation. The basis of the relationship seems to lie in the phototoxicity of chloroquine and related drugs.

Because malaria is a disease most prevalent in regions of high light intensity, protective measures (clothing, sunblock, sunglasses or eye wraps) should be recommended whilst taking antimalarial drugs.

Amiodarone

Amiodarone hydrochloride is a benzofurane derivative used for cardiac abnormalities. Its use is commonly associated with an asymptomatic keratopathy. The antiarrhythmic drug also produces anterior subcapsular lens opacities that are usually asymptomatic. Anterior subcapsular lens opacities were observed in 7 of 14 patients treated with moderate to high doses of amiodarone at the Veterans Administration Medical Center in San Francisco in 1982. In 1993, a report was published that summarized the status of these same 14 patients 10 years later. Anterior subcapsular lens opacities developed or progressed in all patients continuing treatment with this antiarrhythmic agent during the ensuing 10-year interval. Although Snellen visual acuities were not decreased, subtle visual impairment was present as measured by contrast sensitivity measurements with and without glare. The authors of the report concluded that decrease in visual acuity should not be a contraindication for therapy with this potentially life-saving drug.

Hypocholesterolemic Drugs

Cataract in animals and men are in some instances associated with genetic defects in enzymes that regulate cholesterol metabolism and the use of drugs which inhibit lens cholesterol biosynthesis. The basis of this relationship apparently lies in the need of the lens to satisfy its sustained requirement for cholesterol by on-site synthesis, and impairing this synthesis can lead to alteration of lens membrane structure. The lens membrane contains the highest cholesterol content of any known membrane. The genetic defects Smith-Lemli-Opitz syndrome, mevalonic aciduria, and cerebrotendinous xanthomatosis all involve mutations in enzymes of cholesterol metabolism, and affected patients can develop cataract. Questions about the ocular safety of drugs, which can inhibit lens cholesterol biosynthesis, persist. Concern over potential damage to the lens from the use of hypocholesterolemic drugs stems from the reports in 1962 by Kirby et al and Laughlin et al that treatment of patients with Triparanol (Mer 29, Wm S Merrel Co.) to lower blood cholesterol was associated with development of cataract. Drugs used to lower blood cholesterol are among the most widely prescribed medicines. One drug in

the group, lovostatin (Mevacor, Merck), is alone the third most prescribed drug in the United States. This drug can inhibit cholesterol synthesis in lens and produce cataract in dogs. Whether these drugs inhibit cholesterol biosynthesis in human lenses at therapeutic doses is unknown.

The clinical safety trials indicate that treatment with lovastatin for up to five years does not significantly increase the development of cataract or grossly alter visual function. The ocular safety in an older patient population (>50 years) appears high. This seems also to apply to simvastin, except that one clinical trial showed a significant increase in cortical opacities with the use of this drug (**Figure 1.15**).

An unpublished study conducted at the University of Stellenbosch Medical School found that the rate at which opacification occurs in dyslipidemic patients on Cerivastatin was 4.5% per year (**Figure 1.15**). Although this rate of opacification is not statistically noteworthy it would seem that if these data are projected over a period of 20 years and compared the normal rate of opacification reported by Boccuzzi and Leino et al, an alarming amount of opacities would be present in the group of patients on cerivistatin.

Hypolipidemic drugs are intended for life-long use and patients as young as 18 years can receive these drugs. Although the human lens grows throughout life, the rate of growth is slow after 10 years of age. About 40 years are required for the lens cortex to double in width. The size of the nucleus remains essentially constant after 10 years of age. Thus, the consequences of inhibiting lens growth due to block of cholesterol biosynthesis may be difficult to assess in only a 1 to 5 years period. A considerable body of evidence indicates that sustained alteration of lens sterol content and composition due to genetic mutations or exposure to drugs can lead to altered lens clarity. Long-term ocular safety of the vastatin drugs should perhaps be viewed in units of 10 to 20 years. Certainly a 20-year-old person required to have cataract surgery at age 40 because of some chronic treatment would constitute a medical crisis for this individual, particularly if a less toxic treatment had

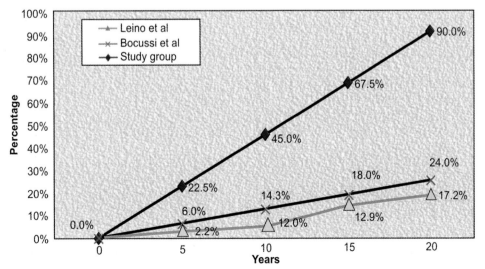

FIGURE 1.15: Tempo of lens opacification with Vastatin therapy

been available. The question of whether the vastatin drugs inhibit lens cholesterol biosynthesis in humans treated with standard therapeutic doses is unanswered. Since very low concentrations of lovastatin and simvastatin are required to inhibit cholesterol synthesis in animal lenses (3–22 nM), and only five times the therapeutic dose of lovostatin decreased cholesterol accumulation by the rat lens, it at least appears possible that therapeutic doses could inhibit lens cholesterol biosynthesis in humans.

CONCLUSION

Human lenticular opacification leading to the clinical challenge of cataract formation is etiologically multi-factorial. It does seem, however, that evidence is slowly mounting to encourage clinicians to consider cataract as belonging to the growing list of preventable ocular diseases.

FURTHER READING

1. Adler NE, Boyce T, Chesney MA, et al. Socioeconomic inequalities in health. No easy solution. JAMA 1993;269: 3140-5.
2. Alden ER, Ralina RE, Hodson WA. Transient cataract in low-birth-weight infants. J Pediatr 1973;82: 318-31.
3. Amaya LG, Speedwell L, Taylor D. Contact lenses for infant aphakia. Br J Ophthalmol 1990;74: 154-6.
4. Ames GM, Janes CR. Heavy and problem drinking in an American blue-collar population: implications for prevention. Soc Sci Med 1987;8: 949-60.
5. Ansari NH, Awasthi YG, Srivastava SK. Role of glycosy-lation in protein disulphide formation and cataracto-genesis. Exp Eye Res 1980;31: 9-19.
6. Armitage MM, Kivun JD, Farrell RE. A progressive early onset cataract gene maps to human chromosome 17q24. Nature Facet 1995; 937-40.
7. Assmann, et al. Lipid Metabolism Disorders and Coronary Heart Disease. MMV-Medizin-Verl (2nd ed), 1993.
8. Baghdassarian SA, Tabbara KF. Childhood blindness in Lebanon. Am J Ophthalmol 1975;79: 827-30.
9. Bandmann O, Vaughan J, Holmans P, et al. Association of slow acetylator genotype for N-Acetyltransferase 2 with familial Parkinson's disease. Lancet 1997;350: 1136-9.
10. Barnes PJ. Anti-inflammatory mechanisms of glucocorticoids. Biochem Soc Trans 1995;23: 940-5.
11. Behrens-Baumann W, Thiery J, Wieland E, et al. 3-Hydroxy-3-methylglutaryl coenzyme—a reductase inhibitor simvastatin and the human lens: clinical results of 3-year follow-up. Arzneim-Forsch 1992;42(11): 1023-4.
12. Beigi B, O'Keefe M, Bowell R, et al. Ophthalmic findings in classical galactosaemia—prospective study. Br J Ophthalmol 1993;77: 1624-64.
13. Belpoliti M, Maraini G. Sugar alcohols in the lens epithelium of age-related cataract. Exp Eye Res 1993;56: 3-6.
14. Benos DJ. Amiloride: a molecular probe of sodium trans-port in tissues and cells. Am J Physiol 1982;242: C131-45.
15. Benson WH, Farber ME, Caplan RJ. Increased mortality rates after cataract surgery: a statistical analysis. Ophthalmology 1988;95: 1288-92.
16. Berger J, Shepard D, Morrow F, et al. Relationship between dietary intake and tissue levels of reduced and total vitamin C in the guinea pig. J Nutr 1989;119: 1-7.
17. Bernstein HN. Chloroquine ocular toxicity. Surv Ophthalmol 1967;12(5): 415-47.
18. Bhatnagar R, West KP (Jr), Vitale S, et al. Risk of cataract and history of severe diarrheal disease in Southern India. Arch Ophthalmol 1991;109: 696-99.
19. Bhuyan KC, Bhuyan DK, Podos SM. Free radical enhancer xenobiotic is an inducer of cataract in rabbit. Free Radical Res Comm 1991;12-13: 609-20.
20. Bhuyan KC, Bhuyan DK, Podos SM. Lipid peroxidation in cataract of the human. Life Sci 1986;38: 1463-71.
21. Bialas MC, Routledge PA. Adverse effects of cortico-steroids. Adverse Drug React Toxicol Rev 1998;17(4): 227-35.
22. Björkhem, I Boberg KM. Inborn errors in bile biosynthesis and storage of sterols other than cholesterol. Metabolic Basis of Inherited Disease; New York, McGraw-Hill 1995;7: 2073-99.
23. Blondin J, Baragi VJ, Schwartz E, et al. Delay of UV-induced eye lens protein damage in guinea pigs by dietary ascorbate. Free Radic Biol Med 1986;2: 275-81.
24. Boccuzzi SJ, Bocanegra TS, Walker JF, et al. Long-term safety and efficiency profile of simvastatin. Am J Cardiol 1991;86: 1127-31.
25. Bochow TW, West SK, Axar A, et al. Ultraviolet light exposure and risk of posterior subcapsular cataract. Arch Ophthalmol 1989;107: 369-72.
26. Bonting SJ. Na'K' activated adenosine triphosphatase and active cation transport in the lens. Invest Ophthalmol 1965;4: 723.
27. Brauweiler PH, Wehler T, Busin M. High incidence of cataract formation after implantation of a silicone posterior chamber lens in phakic, highly myopic eyes. Ophthalmology 1999;106(9):1651-5.
28. Brilliant LB, Grasset NC, Pokrel RP, et al. Associations among cataract prevalence, sunlight hours and altitude in the Himalayas. Am J Epidemiol 1983;118: 250-64.
29. Brown CA, Burman D. Transient cataract in a diabetic child with hyperosmolar coma. Br J Ophthalmol 1973;57: 429-33.
30. Burke JP, O'Keefe M, Bowell R, et al. Ophthalmic findings in classical galactosemia: a screened population. Pediatr Ophthal Strabismus 1989;26: 165-8.
31. Caird Fl, Pirie A, Ramsell TG. Diabetes and the Eye. Blackwell Scientific: Oxford 1969.
32. Caird Rl, Hutchinson M, Pirie A. Cataract and diabetes. BMJ 1964;2: 665-8.
33. Cenedella RJ. Cholesterol and cataract. Surv Ophthalmol 1996;40: 320-37.
34. Chatterjee A, Milton RC, Thyle S. Prevalence and aetiology of cataract in Punjab. Br J Ophthalmol 1982;66: 35-42.
35. Chiba M, Masironi R. Toxic and trace elements in tobacco and tobacco smoke. Bull World Health Organ 1992;70: 270-6.
36. Christen WG, Manson JE, Seddon JM, et al. A prospective study of cigarette smoking and risk of cataract in men. JAMA 1992;268: 989-93.
37. Chylack LT Jr, Henriques H, Tung W. Inhibition of sorbitol production in human lenses by an aldose reductase inhibitor. Invest Ophthalmol Vis Sci 17: ARVO (Suppl): 1978;300.
38. Cigala O, Pancallo MT, Della Valle M, et al. La simvastatina nel trattamento delle piercolesterolemie. La Clinica Terapeu 1991;137: 333-7.
39. Clair WK, Chylack LTJ, Cook EF, et al. Allopurinol use and the risk of cataract formation. Br J Ophthalmol 1989;73: 173-6.
40. Clayton RM, Cuthbert J, Duffy J, et al. Some risk factors associated with cataract in SE Scotland: a pilot study. Trans Ophthalmol Soc UK 1982;102: 331-6.

41. Clayton RM, Cuthbert J, Philips CJ, et al. Analysis of individual cataract patients and the lenses: a progress report. Exp Eye Res 31: 553-66.

42. Clayton RM, Cuthbert J, Philips CJ, et al. Epidemiological and other studies in the assessment of factors contributing to cataractogenesis. Ciba Fdn Symp 1984;106: 25-47.

43. Clayton RM, Cuthbert J, Philips CJ, et al. Some risk factors associated with cataract in SE Scotland: A pilot study. Trans Ophthalmol Soc UK, 1982;102: 331-6.

44. Clayton RM, CuthbertJ, Phillios CI, et al. Analysis of individual cataract patients and their lenses: a progress report. Exp Eye Res 1980; 31: 553-6.

45. Cohen DL, Neil HA, Sparrow J, et al. Lens opacity and mortality in diabetes. Diabetic Med 1990;7: 615-7.

46. Collman GW, Shore DL, Shy CH, et al. Sunlight and other risk factors for cataract: an epidemiological study. Am J Public Health 1988;78: 1459-62.

47. Cooperative Study of Lipoproteins and Atherosclerosis. Evaluation of serum lipoprotein and cholesterol measurements as predictors of clinical complications of atherosclerosis. Circulation 1956;14.2: 691-741.

48. Cotlier E, Kwan B, Beatty C. The lens as an osmometer. Bioctfm Biophys Acta 1968;150: 705.

49. Cotlier E, Rice P. Cataract in the Smith-Lemli-Opitz syndrome. Am J Ophthalmol 1971;72: 955-9.

50. Cotlier E. Congenital rubella cataract. In Cotlier E, Lam-bert SR, Taylor D (Eds): Congenital Cataract. RG Landes/CRC: Boca Raton, 1994;65-76.

51. Cotlier E. Congenital varicella cataract. Am Ophihalmol 1978;86: 627-9.

52. Cruickshanks KI, Klein BEK, Klein R. Ultraviolet light exposure and lens opacities: the Beaver Dam Eye Study. Am J Public Health 1992;82: 1658-62.

53. Cuthbert J, Clayton RM, Philips. Cuneiform cataract: a special case? Colloq D'INSERM, 147: 387-96.

54. Dawber TR. The Framingham Study: The Eipidemiology of Atherosclerotic Disease. Cambridge Harvard University Press: London 1980.

55. de Vries ACJ, Cohen LH. Different effects of the hypo-lipidemic drugs pravastatin and lovastatin on the cholesterol biosynthesis of the human ocular lens in organ culture and on the cholesterol content of the rat lens in viva. Biochim Biophys Acta 1993;1167: 63-69.

56. Dohi K, Fukuda K, et al. Cataract in kidney transplant patients. Horishima J Med Sci 1984;33: 275-8.

57. Dolan BJ, Flach AJ, Peterson JS. Amiodarone keratopathy and lens opacities. J Am Optom Assoc 1985;56(6): 468-70.

58. Donahue RP, Bias WB, Renwickj H, et al. Probable assignment of the Duffy blood group locus to chromosome I in man. Proc Natl Acad Sci USA 1968;61: 949-55.

59. Dorland's Illustrated Medical Dictionary (28th edn) WB Saunders: Philadelphia 276.

60. Drack AV, Burke JP, Pulido JS, et al. Transient punctate lenti-cular opacities as a complication of argon laser photo-ablation in an infant with retinopathy of prematurity. Am J Ophthalmol 1992;113: 583-4.

61. Drews RC. Alcohol and cataract. Arch Ophthalmol 1993; 111:1312.

62. Drews RC. Ethanol cataract. In Solanes M (Ed): XXI Concilium Ophthalmologicum Mexico 1970. Amsterdam: the Netherlands Exerpta Medica 1970;753-8.

63. Duncan G, Hightower KR, Gandolfi SA, Tomlinson J, Maraini G. Human lens membrane cation permeability increases with age. Invest Ophthalmol Vis Sci 30: 1989;1855-9.

64. Dunn JP, Jabs DA, Wingard JC, et al. Bone marrow trans-plantation and cataract development. Arch Ophthalmol 1993; 11:1367-73.

65. Duthie GG, Arthur JR, James WP. Effects of smoking and vitamin E on blood antioxidant status. Am J Clin Nutr 1991;53(Suppl):1061S-64S.

66. Ederer F, Hiller R, Taylor HR. Senile lens changes and diabetes in two population studies. Am J Ophthalmol 1981;91: 381-95.

67. Eiberg H, Marner E, Rosenberg T, et al. Marner's cataract (AM) assigned to chromosome 16: linkage to haptoglobin. Clin Cenet 1988;34: 272-5.

68. Elsas U II, Fridovich-Keil JL, Leslie ND. Galactosemia: a mole-cular approach to the enigma. Pediatr 1993;8: 101-09.

69. Elsas U, Dembure PP, Langley S, et al. A common mutation asso-ciated with the Duarte galactosemia allele. Am J Hum Cenet 1994;54: 1030-36.

79. El-Yazigi A, Johansen K, Raines DA, et al. N-Acetylation Poly-morphism and diabetes mellitus among Saudi-Arabians. J Clin Pharmacol 1992;32(10): 905-10.

71. Emmelot P. The organization of the plasma membrane of mam-malian cells: structure in relation to function. In Jamieson GA, Robinson DM (Eds): Mammalian Cell Membranes, Butterworths: Boston, 1977;2: 1-54.

72. Emmerson BT. The management of gout. N Engl J Med 1996;446: 445-51.

73. Epstein FH. Cardiovascular Disease Epidemiology; A Journey from the Past Into the Future. Circulation 1996;93: 1755-64.

74. Erdman J. The physiologic chemistry of carotenes in man. Am J Clin Nutr 1988;7: 101-6.

75. Fechner PU. Cataract formation with a phakic IOL. J Cataract Refract Surg 1999;25(4): 461-2.

76. Fink AM, Gore C, Rosen E. Cataract development after implanta-tion of the Staar Collamer posterior chamber phakic lens. J Cataract Refract Surg 1999;25(2): 278-82.

77. Finley SC, Finley WH, Monsky DM. Cataract in girl with features of Smith-Lemli-Opitz syndrome. J Pediatr 1969;75: 706-07.

78. Flach AJ, Dolan BJ, Sudduth B, et al. Amiodarone-induced lens opacities. Arch-Ophthalmol 1983;101(10): 1554-6.

79. Flach AJ, Dolan BJ. Progression of amiodarone induced cataract. Doc Ophthalmol 1993;83(4): 323-9.

80. Flaye DE, Sullivan KN, Cullinan TR, et al. Cataract and cigarette smoking: the City Eye Study. Eye 1989;3: 379-84.

81. Francois J. Congenital Cataract, Charles C Thomas (Ed): Springfield, 1963.

82. Francois J. Late results of congenital cataract surgery. Ophthalmol 1979;86: 1586-98.

83. Franfelder FT. Do inhaled corticosteroids significantly increase cataract surgery in elderly patients? Arch Ophthalmol 1998;116: 1369.

84. Fraunfelder FT, Hanna C, Dreis MW, et al. Cataract associated with allopurinol therapy. Am J Ophthalmol 1982;94: 137-40.

85. Friend J, Chylack LT, Khu P, et al. The MSDRL Study Group: Lack of human cataractogenic potential of lovastatin: results of three-year study. Invest Ophthalmol Vis Sci 1992;33: 1301.

86. Garbe E, Suissa S, LeLorier J. Exposure to allopurinol and the risk of cataract extraction in elderly patients. Arch Ophthalmol 1998;116: 1652-6.

87. Garner MH, Spector A. ATP hydrolysis kinetics by Na, K-ATPase in cataract. Exp Eye Res 198642: 339-48.

88. Gibbs ML, Jacobs M, Wilkie AOM, et al. Posterior lens. Surv Ophthalmol 1996;40(6).

89. Giblin FJ, Padgaonkar VA, Leverenz VR, et al. Nuclear light scattering, disulfide formation and membrane damage in lenses of older guinea pigs treated with hyperbaric oxygen. Exp Eye Res 1995;60: 219-35.

90. Giblin FJ, Schrimscher L, Chakrapani B, et al. Exposure of rabbit lens to hyperbaric oxygen in vitro: regional effects on GSH level. Invest Ophthalmol Vis Sci 1988;29: 1312-9.

91. Glynn RJ, Christen WG, Manson JE, et al. Body Mass Index—an independent predictor of cataract. Arch Ophthalmol 1995;113: 1131-7.

92. Gofman, et al. The role of lipids and lipoproteins in atherosclerosis. Science 1950;111: 166-71.

93. Gretton C. Like falling off a cliff. Med Ad News 1994;3-25.

94. Grundy SM. HMG-KoA reductase inhibitors for treatment of hypercholesterolemia. N Engl J Med 1988;319: 24:33.

95. Gumming RG, Mitchell P, Leeder SR. Use of inhaled corticosteroids and the risk of cataract. N Engl J Med 1997;337: 8-14.

96. Hankinson SE, Seddon JM, Colditz, et al. A prospective study of aspirin use and cataract extraction in women. Arch Ophthalmol 1989;111: 503-8.

97. Hankinson SE, Stampfer MJ, Seddon JM, et al. Intake and cataract extraction in women: a prospective study. Br Med J 1992;305: 335-9.

98. Hankinson SE, Willet WC, Colditz GA, et al. A prospective study of cigaret smoking and risk of cataract surgery in woman. JAMA 1992;268: 994-8.

99. Harding J. Cataract: Biochemistry, Epidemiology and Pharmacology. Chapman and Hall: London, 1991;122-3.

100. Harding JJ, Crabe MJC. The lens: development, proteins, metabolism and cataract. In Davidson H (Ed): The Eye, Academic Press: London, 207-492.

101. Harding JJ, Egerton M, Harding RS. Protection against cataract by aspirin, paracetamol and ibuprofen. Acta Ophthalmol 1989;67: 518-24.

102. Harding JJ, Harding RS, Egerton M. Risk factors for cataract in Oxfordshire: diabetes, peripheral neuropathy, myopia, glaucoma and diarrhoea. Acta Ophthalmol 1989;67: 510-17.

103. Harding JJ, van Heyningen R. Beer, cigarets and military work as risk factors for cataract. Dev Ophthalmol 1989;17: 13-16.

104. Harding JJ, van Heyningen R. Drugs including alcohol that act as risk factors for cataract and possible protection against cataract by aspirin like drugs. Br J Ophthalmol 1989;73: 579-80.

105. Harding JJ, van Heyningen R. Drugs including alcohol, that act as risk factors for cataract, and possible protection against cataract by aspirin-like analgesics and cyclopenthiazide. Br J Ophthalmol 1988;72: 809-14.

106. Harding JJ. Cataract Biochemistry, Epidemiology and Pharma-cology. Chapman and Hall 1991: 116-8.

107. Harding JJ. Physiology, biochemistry, pathogenesis, and epidemiology of cataract. Curr Opinion Ophthalmol 1992;3: 3-12.

108. Harding JJ. Possible causes of the unfolding of proteins in cata-ract and a new hypothesis to explain the high prevalence of cataract in some countries. In Regnault F, Hockwin O, Courtois Y (Eds): Ageing of the lens. Procee-dings of the symposium on the aging of the lens held in Paris, September 1979. Biomedical Press: Amsterdam, 1980;71-80.

109. Havel, et al. Lovastatin (Mevolin) in the treatment of heterozygous familial hypercholesterolemia. Ann Intern Med 1987;107: 609-15.

110. Hayes RB, Bi W, Rothman N, et al. N-Acetylation phenotype and genotype and risk of bladder cancer in benzidine-exposed workers. Carcinogenesis (United States); 1993;14(4): 675-8.

111. Henkj M, Whitelocke RAF, Warrington AlP, et al. Radiation dose to the lens and cataract formation. Radiat Oncol Biol Phys 1993;25: 815-20.

112. Hesker H. Antioxidative vitamins and cataract in the elderly. Z Ernahrungswiss 1995;34: 167-76.

113. Hiller R, Giacometti L, Yuen K. Sunlight and cataract—an epidemiologic investigation. Am J Epidemiol 1977;105.

114. Hiller R, Sperduto RD, Ederer F. Epidemiologic associations with cataract in the 1971-1972 National Health and Nutrition Examination Survey. Am J Epidemiol 1983;118: 239-49.

115. Hiller R, Sperduto RD, Ederer F. Epidemiologic associa-tions with nuclear, cortical, and posterior subcapsular cataract. Am J Epidemiol 1986;124: 916-25.

116. Hiller R, Yuen K. Sunlight and cataract: an epidemiological investigation. Am J Epidemiol 1977;105: 450-9.

117. Hing S, Speedwell L, Taylor D: Lens surgery in infancy and childhood. Br J Ophthalmol 1990;74: 73-7.

118. Hockwin O, Koch H. Cataract of toxic etiology. In Bellows (Ed): Cataract and Abnormalities of the Lens. Grune and Stratton 1975;234-45.

119. Hoffmann G, Gibson KM, Brandt IK, et al. Mevalonic aciduria: an inborn error of cholesterol and nonsterol isoprene biosynthesis. N Engl J Med 1986;314: 1610-14.

120. Holowich F, Boateng A, Kolck B. Toxic Cataract. In Bellows JG (Ed): Cataract and Abnormalities of the Lens. Grune and Stratton: New York 1975;230-43.

121. Hunninghake, et al. Lovastatin—follow up ophthalmo-logical data. JAMA 1988;259: 354-5.

122. Hyman L. Epidemiology of eye disease in the elderly. Eye 1987;1: 330-41.

123. Jaafar MS, Robb RM. Congenital anterior polar cataract. Ophthalmology 1984;91: 249-54.

124. Jackson RC. Temporary cataract in diabetes mellitus. Br J Ophthalmol 1955;39: 629-31.

125. Jacques PF, Chylack LT (Jr). Epidemiologic evidence of a role for the antioxidant vitamins and carotenoids in cataract prevention. Am J Clin Nutr 1991;53: 352S-55S.

126. Jacques PF, Taylar A, Hankinson SE, et al. Long-term vitamin C supplement use and prevalence of early age-related lens opacities. Am J Clin Nutr 1997;66: 911-6.

127. Jahn CE, Janke M, Winowski H, et al. Identification of metabolic risk factors for posterior subcapsular cataract. Ophthalmic Res 1986;18: 112-6.

128. Jay B, Black RE, Wells RS. Ocular manifestations of ichthyosis. Br J Ophthalmol 1968;52: 217-26.

129. Jedziniak JA, Chylack LT Jr, Cheng HM, et al. The sorbitol path-way in the human lens: aldose reductase and polyol dehydro-genase. Invest Ophthalmol Vis Sci 1981;20: 314-26.

130. Jick H, Brandt DE. Allopurinol and cataract. Am J Ophthalmol 1984;98: 355-8.

131. Kahn HA, Leibowitz HM, Ganley JP, et al. The Framingham Eye Study. II—Association of ophthalmic pathology with single variables previously measured in the Framingham Heart Study. Am J Epidemiolo 1977;106: 33-41.

132. Kahn MU, Kahn MR, Sheikh AK. Dehydrating diarrhoea and cataract in rural Bungladesh. Ind J Med Res 1987;85: 311-5.

133. Kallner AB, Hartmann D, Horning DH. On the require-ments of ascorbic acid in men: steady-state turnover and blood pool in smokers. Am J Clin Nutr 1981;34: 1347-55.

134. Kanski JJ. Clinical Ophthalmology (3rd edn). Butterworth-Heineman: Oxford. 1994;289.

135. Kasai K, Nakamura T, Kase N et al. Increased glycosylation of proteins from cataractous lenses in diabetes. Dia-betologia 1983;25: 36-8.

136. Kench PS, Kendall EC, Slocumb CH, Polley HF. The effect of a hormone of the adrenal cortex (17-hydroxy-11-dehydrocortico-sterone; compound E) and of pituitary and adrenocorticotrophic hormone on rheumatoid arthritis. Mayo Clin Prvc 1949;4: 181-97.

137. Keys A. Atherosclerosis: a problem in newer public health. J Mt Sinai Hosp 1953;20:118-39.

138. Kirby TJ, Achor RWP, Perry HO, et al. Cataract formation after triparanol therapy. Arch Ophthalmol 1962;68: 486-9.

139. Klein BEK, Klein R, Jensen SC, et al. Hypertension and lens opacities from the Beaver Dam Eye Study. Am J Ophthalmol 1995;119: 640-6.

140. Klein BEK, Klein R, Lee KE. The incidence of age-related cataract, the Beaver Dam Eye Study. Arch Ophthalmol 1998;116: 219.

141. Klein BEK, Klein R, Linton KL, et al. Cigaret smoking and lens opacities: the Beaver Dam Eye Study. Am J Prev Med 1993;9: 27-30.

142. Klein BEK, Klein R, Linton KL, et al. The Beaver Dam Eye Study: the relation of age-related maculopathy to smoking. Am J Epidemiol 1993;137: 190-200.

143. Klein BEK, Klein R, Moss SE. Prevalence of cataract in a popu-la-tion-based study of persons with diabetes mellitus. Ophthalmology 1985;92: 1191-6.

144. Klein BEK, Klein R, Ritter LL. Is there evidence of an estrogen effect on age-related lens opacities? The Beaver Dam Eye Study. Arch Ophthalmol 1994;112: 85-91.

145. Klein R, Klein BEK, Jenses SC, et al. The relation of socioeconomic factors to age-related cataract, maculopathy, and impaired vision. Ophthalmology 1969-79;101(21).

146. Klein R, Klein BEK, Moss SE. Visual impairment in diabetes. Ophthalmology 1984;91:1-8.

147. Klein R, Moss SE, Klein BE, et al. Relation of ocular and systemic factors to survival in diabetes. Arch Intern Med 1989;149: 266-72.

148. Kleinman NJ, Spector A. The relationship between oxi-dative stress, lens epithelial cell DNA and cataractogenesis. Exp Eye Res 1992;55(Suppl): 1 (abstract 807).

149. Koga T, Shimada Y, Kuroda M, et al. Tissue-selective inhibition of cholesterol synthesis in viva by pravastatin sodium, a 3-hydroxy-3-methylglutaryl coenzyme: a reductase inhibitor. Biochim Biophys Acta 1990;1045:115-20.

150. Köhler L, Stigmar G. Vision screening of four-year-old children. Acta Paediatr Scand 1973;62:17-27.

151. Kreines K, Rowe KW. Cataract and adult diabetes. Ohio Med J 1979;75: 782-6.

152. Kretzer FL, Hittner HM, Mehta RS. Ocular manifestations of the Smith-Lemli-Opitz syndrome. Arch Ophthalmol 1981;99: 2000-6.

153. Kuchle M, Schonherr U, Dieckmann U. Risk factors for capsular rupture and vitreous loss in extracapsular cataract extraction. The Erlangen Ophthalmology Group. Fortschr Ophthalmol 1989;86: 417-21.

154. Kuriyama M, Fujiyama J, Yoshidome H, et al. Cerebro-tendinous xanthomatosis: clinical and biochemical evaluation of eight patients and review of the literature. J Neurol Sci 1991;102: 225-32.

155. Kuzma JW, Kissinger DG. Patterns of alcohol and cigarette use in pregnancy. Neurobehav Toxicol Teratol 1981;3: 211-21.

156. Lambert SR, Taylor D, Kriss A, et al. Ocular manifestations of the congenital varicella syndrome. Arch Ophthalmol 1989;107: 52-6.

157. Laqua H. Kataract bei chronisher Nierensuffinzeinz und Dialysebehanlung. Klin MBl Augenheilk 1972;160: 346-9.

158. Laties AM, Shear CL, Lippa EA, et al. Expanded clinical evaluation of lovastatin (EXCEL) study results II. Assess-ment of the human lens after 48 weeks of treatment with lovastatin. Am J Cardiol 1991;67: 447-53.

159. Laughlin RC, Carey TF. Cataract in patients treated with triparanol. JAMA 1962;181: 339-40.

160. Laurent M, Kern P, Regnault F. Thickness and collagen metabolism of lens capsule from genetically prediabetic mice. Ophthalmic Res 1981;13: 93.

161. Law MR, Wald NJ. An ecological study of serum cholesterol and ischeamic heart disease between 1950 and 1990. Eur J Clin Nutr 1994;48: 305-25.

162. Leino M, Pyorala K, Lehto S, et al. Lens opacities in patients with hypercholesterolemia and ischemic heart disease. Doc Ophthalmol 1992;80: 309-15.

163. Lerman S, Megaw JM, Fraunfelder FT. Further studies on allopurinol therapy and human cataractogenesis. Am J Ophthalmol 1984;97: 205-9.

164. Lerman S, Megaw JM, Gardner K. Allopurinol therapy and cataractogenesis in humans. Am J Ophthalmol. 1982;94: 141-6.

165. Lerman S, Moran M. Sorbitol generation and its inhibition by Sorbinil in the aging normal human and rabbit lens and human diabetic cataract. Ophthalmic Res 1988;20: 348-52.

166. Leske MC, Chylack LT (Jr), He Q, et al. The LSC Group: Anti-oxidant vitamins and nuclear opacities—The longi-tudial study of cataract. Ophthalmology 1998;105: 831-6.

167. Leske MC, Chylack Lt (Jr), Wu S. The lens opacities case-control study: Risk factors for cataract. Arch Ophthalmol 1991;109: 244-51.

168. Leske MC, Connel AMS, Schadat A. Prevalence of lens opacities in the Barbados Eye Study. Arch Ophthalmol 1997;115: 105.

169. Lessel S, Forbes AP. Eye signs in Turner's syndrome. Arch Ophthalmol 1966;76: 211-3.

170. Letson RD, Desnick RJ. Punctate lenticular opacities in Type II mannosidosis. Am J Ophthalmol 1978;85: 218-24.

171. Leveille PJ, Weidruch R, Walford RL, et al. Dietary restriction retards age-related loss of gamma crystalline in the mouse lens. Science 1998;224: 1247-9.

172. Liang J, Chakrabarti B. Sugar-induced change in near ultraviolet circular dichroism of alpha-crystallin. Biochem Biophys Res Commun 1981;102: 180.

173. Libondi T, Menzione M, Auricchio G. In vitro effect of alpha-tocopherol on lysophosatiphatidylcholine-induced lens damage. Exp Aye Res 1985;40: 661-6.

174. Lim R, Mitchell P, Cumming RG. Refractive associations with cataract: the Blue Mountains Eye Study. Invest Ophthalmol Vis Sci 1999;40(12): 3021-6.

175. Lin LR, Reddy VN, Giblin FJ, et al. Polyol accumulation in cultured human lens epithelial cells. Exp Eye Res 1991;52: 93-100.

176. Liu CS, Brown NA, Leanard TJ, et al. The prevalence and morpho-logy of cataract in patients on allopurinol treatment. Eye 1988;2: 600-6.

177. Lovastatin Study Group II. Therapeutic response to lovastatin (mevolin) in non-familial hypercholesterolemia. JAMA 1988;260: 359-66.

178. Lovastatin Study Group III. A multicenter comparison of lovastatin and cholestyramine therapy for severe primary hypercholesterolemia. JAMA 1988;260: 359-66.

179. Lovastatin Study group IV. A multicenter comparison of lovastatin and probucol for treatment of severe primary hypercholesterolemia. Am J Cardiol 1990;66: 22B-30B.

180. Lubkin VL. Steroid cataract—a review and conclusion. J Asthma Res 1977;14: 55-9.

181. Lubsen NH, Renwickjfl, Tsui LC, et al. A locus for a human hereditary cataract is closely linked to the gamma-crystallin gene family. Proc NatI Acad Sri USA 1987;84: 489-92.

182. Machlin LJ, Bendich A. Free radical tissue damage: protective role of antioxidants. FASEB J 1987;1: 441-5.

183. Marais JS. The Cape Coloured People 1652 to 1932 (1st edn) 1-31. Witwatersrand University Press: Johannesburg, 1957.

184. Mares-Perlman JA, Brady WE, Klein BEK, et al. Diet and nuclear lens opacities. Am J Epidemiol 1995b ;141: 322-34.

185. Mares-Perlman JA, Klein BEK, Klein R, et al. Relation between lens opacities and vitamin and mineral supplement use. Ophthalmology 1994;101: 315-25.

186. Marinho A, Neves MC, Pinto MC, et al. Posterior chamber silicone phakic intraocular lens. J Refract Surg 199713(3): 219-22.

187. Marmot MG, Kogevinas M, Elston MA. Social/economic status and disease. Ann Rev Public Health 1987;8: 111-35.

188. Marmot MG, Smith GD, Stansfeld S, et al. Health inequalities among British civil servants: the Whitehall II study. Lancet 1991;337: 1387-93.

189. Matthews KA, Kelsy SF, Meilahn EN, et al. Educational attainment and behavioral and biologic risk factors for coronary heart disease in middle-aged women. Am J Epidemiol 1989;129: 1132-44.

190. McCarty CA, Mukesh BN, Fu CL, et al. The epidemiology of cataract in Australia. Am J of Ophthal 1999;128(4): 446-65.

191. McCornsick AQ. Transient cataract in prensature infants:a new clinical entity. Can J Ophthalmol 1968;3: 302-8.

192. Meltzer EO. Prevalence, economic, and medical impact of tobacco smoking. Ann Allergy 1994;73: 381-91.

193. Merin S, Crawbird S: The etiology of congenital cataract. Can J Ophthalmol 1971;6: 1782-4.

194. Merits S, Craw S. Hypoglycemia and infantile cataract. Arch Ophthalmol 1993;86: 495-8.

195. Micozzi MS, Beecher GR, Taylor HR, et al. Carotenoid analyses of selected raw and cooked foods associated with a lower risk for cancer. J Natl Cancer Inst 1990;82: 282-5.

196. Minassian DC, Mehra V, Jones BR. Dehidrational crisis from severe diarrhoea or heatstroke and risk factor for cataract. Lancet 1984;1: 751-3.

197. Minassian DC, Mehra V, Jones BR. Dehidrational crisis: a major risk factor in the risk of blinding cataract. Br J Ophthalmol 1989;73: 100-5.

198. Minchin RF, Kadlubar FF, Ilett KF. Role of acetylation in colorectal cancer. Mutat Res 1993;290(1): 35-42.

199. Mitchell RN, Cotran RS: In Kumar V, Cotran RS, Robinson SL (Eds). Basic Pathology (6th edn): WB Saunders Company.

200. Mohan M, Sperduto RD, Angra SK, et al. India US case control study of age-related cataract. Arch Ophthalmol 1989;107: 670-6.

201. Molgaard J, Lundh B, van Schenck H, et al. Long- term efficacy and safety of simvastatin alone and in combination therapy in treatment of hypercholesterolemia. Atherosclerosis 1991;91: S21-24.

202. Mosley ST, Kalinowski SS, Schafer BL, et al. Tissue-selective acute effects of inhibitors of 3-hydroxy-3-methyl- glutaryl coenzyme: a reductase on cholesterol biosynthesis in lens. J Lipid Res 1989;50: 1411-20.

203. Mostafa MSE, Teintamy S, EI-Gammal MY, et al. Genetic studies of congenital cataract. Metah Pediatr Ophthalmol 1981;5: 233-42.

204. Motten AG, Martinez LJ, Holt N, et al. Photophysical studies on antimalarial drugs. Photochem Photobiol 1999;69(3): 282.

205. Mune M, Meydani M, Jahngen-Hodge J, et al. Effect of calorie restriction on liver and kidney glutathione in aging emory mice. AGE 1995;18: 49.

206. Munoz B, Tajchman U, Bochow T, et al. Alcohol use and risk of posterior subcapsular opacities. Arch Ophthalmol 1993;111: 110-12.

207. Nagata M, Hohmann TC, Nisihimura C, et al. Polyol and vacuole formation in cultured canine kens epithelial cells. Exp Eye Res 1989;48: 667-77.

208. Nakamura B, Nakamura O. Ufer das vitamin C in der linse und dem Kammerwasser der menschliche katarakte. Graefes Arch Clin Exp Ophthalmol 1935;134: 197-200.

209. Neilson NV, Vinding T. The prevalence of cataract in insulin-dependent and non-insulin-dependent diabetes mellitus: an epidemiological study of diabetics treated with insulin and oral hypoglycaemic agents (OHA). Acta Ophthalmol 1984;62: 591-602.

210. O'Neil WM, Gilfix BM, DiGirolamo A, et al. N-acetylation among HIV-positive patients and patients with AIDS: when is fast, fast and slow, slow? Clin Pharmacol Ther 1997;62(3): 261-71.

211. Orzechowska-Juzwenko K, Milejski P, Patkowski J, et al. Acetylator phenotype in patients with allergic diseases and its clinical significance. Int J Clin Pharmacol Ther Toxicol 1990;28(10): 420-5.

212. Oshima Y, Emi K, Motokura M, et al. Survey of surgical indications and results of primary pars plana vitrectomy for rhegmatogenous retinal detachments. Jpn J Ophthalmol 1999;43(2): 120-6.

213. Oxman TE, Berkman LF, Kasl S, et al. Social support and depres-sive symptoms in the elderly. Am J Epidemiol 1992;135: 356-68.

214. Pacurariu I, Marin C: Changes in the incidence of ocular disease in children and old people. Ofhalmologia (Buchuresti). 1973;17: 289-308.

215. Palmquist BM, Phillipson B, Barr PO. Nuclear cataract and myopia during hyperbaric oxygen therapy. Br J Ophthalmol 1984;60: 113-7.

216. Pande A, Gamer WH, Spector A. Glucosylation of human lens protein and cataractogenesis. Biochem Biophys Res Commun 1979;89:1260-6.

217. Petrohelos MA: Chloroquine-induced ocular toxicity. Ann Ophthalmol 1974;6(6): 615.

218. Pirie A, van Heyningen R. The effect of diabetes on the content of sorbitol, glucose, fructose and inositol in the human lens. Exp Eye Res 1964;3: 124-31.

219. Probst-Hensch NM, Haile RW, Ingles SA, et al. Acetylation polymorphism and prevalence of colorectal adenomas. Cancer Res (US) 1995;55(10): 2017-20.

220. Pruett RC. Ritinitis pigmentosa: clinical observations and correlations. Trans Am Ophthalmol Soc 1983;81: 693-35.

221. Racz P, Erdohelyi A. Cadmium, lead and copper concentrations in normal and senile cataractous human lenses. Ophthalmic Res 1988;20: 10-13.

222. Rafferty iVS. Lens morphology. In Maisel H (Ed): The Ocular Lens: Structure, Function and Pathology. Marcel Dekker: New York 1985;1-60.

223. Ramsay RC, Barbosa JJ. The visual status of diabetic patients after renal transplantation. Am J Ophthalmol 1979;87: 305-10.

224. Reddy VN. Glutathione and its function in the lens—an overview. Exp Eye Res 1990;150: 771-8.

225. Renwick JH, Lawler SD. Probably linkage between a congenital cataract locus and the Duffy blood group locus. Ann Ham Genet 1963;27: 67-84.

226. Resnikoff S, Filliard G, Dell'Aquila B. Climatic droplet kera-topathy, exfoliation syndrome, and cataract. Br J Ophthalmol 1991;75: 734-6.

227. Risch A, Wallace DM, Bathers S, et al. Slow N-Acetylation genotype is a susceptibility factor in occupational and smoking related bladder cancer. Hum Mol Genet (Feb 1995);4(2): 231-6.

228. Ritter LL, Klein EK, Klein R, et al. Alcohol use and lens opacities in the Beaver Dam Eye Study. Arch Ophthalmol 1993;111: 113-17.

229. Robertson J McD, Donner AP, Trevithick JR. Vitamin E intake and risk for cataract in humans. Ann NY Acad Sci 1989;570: 372-82.

230. Rouhianen P, Rouhiainen H, Salonen TJ. Association between low plasma vitamin E concentration and progression of early cortical lens opacities. Am J Epidemiol 1996;144: 496-500.

231. Rubb RM. Cataract acquired following varicella infectims. Ault Ophthalmol 1972;873-2254.

232. Sabiston DW. Cataract, Dupuytren's contracture, and Alcohol Addiction. Am J Ophthalmol 1973;76: 1005-7.

233. Sacanove A. Pigmentation due to phenothiazines in high and prolonged dosage. JAMA 1965;19I: 263-8.

234. Salive ME, Guralnik J, Christen W, et al. Functional blindness and viusal impairment in older adults from three communities. Ophthalmology 1992;99: 1840-7.

235. Salmon JF, Wallis CE, Murray ADN. Variable expressivity of autosomal dominant microcornea with cataract. Arch Ophthalmol 1988;106: 505-10.

236. Scales DK. Immunomodulatory agents. In Mauger TF, Craig EL (Eds): Haveners Ocular Pharmacology (Mosby-Yearbook: St Louis 1994;402-14.

237. Schein OD, West S, Mlnoz B, et al. Cortical lenticular opacification: distribution and location in a longitudinal study. Invest Ophthalmol Vis Sci 1994;35: 363-6.

238. Schocket SS, Esterson J, Bradford B, et al. Induction of cataract in mice by exposure to oxygen. Israel J Med 1972;8: 1596-1601.

239. Scott MR, Hejtmaucik F, Wozencraft LA, et al. Autosomal dominant congenital cataract; interocular phenotypic variability. Ophthalmol 1994;101: 866-71.

240. Shun Shin GA, Ratcliffe P, Bron AJ, et al. The lens after renal transplantation. Br J Ophthalmol 1990;73: 522-27.

241. Siddall JR. The ocular toxic findings with prolonged and high dosage chlorpromazine intake. Arch Ophthalmol 1965;74: 460-4.

242. Siegmund W, Fengler JD, Frane G, et al. N-Acetylation and debrisoquine hydroxylation polymorphisms in patients with Gilbert's syndrome. Br J Clin Pharmacol 1991;32(4): 467-72.

243. Simonelli F, Nesti A, Pensa M, et al. Lipid peroxidation and human cataractogenesis in diabetes and severe myopia. Exp Eye Res 1989;49: 181-7.

244. Simons LA. Interrelations of lipids and lipoproteins with coronary artery disease mortality in 19 countries. Am J Cardiol 1985;57: 5G-10G.

245. Sirtori CR. Tissue selectivity of hydroxymethylglutaryl co-enzyme A (HMG CoA) reductase inhibitors. Pharmacol Ther 1993;60: 431-59.

246. Solberg Y, Rosner M, Belkin M. The association between cigaret smoking and ocular diseases. Surv Ophthalmol 1998;42: 535-57.

247. Spector A, Garner WH. Hydrogen peroxide and human cataract. Exp Eye Res 33: 673-81, 1981.

248. Sperduto RD, Hu T-S, Milton RC, et al. The Linxian Cataract Studies: two nutrition intervention trials. Arch Ophthalmol 1993;111: 1246-53.

249. Srivastava S, Ansari NH. Prevention of sugar induced cata-ractogenesis in rats by mutilated hydroxytoluene. Diabetes 1988;37: 1505-8.

250. Stambolian D. Galactose and cataract. Surv Ophthalmol 1988;32: 333-49.

251. Stayte M, Reeves B, Wortham C. Ocular and vision defects in preschool children. Br J Ophthalmol 1993;77:228-32.

252. Steele G, Peters R. Persistent hyperplastic primary vitreous with myopia: a case study. J Am Optom Assoc 1999;70(9): 593-7.

253. Stewart Brown SL, Raslum MN. Partial sight and blindness in children of the 1970 birth cohort at 10 years of age. J Epidemiol Community Health 1988;42:17-23.

254. Stoll C, Alembik Y, Dott B, Roth MP. Epidemiology of con-genital eye malformations in 131,760 consecutive births. Ophthalmic Pediatr Genet 1993;39:433-5.

255. Stryker WS, Kaplan LA, Stein EA, et al. The relation of diet, cigaret smoking, and alcohol consumption to plasma beta-carotene and alpha-tocopherol levels. Am J Epidemiol 1988;127: 283-296.

256. Subar AF, Block G. Use of vitamin and mineral supplements: demographics and amounts of nutrients consumed—the 1987 Health Interview Survey. Am J Epidemiol 1990;132: 1091-1101.

257. Summers CG, Letson RD. Is the phakic eye normal in mo-nocular pediatric aphakia? J Pediatr Ophthalmol Strabismus 1992;29: 324-7.

258. Szmyd L Jr, Schwartz B. Association of systemic hypertension and diabetes mellitus with cataract extraction: A case-control study. Ophthalmology 1989;96: 1248-52.

259. Takemoto L, Takehana M, Horwitz J. Covalent changes in MIP 26K during aging of the human lens membrane. Invest Ophthalmol Vis Sci 1986;27: 443-6.

260. Tavani A, Negri E, La Vecchia C. Selected diseases and risk of cataract in Women. A case-control study from northern Italy. Ann Epidemiol 1995;5(3): 234-8.

261. Taylor A, Jacques P, Nadler D, et al. Relationship in humans between ascorbic acid consumption and levels of total and reduced ascorbic acid in lens, aqueous humor , and plasma. Curr Eye Res 1997;16: 857-64.

262. Taylor A, Jacques PF, Nadler D et al. Relationship in humans between ascorbic acid consumption and levels of total and reduced ascorbic acid in lens, aqueous humor, and plasma. Curr Eye Res 1991;10: 751-9.

263. Taylor A, Jaques PF, Epstein EM. Relations among aging, antioxidant status, and cataract. Am J Clin Nutr 1995;62(Suppl):1439S-47S.

264. Taylor A. Nutritional and Environmental Influences on the Eye. CRC Press, London; 1999;1-5.

265. Taylor A. Nutritional and Environmental Influences on the Eye. CRC Press: London. 1999;56-81.

266. Taylor D, Rice NSC. Congenital cataract, a cause of preventable child blindness. Arch Dis Child 1982;57: 165-7.

267. Taylor HR, West S, Munoz B, et al. The long-term effects of visible light on the eye. Arch Ophthalmol 1992;110: 99-104.

268. Taylor HR. The environment and the lens. Br J Ophthalmol 1980;64: 303-10.

269. Taylor HR. Ultraviolet radiation and the eye: an epidemiologic study. Trans Am Ophthalmol Soc 1989;87: 802-53.

270. Teramoto S, Fukuchi Y, Uejima Y. Influences of chronic tobacco smoke inhalation on ageing and oxidant-antioxidant balance in the senescence-accelerated mouse (SAM)-P/2. Exp Gerontol 1993;28: 87-95.

271. Thaler JS, Curinga R, Kiracofe G. Relation of graded ocular anterior chamber pigmentation to phenothiazine intake in schizophrenics: quantification procedures. Am J Optom Physiol Optics 1985;62: 600-04.

272. The Italian-American Cataract Study Group: Risk factors for age-related cortical, nuclear, and posterior subcapsular cataract. Am J Epidemiol 1991;133: 541-53.

273. Tielsch JM, Sommer A, Katz J, et al. Socioeconomic status and visual impairment among urban Americans. Arch Ophthalmol 1991;109: 637-41.

274. Tint, et al. Defective cholesterol biosynthesis associated with the Smith-Lemli-Opitz syndrome. N Engl J Ed 1994;330: 107-13.

275. Tobert JA. New developtments in lipid-lowering therapy: the role of inhibitors of hydroxymethylglutaryl-coenzyme A reductase. Circulation 1987;76: 534-8.

276. Traboulsi El, Weinberg RJ. Familial congenital cornea gut-tata with anterior polar cataract. Am J Ophthalmol 1989;108: 123-5.

277. Trindade F, Pereira F. Cataract formation after posterior chamber phakic intraocular lens implantation. J Cataract Refract Surg 1998;24(12): 1661-3.

278. Tsutomu Y, Mihori K, Yoshito H. Traumatic cataract with ruptured posterior capsule from a nonpenetrating ocular injury.

279. Tuormaa TE: The adverse effects of tobacco smoking on reproductive and health: A review from the literature. Nutr Health 1995;10: 105-120.

280. Ughade SN, Zodpey SP, Khanolkar VA. Risk factors for cataract: a case control study.

281. Urban RC (Jr), Cotlier E. Corticosteroid-induced cataract. Surv Ophthalmol 1986;31: 102-10.

282. Vadot E, Guibal JP. Pathogenic de la cataracte diabetique. Bull Soc Ophthalmol Fr 1982;82: 1513-4.

283. Vajpayee RB, Angra SK, Honavar SG, et al. Pre-existing posterior capsular breaks from penetrating ocular injuries. J Cataract Refract Surg 1994;20: 991-94.

284. Van Heyningen R, Harding JJ. A case-control study of cataract in Oxford: some risk factors. Br J Ophthalmol 1988;72: 804-08.

285. van Heyningen R, Harding JJ. Do aspirin-like analgesics protect against cataract? Lancet i: 1986;1111-3.

286. van Heyningen R. The human lens. I—a comparison of cataracts extracted in Oxford (England) and Shikarpur (W Pakistan). Exp Eye Res 1972;13: 136-47.

287. Varma S, Schocket SS, Richards RD. Implications of aldose reductase in cataract in human diabetes. Invest Ophthalmol Vis Sci 1979;18: 237-41.

288. Vesti E. Development of cataract after trabeculectomy. Acta Ophthalmol 1993;71(6): 777-81.

289. Vidal P, Fernandez-Vigo J, Cabezas-Cerrato J. Low glycation level and browning in human cataract. Acta Ophthalmol 1988;66: 220–22.

290. Vitale S, West S, Hallfrisch J, et al. Plasma antioxidants and risk of cortical and nuclear cataract. Epidemiol 1994;4: 195-203.

291. Waxman SL, Bergen RL. Wagner's vitreoretinal degene-ration. Ann Ophthalmol 1980;12(10): 1150-51.

292. Weale R: A note on a possible relation between refraction and a dis-position for senile nuclear cataract. Br J Ophthalmol 1980;64: 311-4.

293. Weber WW. Acetylation. Birth Defects Orig Artic Ser 1990;26(1): 43-65.

294. Wensor MD, McCarty CA, Taylor HR. The prevalence and risk factors of myopia in Victoria, Australia. Arch Ophthalmol 1999;117: 658-63.

295. West S, Munoz B, Emmett EA, et al. Cigaret smoking and risk of nuclear cataract. Arch Ophthalmol 1989;107: 1166-9.

296. West S, Munoz B, Schein OD, et al. Cigaret smoking and risk for progression nuclear opacities. Arch Ophthalmol 1995;113: 1377-80.

297. Wiechens B, Winter M, Haigis W, et al. Bilateral cataract after phakic posterior chamber top hat-style silicone intraocular lens. J Refract Surg 1997;13(4): 392-7.

298. Wilczek M, Zygulska-Machowa H. Zawartosc witaminy C W.roznych typackzaem. J Klin Oczna 1968;38: 477-80.

299. Winkleby MA, Fortmann SP, Barret DC. Social class disparities in risk factors for disease: eight-year prevalence patterns by level of education. Prev Med 1990;19: 1-12.

300. Wolff SM. The ocular manifestations of congenital rubella. Sri Am Ophthalmol Soc 1972;70: 577-14.

301. World Health Organization. Management of Cataract in Primary Health Care Services. WHO: Geneva 1990.

302. Ye JJ, Zadunaisky JA. A Na+/H+ exchanger and its relation to oxidative effects in plasma membrane vesicles from lens fibers. Exp Eye Res 1992;55: 251-60.

303. Young RW. Optometry and the preservation of visual health. Optom Vis Sd 1993;70: 255-62.

304. Zadok D, Chayet A. Lens opacity after neodymium: YAG iridectomy for phakic intraocular lens implantation. J Cataract Refract Surg 1999;25(4): 592-3.

305. Zelenka PS. Lens lipids. Curr Eye Res 1984;3: 1337-59.

CHAPTER 2

Biochemistry of the Lens

Ashok Garg

INTRODUCTION

The crystalline lens which is positioned behind the iris is the chief refractive medium of the eye having the maximum refractory power. It is a transparent, elastic and biconvex lens enclosed in a capsule. It refracts the light entering the eye through the pupil and focuses it on the retina.

BIOCHEMISTRY OF THE LENS

The human lens is the least hydrated organ of the body. It contains 66% water, and the 33% remaining bulk is composed mainly of protein. The lens cortex is more hydrated than the lens nucleus. **Lens dehydration is maintained by an active Na^+ ion water pump that resides within the membranes of cells in the lens epithelium and each lens fiber.**

The inside of the lens is electronegative. There is a –23 mV difference between anterior and posterior surfaces of the lens. Thus, the flow of electrolytes into the lens is directed by an electrical gradient.

CRYSTALLINE LENS AS AN OSMOMETER

The capsule of the lens acts as an intact cell and induces properties like swelling in hypotonic media and dehydration in hypertonic media. The osmolarity of the human lens is 302 mOsm and equals the osmolarity of aqueous. Cations like sodium and potassium with concentration of 145 mEq/L and anions (chloride, bicarbonate, sulfate, ascorbate and glutathione) with concentration of 50 to 60 mEq/L contribute to lens osmolarity. An anionic deficit of 90 mEq/L is probably made by acidic groups of lens protein and glycoproteins.

The water equilibrium between the lens and the surrounding fluids is disrupted if the concentration of osmotically active compounds (Na^+, K^+, etc.) increases inside the lens. Increase in Na^+ and K^+ levels also follows lens exposure to surface active detergents or antibiotics. When retained inside the cell, abnormal products of sugar metabolism such as sorbitol can exert osmotic effects and result in water influx and lens swelling.

LENS PROTEINS

The human lens contains the highest concentration of proteins (33%) of any tissue in the body. Proteins are synthesized in the anterior epithelium and the equatorial region. The perfect physiochemical arrangement of the lens protein living in an optimum environment of water, electrolytes and sulfhydryl gives transparency to the lens. Amino acids which are actively transported by the anterior lens epithelium are used by the lens to synthesize lens proteins. **Since lens protein is sequestered from the body immune system during embryonic life, later exposure of the lens protein can result in an autoimmune reaction.** The separation of lens proteins is based initially on their solubility of water. Fifteen percent of the lens proteins are insoluble in water. These form the albuminoid fraction which is thought to include membrane bound protein and aggregated crystallins. The remaining 85% are soluble in water and are classified as alpha, beta and gamma crystallins on the basis of molecular weight, electrophoretic mobility and presence or absence of subunits as shown in **Figure 2.1**. The soluble alpha and gamma crystallins leak into the aqueous humor during cataract formation causing a reduction in total lens protein.

The water soluble lens proteins are grouped as: (i) α-crystallins (15%), (ii) β-crystallins (55%), and (iii) γ-crystallins (15%). On the basis of their electrophoretic mobility towards the anode, α-crystallin is fastest, β-crystallin is intermediate and γ-crystallins is slowest. The molecular weight of crystallins in daltons is α-crystallin 1,000,000, β-crystallin 50,000-100,000 and γ-crystallin 20,000. α and β-crystallins are made of subunits and aggregation or separation of these subunits determines the physiochemical characteristics of each crystallin. The protein subunits are assembled by the alignment of amino acids through ribonucleic acid (RNA) as specified by the genetic code **(Figure 2.2)**. Lens proteins are degraded by proteases and amino peptidases. In the normal lens the membrane of lens fibers and lens capsule do not allow the passage of protein molecules from the lens to the aqueous humor. **When a mature cataract develops, the membranes of the lens fibers are lysed, the capsule becomes more permeable and protein can leak out of the lens. Lens proteins in the anterior chamber can act as an antigen which lead to inflammation of the uveal tissues known as lens induced or phacogenic uveitis.**

Sometimes degraded lens proteins leak through the capsule into the aqueous humor and are engulfed by macrophages which plug up the trabecular meshwork thus blocking aqueous humor outflow and producing increased intraocular pressure (IOP)—phacolytic glaucoma.

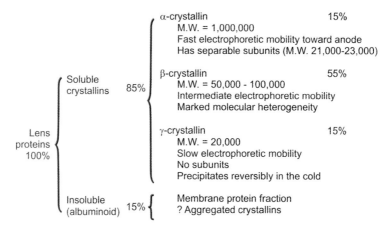

FIGURE 2.1: Human lens protein composition

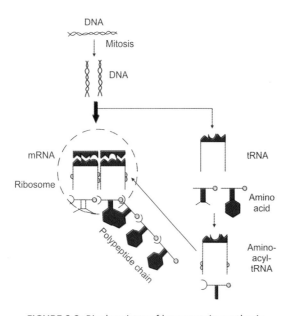

FIGURE 2.2: Biochemistry of lens protein synthesis

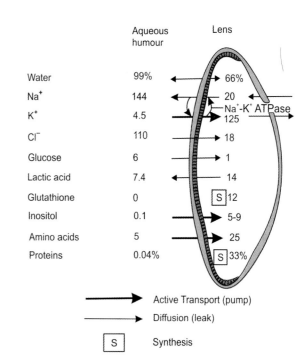

FIGURE 2.3: Chemical composition of human lens. (All values in mmol/kg of lens water), unless otherwise stated

ACTIVE TRANSPORT PROCESSES

WATER AND ELECTROLYTE TRANSPORT

The electrolyte and water content of the lens resembles that of an intact cell as shown in **Figure 2.3**. Whereas the Na^+, Cl^- and K^+ ion and water content of aqueous and vitreous is similar to that in plasma or extracellular fluids. To maintain electrolyte and water gradients against the surrounding fluids, the lens generates chemical and electrical energy. Chemical energy extrudes Na^+ ions and water is provided by ATP through glucose metabolism.

CATION TRANSPORT

The energy dependent cation pump in the lens accumulates K^+ intracellularly and extrudes sodium (Na^+). The influx of K^+ and efflux of Na^+ are thought to be linked and mediated by the membrane bound enzyme, Na^+-K^+-ATPase which degrades ATP to adenosine diphosphate (ADP)

inorganic phosphate and energy with which to power this cation pump. The action of Na^+-K^+-ATPase of lens can be inhibited by cardiac glycoside such as digitalis thereby stopping the cation pump.

It is generally believed that the cation pump of the lens functions at the anterior epithelial surface because the concentration of Na^+-K^+-ATPase is greater in this area than elsewhere. When K^+ is pumped into the lens and Na^+ is pumped out at the anterior surface, a chemical gradient is generated that stimulates a diffusion of Na^+ into the lens and K^+ out of the primarily through the posterior surface. This process of active transport (pump) stimulating passive diffusion (leak) has been termed as "pump and leak" theory of cation transport **(Figure 2.4)**. This cation transport system performs three important functions.

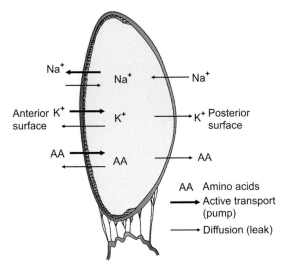

FIGURE 2.4: Active transport process of lens (pump-leak) mechanism

- It regulates the water content of the lens, thereby allowing the lens to act as a perfect osmometer. This prevents colloid osmotic swelling.
- It produces and maintains an electrical potential difference (approximately – 70 mV) between the lens and the medium surrounding it.
- It promotes the proper physiochemical environment within the lens to maintain transparency and optimal enzymatic activity.

Surface active agents (antibiotics, detergents, lysophospholipids and fatty acids) disrupt the physiochemical integrity of the membrane and Na^+ extrusion pump with subsequent gain of Na^+ ions and water by the lens, lens swelling and eventually complete loss of lens transparency follow.

AMINO ACIDS

Amino acids and inositol are actively transported into the lens at the anterior epithelial surface **(Figure 2.5).** Once in the lens, free amino acids are incorporated into RNA to

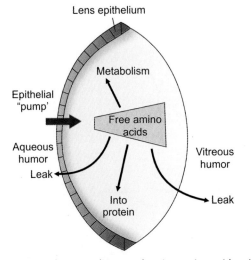

FIGURE 2.5: Schematic diagram showing amino acid active transport into the lens (epithelial pump)

form lens protein, can be metabolized with formation of CO_2, or can efflux from the lens. The turnover of free amino acids in the lens is very rapid, the renewal rate for lysine being 16% of the total in the lens per hour. There are three separate pumps for acidic, basic and neutral amino acids. Once in the lens these amino acids are metabolized and used for energy.

GLUTATHIONE-SULFHYDRYL PROTEINS

Glutathione, a polypeptide is actively synthesized in the lens. It is a tripeptide containing glycine, cysteine and glutamic acid. The levels of glutathione in the lens are high and in most of lens glutathione is in the reduced form (GSH). Only 6.8% of all lens glutathione is in the oxidized form (GSSG). GSH and GSSG are in equilibrium.

$$2GSH + \frac{1}{2} O_2 \rightleftharpoons = GSSG + H_2O$$

GSH concentrations are 12.0 micromoles/gm in the human lens. GSH levels are much higher in the cortex than in the nucleus of the lens. A reducing agent by virtue of its free sulfhydryl group, glutathione maintains membrane stability in the lens by supporting the protein complexes of the membrane. GSH levels decrease slightly with age. One of the earliest changes noted in the lens in different types of cataracts is the loss of glutathione. This allows the cross-linkage of proteins by the formation of disulfide bonds through sulfhydryl oxidation.

Another polypeptide ophthalmic acid is also found in the lens in concentrations of 1/10 to 1/100 those of GSH.

The pentose shunt of glucose metabolism active in the lens generates NADPH (reduced nicotinamide-adenine dinucleotide phosphate) that maintains glutathione in the reduced state by the following reductase:

$$GSSH + NADPH + H^+ \rightleftharpoons 2GSH + NADP.$$

Lens proteins contain reduced sulfhydryl groups (PSH) and oxidized disulfide groups (PSSP) maintaining high levels of GSH as shown in the following reaction:

$$2PSH + GSSG — 2GSH + PSSP$$

Thus, decreased GSH or increased GSSG will result in PSH oxidation and alterations in protein linkages, their solubility and their transparency.

The main functions of lens GSH are:
- To preserve the physiochemical equilibrium of lens proteins by maintaining high levels of reduced sulfhydryl (SH^-) groups.
- To maintain transport pumps and the molecular integrity of lens fiber membranes.

Synthesis of lens glutathione proceeds via α-glutamylcysteine synthetase which is markedly decreased in human senile cataracts. The enzyme glutathione peroxidase removes H_2O_2 or toxic lipid peroxides but decreases rapidly with age and in senile cataracts. Thus, the ability of lens to remove toxic oxygen appears impaired in early senile cataracts.

LIPIDS

The lipids of human lens are unique and differ markedly from those of other species. Lipids represent about 3 to 5% of the dry weight of lens. In human lens cholesterol is about 50% of lipids followed by phospholipids (45%) and glycosphingolipids and ceramides (5%). The lipids are major components of the lens fiber membranes and either decrease in their synthesis or impaired degradation brings about lens membrane damage and lens opacities. Cataracts develop in humans if treated with anticholesterolemic agents such as triparanol. Esterification of cholesterol takes place in human lens where 25% of total cholesterol is in the ester form. Among phospholipids, the human lens is specially rich in sphingomyelin and its precursor ceramides may increase in senile cataracts. Ceramide synthesis proceeds via fatty acids and sphingosine. Its degradative enzyme ceramidase is present in the human lens. Sphingomyelin is degraded by sphingomyelinase which is somewhat decreased in senile cataract.

The cholesterol-phospholipid ratio of human lens fiber membranes is the highest among cell or organelle membranes, thus conferring the lens resistance to deformation. Lipids as structural components of lens fiber membranes are associated with the insoluble lens proteins. The increased insolubility of the proteins with age or during cataract formation may be due to derangements in the stereochemical arrangement between lipids and proteins in the membrane and soluble proteins inside the fibers.

ASCORBIC ACID

In human lens ascorbic acid values are higher in the lens than in the aqueous. The role of ascorbic acid in the lens is not clear, but it could participate in oxidation-reduction reactions alone or coupled to glutathione.

GLUCOSE METABOLISM

Lens is avascular and surrounded by aqueous and vitreous humors. Both of which are rich in glucose and poor in oxygen. Glucose used by the lens is metabolized through following four main pathways.
- The glycolytic pathway
- The Krebs (oxidative) cycle
- The hexose monophosphate (pentose) shunt
- The sorbitol pathway.

End products of glucose metabolism are lactic acid, carbon dioxide and water. Lactic acid from the lens diffuses to the aqueous and is eliminated via this circulating fluid.

About 80% of glucose used by the lens is metabolized anaerobically by the glycolytic pathway to produce lactic acid and adenosine triphosphate (ATP). A small proportion of lens glucose may be metabolized via oxidative Krebs' citric acid cycle which is 18 times more efficient in producing ATP than glycolysis **(Figure 2.6)**. About 15% of the glucose consumed by the lens is metabolized by the pentose or hexose monophosphate shunt. Although this pathway produces no energy in the form of ATP it does provide five carbon sugars (pentoses) for the synthesis of RNA and NADPH to maintain glutathione in a reduced state.

The sorbitol pathway in which glucose is converted to sorbitol by aldose reductase in the normal lens is relatively insignificant, but it is extremely important in the production of cataracts in diabetic and galactosemic patients **(Figure 2.7)**.

The lens uses the energy of metabolism for two principle processes, reproduction and growth and active transport processes.

The synthesis of RNA, DNA, lens fiber membrane constituents, enzymes and other lens proteins occurs mainly at the anterior surface and equatorial region of the lens.

Glucose metabolism generates adenosine triphosphate. ATP breakdown is required for active transport of ions and

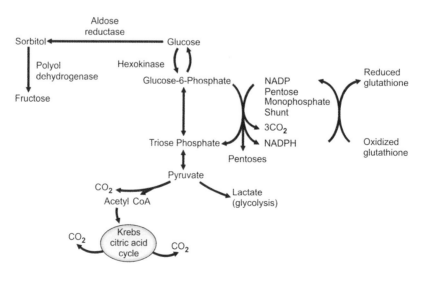

FIGURE 2.6: Lens glucose metabolism pathway (Krebs' cycle)

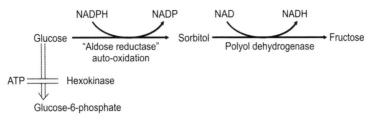

FIGURE 2.7: Lens glucose metabolism (sorbitol pathway)

amino acids, maintenance of lens dehydration, lens transparency and for continuous protein and GSH synthesis. The pentose shunt does not generate ATP, but it forms pentoses required for RNA synthesis. NADPH generated from the shunt is needed to maintain lens glutathione in the reduced state. The pentose shunt is extremely active in the lens. In addition, an active mechanism for pyruvate decarboxylation exists in the lens which results in formation of carbon dioxide and acetaldehyde. The latter is metabolized through lens aldehyde dehydrogenase. The carbon dioxide combination with water to form bicarbonate (HCO_3^-) may be partially active in the lens nucleus where the levels of carbonic anhydrase exceed those in lens cortex. However, carbonic anhydrase inhibitors do not produce cataracts.

The enzymes hexokinase and phosphofructokinase regulate the rate of glucose metabolism by the lens whereas oxygen is not essential for glucose metabolism. Conversion of glucose to amino acids such as glutamic acid, aspartic acid, glycine and others may account for 6 to 8% of glucose metabolism. Oxygen consumption by the lens is minimal 0.5 μmol/glens/hour. The Krebs' cycle requires oxygen and it is very inactive in the lens as there is paucity of mitochondria and oxidative enzymes. If the lens is deprived of glucose, it will utilize its own endogenous energy reserves.

When deprived of glucose the lens will gain water and lose transparency. In infantile hypoglycemia, cataract develops because of the low plasma glucose level are present.

The levels of glucose are higher in the aqueous (5.5 μmol/ml) than in the lens (1 μmol/ml) and glucose diffuses readily into the lens. Transport of glucose into the lens is not affected by the absence of sodium or calcium ions. However, other sugars or phloretin can inhibit lens glucose transport.

Studies of intact lens metabolism or protein structure can be done by noninvasive techniques. The ^{31}P nuclear magnetic resonance (NMR) spectra of intact lens sugar phosphates and dinucleoside phosphate are among the best resolved in biological tissues. For lens protein analysis, laser spectroscopy techniques are available. The Raman laser signals allow determination of the axial distribution of protein subgroups such as tryptophan, sulfhydryl and disulfide which suffer modifications during cataract formation.

APPLIED PHYSIOLOGY

CHEMICAL CHANGES IN LENS PROTEINS IN SENILE CATARACTOGENESIS

Lens proteins glycosylation happens on exposure to high glucose levels. These high glucose levels lead to protein conformational changes, near similar to those that occurs in glycosylated hemoglobin. The amino acid terminals of lens α- and β-crystallins are acetylated. Thus, sugar attachment in lens proteins occurs primarily by binding to amino groups of lysine and formation of covalent sugar-lysine bonds. Glucosyl-lysine combination results in conformational protein changes, protein formation of S-S bonds through oxidation of adjacent sulfhydryl groups, protein aggregation and opacification. These findings explain in part the protein aggregation in human cataracts. Levels of Σ-amino acids in diabetic senile cataracts are substantially reduced as compared to age-related cataract. Another chemical modification of lens protein includes carbamylation, i.e. addition of cyanate which occurs secondary to accumulation of urea cycle metabolites in uremia or secondary to dehydration. Urea cycle enzymes are active in human lens and cataracts.

Research studies have now clearly shown that formation of protein S-S bonds is the major primary or secondary event associated in senile cataracts. Oxidation of lens protein SH groups with H_2O_2 induces protein conformation changes leading to opacification.

Protection against oxidation of protein SH groups is vital. Cysteine and glutathione have proven effective to prevent formation of S-S protein bonds. Protein unfolding due to primary modification of exposed lysine amine groups can be prevented by lysine acetylation. Lysine acetylation of protein prevents attachment of glycosyl, cyanate or other reactive groups like keto groups of steroids.

BIOCHEMISTRY OF CORTICAL CATARACTS

Cortical cataract is characterized by abnormalities in fiber permeability that causes vacuoles or clefts in the lens cortex. Damage to the membranes of lens fibers represents the initial insult due to X-rays, diabetes, galactosemia, arachidonic acid or other surface active agents. The various chemical changes some of which develop prior to clinical cortical changes include :

- Loss of glutathione with compensatory increase in NADPH synthesis
- Increase K^+ ion efflux
- Loss of K^+ ions, inositol and amino acids from lens
- Gain in Na^+ ions
- Decrease lens protein synthesis with decrease in the proportional of soluble protein and increase in insoluble protein
- Increase in protein S-S groups and in Ca^{++} ions.
- Decreased activity of most enzymes and increased activities of hydrolytic enzymes
- Decreased ATP content.

The majority of cataractogenic agents damage the ability of the lens to maintain GSH synthesis or increase its efflux through more permeable membranes. Thus, a cycle of increased exudation of K^+ ions, amino acids and inositol is initiated. The lens epithelium tries to maintain the concentration of these compounds by increased pumping. Depending upon the magnitude of cataractogenic stimuli, the GSH leak out may continue or stop. To maintain normal levels of NADPH is required which in turn stimulate the glucose metabolism through the pentose shunt. If the epithelium or lens fibers are structurally damaged and are unable to extrude Na^+ ions water gain will occur. This is followed by a decrease in protein synthesis which manifest itself by decreased levels of soluble lens proteins. This is compounded by the retention of cations and formation of disulfide S-S bonds with increased turbidity and protein insolubility. At this stage of cataractogenesis, the increased activity of glycolysis and other enzymes is detected. The generalized disarray of lens metabolism is accompanied by ATP loss. The end result is a total opaque or cataractous lens.

NUCLEAR SCLEROSIS

The human lens normally undergoes changes with age. It slowly increases in size as new lens fibers develop throughout life. Older lens fibers in the center of the lens become dehydrated and compacted. The cross-linking of proteins in the nucleus increases its optical density and decreases its transparency. Clinically this condition is known as nuclear sclerosis which may cause refractive changes. Simultaneously splits in sutures or clefts in the cortical fibers are visible causing damage to the permeability of the lens. The nucleus of the lens becomes more compact and resists mechanical disruption with aging. There is extensive cross-linkage of the lens protein. The cataract protein cross-linkage is accompanied by increased pigmentation in certain cases. In senile cataracts, changes in lens color to dark yellow, yellow brown or brown and hardening of the nucleus parallel lead to decreased transparency. Three major types of cross-links are identified in senile cataracts.

- Disulfide cross-links (S-S)
- Lysine modification
- Dityrosine cross-links.

Protein SH groups are oxidized and noncovalent S-S protein cross-links are formed in senile cataracts.

These S-S bonds are susceptible to dissociation by a variety of reducing agents. The origin of oxidative insult is attributed to either the loss of lens glutathione, excessive H_2O_2 or lipid peroxidase in aqueous humor, increased permeability to oxygen into the aqueous or lack of oxygen detoxifying enzymes. S-S cross-links may explain the conformational changes in protein causing opacity, the presence of covalent bonds is a feature of senile cataracts.

Superoxide anion-free radicals (O_2^-) or its derivative peroxide (H_2O_2), singlet, oxygen ($^1O_2$) and OH^- induce oxidative damage to a variety of cells. The lens is highly susceptible to these radicals. Peroxide (H_2O_2) is catalyzed through catalase and peroxidase and synthesized through superoxide dismutase. This oxidative damage as a result of free radicals to human lens leads to cataract formation **(Figure 2.8)**.

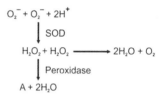

FIGURE 2.8: Oxidative damage of lens (by free radicals)

DIABETIC CATARACT

Snow flake cortical lens opacities also known as metabolic cataract is found in diabetic patients.

Increased levels of glucose in the aqueous and lens are found in patients with diabetes mellitus. In general glucose concentration in the aqueous is similar to concentrations in the plasma. From the aqueous glucose diffuses rapidly into the lens. The lens metabolizes glucose through the four main pathways as already mentioned in this chapter. In diabetes excessive glucose in the lens (more than 200 mg/100 ml) saturates hexokinase. Excessive glycosylation of lens proteins takes place and glucose is converted to sorbitol by auto-oxidation and protein binding (aldose reductase). These chemical changes are present in human diabetic cataract. However, glucose oxidation to sorbitol plays a more important role in the rapidly developing diabetic cataract. Whereas abnormal protein glycosylation is of greater significance in the slowly developing senile cataracts in patients with diabetes.

CHAPTER 3

History of Phacoemulsification

Charles D Kelman

INTRODUCTION

A resident in ophthalmology today, seeing his first cataract performed by a surgeon who uses Kelman phacoemulsification, might wonder how it could be performed any other way. Seated comfortably at the operating microscope, the surgeon makes a tiny incision, neatly peels open the anterior capsule, emulsifies and aspirates the lens within the remaining capsule, and then, through the same incision inserts a foldable lens. On the first postoperative day, in most cases, it is difficult to tell with the naked eye, which eye has been operated.

In contrast, in 1960, when the author finished his residency at Wills Eye Hospital, general anesthesia was common, no microscopes were used for any ophthalmic surgery anywhere in the world (except for a surgeon in Chicago, Richard Peritz). A 180-degree incision was made, a large sector iridectomy was performed, and then the lens was grasped by a capsule forceps, and the entire lens was pulled from the eye. Eight or more sutures closed the incision, and the patient remained hospitalized for 7 to 10 days. The eyes were red, the lids swollen, and irritated for up to six weeks.

One might ask how the idea for phaco came to the author. Did he one day thought, "I'll just take an ultrasonic needle and remove the cataract that way?" As brilliant as that leap of thought would have been, the author cannot pretend to claim credit for making it. Actually, it is so far from the truth that the real answer serves to illustrate a point—the final solution to a problem is usually far afield from the first attempts at its solution.

First, the impetus for wanting to find a better way to remove cataracts:

The author was in the process of writing a grant application to the John A Hartford Foundation to investigate the effects of freezing on the eye, and after finishing the final draft, he went to bed, but he could not sleep. The application seemed "boring" and he knew that the foundation looked to support breakthrough procedures, not boring scientific studies. The author knew in his heart that the application would be rejected. The author needed something exciting, but he did not know what. Without knowing what he was doing, he put his subconscious mind to work, and went to bed.

Sometime in the night, the author got out of bed and wrote a phrase, which would forever change his life, and would forever change the practice of cataract surgery. That phrase was, "The author will also find a way to remove a cataract through a tiny incision, eliminating the need for hospitalization, general anesthesia, and dramatically shortening the recovery period." That statement looked well on paper. The author had no idea how he would accomplish this feat. He was, however, confident that he could do so easily—this confidence sprang from three factors: (i) The author had quite easily discovered cryoretinopexy and had published the first paper on that subject,[1] (ii) The author had quite easily codiscovered (Krwawicz, in Poland had also, independently discovered the same thing) cryoextraction of cataracts,[2] and (iii) The author was blissfully and naively unaware of the complexity of the task he had set out for himself. It is certainly possible, that had he known the number of problems he would have to solve, he would have been intimidated, and might have never started. It is for this reason that often people outside of a particular discipline are able to make breakthroughs. Those more knowledgeable are too aware of the difficulties.

The Hartford Foundation director, E Pierre Roy, called the author a few days later to tell him that he was not interested in the effects of freezing on the eye, but that he would give the grant for the new cataract operation. The author was ecstatic! This was going to be easy!

The first "method" for removing the lens through a small incision revolved around a collapsible "butterfly net" **(Figure 3.1)**, the net portion being made out of condom thin latex. The idea that the author had was to dilate the pupil, instill an enzyme to loosen the zonule, turn the patient over on his or her face and vibrate his or her head with a manual vibrator, until the lens fell into the anterior chamber, then instill acetylcholine to constrict the pupil. Once the cataract would be trapped in the anterior chamber, the

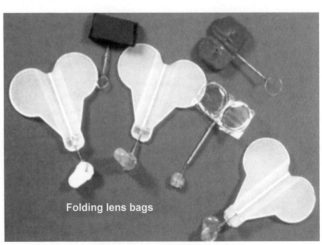

Folding lens bags

FIGURE 3.1: Folding lens bags

collapsed latex net would be introduced to trap the cataract, which would then be simply mushed up with a needle, until the net and the squashed cataract could be pulled through the small incision. It is important for the reader to note how far from the sophisticated phaco machines this original, naive idea was. It would have been so easy to listen to those who said to the author, "I told you, you could not do it," and admit defeat, just as it may be easy for the readers to abandon their first idea on a subject, and never get to the second generation, the third, the fourth, the fifth, the sixth, etc. until the readers come up with a solution totally unrelated to author's original idea.

This "cat in the bag method" could not be made to work (all attempts with this device were made on animal and eye bank eyes). It was too traumatic to the cornea, the bag was too thick, took too much volume in the anterior chamber, and the bag kept breaking. It had taken six months for the author to fabricate this "butterfly net" and to test it. He had used up one-sixth of his three-year grant and he began to worry.

He then began investigating devices, which would break up a cataract, so that it could be irrigated and aspirated from the eye.

Various drills, rotary devices and several types of microblenders were constructed and tried **(Figures 3.2 to 3.4)**. Each failed for several reasons. If the iris was touched with a rotating tip, it would immediately become completely ensnared and a total 360 iridodialysis would inadvertently be performed. Usually, uncontrollable hemorrhage would ensue. Furthermore, the iris did not even have to be close to the rotating tip. The eddy currents set up within the chamber were enough to draw the iris to the rotating tip and instantaneously disinsert and remove it.

The second obstacle to fast rotating devices was that the eddy currents set up in the anterior chamber would throw lens particles against the corneal endothelium and completely denude it in a few seconds, leading to permanent opacification. Thirdly, the lens itself when caught on the rotating tip would also spin in the chamber with the consequent destruction of the endothelium. The

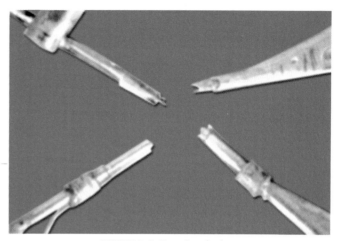

FIGURE 3.3: Rotating devices

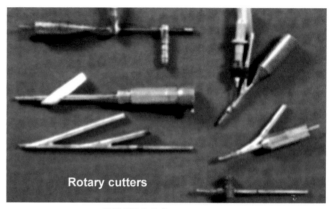

FIGURE 3.4: Rotary cutters

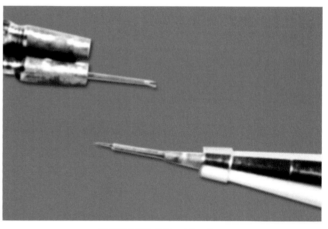

FIGURE 3.5: Microblenders

microblender **(Figure 3.5)** with needles rotating in opposite directions was intended to prevent the lens from spinning, but it was unsatisfactory. It also increased the chances of incarcerating the iris in the two rotating tips. Slow-turning drills **(Figure 3.6)** were designed, but these, too, were unable to prevent the lens from turning. Rocking vibrators still rubbed off endothelium. These abandoned devices are similar to the rotorooter-type devices, which others are reevaluating at present. Steps were taken to fix the lens from the opposite side with the use of the prongs. The sharp tips, however, endangered the posterior capsule. Low-frequency vibrators were tried, but the lens merely vibrated with the

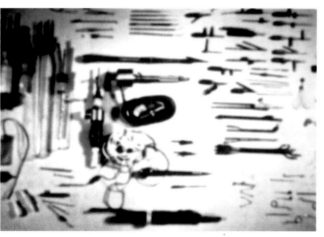

FIGURE 3.2: Various unsuccessful devices

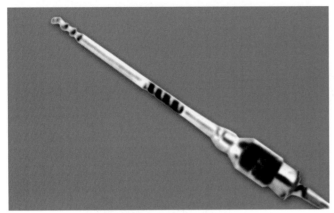

FIGURE 3.6: Worm gear feeder

tip. None of the aforementioned devices were ever used clinically, as they were considered dangerous and ineffective.

Two years and most of the grant money had now elapsed. The solution of this problem had become more than a challenge—it had become an obsession.

In analyzing the difficulties, the author had so far become clear that the main problem was that the lens was moving, rotating, or vibrating inside of the anterior chamber and, therefore, rubbing against the endothelium. This realization eventually led to the solution only a few months before the expiration of the grant. At this time, it became obvious that in order to let the lens remain stationary in the chamber, the acceleration of the moving tip against it had to be high enough so that the standing inertia of the lens would not be overcome. In other words, high enough acceleration was required so that the lens could not back away, vibrate, or rotate with the tip. To demonstrate this principle, imagine a sharp knife slowly punching against a punching bag. The punching bag will move with the knife. If, however, the knife is quickly plunged against the bag, the knife will enter and the bag will not move. In this analogy, the punching bag represents the lens, and the knife represents the tool used to enter the lens. The high acceleration could only be achieved with an ultrasonic frequency. Early experiments with a dental ultrasonic unit using irrigation only and a nonlongitudinal motion were encouraging, but were clinically unsuccessful because of the high energy radiated and the relative inefficiency requiring many minutes of ultrasonic time in the anterior chamber. Substitution of a longitudinal motion at the tip was introduced to prevent disinsertion of the iris and to reduce radiation. This type of motion also significantly reduced flaking (originally published in 1974, courtesy of the American Academy of Ophthalmology[3]).

Once the author had discovered the method of breaking up the lens, he thought the rest would be easy, but it was not. There were three types of problems lurking ahead, which as they were discovered, had to be overcome:

   i. Surgical problems,
   ii. Instrument problems, and
   iii. Political problems.

SURGICAL PROBLEMS

PUPIL CONSTRICTION

In the first attempt to do phacoemulsification, the pupil constricted during the surgery. There had to be new drugs and methods to maintain dilatation.

In the early cases, the pupil constricted rapidly in the procedure, since there were no potent mydriatics at that time. At first, the author performed large sector iridectomies so that he could see behind the iris. However, in many cases, the iris became aspirated into the tip and became badly frayed. Because of this problem, the author began to bring the lens into the anterior chamber before performing the phaco, and before the pupil constricted. For several years he taught anterior chamber phaco, which he believe is still a viable alternative to posterior chamber phaco, for those less skilled. There is a slight increase in endothelial cell loss over the posterior chamber phaco, but not enough to be significant.

After a few years, mydriatics were placed in the irrigating solution, and anti-inflammatory drops were used on the cornea in combination with more powerful mydriatics. Once viscoelastics came into use, they too aided in pupillary dilation, and posterior chamber phaco became much easier. For those pupils, which are fibrotic, several models of iris hooks are available.

ANTERIOR CAPSULAR OPENING

A method of opening the anterior capsule had to be developed which would be consistent, exposing the lens, but not extending to the zonules.

The author's first attempts to incise the anterior capsule in several directions, with criss-crossing lines taught him that these incisions in the capsule, if subjected to traction, could extend around the anterior surface of the lens into the zonule, and perhaps even onto the posterior capsule. One day, the author observed on an animal eye, that if he used a dull cystotome rather than a sharp one, instead of cutting the capsule, the cystotome tore it. And that tear was always in the form of a triangle. The author named this technique the Christmas tree opening **(Figure 3.7).** If he could rewrite history, he would call it a triangular capsulorhexis, a more accurate description, and one that would place it in its proper historical position, the forerunner of the continuous tear capsulorhexis. Once the triangular tear was made, the pie-shaped flap would be grasped with a forceps, gently extracted, and then cut at its base. This method was in general use until the "can opener technique" was introduced, and then finally the continuous tear technique widely used today.

MAGNIFICATION AND VISUALIZATION

Using loups (the standard method of magnification at that time), the magnification was not adequate. Using existing surgical microscopes gave no depth perception, since the lighting was flat, and there was no red reflex.

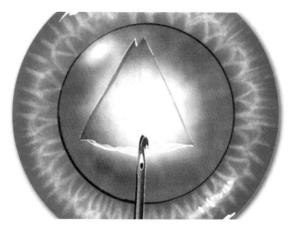

FIGURE 3.7: Christmas tree opening

This technique involved acute visualization of the intraocular structures never really seen before. No surgeon had ever really seen at surgery, cortical material lying on top of a capsule, or a tiny zonular dehiscence, or a minute opening in the capsule, and yet this type of visualization was required if phaco was ever going to be successful.

The first microscopes the author tried were tabletop dissecting microscopes, and they had inadequate side illumination. In examining other types of microscopes, he came upon an exciting discovery. Using an ENT microscope, the red reflex from the coaxial light gave him an incredible depth perception intraocularly. From then on, only ENT microscopes were used until Zeiss finally made one more suitable for ophthalmology.

PROTECTION OF THE POSTERIOR CAPSULE

The posterior capsule is not a strong membrane. Techniques had to be developed which would protect it during the lens removal.

It became evident to the author very early on that the big obstacle to phaco would be the rupture of the posterior capsule. The early phaco machines did not have the power or the suction that present models have, and the tip had to be pushed into a hard nucleus in order to emulsify it. Like a dull knife must be pushed harder onto tissue than a sharp one. This pushing often broke the capsule. One must remember that there were no viscoelastics at that time. In order to make the procedure safer for the author, and especially for others learning it, he devised a technique for prolapsing the entire nucleus into the anterior chamber, where it could be emulsified at some distance from the capsule. This method remained in vogue until the equipment was improved, at which time phaco in the posterior chamber (where phaco began) was reintroduced.

PROTECTION OF IRIS AND CORNEA

A technique of surgery had to be developed which would allow the surgeon to safely emulsify the nucleus without damaging the endothelium, or the iris.

In the early cases, the corneas collapsed many times against the vibrating needle, and the corneas had severe striate for sometimes up to one month. There was no method at this time of counting endothelial cells, but later studies showed up to 50% cell loss in these first cases. It is interesting to note that these corneas eventually cleared, giving the patients good vision.

CORTICAL CLEAN-UP

A technique would be needed to safely pull the cortex out of the fornices of the capsule, and then to aspirate it.

In the early cases, the same phaco tip and sleeve were used to remove cortex, but it became obvious that this terminal opening endangered the capsule. The author modified the tip, so that it had a closed terminal end, with the lumen on the side, so that it could be directed away from the capsule.

INSTRUMENT PROBLEMS

An instrument powerful enough to emulsify all types of cataracts, without damaging adjacent structures would have to be developed.

The first phacoemulsifier used on animals and patients consisted of a table with various parts and devices connected to each other. One of the parts was a dental apparatus used to remove tartar from the teeth. This was modified, so as to add suction and irrigation. The ultrasonic stroke was not only too small to act on hard cataracts, but it got dampened even further when a load (the cataract) was put on. The author found that with piezoelectric crystals, rather than magnetostrictive stacks, a greater stroke could be achieved, and that dampening could be prevented. Today there is no cataract too hard to be emulsified.

HEAT BUILD-UP

Ultrasonic frequencies build-up sufficient heat to denature tissue. Cooling would have to be guaranteed.

After actually cooking and denaturing the protein of the lens in some animal eyes, it became clear to the author that constant irrigation of the vibrating tip had to be assured. His original idea of having a watertight, close-fitting incision was not going to work, since when the tip was occluded, the outflow through the tip was blocked, and since the incision was tight around the tip, no fluid could escape. It then became necessary to have the incision slightly larger than the tip so that fluid could always escape from the eye, and also to insure that the amount of fluid flowing into the eye always exceeded the amount being aspirated. Once these concepts were put into effect, heat build-up ceased to be a problem.

ANTERIOR CHAMBER COLLAPSE

Considerable suction was necessary to hold lens material onto the vibrating tip. Once this material was aspirated in a few milliseconds, there was enough suction build up to collapse the chamber. The result of this collapse was to see the cornea touching the vibrating tip, with the endothelium being emulsified. A method had to be found to prevent this.

In order for the lens material (especially if it is hard nucleus) to remain fixed to the tip while that tip is vibrating, a fairly high level of vacuum must be achieved. If starting is done with the high level of vacuum, copious amounts of fluid would always be entering and leaving the eye. Also, if the capsule or iris were inadvertently engaged, these tissues would be more susceptible to damage, than if the suction were lower. It became obvious that a peristaltic type pump could apply minimum suction until such a time as the tip became occluded, at that time the suction would rise, holding the lens material onto the tip while it was being emulsified. The problem created with this system was that as soon as the lens material became suddenly aspirated, the high level of suction in the system would collapse the chamber. For the first 50 or so cases, the author had no other solution to this problem rather than that of trying to anticipate the collapse, and just before the morcel would be aspirated, he would take the foot off the foot pedal. This was very ineffective, and many times during the first cases, the cornea would collapse onto the vibrating tip. Although the author was sure that the endothelium was damaged, to his good fortune, these eyes always cleared after a few days, permitting him to continue developing the instrument and technique.

After much searching, the author finally found a fluid control system, which monitored flow in arteries by creation of an electrical current from the ions as they rushed through the arteries. He adapted this system so that the fluid flow through the aspiration line was monitored. When it stopped (tip occlusion), a valve was put into the alert position. Within a few milliseconds after flow started up again (aspiration of the morcel), this valve would open to the atmosphere, killing the suction. This was a very satisfactory system, and was used for several generations of phacoemulsifiers.

After having suffered through hundreds of actual collapses on his first cases, the author still remember the joy of seeing the tiny "beat" of the cornea, instead of a collapse, once the system was working.

HANDPIECE DESIGN

The early handpieces were extremely heavy and cumbersome. The original procedures took up to four hours, with over one hour of ultrasonic time. A special three-dimensional parallelogram had to be invented and constructed to hold the handpiece.

Ophthalmic surgeons are used to tiny instruments, which fit into the fingers. The original phaco handpiece was about the size of a large flashlight, and weighed almost a pound. The author was willing to use it while he was developing the techniques, but he knew no one else would be willing. While looking for ways to make the handpiece lighter and smaller, he developed the three-dimensional parallelogram to hold the handpiece with all the axes of rotation around the incision **(Figure 3.8)**.

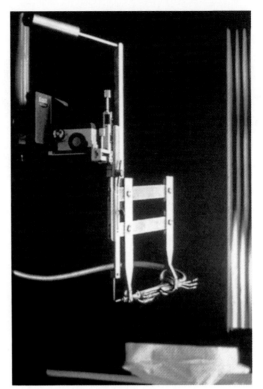

FIGURE 3.8: Three-dimensional parallelogram support for handpiece

The original handpiece was magnetostrictive and had a frequency of 25,000 cycles. By substituting piezoelectric crystals for the heavy magnetostrictive plates, the size and weight were greatly reduced, and the frequency was raised to 40,000 cycles. he now had a handpiece that others might be willing to try.

HANDPIECE HEAT BUILD-UP

The original handpiece was magnetostrictive and had to be water cooled. This cooling water had to be isolated from the sterile end of the handpiece.

The original handpiece was water cooled, as nonsterile water flowed in, around and out of the magnetostrictive plates. The first handpiece had a set of O-rings to isolate this nonsterile water from the sterile irrigation fluid, but in one instance the O-rings failed, causing an infection. The interim solution was to add a second set of O-rings, but finally, when the piezoelectric crystal replaced the magnetostrictive, air cooling was sufficient, and no O-rings were needed.

FLAKING OF THE TIPS

The original tips were steel, and flaking was a problem, with the possibility of leaving iron shavings inside the eye.

Titanium is a completely inert metal, and is silent in tissue. It is also less friable than steel, and therefore the steel tips were replaced with this metal, and in millions of cases now, there has not been any report of adverse effects from this material. It is extremely rare to see any particle in any operated eye.

INSULATING THE VIBRATING TIP

The vibrating tip had to be insulated from the corneoscleral wound to prevent heating. Various materials were tried and the two best found were silicon and Teflon. Since silicon was softer, it was the final choice.

IRRIGATING SOLUTION

Since a fair amount of solution would be washing over the cornea during the procedure, it was important to find the best possible irrigating solution. Rather than embark on a scientific quest as to which solution would be the safest, the author had observed in Barcelona, that Joaquin Barraquer employed a solution, made in Spain, which closely approximated the fluid in the anterior chamber. He began importing and using this solution.

POLITICAL PROBLEMS

It is difficult enough for a serious scientist to introduce a dramatic change in a procedure, which everyone thinks is already ideal. But when this new technique involves considerable training, using an operating microscope when one has never used one before; when those who are unable to perform the new technique announce that you have to lose a "bucketful of eyes" before you are adept at it; and when that technique is developed by a saxophone player who is still appearing in Carnegie Hall; and doing stand-up comedy in the casinos of Atlantic city; it sounds like getting this procedure accepted would be a hopeless proposition.

At this point, the author must say again, that if he had known in advance how many problems there were, he might well never have started the project. The Chinese proverb is appropriate here, "The longest journey in the world begins with the first step."

Although the surgical and instrument problems outlined above were difficult to solve, they were a constant challenge and their solution brought a great deal of satisfaction. Not so for the political problems! When the author first introduced phacoemulsification and aspiration, it was met with more than scientific reserve, it was met with scorn. How dare I, a young nobody presume to change what the University professors were proclaiming the safest and most sophisticated surgical procedure ever devised (intracapsular surgery)? At meetings where the author presented the concept, there was considerable derision, mockery and hostility in the questions from the floor.

At Manhattan Eye and Ear Hospital where the author was assistant attending surgeon, the hospital voted to allow only one case per week, for every year an attending was on the staff. This vote cut down on the number of cataract cases he could do. Since that edict only affected the author, he was, after a great battle, able to get this ruling considered "restraint of trade," and the hospital had to withdraw that ruling. When he began doing phacoemulsification, the surgeon directors advised him that he would have to stop immediately if he had even one case of serious complications. When you put that sword of Damocles together with the problems outlined above with the technique and instrument, one can imagine the pressure involved in every procedure.

Once the technique had been taken up by several others in various parts of the country, each investigator was met with the same hostility that the author had encountered. Once it began to be accepted by several dozen surgeons, the political forces against it had the operation declared "experimental" by Medicare, meaning that there would be no reimbursement for the procedure. It took several months, and letters from a thousand patients from all over the country to get this ruling by the government reversed.

The American Academy of Ophthalmology then commissioned one of the most vociferous antagonists to the procedure to do an "unbiased" study comparing the results of phaco to intracapsular surgery. The author was put on the panel, but was never allowed to see any of the results of this study until they were ready to be submitted. It came as no surprise to find that intracapsular surgery was found to be infinitely superior to phacoemulsification. Since the justification of this conclusion was rather suspect, he was able to engage the professor of statistics at Columbia Presbyterian University to examine the methods and conclusions drawn. His report was so scathing, that the original report was discarded, and the final verdict submitted to the Academy was that phaco was at least as safe and effective as intracapsular surgery.

The increase in the percentage of cases done with phaco slowly increased over the years, until foldable lenses were introduced. At that time, Phaco cases increased dramatically, until today, more than 85% of cataracts removed use phacoemulsification and aspiration.

The author is grateful to the early pioneers who stood with him, and grateful to all those who even today are improving this technique.

REFERENCES

1. Kelman CD. Cryosurgery of retinal detachment and other ocular conditions. Eye Ear Nose Throat Mon. 1963;42:42-6.
2. Irving S. Cooper, MD. Cryogenic Surgery — A New Method of Destruction or Extirpation of Benign or Malignant Tissues. N Engl J Med. 1963;268: 743-9.
3. Kelman CD. Symposium; phacoemulsification. History of emulsification and aspiration of senile cataracts. Trans Am Acad Ophthalmol Otolaryngol. 1974;78(1):OP5-13.

CHAPTER 4

Intraocular Lens Power Calculations

Li Wang, Douglas D Koch

INTRODUCTION

Accurate intraocular lens (IOL) power calculation is crucial to meet the high expectations of patients undergoing cataract surgery. With current technological advances, IOL power calculation in normal eyes is relatively straightforward. However, it is problematic in eyes that have undergone corneal refractive surgery.

AXIAL LENGTH MEASUREMENT

Precise biometry of intraocular distances is essential. By A-scan biometry, errors in axial length measurement account for 54% of IOL power error when using two-variable formulas.[1] Because of this, much research has been dedicated for achieving more accurate and reproducible axial lengths. Although ultrasound biometry is a well-established method for measuring ocular distances, optical coherence biometry has been shown to be significantly more accurate and reproducible and is rapidly becoming the prevalent methodology for the measurement of axial length.

ULTRASOUND

Axial length has traditionally been measured using ultrasound biometry. A fraction of the signal echoes back when sound waves encounter an interface of differing densities. Greater differences in density produce a greater echo. By measuring the time required for a portion of the sound beam to return to the ultrasound probe, the distance can be calculated ($d = v \times t$). Because the human eye is composed of the structures of varying densities (cornea, aqueous, lens, vitreous, retina, choroid, scleral and orbital fat), the axial length of each structure can be indirectly measured using ultrasound. Clinically, applanation and immersion techniques have been most commonly used.

APPLANATION TECHNIQUE

With the applanation technique, the ultrasound probe is placed in direct contact with the cornea. After the sound waves exit the transducer, they encounter each acoustic interface within the eye and produce a series of echoes that are received by the probe. Based on the timing of the echo and the assumed speed of the sound wave through the various structures of the eye, the biometer's software is able to construct a corresponding echogram. The axial length is

the summation of the anterior chamber depth, the lens thickness, and the vitreous cavity.

Because the applanation technique requires direct contact with the cornea, compression will typically cause the axial length to be falsely shortened. During applanation biometry, the compression of the cornea has been shown to range from 0.14 to 0.33 mm.[2-4] At normal axial lengths, compression by 0.1 mm results in roughly 0.25 D of post-operative myopic refractive error. Additionally, this method of ultrasound biometry is highly operator dependent. Because of the extent of error produced by direct corneal contact, applanation biometry has given way to noncontact methods, which have been shown to be more reproducible.

IMMERSION TECHNIQUE

Immersion technique is the currently preferred A-scan method, which, if properly performed, eliminates compression of the globe. Although the principles of immersion biometry are the same as with applanation biometry, the technique is slightly different. The patient lies supine with a clear plastic scleral shell placed over the cornea and between the eyelids. The shell is filled with coupling fluid through which the probe emits sound waves.

Although the immersion technique has been shown to be more reproducible than applanation technique, both use the properties of ultrasound. Axial length is calculated from the measured time and the assumed average speed that sound waves travel through the eye. Because the speed of ultrasound varies in different media, the operator must account for prior surgical procedures involving the eye such as IOL placement, aphakia, or the presence of silicone oil in the vitreous cavity. For pseudophakia, using a single instrument setting may also lead to significant errors because IOL implants vary in sound velocity and thickness. To account for these special situations, the operator must alter ultrasound speed settings for eyes that are pseudophakic or aphakic or contain silicone oil in the vitreous cavity.

Another source of axial length error is that the ultrasound beam has a larger diameter than the fovea. If most of the beam reflects off a raised parafoveal area and not the fovea itself, this will result in an erroneously short axial length reading. The parafoveal area may be 0.10 to 0.16 mm thicker compared to the fovea. In addition to compression and beam width, an off-axis reading may also result in a falsely shortened axial length. The probe should be positioned so that the magnitude of the peaks is greatest. If the last two spikes are not present (sclera and orbital fat), the beam may be inadvertently directed to the optic nerve instead of the fovea.

The incidence of posterior staphyloma increases with growing axial length, and it is likely that nearly all eyes with pathologic myopia have some form of posterior staphyloma. When the fovea is situated on the sloping wall of the staphyloma, it may only be possible to display a high-quality retinal spike when the sound beam is directed eccentric to the fovea, toward the rounded bottom of the staphyloma. This will result in an erroneously long axial length reading.

An immersion A/B-scan approach to axial length measurement in the setting of a posterior staphyloma has been proposed.[5,6] Using a horizontal axial B-scan, an immersion echogram through the posterior fundus is obtained with the cornea and lens echoes centered while simultaneously displaying the optic nerve void. The A-scan vector is then adjusted to pass through the middle of the cornea as well as the anterior and posterior lens echoes to assure that the vector will intersect the retina in the region of the fovea. Alternatively, if it is possible to visually identify the center of the macula with a direct ophthalmoscope, the cross-hair reticule can be used to measure the distance from the center of the macula to the margin of the optic nerve head. The A-scan is then positioned that measured distance temporal to the void of the optic nerve on simultaneous B-scan.

OPTICAL COHERENCE BIOMETRY

Optical coherence biometry was introduced in 2000 and has proved to be an exceptionally accurate and reliable method of measuring axial length. The IOLMaster® (Carl Zeiss Meditec) is the first optical biometer on the market. Recently, the Lenstar LS 900 optical biometer (Haag-Streit AG) became available for clinical use.

The IOLMaster® optical biometer (Carl Zeiss Meditec) uses partial coherence interferometry with a 780 μm laser diode infrared light to measure AL. The technology used by the Lenstar is based on optical low-coherence reflectometry with an 820 μm superluminescent diode. In addition to axial length, anterior chamber depth and keratometry, the Lenstar also displays other parameters including the crystalline lens thickness, central corneal thickness, aqueous depth (corneal endothelium to the anterior lens surface), size and centricity of the pupil.

Studies comparing the biometric measurements with the IOLMaster and the Lenstar showed high correlations for axial length and keratometry measurements between the two devices.[7-9] The Lenstar unit measured a slightly longer AL in the cataract group and clear lens group (mean difference 0.026 mm and 0.023 mm, respectively), a deeper ACD (0.128 mm and 0.146 mm, respectively), and a flatter K (-0.107 D and -0.121 D, respectively). The mean absolute errors in IOL power prediction were similar (0.461 ± 0.31 D with the IOLMaster and 0.455 ± 0.32 D with the Lenstar).[7]

Compared to A-scan biometry, there are several advantages to optical coherence biometry. The optical coherence biometer can readily measure pseudophakic, aphakic, and phakic IOL eyes and, if the cataract is not too dense, accurate measurements can be made through silicone oil without the need for the use of conversion equation. Because optical coherence biometry uses a partially coherent light source of a much shorter wavelength than ultrasound, axial length can be more accurately obtained. Optical coherence biometry has been shown to reproducibly measure axial length with an accuracy of 0.01 mm. It permits accurate measurements when posterior staphyloma are present. Since the patient fixates along the direction of the measuring beam, the instrument is more likely to display an accurate axial length to the center of the macula. Additional measurements of corneal power, anterior chamber depth, and crystalline lens thickness enable the devices to perform IOL calculations using newer generation formulas such as Haigis and Holladay 2.

The primary limitation of optical biometry is its inability to measure through dense cataracts and other media opacities that obscure the macula; due to such opacities or fixation difficulties, approximately 10% of eyes cannot be accurately measured using the IOL Master.[10]

KERATOMETRY

Errors in corneal power measurement can be an equally important source of IOL power calculation error, as the error in keratometry will result in same amount of postoperative error at the spectacle plane. A variety of technologies are available to measure corneal power, including manual keratometry, automated keratometry and corneal topography. These devices measure the radius of curvature and provide the corneal power in the form of keratometric diopters using an assumed index of refraction of 1.3375. The obtained values should be compared to the patient's manifest refraction, looking for large inconsistencies in the magnitude or meridian of the astigmatism that should prompt further evaluation of the accuracy of the corneal readings.

The keratometry readings with the IOLMaster are calculated by analyzing the anterior corneal curvature at six reference points in a hexagonal pattern at approximately 2.3 mm optical zone. With the Lenstar, the keratometry readings are calculated by analyzing the anterior corneal curvature at 32 reference points orientated in two circles at approximately 2.30 mm and 1.65 mm optical zones.

Important sources of error are corneal scars or dystrophies that create an irregular anterior corneal surface. While these lesions can often be seen with slit lamp biomicroscopy, their impact on corneal power measurements can best be assessed by examining keratometric or topographic mires. The latter in particular gives an excellent qualitative estimate of corneal surface irregularity (**Figure 4.1**). In the authors' practice, if the irregularity is considered to be

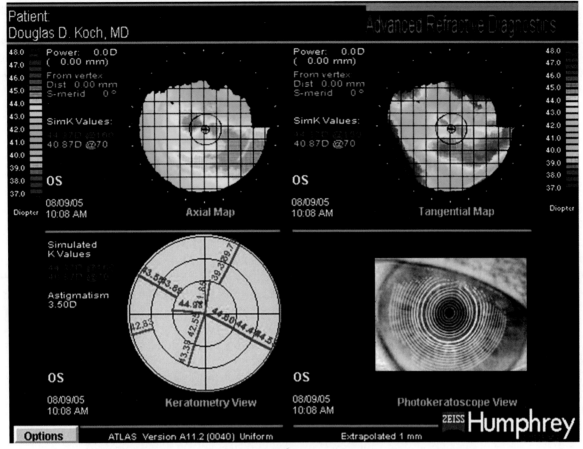

FIGURE 4.1: Corneal surface irregularity shown on the Humphrey topographic map of an eye with epithelial basement disease

clinically important, they try to correct it whenever feasible before proceeding with cataract surgery. Examples would include epithelial debridement in corneas with epithelial basement disease, and superficial keratectomy in eyes with Salzmann's nodular degeneration.

When the patient has undergone prior corneal refractive surgery or corneal transplantation, standard keratometric and topographic values cannot be used. This topic will be further discussed later.

ANTERIOR CHAMBER DEPTH MEASUREMENT

A-scan biometers calculate anterior chamber depth (ACD) as the distance from the anterior surface of the cornea to the anterior surface of the crystalline lens. The IOLMaster measures the ACD through a lateral slit-illumination and is defined as the measurement between the corneal epithelium and the anterior lens surface. The Lenstar uses optical low-coherence reflectometry to measure central corneal thickness (CCT) and aqueous depth, defined as the measurement from the corneal endothelium to the anterior lens surface, and the sum of the CCT and aqueous depth equals the ACD. In some IOL calculation formulas, the measured anterior chamber depth is used to aid in the prediction of the final postoperative position of the IOL (known as the effective lens position or the ELP).

INTRAOCULAR LENS CALCULATION FORMULAS

Currently, there are two major types of IOL formulas: empirical and theoretical. The empirical formulas are derived from linear regression analysis of a large number of cases, while the theoretical formulas are derived from a mathematical consideration of the optics of the eye.

The first IOL power formula was published by Fyodorov in 1967 based on schematic eyes.[11] Subsequent formulas based on regression analysis were introduced by several investigators.[12-16] All of these formulas depended on a single constant for each IOL that represented the predicted IOL position. In the 1980s, further refinement of IOL formulas occurred with the incorporation of relationships between the position of an IOL and the axial length as well as the central power of the cornea.

THE SECOND AND THIRD GENERATION OF IOL FORMULAS

The IOL constants in the second- and third-generation IOL formulas work by simply moving up or down the position of an IOL power prediction curve for the utilized formula. The shape of this power prediction curve is mostly fixed for each formula and, other than the lens constant, these formulas treat all IOLs the same and make a number of broad assumptions for all eyes regardless of individual differences.

Popular third-generation, two-variable formulas (SRK/T, Hoffer Q and Holladay 1) also assume that the distance from the principal plane of the cornea to the thin lens equivalent of the IOL is, in part, related to the axial length. That is to say, short eyes may have a shallower anterior chamber and long eyes may have a deeper anterior chamber. In reality, this assumption may be invalid. Short eyes and many long eyes typically have perfectly normal anterior chamber anatomy with normal anterior chamber depth. The error in this assumption accounts for the characteristic limited axial length range of accuracy of each third-generation, two-variable formula. The Holladay 1 formula, for example, works well for the eyes of normal to moderately long axial lengths, while the Hoffer Q has been reported to be better suited for normal and shorter axial lengths.[17]

Optimization of lens constants for each surgeon plays a critical role in improving the accuracy of refractive prediction. Variations in keratometers, ultrasound machine settings and surgical techniques (such as the creation of the *capsulorrhexis*) can impact the refractive outcome. "Personalizing" the lens constant for a given IOL and formula can make global adjustments and eliminate systematic errors (such as systematic myopic or hyperopic outcomes) for a variety of practice-specific variables.

THE FOURTH GENERATION OF IOL FORMULAS

Popular fourth-generation IOL formulas are Holladay 2 formula and Haigis formula.

The Holladay 2 formula uses an innovative approach to improve the accuracy of IOL power calculation by including various parameters (corneal power, corneal diameter, ACD, lens thickness, refractive error and axial length) to further refine the effective lens position estimation. The Holladay 2 formula is based on previous observations from a large research data set and has been shown to be advantageous in both long and short eyes.

Rather than moving a fixed formula-specific IOL power prediction curve up or down, the Haigis formula[18] uses three constants (a_0, a_1 and a_2) to set both the position and the shape of a power prediction curve:

$$d = a_0 + (a_1 \times ACD) + (a_2 \times AL)$$

where d is the effective lens position, ACD is the measured anterior chamber depth of the eye (corneal vertex to the anterior lens capsule), and AL is the axial length of the eye (the distance from the cornea vertex to the vitreoretinal interface). The a_0 constant basically moves the power prediction curve up, or down, in much the same way that the A-constant, Surgeon Factor, or pACD does for the SRK/T, Holladay 1 and Hoffer Q formulas. The a_1 constant is tied to the measured anterior chamber depth, and the a_2 constant is tied to the measured axial length. In this way,

the value for d is determined by three constants, rather than a single number.

With optimization of the lens constants, the a_0, a_1 and a_2 constants are derived by regression analysis for each IOL type. It is recommended including large sample size with a wide range of axial lengths and anterior chamber depths in the optimization process.

INTRAOCULAR LENS POWER CALCULATION FOLLOWING CORNEAL REFRACTIVE SURGERY

Accurate IOL power calculation in eyes following laser corneal refractive surgery is known to be very complicated.[19,20] There are two major causes of error in IOL calculations in these eyes: inaccurate corneal power measurements obtained from standard keratometers or computerized videokeratography (CVK), and incorrect estimation of effective lens position (ELP) calculated by most third- or fourth-generation IOL power calculation formulas.

Standard keratometry and simulated K readings from CVK measure only four points or small zones on the anterior cornea in a paracentral region, ignoring more central region altered by ablation. Furthermore, standard keratometry and CVK only measure the anterior corneal surface and the power of the posterior corneal surface needs to be assumed. Therefore, these devices use a standardized corneal refractive index, which is 1.3375 in most devices, to convert the anterior corneal measurement to an estimation of total corneal refractive power. Because LASIK/PRK alters the relationship between anterior and posterior corneal surface, this index is no longer valid. More recently, several technologies that measure both anterior and posterior corneal surfaces are commercially available: Scheimpflug imaging-the Pentacam and Galilei, slit-scanning -Orbscan, and optical coherence tomography-RTVue. Studies have shown that the Orbscan II is not sufficiently reliable in its measurements of posterior corneal curvature in post-LASIK eyes.[21,22] Promising results have been reported for the repeatability of posterior corneal surface with the Pentacam and Galilei.[23-25] Huang et al reported that the reproducibility of the total corneal power measurements with the RTVue was 0.26 D for the post-LASIK eyes (Presented at ARVO 2008).

Except for Haigis formula, third- and fourth-generation IOL formulas use corneal power to predict the ELP. The flattened K values after myopic LASIK/PRK will cause these formulas to predict a falsely shallower ELP and calculate insufficient IOL power, yielding a postoperative hyperopic surprise. The authors found that the magnitude of the ELP-related error varies according to the particular formula, the amount of refractive correction and the axial length (AL).[26,27] To solve this problem, Aramberri proposed the double-K method,[14] which uses two different K-values:

the preoperative-K value for the estimation of ELP and the postoperative-K value for the calculation of IOL power in vergence formula. This approach was previously developed by Holladay in the Holladay 2 formula. Several studies have shown that the double-K method improves the accuracy of IOL power calculation after LASIK/PRK.[28-30] Nomograms proposed in the authors' study can be used to adjust the IOL power when the modified corneal powers are used for these formulas.[27] With the Holladay 2 formula, one can enter preoperative-K value to predict the ELP or if previous data are not available, one can check the "previous RK/PRK/LASIK" box, which will instruct the formula to use the default corneal power of 43.86 D.

IOL POWER CALCULATION IN POST-LASIK/PRK EYES

Several methods have been proposed to improve the accuracy of IOL power calculation in eyes following corneal refractive surgery; these can be divided into three categories depending on the requirement for preoperative data.

Methods Requiring Historical Data

These methods require the preoperative-K readings and manifest refraction (MR) and the surgically induced change in MR (ΔMR). In these approaches, care should be taken to obtain accurate historical data, including measurement of the post-LASIK stable refraction and before the cataract has begun to develop.

The concern with this category is their dependence on the accuracy of preoperative data. There is a one-to-one diopter error, if any of the historical data are incorrect. Historical data are often obtained from another office where one cannot verify the calibration of the keratometer, etc. Also, it is often difficult to accurately determine when the post-LASIK refraction has stabilized before the cataract has begun to alter the refractive error. For all of these reasons, the authors have found that methods using historical data are less accurate, compared to the other two types of methods as described below:

Clinical history method: With this method, postoperative corneal power is calculated by subtracting the change in manifest refraction at the corneal plane induced by the refractive surgical procedure from the corneal power values obtained prior to refractive surgery. Several studies have suggested that the clinical history method is the best for calculating corneal power after refractive surgery; however, the numbers of the eyes in these studies were relatively small and the accuracy of this method varied largely.[31-33]

Feiz-Mannis method: This method[34] calculates the IOL power by using pre-LASIK/PRK K as if the patients had not undergone LASIK/PRK. Intraocular lens power is calculated using pre-LASIK corneal power values and the axial length measured just prior to cataract surgery. To this value, the LASIK-induced change in refractive error divided by 0.7 is added.

Corneal bypass method: This method[35] uses pre-LASIK/PRK K values, pre- and post-LASIK/PRK refractions, and current AL measurement. It assumes that the patient had no LASIK/PRK procedure and calculates the IOL power by targeting refraction at the pre-LASIK/PRK refraction or the net refractive correction if the post-LASIK/PRK refraction is not plano.

Methods Using Historical Refraction Data and Current Corneal Power Measurements

There are several methods that modify corneal power measurements or IOL powers based on the amount of refractive change induced by the LASIK surgery. The advantages of methods in this category are that they use corneal data obtained at the time the patient presents for cataract surgery, as well as by multiplying the change in manifest refraction by some fraction, typically less than 0.3, they avoid the one-for-one error involved in the approaches that rely entirely on historical data.

Adjusted EffRP: The EffRP from the EyeSys topographer is the mean corneal power over the central 3-mm zone, accounting for the Stiles-Crawford effect. Hamed et al proposed adjusted EffRP, which is modified according to ΔMR:[36,37]

Adjusted EffRP in post myopic LASIK/PRK = EffRP – 0.152 × (ΔMR) – 0.05

Adjusted EffRP in post hyperopic LASIK/PRK = EffRP + 0.162 × (ΔMR) – 0.279

Adjusted AnnCP: The AnnCP from the Atlas topographer is the average corneal powers of the 0-, 1-, 2- and 3-mm annular zones. AnnCP is modified according to ΔMR. With this method, the authors found that the accuracy of the IOL power calculation in eyes following hyperopic LASIK/PRK significantly improved:[37]

Adjusted AnnCP in post-hyperopic LASIK/PRK = AnnCP + 0.191 × (ΔMR) – 0.396

Adjusted AnnCP in post-myopic LASIK/PRK = AnnCP – 0.2 × (ΔMR),

where AnnCP is the average of powers at the 0-, 1-, 2-, and 3-mm annular zones from the Atlas.

Adjusted K: Adjusted keratometry values can be obtained as follows, in the absence of EffRP or other CVK value.[36] However, this method is not as accurate as the adjusted EffRP and adjusted AnnCP methods:

Adjusted K = K – 0.24 × (ΔMR) + 0.15

Adjusted ACCP: The ACCP from the TMS topographer is the average corneal power within the central 3-mm of the topographical map. Adjusted ACCP is modified according to ΔMR. Awwad et al[38] reported that this method accurately predicted the corneal refractive power after myopic LASIK:

Adjusted ACCP in post-myopic LASIK/PRK = ACCP – 0.16 × (ΔMR)

Latkany formula: This method[39] uses SRK/T formula with flattest or average K values to adjust IOL power. It requires pre-LASIK/PRK MR:

Adjustment of IOL for flat K= – (0.47 × pre-LASIK/PRK refraction + 0.85)

Adjustment of IOL for average K = – (0.46 × pre-LASIK/PRK refraction + 0.21)

Masket formula: With this method,[40] the IOL power is calculated using the IOLMaster's K and SRK/T formula as if LASIK/PRK had not been done, and then adjusted by around 33% of the refractive correction.

Adjustment of IOL = [(ΔMR) × 0.326] + 0.101

Modified Masket formula: The Masket formula was modified by Hill [Presented at the American Society of Cataract and Refractive Surgery (ASCRS) 2006].

Adjustment of IOL = [(ΔMR) × 0.4385] + 0.0295

Methods Using No Prior Data

These methods are obviously essential, as one often encounters patients for whom no prior data are available. The advantage of these methods is that they require no historical data and have a low variance when used with either the Holladay 2 formula or a modern third generation 2-variable formula combined with the "double K method" proposed by Aramberri and the correction nomograms published by Koch and Wang.[27,28]

Contact lens over-refraction method: This method does not require historical data; however it can be only used for eyes with visual acuity of 20/70 or better: [34]

$$K_{CL} = BC + D + (OR_{CL} – MR)$$

Where K_{CL} is estimated corneal power following refractive surgery, BC is base curvature of contact lens in diopters, D is refractive power of contact lens in diopters, OR_{CL} is SE of over-refraction, and MR is SE of manifest refraction without contact lens.

Previous reports[29,33,41] found poorer accuracy for the contact lens method compared to other methods. The authors believe that this is at least partially due to the poor fit of the trial lenses typically used in this setting. Contact lenses with a special back surface and better fitting on the post-LASIK/PRK corneas might improve the accuracy and precision of this method.[42,43]

Modified Maloney method: This method converts the central corneal power from the Atlas back to the anterior corneal power and then subtracts an assumed posterior corneal power of 5.51D.

Post-LASIK K = Central power × (376.0/337.5 or 1.114) – 5.51

Wang et al[29] originally suggested using the assumed posterior corneal power of 6.1D in this method. Using a different series of 11 post-myopic LASIK cases that had cataract surgery, the original method resulted in myopic outcome in 10 out of 11 cases (average refractive prediction error of -0.57D, unpublished data). When used with double-K version of either the Holladay 2 formula or third-generation formulas, the modified Maloney method provided more consistent results than the clinical history method.

Wang-Koch-Maloney method: The Wang-Koch-Maloney method converts the average corneal power of 0-, 1-, 2-, and 3-mm annular zones from Atlas back to the anterior corneal power and then subtracts an assumed posterior corneal power of 5.59D (Presented at ASCRS 2007).

Post-LASIK K = Atlas$_{0-3}$ × (376.0/337.5 or 1.114) – 5.59

where the Atlas$_{0-3}$ is the average of powers at the 0-, 1-, 2-, and 3-mm annular zones from the Atlas.

Shammas method: This method[44] is based on a regression equation between post-LASIK K values and corneal powers obtained from the clinical history method.

Corrected Post-LASIK corneal power = $1.14K_{post}$ – 6.8

where K_{post} is the post-LASIK K value.

Haigis-L formula: The Haigis-L formula is included into the IOLMaster.[45] This formula uses a regression equation to correct post-LASIK corneal radius obtained from the IOLMaster based on the corneal powers calculated from the historical method.

Corrected corneal radius = 331.5/ (-5.1625 × post-LASIK corneal radius with the IOLMaster + 82.2603 - 0.35)

Intraocular lens power is then calculated using the Haigis formula.

Galilei total corneal power (TCP) method: The TCP obtained from the Galilei is the total corneal power averaged over the central 4-mm zone calculated by the ray-tracing through the anterior and posterior corneal surfaces using the Snell's law.

This method is based on the regression equation between the TCP values and the corneal powers derived from the historical method (unpublished data).

Adjusted corneal power in myopic LASIK eyes = 1.0887 × TCP – 1.8348

A study of 17 post-myopic LASIK eyes found that the Galilei TCA had comparable performance to other methods requiring no prior data and was superior to methods based on historical data (unpublished data).

Intraoperative refraction: There have been two reports that proposed performing the refraction during cataract surgery in post-LASIK/PRK eyes.

a. Optical refractive biometry method: This method[46] performs aphakic retinoscopy after removal of the cataract and before implantation of the IOL. It does not require AL and K reading.

$$IOL \ power = 2.01449 \times intraoperative \ SE$$

b. Aphakic refraction technique: This method performs the manifest aphakic refraction at 30 minutes after the removal of the cataract.[47] The formula is as follow:

$$IOL \ power = 1.75 \times aphakic \ refraction \ (SE)$$

Although the advantage of these intraoperative refraction methods is that they avoid many of the pitfalls of other methods by eliminating the need for historical data and not requiring precise determination of corneal refractive power, the authors' concern is whether refraction can be accurately determined in this setting. Further studies with large number of eyes are needed before the clinical use of these methods.

Gaussian optics formula: The Gaussian optics formula calculates the total corneal power using the anterior and posterior corneal powers, and the corneal thickness.

$$Fe = F1 + F2 - (d/n) \ (F1 \times F2)$$

where Fe, F1, and F2 are the powers of total, anterior, and posterior corneal surfaces in diopters, respectively, d is pachymetry, and n is the corneal refractive index.

With this formula, two approaches with the Pentacam have been reported to estimate the total corneal power.

a. Equivalent K-readings (EKR; 4.5 mm zone): The EKR is displayed on the Holladay Report of the Pentacam. To obtain EKR, the Pentacam calculates the anterior and posterior central powers and adjusts them for the mean of the population.[48] Because the EKR is intended to improve corneal power estimation, especially in eyes after LASIK/PRK, it can be used in IOL calculation formulas without adjustment.

b. BESSt formula: This formula is based on the Gaussian optics formula.[49] In 143 virgin corneas, Borasio et al found that the Gaussian optic formula consistently provided smaller corneal powers than CVK. To compensate for this underestimation, they developed the BESSt_vc formula (vc= virgin corneas) using regression analysis. For post-LASIK eyes, they also performed regression analysis between the corneal powers with the BESSt_vc formula and those with the clinical history method.

$$K\text{-values BESSt\_vc} = 0.2431 + 0.9942 \times K\text{-values Gaussian optics}$$

$$K\text{-values BESSt} = 7.8385 + 0.7458 \times K\text{-values BESSt\_vc}$$

IOL Power Calculation in Post-radial Keratotomy (RK) Eyes

In post-RK eyes, unlike post-LASIK/PRK eyes, posterior corneal curvature also changes, presumably more closely preserving the ratio between the anterior and posterior corneal surface. Therefore, an average corneal power over the central 2–3 mm provided by any topographers can be used for post-RK eyes. In the ASCRS post-refractive surgery calculator (mentioned later in the chapter), one can enter the average corneal powers from the Atlas for the 1-, 2-, 3-, and 4-mm annular zones, the EffRP from the EyeSys, and the central total corneal power from the Galilei. Presumably, topographers that provide average values over the central 2 or 3 mm can also be used. Compensation for potential error in ELP is still required by using double-K version of IOL formulas, and the double-K Holladay 1 formula is used by the ASCRS online calculator.

In 22 eyes with prior RK, the authors compared the accuracy of four devices for IOL power calculation: IOLMaster, EyeSys, Atlas and Galilei. With the Galilei, they studied the performance of TCP average over central 2-, 3-, 4-, and 5-mm zones, and TCP average of 1-, 2- and 3-mm annuli, and 1-, 2-, 3- and 4-mm annuli. The variance of IOL power prediction error was the smallest with the TCP 1–4 mm annuli, indicating the best consistency of performance with the TCP 1–4 mm annuli. When comparing the accuracy of four devices, Galilei TCP 1–4 mm annuli tended to produce the smallest refractive mean absolute error (MAE) of 0.59 D. It is followed by the MAE of 0.68 D with the IOLMaster keratometry, 0.74 D with the EyeSys EffRP and 0.78 D with the Atlas central 3-mm zone value, although there were no significant differences among devices.

The authors also find relatively poor accuracy in post-RK eyes compared to virgin eyes. This may in part be due to greater variability in anterior corneal curvature and posterior curvature changes that deviate from those estimated by using the standardized refractive index. In addition, it has been reported that 20% to 50% of RK eyes have a gradual hyperopic shift.[50-52] For these reasons, the authors usually target IOL power calculations for -0.75 to -1.00 D.

WEB-BASED IOL POWER CALCULATOR

It is time consuming to perform calculations with various methods. To save time, in collaboration with Dr Warren

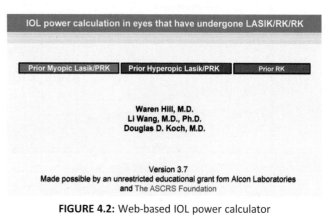

FIGURE 4.2: Web-based IOL power calculator

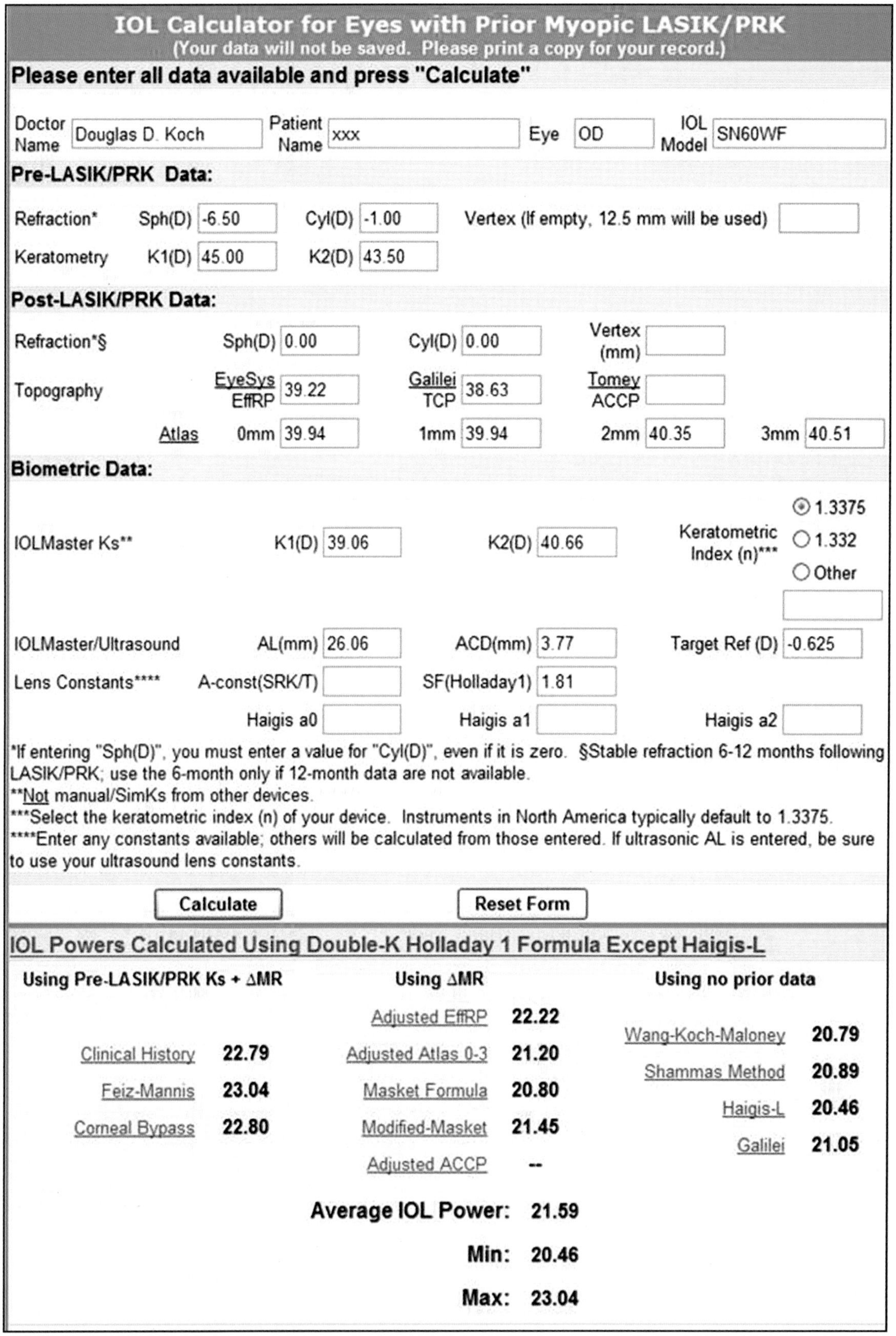

IOL Calculator for Eyes with Prior Myopic LASIK/PRK
(Your data will not be saved. Please print a copy for your record.)

Please enter all data available and press "Calculate"

| Doctor Name | Douglas D. Koch | Patient Name | xxx | Eye | OD | IOL Model | SN60WF |

Pre-LASIK/PRK Data:

Refraction*	Sph(D) -6.50	Cyl(D) -1.00	Vertex (If empty, 12.5 mm will be used)		
Keratometry	K1(D) 45.00	K2(D) 43.50			

Post-LASIK/PRK Data:

Refraction*§		Sph(D) 0.00	Cyl(D) 0.00	Vertex (mm)		
Topography		EyeSys EffRP 39.22	Galilei TCP 38.63	Tomey ACCP		
	Atlas	0mm 39.94	1mm 39.94	2mm 40.35	3mm 40.51	

Biometric Data:

Keratometric Index (n)***
- ⊙ 1.3375
- ○ 1.332
- ○ Other

IOLMaster Ks**	K1(D) 39.06	K2(D) 40.66	
IOLMaster/Ultrasound	AL(mm) 26.06	ACD(mm) 3.77	Target Ref (D) -0.625
Lens Constants****	A-const(SRK/T)	SF(Holladay1) 1.81	
	Haigis a0	Haigis a1	Haigis a2

*If entering "Sph(D)", you must enter a value for "Cyl(D)", even if it is zero. §Stable refraction 6-12 months following LASIK/PRK; use the 6-month only if 12-month data are not available.
**Not manual/SimKs from other devices.
***Select the keratometric index (n) of your device. Instruments in North America typically default to 1.3375.
****Enter any constants available; others will be calculated from those entered. If ultrasonic AL is entered, be sure to use your ultrasound lens constants.

| Calculate | Reset Form |

IOL Powers Calculated Using Double-K Holladay 1 Formula Except Haigis-L

Using Pre-LASIK/PRK Ks + ΔMR		Using ΔMR		Using no prior data	
		Adjusted EffRP	22.22		
				Wang-Koch-Maloney	20.79
Clinical History	22.79	Adjusted Atlas 0-3	21.20	Shammas Method	20.89
Feiz-Mannis	23.04	Masket Formula	20.80		
				Haigis-L	20.46
Corneal Bypass	22.80	Modified-Masket	21.45		
				Galilei	21.05
		Adjusted ACCP	--		

Average IOL Power: 21.59

Min: 20.46

Max: 23.04

FIGURE 4.3: IOL power calculator for eyes with prior myopic LASIK/PRK

Hill, the authors developed the web-based IOL power calculator (www.ascrs.org) **(Figure 4.2)**. This calculator has three modules: (1) prior myopic LASIK/PRK, (2) prior hyperopic LASIK/PRK, and (3) prior RK.

When one uses the IOL calculator for eyes with prior myopic or hyperopic LASIK/PRK, pre- and post-LASIK/PRK data, and biometric data may be entered. By clicking the "Calculate" button, the results are shown in the bottom **(Figure 4.3)**. Depending on the availability of historical data, the IOL calculator categorizes the various calculation methods into three groups: (1) methods using Pre-LASIK/PRK Ks and ΔMR, (2) methods using ΔMR and corneal measurements at the time of cataract surgery, and (3) methods using no prior data. The IOL power is calculated using the double-K Holladay 1 formula, except for the Haigis-L method. In the double-K Holladay 1 formula, pre-LASIK/PRK K is used to estimate the ELP. If pre-LASIK/PRK K is not available, 43.86 D is used. The average and range of IOL powers from all methods available for that case are also displayed.

Using this calculator, the authors' study of 72 post-LASIK/PRK eyes that had cataract surgery found that compared to methods requiring pre-LASIK/PRK Ks and ΔMR, methods using ΔMR or using no prior data had smaller IOL prediction errors, smaller variances, and greater percent of eyes within 0.5 and 1.0 D of refractive prediction errors.[53] Further studies, especially using post-hyperopic LASIK/PRK eyes are desirable.

Another excellent resource is a comprehensive spreadsheet developed by Kenneth Hoffer and Giacomo Savini (http://www.eyelab.com/).

CONCLUSION

The methodology for accurately calculating IOL power in normal and complex eyes has improved dramatically in recent years. Future advances are needed in all areas, including methods of measuring corneal power, predicting effective lens position and perhaps even measuring axial length. The "Holy Grail" in this field may be an adjustable IOL, which could facilitate correction of residual spherical and astigmatic refractive errors and residual higher order aberrations. Ideally, such an IOL could be modified multiple times to adapt to the patient's changing visual needs and to compensate for aging changes of the cornea.

REFERENCES

1. Olsen T. Sources of error in intraocular lens power calculation. J Cataract Refract Surg. 1992;18:125-9.
2. Olsen T, Nielsen PJ. Immersion versus contact technique in the measurement of axial length by ultrasound. Acta Ophthalmol (Copenh). 1989;67:101-2.
3. Schelenz J, Kammann J. Comparison of contact and immersion techniques for axial length measurement and implant power calculation. J Cataract Refract Surg. 1989;15:425-8.
4. Shammas HJ. A comparison of immersion and contact techniques for axial length measurement. J Am Intraocul Implant Soc. 1984;10:444-7.
5. Zaldiver R, Shultz MC, Davidorf JM, et al. Intraocular lens power calculations in patients with extreme myopia. J Cataract Refract Surg. 2000;26:668-74.
6. Byrne SF, Green RL. Ultrasound of the Eye and Orbit. Mosby Year-Book; 1992;234-6.
7. Hoffer KJ, Shammas HJ, Savini G. Comparison of 2 laser instruments for measuring axial length. J Cataract Refract Surg. 2010;36:644-8.
8. Holzer MP, Mamusa M, Auffarth GU. Accuracy of a new partial coherence interferometry analyser for biometric measurements. Br J Ophthalmol. 2009;93:807-10.
9. Rabsilber TM, Jepsen C, Auffarth GU, et al. Intraocular lens power calculation: clinical comparison of 2 optical biometry devices. J Cataract Refract Surg. 2010;36:230-4.
10. Lege BA, Haigis W. Laser interference biometry versus ultrasound biometry in certain clinical conditions. Graefe's Arch Clin Exp Ophthalmol. 2004;242:8-12.
11. Fyodorov SN, Kolonko AI. Estimation of optical power of the intraocular lens. Vestnik Oftalmologic (Moscow). 1967;4:27.
12. Binkhorst RD. The optical design of intraocular lens implants. Ophthalmic Surg. 1975;6:17-31.
13. Colenbrander MC. Calculation of the power of an iris clip lens for distant vision. Br J Ophthalmol. 1973;57:735-40.
14. Hoffer KJ. Intraocular lens calculation: the problem of the short eye. Ophthalmic Surg. 1981;12:269-72.
15. Retzlaff J. A new intraocular lens calculation formula. J Am Intraocul Implant Soc. 1980;6:148-52.
16. Sanders D, Retzlaff J, Kraff M, et al. Comparison of the accuracy of the Binkhorst, Colenbrander, and SRK implant power prediction formulas. J Am Intraocul Implant Soc. 1981;7:337-40.
17. Hoffer KJ. The Hoffer Q formula: a comparison of theoretic and regression formulas. J Cataract Refract Surg. 1993;19:700-12.
18. Haigis W, Lege B, Miller N, et al. Comparison of immersion ultrasound biometry and partial coherence interferometry for intraocular lens calculation according to Haigis. Graefes Arch Clin Exp Ophthalmol. 2000;238:765-73.
19. Koch DD, Liu JF, Hyde LL, et al. Refractive complications of cataract surgery after radial keratotomy. Am J Ophthalmol. 1989;108:676-82.
20. Seitz B, Langenbucher A, Nguyen NX, et al. Underestimation of intraocular lens power for cataract surgery after myopic photorefractive keratectomy. Ophthalmology. 1999;106:693-702.
21. Maldonado MJ, Nieto JC, Diez-Cuenca M, et al. Repeatability and reproducibility of posterior corneal curvature measurements by combined scanning-slit and placido-disc topography after LASIK. Ophthalmology. 2006;113:1918-26.
22. Hashemi H, Mehravaran S. Corneal changes after laser refractive surgery for myopia: comparison of Orbscan II and Pentacam findings. J Cataract Refract Surg. 2007;33:841-7.
23. Ciolino JB, Belin MW. Changes in the posterior cornea after laser in situ keratomileusis and photorefractive keratectomy. J Cataract Refract Surg. 2006;32:1426-31.
24. Jain R, Dilraj G, Grewal SP. Repeatability of corneal parameters with Pentacam after laser in situ keratomileusis. Indian J Ophthalmol. 2007;55:341-7.
25. Wang L, Shirayama M, Koch DD. Repeatability of corneal power and wavefront aberration measurements with a dual-Scheimpflug Placido corneal topographer. J Cataract Refract Surg. 2010;36:425-30.

26. Koch DD, Wang L, Booth M. Intraocular lens calculations after LASIK. In: LASIK – advances, controversies and custom. Louis Probst (Ed). Thorofare, NJ: Slack Inc.; 2004;259-67.

27. Koch DD, Wang L. Calculating IOL power in eyes that have had refractive surgery. J Cataract Refract Surg. 2003;29:2039-42.

28. Aramberri J. Intraocular lens power calculation after corneal refractive surgery: double-K method. J Cataract Refract Surg. 2003;29:2063-8.

29. Wang L, Booth MA, Koch DD. Comparison of intraocular lens power calculation methods in eyes that have undergone LASIK. Ophthalmology. 2004;111:1825-31.

30. Chan CC, Hodge C, Lawless M. Calculation of intraocular lens power after corneal refractive surgery. Clin Experiment Ophthalmol. 2006;34:640-4.

31. Gimble HV, Sun R. Accuracy and predictability of intraocular lens power calculation after laser in situ keratomileusis. J Cataract Refract Surg. 2001;27:571-6.

32. Randleman JB, Loupe DN, Song CD, et al. Intraocular lens power calculations after laser in situ keratomileusis. Cornea. 2002;21:751-5.

33. Argento C, Cosentino MJ, Badoza D. Intraocular lens power calculation after refractive surgery. J Cataract Refract Surg. 2003;29:1346-51.

34. Feiz V, Mannis MJ, Garcia-Ferrer F, et al. Intraocular lens power calculation after laser in situ keratomileusis for myopia and hyperopia: a standardized approach. Cornea. 2001;20:792-7.

35. Walter KA, Gagnon MR, Hoopes PC, et al. Accurate intra-ocular lens power calculation after myopic laser in situ kerato-mileusis, bypassing corneal power. J Cataract Refract Surg 2006;32:425-9.

36. Hamed AM, Wang L, Misra M, et al. A comparative analysis of five methods of determining corneal refractive power in eyes that have undergone myopic laser in situ keratomileusis. Ophthalmology. 2002;109:651-8.

37. Wang L, Jackson DW, Koch DD. Methods of estimating corneal refractive power after hyperopic laser in situ keratomileusis. J Cataract Refract Surg. 2002;28:954-61.

38. Awwad ST, Manasseh C, Bowman RW, et al. Intraocular lens power calculation after myopic laser in situ keratomileusis: Estimating the corneal refractive power. J Cataract Refract Surg. 2008;34:1070-6.

39. Latkany RA, Chokshi AR, Speaker MG, et al. Intraocular lens calculations after refractive surgery. J Cataract Refract Surg. 2005;31:562-70.

40. Masket S, Masket SE. Simple regression formula for intraocular lens power adjustment in eyes requiring cataract surgery after excimer laser photoablation. J Cataract Refract Surg. 2006;32:430-4.

41. Haigis W. Corneal power after refractive surgery for myopia: contact lens method. J Cataract Refract Surg. 2003;29:1397-411.

42. Joslin CE, Koster J, Tu EY. Contact lens overrefraction variability in corneal power estimation after refractive surgery. J Cataract Refract Surg. 2005;31:2287-92.

43. Gruenauer-Kloevekorn C, Fischer U, Kloevekorn-Norgall K, et al. Varieties of contact lens fittings after complicated hyperopic and myopic laser in situ keratomileusis. Eye Contact Lens 2006;32:233-9.

44. Shammas JH, Shammas MC, Garabet A, et al. Correcting the corneal power measurements for intraocular lens power calculations after myopic laser in situ keratomileusis. Am J Ophthalmol. 2003;136(3):426-32.

45. Haigis W. Intraocular lens calculation after refractive surgery for myopia: Haigis-L formula. J Cataract Refract Surg. 2008;34:1658-63.

46. Ianchulev T, Salz J, Hoffer K, et al. Intraoperative optical refractive biometry for intraocular lens power estimation without axial length and keratometry measurements. J Cataract Refract Surg. 2005;31:1530-6.

47. Mackool RJ, Ko W, Mackool R. Intraocular lens power calculation after laser in situ keratomileusis: Aphakic refraction technique. J Cataract Refract Surg. 2006;32:435-7.

48. Holladay JT, Hill WE, Steinmueller A. Corneal power measurements using Scheimpflug imaging in eyes with prior corneal refractive surgery. J Refract Surg. 2009;25:862-8.

49. Borasio E, Stevens J, Smith GT. Estimation of true corneal power after keratorefractive surgery in eyes requiring cataract surgery: BESSt formula. J Cataract Refract Surg. 2006; 32: 2004-14.

50. Arrowsmith PN, Marks RG. Visual, refractive, and keratometric results of radial Keratotomy. Five-year follow-up. Arch Ophthalmol. 1989;107:506-11.

51. Deitz MR, Sanders DR, Raana MG, et al. Long term (5- to 12-year) follow-up of metal-blade radial keratotomy procedures. Arch Ophthalmol. 1994;112:614-20.

52. Waring GO, Lynn MJ, Gelender H, et al. Results of the prospective evaluation of radial Keratotomy (PERK) study one year after surgery. Ophthalmology. 1983;92:177-98.

53. Wang L, Hill WE, Koch DD. Evaluation of intraocular lens power prediction methods using the American Society of Cataract and Refractive Surgeons Post-Keratorefractive Intraocular Lens Power Calculator. J Cataract Refract Surg. 2010; 36(9):1466-73.

CHAPTER 5

IOL Power Calculation in Complex Cases

Benjamin F Boyd, L Samuel Boyd, Luis W Lu

INTRODUCTION

Determination of intraocular lens power through meaningful keratometer readings, a topographer and axial length measurement through A-Scan ultrasonography has become a "standard of care." It is a challenging technique and crucial to the visual result and patient satisfaction. In small incision techniques, cataract surgery has attained the status of refractive surgery. Therefore, exact determination of the IOL power to end up with the specific planned post-operative refraction is essential. The advent of multifocal foldable IOLs makes this even more of an important, though complex subject, as well as operating on eyes with different axial lengths: normal (**Figure 5.1**), short as in hyperopia (**Figure 5.2**), long as in myopia (**Figure 5.3**).

SPECIFIC METHODS TO USE IN COMPLEX CASES

Considering that there are no specific methods on which there is full agreement as to what to do in these patients, and after consulting different authorities in this field, the authors hereby recommend the use of third- or fourth-generation formulas, preferably more than one and that the highest resulting intraocular lens (IOL) power should be used for the implant. These formulas are preferably the Holladay 2, the SRK/T or the Hoffer formulas. Do not use a regression formula (e.g. SRK I or SRK II). The authors also recommend that you use central topography's flattest curve as a keratometric method unless you are fortunate to have all the information needed in order to use the "historical method." This reading is fed to the computer utilizing the selected formulas. The computer will then provide you with the power of the IOL to use.

The modern formulas hereby recommended are already available in most of the computers available today to calculate IOL power. You just select the formulas you believe adequate which should be present within your equipment.

METHOD FOR CHOOSING FORMULAS BASED UPON THE AXIAL LENGTH

From a practical standpoint, if several formulas are available to the clinician, the first choice is as follows:

- Short eyes: L <22.00 mm: Holladay 2 or Hoffer Q, Haigis and Hoffer-Colenbrander. These constitute 8% of cases.
- AL (axial length) between 22.00 and 24.50 mm; 72% of the cases: mean of the three formulas: Hoffer, Holladay and SKR/T.
- AL higher than 24.00 mm; 20% of the cases: SRK/T formula.

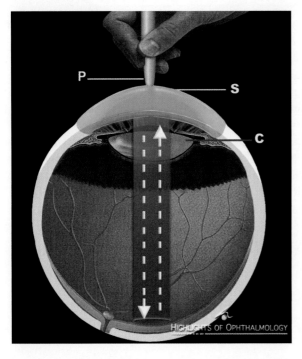

FIGURE 5.1: Determination of IOL power in patients with normal axial length (normal eyes)—mechanism of how ultrasound measures distances and determines axial length. The use of ultrasound to calculate the intraocular lens power takes into account the variants that may occur in the axial diameter of the eye and the curvature of the cornea. The ultrasound probe (P) has a piezoelectric crystal that electrically emits and receives high frequency sound waves. The sound waves travel through the eye until they are reflected back by any structure that stands perpendicularly in their way (represented by arrows). These arrows show how the sound waves travel through the ocular globe and return to contact the probe tip. Knowing the speed of the sound waves, and based on the time it takes for the sound waves to travel back to the probe (arrows), the distance can be calculated. The speed of the ultrasound waves (arrows) is higher through a dense lens (C) than through a clear one. Soft-tipped transducers (P) are recommended to avoid errors when touching the corneal surface (S). The ultrasound equipment computer can automatically multiply the time by the velocity of sound to obtain the axial length. Calculations of intraocular lens power are based on programs such as SRK-II, SRK-T, Holladay or Binkhorst among others, installed in the computer (*Source:* Highlights of Ophthalmology)

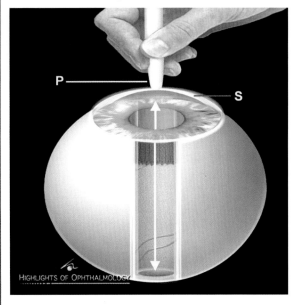

FIGURE 5.2: IOL power calculation in patients with very short axial length (hyperopia). In eyes with short or very short axial lengths, the third-generation formulas such as **Holladay 2** and **Hoffer-Q** seem to provide the best results. **Holladay** has discovered that the size of the anterior and posterior segments is not proportional in extremely short eyes (<20.0 mm). Only 20% of short eyes present a small anterior segment (nanophthalmic eyes); 80% present a normal anterior segment and it is the posterior segment that is abnormally short as shown here. P represents probe, S represents corneal surface. (*Source:* Highlights of Ophthalmology)

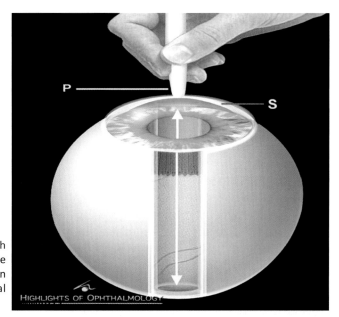

FIGURE 5.3: IOL power calculation in high myopia. In high myopia with axial lengths higher than 27.0 mm, the use of the SRK II formula with an individual surgeon's factor has shown good predictability of the refractive target. Probe (P), corneal surface (S). (*Source:* Highlights of Ophthalmology)

HIGH HYPEROPIA

There are two main difficulties in measuring the axial length in these eyes, the utilization of the correct ultrasound velocity (Hoffer has recommended using 1560 m/sec) and dealing with the errors induced by the ultrasound contact techniques in these short eyes (Perhaps is more convenient to use immersion techniques).

In eyes with short or very short axial lengths (**Figure 5.2**), the third-generation formulas such as Holladay 2 and Hoffer-Q seem to provide the best results. Observing high refractive errors in extremely short eyes (< 20.0 mm), Holladay has discovered that the size of the anterior and posterior segments is not proportional, and has devised certain measurements to be used to calculate the parameters in these eyes. Assembling data from 35 international researchers, Holladay concluded that only 20% of short eyes present a small anterior segment (nanophthalmic eyes); 80%

present a normal anterior segment and it is the posterior segment that is abnormally short. This means that the formulas that predict a small anterior segment in a short eye provoke an 80% error margin, as they will predict an abnormally shallow anterior chamber, which in turn can lead to hyperopic errors of up to 5 diopters. The Holladay 2 formula comprises the seven parameters previously described for IOL calculation: axial length, keratometry, anterior chamber depth (ACD), lens width, white-to-white corneal horizontal diameter, preoperative refraction and age. This new formula has reduced 5 D errors to less than 1 D in eyes with high hyperopia.

THE USE OF PIGGYBACK LENSES IN VERY HIGH HYPEROPIA

For very short eyes (< 22.00 mm in length) even though the Holladay 2 or the Hoffer Q formulas are a significant

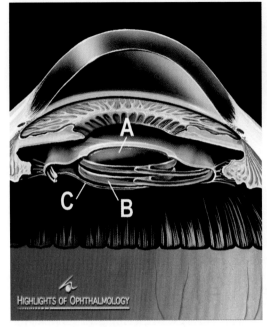

FIGURE 5.4: Concept of the piggyback high plus intraocular lenses. In cases of very high hyperopia, a clear lens extraction may be done combined with the use of piggyback high-plus intraocular lenses. One (A), or two (B) or, some surgeons suggest, three or more intraocular lenses can be implanted inside the capsular bag (C). This piggyback implantation technique may solve the problems of having to implant a lens of over +30 diopters with its consequent optical aberrations, but the procedure may give rise to postoperative complications. Some prestigious surgeons have their reservations (see text) (*Source:* Highlights of Ophthalmology)

advance in calculating the IOL power needed. The author do not have IOLs easily available with a power higher than +40 diopters because a higher diopter lens would have a marked, almost spherical curvature, that would cause major optical aberrations. Such lenses can be customized but still may cause undesirable optical aberrations. In these cases, the piggyback method is employed, i.e. the implantation of more than one IOL in a single eye, dividing the total power among the different lenses, placing two-third of the power in the posterior lens and one-third in the anterior lens **(Figure 5.4)**.

Gayton (1994) was the first to place two lenses in a single eye. He observed that placing multiple lenses in a single eye produces improved optical quality because there are fewer spherical aberrations than with very high diopter lenses.

Measuring the position of piggyback lenses, Holladay observed that contrary to what he supposed — that the anterior lens would occupy a more anterior position — what effectively happens is that the anterior lens preserves its normal position while the posterior lens moves backwards because of the distensible nature of the capsular bag. The latter may accommodate more than two IOLs and there are cases of patients with four piggyback lenses in the same eye.

The total power of the piggyback IOL implantation is calculated more precisely with the Hoffer-Colenbrander, or with a modification of the Holladay 2 formula.

Gayton and Apple described the presence of inter-lenticular opacification (ILO) in endocapsular piggyback implantation. The mentioned tissue consisted of retained/proliferative lens epithelial cells mixed with lens cortical material. They recommended three surgical means that may help to prevent this complication:

i. Meticulous cortical cleanup, especially in the equatorial region.

ii. Creation of a relatively large continuous curvilinear capsulorhexis to sequester retained cells peripheral to the IOL optic within the equatorial fornix.

iii. Insertion of the posterior IOL in the capsular bag and the anterior IOL in the ciliary sulcus to isolate retained cells from the interlenticular space.

Echobiometry in highly hyperopic eyes, especially microphthalmic and nanophthalmic eyes, is still far from desirable.

HIGH MYOPIA

According to Zacharias and Centurion's experience, results of cataract surgery in highly myopic eyes with axial lengths higher than 31.0 mm with the implantation of low or negative power IOLs may be successful, without any more operative or postoperative complications than normal eyes. The use of the SRK II formula with an individual surgeon's factor showed good predictability of the refractive target **(Figure 5.3)**. However, better formulas without the use of a personalized correction factor have yet to be developed. Zacharias and Centurion emphasize that there are technical difficulties in performing the echobiometry of patients with high myopia, especially when they have a posterior staphyloma. In those cases, they obtain extremely irregular retinal echoes that cannot provide certainty in the terms of really correct results of the IOL calculation. In addition, a posterior staphyloma may not always coincide with the macula, so the higher measurement is not necessarily the correct one, as is the case with normal eyes.

In these patients, it is useful to perform B type ultrasound to identify the existence of a staphyloma and its relation with the macula. Equally important is to have an ultrasound probe with a fixation light. The patient is asked to fixate at the light, which he will do with the macula, facilitating the measurement.

DETERMINING IOL POWER IN PATIENTS WITH PREVIOUS REFRACTIVE SURGERY

Patients who have undergone excimer laser procedures, radial keratotomy or intracorneal segment rings, have had modifications to their corneal curvatures (**Figures 5.5 to 5.7**). Accurate keratometric readings are fundamental in calculating IOL power. Intraocular lens power calculation for cataract surgery in patients previously submitted to refractive surgery by modification of the corneal curvature is a new challenge for the cataract surgeon because of two features: (1) Patients who previously decided to undergo refractive surgery are more psychologically resistant to using spectacles to correct residual ametropia. Consequently, their expectations for cataract surgery are unusually high. (2) So far there is no universally accepted formula to calculate these patients' IOL power accurately. Routine keratometry readings do not accurately reflect the true corneal curvature in these cases and may result in errors if used for IOL calculations. Therefore, standard keratometry readings should not be used for IOL calculations in these patients. If done, the standard IOL power-predictive formulas based on such readings commonly result in substantial undercorrection with postoperative hyperopic refraction or anisometropia both of which are very undesirable.

COMMONLY USED METHODS

There are three methods to determine the effective power of the cornea in these complex cases: (1) the clinical history

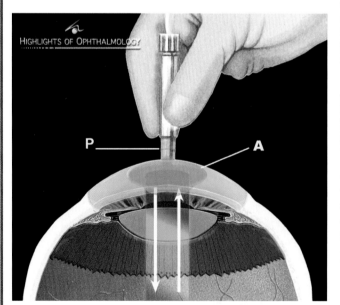

FIGURE 5.5: IOL power calculation in patients after excimer laser procedure. In this group of patients even with the most advanced ultrasonic equipment, there is a degree of variation in the results of the IOL power calculation. This is the result of the varying modification in the curvature of the cornea after the excimer laser ablation (A). Ultrasound transducer (P) (*Source:* Highlights of Ophthalmology)

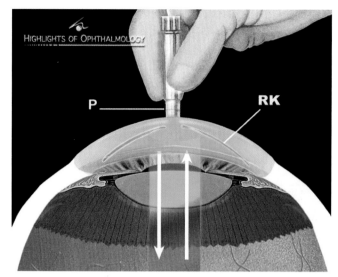

FIGURE 5.6: IOL power calculation in patients after radial keratotomy. Patients operated of radial keratotomy with an used optical zone smaller than 4.0 mm, cannot have their central corneal curvature measured reliably with the standard keratometric methods. Ultrasound transducer (P), radial keratotomy incisions (RK) (*Source:* Highlights of Ophthalmology)

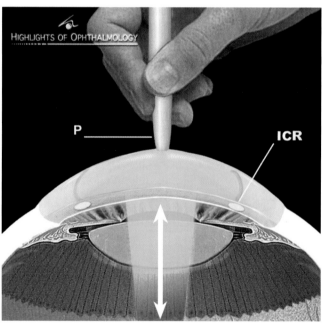

FIGURE 5.7: IOL power calculation after an intracorneal ring segment procedure. As with other refractive procedures on the cornea, this technique for correction of low myopia also modifies the central corneal curvature (arrows). Topography determines the present corneal curvature. The surgeon uses the central flattest keratometric reading as a reference in cases where the pre-refractive procedure keratometry cannot be obtained. Ultrasound transducer (P), intracorneal rings (ICR) (*Source:* Highlights of Ophthalmology)

method, also termed by Holladay "the calculation method"; (2) the contact lens method; and (3) the topography method. Holladay believes that the calculation or "clinical history" method and the hard contact lens trial are the two more reliable of the three, because the corneal topography instruments presently available do not provide accurate central corneal power following PRK, LASIK and RKs with optical zones of 3 mm or less. In RKs with larger optical zones, the topography instruments become more reliable. The great majority of cases, however, have had RK with an optimal zone larger than 3 mm, so they should also qualify for this method.

The Clinical History Method

Holladay proposed this method based on the idea that refractive surgery has changed the corneal power and that this refractive change must be substracted to the presurgical power of the cornea in order to estimate its present power. You need to obtain:

- A preoperative average K reading (Kp)
- A preoperative spherical equivalent refractive error (Rp, before refractive corneal surgery).
- A postoperative spherical equivalent refractive error (Ro, after the eye has healed following refractive surgery and visual acuity has stabilized but before cataract formation)

To calculate the eye's estimated corneal power (K), use the Hoffer formula:

$$K = Kp + (Rp) - (Ro)$$

Remember to add algebraically and to change the sign when opening the second parenthesis.

Vertex correcting the refractions is no longer recommended.

The Trial Hard Contact Lens Method

The method is based on the concept that, if a hard PMMA contact lens of known base curve (i.e. 36.00 D) and known power (i.e. Plano) is placed on the cornea and the refraction does not change, the effective power of the cornea must be 36.00 D. If the power is different from plano and/or the difference in refraction is not zero, the formula will calculate the power. This method is limited to those cataractous eyes with a minimum best corrected visual acuity of 20/80. The method will not work in eyes that are not able to be refracted.

You need to obtain:
- A hard PMMA (not RGP) contact lens with a base curve (B) close to the estimated K reading and with a known power (P, easier if plano).
- A bare manifest refraction without a contact lens (Rb).
- A manifest overrefraction with a contact lens (Rc).

To calculate the eye's estimated corneal power (K), use the formula:

$$K = B + P + Rc - Rb.$$

Remember to add algebraically and that is no longer recommended to vertex correcting the refractions.

The Corneal Topography Method

When information is not available for the Clinical History Method, it has been recommended by Zacharias and Centurion, as well as by Torres and Suarez, that the keratometric reading be taken with the topography unit, using the flattest K found in the central 3 mm of the corneal mapping.

Hoffer has suggested that after looking at the preceding methods, the author should choose the lowest K reading from those you have calculated to use in the formula and then employ the Aramberri Double-K Method.

Aramberri Double-K Method

In 2001, Dr Jaime Aramberri had the idea that the postsurgical flatter K reading should not be used in modern, theoretic formulas to calculate the estimated position of the IOL (estimated lens position, ELP, the visual axial distance from the apex of the cornea to the principal plane of the IOL, or anterior chamber depth). This concept is based on the fact that the flattening and thinning of the cornea has not changed the biometric measurements of the anterior chamber structures; that is, the cornea has not changed its distance relationship with the crystalline lens and iris. Hoffer calls it the Aramberri Double-K Method.

What you need to do is:
- Use the preoperative K reading (Kp., e.g. 43.50 D) in the part of the formula that predicts the estimated lens position (anterior chamber depth)
- Use the postoperative (Ko, e.g. 35.00 D) in the part of the formula that calculates the IOL power.

Presently this option is only available on the Hoffer Programs version 2.5. This method has not been tested for accuracy on a large reported series.

K-Method in Previous Radial Keratotomy

For patients with previous RK with optical zone (OZ) of less than 4.0 mm, use the clinical history method if possible, otherwise use the flattest K of the central 3.0 mm in the topographic map or both. Check the IOL power with the SRK/T formula of the Hoffer 2.5 software. If the OZ is larger than 4.0 mm, use the measured K obtained with the keratometer as it will not be affected.

In conclusion, in patients with previous Myopic Lasik / Lasek / PRK, use the clinical history method if possible, otherwise use the flattest K of the central 3.0 mm of the topographic map. In hyperopic lasik/PRK, conductive keratoplasty (CK) and intracorneal rings, the central corneal thickness is basically unaffected. In these cases, the K readings obtained can be used for the IOL power calculation. The clinical history method is utilized to double-check the corneal power.

THE IMPORTANCE OF DETECTING IRREGULAR ASTIGMATISM

Holladay has strongly recommended that biomicroscopy, retinoscopy, corneal topography and endothelial cell counts be performed in all of these complex cases. The first three tests are primarily directed at evaluating the amount of irregular astigmatism. This determination is extremely important preoperatively because the irregular astigmatism may be contributing to the reduced vision as well as the cataract. The irregular astigmatism may also be the limiting factor in the patient's vision following cataract surgery. The endothelial cell count is necessary to recognize any patients with low cell counts from the previous surgery who may be at higher risk for corneal decompensation or prolonged visual recovery.

The potential acuity meter (PAM), super pinhole and hard contact lens trial are often helpful as secondary tests in determining the respective contribution to reduced vision by the cataract and the corneal irregular astigmatism. The patient should be informed that only the glare from the cataract would be eliminated. Any glare from the kerato-refractive procedure will essentially remain unchanged.

IOL POWER CALCULATION IN PEDIATRIC CATARACTS

How to optically correct patients with bilateral congenital cataracts and monocular congenital cataract has been a major subject of controversy for many years. Twenty years ago, some distinguished ophthalmic surgeons were strongly against performing surgery in monocular congenital cataract followed by the treatment of amblyopia with a contact lens. Visual results were so bad that children with this problem must be amblyopic by nature, they thought, and the psychological damage to the children and the parents by forcing such treatment was to be condemned.

Surgery of bilateral congenital cataracts at a very early age followed by correction with spectacles and sometimes with contact lenses usually ended with no better than 20/60 vision bilaterally. This was again a source for belief that congenital cataracts either unilateral or bilateral were by nature associated with amblyopia, profound in the cases of monocular cases and fairly strong in bilateral cataracts.

When posterior chamber IOL implantation in adults became established as the procedure of choice, strong influences within ophthalmology were adamantly opposed to their use in children for the following reasons: (1) the eye grows in length with consequent significant change in refraction. It was considered impossible to predict such change and consequently, the accurate IOL power adequate for each child. (2) There was opacification of posterior capsule in most cases. This required a second operation for posterior capsulotomy in the presence of an IOL.

The situation has now significantly changed. The previous failures with spectacles and contact lenses, the new developments in technology and surgical techniques and the fresh insight of surgeons of a new generation has led us to discard the previous thinking and very definitely implant posterior chamber IOLs in children. This has been

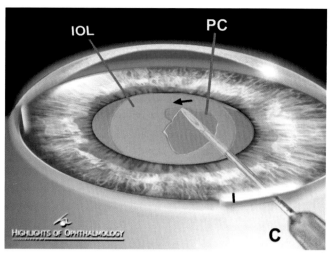

FIGURE 5.8: Posterior capsulorhexis in pediatric patients. Following the conventional steps of phacoemulsification, an appropriate intraocular lens for children is inserted (IOL) with the required power in compliance with the criteria of the practitioner following the guidelines in the text. Once the intraocular lens is located in the bag and properly protecting the tissues with viscoelastics, a cystotome (C) is introduced through the limbal incision (I), and directed behind the IOL to perform a posterior capsule tear or posterior capsulorhexis (PC). This opening in the posterior capsule at the time of the phaco procedure can provide permanent improved vision to the child (*Source:* Highlights of Ophthalmology)

made possible because of new medications that effectively prevent and/or control inflammation; the introduction of posterior capsule capsulorhexis (**Figure 5.8**); high viscosity viscoelastics to facilitate intraocular surgery in smaller eyes; new, more appropriate IOLs and more refined technology that leads to a less difficult calculation of the IOL power.

DIFFERENT ALTERNATIVES

The limitations in calculating these lenses power (**Figure 5.9**) is due to the fact that the eye grows after cataract surgery and therefore refraction will change. Two main methods of choosing an IOL power for pediatric patients are available: (1) Make the eye emmetropic at the time of surgery and thereby treat amblyopia immediately taking advantage of a much better visual acuity. This is followed later by an IOL exchange or a secondary piggyback IOL implantation of a negative power or other means of treatment for the residual eventual myopia. (2) Proceed with incomplete correction of the eye at the time of surgery (treated with glasses or contact lenses) taking advantage of the trend toward emmetropization, which will occur as the eye grows. By "incomplete" the author mean leaving the eyes hyperopic. As the eye grows in length with age (axial growth), the myopization that takes place in an eye artificially rendered hyperopic will lead to emmetropia or close to normal refraction. This measure avoids myopic anisometropia that may lead to an undesirable change of IOL surgically. In the meantime, the temporary hyperopia is managed with standard spectacles or contact lenses.

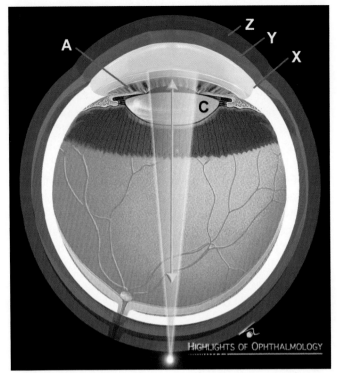

IOL POWER CALCULATION FOLLOWING VITRECTOMY

For the most part, IOL power calculation in eyes that develop a cataract following vitrectomy is very straightforward. The intravitreal gas is reabsorbed and slowly replaced by aqueous. If silicone oil is used, once it is removed aqueous fills the vitreous cavity. Since the refractive indices of aqueous and vitreous are identical (1.336), no corrections are needed in the IOL power calculation.

For patients who may undergo a silicone oil procedure at some point, it is wise to consider obtaining bilateral baseline axial length measurements by immersion A-scan biometry or by Optical Coherence Biometry—OCB (IOL Master). This category would include any patient with a prior retinal detachment, moderate-to-high axial myopia, proliferative vitreoretinopathy, proliferative diabetic retinopathy, acquired immunodeficiency syndrome, giant retinal tear, or history of a perforating ocular injury (**Figure 5.10**).

FIGURE 5.9: IOL power calculation in pediatric cataract. The growth of the ocular globe is ecographically registered until 18 years of age. However, the lens continues growing throughout the life of the individual. In normal conditions, anterior chamber (A) depth is reduced as the lens increases in size. In pathological conditions such as the presence of cataracts, the opposite may happen: the anterior chamber depth may increase due to reduction in the volume of the lens (C). In this illustration, we can see the changes in the size of the globe through the shaded images that outline the growth of the eye by stages. At birth, the axial diameter in the normal patient may measure approximately 17.5 mm, at three years of age it may measure 21.8 mm (X), at ten years 22.5 mm identified in (Y) and in normal adulthood nearly 24 mm (Z). In selecting the lens power to be used, some surgeons choose to make the child hyperopic (arrows) with the intention that his growth will compensate hyperopia with the passage of time and will be eventually closer to achieving an emmetropic eye. Others prefer to calculate an intraocular lens closer to emmetropia with the intention of keeping the child emmetropic during his growing years and prescribing eyeglasses in the future (*Source:* Highlights of Ophthalmology)

ALTERNATIVES OF CHOICE

In the IOL power calculation in children younger than 1 year, keratometry is difficult and fortunately less important because the values change very rapidly during the first six months. Thus keratometry may be replaced by the mean adult average keratometry value of 44.00 D. Children less than two years old may be incompletely corrected +3.00 D to even +4.00 D; between three and four years old incompletely correct them +3.00 D in those closer to three and +2.50 D in those closer to four. In children closer to six or seven, who have little chance of recovering from any amblyopia present but who are the ones that more frequently suffer from a unilateral traumatic cataract, overcorrect them by +1.00 D.

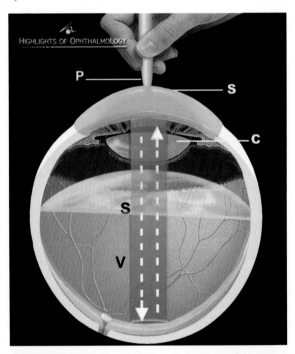

FIGURE 5.10: IOL power calculation in patients after vitrectomy procedure with silicone. If the patient is in the process of undergoing this procedure, it is recommended to calculate the intraocular lens before using silicone in the vitreous cavity (V) and extracting the lens (C). Polymethylmethacrylate lenses (PMMA) are recommended. Silicone foldable IOLs are not recommended because the silicone oil in the vitreous cavity sticks to the intraocular lens and sometimes causes opacities. In the calculation of these lens powers there may be differences in excess of 5–7 diopters. Errors can be frequent because if the vitreous cavity (V) is not filled completely with silicone (S), the movement of the bubble can induce errors in the calculation of the lens. In addition, in the eye filled with silicone, the ultrasound waves travel slower (arrows). This affects the axial diameter measurement during IOL power calculation. For alternative methods of IOL power calculation, see text (*Source:* Highlights of Ophthalmology)

Eyes that have undergone complicated retinal detachment repair with silicone oil placed in the vitreous cavity often require subsequent cataract surgery. Accurate A-scan biometry can be very difficult in these eyes because silicone oil has a slower sound velocity than vitreous and often produces strong sound attenuation. These factors may prevent the display of a high-quality retinal spike and can contribute to significant measurement errors. Therefore, it is best to use OCB to measure theses eyes whenever possible.

Two densities of silicone oil are presently in use, each of which has a slower sound velocity than vitreous (1532 m/sec). The 1000 centistokes (cSt) silicone oil (eq. Silikon 1000, Alcon Laboratories, Ft. Worth, Texas) has a sound velocity of 980 m/sec. The higher density 5000 cSt silicone oil (eq. Adato Sil-Ol 5000, Bausch & Lomb Surgical, Irvine, California) produces a velocity of 1040m/sec. It is important to know which density of silicone oil is present in the vitreous cavity before A-scan biometry so that the correct velocity setting can be used.

For eyes containing silicone oil, A-scan axial length measurements are best carried out with the patient seated as upright as possible. This is especially important if the vitreous cavity is only partly filled with silicone oil. In the upright position, silicone oil is more likely to remain in contact with the retina during the examination. Because of its lighter density with the patient fully recumbent, the entire mass of silicone oil often shifts away from the retina, towards the anterior segment, leading to confusion as to the true position of the retinal spike.

If an incorrect sound velocity is used to measure the axial length of an eye containing silicone oil, the measurement displayed usually will be erroneously long. Measuring each component of the eye individually, using the correct corresponding sound velocity avoids errors and gives good approximation of the true axial length. Examples of sound velocities include anterior chamber depth at 1532 m/sec, crystalline lens thickness at 1641 m/sec, and vitreous cavity length at either 980 m/sec (for 1000 cSt silicone oil) or 1040 m/sec (for 5000 cSt silicone oil). Ideally, the biometer should have four electronic measuring gates and should allow the sound velocity to be modified when necessary. This allows for independent measurement of the individual components of the eye at the appropriate sound velocity. When the biometer provides only two gates and the sound velocities are not adjustable, a more complex approach is required.

The easiest way to measure the axial length of an eye containing silicone oil is to use optical coherence biometry (OCB). Measurements can be made, without any special corrections, in phakic and aphakic eyes containing silicone oil. However, a large posterior subcapsular plaque or a dense nuclear cataract may make a reliable measurement impossible with this technique.

If the silicone oil is to be removed at some point, standard IOL power calculations can be performed after the true axial length has been determined. However, if the silicone oil is to remain in the eye indefinitely, a power adjustment must be made to prevent significant postoperative hyperopia.

When silicone oil is placed in the vitreous cavity, a higher-power IOL is required to achieve the same refractive result. This is because the index of refraction for silicone is higher than that of normal vitreous. In addition, it is recommended that these patients receive a polymethylmethacrylate (PMMA) convex-plano lens; with the plano side oriented toward the vitreous cavity (and preferably over an intact posterior capsule). This approach prevents the silicone oil from altering the refractive power of the posterior surface of the IOL. The Holladay IOL Consultant software is very helpful for these cases as it has the ability to compensate for the different index of refraction of silicone oil compared to that of the vitreous.

For an average-length eye in which the vitreous cavity is filled with silicone oil, the additional power needed for a convex-plano PMMA IOL is typically between + 3.0 D to + 3.5 D. For example, the true axial length (TALs) of an eye with 1000 cSt silicone oil filling the vitreous cavity is 25.17 mm. The anterior chamber depth is measured at 3.21 mm and the IOL power calculation calls for a plus 20.0 D convex-plano lens. In this circumstance, plus 3.07 D of additional IOL power must be added at the level of the capsular bag to compensate for the differing refractive index of silicone oil. This will result in the implantation of a plus 23.0 D lens.

If, however, removal of the silicone oil at a later date is anticipated, a possible alternative is to implant a plus 20.0 D convex-plano PMMA IOL in the capsular bag and a plus 3.0 D PMMA lens temporarily in the ciliary sulcus. The silicone oil and the ciliary sulcus lens could then be removed at the same time, this avoiding a more complicated IOL exchange.

Meldrum, Aaberg, Patel and Davis make the following recommendations:
- Measure the axial length using the velocity of sound in silicone oil.
- Calculate the IOL power to achieve emmetropia using the traditional formulas. To this IOL power, a correction factor must be added to obtain the IOL power to achieve emmetropia in silicone oil. The correction factors range from 2.79 D to 3.94 D, for axial lengths from 20 mm to 30 mm.
- Choose a convex-plano IOL if possible. If another type of lens is used, another correction factor must be added to obtain the total power of the IOL in the presence of silicone oil. For a convex-plano lens no additional correction factor is required.

For instance, let us suppose that a patient requires indefinite intraocular tamponade with silicone oil and develops a cataract. Using the traditional formulas, assuming that the IOL power is calculated to be 22 D based on a measured axial length of 23 mm. To this 22 D, the author must add a correction factor of 3.64 D (Meldrum et al.) to correct for the axial length. Thus, for this patient a 25.5 D convex-plano lens should be implanted to achieve emmetropia in the presence of silicone oil. No additional correction factor for the IOL design is necessary.

RECOMMENDED READINGS

1. Lu LW, Fine IH. Phacoemulsification in Difficult and Challenging Cases. New York: Thieme; 1999.
2. Mendicute J, Cadarso L, Lorente R., et al. Facoemulsificación. 1999.

BIBLIOGRAPHY

1. Aramberri J. Intraocular lens power calculation after corneal refractive surgery: Double K method. J Cataract Refract Surg. 2003;29:2063-8.
2. Boyd BF. Undergoing cataract surgery with a master surgeon: a personal experience. Highlights of Ophthalm. Bi-monthly Journal. 1999;27(1);3.
3. Brady KM, Atkinson CS, Kilty LA, et al. Cataract surgery and intraocular lens implantation in children. Am J Ophthalmol, 1995;120:1-9.
4. Buckley EG, Klombers LA, Seaber JH, et al. Management of the posterior capsule during intraocular lens implantation. Am J Ophthalmol 1993;115:722-8.
5. Celikkol L, Pavlopoulos G, Weinstein B, et al. Calculation of intraocular lens power after radial keratotomy with computerized videokeratography. Am J Ophthalmol. 1995; 120:739-50.
6. Chen L, Mannis MJ, Salz JJ, et al. Analysis of intraocular lens power calculation in post-radial keratotomy eyes. J Cataract Refract Surg. 2003;29:65-70.
7. Dahan E, Drusedan MU. Choice of lens and dioptric power in pediatric pseudophakia. J Cataract Refract Surg. 1997;23:618-23.
8. Gayton JL. Implanting two posterior chamber intraocular lenses in microphthalmos. Ocular Surgery News. 1994:64-5.
9. Gayton JL, Apple DJ, Peng Q, et al. Interlenticular opacification: Clinicopathological correlation of a complication of posterior chamber piggyback intraocular lenses. J Cataract Refract Surg. 2000; 26:330-6.
10. Gimbel HV. Posterior continuous curvilinear capsulorhexis and optic capture of the intraocular lens to prevent secondary opacification in pediatric cataract surgery. J Cataract Refract Surg. 1997;23:652-6.
11. Gimbel HV, Basti S, Ferensowicz MA, et al. Results of bilateral cataract extraction with posterior chamber intraocular lens implantation in children. Ophthalmology. 1997;104:1737-43.
12. Grinbaum A, Treister G, Moisseiev J. Predicted and actual refraction after intraocular lens implantation in eyes with silicone oil. J Cataract Refract Surg 1996;22:726-9.
13. Grusha YO, Masket S, Miller KM. Phacoemulsification and lens implantation after pars plana vitrectomy. Ophthalmology. 1998;105:287-94.
14. Holladay JT. Intraocular lens power in difficult cases. In: Masket S, Crandal AS (Eds). Atlas of Cataract Surgery. London: Martin Dunitz; 1999; 147-58.
15. Holladay JT, Gills JP, Leidlein J, et al. Achieving emmetropia in extremely short eyes with two piggyback posterior chamber intraocular lenses. Ophthalmology. 1996;103:1118-23.
16. Hoffer KJ. Intraocular lens power calculation for eyes after refractive keratotomy. J Refract Surg. 1995;11:490-3.
17. Hoffer KJ. The Hoffer Q formula: a comparison of theoretic and regression formulas. J Cataract Surg. 1993;19:700-12.
18. Hoffer KJ. Ultrasound velocities for axial eye length measurement. J Cat Refract Surg. 1994;20:554-62.
19. Kora Y, Shimizu K, Inatomi M, et al. Eye growth after cataract extraction and intraocular lens implantation in children. Ophthalmic Surg. 1993;24:467-75.
20. Lacava AC, Centurion V. Cataract surgery after refractive surgery. Faco Total, Editora Cultura Medica. 2000;269-76.
21. Lyle WA, Jin GJ. Intraocular lens power prediction in patients who undergo cataract surgery following previous radial keratotomy. Arch Ophthalmol. 1997;115:457-61.
22. Maeda N, Klyce SD, Smolek MK, et al. Disparity between keratometry-style reading and corneal power within the pupil after refractive surgery for myopia. Cornea. 1997;16:517-24.
23. McCartney DL, Miller KM, Stark WJ, et al. Intraocular lens style and refraction in eyes treated with silicone oil. Arch Ophthalmol. 1987;105:1385-7.
24. Meldrum LM, Aaberg TM, Patel A, et al. Cataract extraction after silicone oil repair of retinal detachments due to necrotizing retinitis. Arch Ophthalmol. 1996;114:885-92.
25. Olsen T, Thim K, Corydon L. Theoretical versus SRK I and SRK II calculation of intraocular lens power. J Cataract Refract Surg. 1990;16:217-25.
26. Sanders DR, Retzlaff J, Kraff MC, et al. Comparison of the SRK/T formula and other theoretinal and regression formulas. J Cataract Refract Surg. 1990; 16(3):341-6.
27. Zacharias W, Centurion V. Biometry and the IOL calculation for the cataract surgeon: Its importance. Faco Total. 2000;66-88.
28. Zaldivar R, Schultz MC, Davidorf JM, et al. Intraocular lens power calculations in patients with extreme myopia. J Cataract Refract Surg. 2000; 26:668-74.

CHAPTER 6

IOLMaster for Determining the IOL Power at the Time of Surgery

Hampton Roy, Warren E Hill

INTRODUCTION

The Zeiss IOLMaster is a noncontact optical device that measures axial length of the eye by partial coherence interferometry, with a consistent accuracy of 0.02 mm (less than 0.10 diopter), or better. It also does automated keratometry, measures anterior chamber depth, the horizontal corneal diameter, and calculates intraocular lens powers, all in a single sitting.[1-6]

The IOLMaster employs a modified Michelson interferometer to divide, and phase delay, a 780 nm partially coherent beam of light. One beam is reflected from the corneal surface, while the other is reflected from the retinal pigment epithelium. A photodetector and on-board computer translate the interference pattern produced by the two beams into a highly accurate measurement of axial length. Calibrated against the ultra-high resolution 40-MHz Greishaber Biometric System, an internal algorithm then approximates the distance to the vitreo-retinal interface, for the equivalent of the ultrasonic axial length. Considering the fact that axial length measurements by A-scan ultrasonography (using a standard 10-MHz transducer) have a typical resolution of 0.10 to 0.12 mm, axial length measurements by the IOLMaster represent a fivefold increase in accuracy.

Using the instrument is straightforward. The patient is placed in the chin rest and looks straight ahead at a small red fixation target. The eye is viewed on a video screen by the technician during all phases of measurement, allowing for proper alignment.

MODES

The following modes are useful:

Overview mode
This allows the technician to grossly align the instrument.

Axial length mode
The axial length can be determined in most eyes with a high degree of precision, including high myopes with posterior staphyloma, aphakia, pseudophakia and even for eyes filled with silicon oil. The machine displays a signal-to-noise ratio for each measurement, as one indication of reliability, and also compares multiple measurements. If the measurements are all within 0.1 mm, the machine displays an average axial

length. If the measurements fall outside this range, the technician is instructed to evaluate the series of measurements before concluding the examination.

The characteristics of a proper axial length display are the following:
- Signal-to-noise ratio greater than 2.0
- Tall and narrow primary maxima with a thin well-centered termination
- At least one set of secondary maxima. However, if the ocular media is poor, secondary maxima may not be displayed
- At least four of the 20 measurements taken should be within 0.02 mm of one another and show the characteristics of a good axial length display.

Automated keratometry mode
IOLMaster uses an integrated autokeratometer to determine the corneal curvature of the principal meridians with corresponding axes, displayed in diopters, or in millimeters. The instruments take five measurements within 0.5 seconds and averages them. The latest software revision (version 3.01) has an improved keratometry algorithm and will alert the operator if a keratometry measurement is questionable.

Anterior chamber depth mode
The distance between the optical section of the cornea, and the crystalline lens, is measured using a lateral slit illumination at approximately 30 degrees to the optical axis. This measurement is helpful for intraocular lens power calculation formulas, such as Haigis and Holladay 2, which require a measured anterior chamber depth.

Intraocular lens power calculation mode
The collected data can be transferred to the intraocular lens power calculation area. Five intraocular lens power calculation formulas (Haigis, Hoffer Q, Holladay 1, SRK II, SRK/T) are included with the IOLMaster software. The surgeons selects the calculation formula that he wishes to use, the target refraction, and the IOLMaster will calculate the power of up to four intraocular lenses in the physician database.

The IOLMaster can accommodate as many as 20 surgeons, each with up to 20 preferred intraocular lenses, and corresponding personalized lens constants.

The IOLMaster is easy to use, accurate and has excellent reproducibility.

NEW INTRAOCULAR LENS CONSTANTS

Some lenses, like the Alcon SA60AT, show very little difference when compared to immersion A-scan ultrasonography, while others, like the Bausch and Lomb U940A show a larger difference. In order to determine the best initial IOLMaster constant, Dr. Wolfgang Haigis, at the University of Würzburg in Germany has recommended the following approach for calculating the initial A-constant.

$A_{IOLMaster} = A_{Ultrasound} + 3 * (AL_{IOLMaster} - AL_{Ultrasound})$

$A_{IOLMaster}$ = Optimized A – constant for IOLMaster
$A_{Ultrasound}$ = Optimized A – constant for ultrasonography
$AL_{IOLMaster}$ = Average IOLMaster axial length
$AL_{Ultrasound}$ = Average ultrasound axial length

ADVANTAGES

- No topical anesthetic is needed.
- Multiple measurements, at different instrument stations, are not necessary.
- Patients sit upright.
- Using the IOLMaster is quick, accurate, and requires minimal training, although some Interpretation by the operator is necessary.
- Noncontact technique precludes the occurrence of corneal epithelial injuries, and the transmission of infections.

DISADVANTAGES

- Unable to use for dense nuclear cataracts, posterior subcapsular plaques, corneal scars and vitreous hemorrhages. In any case in which the axial opacity interferes with the partially coherent light beams, IOLMaster cannot be used.
- Unable to use on patients that cannot fully cooperate because of physical or psychological reasons. Approximately 95 percent of patients can be measured successfully using the IOLMaster.

RESULTS

The accuracy of intraocular lens power predictions from the IOLMaster measurements have been found to be as good, or better, than immersion A-scan ultrasonography. With a combination of the IOLMaster, and the Holladay 2 formula, Warren E Hill, MD has been able to consistently achieve refractive outcomes with a mean absolute prediction error of better than ±0.25 diopters. This approaches the theoretic limit of the exercise, given the fact that intraocular lens implants come in 0.50 diopter steps.

SUMMARY

Think of the IOLMaster (**Figure 6.1**) as a form of ultra high-resolution immersion A-scan ultrasonography, giving the refractive axial length, rather than the anatomic axial length.

Because the IOLMaster is an optical device, measurements may not be possible in the presence of significant

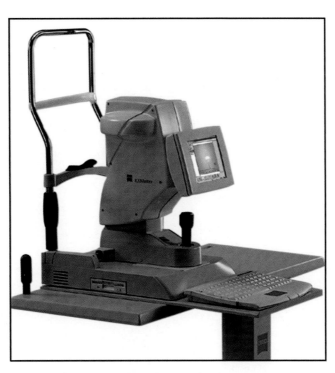

FIGURE 6.1: IOLMaster

axial opacities, such as a corneal scar, mature cataract, vitreous hemorrhage, or dense PSC plaque, etc.

IOL constants for the IOLMaster will often be slightly higher than the manufacturer's suggested numbers and are very close to those used for immersion A-scans. It is suggested that IOLMaster-specific intraocular lens constants be used with the various popular intraocular lens power calculation formulas.

The IOLMaster is a highly reliable tool for determining the intraocular lens power prior to surgery.

REFERENCES

1. Vogel A, Dick B, Krummenauer F. Reproducibility of optical biometry using partial coherence interferometry. Intraobserver and interobserver reliability. J Cataract Refract Surg. 2001;27: 1961-8.

2. Schachar RA, Levy NS, Bonney RC. Accuracy of intraocular lens powers calculated from A-scan biometry with the Echo-Oculometer. Ophthalmic Surg. 1980;11: 856-8.

3. Drexler, W, Findl O, Menapace R, et al. Partial Coherence Inferometry: A Novel Approach to Biometry in Cataract Surgery. Am J Ophthalmol. 1998;126: 524-34.

4. Holladay JT, Musgrove KH, Praeger TC, et al. A three-part system for refining intraocular lens power calculations. J Cataract Refractive Surgery. 1988; 14: 17-24.

5. Wallace RB. IOLMaster Optical Coherence Biometry: Accurate Axial Length Measurement for Cataract Surgery and Refractive Lensectomy. Refractive Eyecare for Ophthalmologists. 2000;4: 17-20.

6. Retzlaff J, Sanders DR, Kraff MC. Development of the SRK/T intraocular lens implant power calculation formula. J Cataract Refractive Surgery. 1990;16: 333-40.

CHAPTER 7

Corneal Topography in Cataract Surgery

Athiya Agarwal, Amar Agarwal

INTRODUCTION

Topography is defined as the science of describing or representing the features of a particular place in detail. In corneal topography, the place is the cornea, i.e. the features of the cornea are described in detail.

The word "topography" is derived[1,2] from two Greek words:

Topos meaning *place* and Graphien meaning to *write*.

CORNEA

The cornea is the most important plane or tissue for refraction. This is because it has the highest refractive power (which is about + 45 D) and it is easily accessible to the surgeon without going inside the eye.

To understand the cornea, one should realize that the cornea is a parabolic curve — its radius of curvature differs from center to periphery. It is steepest in the center and flatter in the periphery. For all practical purposes, the central cornea that is the optical zone is considered when a refractive surgery is performed. A flatter cornea has less refraction power and a steeper cornea has a higher refraction power. If the refraction is to be changed then the steeper diameter has to be flattened and the flatter diameter has to be steepened.

KERATOMETRY

The keratometer was invented by Hermann von Helmholtz and modified by Javal-Schiotz, et al. If the object is placed in front of a convex mirror, then a virtual, erect and minified image is obtained (**Figure 7.1**). A keratometer in relation to the cornea is just like an object in front of a convex reflecting mirror. Like in a convex reflecting surface, the image is located posterior to the cornea. The cornea behaves as a convex reflecting mirror and the mires of the keratometer are the objects. The radius of curvature of the cornea's anterior surface determines the size of the image.

The keratometer projects single mire on the cornea and the separation of the two points on the mire is used to determine corneal curvature. The zone measured depends upon corneal curvature—the steeper the cornea, the smaller the zone. For example, for a 36 D cornea, the keratometer measures a 4 mm zone and for a 50 D cornea, the size of the cone is 2.88 mm.

Keratometers are accurate only when the corneal surface is a sphere or a spherocylinder. Actually, the shape of the

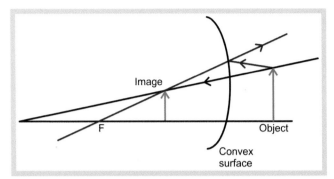

FIGURE 7.1: Physics of a convex mirror. Note the image is virtual, erect and minified. The cornea acts like the convex mirror and the mire of the keratometer is the object

anterior surface of the cornea is more than a sphere or a spherocylinder. However, keratometers measure the central 3 mm of the cornea, which behaves like a sphere or a spherocylinder. This is the reason why Helmholtz could manage with the keratometer (**Figure 7.2**). This is also the reason why most ophthalmologists can manage management of cataract surgery with the keratometer. However, the ball game has changed with refractive surgery today. This is because when the cornea has complex central curves like in keratoconus or after refractive surgery, the keratometer cannot give good results and becomes inaccurate. Thus, the advantages of the keratometer like speed, ease of use, low cost and minimum maintenance are obscured.

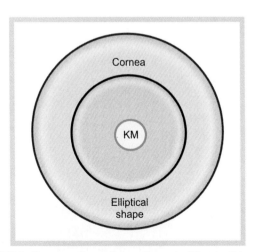

FIGURE 7.2: Keratometers measure the central 3 mm of the cornea, which generally behaves like a sphere or a spherocylinder. This is the reason why keratometers are generally accurate. However, in complex situations like in keratoconus or refractive surgery they become inaccurate

The objects used in the keratometer are referred to as mires. Separation of two points on the mire are used to determine corneal curvature. The object in the keratometer can be rotated with respect to the axis. The disadvantages of the keratometer are that they measure only a small region of the cornea. The peripheral regions are ignored. They also lose accuracy when measuring very steep or flat corneas. As the keratometer assumes the cornea to be symmetrical, it becomes a disadvantage if the cornea is asymmetrical as after refractive surgery.

KERATOSCOPY

To solve the problem of keratometers, scientists worked on a system called keratoscopy. In this, they projected a beam of concentric rings and observed them over a wide expanse of the corneal surface. However, this was not enough and the next step was to move into computerized videokeratography.

COMPUTERIZED VIDEOKERATOGRAPHY

In this some form of light like a placido disk is projected onto the cornea. The cornea modifies this light and this modification is captured by a video camera. This information is analyzed by computer software and the data is then displayed in a variety of formats. To simplify the results to an ophthalmologist, Klyce in 1988 started the corneal color maps. The corneal color maps display the estimate of corneal shape in a fashion that is understandable to the ophthalmologist. Each color on the map is assigned a

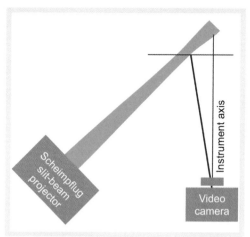

FIGURE 7.3: Principle of the Orbscan (*Courtesy:* Dr Agarwal's Eye Hospital, India)

defined range of measurement. The placido type topographic machines do not assess the posterior surface of the cornea. The details of the corneal assessment can be done only with the Orbscan (Bausch & Lomb) as both anterior and posterior surface of the cornea are assessed.

ORBSCAN

The Orbscan (Bausch & Lomb) corneal topography system **(Figures 7.3 and 7.4)** uses a scanning optical slit scan that is fundamentally different from the corneal topography that analyzes the reflected images from the anterior corneal surface. The high-resolution video camera captures 40 light slits at 45 degrees angle projected through the cornea

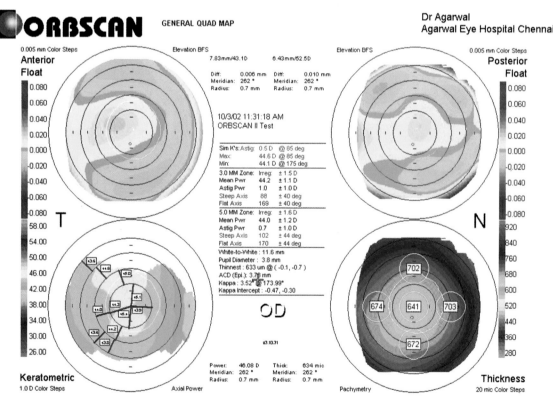

FIGURE 7.4: Orbscan printout of a normal patient (*Courtesy:* Dr Agarwal's Eye Hospital, India)

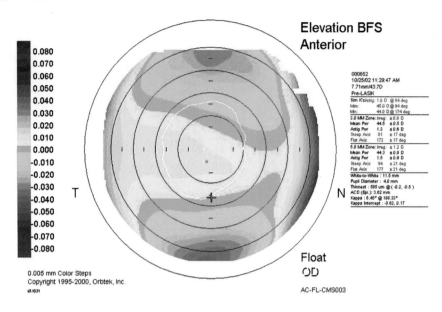

FIGURE 7.5: Topography of a normal cornea

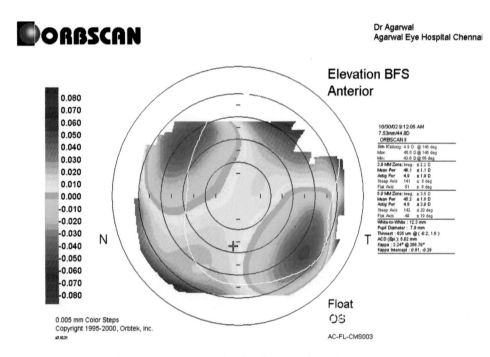

FIGURE 7.6: Topography showing an astigmatic cornea

similarly as seen during the slit lamp examination. The slits are projected on to the anterior segment of the eye: the anterior cornea, the posterior cornea, the anterior iris and anterior lens. The data collected from these four surfaces are used to create a topographic map.

NORMAL CORNEA

In a normal cornea (**Figure 7.5**), the nasal cornea is flatter than the temporal cornea. This is similar to the curvature of the long end of an ellipse. In **Figure 7.5**, the values written on the right end of the picture indicates the astigmatic values. In the figure, Max K is 45 at 84 degrees and Min K is 44 at 174 degrees. This means the astigmatism is + 1.0 D at 84 degrees. This is with the rule astigmatism as the astigmatism is Plus at 90 degrees axis. If the astigmatism was Plus at 180 degrees then it is against the rule astigmatism. The normal corneal topography can be round, oval, irregular, symmetric bow tie or asymmetric bow tie in appearance. **Figure 7.6** shows a case of astigmatism in which the astigmatism is + 4.9 D at 146 degrees. These figures show the curvature of the anterior

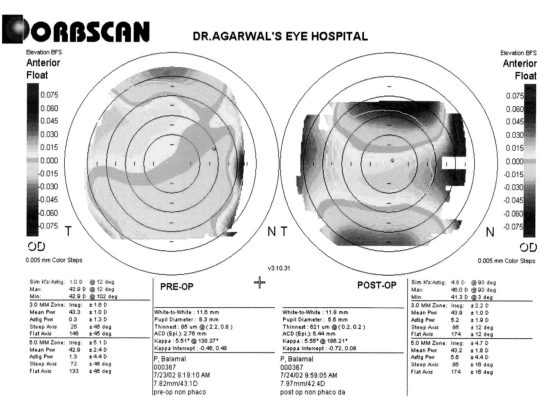

FIGURE 7.7: Topography after extracapsular cataract extraction (ECCE). The figure on the left shows astigmatism of + 1.1 D at 12 degrees preoperatively. The astigmatism has increased to + 4.8 Das seen in the figure on the right

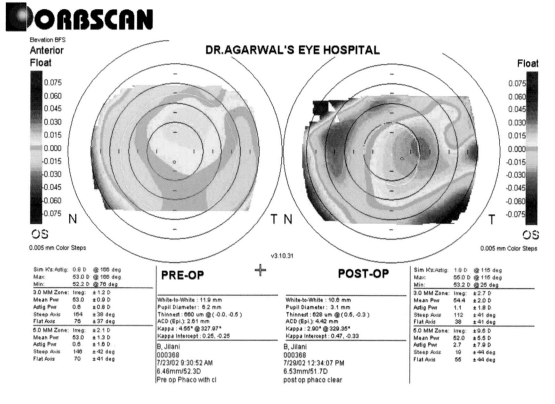

FIGURE 7.8: Topography of a non-foldable IOL implantation

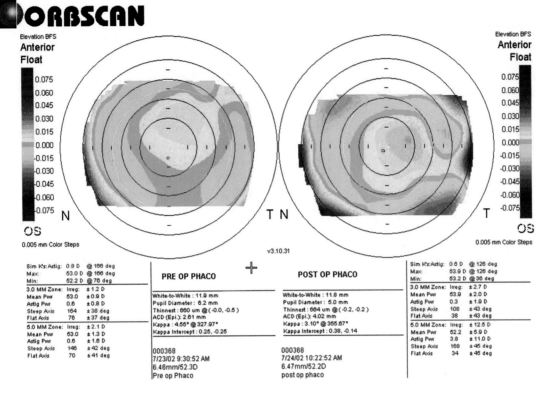

ORBSCAN

Elevation BFS
**Anterior
Float**

0.075
0.060
0.045
0.030
0.015
0.000
-0.015
-0.030
-0.045
-0.060
-0.075

N   T N

OS
0.005 mm Color Steps

Elevation BFS
**Anterior
Float**

0.075
0.060
0.045
0.030
0.015
0.000
-0.015
-0.030
-0.045
-0.060
-0.075

T

OS
0.005 mm Color Steps

v3.10.31

Sim K's: Astig:	0.8 D @ 166 deg
Max:	53.0 D @ 166 deg
Min:	52.2 D @ 76 deg

3.0 MM Zone:	Irreg:	± 1.2 D
Mean Pwr	53.0	± 0.9 D
Astig Pwr	0.6	± 0.8 D
Steep Axis	164	± 38 deg
Flat Axis	76	± 37 deg

5.0 MM Zone:	Irreg:	± 2.1 D
Mean Pwr	53.0	± 1.3 D
Astig Pwr	0.6	± 1.6 D
Steep Axis	146	± 42 deg
Flat Axis	70	± 41 deg

PRE OP PHACO

White-to-White : 11.9 mm
Pupil Diameter : 6.2 mm
Thinnest : 660 um @ (-0.0, -0.5)
ACD (Epi.): 2.61 mm
Kappa : 4.55° @ 327.97°
Kappa Intercept : 0.25, -0.25

000368
7/23/02 9:30:52 AM
6.46mm/52.3D
Pre op Phaco

POST OP PHACO

White-to-White : 11.8 mm
Pupil Diameter : 5.0 mm
Thinnest : 664 um @ (-0.2, -0.2)
ACD (Epi.): 4.02 mm
Kappa : 3.10° @ 355.67°
Kappa Intercept : 0.38, -0.14

000368
7/24/02 10:22:52 AM
6.47mm/52.2D
post op phaco

Sim K's: Astig:	0.6 D @ 126 deg
Max:	53.9 D @ 126 deg
Min:	53.2 D @ 36 deg

3.0 MM Zone:	Irreg:	± 2.7 D
Mean Pwr	53.9	± 2.0 D
Astig Pwr	0.3	± 1.9 D
Steep Axis	108	± 43 deg
Flat Axis	38	± 43 deg

5.0 MM Zone:	Irreg:	± 12.5 D
Mean Pwr	52.2	± 5.9 D
Astig Pwr	3.8	± 11.0 D
Steep Axis	169	± 45 deg
Flat Axis	34	± 45 deg

FIGURE 7.9: Topography of phaco cataract surgery with a foldable IOL implantation

surface of the cornea. It is important to remember that these are not the keratometric maps. Therefore, the blue/green color denotes steepening and the red color denotes flattening. If the red color is denoted for steepening then the colors can be inverted.

CATARACT SURGERY

Corneal topography is extremely important in cataract surgery. The smaller the size of the incision lesser the astigmatism and earlier stability of the astigmatism will occur. One can reduce the astigmatism or increase the astigmatism of a patient after cataract surgery. The simple rule to follow is that wherever you make an incision that area will flatten and wherever you apply sutures that area will steepen.

EXTRACAPSULAR CATARACT EXTRACTION

One of the problems in extracapsular cataract extraction (ECCE) is the astigmatism, which is created as the incision size is about 10–12 mm. In **Figure 7.7**, you can see the topographic picture of a patient after ECCE. You can see the picture on the left is the preoperative photo and the picture on the right is a postoperative day one photo. Preoperatively one will notice the astigmatism is + 1.0 D at 12 degrees and postoperatively it is + 4.8 D at 93 degrees. This is the problem in ECCE. In the immediate post-operative period, the astigmatism is high that would reduce with time. However, the predictability of astigmatism is not there which is why smaller incision cataract surgery is more successful.

NON-FOLDABLE IOL

Some surgeons perform phaco and implant a non-foldable IOL in which the incision is increased to 5.5 to 6 mm. In such cases, the astigmatism is better than in an ECCE. In **Figure 7.8**, the pictures are of a patient who has had a non-foldable IOL. Notice in this, the preoperative astigmatism is + 0.8 D at 166 degrees. This is the left eye of the patient. If phaco is done with a foldable IOL, the astigmatism would have been nearly the same or reduced as the incision would have come in the area of astigmatism. However, in this case after a phaco, a non-foldable IOL was implanted. The postoperative astigmatism one week postoperative is + 1.8 D at 115 degrees. The two pictures clearly show that the astigmatism has increased.

FOLDABLE IOL

In phaco with a foldable IOL the amount of astigmatism created is much less than in a non-foldable IOL. In **Figure 7.9**, the patient has negligible astigmatism in the left eye and the picture on the left shows a preoperative astigmatism of + 0.8 D at 166 degrees axis. A temporal clear corneal approach is used generally, and so the incision is made at the area of the steepend axis in the left eye. This will reduce the astigmatism. The postoperative photo of day one shows the astigmatism is only + 0.6 D at 126 degrees. This means that after a day, the astigmatism has not changed much and this shows a good result. This patient had a foldable IOL implanted under the no anesthesia cataract surgical technique after a phaco cataract surgery with the size of the incision being 2.8 mm.

ASTIGMATISM INCREASED

If one is not careful enough in selecting the incision depending upon the corneal topography, hands can be burnt. **Figure 7.10** illustrates a case in which astigmatism has increased due to the incision being made in the wrong meridian. The patient had a 2.8 mm incision with a foldable IOL implanted after a phaco cataract surgery under the no anesthesia cataract surgical technique. Both the pictures are of the right eye. In **Figure 7.10**, look at the picture on the left. In the picture on the left, you can see the patient has an astigmatism of + 1.1 D at axis 107 degrees. As this is the right eye with this astigmatism, a superior incision to reduce the preoperative astigmatism can be made. However, if by mistake a temporal clear corneal incision is made, it can lead to increased astigmatism. In order to flatten this case, the incision should have been made at the 105 degrees axis where the steeper meridian was. However, the incision is made in the opposite axis because earlier temporal clear corneal incisions were done routinely. Now look at the picture on the right. The astigmatism has increased from + 1.1 D to + 1.7 D. This shows a bad result. If the incision was made superiorly at 107 degrees axis, it would have flattened that axis and the astigmatism would have been reduced.

BASIC RULE

The basic rule, which the ophthalmologists must follow is to look at the number written in red. The red numbers indicate the plus axis. If the difference in astigmatism is say 3 D at 180 degrees, it means the patient has + 3 D astigmatism at axis 180 degrees. This is against the rule astigmatism. In such cases, make your clear corneal incision at 180 degrees so that you can flatten this steepness. This will reduce the astigmatism.

UNIQUE CASE

In **Figure 7.11**, the patient had a temporal clear corneal incision for phaco cataract surgery under no anesthesia with a non-foldable IOL. Both the pictures are of the left eye. The figure on the left shows the postoperative topographic picture. The postoperative astigmatism was + 1.8 D at axis 115 degrees. This patient had three sutures in the site of the incision. These sutures were put as a non-foldable IOL and had been implanted in the eye with a clear corneal incision. The sutures were removed in the follow-up session and the patient faced loss of vision on the next day. On examination, it was found that the astigmatism had increased and another topography was done. The picture on the right is of the topography after removing the sutures. The astigmatism increased to + 5.7 D. So, one should be very careful in analyzing the corneal topography when one does suture removal also. To solve this problem one can do an astigmatic keratotomy.

PHAKONIT

Phakonit is a technique devised by Dr Amar Agarwal in which the cataract is removed through a 0.9 mm incision. The advantage of this is obvious. The astigmatism created

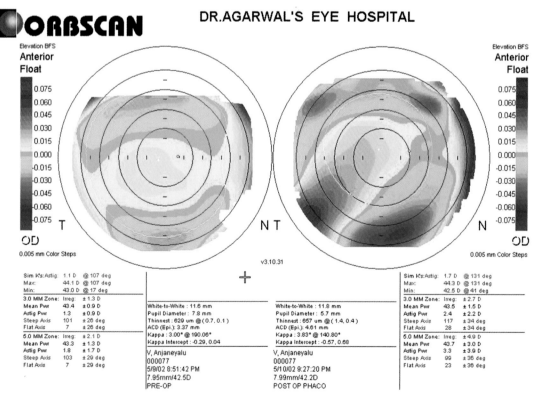

FIGURE 7.10: Increase in astigmatism after cataract surgery due to incision being made in the wrong meridian. Topography of a phaco with foldable IOL implantation

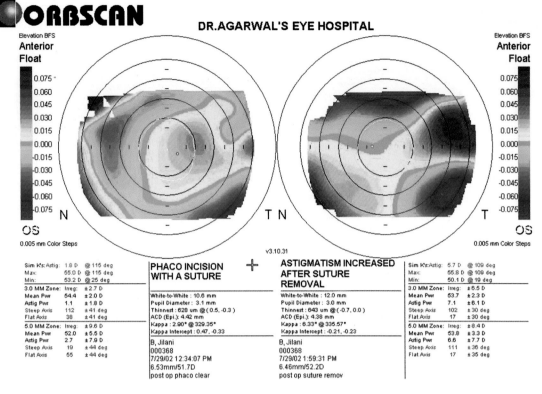

FIGURE 7.11: Unique case—topographic changes after suture removal

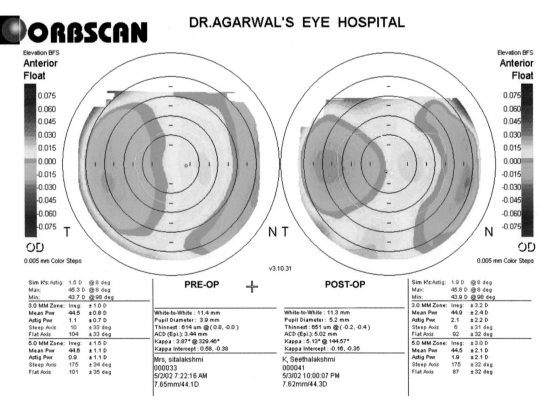

FIGURE 7.12: Topography of a phakonit with a rollable IOL

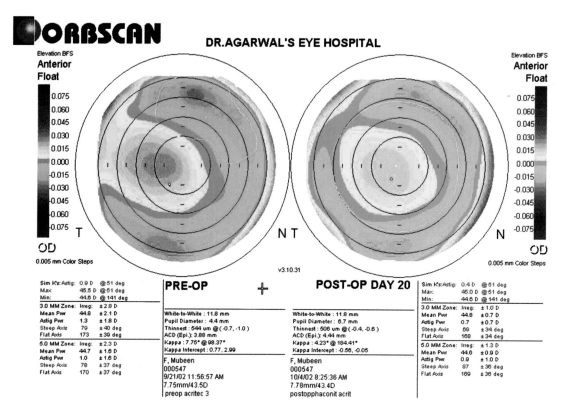

ORBSCAN

DR.AGARWAL'S EYE HOSPITAL

Elevation BFS
Anterior
Float

0.075
0.060
0.045
0.030
0.015
0.000
-0.015
-0.030
-0.045
-0.060
-0.075

T

OD
0.005 mm Color Steps

Elevation BFS
Anterior
Float

0.075
0.060
0.045
0.030
0.015
0.000
-0.015
-0.030
-0.045
-0.060
-0.075

N

OD
0.005 mm Color Steps

v3.10.31

NT

PRE-OP + **POST-OP DAY 20**

Sim K's:Astig:	0.9 D	@51 deg
Max:	45.5 D	@51 deg
Min:	44.6 D	@141 deg

3.0 MM Zone:	Irreg:	±2.8 D
Mean Pwr	44.8	±2.1 D
Astig Pwr	1.3	±1.8 D
Steep Axis	79	±40 deg
Flat Axis	173	±39 deg

5.0 MM Zone:	Irreg:	±2.3 D
Mean Pwr	44.7	±1.6 D
Astig Pwr	1.0	±1.6 D
Steep Axis	78	±37 deg
Flat Axis	170	±37 deg

White-to-White : 11.8 mm
Pupil Diameter : 4.4 mm
Thinnest : 544 um @ (-0.7, -1.0)
ACD (Epi.): 3.88 mm
Kappa : 7.75° @98.37°
Kappa Intercept : 0.77, 2.99

F, Mubeen
000547
9/21/02 11:56:57 AM
7.75mm/43.5D
preop acritec 3

White-to-White : 11.8 mm
Pupil Diameter : 6.7 mm
Thinnest : 506 um @ (-0.4, -0.6)
ACD (Epi.): 4.44 mm
Kappa : 4.23° @ 184.41°
Kappa Intercept : -0.56, -0.05

F, Mubeen
000547
10/4/02 8:25:36 AM
7.78mm/43.4D
postopphaconit acrit

Sim K's:Astig:	0.4 D	@51 deg
Max:	45.0 D	@51 deg
Min:	44.6 D	@141 deg

3.0 MM Zone:	Irreg:	±1.0 D
Mean Pwr	44.8	±0.7 D
Astig Pwr	0.7	±0.7 D
Steep Axis	89	±34 deg
Flat Axis	168	±34 deg

5.0 MM Zone:	Irreg:	±1.3 D
Mean Pwr	44.6	±0.9 D
Astig Pwr	0.9	±1.0 D
Steep Axis	87	±36 deg
Flat Axis	169	±36 deg

FIGURE 7.13: Topography of a phakonit with an acritec IOL

by a 0.9-mm incision is very little compared to a 2.6 mm phaco incision. Today with the rollable IOL and the Acritec IOLs, which are ultra-small incision IOLs one can pass IOLs through sub 1.4 mm incisions. This is seen clearly in **Figures 7.12 and 7.13**. **Figure 7.12** shows the comparison after Phakonit with a Rollable IOL and **Figure 7.13** with an Acritec IOL. If you will see the preoperative and the postoperative photographs in comparison, you will see there is not much difference between the two. In this case, a rollable IOL was implanted. The point to be noticed in this picture is that the difference between the preoperative photo and the one-day postoperative photo is not much.

SUMMARY

Corneal topography is an extremely important tool for the ophthalmologist. It is not only the refractive surgeon

who should utilize this instrument but also the cataract surgeon. The most important refractive surgery done in the world is cataract surgery and not laser in-situ keratomileusis (Lasik) or photorefractive keratectomy (PRK). With more advancements in corneal topography, topographic-assisted lasik will become available to everyone with an excimer laser. One might also have the corneal topographic machine fixed onto the operating microscope so that one can easily reduce the astigmatism of the patient.

REFERENCES

1. Gills JP. Corneal topography: the state-of-the-art. New Delhi: Jaypee Brothers Medical Publishers; 1996.
2. Agarwal S, Agarwal A, Sachdev MS, et al. Phacoemulsification, Laser Cataract Surgery & Foldable IOL's (2nd edn). New Delhi: Jaypee Brothers Medical Publishers; 2000.

Instrumentation, Medication and Machines

CHAPTER 8

The Phaco Machine: How It Acts and Reacts

William J Fishkind

INTRODUCTION

All phaco machines consist of a computer to generate ultrasonic impulses, and a transducer, piezoelectric crystals, to turn these electronic signals into mechanical energy. The energy thus created is then harnessed within the eye to overcome the inertia of the lens and emulsify it. Once turned into emulsate, the fluidic systems remove the emulsate replacing it with balanced salt solution. The recent trend in phaco surgery is to minimize power utilizing new power modalities, and maximize the use of fluidics to remove the cataractous lens.

POWER GENERATION

Power is created by the interaction of frequency and stroke length. Frequency is defined as the speed of the needle movement. It is determined by the manufacturer of the machine. Presently, most machines operate at a frequency of between 35,000 cycles per second (Hz) to 45,000 cycles per second. This frequency range is the most efficient for nuclear emulsification. Lower frequencies are less efficient and higher frequencies create excess heat.

Frequency is maintained constantly by tuning circuitry designed into the machine computer. Tuning is vital because the phaco tip is required to operate in varied media. For example, the resistance of the aqueous is less than the resistance of the cortex, which in turn, is less than the resistance of the nucleus. As the resistance to the phaco tip varies to maintain maximum efficiency, small alterations in frequency are created by the tuning circuitry in the computer. The surgeon will subjectively appreciate good tuning circuitry by a sense of smoothness and power.

Stroke length is defined as the length of the needle movement. This length is generally 2 to 6 mils (thousandth of an inch). Most machines operate in the 2 to 4 mil range. Longer stroke lengths are prone to generate excess heat. The longer the stroke length, the greater the physical impact on the nucleus. In addition, the greater the generation of cavitation forces. Stroke length is determined by foot pedal excursion in position three during linear control of phaco.

ENERGY AT THE PHACO TIP

The actual tangible forces, which emulsify the nucleus, are thought to be a blend of the "jackhammer" effect and cavitation. The "jackhammer" effect is merely the physical striking of the needle against the nucleus. The cavitation effect is more convoluted. Recent studies indicate that there are two kinds of cavitational energy. One is transient cavitation and the other is sustained cavitation.

TRANSIENT CAVITATION

The phaco needle, moving through the liquid medium of the aqueous at ultrasonic speeds, creates intense zones of high and low pressure. Low pressure created with backward movement of the tip, literally pulls dissolved gases out of solution thus giving rise to microbubbles. Forward tip movement then creates an equally intense zone of high pressure. This produces compression of the microbubbles until they implode. At the moment of implosion, the bubbles create a temperature of 13,000 degrees and a shock wave of 75,000 PSI. Of the microbubbles created 75% implode, amassing to create a powerful shock wave, radiating from the phaco tip in the direction of the bevel with annular spread. However, 25% of the bubbles are too large to implode. These microbubbles are swept up in the shock-wave and radiate with it. Transient cavitation is a violent event. The energy created by transient cavitation exists for no more than 6 to 25 milliseconds. It is this form of cavitation that is thought to generate the energy responsible for the emulsification of cataractous material (**Figure 8.1**).

The cavitation energy thus created can be directed in any desired direction as the angle of the bevel of the phaco needle governs the direction of the generation of the shockwave and microbubbles.

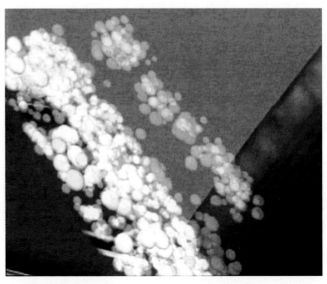

FIGURE 8.1: Microbubbles generated at the phaco tip

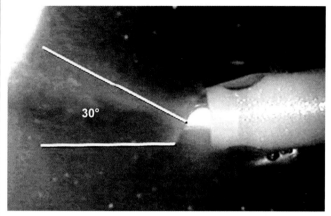

FIGURE 8.2: 30° tip. Enhanced cavitation shows ultrasonic wave focused 1 mm from the tip, spreading at an angle of 30°

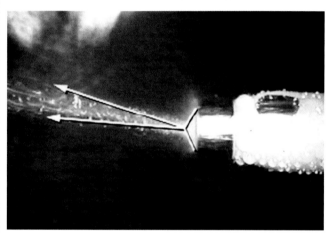

FIGURE 8.3: 0° tip. Enhanced cavitation shows ultrasonic wave focused ½mm in front of the tip spreading directly in front of it

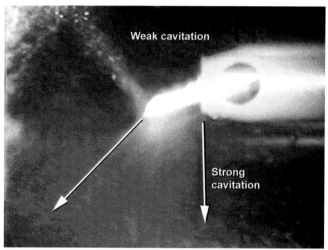

FIGURE 8.4: Kelman tip. Enhanced cavitation shows a broadband of enhanced cavitation spreading inferiorly from the angle of the tip. A weak band of cavitation spreads from the tip

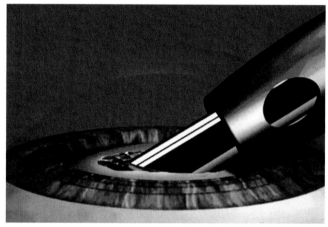

FIGURE 8.5: 30° tip bevel down.Turning the bevel of the phaco tip toward the nucleus focuses cavitation and jackhammer energy into the nucleus

The author has developed a method of visualization of these forces, called "enhanced cavitation." Using this process, it can be seen that with a 45° tip, the cavitation wave is generated at 45° from the tip and comes to a focus 1 mm from it. Similarly, a 30° tip generates cavitation at a 30° angle from the bevel, and a 15° tip — 15° from the bevel (**Figure 8.2**). A 0° tip creates the cavitation wave directly in front of the tip and the focal point is 0.5 mm from the tip (**Figure 8.3**). The Kelman tip has a broad band of powerful cavitation, which radiates from the area of the angle in the shaft. A weak area of cavitation is developed from the bevel but is inconsequential (**Figure 8.4**).

The analysis of enhanced cavitation is taken into consideration because it can be concluded that phacoemulsification is most efficient when both the jackhammer effect and cavitation energy are combined. To accomplish this, the bevel of the needle should be turned toward the nucleus or nuclear fragment. This simple maneuver will cause the broad bevel of the needle to strike the nucleus. This will enhance the physical force of the needle striking the nucleus. In addition, the cavitation force is then concentrated into the nucleus rather than away from it. Finally, in this configuration, the vacuum force can be maximally exploited as occlusion is encouraged (**Figure 8.5**). It causes this energy to emulsify the nucleus and be absorbed by it.

A zero degree tip automatically focuses both the jackhammer and cavitational energy directly in front of it (**Figure 8.6**). When the bevel is turned away from the nucleus, the cavitational energy is directed up and away from the nucleus toward the iris and endothelium (**Figure 8.7**).

SUSTAINED CAVITATION

If phaco energy is continued beyond 25 milliseconds, transient cavitation with generation of microbubbles and shock waves ends. The bubbles then begin to vibrate, without implosion. No shock wave is generated. Therefore, there is no emulsification energy produced. Sustained cavitation is ineffective for emulsification of the cataractous lens (**Figure 8.8**).

Water bath, hydrophonic studies indicate that transient cavitation is significantly more powerful than sustained cavitation. With this information in mind, it would appear that continuous phaco is best used to emulsify the intact nucleus, held in place by the capsular bag, as one does

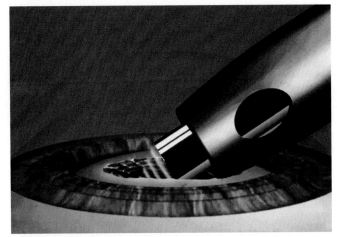

FIGURE 8.6: The 0° tip, by its design, focuses both jackhammer and cavitation forces directly ahead, and into the nucleus

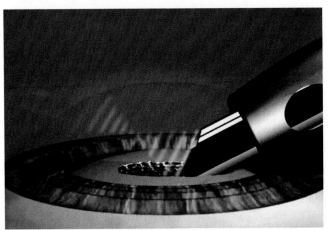

FIGURE 8.7: 30° Tip bevel up. The bevel is turned away from the nucleus. Cavitation energy is wasted and may damage iris and endothelium

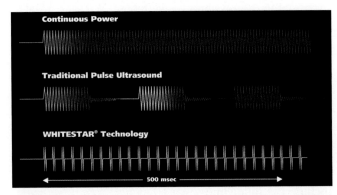

FIGURE 8.8: Transient cavitation energy is shown in red and stabilized cavitational energy is shown in blue. Continuous power: Only the initial energy is transient. The remainder is stabilized energy. In a 50-millisecond pulse, only the initial 25 milliseconds is transient. In micropulse phaco, the entire pulse is transient energy (*Photo Source:* Mark E Schafer, PhD, AMO)

during the sculpting phase of divide and conquer or stop and chop. Transient cavitation is maximized during micropulse phaco. This is best used during phaco of the nuclear fragments in the later phase of the above two procedures, or during phaco chop procedures.

MODIFICATION OF PHACO POWER INTENSITY

Application of the minimal amount of phaco power intensity necessary for emulsification of the nucleus is desirable. Unnecessary power intensity is a cause of heat with subsequent wound damage, endothelial cell damage, and iris damage with alteration of the blood-aqueous barrier. Phaco power intensity can be modified by: (1) Alteration in stroke length, (2) Alteration of duration, and (3) Alteration of emission.

Alteration of Stroke Length

Stroke length is determined by foot pedal adjustment. When set for linear phaco, depression of the foot pedal will increase stroke length and therefore power. New foot pedals, such as those found in the Allergan Sovereign and the Alcon INFINITI, permit surgeon adjustment of the throw length of the pedal in position three. This can refine power application. The Bausch & Lomb Millennium dual linear foot pedal permits the separation of the fluidic aspects of the foot pedal from the power elements.

Alteration of Duration

The duration of application of phaco power has a dramatic effect on overall power delivered. Usage of pulse or burst mode phaco will considerably decrease overall power delivery. New machines allow for a power pulse of duration alternating with a period of aspiration only. Burst mode (parameter is machine dependant) is characterized by 80 or 120 millisecond periods of power combined with fixed short periods of aspiration only. Pulse mode utilizes fixed pulses of power of 50 or 150 milliseconds with variable short periods of aspiration only.

Micropulse

Recently, through the development of highly responsive and low mass piezo crystals, combined with software modifications, the manufacturers of phaco machines have shortened the cycle of on and off time. This process, patented by Advanced Medical Optics now known as Abbott Medical Optics (AMO) is called "micropulse." This technology is now available in most phaco machines.

A duty cycle is defined as the length of time of power on combined with power off. The short bursts of phaco energy followed by a short period without phaco energy allow two events to occur. First, the period without phaco energy permits the nuclear material to be drawn towards the phaco tip with increased efficiency. Second, the absence of power allows for cooling of the phaco tip. This cool phaco tip has been termed "cold phaco." This is a misnomer as the phaco tip is not cold, but warm. However, studies indicate that it will not develop a temperature greater than 55° celsius, the temperature required to create a wound burn.

Phaco techniques, such as phaco chop, utilize minimal periods of power in pulse mode or micropulse mode to reduce power delivery to the anterior chamber. In addition, the use of pulse mode or micropulse mode to remove the epinucleus provides for an added margin of safety. When the epinucleus is emulsified, the posterior capsule is exposed to the phaco tip and may move forward towards it due to surge. Activation of pulse phaco or micropulse phaco will create a deeper anterior chamber to work within. This occurs because, as noted previously, each period of phaco energy is followed by an interval of no energy. During the interval of absence of energy, the epinucleus is drawn towards the phaco tip, producing occlusion and interrupting outflow. This allows inflow to deepen the anterior chamber immediately prior to the onset of another pulse of phaco energy. The surgeon will recognize the outcome as operating in a deeper, more stable anterior chamber.

Alteration of Emission

The emission of phaco energy is modified by tip selection. Phaco tips can be modified to accentuate (1) power, (2) flow or (3) a combination of both.

1. Power intensity is modified by altering bevel tip angle. Noted previously, the bevel of the phaco tip will focus power in the direction of the bevel. The Kelman tip will produce broad powerful cavitation directed away from the angle in the shaft. This tip is excellent for the hardest of nuclei. New flare and cobra tips direct cavitation into the opening of the bevel of the tip. Thus, random emission of phaco energy is minimized. Designer tips such as the "flathead" designed by Dr Barry Seibel and power wedges designed by Douglas Mastel modify the direction and focus delivery of phaco energy intensity.

2. Power intensity and flow are modified by utilizing a 0° tip. This tip will focus power directly ahead of the tip and enhance occlusion due to the smaller surface area of its orifice. Small diameter tips, such as 21 ga tips, change fluid flow rates. Although they do not actually change power intensity, they appear to have this effect, as the nucleus must be emulsified into smaller pieces for removal through the smaller diameter tip.

   The Alcon Aspiration Bypass System (ABS) tip modification is available with a 0° tip, a Kelman tip or a flare tip. The flare is a modification of power intensity and the ABS a flow modification. In the ABS system, a 0.175 mm hole in the shaft permits a variable flow of fluid into the needle, even during occlusion. Therefore, occlusion is never allowed to occur (**Figure 8.9**). This flow adjustment serves to minimize surge.

3. Finally flow can be modified by utilizing one of the microseal tips. These tips have a flexible outer sleeve to seal the phaco incision. They also have a rigid inner sleeve or a ribbed shaft configuration to protect cooling irrigant inflow. Thus a tight seal allows low-flow phaco without the danger of wound burns. Phaco power intensity is the energy that emulsifies the lens nucleus. The phaco tip must operate in a cool environment and with adequate space to isolate its actions from delicate intraocular structures. This portion of the action of the machine is dependent upon its fluidics.

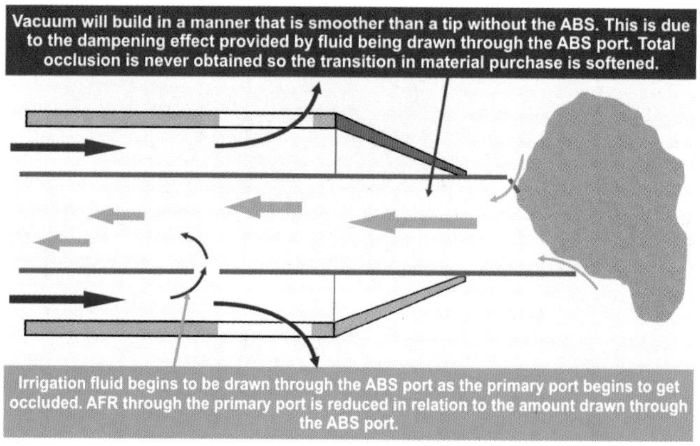

FIGURE 8.9: A 0.175 mm hole drilled in the shaft of the ABS tip provides an alternate path for fluid to flow into the needle when there is an occlusion at the phaco tip (*Photo Source:* Alcon)

FLUIDICS

The fluidics of all machines are fundamentally a balance of fluid inflow and fluid outflow. Inflow is determined by bottle height above the eye of the patient and irrigating tubing diameter. It is important to recognize that with recent acceptance of temporal surgical approaches and modifications of the surgical table, the eye of the patient may be physically higher than in the past. This then requires that the irrigation bottle be adequately elevated. A shallow, unstable anterior chamber will otherwise result.

Outflow is determined by the sleeve-incision relationship, as well as the paracentesis size, aspiration rate and vacuum level commanded. The incision length selected should create a snug fit with the phaco tip selected. This will result in minimal uncontrolled wound outflow with resultant increased anterior chamber stability.

Aspiration rate or flow is defined as the flow of fluid, measured in cc/min, through the tubing. With a peristaltic pump, it is determined by the speed of the pump. Flow determines how well particulate matter is attracted to the phaco tip. Aspiration level or vacuum is a level and measured in mm Hg. It is defined as the magnitude of negative pressure created in the tubing. Vacuum is the determinant of how well, once occluded on the phaco tip, particulate material will be held to the tip.

VACUUM SOURCES

The three categories of vacuum sources or pumps include the following:

1. *Flow pumps:* The primary example of the flow pump type is the peristaltic pump. These pumps allow for independent control of both aspiration rate (flow) and aspiration level (vacuum).

2. *Vacuum pumps:* The primary example of the vacuum pump is the venturi pump. This pump type allows direct control of only vacuum level. Flow is dependent upon vacuum level setting. Additional examples are the rotary vane and diaphragmatic pumps.

3. *Hybrid pumps:* The primary example of the hybrid pump is the AMO Sovereign peristaltic pump or the Bausch

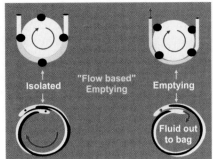
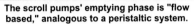
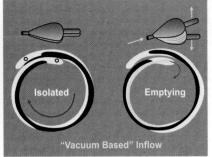

The scroll pumps' emptying phase is "flow based," analogous to a peristaltic system.

During the inflow phase, the male scroll opens like a bellows, creating vacuum response similar to a venturi system.

FIGURE 8.10: Concentrix pump showing flow-based mechanics
(*Photo Source:* Bausch & Lomb)

& Lomb Concentrix pump (**Figure 8.10**). These pumps are interesting as they are able to act like either a vacuum or flow pump dependent upon programming. They are the most recent supplement to pump types. They are generally controlled by digital inputs creating incredible flexibility and responsiveness. They are rapidly becoming the standard type of pump for modern phaco.

The challenge to the surgeon is to balance the effect of phaco intensity, which tends to push nuclear fragments off the phaco tip; with the effect of flow, which attracts fragments toward the phaco tip; and vacuum, which holds the fragments on the phaco tip. Generally, low flow slows down intraocular events and high vacuum speeds them up. Low or zero vacuum is helpful during the sculpting of hard or large nucleus, where the high power intensity of the tip may be applied near the iris or anterior capsule. Zero vacuum will prevent inadvertent aspiration of the iris or capsule preventing significant morbidity.

SURGE

A principal limiting factor in the selection of high levels of vacuum or flow is the development of surge. When the phaco tip is occluded, flow is interrupted and vacuum builds to its preset level (**Figure 8.11**). Emulsification of the occluding fragment then clears the occlusion. Flow immediately begins at the preset level in the presence of the high vacuum level. In addition, if the aspiration line tubing is not reinforced to prevent collapse (tubing compliance), the tubing will be constricted during the occlusion. It then expands on occlusion break. The expansion is an additional source of vacuum production. These factors cause a rush of fluid from the anterior segment into the phaco tip. The fluid in the anterior chamber may not be replaced rapidly enough by infusion to prevent shallowing of the anterior chamber. Therefore, there is subsequent rapid anterior movement of the posterior capsule. This abrupt forceful stretching of the bag around nuclear fragments may be a cause of capsular tears. In addition, the posterior capsule can be literally sucked into

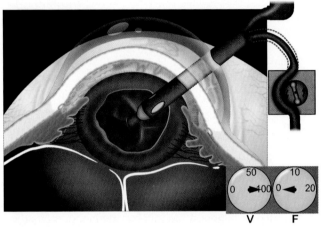

FIGURE 8.11: Occlusion: Vacuum builds, flow falls toward zero, tubing collapses (*Photo Source:* Thieme Medical Publishers, NY)

the phaco tip, tearing it. The magnitude of the surge is contingent on the presurge settings of flow and vacuum (**Figure 8.12**).

Surge is therefore modified by selecting lower levels of flow and vacuum. The phaco machine manufacturers help to decrease surge by providing non-compliant aspiration tubing. This will not constrict in the presence of high levels of vacuum. More important are new technologies, which are noteworthy:

1. *AMO Sovereign:* Microprocessors sample vacuum and flow parameters 50 times a second creating a "virtual" anterior chamber model. At the moment of surge, the machine computer senses the increase in flow and instantaneously slows or reverses the pump to stop surge production. The Alcon INFINITI works in a similar manner.

2. *Bausch & Lomb Millennium:* The dual linear foot pedal can be programmed to separate both the flow and vacuum, from power. In this way, flow or vacuum can be lowered before beginning the emulsification of an occluding fragment. The emulsification therefore occurs in the presence of a lower vacuum or flow so that surge is minimized.

THE PHACO MACHINE: HOW IT ACTS AND REACTS

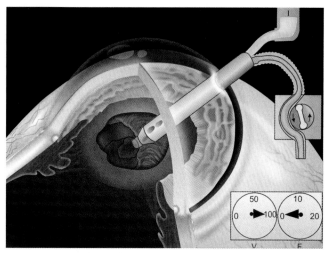

FIGURE 8.12: Occlusion break: Vacuum drops to zero. Flow rapidly increases to preset. Tubing expands. Outflow exceeds inflow. Anterior chamber begins to shallow (*Photo Source:* Thieme Medical Publishers, NY)

3. *Alcon INFINITI/Legacy:* The Aspiration Bypass System (ABS) Tips have mm holes drilled in the shaft of the needle. During occlusion, the hole provides for a continuous alternate fluid flow. This will cause dampening of the surge on occlusion break.

Preocclusion Phaco

Another way to avoid surge is to prevent occlusion entirely. By definition, a surge requires occlusion. In preocclusion phaco utilizing micropulse, the nuclear fragment is emulsified before it can occlude the phaco tip. Therefore, vacuum never builds to maximum and surge is avoided. This appears to be an extremely efficient method of emulsification. It allows for fragment removal with minimal energy level and duration, in a deep and controlled anterior chamber.

NeoSoniX technology (Alcon) also creates preocclusion phaco. The oscillatory movement of the phaco tip mechanically knocks the fragments off the phaco tip. This will prevent occlusion.

PHACO TECHNIQUE AND MACHINE TECHNOLOGY

The patient will have the best visual result when total phaco energy delivered to the anterior segment is minimized. Additionally, phaco energy should be focused into the nucleus. This will prevent damage to iris blood vessels and endothelium. Finally, proficient emulsification will lead to shorter overall surgical time. Therefore, a lesser amount of irrigation fluid will pass through the anterior segment. The general principles of power management are to focus phaco energy into the nucleus, vary fluid parameters for efficient sculpting and fragment removal, and minimize surge.

Divide and Conquer Phaco

Sculpting: To focus cavitation energy into the nucleus a zero degree tip or a 15°, or 30° tip turned bevel down should be utilized. Zero or low vacuum (dependent upon the manufacturer's recommendation) is mandatory for bevel down phaco. This will prevent occlusion. Occlusion, at best, will cause excessive movement of the nucleus during sculpting. At worst, occlusion occurring near the equator is the cause of tears in the equatorial bag early in the phaco procedure, and occlusion at the bottom of a grove will cause phaco through the posterior capsule. Once the grove is judged to be adequately deep, the bevel of the tip should be rotated to the bevel up position to improve visibility and prevent the possibility of phaco through the posterior nucleus and posterior capsule. If micropulse phaco is used, duty cycles with longer power on than off should be selected. This will allow phaco to proceed with clean emulsification and avoid pushing the nucleus away from the phaco tip potentially damaging zonules.

Quadrant and fragment removal: The tip selected, as noted above, is retained. Vacuum and flow are increased to reasonable limits subject to the machine being used. The limiting factor to these levels is the development of surge. The bevel of the tip is turned towards the quadrant or fragment. Low pulsed or burst power is applied at a level high enough to emulsify the fragment without driving it from the phaco tip. *Chatter* is defined as a fragment bouncing from the phaco tip due to aggressive application of phaco energy.

Epinucleus and cortex removal: For removal of epinucleus and cortex the vacuum is decreases while flow is maintained. This will allow for grasping of the epinucleus just deep to the anterior capsule. The low vacuum will help the tip hold the epinucleus on the phaco tip, without breaking off chunks due to high vacuum, so that it scrolls around the equator and can be pulled to the level of the iris. There, low power pulsed phaco is employed for emulsification. If cortical cleaving hydrodissection has been performed, the cortex will be removed concurrently.

Stop and Chop Phaco

Groove creation is performed as noted above under divide and conquer sculpting techniques. Once the groove is adequate, vacuum and flow are increased to improve holding ability of the phaco tip. The tip is then burrowed into the mass of one hemi nucleus using pulsed linear phaco. The sleeve should be 1 mm from the base of the bevel of the phaco tip to create adequate exposed needle length for sufficient holding power. Excessive phaco energy application is to be avoided, as this will cause nucleus immediately adjacent to the tip to be emulsified. The space thus created in the vicinity of the tip is responsible for interfering with the seal around the tip and therefore the capability of vacuum to hold the nucleus. The nucleus will then pop off the phaco tip making chopping more difficult. With a good seal, the hemi nucleus can be drawn toward the incision and the chopper can be inserted at the endo nucleus-epinucleus junction. After the first chop a second similar chop is performed. The pie-shaped piece of nucleus thus created is removed with low power pulsed phaco as discussed in the divide and conquer section. Epinucleus and cortex removal is also performed as noted above.

Phaco Chop

Phaco chop requires no sculpting. Therefore, the procedure is initiated with high vacuum and flow and linear pulsed phaco power. For a 0° tip, when emulsifying a hard nucleus, a small trough may be required to create adequate room for the phaco tip to borrow deep into the nucleus. For a 15° or a 30° tip, the tip should be rotated bevel down to engage the nucleus. The phaco tip should be buried into the endonucleus with the minimal amount of power necessary. If the phaco tip is inserted into the nucleus with excess power, the adjacent nucleus will be emulsified creating a poor seal between nucleus and tip. This will make it impossible to remove fragments as the tip will just "let go" of the nuclear material (**Figures 8.13A and B**). Additionally, the bevel should be turned toward the fragment to create a seal between tip and fragment, allowing vacuum to build and create holding power (**Figures 8.14A and B**)

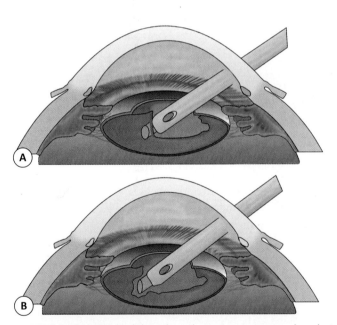

FIGURES 8.13A AND B: (A) Power adequate to enter nucleus but maintain seal between the tip and nucleus. This will allow the tip to maneuver the nucleus. (B) Excessive power causes the nucleus around the tip to be emulsified. There is no seal around the phaco tip. The nucleus cannot be maneuvered by the tip (*Photo Source:* Thieme Medical Publishers, NY)

Horizontal Chop (*Figure 8.15*)

A few bursts or pulses of phaco energy will allow the tip to be buried within the nucleus. It then can be drawn toward the incision to allow the chopper access to the epi-endonuclear junction. If the nucleus comes off the phaco tip,

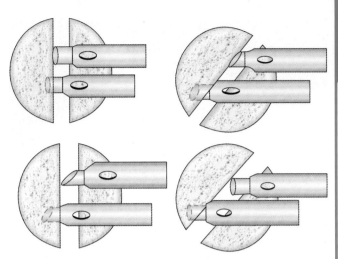

FIGURES 8.14A AND B: (A) Correct position of nucleus in relation to the phaco tip. Occlusion is effortless. (B) Incorrect orientation. Occlusion is difficult (*Photo Source:* Thieme Medical Publishers, NY)

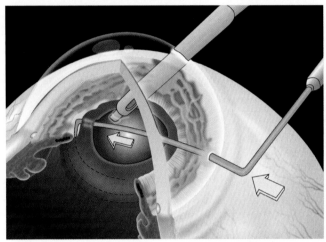

FIGURE 8.15: Horizontal chop. The phaco tip is drawn toward the wound and the chopper is placed into the epinucleus-endonucleus junctions, under the anterior capsule (*Photo Source:* Thieme Medical Publishers, NY)

excessive power has produced a space around the tip impeding vacuum holding power as noted above. The first chop is then produced. Minimal rotation of the nucleus will allow for the creation of the second chop. The first pie-shaped segment of nucleus is mobilized with high vacuum and elevated to the iris plane. There it is emulsified with low linear power, high vacuum and moderate flow. The process of chopping and segment removal is continued until the endonucleus is removed.

Vertical Chop (*Figure 8.16*)

Once the phaco tip is embedded within the nucleus, a sharp chopper (Nichamin made by Katena) is pushed down into the mass of the nucleus at the same time the phaco tip is elevated. The chopper is then advanced down and left and the phaco tip is up and right. This creates a cleavage in the nucleus. The process is repeated until the entire nucleus is chopped. The segments thus created are then elevated to the plane of the pupil and emulsified.

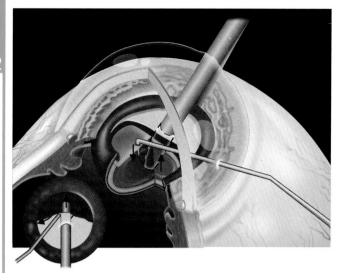

FIGURE 8.16: Vertical chop. The sharp chopper is placed adjacent to the phaco tip and plunged into the substance of the endonucleus (*Photo Source:* Thieme Medical Publishers, NY)

Bimanual Micro Incisional Phaco

The development of micropulse, "cold phaco," has led to the performance of phaco with an unsleeved tip. This allows for two 20 gauge 1.4 mm incisions or 21 gauge 1.2 mm incisions. The instrumentation for this procedure is important and the relationship between the instrument and incision size is essential. If there is too tight a wound, it is difficult to manipulate the instruments. If the wound is too large excessive outflow permits chamber shallowing. Microincision phaco is reportedly more efficient than standard as the flow from irrigating chopper in the direction of the phaco tip captures fragments and carries them toward the phaco tip. The small incisions cause less disruption of the blood aqueous barrier, and are more stable and secure. With insertion of an IOL through the 1.4 mm incision, there is less disruption of ocular integrity with immediate return to full activities and less risk of postoperative wound complications.

Irrigation and Aspiration (I&A)

Similar to phaco anterior chamber stability during I&A is due to a balance of inflow and outflow. Wound outflow can be minimized by employing a soft sleeve around the I&A tip. Combined with a small incision (2.8 to 3 mm) a deep and stable anterior chamber will result. Generally, a 0.3 mm I&A tip is used. With this orifice, a vacuum of 500 mm Hg and flow of 20 cc/min is excellent to tease cortex from the fornices. Linear vacuum allows the cortex to be grasped under the anterior capsule and drawn into the center of the pupil at the iris plane. There, in the safety of a deep anterior chamber, vacuum can be increased and the cortex aspirated. Alcon has developed a steerable silicone I&A tip. This tip allows for maneuverability in the anterior chamber to remove hard to reach cortex, such as subincisional cortex. Additionally, the soft orifice will not tear the posterior capsule even if it is aspirated.

Vitrectomy

Most phaco machines are equipped with a vitreous cutter, which is activated by compressed air or by electric motor. As noted previously, preservation of a deep anterior chamber is dependent upon a balance of inflow and outflow. For vitrectomy, a 23 ga cannula or chamber maintainer, inserted through a paracentesis, provides inflow. Bottle height should be adequate to prevent chamber collapse. The vitrector should be inserted through another paracentesis. If equipped with a Charles Sleeve, this should be removed and discarded. Utilizing a flow of 20 cc/min, vacuum of 250 mm Hg, and a cutting rate of 250 to 350 cuts/min; the vitrector should be placed through the tear in the posterior capsule, orifice facing upward, pulling vitreous out of the anterior chamber. The vitreous should be removed to the level of the posterior capsule **(Figure 8.17)**.

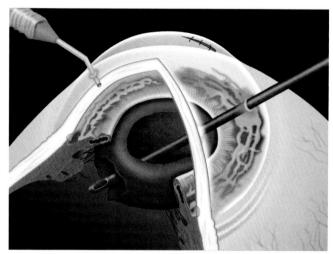

FIGURE 8.17: The vitrector is placed through a new paracentesis deep to the rent in the posterior capsule. Irrigation is via a cannula (*Photo Source:* Thieme Medical Publishers, NY)

Alternatively, the vitrector can be inserted through a pars plana incision 3 mm, posterior to the limbus. In an effort to better visualize the vitreous for thorough vitrectomy, unpreserved sterile prednisone acetate (Kenalog) can be injected into the vitreous. The prednisone particles adhere to the vitreous strands making the invisible, visible.

CONCLUSION

It has been said that the phaco procedure is blend of technology and technique. Awareness of the principles, which influence phaco machine settings, is requisite for the performance of a proficient and safe operation. Additionally, often during the procedure, there is a demand for modification of the initial parameters. A thorough understanding of fundamental principles will enhance the capability of the surgeon for appropriate response to this requirement. It is a fundamental principle that through relentless evaluation of the interaction of the machine and the phaco technique, the skillful surgeon will find innovative methods to enhance technique.

BIBLIOGRAPHY

1. Buratto L, Osher RH, Masket S. Cataract Surgery in Complicated Cases. Thoroughfare, NJ: Slack Inc.; 2001.
2. Fishkind WJ. Complications in Phacoemulsification: Recognition, Avoidance, and Management. New York City: Thieme; 2001.
3. Fishkind WJ. Pop Goes the Microbubbles, ESCRS Film Festival Grand Prize Winner, 1998.
4. Fishkind WJ, Neuhann TF, Steinert RF. The Phaco Machine, in Cataract Surgery, Technique Complications & Management. Chapter 6, Second Edition. Philadelphia, PA: WB Saunders; 2004. pp. 61-77.
5. Seibel BS, Phacodynamics, mastering the tools and techniques of phacoemulsification surgery Third Edition. Thoroughfare, NJ: Slack Inc.; 2000.

CHAPTER 9

The Fluidics and Physics of Phaco

Barry S Seibel

INTRODUCTION

Phacoemulsification is comprised of two basic elements: (i) ultrasound energy is used to emulsify the nucleus, and (ii) a fluidic circuit is employed to remove the emulsate through a small incision while maintaining the anterior chamber **(Figure 9.1)**. This circuit is supplied by an elevated irrigating bottle, which supplies both the fluid volume and pressure to maintain the chamber hydrodynamically and hydrostatically, respectively; anterior chamber pressure is directly proportional to the height of the bottle. The fluid circuit is regulated by a pump, which not only clears the chamber of the emulsate, but also provides significant clinical utility. When the phaco tip is unoccluded, the pump produces currents in the anterior chamber, measured in cc per minute, which attract nuclear fragments. When a fragment completely occludes the tip, the pump provides holding power, measured in mm Hg vacuum, which grips the fragment. In order to fully exploit the potential of a phaco machine, the surgeon must understand the logic behind setting the parameters of ultrasound power, vacuum and flow.

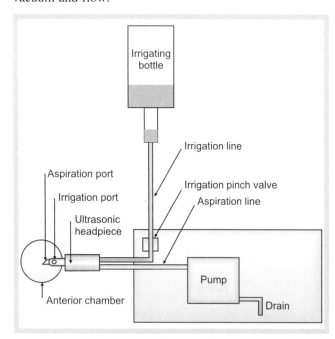

FIGURE 9.1: Phacoemulsification

CATEGORIZATION OF PUMPS

A discussion of flow and vacuum in phaco surgery must begin with a categorization of the various pumps, which are utilized. There are two basic types of pumps in phaco: (i) the flow pump, and (ii) the vacuum pump.

FLOW PUMP

The flow pump, also known as a positive displacement pump, physically regulates the fluid in the aspiration line via direct contact between the fluid and the pump mechanism. Although the scroll pump is the newest example of a flow pump, the peristaltic pump is most commonly employed in current phaco machines and serves as a good schematic example of the flow pump's principles **(Figure 9.2)**.

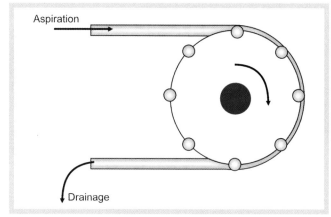

FIGURE 9.2: Scroll pump

One important characteristic of a flow pump is its ability to independently control flow and vacuum. Flow rate, also known as aspiration flow rate, is measured in cc per minute and is directly proportional to the rotational speed of the pump head, measured in revolutions per minute (rpm). Note that because the pump head physically interdigitates with the fluidic circuit via the aspiration line tubing, it regulates the flow rate independently of the amount of pressure in the line via the elevated irrigating bottle. Therefore, flow rate is independent of bottle height when using flow pumps.

However, actual fluid flow rate is very dependent on the degree of phaco tip occlusion. Flow rate decreases with increasing tip occlusion (i.e. decreased effective aspiration port surface area) until flow ceases completely with complete tip occlusion. Note that in **Figure 9.3**, the irrigation bottle's drip chamber mirrors the activity in the anterior chamber. Aspiration flow control on the phaco machine is still important with complete tip occlusion in that it controls the rotational speed of the pump head. Even

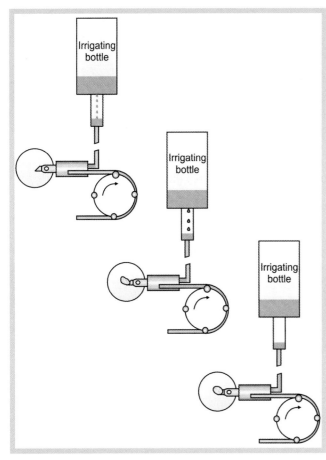

FIGURE 9.3: The irrigation bottle's drip chamber mirrors the activity in the anterior chamber

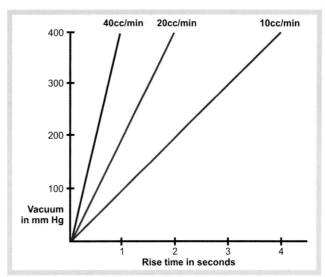

FIGURE 9.4: Graph showing that the rise time is inversely proportional to the rotational speed of the pump head

though no actual flow exists with complete occlusion, the surgeon can control the speed of vacuum build-up via pump speed control. The amount of time required to reach a given vacuum preset, assuming complete tip occlusion, is defined as rise time.

Rise time is inversely proportional to the rotational speed of the pump head **(Figure 9.4)**. All graphs represent the same machine, but note that when the flow rate is cut in half (from 40 to 20 cc per minute), the rise time is doubled (from one second to two seconds). Rise time is doubled again to four seconds when flow rate is halved again to 10 cc per minute. A longer rise time gives the surgeon more time to react in the cases of inadvertent incarceration of iris, capsule or other unwanted material, although a useful setting for training residents, even experienced surgeons appreciate the enhanced safety margin afforded by a longer rise time.

Several points should be made about the preceding discussion on rise time. First, rise time was adjusted via manipulation of the machine's flow rate control. However, as discussed previously, no actual flow exists with complete occlusion, which is necessary to efficiently build vacuum at the phaco tip. Adjusting the machine's flow parameter, measured in cc per minute, actually directly affects the rotational speed of the pump head. Vacuum builds more quickly as the rollers more rapidly traverse the aspiration

line tubing in the pump head, even though no additional fluid is removed from the anterior chamber through the occluded phaco tip.

The second point regarding the rise time discussion concerns the fact that although no fluid flows from the eye with tip occlusion, a minute amount of fluid is pumped from the aspiration line tubing as vacuum is built up, thus, accounting for the relation of pump speed to rise time. Because fluid is noncompressible and nonexpansible, theoretically no change in aspiration line fluid volume would occur as the pump head exerted pressure on the fluid. However, two factors account for this not being true with peristaltic pumps: (i) the use of the aspiration line tubing as a conduit for transmitting the pump rollers' force results in some inefficiency in the form of slippage, both between the pump rollers and the tubing, as well as in between the opposed internal surfaces of the aspiration line tubing, and (ii) the mechanism of action of a peristaltic pump requires enough aspiration line tubing compliance to allow for collapse by the pump rollers. This compliance must be overcome during rise time in the form of some tubing constriction as some fluid is removed from the line (not the eye) by the pump even with complete tip occlusion **(Figure 9.5)**. The most modern peristaltic pumps minimize the system's compliance to the minimum level compatible with the functioning of the pump, thereby, attaining fairly rapid potential rise times. By placing the pump element directly into aspiration fluid path, a scroll pump further reduces the need for aspiration line compliance to the minimum amount required for ergonomic handpiece control. This type of pump can therefore achieve the tightest potential control of rise time with the most rapid vacuum build-up attainable.

The final point concerning rise time and flow pumps is the fact that a maximum attainable vacuum can be preset on the machine. In order to prevent vacuum build-up past this level, a variety of methods are employed. For example,

THE FLUIDICS AND PHYSICS OF PHACO

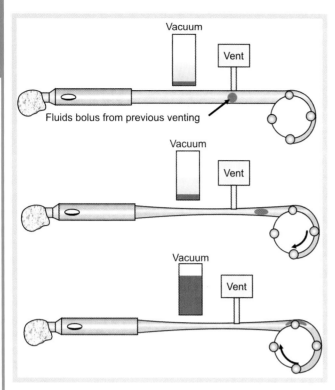

FIGURE 9.5: Removal of the fluid from the line by the pump

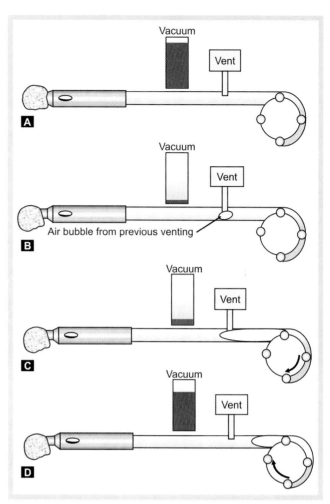

FIGURE 9.6: Figure showing that higher compliance increases rise time and decreases the machine's responsiveness to foot-pedal vacuum control

the pump head can be stopped when the preset value is reached. Alternatively, vacuum can be regulated with a moving pump head by venting air or fluid into the aspiration line if the preset value is exceeded. Venting is also employed if the surgeon wishes to release material, which is held to the phaco tip with vacuum. Air venting has the disadvantage of increasing the fluidic circuit's compliance relative to fluid venting. Higher compliance increases rise time and decreases the machine's responsiveness to foot-pedal vacuum control. **Figure 9.6** illustrates this principle, whereby an air-bubble, which was vented into the circuit to decrease vacuum must be first stretched out by the pump before vacuum can begin to build in the aspiration line again. By employing either air or fluid venting to regulate vacuum build-up, a flow pump therefore not only directly controls flow but also allows indirect control of vacuum.

VACUUM PUMP

In contrast, a vacuum pump directly controls vacuum although it can indirectly control flow. Vacuum pumps represent the second main category of phaco pump, with examples being the rotary vane pump, the diaphragm pump, and the venturi pump. Vacuum pumps have in common a rigid drainage cassette attached to the aspiration line tubing. The various pumps are linked to the cassette and produce vacuum in it, which in turn proportionately produces flow when the aspiration port is unoccluded (**Figure 9.7**). When the tip is occluded, flow ceases and vacuum is transferred from the cassette down the aspiration line to the occluded tip (**Figure 9.8**). Because no rollers are required to collapse the tubing as with peristaltic pumps, vacuum pumps can

employ more rigid tubing with less compliance. This lower compliance coupled with the short times needed for vacuum transfer from the cassette to the phaco (or IA) tip result in low-rise times with vacuum pumps.

Low-rise times can be a potential liability when using high vacuum techniques, if unwanted material is inadvertently incarcerated in the aspiration port, the surgeon has little time to react before potentially permanent damage occurs. Recall that when using a flow pump with a high vacuum preset, low flow rate can be set to produce longer rise times, which give the surgeon more time to react to unwanted occlusions. Most vacuum pumps do not allow the attenuation of rapid rise times, although the Storz Millennium and Premiere machines are exceptions. These pumps allow the surgeon to set at time delay for full commanded vacuum build-up, which starts when the surgeon enters pedal position two. However, once this delay has elapsed, any subsequent engagement of material will be exposed to a typically rapid vacuum pump rise time. An even better, if not elegant, solution to this issue is the dual linear foot control on the millennium (**Figure 9.9**), this separates simultaneous linear control of vacuum and ultrasound in two planes of pedal movement (pitch and

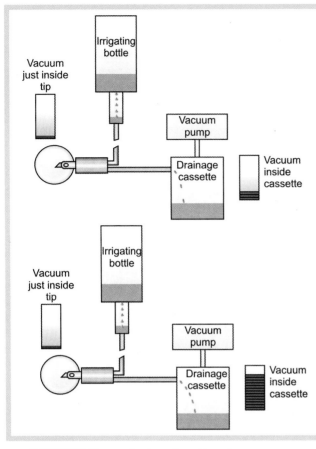

FIGURE 9.7: The mechanism of working of vacuum pump

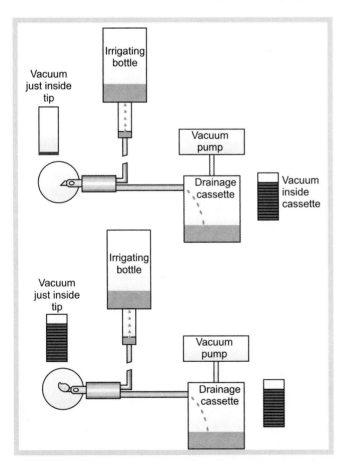

FIGURE 9.8: Vacuum is transferred from the cassette down the aspiration line to the occluded tip

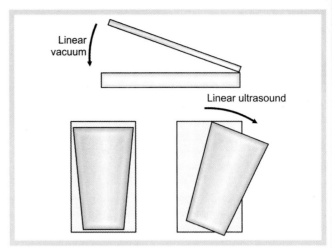

FIGURE 9.9: Dual linear foot control on the millennium

yaw). With linear control of vacuum in phaco mode, the surgeon can approach material with safer lower vacuum levels and increase it only after desired material is positively engaged.

Direct linear control of vacuum has another advantage with vacuum pumps in that it allows subsequently indirect linear control of aspiration flow rate when the tip's aspiration port is unoccluded (**Figure 9.7**). However, because flow is thus indirectly controlled by these pumps, it is more sensitive to resistive variances in the fluidic circuit. For example (**Figure 9.10**), a vacuum pump will produce a certain flow rate at a particular vacuum when using a phaco tip; this same flow rate could also be produced on a flow pump. However, changing to an IA tip (with its smaller surface are aspiration port and subsequently higher fluidic resistance) will decrease actual flow in both systems, but to a greater degree in the vacuum pump. This indirect control of flow by a vacuum pump has another important clinical corollary with regard to bottle height.

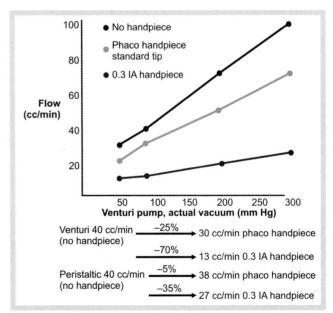

FIGURE 9.10: Vacuum pump producing a certain flow rate at a particular vacuum when using a phaco tip

Unlike a flow pump, a vacuum pump's flow rate is affected by bottle height as a result of a higher pressure head from a higher bottle height pushing fluid through the open circuit more rapidly (compare the fluidic schematics in **Figures 6.2 and 6.7**, noting again the interdigitation of the flow pump in its fluidic circuit).

APPLICATION OF ULTRASOUND POWER

Besides setting fluidic parameters, the surgeon must also decide on the application of ultrasound power, which is produced most often by a piezoelectric crystal oscillating between approximately 20,000 and 60,000 times a second for most machines. This frequency is fixed on a given machine. Ultrasound power is varied by changing the amplification voltage of the handpiece. Increased voltage translates to increased stroke length at the phaco needle tip, up to a maximum of about five microns on most machines (**Figure 9.11**). Usually, a maximum ultrasound limit is preset on the machine's front panel, and the surgeon then titrates with linear pedal control the percentage of this preset maximum, which is appropriate to a given intraoperative instant.

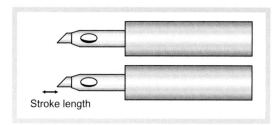

FIGURE 9.11: Increased voltage translates to increased stroke length at the phaco needle tip

The actual mechanism of action of ultrasonic phacoemulsification is somewhat controversial. One school of thought centers around the acoustic break-down of lenticular material as a result of sonic wave propagation through the fluid medium. Another theory concerns the microcavitation bubbles produced at the distal phaco tip, the implosion of these bubbles produces brief instances of intense heat and pressure, which is thought to emulsify adjacent lens material. Yet another potential mechanism of action is via the tips axial oscillations through its stroke length, this resultant jackhammer affect is thought to mechanically break down lens material. This last mechanism also explains the clinical phenomenon of repulsion of free-floating lens material with high ultrasound power levels, these levels need appropriate fluidic titration of the attractive parameters of flow and vacuum to counteract this repulsion.

Ultrasonic phaco needles are available in a variety of configurations. One basic design parameter is the distal bevel angle, which is most commonly 0°, 15°, 30°, or 45° as shown in **Figure 9.12**. The sharper 45° angle is thought

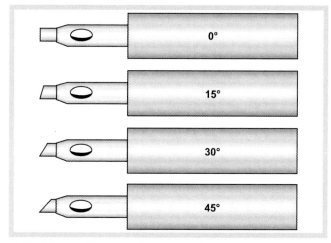

FIGURE 9.12: Different configurations of ultrasonic phaco needles

to carve dense nuclei more efficiently to the extent that the jackhammer mechanism of action is valid, whereas the 0° tip would be more efficient to the extent that the microcavitation theory is valid (the 0° tip has more frontal surface area perpendicular to the axis of oscillation, thereby, producing more cavitation bubbles). In practice, it is difficult to quantitatively compare these efficiencies on a standard density nucleus. Another traditional teaching regarding tip angulation is that a 0° tip occludes more readily than 45° tip, this observation is correct only in that the smaller surface area and perimeter of the 0° tip does seal more readily than does the tip with a larger bevel. However, this axiom is less relevant intraoperatively. A tip occludes readily when the surface to be occluded is parallel to the needle bevel, the surface can and should be manipulated as necessary to achieve this configuration (**Figure 9.13**, which illustrates the attempted gripping of a heminucleus during a stop and chop maneuver).

When titrating ultrasound power, the surgeon must be aware of interrelated clinical variables affecting the resistance to emulsification, especially sculpting. This resistance is directly proportional to both the linear speed of sculpting as well as the amount of the tip engaged. In **Figure 9.14**, it can be noted that for the increased resistive load caused by the increased tip engagement, the surgeon must compensate by either increasing phaco power or decreasing in linear speed of sculpting. Either solution is satisfactory, as long as the interrelationship among the above variables is respected, so as to facilitate the needle carving through the nucleus instead of pushing it and stressing the zonules or capsule.

ADJUSTMENT OF MACHINE PARAMETERS

In order to appropriately adjust the machine parameters for various stages of surgery, it is necessary to analyze the function of those parameters for a given stage. For example, sculpting requires titration of ultrasound power as described

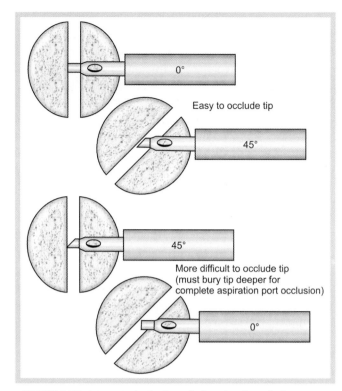

FIGURE 9.13: Attempted gripping of a heminucleus during a stop and chop maneuver

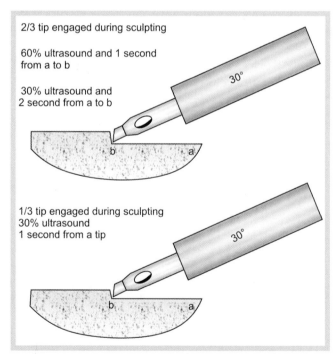

FIGURE 9.14: Compensation by the surgeon in the form of increasing phaco power or decreasing linear speed of sculpting

in the previous paragraph. Furthermore, it requires enough flow to clear the anterior chamber of the emulsate produced by ultrasound as well as sufficient flow to cool the phaco tip, a modest flow of 18 cc/min is usually adequate for these functions. There is little need for vacuum during sculpting, as there are not yet any fragments, which need to be occluded and gripped. Furthermore, vacuum is not needed

to counteract the repulsive action of ultrasound since the nucleus is held stationary by the capsule, zonules, and its intact structure at this point. Therefore, a low vacuum is adequate for sculpting. Although 0 mm Hg is advocated by some surgeons, a slightly higher level of 15 to 30 mm Hg still provides significant safety (in case of contra-incisional peripheral epinuclear or capsule incarceration) while decreasing the likelihood of a clogged aspiration line.

Once the nucleus is debulked or grooved, it then needs manipulation such as rotation or cracking. These maneuvers should be performed in pedal position one so that the chamber will be pressurized without any pump action, which might inadvertently aspirate unwanted material. Once the nucleus is debulked or cracked into fragments, machine parameters need to adapt to the needs to emulsifying these fragments. Ultrasound power requirements are lower at this stage relative to sculpting because of the increased efficiency of phaco aspiration with complete or almost complete tip occlusion. Even with only moderate ultrasound levels, though, flow rate and vacuum usually must be increased from their sculpting levels in order to overcome the repulsive action of ultrasound at the axially vibrating needle tip. Although 26 cc/min flow rate and 120 mm Hg vacuum are reasonable baseline values at this stage, these parameters should ideally be linearly titrated intra-operatively to a given ultrasound level and nuclear density. This level of control has only recently been available to the surgeon with the advent of the dual linear pedal as previously described.

Chopping maneuvers often require further manipulation of parameters. The actual chop may require only moderate vacuum because the nucleus is mechanically fixated between the phaco tip and the chopper. However, higher vacuum levels of 200 to 250 mm Hg can be used advantageously to grip and manipulate the nucleus. For example, the gripped nucleus can be displaced so that the chopper is more centrally located when engaging the nuclear periphery. This maneuver is especially effective if the nucleus was previously grooved and hemisected as has been described by Drs Paul Koch and Ron Stasiuk **(Figure 9.15).** If a flow pump is used, 26 cc/min is a useful compromise between a reasonably rapid rise time and a reasonable safety margin against surge. If a vacuum pump is used at 200 to 250 mm Hg, the surge potential is especially high. When the chop is completed and the occlusion breaks, the subsequent induced flow with a standard needle would be over 60 cc/min. A Microflow or similar needle with a reduced inner diameter (therefore increased fluidic resistance) reduces this flow by about 40% to a safer level. The safest technique, though, would be to use the high vacuum level during the actual manipulation and chop when gripping the nucleus and then to dynamically decrease the vacuum with pedal control just as the chop is completed to minimize the surge potential.

Surge, as has been discussed, occurs when an occluded fragment is held by high vacuum and is then abruptly

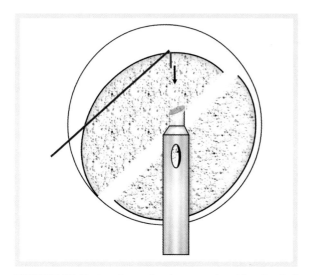

FIGURE 9.15: Nucleus is previously grooved and hemisected before carrying out chopping maneuvers

aspirated (i.e. with a burst of ultrasound), fluid tends to rush into the tip to equilibrate the built-up vacuum in the aspiration line with potentially consequent shallowing or collapse of the anterior chamber **(Figure 9.16)**. In addition to the preventive measures mentioned in the previous paragraph, phaco machines employ a variety of methods to combat surge. Fluidic circuits are engineered with minimal compliance, which will still allow adequate ergonomic manipulation of the tubing as well as functioning of the pump mechanism, the latter being primarily important for peristaltic pumps. Small-bore aspiration line tubing, utilized by Allergan and Alcon, provide increased fluidic resistance, which obtunds surges in a manner similar to that of the MicroFlow needle previously discussed. The Surgical Designs machine incorporates a second, higher irrigating bottle whose fluidic circuit is engaged upon detection of a surge. While all of these designs are helpful, it is ultimately up to the surgeon to set parameters, which optimize a given machine for a given patient with regard to surge prevention.

The parameter of bottle height has a constant function during all phases of surgery—to keep the chamber safely formed without overpressurization which might stress zonules, misdirect aqueous into the vitreous, or cause excessive incisional leakage. Approximately, 10 mm Hg hydrostatic pressure is produced intraocularly for every 15 cm bottle height above the eye.

However, it is vital that the appropriate bottle height be set hydrodynamically with the pump operating (pedal position two or three) and the tip unoccluded so that an adequate pressure head will be established to keep up with the induced aspiration outflow from the eye.

This chapter has stressed the importance of appropriate machine parameter settings. It should also be stressed, of course, that surgical technique is not only just as important, but is moreover integrally related. For example, if a surgeon wishes to grip and pull a heminucleus in preparation for chopping yet finds that the tip instead pulls away from the lens material, the tendency would be to increase the vacuum parameter to give a stronger grip. However, it is critical to remember that the full preset vacuum can be produced at the phaco tip only with complete tip occlusion. Therefore, if an adequate vacuum seal is not obtained, the preset value will not be reached. Increasing the vacuum preset will not affect the clinical performance in the absence of a good vacuum seal, which is obtained by embedding the phaco tip at least 1 to 1.5 mm with light ultrasound energy so as to avoid excessive cavitation **(Figure 9.17)**. The tip is also embedded in the central densest nucleus as opposed to more peripheral, softer material, which might irregularly aspirate, again causing a loss of the vacuum seal **(Figure 9.18)**. This subtle attention to technique pays off with the machine being used to its most effective potential.

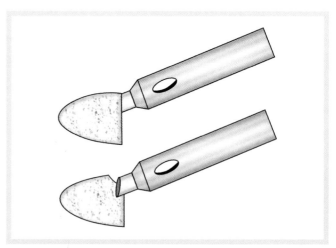

FIGURE 9.17: Embedding the phaco tip at least 1 to 1.5 mm with light ultrasound energy so as to avoid excessive cavitation

SUMMARY

Modern phaco machines offer unprecedented levels of control and safety. In order to fully exploit these values, a

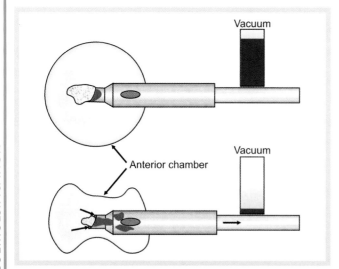

FIGURE 9.16: Fluid rushing into the tip to equilibrate the built-up vacuum in the aspiration line

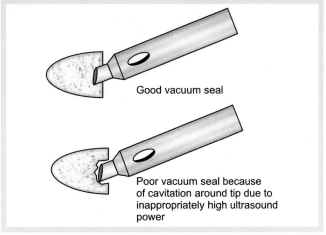

Good vacuum seal

Poor vacuum seal because
of cavitation around tip due to
inappropriately high ultrasound
power

FIGURE 9.18: Embedding the tip in central densest nucleus as
opposed to more peripheral, softer material

thorough understanding of the principles by which the machines operate is essential. In particular, the surgeon must appropriately adjust flow rate, vacuum, ultrasound power, and bottle height as necessary for a given patient and for a given stage in the operation. This vigilance and attention, coupled with meticulous technique designed to optimize the machine's performance, will result in the safest, most efficient phacoemulsification surgery.

CHAPTER 10

Air Pump and Gas-Forced Infusion

Smita Narasimhan, Amar Agarwal

HISTORY

The main problem the authors had in bimanual phaco/phakonit was the destabilization of the anterior chamber during surgery. They solved it to a certain extent by using an 18-gauge irrigating chopper. Then Dr Sunita Agarwal suggested the use of an antichamber collapser, which injects air into the infusion bottle (**Figure 10.1**). This pushes more fluid into the eye through the irrigating chopper and also prevents surge.[1-11] Thus, the authors were able to use a 20-gauge or 21-gauge irrigating chopper, as well as solve the problem of destabilization of the anterior chamber during surgery. Now with microphakonit because of gas-forced infusion, they are able to remove cataracts with a 0.7 mm irrigating chopper (22 gauge). Subsequently they used this system in all their coaxial phaco cases including microincisional coaxial phaco to prevent complications like posterior capsular ruptures and corneal damage.

INTRODUCTION

Since the introduction of phacoemulsification by Kelman,[1] it has been undergoing revolutionary changes in an attempt to perfect the techniques of extracapsular cataract extraction surgery. Although advantageous in many aspects, this technique is not without its attending complications. A well maintained anterior chamber without intraocular fluctuations is one of the prerequisites for safe phacoemulsification and phakonit.[2]

When an occluded fragment is held by high vacuum and then abruptly aspirated, fluid rushes into the phaco tip to equilibrate the built-up vacuum in the aspiration line, which causes surge.[3] This leads to shallowing or collapse of the anterior chamber. Different machines employ a variety of methods to combat surge. These include usage of noncompliant tubing,[4] small bore aspiration line tubing,[4] microflow tips,[4] aspiration bypass systems,[4] dual linear foot pedal control[4] and incorporation of sophisticated microprocessors[4] to sense the anterior chamber pressure fluctuations.

The surgeon dependent variables to counteract surge include good wound construction with minimal leakage,[5] and selection of appropriate machine parameters depending on the stage of the surgery.[5] An anterior chamber maintainer has also been described in literature to prevent surge, but an extra side port makes it an inconvenient procedure.

The authors started a simple and effective method to prevent anterior chamber collapse during phacoemulsification and phakonit in 1999 by increasing the velocity of the fluid inflow into the anterior chamber. This is achieved by an automated air pump, which pumps atmospheric air through an air filter into the infusion bottle thereby preventing surge. The authors stumbled upon this idea when they were operating cases with phakonit,[7] where they wanted more fluid entering the eye, but now also use it in all their phaco cases.[8]

AIR PUMP

An automated air pump is used to push air into the infusion bottle thus increasing the pressure with which the fluid flows into the eye. This increases the steady-state pressure of the eye making the anterior chamber deep and well maintained during the entire procedure. It makes phakonit and phacoemulsification a relatively safe procedure by reducing surge even at high vacuum levels.

TECHNIQUE

A locally manufactured automated device, used in fish tanks (aquariums) to supply oxygen, is utilized to forcefully pump air into the irrigation bottle. This pump is easily available in aquarium shops. It has an electromagnetic motor, which moves a lever attached to a collapsible rubber cap. There is an inlet with a valve, which sucks in atmospheric air as the cap expands. On collapsing, the valve closes and the air is pushed into an intravenous (IV) line connected to the infusion bottle (**Figure 10.1**). The lever vibrates at a frequency of approximately 10 oscillations per second. The

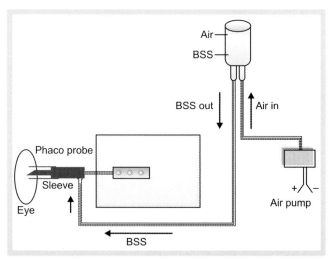

FIGURE 10.1: Diagrammatic representation of the connection of the air pump to the infusion bottle

electromagnetic motor is weak enough to stop once the pressure in the closed system (i.e. the anterior chamber) reaches about 50 mm Hg. The rubber cap ceases to expand at this pressure level. A millipore air filter is used between the air pump and the infusion bottle so that the air pumped into the bottle is clean of particulate matter.

METHOD

1. First of all, a balanced salt solution (BSS) bottle is taken and put in the IV stand.
2. Now the authors take an air pump. This air pump is the same air pump, which is used in fish tanks (aquariums) to give oxygen to the fishes. The air pump is plugged on to the electrical connection.
3. An IV set now connects the air pump to the infusion bottle. The tubing passes from the air pump and the end of the tubing is passed into one of the infusion bottles.
4. What happens now is that when the air pump is switched on, it pumps air into the infusion bottle. This air goes to the top of the bottle and because of the pressure, it pumps the fluid down with greater force. With this, the fluid now flows from the infusion bottle to reach the phaco handpiece or irrigating chopper. The amount of fluid now coming out of the handpiece is much more than what would normally come out and with more force.
5. A millipore air filter is connected between the air pump and the infusion bottle so that the air, which is being pumped into the bottle is sterile.
6. This extra amount of fluid coming out compensates for the surge, which would otherwise occur.

CONTINUOUS INFUSION

Before the authors enter the eye, they fill the eye with viscoelastic. Then once the tip of the phaco handpiece in phaco or irrigating chopper in phakonit is inside the anterior chamber, they shift to continuous irrigation. This is very helpful especially for surgeons who are starting phaco or phakonit. This way, the surgeon never comes to position zero and the anterior chamber never collapses. Even for excellent surgeons this helps a lot.

Advantages

1. With the air pump, the posterior capsule is pushed back and there is a deep anterior chamber.
2. The phenomenon of surge is neutralized. This prevents the unnecessary posterior capsular rupture.
3. Striate keratitis is reduced postoperatively, as there is a deep anterior chamber.
4. One can operate hard cataracts also quite comfortably, as striate keratitis does not occur postoperatively.
5. The surgical time is shorter as one can emulsify the nuclear pieces much faster as surge does not occur.
6. One can easily operate cases with the phakonit technique as quite a lot of fluid now passes into the eye. Thus, the cataract can be removed through a smaller opening.

7. It is quite comfortable to do cases under topical or no anesthesia.

TOPICAL OR NO ANESTHESIA CATARACT SURGERY

When one operates under topical or no anesthesia, the main problem is sometimes the pressure is high especially if the patient squeezes the eye. In such cases, the posterior capsule comes up anteriorly and one can produce a posterior capsular rupture. To solve this problem, surgeons tend to work more anteriorly, performing supracapsular phacoemulsification/phakonit. The disadvantage of this is that striate keratitis tends to occur.

With the air pump, this problem does not occur. When the authors use the air pump, the posterior capsule is quite back, as if they are operating a patient under a block. In other words, there is a lot of space between the posterior capsule and the cornea, preventing striate keratitis and inadvertent posterior capsular rupture.

INTERNAL GAS-FORCED INFUSION

Internal gas-forced infusion was started by Arturo Pérez-Arteaga from Mexico. The anterior vented gas-forced infusion system (AVGFI) of the accurus surgical system is used.

This system is incorporated in the Accurus machine that creates a positive infusion pressure inside the eye; it was designed by the Alcon engineers to control the intraocular pressure (IOP) during posterior segment surgery. It consist of an air pump and a regulator which are inside the machine; then the air is pushed inside the bottle of intraocular solution, and so the fluid is actively pushed inside the eye without raising or lowering the bottle. The control of the air pump is digitally integrated in the Accurus panel; it also can be controlled via the remote. In addition, the footswitch can be preset with the minimal and maximum of desired fluid inside the eye and go directly to this value with the simple touch of the footswitch. Arturo Pérez-Arteaga recommends to preset the infusion pump at 100 mm Hg; it is enough strong irrigation force to perform a microincision phaco. This parameter is preset in the panel and also as the minimal irrigation force in the footswitch. Then it is recommended to preset the maximum irrigation force at 130 to 140 mm Hg in the foot pedal, so if a surge exist during the procedure, the surgeon can increase the irrigation force by the simple touch of the footswitch to the right. With the AVGFI, the surgeon has the capability to increase even more than these values. A millipore filter is used again between the tubing and the air pump (**Figure 10.2**).

STELLARIS PRESSURIZED INFUSION SYSTEM

Bausch & Lomb installed the air pump in their Stellaris machine in 2009. The advantage of this is that one has an

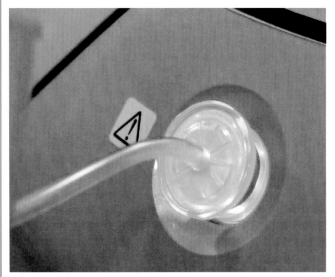

FIGURE 10.2: Millipore filter to connect the air pump to the tubing. Air pump in the Stellaris (Bausch and Lomb) machine

internal gas-forced infusion now as the air pump, which was an external gas-forced infusion system is now inside the machine **(Figure 10.3)**. Another advantage is that there is a monitor in the panel of the machine and one can lower or raise the pressure of the air pump.

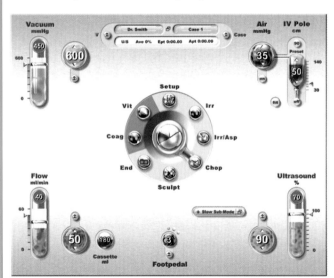

FIGURE 10.3: Stellaris (Bausch and Lomb) pressurized infusion system. Note in the upper right corner IV pole height in cm and next to it shows the air pump (gas-forced infusion pressure) in mm Hg

AIR PUMP-ASSISTED PHACO FOR MANAGING CASES WITH INCOMPLETE RHEXIS

The idea of the concept that air pump-assisted phaco for managing cases with incomplete rhexis was given by Dr Smita Narasimhan. In the event of a runaway capsulorhexis, continuing with phacoemulsification carries the risk of extension of the capsular tear through the equator onto the posterior capsule. This can potentially lead to

nucleus drop, vitreous loss and reduces the chances of a stable in the bag IOL implantation. Multiple techniques can be used in the event of a tear. These include starting of capsulorhexis from the opposite side to include the tear, backward traction on the base of the capsular flap, but are not always successful. The authors describe a novel technique to complete phacoemulsification following an irretrievable anterior capsular tear with the assistance of an air pump (gas-forced infusion) in cataracts with nuclear sclerosis grade 1–3 or white cataracts in patients under 60 years of age.

The anterior capsulorhexis is started as a capsular nick from the center, which is then moved to the right. The capsular flap is then lifted off and teased downwards **(Figure 10.4)**. As the maximum tendency to lose the capsulorhexis is near its completion, the authors are usually left with an incomplete capsulorhexis superiorly and to the right. Since all manipulations will be directed down and to the left, the chances of the capsulorhexis extending will be less. For a left-handed surgeon, one should start from the center and move to the left. Following an irretrievable anterior capsular tear **(Figure 10.5)**, the authors refrain from

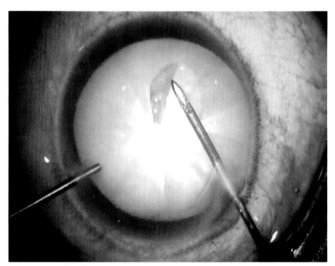

FIGURE 10.4: Rhexis started in a mature cataract

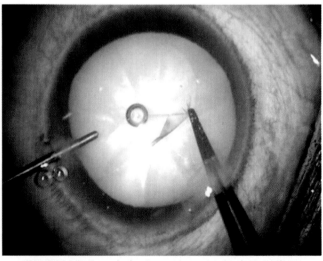

FIGURE 10.5: Capsulorhexis running away to the periphery

making further manipulations, which may extend the tear to the posterior capsule. If there is suspicion of posterior capsular extension of the tear, the authors prefer to convert the surgery to an extracapsular cataract extraction (ECCE). The anterior capsule is then flattened with the help of viscoelastics and they make a nick from the opposite side using a cystitome or vannas scissor and complete the capsulorhexis. The viscoelastic in the anterior chamber (AC) is then expressed out to make the globe hypotonus, following which a gentle hydrodissection (**Figure 10.6**) is done at a site 90 degrees from the tear while pressing the posterior lip of the incision to prevent any rise in IOP. No attempt is made to press on the center of the nucleus to complete the fluid wave. The fluid is usually sufficient to prolapse one pole of the nucleus out of the capsular bag (**Figure 10.7**); else it is removed by embedding the phacoemulsification probe, making sure not to exert any downward pressure and then gently pulling the nucleus anteriorly. The whole nucleus is brought out into the AC and no nuclear division techniques are tried in the bag.

Phacoemulsification can be started at this stage for cataracts with nuclear sclerosis 1–3, but it is safer to convert

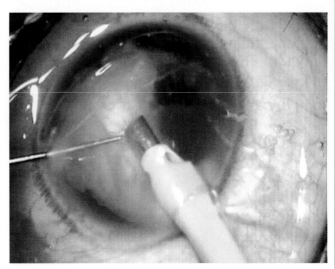

FIGURE 10.8: Nucleus being removed by phacoemulsification in the supracapsular area after prolapsing it into the anterior chamber. The air pump is one so no damage occurs to the corneal endothelium as the chamber is quite deep

to an ECCE for nuclear sclerosis grade 4. Phacoemulsification is started with the gas-forced infusion in place and the bottle height 75 cm above eye level (**Figure 10.8**). The infusion is kept on continuous mode at all times. This prevents the AC from collapsing even if the surgeon takes the foot off the machine. As the entire nucleus is prolapsed into the anterior chamber and emulsified, it prevents any stretch on the torn capsulorhexis. The gas-forced infusion provides for a deep anterior chamber, pushes the posterior capsule back and prevents surge to allow safe anterior chamber phacoemulsification. While withdrawing the probe, viscoelastic is injected simultaneously through the side port incision. Irrigation aspiration is performed in the "Cap Vac" mode with the aspiration set at 5 mm Hg and the flow rate at 6 ml/min and the gas-forced infusion pump on (**Figures 10.9 and 10.10**). In the presence of a thick epinucleus, the authors first inject viscoelastic between the capsule and the cortical matter, 90 degrees from the site of

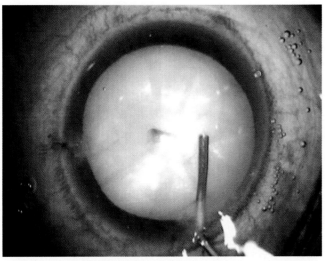

FIGURE 10.6: Hydrodissection done

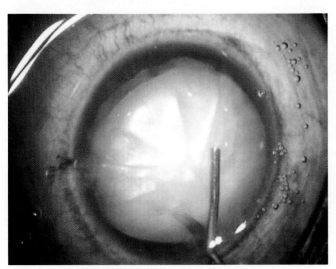

FIGURE 10.7: Nucleus prolapsed into the AC

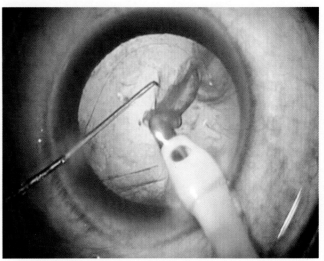

FIGURE 10.9: Irrigation aspiration being performed in the "Cap Vac" mode

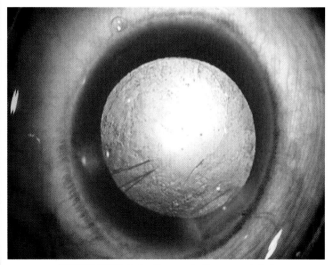

FIGURE 10.10: Irrigation aspiration completed

the tear, to express the epinuclear plate into the anterior chamber. The epinucleus is then aspirated in the anterior chamber keeping the vacuum at 120 mmHg and flow rate at 20 ml/min. The cortex in the region of the capsular tear is aspirated out last. The anterior chamber and bag are partially filled with a viscoelastic and the IOL is injected introducing the leading haptic into the bag but pointing away from the area of the tear and not directing the IOL too posteriorly **(Figure 10.11)**. The IOL is gently manipulated into the capsular bag with the help of a Y rod (Katena, USA- Agarwal globe stabilization rod) giving a final orientation of the haptics 90 degrees away from the anterior capsular tear .

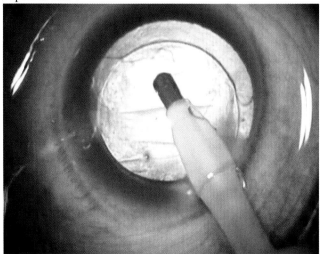

FIGURE 10.11: Foldable PC IOL implanted

DISCUSSION

Surge is defined as the volume of the fluid forced out of the eye into the aspiration line at the instant of occlusion break. When the phacoemulsification handpiece tip is occluded, flow is interrupted and vacuum builds up to its preset values. Additionally the aspiration tubing may collapse in the presence of high vacuum levels. Emulsification of the occluding fragment clears the block and the fluid

rushes into the aspiration line to neutralize the pressure difference created between the positive pressure in the anterior chamber and the negative pressure in the aspiration tubing. In addition, if the aspiration line tubing is not reinforced to prevent collapse (tubing compliance), the tubing constricted during occlusion, then expands on occlusion break. These factors cause a rush of fluid from the anterior chamber into the phaco probe. The fluid in the anterior chamber is not replaced rapidly enough to prevent shallowing of the anterior chamber.

The maintenance of intraocular pressure (steady–state IOP)[2] during the entire procedure depends on the equilibrium between the fluid inflow and outflow. The steady state pressure level is the mean pressure equilibrium between inflow and outflow volumes. In most phacoemulsification machines, fluid inflow is provided by gravitational flow of the fluid from the balanced salt solution (BSS) bottle through the tubing to the anterior chamber. This is determined by the bottle height relative to the patient's eye, the diameter of the tubing and most importantly by the outflow of fluid from the eye through the aspiration tube and leakage from the wounds.[2]

The inflow volume can be increased by either increasing the bottle height or by enlarging the diameter of the inflow tube. The intraocular pressure increases by 10 mm Hg for every 15 centimeters increase in bottle height above the eye.[5]

High steady-state IOPs increase phaco safety by raising the mean IOP level up and away from zero, i.e. by delaying surge-related anterior chamber collapse.[2]

Air pump increases the amount of fluid inflow thus making the steady-state IOP high. This deepens the anterior chamber, increasing the surgical space available for maneuvering and thus prevents complications like posterior capsular tears and corneal endothelial damage. The phenomenon of surge is neutralized by rapid inflow of fluid at the time of occlusion break. The recovery to steady-state IOP is so prompt that no surge occurs and this enables the surgeon to remain in foot position 3 through the occlusion break. High vacuum phacoemulsification/phakonit can be safely performed in hard brown cataracts using an air pump. Phacoemulsification or phakonit under topical or no anesthesia[6,7] can be safely done neutralizing the positive vitreous pressure occurring due to squeezing of the eyelids.

SUMMARY

The air pump is a new device, which helps to prevent surge. This prevents posterior capsular rupture, helps deepen the anterior chamber and makes phacoemulsification and phakonit safe procedures even in hard cataracts.

REFERENCES

1. Kelman CD. Phacoemulsification and aspiration; a new technique of cataract removal; a preliminary report. Am J Ophthalmol. 1967;64:23-5.

2. Wilbrandt RH. Comparative analysis of the fluidics of the AMO Prestige, Alcon Legacy, and Storz Premiere phacoemulsification systems. J Cataract Refract Surg. 1997;23:766-80.

3. Seibel SB. Phacodynamics. Thorofare, NJ: Slack Inc; 1995. p. 54.

4. Fishkind WJ. The Phaco Machine: How and why it acts and reacts? In: Agarwal's Four volume Textbook of Ophthalmology. Jaypee Brothers Medical Publishers: New Delhi; 2000.

5. Seibel SB. The fluidics and physics of phaco. In: Agarwal's et al. Phacoemulsification, Laser Cataract Surgery and Foldable IOLs, Second edition. Jaypee Brothers Medical Publishers: New Delhi; 2000. p. 45-54.

6. Agarwal A. No anaesthesia cataract surgery with karate chop; In: Agarwal's Phacoemulsification, Laser cataract surgery and foldable IOLs, Second edition. Jaypee Brothers Medical Publishers: New Delhi; 2000. p. 217-26.

7. Agarwal A. Phakonit and laser phakonit. In: Agarwal's Phacoemulsification, Laser Cataract Surgery and Foldable IOLs. Second edition. Jaypee Brothers Medical Publishers: New Delhi; 2000. 204-16.

8. Agarwal A, Agarwal S, Agarwal A. Antichamber collapser. J Cataract Refract Surg. 2002;28(7):1085-6.

9. Agarwal A, Agarwal S, Agarwal A. Phakonit: phacoemulsification through a 0.9 mm incision. J Cataract Refract Surg. 2001; 27(10):1548-52.

10. Agarwal A, Trivedi RH, Jacob S, et al. Microphakonit: 700 micron cataract surgery. Clinical Ophthalmology. 2007;1(3): 323-5.

11. Agarwal A, Kumar DA, Jacob S, et al. In vivo analysis of wound architecture in 700 micron microphakonit surgery. J Cataract Refract Surg. 2008;34(9):1554-60.

AIR PUMP AND GAS-FORCED INFUSION

CHAPTER 11

Torsional Phacoemulsification

Sunil Thadani, Bonnie An Henderson

BACKGROUND AND INTRODUCTION

Since the introduction of phacoemulsification technology in 1967, technological improvements in nuclear fragmentation and improved pump systems have helped to reduce the amount of energy needed to remove cataracts. Energy delivery in cataract surgery may be mechanical, fluidic and through the use of ultrasound. The ultrasound component is one that is likely to have the most direct negative effect on ocular structures.[1]

Ultrasound energy delivery has gone through several advances. Originally power was delivered in a fixed or "on and off" fashion, then advances were made to include linear continuous power and then burst technology, which involved the use of pulses to deliver phacoemulsification energy.

This ultrasound power has conventionally been delivered through longitudinal movement of the phaco needle tip. That is, forward and backward movement of the needle allows for energy to be delivered directly in front of the tip. One negative effect of this type of energy delivery involves repulsion, which occurs as the tip pushes nuclear fragments away as it goes through forward motion. Additionally there may be a "chattering effect" as the nuclear fragments move back and forth with the delivery of the energy from the tip.

Torsional ultrasound was incorporated as the OZil® torsional handpiece for the INFINITI Vision System in 2006 (Alcon Laboratories, Fort Worth, TX). This change to the INFINITI Vision System included upgrade to both the handpieces and the machine software. The OZil® handpiece produces rotary movement through oscillations at the phacoemulsification tip with a frequency of 32 Kz **(Figure 11.1)**. This movement is thought to reduce the repulsion and "chattering effect" that occur during conventional longitudinal ultrasound delivery and allow bidirectional horizontal emulsification.

In this chapter, the authors will discuss torsional ultrasound with respects to temperature and heat production, tip travel and followability, application in various cataract density and morphology settings, and finally comparisons of overall efficiency to longitudinal ultrasound. They will also discuss the Intelligent Phaco, IP© software upgrade and how this has incorporated the use of both torsional and longitudinal ultrasound.

HEAT PRODUCTION

Heat generation occurs at the tip of the phacoemulsification handpiece is a result of frictional forces that are created

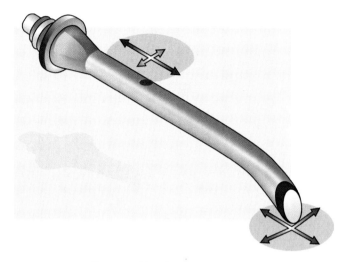

FIGURE 11.1: OZil® torsional handpiece for the INFINITI Vision System in 2006 (Alcon Laboratories, Fort Worth, TX) (Source: Han YK, Miller KM. J Cataract Refract Surg. 2009; 35:1799-805)

between the moving needle and the surrounding silicone sleeve. This may result in corneal wound burns that result in difficult closure and irregular astigmatism. Han and colleagues[2] used thermal infrared cameras to evaluate focal heat production in phacoemulsification tips inserted into silicone test chambers. After clamping aspiration lines to simulate occlusion, longitudinal and torsional tips were allowed to run on continuous ultrasound power for 0, 10, 30, 60 and 120 seconds. Heat production was higher in the longitudinal tips and this was more pronounced with longer phacoemulsification times. In **Figure 11.2**, the same tests were repeated with comparisons of equivalent stroke length and applied energy and torsional phacoemulsification was found to have lower heat generation at each time point.

TIP TRAVEL

As stated earlier, longitudinal phacoemulsification employs a forward and backward motion at the tip of the handpiece, whereas torsional phacoemulsification utilizes an oscillating or side-to-side motion. Decreases in tip travel and improvements in followability are thought to occur as a result of the inherent side to side motion of the torsional tip. A study by Davison[3] used measurement software to evaluate a series of same surgeon surgical videos in which torsional and longitudinal tips were measured for movement during cataract surgery **(Figure 11.3)**. Both angled and straight tips were used in each of the handpieces. Tip travel was found to be significantly reduced in the angled/torsional subgroup

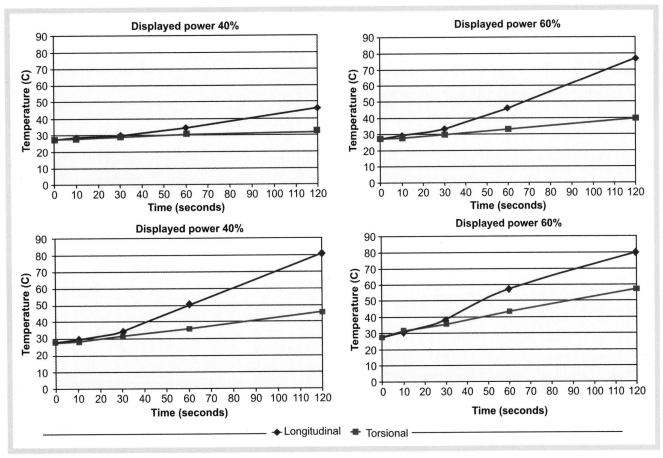

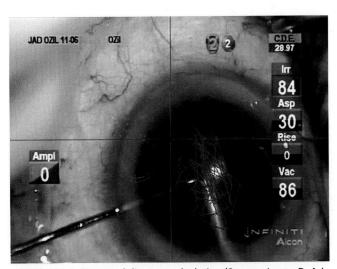

FIGURE 11.2: Heat production in phacoemulsification tips (Source: Han YK, Miller KM. J Cataract Refract Surg. 2009; 35:1799-805)

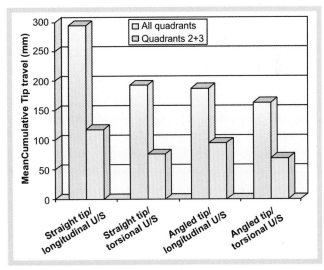

FIGURE 11.3: Tip travel distance calculation (Source: James D. A J Cataract Refract Surg. 2008;34:986-90)

FIGURE 11.4: Tip travel comparison (Source: James D. A J Cataract Refract Surg. 2008;34:986-90)

compared to all the other subgroups (**Figure 11.4**). There was also a reduction in phacoemulsification time in the angled/torsional combination when compared to all other subgroups.

COMPARISONS OF TORSIONAL AND LONGITUDINAL ULTRASOUND SYSTEMS

Comparisons of torsional and conventional longitudinal phacoemulsification were evaluated by a randomized study

by Liu and colleagues.[4] In this comparative study, approximately 525 eyes undergoing cataract surgery were assigned to phacoemulsification by torsional or longitudinal modes. Outcomes evaluated included ultrasound time, dissipated energy, visual acuity, changes in corneal clarity, central thickness and endothelial cell count.

Another study by Rekas and colleagues[1] evaluated approximately 400 eyes randomly assigned to phaco-

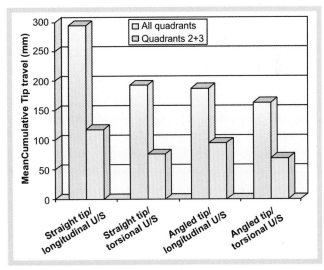

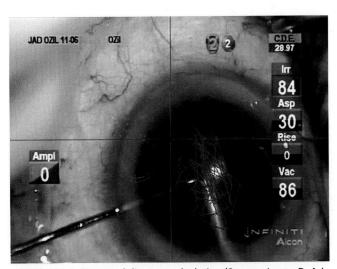

emulsification by either torsional or longitudinal ultrasound modes. The outcome measures that were evaluated include ultrasound time and power, torsional amplitude and aspiration time.

ULTRASOUND TIME AND ENERGY DISSIPATION

Ultrasound time was classified as the duration in which the foot pedal remained in the third position. This was evaluated using four categories of progressively increased cataract density using the Lens Opacities Classification System II (LOCS II).[5] Liu and colleagues found significantly lower ultrasound times in each of the four nucleus density grades for torsional ultrasound when compared to longitudinal ultrasound (**Figure 11.5**).

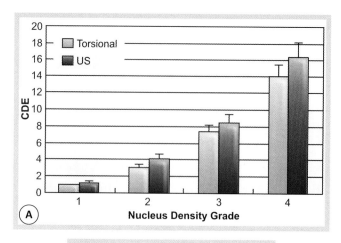

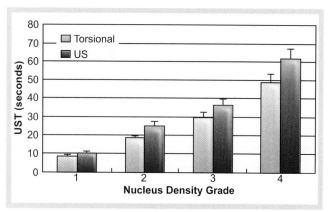

FIGURE 11.5: Ultrasound time (Source: Liu Y, et al. J Cataract Refract Surg. 2007;33:287-92)

Dissipated energy was evaluated as a function of ultrasound power and ultrasound time. Liu and colleagues found that torsional ultrasound resulted in lower dissipated energy for each nuclear density grade (**Figures 11.6A and B**).

Rekas and colleagues also found a consistently lower amount of dissipated energy among individuals undergoing torsional phacoemulsification. However, the difference between the two groups decreased as the nuclear density increased. Interestingly, the dissipated energy was not statistically significant in grade IV cataracts.

CORNEAL EDEMA AND ENDOTHELIAL CELL COUNT

Liu and colleagues found corneal edema and striae to be higher in the conventional ultrasound group than the torsional group at postoperative day one and postoperative day seven. However when followed out to day 30, neither group had any corneal edema.

Endothelial cell counts were evaluated preoperatively, and at 7 and 30 days after surgery. Postoperative day seven mean endothelial cell counts decreased 17.6 % for the ultrasound group compared to 10.4% for the torsional group. At postoperative day 30, cell counts decreased by 19.1% in the ultrasound group and 12.5% in the torsional group.

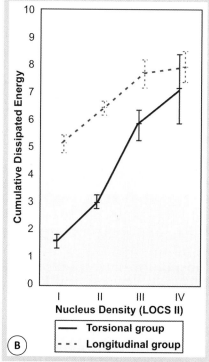

FIGURES 11.6A AND B: Dissipated energy (Sources: (A) Liu Y, et al. J Cataract Refract Surg. 2007;33:287-92. (B) Rekas M, et al. J Cataract Refract Surg. 2009;35:1719-24)

VISUAL ACUITY

One study showed that at postoperative day one and seven, there were statistically significant differences in visual acuity favoring torsional phacoemulsification. This difference, however, was not seen at postoperative day 30. Rekas and colleagues did not find a significant difference in visual acuity at day one, seven or day thirty. However, significant improvements in visual acuity compared to preoperative visual acuities were seen in both groups.

TORSIONAL ULTRASOUND AND CATARACT DENSITY

Wang and colleagues[6] showed that increased vacuum levels improved the efficiency of torsional phacoemulsification at all cataract density levels resulting in reduced ultrasound time, decreased cumulative dissipated energy and lower endothelial cell loss. Increased vacuum levels, however, may result in higher levels of post-occlusion surge.

At higher levels of cataract density, similar cumulative dissipated energy values are seen in torsional phacoemulsification and conventional ultrasound phacoemulsification. Thus, the favorable advantage afforded by torsional ultrasound becomes less apparent with the cataracts of higher density and mass. Additional parameter settings have been implemented, specifically using a combination of torsional and linear phacoemulsification to address the challenges seen in cataracts of increased density and mass.

INTELLIGENT PHACOEMULSIFICATION IP©

The OZil® IP (Intelligent Phaco) software (Alcon Laboratories, Fort Worth, TX) is a recent addition to improve the efficiency of the torsional phacoemulsification system. It allows continuous monitoring of the tip for evidence of increased pressure indicating an occlusion. At the time of occlusion, a change in the phacoemulsification parameters allow a burst of longitudinal phacoemulsification power resulting in fragment repositioning, which results in fragments being maintained at an optimal position for torsional movement. This is thought to improve efficiency and minimize post-occlusion surge.

The benefits of combining longitudinal and torsional phacoemulsification systems were demonstrated in a study by Zeng and colleagues.[7] Torsional phacoemulsification was combined with the short bursts of conventional ultrasound. This was found to be effective and safe for hard nucleus extraction and resulted in less ultrasound time and cumulative dissipated energy than conventional ultrasound alone.

CONCLUSION

Advances in mechanical techniques, fluidics and ultrasound delivery have helped improve the efficiency of cataract extraction over the last two decades. The advent of torsional phacoemulsification represents another important tool in cataract surgery allowing improved efficiency of cataract extraction while decreasing damage to ocular structures.

REFERENCES

1. Rekas M, Montés-Micó R, Krix-Jachym K, et al. Comparison of torsional and longitudinal modes using phacoemulsification parameters. J Cataract Refract Surg. 2009;35:1719-24.
2. Han YK, Miller KM. Heat production: Longitudinal versus torsional phacoemulsification. J Cataract Refract Surg. 2009;35:1799-805.
3. Davison JA. Cumulative tip travel and implied followability of longitudinal and torsional phacoemulsification. J Cataract Refract Surg. 2008;34:986-90.
4. Liu Y, Zeng M, Liu X, et al. Torsional mode versus conventional ultrasound mode phacoemulsification: randomized comparative clinical study. J Cataract Refract Surg. 2007;33: 287-92.
5. Chylack LT, Leske MC, McCarthy D, et al. Lens opacities classification system II (LOCS II). Arch Ophthalmol. 1989;107:991-7.
6. Wang Y, Xia Y, Zeng M, et al. Torsional ultrasound efficiency under different vacuum levels in different degrees of nuclear cataract. J Cataract Refract Surg. 2009;35:1941-5.
7. Zeng M, Liu X, Liu Y, et al. Torsional ultrasound modality for hard nucleus phacoemulsification cataract extraction. Br J Ophthalmol. 2008;92(8):1092-6.

CHAPTER 12

Viscoelastics and Ophthalmic Viscosurgical Devices (OVDs) in Ophthalmic Surgery

Guillermo L Simón-Castellví, Sarabel Simón-Castellví, José María, Simón-Castellví Simón-Tor, Esteban Pertejo-Fernández

INTRODUCTION

When the authors started their first modern cataract surgeries in the early 1980s after decades of intracapsular lens extraction, anterior capsulotomy, either can-opener capsulotomy or envelope capsulotomy, was performed by the means of an insulin bent needle, under an air bubble or entering anterior chamber with the needle, avoiding the leakage of aqueous humor outside the anterior chamber.

The authors soon discovered that the three major advances in modern cataract surgery were:
1. The invention of intraocular lenses (IOLs) by Sir Harold Ridley (July 10, 1906 Kibworth, Harcourt, Beauchamp in Leicestershire – May 25, 2001, United Kingdom),
2. The introduction of viscoelastics (by the Hungarian Dr Endre Balazs) and
3. The practice of a continuous curvilinear capsulotomy, now called capsulorhexis, introduced by Howard Gimbel, MD (Calgary, Canada), Thomas Neuhann, MD, (Munich, Germany), Calvin Fercho, MD (Fargo, North Dakota, USA) and Kimiya Shimizu, MD (Kanagawa, Japan).

Later, the authors also realized that the next giant step in modern cataract surgery was the introduction of ultrasonic lens emulsification (phacoemulsification) by the American ophthalmologist, Dr Charles D Kelman (1930-2004) in 1967.

In the late 1970s, the advent of first anterior and posterior intraocular lenses, and the move from intracapsular to extracapsular cataract extraction resulted in a dramatic increase in the number of postoperative corneal decompensations (irreversible corneal edemas) that ended in full thickness corneal grafts. A huge preventive leap forward was the advent of viscoelastic substances as a result of the research conducted by Dr Endre A Balazs, MD (Budapest, Hungary). He distinguished himself through pioneering work on the structure and biological activity of hyaluronan, a viscoelastic polysaccharide present in all tissues of the human body, and in large amounts in the vitreous humor of the eye and the soft tissues of joints and skin.

The subsequent licensing of the noninflammatory fraction (NIF) of hyaluronan (hyaluronic acid) to the Swedish Pharmacia® led to the development of modern ophthalmic viscosurgery using Healon®, the first commercially available ophthalmic viscosurgical device (OVD). Ove Wik and his wife Hege Bothner Wik tested various formulations of Balazs's NIF hyaluronic acid, and began using it in ophthalmic surgery. Miller and Stegman were the first to use Healon® in human cataract surgery. In 1980, Healon® was commonly used around the world in ophthalmic surgery. Since then, a large number of viscoelastic substances for intraocular use have appeared, being modified copies of the originals Healon®, Healon® GV and, later, Healon® 5. Their generic name has changed: once called viscoelastic substances, they are now referred as OVDs following the suggestion from Steve Arshinoff, MD (2000) and the recommendations of the International Standards Organization (ISO).[1-5]

Ophthalmic viscosurgical devices are transparent, gel-like substances that have viscous and elastic properties. Composed of sodium hyaluronate, chondroitin sulfate (CDS) and hydroxypropyl methylcellulose, they vary in molecular weights, concentrations and viscosities. These devices can be classified into three main general categories: dispersive, cohesive and viscoadaptatives.

USE OF OPHTHALMIC VISCOSURGICAL DEVICES IN THE OPERATING THEATER

First used in ophthalmic surgery in 1972 as a replacement for vitreous and aqueous humor, OVDs have revolutionized the way cataract surgery is performed, dramatically increasing the safety of modern intraocular surgery.

Ophthalmic viscosurgical devices are used to coat and protect intraocular tissues form mechanical injury, to increase, maintain or preserve the space available for intraocular manipulations, and to displace and stabilize intraocular tissues.

Later, the indications for ophthalmic viscosurgical devices have expanded with the introduction of newly developed ophthalmic viscosurgical devices. In complicated surgeries, modern OVDs can result in ophthalmic surgeons' best friend (like in case of a plane anterior chamber during hyperopic cataract surgery) and have become essential tools in modern mechanized intraocular surgery to facilitate immediate or fast ocular recovery. There are various different OVDs in the operating room, and how to choose the right one as needed during the operation is depended on each special case.

INDICATIONS OF OVDs

Ophthalmic surgery: In ophthalmic surgery (cataract, glaucoma posterior segment) OVDs are used to protect and lubricate the cornea.

In cataract surgery:
- To maintain the anterior chamber during the capsulorhexis and IOL insertion
- To maintain mydriasis and media clarity
- To prevent iris prolapse and trapping nuclear fragments
- To protect the corneal endothelium from turbulences, lens material, and ultrasound energy (placed intracamerally before cataract removal results in significantly decreased endothelial cell loss)
- To enlarge and stabilize the size of the pupil (specific dense ophthalmic viscosurgical devices are used in patients with small pupils or intraoperative floppy iris syndrome)
- To coat the interior of IOL injection cartridge (avoiding the damage of soft IOL's material).

Filtering procedures: In filtering procedures, the use of intracameral and subconjunctival Healon® (Abbott Medical Optics Inc., Santa Clara, CA) promotes superior bleb formation while still maintaining chamber depth postoperatively. In non-perforating procedures, OVDs placed under the scleral flap reduce the risk of early healing and fibrosis. Ophthalmic viscosurgical devices can help to control anterior chamber bleeding. During the whole procedure, they actively participate in corneal wetting and reduce the risk of epithelial damage. A new special injectable cross-linked OVD implant (HealaFlow®, Anteis, Geneva, Switzerland) is described later in this chapter.

Corneal grafts performed over intracameral OVDs receive maximal endothelial protection and show striking postoperative clarity.

Vitreoretinal surgery: In vitreoretinal surgery, OVDs protect corneal epithelium from surgical contact lenses.

In combined cataract-vitrectomy surgery, once the anterior chamber is filled with an OVD, it dramatically reduces the risk of IOL/iris-endothelium contact if gas tamponade is needed, or vitrectomy has to be done under high intraocular pressure to avoid bleeding. Vitreoretinal surgeons should take care to completely remove the OVD at the end of surgery to avoid increased intraocular pressure (IOP). If needed, hyaluronic acid-based OVDs can temporarily replace vitreous (not hydroxypropyl methylcellulose-based OVDs, which may promote vitritis).

CHEMICAL PROPERTIES OF OVDs

The ideal OVD has to fulfill some basic requirements: be easy to inject and easy to remove, maintain volumes, be transparent, give adequate endothelial protection, be sterile, be nontoxic, biologically inert and apyrogenic, be contaminant-free and particle-free, and have a pH similar to that of aqueous humor.

To achieve these goals, three families of molecules are currently used:

i. Sodium hyaluronate (Na-HA) or Hyaluronic acid: A linear polysaccharide molecule of sodium glycuronate and N-acetylglucosamine, which is commonly used in eyedrops and contact lens solutions because of its high wetting and water binding properties. It is a biopolymer found throughout our bodies in connective tissues, including the trabecular meshwork, aqueous and vitreous humors. Hyaluronic acid is also found in cartilage and in the synovial fluid that lubricates the joints: in some patients periodic injections of hyaluronic acid inside the joint temporarily reduce the friction of the worn joints of osteoarthritis, thus greatly helping to reduce pain. Intra-articular HA injections have anti-inflammatory effects: they suppress the synthesis of inflammatory cytokines and of cartilage-degrading proteinases, which are of particular concern in worn and damaged joints.

Hyaluronic acid is derived from "hyalos" (the Greek name for vitreous) and uronic acid, because it was first isolated from the vitreous humor and possesses a high uronic acid content. The term "hyaluronate" refers to the conjugate base of hyaluronic acid. It is the first and oldest OVD and has proved over decades that it will not be easy to substitute. It can be extracted from the dermis of rooster combs, umbilical cords or biosynthesized in bacterial cultures (streptococci) through genetic engineering. Manufacturers emphasize the importance of the product's purity and claim for their proprietary method used to ensure the quality. It is sometimes combined with chondroitin sulfate (e.g. Viscoat®, Alcon Laboratories, Inc., Fort Worth, TX). However, its use is limited in ophthalmic surgeries **(Figure 12.1)**.

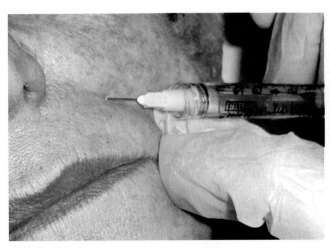

FIGURE 12.1: Hyaluronic acid used in cosmetics to correct moderate-to-severe wrinkles and folds cannot be used for intraocular surgery. The molecules are cross-linked (reticulated) and last for months; most products incorporate an anesthetic to ease intradermal injection, and they are not approved for intraocular use

ii. Chondroitin sulfate (CS): Like hyaluronic acid, chondroitin sulfate is a biopolymer found in the extracellular matrix, mainly in solid tissue parts (like cartilage or corneal stroma). Two chondroitin sulfate proteoglycans are found in the vitreous: Type IX collagen and versican.

It is mainly extracted from shark fin cartilage and bovine or porcine cartilages. The degradation of chondroitin sulfate is also involved in the clinical progression of osteoarthritis: as it degrades, the joint's cartilage loses its ability to resist compression and joint pain, and swelling does occur. Traumatologists have observed in clinical practice the ability of intra-articular chondroitin sulfate injections to reduce the pain and swelling associated with arthritis.

In ophthalmology, at low concentrations it is useful for coating tissues but fails in maintaining spaces because of its low viscosity. By increasing concentration, viscosity is increased but CS causes endothelial dehydration and endothelial cells toxicity. The combination of two biological polymers, 3% sodium hyaluronate and 4% chondroitin sulfate results in a unique chemical structure with good coating ability and good cell protection. In some countries, there is a combination of CS and hydroxypropyl methylcellulose.

iii. Hydroxypropyl methylcellulose (HPMC): It is a disaccharide with side chains that make the molecule more hydrophilic. It is synthesized from methylcellulose, a component of plant fibers like cotton and wood pulp. It is not found in humans or animals. In ophthalmology, methylcellulose is used as a lubricant because of its wetting and coating capacity. Once injected in the human body, methylcellulose shows a significant inflammatory potential, and it is not fully metabolized. It is relatively difficult to completely remove HPMC from the eye: irrigating/aspirating maneuvers may result in corneal damage in compromised corneas.

Polyacrylamide and collagen of porcine origin and other substances have also been evaluated as OVDs, but have only historical interest since they did not show clinical evidence and proved some safety concerns.

Each OVD has unique properties in function of a number of variables that include concentration, molecular weight and size of molecular building blocks of the material (**Table 12.1**). Some products combine two different molecules in the same syringe (like Viscoat®, 3% sodium hyaluronate and 4% chondroitin sulfate, Alcon Laboratories, Inc., Fort Worth, TX) and some manufacturers offer combined packages (two syringes with two different products inside, like Duovisc® from Alcon Laboratories, Inc., that combines Viscoat® and Provisc®). The reader is invited to read further to discover physical-rheological properties and advantages and disadvantages of commercially available presentations.

MOLECULAR ORGANIZATION OF OVDs

Composed of sodium hyaluronate, chondroitin sulfate and methylcellulose, OVDs vary in molecular weights (long chains have high molecular weight) and viscosities. The same way proteins are composed of amino acids, sodium hyaluronate, chondroitin sulfate and hydroxypropyl methylcellulose are composed of different disaccharide units, binded together to form long chains of semi-rigid molecules freely organized in space. When found in a liquid solution, they form long flexible chains, easily injectable through a cannula into the anterior chamber (imagine them as cooked spaghetti pasta, deformable). The higher the molecular weight, the more deformable the molecules are. On the opposite, low-molecular weight products (imagine them as cooked tortellini pasta, nondeformable) need to be injected through a larger cannula because their molecules do not deform while being injected.

Longer chains (high molecular weight) are strongly binded together (high cohesion) and will be easily removed from the eye as a whole, in block: they are easier to remove from the eye since they stick together and are aspirated as long pieces.

PHYSICAL OR RHEOLOGICAL PROPERTIES OF OVDs

Ophthalmic viscosurgical devices were formerly called viscoelastic substances (viscoelastics) because they respond to deforming forces with both elastic and viscous properties. Ophthalmic viscosurgical devices have properties of both fluids and solids, and vary among each other with respect to their molecular composition and the resulting physical and rheological properties. According to these properties, OVDs have different clinical applications in ophthalmic surgery. The rheological properties of viscoelastics

TABLE 12.1 Ophthalmic surgeons and their assistants should be very careful and fulfill every product's conservation needs: some require refrigeration, others do not			
	Sodium hyaluronate (Na-HA) hyaluronic acid	Chondroitin sulfate (CS)	Hydroxypropyl methylcellulose (HPMC)
Requires refrigeration	YES NO: Vitrax II® = 3% Na-Ha (Abbott Medical Optics, Santa Clara, CA)	YES	NO
	Needs acclimatation to room temperature prior to use	Needs acclimatation to room temperature prior to use	Room-temperature storage

TABLE 12.2	Pseudoplasticity is the ability of a solution to change viscosity under various shear (applied forces) conditions	
Low shear	**Medium shear**	**High shear**
Substance at rest Viscosity increases Gel	**Example:** Instruments moving in eye	Substance under force Viscosity decreases Liquid **Example:** Injection through the cannula

determine the classification (read later in this chapter), behavior and utility of each OVD. These properties include viscosity, pseudoplasticity, elasticity, ability to coat (coatability or surface tension) and cohesiveness. Understanding the physical concepts is very useful to understand when making the right choice for use in ophthalmic surgery.

1. *Viscosity:* It can be described as the internal friction caused by molecular attraction that leads to a solution's resistance to flow. It describes the resistance to flow: it is primarily determined by the molecular weight and concentration of an OVD, so that substances with high molecular weight and high concentration have the highest viscosity. Viscosity denotes the protective and lubricating property of a viscoelastic. It varies inversely with temperature.

   The viscosity of OVDs changes with different flow rates: OVDs flow properties are not single and constant (as they are in solutions like water). Water, silicone oil or chondroitin sulfate have viscosities that remain constant when they are exposed to shear forces (shear is defined as the stress that is applied parallel to the material): they are referred as Newtonian substances. Ophthalmic viscosurgical devices become less viscous as shear rate increases, they are pseudoplastic.

   The faster an OVD flows, the greater the decrease in the viscosity, and the easier its injection becomes. Zero flow (or zero shear rate) gives the maximum viscosity of an OVD, which determines the material's stabilizing effect. Medium viscosity occurs at medium flow of fluid or at the velocity at which a surgeon moves instruments through the eye: it describes the mobilizing effects of OVDs. High-viscosity solutions tend to stay within the anterior chamber and separate tissues well.

2. *Pseudoplasticity:* Pseudoplasticity, also called rheofluidity, refers to changes in viscosity with different shear rates (shear being defined as the stress that is applied parallel to the material). It is the ability of a substance to transform when under pressure from a gel-like state to a more liquid state. As mentioned before, some OVDs (chondroitin sulfate) do not have pseudoplasticity because their viscosity is constant regardless of shear rate. Other OVDs (sodium hyaluronate and methylcellulose) demonstrate pseudoplasticity: at higher shear rates, they have lower viscosity. This property enables easy injection and removal of an agent at increasing flow rates. Pseudoplasticity at low shear rates basically depends on molecular weight and concentration of the OVD, but at high shear rates, it becomes independent of molecular weight and concentration **(Table 12.2)**.

3. *Elasticity:* It refers to the ability of a substance or material to return to its original shape after being deformed (i.e. stretched or compressed) **(Figures 12.2A to D)**. Elastic substances are excellent for maintaining space **(Figure 12.3)**. The viscoelasticity of an OVD, determined by its viscosity and molecular structure, allows it to protect ocular tissue from forces such as ultrasound energy and fluid irrigation turbulences. Long molecules (molecules of high molecular weight OVDs) are more elastic than short molecules.

4. *Coatability:* It measures the adhesion capacity of OVDs: it is inversely proportional to surface tension and the contact angle between the OVD and a solid material. It can also be referred as the "lubricating power" of a substance. Thus, an OVD with low surface tension and contact angle is better at coating tissue (i.e. chondroitin sulfate has better coatability than sodium hyaluronate).

   The ability of an OVD to coat the endothelium or the IOL is related to its surface tension, contact angle and molecular charge. Low surface tension, low contact angles and more negatively charged OVDs better coat the endothelium, IOL and instruments. Hydroxypropyl methylcellulose solutions and chondroitin sulfate solutions (alone or in combination with sodium hyaluronate) have lower surface tension and contact angle values than solutions of sodium hyaluronate alone.

5. *Cohesiveness:* Cohesiveness is the degree to which material adheres to itself. It depends on molecular weight, strength of molecular binding and elasticity. The more cohesive an OVD, the lower the flow rate, so cohesive OVDs (e.g. Healon GV®) are good for space maintenance and are easily removed as a bolus during irrigation and aspiration **(Figures 12.4A and B)**. According to cohesiveness parameters, viscoelastics can be classified depending on their point-of-rupture (of the cohesion) and cohesive/dispersive index (CDI) into two main groups: cohesive and dispersive (i.e. not cohesive) substances. The CDI is defined as the percentage of viscoelastic agent aspirated/100 mm Hg; it classifies OVDs in terms of viscosity, cohesion and dispersion. The higher the CDI, the quicker the substance can be aspirated when a certain amount of aspiration is reached. This classification system also accounts for the not so traditional

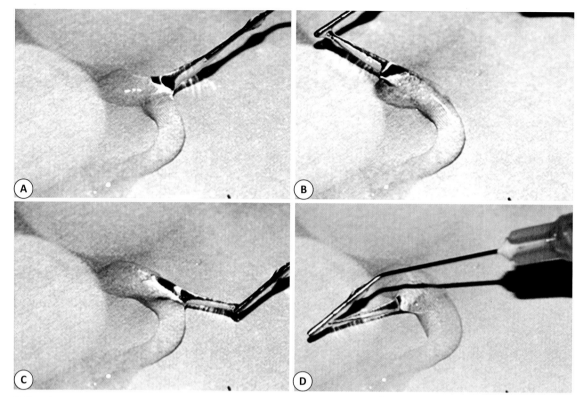

FIGURES 12.2A TO D: Images of an experimental OVD in laboratory: the cannula is being moved around after touching the surface of the substance. Observe the high adhesion power (the OVD is permanently attached to the cannula) and the elasticity of the substance that changes its shape according to the traction forces

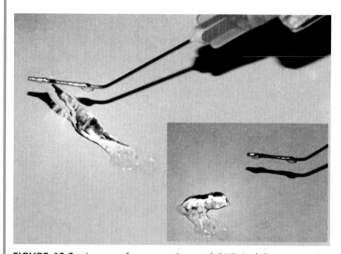

FIGURE 12.3: Image of an experimental OVD in laboratory: the cannula touches the surface of the substance. Observe the high adhesion power (the OVD is attached to the cannula) and the elasticity of the substance. The detail shows the ability of the substance to coat the cannula once adhesion is broken by intense traction

viscoadaptive OVD Healon5®, and viscous-dispersive DisCoVisc® products. The viscoadaptive Healon5® is highly viscous and cohesive at low-flow rate phaco-emulsification but under high-shear conditions, it breaks and acts as a highly dispersive substance. In comparison to traditional cohesive OVDs (like Healon GV®), the viscous-dispersive DisCoVisc® is considered a higher viscosity dispersive, but has a zero-shear viscosity (i.e. viscosity at rest) like more cohesive OVDs **(Figure 12.5).**

6. *Dispersiveness:* It is the tendency of a material to disperse when injected into the anterior chamber. Dispersive viscoelastics (like hydroxypropyl methylcellulose) have low molecular weights and short molecular chains: therefore, they are difficult to remove.

CLASSIFICATION OF OVDs (TABLE 12.3)

The aim of this chapter is to help surgeons to easily understand the full spectrum of OVDs: the abundance of commercial presentations and the confusing variety of marketing strategies make it very difficult to easily decide, which OVD is preferable for each step of a surgery.

To simplify the choice, the authors classify OVDs according to their consistency spectrum, from dispersive to cohesive into four groups:

1. *Dispersive:* They have a low viscosity and the ability to coat intraocular structures. The molecules behave separately and build up a solution (honey-like). They tend to stay in place during the fluidic movements of phacoemulsification surgery.
2. *Cohesive:* They have high viscosity and are able to give pressure to the eye and create and maintain space. They act like a gel: the entire volume of OVD tends to stick together during the fluidic movements of phacoemulsification surgery.
3. *Combination OVDs (dispersive/cohesive):* They are a new generation of viscoelastics. Imagine them as highly viscous dispersive OVDs. They are supposed to combine

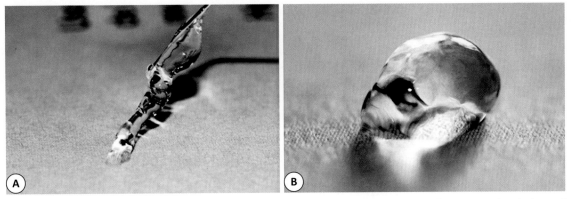

FIGURES 12.4A AND B: A highly cohesive experimental OVD is being injected on a paper surface: notice that during and after injection the molecules remain together in a compact droplet volume that proves the cohesive characteristics of this high molecular weight substance

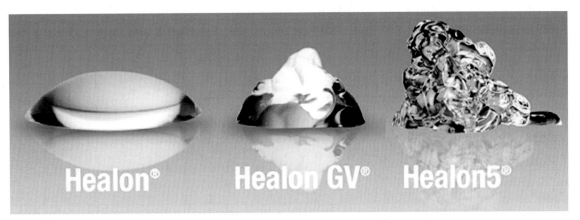

FIGURE 12.5: Image represents the cohesiveness of the Healon® family of OVDs (Abbott Medical Optics, Santa Clara, CA) so that the reader can deduce their ability to create and maintain space. Healon® is a cohesive OVD with some dispersive properties, and Healon GV® is a highly cohesive OVD while Healon5® is an ultra-cohesive OVD with "viscoadaptative" properties that make it unique in the classification of OVDs. Read later in this chapter for explanation of viscoadaptative properties. Source: Abbott Medical Optics

the best of dispersive and cohesives. They have characteristics of both high viscosity cohesive OVDs, as well as low viscosity dispersive OVDs. They are sold as OVDs for every surgical need.

4. *Viscoadaptative OVD:* The rheological properties vary with the fluidics of phacoemulsification surgery. A viscoadaptative OVD changes its behavior at different flow rates. Healon5® (Abbott Medical Optics, Santa Clara, CA) was the first and only product marketed as viscoadaptative (**Figures 12.6A and B**). Imagine it as a pseudodispersive, super-viscous cohesive that behaves as a highly cohesive viscoelastic to pressurize and create space, but can also provide the protection of a dispersive OVD. At low flow rates, it is very viscous and cohesive. At high flow rates, it becomes pseudodispersive and effectively protects endothelial cells.

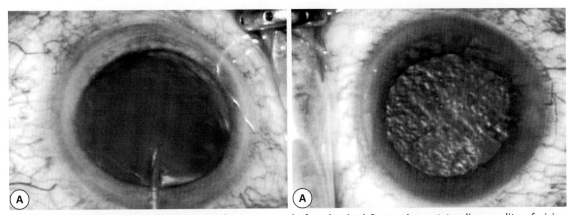

FIGURES 12.6A AND B: Not all OVDs are the same: try before buying! Some give outstanding quality of vision during surgery, while others clearly difficult surgeon's view through the microscope. *Source:* Abbott Medical Optics, Santa Clara, CA. (A) Healon® OVD and (B) Competitive viscoelastic

TABLE 12.3 Simplified classification of OVDs according to their chemical and physical properties

	HPMC (always dispersive)	Dispersive Na-Ha	Cohesive Na-Ha	Super Cohesive Na-Ha	Viscoadaptative Na-Ha (dispersive/cohesive)
Example (more are commercially available)	*Ocucoat®*	*Vitrax II®*	*Healon® (is a cohesive with some dispersive properties)*	*Healon® GV*	*Healon® 5 (viscoadaptative)*
Cohesion degree	-/+	+	++	+++	++/+++++ (varies with flow)
Molecular Weight *The higher the molecular weight, the higher the viscosity*	Low (>80,000 daltons)	Low (500,000-800,000 daltons)	High/Very high (4,000,000 daltons)	Very high (5,000,000 daltons)	High/Very high (4,000,000 daltons)
Concentration	1-2%	3%	1%	1.4%	2.3%
Zero shear viscosity (Viscosity at rest) *The higher the zero-shear viscosity, the more viscous the OVD is at rest*	-/+ (86,000 mPas)	+ (42,000-56,000 mPas)	++ (300,000 mPas)	+++ (3,000,000 mPas)	+++ (7,000,000 mPas)
Pseudoplasticity	-/+	+	++	+++	++/+++
Elasticity	-/+	+	+++	+++	-/++
Cohesion/dispersion index *The higher the – cohesion/dispersion index, the quicker the OVD can be aspirated when a certain value of vacuum is reached*	-	-	(31.2)	(72.3)	-

Summary of "cohesive-versus-dispersive" OVDs rheologic characteristics is shown in **Table 12.4** and advantages and disadvantages of cohesive OVDs are shown in **Table 12.5**. The required OVD properties for each step of modern cataract surgery are shown in **Table 12.6**.

A BUYING GUIDE FOR THE NOVICE SURGEON

Different manufacturers sell different OVDs, with different presentations. Ophthalmic viscosurgical devices are presented in syringes of different volumes (either 0.5 ml, 0.6 ml, 0.85 ml, 1 ml or 2 ml). Modern safe phaco requires larger volumes than old procedures: always try to have as much OVD as possible: it is not rare that an uncomplicated surgery requires a couple of syringes.

Modern presentations include the following:
1. One syringe (of variable volume) of a substance alone (either sodium hyaluronate, chondroitin sulfate or hydroxypropyl methylcellulose, at different concentrations) (e.g. 1% Na-Ha Healon®, Abbott Medical Optics Inc., Santa Clara, CA, is available in 0.4 ml, 0.55 ml and 0.85 ml). They are presented in different concentrations and classified as dispersive or cohesive. The gauge of the cannula is different depending on the molecular weight of the molecules: high molecular weight substances are more deformable and need a thinner cannula. Hydroxypropyl methylcellulose OVDs have the larger cannulas, and since the product is less expensive to produce the syringe contains a larger amount of OVD, typically 2 ml (e.g. while Healon® can be injected through a 27 g cannula, Ocucoat® HMPC, Bausch & Lomb, needs a 20 g cannula because its molecules are less deformable).

2. One syringe with two mixed substances inside (e.g. Viscoat®, Alcon Laboratories, Inc., Fort Worth, TX, contains 3% Na-Ha and 4% CDS). A recently introduced product, Eyefil® DC (Croma-Pharma, Austria) contains a novel combination of 1.37% biofermentative hyaluronic acid and 0.57% HPMC.

3. One syringe with two phases: first phase, which will be first injected, contains an OVD suitable for capsulorhexis and phacoemulsification (**Figures 12.7A and B**), while the second phase (which will be injected later) contains another OVD suitable for IOL implantation (e.g. Ixium Twin®, LCA Pharmaceutical, France: phase one contains 2% Na-Ha and phase 2 contains 1.4% Na-Ha).

TABLE 12.4 Summary of "cohesive-versus-dispersive" OVDs rheologic characteristics

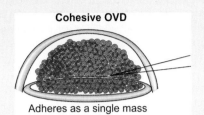
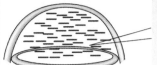

Cohesive OVD	Dispersive OVD
Adheres as a single mass "Jelly-Like"	Spreads out to coat surfaces "Honey-like"
• High molecular weight • High viscosity • Adhere to themselves • Resist breaking apart • High pseudoplasticity • Easy to remove from the eye using irrigation and aspiration	• Low molecular weight • Low viscosity • Adhere to external surfaces • Tend to break apart • Low pseudoplasticity • More difficult to remove from the eye, requiring aspiration

TABLE 12.5 Advantages and disadvantages of cohesive OVDs

Advantages of cohesive OVDs Healon® (Abbott Medical Optics), Healon GV® (Abbott MO), Provisc® (Alcon), Amvisc® (Bausch & Lomb)	Disadvantages of cohesive OVDs Healon® (Abbott Medical Optics), Healon GV® (Abbott MO), Provisc® (Alcon), Amvisc® (Bausch & Lomb)
Create, deepen and maintain space in anterior chamber	They can come out of the eye easily as a whole during surgery or under intense vitreous pressure (specially in case of large incisions)
Clear vision, transparency	They are unwillingly removed during phacoemulsification
Ideal for flattening the anterior capsule to facilitate capsulorhexis	They do not stay attached to corneal endothelium
Ideal to open capsular bag for IOL insertion	Some have a high risk of postoperative IOP peaks if not completely removed (e.g. Healon® 5)
They mechanically enlarge and stabilize the size of the pupil	
Easy to remove at the end of procedure	
Advantages of dispersive OVDs Vitrax® (Abbott Medical Optics), Viscoat (Alcon), and OcuCoat (Bausch & Lomb)	**Disadvantages of dispersive OVDs** Vitrax® (Abbott Medical Optics), Viscoat (Alcon), and OcuCoat (Bausch & Lomb)
Ability to coat intraocular structures	Low viscosity dispersives do not maintain spaces well
They stay adhered to endothelium during the emulsification procedure (Endothelial Protection)	May have air bubbles inside or form microbubbles during surgery
They tend to stay in place during the fluidics of phacoemulsification surgery (high shear rates)	Difficult to remove completely at the end of procedure (risk of postoperative non inflammatory Tyndall in the anterior chamber)
They separate spaces (ability to partition spaces, surgical compartmentalization). They hold vitreous back in case of loose zonules or in case of a small hole in the posterior capsule)	Some may not be completely transparent or can see transparency reduced under ultrasonic waves
Ability to lubricate IOL and injector	They fragment into small pieces during irrigation and aspiration and this may obscure the visualization of posterior capsule during surgery
Removal of dispersive OVDs requires more effort at the end of procedure	

	Main OVD function	Required properties	Category	Our usual choice
TABLE 12.6 There is no perfect OVD that suits every surgical need. This table summarizes the required OVD properties for each step of modern cataract surgery (ultrasonic phacoemulsification). The column "our usual choice" is given to help novice surgeons to choose a good viscoelastic: the authors have learned modern surgery under the "protection" of Pharmacia's Healon® and since then they trust this manufacturer and mainly use viscoelastics from the Healon® family (Abbott Medical Optics, Santa Clara, CA). Other manufacturers (e.g. Alcon Laboratories, Inc., Fort Worth, TX) supply excellent products, like chondroitin-based OVDs for extreme endothelial protection. Not all OVDs are created equal. The reader is invited to try different OVDs and decide which one does better suit his surgical and cost-effectiveness needs				
Endothelial protection (a must in endothelial corneal diseases)	Endothelial coating (the main OVD function, especially in compromised corneas)	High viscosity and adhesion at any shear rate	Dispersive/Cohesive	Vitrax® Healon® (a cohesive with some dispersive properties)
Capsulorhexis	Maintain deep stable anterior chamber	High viscosity at zero or low shear rates	Highly Cohesive	Healon® GV
Ultrasonic lens emulsification	Remain in eye Coat tissues Protect endothelium	Low/medium molecular weight High viscosity at high shear rates	Dispersive/Cohesive Viscoadaptative	Healon® Healon5® (refill anterior chamber with fresh unfractured Healon5® before phaco)
Nuclear cracking with manipulators	Maintain deep stable anterior chamber	High elasticity	Highly Cohesive	Healon® GV
Cortex removal I/A	Endothelial coating at any flow rate	Low surface tension High viscosity and adhesion at any shear rate	Dispersive/Cohesive Viscoadaptative	Healon® Healon5®
IOL lubrication in cartridge (loading and injecting)	IOL protection	High viscosity and adhesion at zero shear rate	Dispersive Dispersive/cohesive	Healon® Any dispersive OVD (including cheaper HMPC)
IOL insertion into the bag	Expand capsular bag Maintain deep and stable anterior chamber	High viscosity and adhesion at low shear rate High elasticity	Cohesive Cohesive/Dispersive	**With vitreous pressure:** Healon GV® **Without vitreous pressure:** Healon®
OVD removal	Easy to remove completely and quickly	High molecular weight High surface tension	Cohesive	*Healon5® complete removal may not be easy or complete, resulting in increased postoperative IOP*

Another available product from Carl Zeiss Meditec, Twinvisc®, presents two OVDs as the other way round. The first product to be injected is dispersive Na-Ha and the second product is cohesive Na-Ha. This combination should be ideally suited for the Arshinoff's soft-shell technique (described later in this chapter), where a dispersive agent (1% Na-Ha) is injected first to isolate and protect the endothelium, and a cohesive (2.2% Na-HA) agent is injected just after to create and maintain space **(Figure 12.8).**

4. A combination package like Duovisc®, Alcon Laboratories, Inc., that includes a couple of syringes, one is the 3% Na-Ha + 4% CS combination Viscoat® and the other one is 1% Na-Ha Provisc®. One such package is usually enough to complete most cataract surgeries. Different syringe volumes may be available in some countries.

5. A combination of a cohesive OVD and an anesthetic product (e.g. Visthesia®, Carl Zeiss Meditec, provides topical an intracameral anesthesia in a single product, combining 1% lidocaine and 1% or 1.5% sodium hyaluronate). Applied preoperatively on the cornea, it provides topical anesthesia and protection and hydration of the cornea. Injected intracamerally it provides intraocular anesthesia, maintains pupil dilation, protects endothelium and provides space for surgical maneuvers and IOL insertion. Visthesia® 1% and Visthesia® 1,5% may not be sold in some countries.

6. For glaucoma surgery: Healaflow® (Anteis, Switzerland) is a slowly resorbable cross-linked sodium hyaluronate injectable implant, indicated for penetrating and non-penetrating glaucoma surgery **(Figures 12.9A and B)**. It is a transparent viscoelastic gel, obtained by biofermentation (nonanimal origin), presented in 0.6 ml

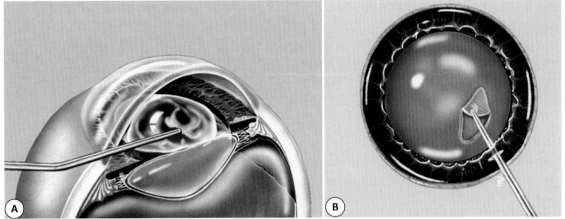

FIGURES 12.7A AND B: Capsulorhexis is an essential step in modern ultrasound phacoemulsification. To safely perform it, either with a cystitome or a forceps, the OVD has to fulfill the following requirements: be transparent and easy to inject, high viscosity to maintain space and volume, must no leave anterior chamber easily, high elasticity to reject tissues (like in case of dealing with a myotic pupil), and a good pseudoplasticity to maintain spaces and the capsular tear. To perform capsulorhexis, the authors prefer cohesive OVDs (like Healon GV®) that are able to pressurize the eye and create space: they are ideal for flattening the anterior capsule to facilitate capsulorhexis creation or for deepening a shallow anterior chamber (e.g. in case of a highly hyperopic cataract). Examples of common cohesive OVDs include Healon® (Abbott Medical Optics Inc., Santa Clara, CA), higher viscosity Healon GV® (Abbott Medical Optics Inc., Santa Clara, CA), Provisc® (Alcon Laboratories, Inc., Fort Worth, TX), and the recent 1.6% Na-Ha Amvisc Plus® (Bausch & Lomb)

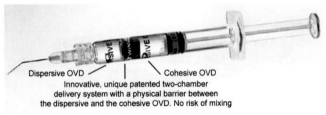

FIGURE 12.8: Twinvisc®, Carl Zeiss Meditec, contains two OVDs: the first product to be injected is dispersive 1% Na-Ha and the second product is cohesive 2.2% Na-Ha. This combination should be ideally suited for the Arshinoff's soft-shell technique, where the dispersive agent is injected first to isolate and protect the endothelium, and the cohesive agent is injected just after to create and maintain space. Source: Carl Zeiss Meditec

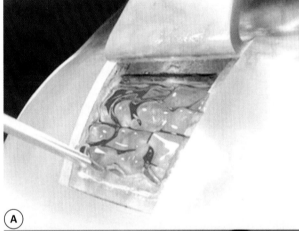

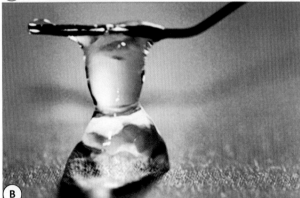

disposable glass syringe with a 25 Gauge 7/8 cannula. Injected under the scleral flap and the conjunctiva, it acts as a drainage implant and limits the postoperative fibrosis thus clearly improving the surgical success rate and in most cases eliminating the need of antifibrotic agents like mitomycin-C. It has a clear anti-inflammatory effect and can be used in any antiglaucoma surgery: in trabeculectomy, deep sclerectomy, viscocanalostomy and after implantation of antiglaucoma shunts, valves or tubes. This particular reticulated OVD can be injected either into the scleral lake, under the scleral flap or under the conjunctiva. It lasts up to 6 months within the surgical site. It is not approved for intraocular use for cataract surgery though being a cross-linked Na-Ha OVD, this would result into dangerous IOP increase.

*** *The products described in this chapter may not be available in every country: the reader is kindly invited to ask local surgical representatives for product availability, presentations and pricing.* ***

FIGURES 12.9A AND B: Healaflow® (Anteis, Switzerland) is a highly cohesive slowly resorbable cross-linked sodium hyaluronate injectable implant indicated for penetrating and non-penetrating glaucoma surgery. Injected under the scleral flap and the conjunctiva, it acts as a drainage implant and limits the postoperative fibrosis. This particular cross-linked OVD can be injected either into the scleral lake, under the scleral flap or under the conjunctiva. Source: Anteis, Geneva, Switzerland

ARSHINOFF'S SOFT-SHELL TECHNIQUE

Steve Arshinoff published the simultaneous use of different categories of OVDs for the first time in 1999 (Arshinoff SA, Dispersive-cohesive viscoelastic soft shell technique. J Cataract Refract Surg. 1999;25:167-73) and this technique has become a standard in advanced surgical facilities.

A low viscosity dispersive (or dispersive/cohesive) agent is first injected into the anterior chamber (Healon®, a dispersive/cohesive agent is mainly used). Then a high-cohesive OVD (e.g. Healon GV®) is injected into the posterior center of the dispersive agent, towards anterior capsule surface. Once the cataract has been extracted, its better to proceed the other-way-round: the cohesive OVD is injected first, and then the low viscosity dispersive viscoelastic is injected in the center of the high viscosity OVD. The cohesive agent will stabilize the intraocular tissues during IOL insertion, and the dispersive agent will be easily aspirated at the end of surgery by placing irrigating/aspirating cannula on the IOL at the pupillary plane. The cohesive OVD will be easily removed as a bolus after that.

Other techniques combining viscoelastics and/or balanced salt solution (BSS®, Alcon Laboratories, Inc. Fort Worth, TX) have been described, like "best-of-both-worlds" or the "ultimate soft-shell-technique," but the original version is still preferred, which has given us unprecedented surgical comfort and endothelial protection.

For example, some surgeons use a shell technique with BSS® on the capsule and under Healon5® OVD. When injecting BSS®, the highly viscous cohesive OVD is forced upward, pressurizing the anterior chamber. Capsulorhexis can then be performed in a watery environment with no resistance. Using this shell technique slows surgery, but provides good condition for controlled capsulorhexis without peripheral extension: the rhexis may be smaller than anticipated.

Another approach may be to inject a bubble of Healon5® centrally on anterior capsule, just smaller than the desired size of capsulorhexis: Healon5® acts as ones finger when a person cut a paper using his/her fingers (without scissors).

OUR PREFERRED OVDs FOR SPECIAL SURGICAL SITUATIONS

In the hands of an experienced surgeon, any OVD will work for an uncomplicated surgery. A cataract surgery is even achieved without using an OVD, but the aim of modern OVDs is to make surgery easier and safer than it was before. The agents that are used have not changed much. The agents are still limited to hyaluronic acid (Na-HA), chondroitin sulfate (CS) and hydroxypropyl methylcellulose (HPMC). What has changed in the last years is the use of various combinations of these substances, and the commercial presentations.

VITAL STAINS IN CATARACT SURGERY

A capsulorhexis may be difficult to perform in the absence of a red fundus reflex (hypermature or white cataracts).

Trypan blue and indocyanine green appear to be the most effective dyes in staining the anterior capsule. Injection strategies should be aimed at reducing uncontrolled dispersion in anterior chamber and especially into the vitreous. Using less than 0.1 ml of trypan blue 0.1% or lissamine green 0.5% to stain the anterior capsule enables us to visualize the capsulorhexis during phacoemulsification.

Vital dyes should be injected in the smallest possible amounts with a 0.1 ml insulin syringe, avoiding their contact with corneal endothelium. To avoid the contact with endothelium, they can be injected in the pupillary plane, under an air-bubble that fills the anterior chamber, or over anterior capsule under a cohesive or –preferably- a viscoadaptive OVD. Make sure that Healon5® fills around 90% on the anterior chamber and does not occlude the incision before injecting the dye under the OVD. To reduce ocular exposure, vital stains should not be injected into an anterior chamber filled with aqueous humor: first empty the anterior chamber's aqueous humor with an air-bubble (or Healon5®) and then inject the vital dye under the air bubble or the OVD. Let the dye stain the anterior capsule during one minute and clean it with BSS®, before filling the anterior chamber with the cohesive OVD to perform the rhexis.

OPHTHALMIC VISCOSURGICAL DEVICES IN MICRO-INCISION CATARACT SURGERY (MICS)

During MICS, the incision is so small that the needs of OVDs are greatly reduced. A cohesive OVD will flatten the anterior capsule for precise capsulorhexis (with a bent needle or a microforceps), and a dispersive is injected before emulsification for endothelial protection. Anterior chamber depth maintenance is not a priority in MICS. During hydrodissection, there is an increased risk of posterior capsule break resulting from excessive pressure (the anterior chamber being almost sealed) **(Figures 12.10A and B)**. Ophthalmic viscosurgical devices must be aspirated or moved by pressing the posterior lip of the incision before hydrodissection or hydrodelineation, and the BSS® (Alcon, Fort Worth, TX) injection must be very careful and progressive with periodic decompression of anterior chamber (also by pressing the posterior lip of the incision).

SMALL PUPIL

In a case of pupil that dilates poorly (e.g. pseudoexfoliation, congenital cataracts, previous irradiation), the eye is prepared preoperatively with topical 1% homatropine eye drops at night-time, 3 days-a-week, starting a couple of months before surgery. On the day of operation, topical combination of 5–10% phenylephrine and tropicamide is used, a part from 0.5–1% cycloplegic drops, instilled every 20 minutes form one and a half hour before surgery. This topical regime works with most cases. Lower concentrations are used in babies and patients at risk of hypertension or heart disease.

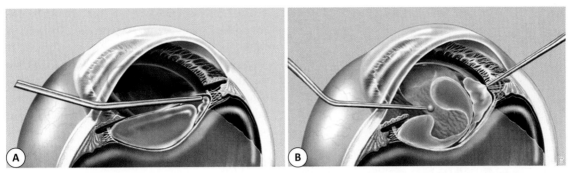

FIGURES 12.10A AND B: Ophthalmic viscosurgical devices are invaluable tools for the novice surgeon confronting surgical difficulties. They greatly help to finish incomplete hydrodissection and nuclear rotation (viscodissection and viscoexpression of the nucleus) and allow to correct positioning of nucleus, or levitation of a cortical shield or remnants to be aspirated/emulsified in the pupillary plane. There are certain indications for using a viscoelastic agent in the capsular bag in the presence of nuclear material, such as loose zonules and difficulty in rotating the lens within the bag. Our residents are always instructed to use OVDs in case of doubt: the use of OVDs always pays despite the fact that the authors do not like wasting viscoelastic substances. Ophthalmic viscosurgical devices are synonyms of surgical safety and surgeon's peace of mind

If mydriasis is still not enough to undergo a safe surgery, superviscous and cohesive OVDs greatly help to mechanically dilate the pupil (e.g Healon GV® and Healon5®, Abbott Medical Optics, Santa Clara, CA) if injected in a circular manner just in front of the pupillary border, in such way that forces move the pupillary border to the periphery. Viscomydriasis is talked about and Healon5® moves the pupil like any other OVD. It moves tissues and maintains space extraordinarily well because of its high molecular weight and concentration.

If present, posterior synechiae could be broken using either a spatula or the OVD cannula (viscosynechialysis).

During surgery, repetitive injections of OVD are needed (together with high infusion levels) to achieve an adequate pupil size until surgery is completed. Healon5® is unique in its ability to effectively dilate a pupil that does not respond to topical or intracameral mydriatics (e.g. lidocaine), and to restore and maintain pupil dilation in case of a progressive intraoperative miosis. Even in cases with shallow anterior chambers (like hyperopic cataract surgery), Healon5® has an extraordinary ability to move tissues and to maintain space providing the surgeon with a stable anterior chamber in which to perform a continuous circular capsulorhexis.

Nevertheless, in some cases iris hooks (e.g. posterior synechiae, patients with uveitis, trabeculectomized patients) are still to be used. Stretching of the iris sphincter, doing small sphincterotomies, and the use of mechanical iris expanders may also be useful in the management of the small pupil.

INTRAOPERATIVE FLOPPY IRIS SYNDROME (IFIS)

Intraoperative floppy iris syndrome is a common cause of progressive pupillary constriction during cataract surgery, caused by a loss of iris rigidity and a reduction of the iris dilator muscle tone. This syndrome is due to the use of a systemic tamsulosin, a selective alpha-1a blocker used in

men to reduce clinical manifestations of prostatic disease. Tamsulosin (Flomax™, Flomaxtra™, Urimax™, Omnic™) is commonly used in the treatment of benign prostatic hyperplasia (prostate adenoma) in men, but is also used as an "off-label" treatment to help managing female urinary retention. Tamsulosin can be used either alone, or in association with dutasteride. The Food and Drug Administration (FDA) has cleared this combination pill in 2010.

During cataract surgery, it presents as an undulating iris with normal intraoperative fluid parameters. The iris has a tendency to prolapse and progressive myosis is observed.

Preoperative cessation of tamsulosin does not eliminate iris dysfunction, and the pupils of patients with IFIS usually dilate normally with pharmacological mydriatics. To reduce the risk of IFIS, 10% phenylephrine eye drops (in combination with other mydriatic agents, either tropicamide or cycloplegic) are always used to dilate pupils for surgery. It is observed that this topical mydriatic regime greatly reduces the risk of IFIS. To reduce the risk of iris prolapse, a tunnelized clear corneal incision (not peripheral) is performed and Healon5® is injected at the angle under the incision to mechanically avoid iris prolapse is injected, making sure not to trap the OVD under the iris. During surgery, the lowest possible infusion and IOP parameters are also used **(Figure 12.11)**.

The progressive pupillary constriction occurs always after surgery has begun. Intraoperative iris stretching and pupillary sphincterotomies are usually ineffective to restore a good dilation. In some cases, iris hooks or ring expanders are necessary, but most of the cases of patients under tamsulosin can be managed safely with an intensive dilating regime that includes phenylephrine and the use of intracameral Healon5®. To maintain pupil size after filling anterior chamber with Healon5®, the aspiration rate and the vacuum level is to be reduced as much as possible, and work in the posterior chamber or the pupillary plane.

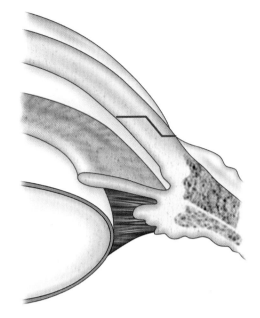

FIGURE 12.11: To reduce the risk of iris prolapse, a tunnelized clear-cornea incision (not peripheral) is performed and Healon5® at the angle under the incision to mechanically avoid iris prolapse is injected, making sure not to trap the OVD under the iris

IRIS HERNIATION OR PROLAPSE

For routine cataract surgeries, a clear-cornea tunnelized incision is almost always perfomed, which makes iris herniation almost impossible. Herniation of the iris during cataract surgery can be avoided by the means of partial elimination of the OVD before hydrodissection, especially if anterior chamber has been intensively deepened with a cohesive OVD for the capsulorhexis. Before hydrodissection, the posterior lip of the incision is slightly pressed with the cannula through which balanced salt solution will be injected for hydrodissection/hydrodelineation, in such a way that the OVD to exit the anterior chamber is forced.

If you use Healon5®, make sure that the OVD does not prevent fluid from escaping out of the incision and check that it does not push the iris towards incision.

If iris herniation persists, excessive OVD can be aspirated through paracentesis, to reduce intraocular pressure. If necessary, a small iridotomy can be performed so that cohesive OVD finds a way out of the posterior chamber.

POSTERIOR CAPSULE TEAR AND VITREOUS PRESENTATION

A dispersive OVD without HPMC is preferable confronting an open capsule with or without vitreous presentation: it protects against vitreous prolapse, coats the anterior chamber, and provides extra protection for the undamaged residual capsule. It allows you to viscoelevate the lens material anteriorly towards pupillary plane or anterior chamber where lens material can be safely aspirated. A dispersive OVD is an indispensable tool for viscoelevation. Additionally, the cannula is useful for manipulating lens material in the anterior chamber. Cohesive OVD may be

useful in case of iris prolapse, but should be injected far from posterior capsule tear or zonular disinsertion to avoid it falling to the vitreous and enlarge the capsule tear.

Hydroxypropyl methylcellulose-based OVDs are "low-cost" dispersives but should not be used in the case of posterior capsule tear: mixed with vitreous they usually produce a certain amount of vitritis (with increased risk of cystoid macular edema).

LOW ENDOTHELIAL CELL COUNTS (E.G. CORNEA GUTTATA)

Most phaco surgeons using common phaco machines with old fluidics (like Bausch & Lomb™ Millennium®), emulsify nuclear material at or just above the pupillary plane to be far enough form posterior capsule. This comprehensible protective attitude endangers endothelial cells. Ultrasonic energy rapidly damages endothelial cells: patients with low preoperative endothelial cell count need absolute endothelial protection. Cohesive agents leave the eye within a couple of minutes after beginning phacoemulsification. They are good in maintaining anterior chamber but not good enough to give endothelial protection. Therefore, if the surgeon does not have a dispersive agent in the eye, the endothelium will suffer intense cellular damage. Turbulences and fluid flow are probably much more traumatic to the endothelium than phaco power and heat.

In most patients, but especially in patients with preoperative endothelial damage (e.g. Fuchs' dystrophy), the dispersive-cohesive Arshinoff's soft-shell technique is always use: a low viscosity dispersive agent is first injected into the anterior chamber (e.g. Vitrax® or Healon®, a cohesive with dispersive properties). Then a high-cohesive OVD (e.g. Healon GV®) is injected into the posterior center of the dispersive agent, towards anterior capsule surface. Once the cataract has been extracted, the surgeons proceed the other-way-round and the cohesive OVD is injected first, and then the low viscosity dispersive viscoelastic is injected in the center of the high viscosity OVD. The cohesive agent will stabilize the intraocular tissues during IOL insertion, and the dispersive agent will be easily aspirated at the end of surgery by placing irrigating/aspirating cannula on the IOL at the pupillary plane. The cohesive OVD will be easily removed as a bolus after that.

In cases with some kind of endothelial disease (or corneal opacity), cornea is not crystal clear and the microscope's optical quality and the choice of the OVD become critical. The transparency of some OVDs decreases as phaco surgery progresses. The reader is invited to perform two cataract surgeries one after the other. For the first one using Healon GV® and for the second using Amvisc Plus® and a clear difference is easily visible. The loss of transparency is more evident if your surgical microscope is not top-notch: if you are in quest for a surgical microscope and you can afford it, do not doubt, buy a Carl Zeiss Meditec™ Lumera®, and you will see details never imagined before.

In order to protect corneas against mechanical, thermal and sonic forces, a dispersive viscoelastic is periodically injected into the anterior chamber (it is done at each surgical step). Cohesive OVDs do not completely protect the cornea against turbulences: a dispersive OVD is required (e.g. Vitrax®, Abbott Medical Optics, Santa Clara, CA). For that purpose, chondroitin sulfate/sodium hyaluronate DisCoVisc® (Alcon Laboratories, Inc., Fort Worth, TX) provides very good endothelial protection at each surgical step.

The HPMC-based OVDs are not used. They are useful to lubricate the corneal epithelium in posterior segment surgeries, to lubricate an IOL in the cartridge, or even to avoid opening a new expensive OVD at the end of a surgery. However, they take too long to remove it from the eye, thus endangering endothelium, which might be critical in a compromised cornea.

CONGENITAL CATARACTS

The newborn eye has some special characteristics that makes cataract surgery very difficult. In the newborn eye, pupil is myotic and dilates poorly (dilator muscle poorly developed) and its endothelium lifetime is supposed to be longer than it is in adults. Its depth of anterior chamber is minimum and the eye is very small (no space to work), the scleral rigidity is very low (important fluctuations of anterior chamber during surgery), vitreous pressure is very intense (dense vitreous) and anterior lens capsule is extremely elastic, making it very difficult to initiate and complete tearing of anterior capsule.

Capsulorhexis is made easier by using highly cohesive OVDs to increase anterior chamber depth and flatten the surface of the anterior capsule. The reduced depth of anterior chamber and the intense vitreous pressure make it very easy to have radial tears and the rhexis to run-away. To reduce the risks, a small rhexis (4–5 mm) is performed and the periphery of anterior chamber is filled with Healon5® before and when doing the procedure, to better control unexpected rhexis run-aways.

The dense cohesive OVD will stabilize posterior capsule and push vitreous back in case a posterior rhexis is needed (e.g. opaque posterior capsule plaque).

ANTERIOR CHAMBER BLEEDING DURING SURGERY

Anterior chamber bleeding is not uncommon in combined glaucoma-cataract surgery, with or without peripheral iridectomy. It is not common with clear corneal incisions, but sometimes intensive deepening of anterior chamber with cohesive OVDs, or IOP changes during surgery result in small bleeding of anterior chamber angle vessels. Risk factors are diabetic patients (with or without iris new-vessels) or patients under platelet aggregation inhibitors.

To effectively cut the bleeding, eye pressure can be raised by means of dispersive OVDs injected over the bleeding vessel, surrounded by the injection of a cohesive

OVD. If necessary, sutures can be placed to close anterior chamber until bleeding cessation.

In combined glaucoma-cataract surgery, OVDs from anterior chamber are not removed till the very end of surgery. The surgery is finished with a comfortable anterior chamber depth and without hypotony bleeding. At the end of surgery, BSS® through the paracentesis is injected to remove OVD from the anterior chamber and the filtering bleb (with a mixture of BSS® and OVD) is obtained and filled.

REMOVAL OF OVDs

At the end of cataract surgery, surgeon's next mission is to completely remove OVDs from anterior chamber as well as from behind the IOL, and that without damaging endothelium or moving IOL form its desired position.

Complete removal of OVD substances from the eye dramatically reduces the risk of postoperative intraocular pressure peaks, which might be extremely dangerous in the case of a damaged optic nerve (e.g. advanced glaucoma patient).

Complete removal of OVD is essential for keeping a toric IOL in the right position at the end of surgery.

Postoperative recovery greatly benefits from careful cleansing of OVDs. It is observed that OVD substances left behind IOL, inside the capsular back, can increase the risk of posterior capsule opacification with the presence of a milky material that reduces visual acuity until posterior Nd-YAG capsulotomy is performed. The milky material is then cleared when mixed with the vitreous body without signs of inflammation (the milky material is not septic). The acute distension of capsular bag has been observed in one patient with incomplete retrolental OVD removal, with intense refraction changes and reduced visual acuity. The patient was successfully treated with a posterior Nd-YAG capsulotomy that rapidly resulted in visual recovery and stable refraction.

Cohesive OVDs, despite the fact that they are responsible of most postoperative intraocular postoperative elevations, are easier to remove than dispersive OVDs. Due to their retentiveness, removal of dispersive OVDs requires more effort at the end of surgery.

Ophthalmic viscosurgical devices can be removed using either bimanual or coaxial irrigation/aspiration handpieces **(Figures 12.12A and B)**.

The unique viscoadaptive properties of Healon5® (Abbott Medical Optics, Santa Clara, CA) deliver a winning combination of protection and control, but extra care must be used to ensure that Healon5® OVD has been completely removed. The removal is started after IOL implantation shifting IOL aside for access to Healon5® from the capsular bag and from behind the IOL. Once Healon5® is removed from the posterior chamber, the irrigation/aspiration (I/A) tip is brought in front of the optic and is continued with high vacuum and the hole of the tip upwards towards the endothelium. Ophthalmic viscosurgical device is removed

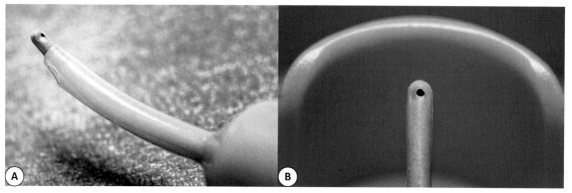

FIGURES 12.12A AND B: If silicone-coated aspiration tips (MST Duet™ System) are used, which make the removal of OVDs more time-consuming (high aspiration rates are needed), but are extremely gentle with posterior capsule and IOL surface, making I/A extremely safe and IOL and capsule-friendly. Notice that the aspiration port (hole) diameter is smaller than in stainless steel I/A cannulas: that is because the silicone sleeve reduces the size of the hole. Removing OVDs with this cannulas is more time-consuming: if necessary, one can change, and use stainless-steel I/A to complete OVD removal at high speed

by circling the tip at the iris plane or on the optic surface. It is important to remember to clean the angles at this stage. It is suggested to opt for Healon5®, as it will not come to the I/A tip.

If remaining OVD is detected after suturing the wound, it is advised to switch to bimanual I/A to avoid removing the suture or modifying the borders' apposition.

If cohesive OVDs (other than Healon5) are mainly used, then IOL centered in place is injected with some acetylcholine into the anterior chamber placing the cannula at the anterior chamber angle opposite to the main incision, slightly pressing the IOL back to posterior capsule. This easy maneuver allows the mass of OVD to easily exit the anterior chamber. After this, the remaining OVD can be delicately removed with a moderate irrigation flow directed towards the back of the IOL, while the aspiration cannula is placed over the IOL, keeping the IOL in place.

The smaller the incisions (2.2 to 2.4 mm or less from the more traditional 2.7 or 2.8 mm) the more time is needed at the end of surgery irrigating fluid through the eye to clear the OVD and any hidden, sulcus-trapped lens fragments. The presence of lens-trapped fragments at sulcus or at anterior chamber angle is more frequent in small incision cataract surgery. Though not much fluid is circulating through the eye during cataract surgery because much smaller incisions are used. The downside of having less fluid in the eye is a slightly greater difficulty removing the viscoelastic agents.

Sometimes, especially in small incision cataract surgeries

(MICS), it is necessary to carefully **go behind the IOL optic** for thorough removal of OVDs.

In case of postoperative IOP increase, a brimonidine tartrate ophthalmic solution (Alphagan® or Combigan®, Allergan Inc., Irvine, CA) is prescribed twice daily, which fastly reduces IOP (IOP reduction can be observed in less than one hour). If necessary (e.g. high intraocular pressure peak with corneal edema), anterior chamber decompression can be done at the slit-lamp with a sterile anterior chamber cannula passed through one of the original corneal incisions (either the main incision or the service paracentesis): aqueous humor and OVD are evacuated from anterior chamber resulting in a dramatic immediate IOP reduction.

REFERENCES

1. Arshinoff SA. The use of ophthalmic viscosurgical devices in cataract surgery. In: Kennedy JF, Phillips GO, Williams PA (Eds). Hyaluronan: Biomedical, Medical and Clinical Aspects, Vol 2. Cambridge, England: Woodhead Publishing Ltd.; 2002.
2. Arshinoff SA, Jafari M. New classification of ophthalmic viscosurgical devices—2005. J Cataract Refract Surg. 2005;31:2167-71.
3. Arshinoff SA, Wong E. Understanding, retaining, and removing dispersive and pseudodispersive ophthalmic viscosurgical devices. J Cataract Refract Surg. 2003;29:2318-23.
4. Arshinoff SA. Using BSS with viscoadaptives in the ultimate soft-shell technique. J Cataract Refract Surg. 2002;28:1509-14.
5. Arshinoff SA. Dispersive-cohesive viscoelastic soft shell technique. J Cataract Refract Surg. 1999;25:167-73.

CHAPTER 13

Local Anesthetic Agents

Ashok Garg

INTRODUCTION

In modern ophthalmology with the preponderance of elderly patients (due to increased life expectancy) and the move towards high-tech outpatient surgical care, there is a growing emphasis and need of local anesthesia.

Local anesthesia is the lifeline of modern ophthalmic surgery and is safer and should always be used unless there are specific indications for general anesthesia. Local anesthesia in the eye may be achieved by topical application of anesthetic drops or by infiltration of the sensory nerves with anesthetic solution (injectables).

LOCAL ANESTHETICS (INJECTABLES)

Local anesthetics prevent the generation and conduction of nerve impulses by reducing sodium permeability, increasing the electrical excitation threshold, slowing the nerve impulses propagation, and reducing the rate of rise of the action potential.

INDICATIONS

Local injectable anesthetics are indicated for infiltration anesthesia in any kind of intraocular surgery.

CONTRAINDICATIONS

Hypersensitivity to local anesthetics, para-amino benzoic acid or parabens. Do not use large doses of local anesthetics in patients with heart block.

PRECAUTIONS DURING LOCAL INJECTABLE ANESTHESIA

- Use local anesthetic with caution when there is inflammation or sepsis in the region of proposed injection.
- Monitor cardiovascular respiratory vital signs and state of consciousness after each injection.
- Local anesthetic should be injected with great care in debilitated or elderly patients, acutely ill patients, children and patients with increased intra-abdominal pressure or patients with severe shock or heart block.
- Many drugs used during local anesthesia are considered potential triggering agents for familial malignant hyperthermia, hence the arrangement for supplemental general anesthesia should be there.
- Use solutions containing a vasoconstrictor with great caution in patients with history of hypertension, peripheral vascular disease, arteriosclerotic heart disease, cerebral vascular insufficiency, heart block, thyrotoxicosis, diabetes. These patients may exhibit exaggerated vasoconstrictor response.
- Watch for hypersensitivity reactions including anaphylaxis to any component of local anesthetics.
- Administer ester type local anesthetics cautiously to patients with abnormal or reduced levels of plasma esterases.
- Some of these anesthetic products contain sulfites which may cause allergic type reactions in certain susceptible patients. Although prevalence of sulfite sensitivity is low.
- Use amide type local anesthetics with care in patients with impaired hepatic function.
- Use local anesthetics with caution in patients with renal disease.
- Exercise caution regarding toxic equivalence when mixtures of local anesthetics are employed.
- Do not use disinfecting agents containing heavy metals for skin (periorbital area) disinfection.
- Do not use local anesthetics in any condition in which a sulfonamide drug is employed.
- Patients should be asked to avoid touching or rubbing the eye until the anesthesia is worn off.

ADVERSE REACTIONS OF LOCAL INJECTABLE ANESTHETICS

The most common acute adverse reactions are related to the CNS and cardiovascular systems. These are generally dose related and may result from rapid absorption from the injection site, from diminished tolerance or from unintentional intravascular injections.

CNS Adverse Reactions

Restlessness, anxiety, dizziness, tinnitus, blurred vision, tremors, convulsions, nausea, vomiting, chills, pupil constriction, excitement may be transient or absent.

Depressive effects These may or may not be preceded by the excitatory symptoms. These are: drowsiness, sedation, generalized CNS depression, unconsciousness, coma, apnea and respiratory depression and even death from respiratory arrest.

Cardiovascular Symptoms of Toxicity

- Peripheral vasodilation
- Hypertension and tachycardia
- Decreased cardiac output

- Hypotension
- Bradycardia
- Methemoglobinemia
- Heart block, ventricular arrhythmias
- Circulatory collapse.

Allergic Adverse Reactions

- Cutaneous lesions of late onset
- Erythema, angioneurotic edema
- Sneezing, syncope
- Excessive sweating
- Elevated temperature and anaphylactoid symptoms.

OVERDOSAGE

Acute emergencies from local injectable anesthetics are generally related to high plasma levels encountered during therapeutic use or to unintended injection overdosage can lead to

- Convulsions, apnea and under ventilation
- Circulatory depression.

If not treated promptly, convulsions and cardiovascular depression can result in hypoxia, acidosis, bradycardia, arrhythmias and cardiac arrest. Various local injectable anesthetics used in ophthalmology are classified as follows.

Esters

- Procaine
- Chloroprocaine
- Tetracaine

Amides

- Lidocaine
- Prilocaine
- Mepivacaine
- Bupivacaine
- Etidocaine
- Centbucridine

Individual drug monographs are described as follows.

ESTERS

PROCAINE

Procaine is para-aminobenzoic acid ester of diethyl-aminoethanol. It was first prepared in 1905. The chemical structure is depicted in **Figure 13.1.**

Indication   Procaine is used for infiltration anesthesia prior to any intraocular surgery. It is not used topically.

Dosage Procaine is available as 1 percent (2 ml) ampoules. It has rapid onset of action (2-5 minutes) with an average duration of action one hour.

Concentrations of 0.5 to 2 percent are used with a maximum dose of 14 mg/kg body weight.

Detoxification occurs by hydrolysis to para-amino benzoic acid and diethylaminoethanol through the enzyme pseudocholinesterase in the plasma.

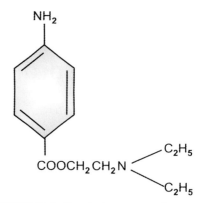

FIGURE 13.1: Chemical structure of procaine

Solution for infiltration anesthesia is freshly prepared. To prepare 60 ml of 0.5 percent solution (5 mg/ml) dilute 30 ml of 1 percent solution with 30 ml sterile distilled water.

Add 0.5 to 1 ml of epinephrine (1:1000 per 100 ml) anesthetic solution for vasoconstrictive effect (1:200000 to 1:100000).

Precautions and adverse reactions have already been described in general monograph section of local injectable anesthetics.

Chloroprocaine

Chloroprocaine is a 2 chloro-4 aminobenzoate ester of B-diethylaminoethanol. It was introduced in 1952 as an analog of procaine. The chemical structure is depicted in **Figure 13.2.**

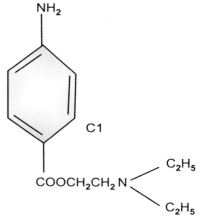

FIGURE 13.2: Chemical structure of chloroprocaine

Chloroprocaine is used for infiltration anesthesia in concentrations of 0.5 to 2 percent. Onset of anesthesia is very rapid (2-5 minutes) and the average duration of action lasts for 1½ hours. It is twice as potent as procaine and has similar pharmacological properties. Metabolism is largely through hydrolysis by pseudo-cholinesterase in the plasma.

Tetracaine (Amethocaine)

Tetracaine is a parabutylaminobenzoic acid ester of dimethylaminoethanol. It was first prepared in 1933. The chemical structure is depicted in **Figure 13.3.**

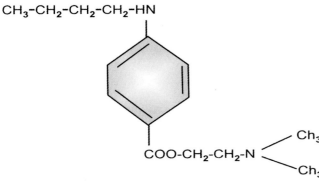

CH₃-CH₂-CH₂-CH₂-HN

COO-CH₂-CH₂-N⟨CH₃ / CH₃⟩

FIGURE 13.3: Chemical structure of tetracaine

Tetracaine is used for infiltration as well as topical anesthesia.

Dosage Tetracaine is available in concentration of 0.25 to 2 percent solutions. Tetracaine is a potent and toxic local anesthetic and dangerous overdosage may occur if it is given in doses higher than 1.5 mg/kg body weight.

It should be given with caution for infiltration anesthesia purpose.

AMIDES

Lidocaine

Lidocaine is one of the most common local injectable anesthetic agents used in ophthalmic surgery worldwide.

Lidocaine is 2-diethylamino-2'-6'-acetoxylidine. It was first prepared in 1948. The chemical structure is depicted in **Figure 13.4.**

Indication Lidocaine 2 percent is used for infiltration anesthesia prior to any type of intraocular surgery.

Dosage Lidocaine is available in concentration of 0.5 to 4 percent as lidocaine hydrochloride (2, 5 ml ampoules and 30 ml and 50 ml vials). For infiltration anesthesia generally 1 percent and 2 percent solutions are used (in 2 ml, 5 ml and 10 ml ampoules; 30 and 50 ml vials). It has rapid onset of action (0.5-2 minute) and average duration of action lasts for 1½ to 2 hours.

Lidocaine is metabolized in the liver to xylidine and diethylaminoacetic acid or is directly excreted into the urine and bile.

For infiltration anesthesia it is generally given with mixture of adrenaline and hyaluronidase to prolong the anesthetic effect and better diffusion to the ocular tissue. Hyaluronidase is an enzyme capable of depolymerizing hyaluronic acid found in interstitial spaces and when it gets depolymerized, fluid passes more easily between the tissues. Preferable 1: 100,000 solution of adrenaline concentration is used and it causes sufficient vasospasm to reduce significantly the rate of removal of local anesthetic agent. A correctly placed retrobulbar or peribulbar injection of this solution causes complete akinesia and anesthesia of the globe. Hyaluronidase is also mixed with 2 percent lidocaine and adrenaline injection for better diffusion of solution into the tissues. It increases the effective area of anesthesia by 40 percent though inevitably of shorter duration.

Various Lidocaine combinations available commercially are:

- Lidocaine HCl 0.5-2 percent with 1:100000 to 1:200000 epinephrine (in 5 ml and 10 ml ampoules, 20, 30 and 50 ml vials).
- Lidocaine HCl 1.5-5 percent with 7.5 percent Dextrose (in 2 ml ampoules).

Safe dose for lidocaine HCl is—7 mg/kg body weight with vasoconstrictors and 2.9 mg/kg body weight without vasoconstrictors. Recently preservative free 1 percent lidocaine hydrochloride (0.5 ml) ampoules have been available commercially for intracameral use during intraocular surgery.

Usual dosage is to inject 0.25 cc of 1 percent preservative free lidocaine into the anterior chamber through the cannula though 1 mm stab incision made in the peripheral cornea, 5 seconds later eye is anesthetized.

Advantages of intracameral injection of lidocaine

- It relieves all discomfort and apprehension of the patient.
- It decreases the need of sedation.
- Surgery is quicker and less tense and patient responds faster with no complications or adverse effects.
- Has an excellent deeper depth of anesthesis.
- Eliminates blocks and their potential complications.
- Has good effect in conjunction with topical anesthesia.

Prilocaine

Prilocaine is α-propyl amino-2-methylproprionic anilide. It was first prepared in 1960. The chemical structure is depicted in **Figure 13.5.**

Its pharmacological properties are similar to those of lidocaine and its onset of action takes 5 to 15 minutes and duration of action lasts for 1 to 3 hours.

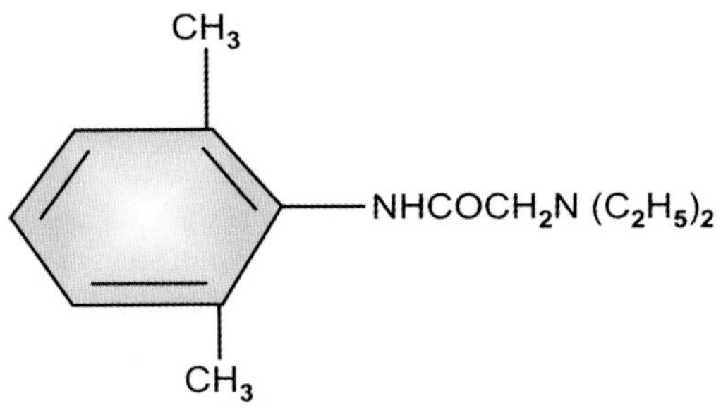

CH₃

CH₃

—NHCOCH₂N (C₂H₅)₂

FIGURE 13.4: Chemical structure of lidocaine

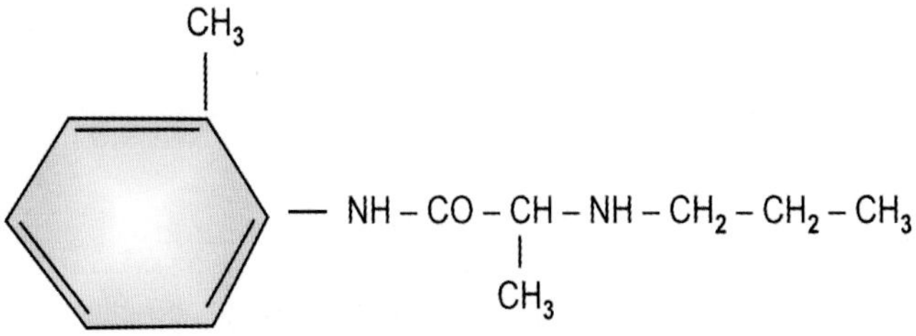

CH₃

— NH – CO – CH – NH – CH₂ – CH₂ – CH₃
|
CH₃

FIGURE 13.5: Chemical structure of prilocaine

Prilocaine is used for infiltration and regional nerve block anesthesia. It is available in concentration of 0.5 to 3 percent. The suggested maximum dose is 10 mg/kg body weight.

Unusual toxic effect seen after administration of large doses (more than 800 mg) is cyanosis due to methemoglobinemia.

Mepivacaine

Mepivacaine is N-methyl pipecolic acid 2,6 dimethyl anilide. It was first prepared in 1956. The chemical structure is depicted in **Figure 13.6**. Mepivacaine has pharmacological properties similar to those of lidocaine. Notable exception is its effect on blood vessels. It is shown to have mild vasoconstrictor effect which reduces its absorption. The effect of mepivacaine on the peripheral circulation is a potentiation of the action of norepinephrine on nerve endings. The onset of action starts within 3 to 5 minutes and duration of action is from 2 to 2½ hours (with epinephrine). The suggested maximum dose is 7.0 mg/kg body weight.

It is used for infiltration and nerve block anesthesia.

Dosage Mepivacaine is commercially available as mepivacaine HCl 1 to 2 percent injectable solutions (in 20, 30 and 50 ml vials). For infiltration anesthesia, 1 percent concentration is used.

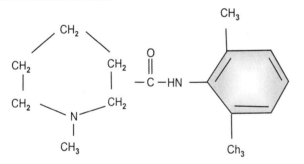

FIGURE 13.6: Chemical structure of mepivacaine

Bupivacaine

Bupivacaine is structurally similar to mepivacaine and is one of the common anesthetic agents used in the ophthalmology for infiltration anesthesia. It was first prepared in 1963. The chemical structure is depicted in **Figure 13.7**.

Bupivacaine is 3 to 4 times more potent than lidocaine. Its onset of action starts within 5 to 10 minutes and duration of action lasts for 3 to 5 hours (with epinephrine).

Dosage Bupivacaine is available as bupivacaine HCl injectable solution in concentration of 0.25 to 0.75 percent (in 2 ml ampoules and 10, 30 and 50 ml vials). For retrobulbar or peribulbar injection 0.75 percent strength solution is used.

Bupivacaine is also available in combination with epinephrine commercially.

Bupivacaine HCl 0.25 to 0.75 percent (in 2 ml ampoules, 10 ml, 30 ml and 50 ml vials).

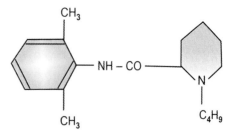

FIGURE 13.7: Chemical structure of bupivacaine

The maximum safe dose is 2.0 mg/kg body weight.

Practically for infiltration anesthesia prior to intraocular surgery it is used in combination of 2 percent lidocaine to produce complete akinesia and anesthesia of globe for more than 2 hours. Usually 50:50 percent of both solutions (0.5% bupivacaine HCl and 2% lidocaine HCl in addition to adrenaline and hylase) are used to produce anesthesia for major ocular surgeries.

Etidocaine

Etidocaine is used for infiltration anesthesia in ophthalmic surgery. It is available as 0.5 to 1 percent injectable solutions (in 30 ml vials and 20 ml ampoules). Its onset of action starts in 5 to 15 minutes and duration of action lasts for 3 to 5 hours. It is also available commercially with epinephrine. Etidocaine HCl 1.0 to 1.5 percent with 1:20000 epinephrine (30 ml vials).

Centbucridine

Centbucridine is 4-N-butylamino-1,2,3,4, tetrahydro-acridine hydrochloride. It is recently introduced anesthetic agent. It has been shown 5 to 8 times more potent than lidocaine.

It is used for infiltration anesthesia and topical anesthesia.

Dosage Centbucridine is available as 0.5 percent centbucridine injectable solution (in 10 ml and 30 ml vials). Its onset of action starts in 2 to 5 minutes and duration of action lasts for 1 to 1½ hours.

LOCAL ANESTHETICS (TOPICAL)

Topical anesthesia is the mainstay of modern ophthalmic surgery. Topical anesthesia is now widely used from superficial minor surgery of conjunctiva and cornea to high-tech phacoemulsification, excimer laser PRK and LASIK surgery. Topical anesthetic agents produce their effect by blocking nerve conduction in the superficial cornea and conjunctiva. The physiological effect of all topical anesthetic agents occurs in a similar fashion. They work at the level of cell membrane by preventing the sodium flux by closing the pores through which the ions migrate in the lipid layer of nerve cell membrane. The anesthetic agents block conduction of afferent nerve impulses thereby abolishing sensation and producing local anesthetic action.

INDICATIONS

Corneal anesthesia of short duration for any diagnostic and surgical procedure on the eye.

CONTRAINDICATIONS

Known hypersensitivity to the drug or to any other ingredient in these preparations. Prolonged used specially for self-medication is not recommended.

PRECAUTIONS

These anesthetic agents are for topical ophthalmic use only. Prolonged use is not recommended as it may diminish duration of anesthesia, retard wound healing and causes epithelial erosions. It may produce permanent corneal opacification with accompanying visual loss, severe keratitis, scarring or corneal perforation, if signs of sensitivity develops, discontinue the use.

- Tolerance varies with the status of the patient. Give debilitated, elderly or acutely ill patients reduced doses commensurate with their weight, age and physical status.
- Use with caution in patients with abnormal or reduced levels of plasma esterases.
- Use with caution in patients with known allergies, cardiac disease or hyperthyroidism.
- Protection of the eye from irritating chemicals, foreign bodies and rubbing during the period of anesthesia is important.

ADVERSE REACTIONS

On topical use these anesthetic agents may cause:
- Mild stinging and burning sensation, vasodilation
- Shortening of tear break-up time
- Decreased blinking
- Corneal edema
- Decreased epithelial mitosis and migration
- Slow epithelial healing
- Punctate epithelial keratitis
- Epithelial desquamation
- Allergic reactions of lid and conjunctiva
- Iritis

Various anesthetic agents used in ophthalmology as topical agents are:
- Benoxinate
- Proparacaine
- Tetracaine
- Lidocaine
- Centbucridine

- Cocaine
- Phenacaine
- Dimethocaine
- Piperocaine
- Dibucaine
- Naepaine
- Butacaine

In today ophthalmic surgery and in diagnostic procedures, proparacaine, benoxinate and tetracaine are commonly used. Their action starts within 15 to 20 seconds and effects last for 15 to 20 minutes.

Other topically applied anesthetic agent is 4 percent Xylocaine, its use is becoming lesser and lesser due to problems with irritation, allergy, etc.

Individual drug monograph of topical anesthetic agent is as follows.

Benoxinate HCl (Oxybuprocaine)

Benoxinate HCl is a para-aminobenzoic acid ester. The chemical structure is depicted in **Figure 13.8.**

It is available as 0.4 percent topical solution. Its action starts within 10 seconds of topical instillation and effect lasts for 15 minutes. 1 to 2 drops of 0.4 percent solution is sufficient to anesthetize the cornea. For deep anesthesia 3 instillations at 90 second interval is sufficient. Because of high degree of safety it is most suitable for topical use.

It is also available as 0.4 percent benoxinate HCl solution with 0.25 percent fluorescein sodium (in 5 ml pack). It is associated with less irritation on instillation.

Another topical anesthetic agent having properties and uses similar to benoxinate is proxymetacaine (0.5%).

Proparacaine

Proparacaine is one of the most common topical anesthetic agents for topical anesthesia in intraocular surgery (phacoemulsification, cataract surgery, excimer laser PRK and LASIK surgery).

It is a benzoic acid ester. The chemical structure is depicted in **Figure 13.9.**

It is available as 0.5 percent and 0.75 percent topical solution. It is used 2 to 5 minutes prior to intraocular surgery.

Its effect starts within 15 to 20 seconds and lasts for 15 minutes. Potency is similar to that of tetracaine. Maximum dose is 10 mg (about 20 crops of 0.5 percent solution on topical instillation).

Due to higher degree of potency and safety it is most appropriate choice for topical ocular anesthesia. It is available as 0.5 percent proparacaine HCl solution and 0.25 percent fluorescein sodium.

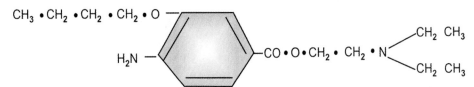

FIGURE 13.8: Chemical structure of benoxinate

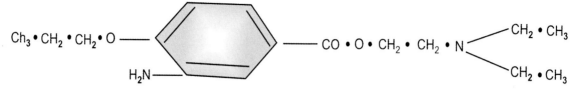

FIGURE 13.9: Chemical structure of proparacaine

Tetracaine

Tetracaine is para-butylaminobenzoic acid ester of dimethylaminoethanol. It is one of the most popular topical anesthetic agents currently used in ophthalmology.

It is available as 0.25 to 1 percent topical solution usually 0.5 percent strength is used for topical anesthesia.

Tetracaine HCl penetrates tissue more deeply than proparacaine and benoxinate.

Its action starts in 20 seconds and lasts for 10 to 12 minutes after topical instillation. It is instilled 2 to 5 minutes prior to the surgery. 1 to 2 drops are instilled topically 2 to 3 times at 60 second duration. Maximum dose is 5 mg (10 drops to each eye of 0.5% solution).

On topical instillation, however, it produces stinging sensation for 30 seconds.

Lidocaine HCl

Lidocaine is 2-diethyl amino, 2, 6 aceto xylidine.

Prior to introduction of topical benoxinate, proparacaine and tetracaine anesthetic agents, 4 percent lidocaine HCl was commonly used for topical anesthesia.

One drop of 4 percent lidocaine solution renders the cornea anesthetized within 30 to 60 seconds and effect lasts for 10 minutes.

It is rapidly acting and does not cause dilation of pupil.

On topical instillation, however, it causes marked stinging sensation for 30 seconds.

Due to its stinging sensation problem, it is now less commonly used for topical anesthesia purpose.

Centbucridine

Centbucridine is recently introduced topical anesthetic agent. It is available as 1 percent topical solution and effect lasts for 15 minutes. It causes very less stinging than 4 percent lidocaine and is safe on topical use. Usual dosage is one drop to be instilled topically and sufficient to produce topical anesthesia.

Cocaine

Cocaine is an alkaloid of erythroxylon coca. It was first introduced in 1884. The chemical structure is given in **Figure 13.10.**

Cocaine was quite extensively used in late fifties of last century. It is available as topical solution in concentration of 1 to 10 percent as cocaine HCl. One drop of 2 percent solution renders the cornea anesthetized within 30 seconds and effect lasts for 12 minutes.

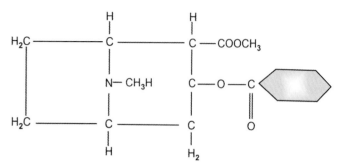

FIGURE 13.10: Chemical structure of cocaine

Maximum dose is 20 mg (about 10 drops to each eye of 2% solution). It is, however, toxic directly to corneal epithelium. It may be used to aid penetration of the other drugs (like cycloplegics) into the cornea and anterior chamber. Cocaine causes mydriasis and when absorbed systemically it may be associated with dangerous drug interactions and hypertensive crisis and CNS stimulation. Toxic doses of cocaine cause fatal circulatory and respiratory collapse. It is now not commonly used for topical purpose as better topical agents are available.

Phenocaine

Phenocaine is derivative of phenetidine. It is N, N, Bis (p-ethoxy-phenyl) acetamidine. The chemical structure is depicted in **Figure 13.11.**

As it is not an ester, it can be considered as an alternative agent for use in patient sensitive to ester group.

It is used as 1 percent topical solution for instillation. Phenocaine is no longer used because it causes excessive irritation and highly toxic.

Dimethocaine

Dimethocaine was first prepared in 1932. It is 3-di-ethylamino, 2, 2 dimethyl propyl p-amino benzoate. The

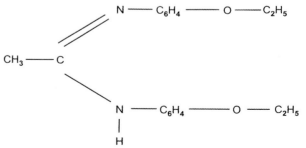

FIGURE 13.11: Chemical structure of phenocaine

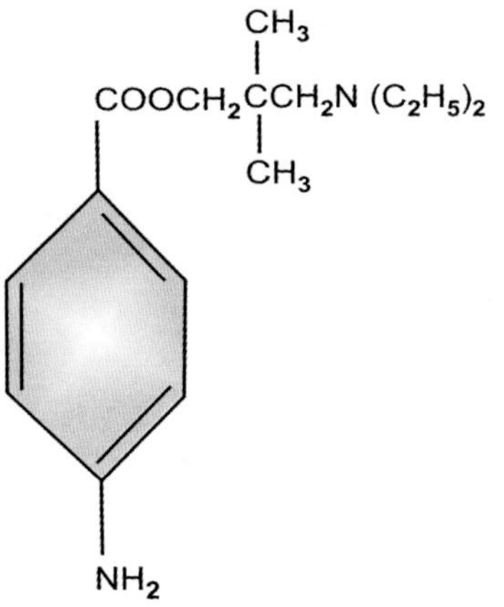

FIGURE 13.12: Chemical structure of dimethocaine

chemical structure is depicted in **Figure 13.12.** It has been used in ophthalmology as topical agent in concentration of 2 to 5 percent. It is derivative of para-aminobenzoic acid.

Piperocaine

Piperocaine is benzoic acid ester of methyl piperidinopropanol. The chemical structure is depicted in **Figure 13.13.** It is used as topical 2 percent solution for topical anesthesia. It has effect of regeneration of corneal epithelium.

Piperocaine along with lidocaine are the only agents associated with normal healing of the cornea.

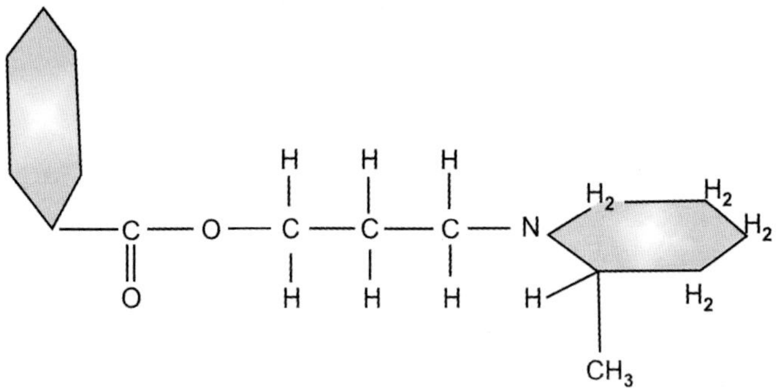

FIGURE 13.13: Chemical structure of piperocaine

Dibucaine

Dibucaine is 2 butoxy-N (2-diethyl aminoethyl) cinchoninamide. It is quinolone derivative and is not an ester. The chemical structure is depicted in **Figure 13.14.**

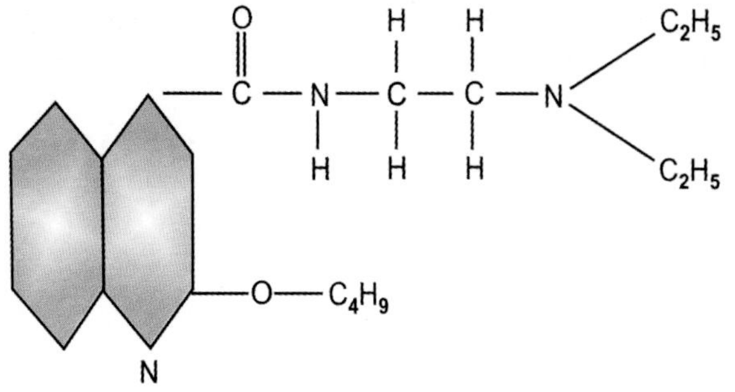

FIGURE 13.14: Chemical structure of dibucaine

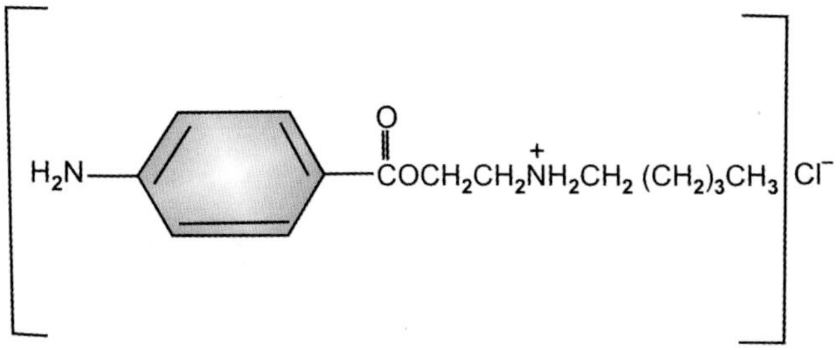

FIGURE 13.15: Chemical structure of naepaine

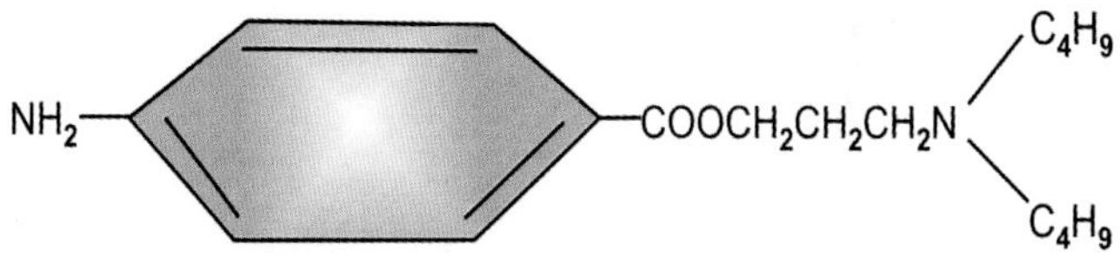

FIGURE 13.16: Chemical structure of butacaine

Dibucaine is probably the most potent local anesthetic agent but its use has declined because of toxicity. It is used as 0.1 percent topical solution for instillation.

Naepaine

Naepaine is mono-n-amylamino ethyl-p-amino benzoate. Its chemical structure is depicted in **Figure 13.15.**

One topical use, it does not cause mydriasis of alteration in intraocular pressure. It is not associated with local irritation. It is derivative of para-aminobenzoic acid and is used 2 to 4 percent topical ophthalmic solution.

Butacaine

Butacaine is para-aminobenzoic acid ester of dibutyl-aminopropanol. The chemical structure is depicted in **Figure 13.16.**

It is used topically as 2 percent solution.

CHAPTER 14

Anesthesia in Cataract Surgery

Ashok Garg

INTRODUCTION

Anesthesia for Cataract Surgery has undergone tremendous changes and advancements in the last century. In 1846, general anesthesia techniques were developed which were not found suitable and satisfactory for ophthalmic surgery. In 1884, Koller discovered surface anesthesia techniques using topical cocaine for cataract surgeries which found favor with the ophthalmologists. However, due to significant complications and side effects of cocaine, Herman Knopp in 1884 described retrobulbar injection as local anesthetic technique for ocular surgery. He used 4% cocaine solution injected into the orbital tissue close to posterior part of the globe to achieve adequate anesthesia but in the subsequent injections, patients experienced pain. In 1914, Van Lint introduced orbicularis akinesia by local injection to supplement subconjunctival and topical anesthesia. However, this technique found favor only after 1930 when procaine (Novocaine) a safer injectable agent made it feasible.

With the development of hyaluronidase as an additive to the local anesthetic solution, Atkinson (1948) reported that large volumes could be injected with less orbital pressure and improved safety injections into the cone (retrobulbar) were recommended and gained rapid favor becoming anesthetic route of choice among ophthalmologists.

In mid 1970s, Kellman introduced an alternative technique of local anesthesia for ocular surgery known as peribulbar injection. However, till 1985 this new technique was not published in ophthalmic literature. In 1985, Davis and Mandel reported local anesthetic injection outside the cone into the posterior peribulbar space (periocular). Further modifications of both retrobulbar and periocular injection techniques were made by Bloomberg, Weiss and Deichaman, Hamilton and colleagues, Whitsett, Murdoch Shriver and coworkers. These modifications consisted of more anterior deposition of anesthetic solution with shorter needles and smaller dosages.

With the introduction of small incision cataract surgery, phacoemulsification and other microsurgical procedures in ophthalmology, use of shorter needles with smaller dosages became more common. Fukasawa and Furata et al reintroduced subconjunctival anesthetic techniques. Fichman in 1992 first reported the use of topical tetracaine anesthesia for phacoemulsification and intraocular lens implantation starting an era of topical anesthesia in ocular surgery.

With the advent of many ocular anesthetic techniques in the past two decades indicates the need for the development of an ideal anesthetic and technique for ocular surgery. Every existing technique has its own advantages and disadvantages. General anesthesia for cataract surgery is virtually out of favor with ophthalmologists. Retrobulbar anesthesia, periocular (peribulbar, subconjunctival, orbital and epidural) and topical anesthesia or a combination of peribulbar and topical are being used in present day ocular surgery. Now with the advent of below 1 mm incision technique, foldable and rollable intraocular lenses, no anesthesia cataract surgery is becoming popular with increased frequency.

ANESTHESIA FOR CATARACT SURGERY

Cataract extraction may be performed under general anesthesia, local anesthesia or topical anesthesia, depending upon condition of patient cataract status and surgeon choice.

GENERAL ANESTHESIA

Usually for cataract surgery, general anesthesia is not given. It is advisable only in highly anxious/nervous patient or when cataract surgery requires a long time for completion. Patients who are extremely apprehensive, deaf, mentally retarded, unstable or cannot communicate well with the surgeon are more suitable for general anesthesia. General anesthetic facilities with expert anesthetist are mandatory.

General Anesthesia Procedure

Preoperative Preparation

A patient who is to be given a general anesthetic needs proper preoperative assessment and examination, preferably on the day before the anesthetic is to be administered, although preparation earlier on the day of surgery may be acceptable in many cases. Patients with cataracts are often elderly and not infrequently have other medical problems that must be considered before anesthesia is induced. These are:

Chronic (Obstructive) Respiratory Disease

These patients require more careful assessment. Their condition in severe cases can be adversely affected by anesthetic drugs and muscle relaxants. On the other hand, the inability to control obstructed respiration can lead to hazardous cataract surgery and a high incidence of failure. Preoperative preparation with antibiotics, bronchodilators, and physiotherapy often enable a sick patient to undergo a safe procedure with the benefit of a general anesthetic.

Cardiovascular Disease
Because many patients with cardiovascular disease will already be on diuretic treatment, preoperative assessment to detect and treat cardiac failure or hypokalemia is most important. The adequate control of hypertension is also an essential safety requirement, especially for the middle aged.

Diabetes Mellitus
Diabetes mellitus is commonly found in those for whom cataract surgery is indicated. Preadmission stabilization is necessary, and when this is in doubt, a longer period of preoperative inpatient assessment and management is required to eliminate any ketonuria or gross hyperglycemia. Oral diabetic medication should be omitted on the day of surgery because the effects may persist for up to 24 hours. During surgery and throughout the early postoperative period, control is effected by using 5 percent glucose intravenously and insulin as required, as shown by the blood glucose levels. When the patient resumes normal oral intake postoperatively, the normal regimen is rapidly resumed.

Dystrophia Myotonica
These patients frequently require cataract surgery while they are quite young. They are particularly sensitive to anesthetic drugs and subject to prolonged respiratory depression. Suxamethonium is contraindicated; minimal doses of other drugs such as atracurium should be used.

Premedication
The aim of premedication is to allow a smooth induction of anesthesia. Most patients appreciate some sedation to alleviate the natural anxiety associated with any eye surgery. Opiates, however, are to be avoided because of their association with respiratory depression and postoperative vomiting. For the aged and anxious, oral premedication with diazepam, 5 to 10 mg, according to fitness and size or lorazepam, 1 to 2 mg, works well. An antiemetic can then be administered during surgery.

For the younger and more robust, one can use a combination of pethidine, promethazine hydrochloride, and atropine. This is also a helpful combination for those with established respiratory disease.

Children over 1 year of age require sedation with trimeprazine tartrate syrup (3 to 4 mg per kg) 2 hours preoperatively. Younger babies should not require sedation. Atropine may be given either intramuscularly (0.2 to 0.6 mg, 30 minutes preoperatively) or intravenously (0.015 to 0.02 mg with induction).

METHOD OF ANESTHESIA

INDUCTION

A smooth induction avoids the problems of increased central nervous pressure with its consequent adverse effect on the intraocular pressure.

The drug most commonly used is thiopentone, which produces a rapid loss of consciousness. When it is used in doses of 3 to 4 mg per kg, the onset is relatively slow in the elderly, who frequently have a slower circulation time. For the very frail, methohexitone is useful, producing less change in blood pressure. More recently, disoprofol (Diprivan) has been found to be useful; it also has a rapid onset of action and induces little nausea and vomiting.

Intubation of the trachea with a non-kinking endotracheal tube is achieved with suxamethonium. Its use is associated with a transient rise in the intraocular pressure due to choroidal expansion. Ventilation with nitrous oxide and oxygen with 0.5 to 1 percent halothane is continued until the effects of the suxamethonium have subsided.

More recently techniques have been described for rapid sequence induction with vecuronium. These methods do not seem to be associated with a significant rise in the intraocular pressure and they avoid the problems of suxamethonium.

MAINTENANCE

A nondepolarizing muscle relaxant is used throughout the surgical procedure, dosages depending on the size, age, and health of the patient. Available drugs include tubocurarine, which is inclined to produce hypotension (occasionally severe), pancuronium, and more recently vecuronium and atracurium. Vecuronium has been demonstrated to lower intraocular pressure. Because both atracurium and vecuronium act and subside rapidly, their effectiveness must be monitored regularly by a peripheral nerve stimulator.

Intermittent positive pressure ventilation is maintained by nitrous oxide, oxygen, and an anesthetic drug. One-half percent halothane has long been considered effective and also lowers the intraocular pressure. Other anesthetic drugs include enflurane (associated with more postoperative vomiting and restlessness, though less hypotension) and isoflurane. The latter does not appear to adversely affect the stability of the cardiovascular system. Its effect on intraocular pressure has not been reported.

Throughout the procedure the pulse, blood pressure, electrocardiographic record, and arterial oxygen saturation must be regularly monitored, along with the nerve stimulation needed for the nondepolarizing muscle relaxant being used. All ventilators should be fitted with an alarm to warn about malfunction.

COMPLETION

Recovery from anesthesia after cataract surgery must be as smooth as the induction, care being taken to avoid gagging, coughing, and of course vomiting. Modern ophthalmic sutures are good but not foolproof! The neuromuscular blockade is reversed with atropine and prostigmine. Gentle extubation is associated with careful pharyngeal suction. Patients are encouraged to resume normal activity as soon as the effects of the anesthetic drugs have worn off.

ANESTHESIA FOR CHILDREN

Adequate premedication and careful handling should ensure a calm and quiet child and allow a smooth induction. Because the cataract is dealt with by using a closed system, the surgical risks of a rise in intraocular pressure are not so severe. Inhalational anesthesia using nitrous oxide and oxygen with halothane is usually sufficient.

COMPLICATIONS OF GENERAL ANESTHESIA

The complications associated with a general anesthetic range from death to the less serious but irritating nuisances of protracted nausea and vomiting or sore throats. This chapter covers only those complications producing serious morbidity or mortality and those peculiar to the patient with eye disease.

- Hypoxemia (insufficient oxygen in the arterial blood to sustain life) is the most common cause of disaster, and failure to ventilate is the most common cause of hypoxemia. Unrecognized esophageal intubation, ventilator disconnection, and, most distressing of all, inability to ventilate after unconsciousness and paralysis have been obtained are all possible causes of failure to ventilate. Delivery of an inadequate oxygen concentration is a less common cause of hypoxemia. Most but not all of the foregoing are preventable with the monitoring and fail-safe devices available today, provided a competent anesthetist is monitoring the devices.

- Aspiration of gastric contents remains a common complication despite such preventive measures as overnight fasting, the use of metoclopramide to enhance gastric emptying, and rapid sequence induction with cricoid pressure in emergency procedures. The two life-threatening results of aspiration are airway obstruction from large food particles and chemical pneumonitis from acidic gastric contents.

- The two most serious cardiovascular complications, aside from cardiovascular collapse secondary to hypoxemia and acute anaphylaxis, are myocardial infarction and cerebrovascular accident. Surgery performed under general anesthesia within 3 months after a myocardial infarction carries a 40 percent incidence of repeat infarction. This figure decreases to about 10 percent at 6 months, after which the incidence is approximately the same as in the general population. All elective surgery is delayed until after 3 months, and a 6-month wait is encouraged unless poor visual acuity seriously limits activities.

- Renal and hepatic toxic effects from anesthetic drugs are seldom seen in our practice. Careful preanesthetic screening identifies all patients with renal and hepatic disease. Halothane, which gained notoriety because of its hepatotoxicity, especially when administered repea-

tedly, is not used in adults and is usually used for induction only in children. The metabolic byproducts of methoxyflurane and enflurane are inorganic fluorides, which can produce nephrogenic diabetes insipidus. We no longer use these drugs because so many of our patients have diabetes and severe renal disease in our population.

- Failure to resume respiration at the end of the surgery occurs often enough to merit mention. The most common causes are simple respiratory depression from the anesthetic drugs or narcotics, electrolyte disturbance (i.e. hypokalemia), hypothermia (particularly in infants), and the use of the combination of mycin antibiotics and nondepolarizing muscle relaxants. It may also occur after the administration of succinyl choline when there is a pseudocholinesterase deficiency. Respirations are maintained until the cause is found and remedied.

Cardiovascular complications are the most commonly seen events in our practice. If diagnosed and treated properly, they need not result in a disaster. Hypertension is the most prevalent problem. The usual causes are apprehension, Neo-synephrine eyedrops, pain, distended bladder if mannitol was given, and autonomic nervous system imbalance secondary to the general anesthetic. Apprehension can be allayed with intravenous injections of 1 to 3 mg of Valium or 0.5 to 2 mg Zolpidem. Nitropaste applied to the skin and sublingual doses of nifedipine have proved invaluable, but an intravenous line should be in place before their use. Hypotension must be treated immediately and vigorously because it is tolerated less well than hypertension. Arrhythmias are the most frequent cause of cancellation on the day of surgery in the elderly patient with eye disease. The sudden onset of atrial fibrillation is the most common arrhythmia. An electrocardiographic monitor is mandatory for eye surgery.

Extrusion of ocular contents during administration of a general anesthetic is a serious complication in eye surgery. The entire anesthetic process is geared to minimize this possibility. Once the eye is opened, patients are kept deeply anesthetized or paralyzed with nondepolarizing relaxants to ensure immobility.

LOCAL ANESTHESIA

Local ocular anesthesia is the mainstay of cataract surgery. Local anesthesia minimizes the risk of wound rupture—a complication frequently associated with coughing during extubation and postoperative nausea and vomiting (in general anesthesia) (**Figure 14.1**). Generally the use of 1:1 mixture of 2% xylocaine and 0.50% bupivacaine alongwith adrenaline and hyaluronidase in facial, retrobulbar and peribulbar blocks achieve rapid anesthesia, akinesia and postoperative analgesia for several hours.

Care should be taken to avoid intravascular injections of anesthetic agents because refractory cardiopulmonary arrest may result from an inadvertent intravenous or intra-arterial injections.

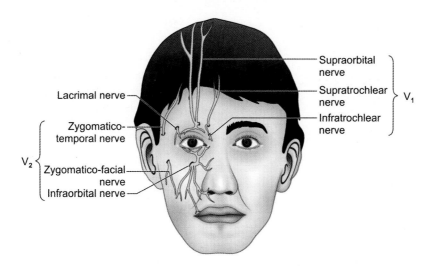

FIGURE 14.1: Diagrammatic surface distribution of sensory nerves. Note branches derived from ophthalmic nerve (V_1) and maxillary nerve (V_2)—a division of the trigeminal nerve

Many patients express pain of facial and retrobulbar injections, so proper preoperative sedation and good rapport with the surgeon make them quite comfortable.

The following techniques are used for giving local anesthesia.

ORBICULARIS OCULI AKINESIA

Temporary paralysis of the orbicularis oculi muscle is essential before making section for the cataract surgery to prevent potential damage from squeezing of the lids. Following methods are used, for getting orbicularis oculi akinesia.

a. *O' Brien's technique:* Usually 10 ml of mixture of 2% lidocaine solution (5 ml) and 0.5% bupivacaine solution (5 ml) with 1:100,000 epinephrine and 150 units of hyaluronidase are infiltrated for local anesthesia.

O'Brien's method is the injection of above mentioned local anesthetic solution down to the periosteum covering the neck of the mandible where the temporofacial division of facial nerve passes forwards and upwards **(Figure 14.2)**. A 10 ml syringe with preferably No. 17 or 18 needle and 2.5 cm in length is used. The patient is asked to open his mouth and the position of the condyle and temporomandibular joint is located by the forefinger of the operators's left hand. After closing the jaw, the injection is given on a horizontal line through the junction of the upper and middle-third of the distance between the zygoma and angle of the mandible. The needle should pass straight down the periosteum. Two to three ml of local anesthetic solution is injected and after withdrawing the needle firm pressure and massage are applied. Paralysis of orbicularis oculi should occur normally within 7 minutes. The injection is unlikely to injure the external carotid artery which lies posterior and at a deeper level. However, damage may be done to posterior facial vein and the transverse facial artery. Movement of jaws is sometimes painful for few days after this injection.

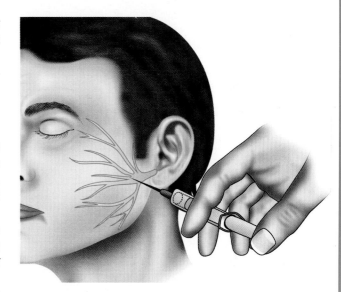

FIGURE 14.2: Diagrammatic presentation of O'Brien's technique of local anesthesia

b. *Van Lint's akinesia:* Van Lint's method is a better alternative. The injection of local anesthetic solution is made across the course of branches of the seventh nerve as they pass over the zygomatic bone **(Figure 14.3)**.

In this technique, a 5 cm in length and 25-gauge needle is passed through the wheal down to the periosteum of the zygomatic bone. The needle is then passed upward towards the temporal fossa without touching the periosteum (as it may be painful) and 4 ml of solution is injected and then forwards medially and downwards towards the infraorbital foramen to inject 2 ml and downwards and backwards along the lower margin of the zygoma for 2.5 cm where 3 ml of solution is injected. It is essential to massage the infiltrated area with a gauze swab. Motor nerves are less susceptible than sensory nerves to a block with local anesthetic agents.

The advantage of Van Lint's method is that it provides regional anesthesia as well as paralysis of the orbicularis muscle. After waiting for 5 to 7 minutes, akinesia is

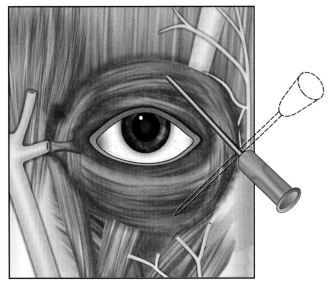

FIGURE 14.3: Needle position for Van Lint's akinesia (*Courtesy:* Ciba Geigy Clinical Symposia)

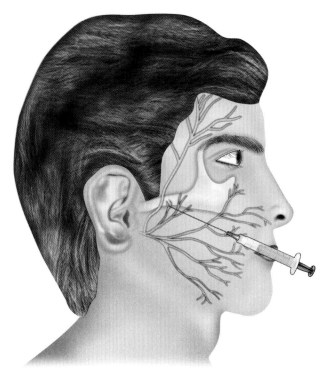

FIGURE 14.4: Atkinson akinesia (intercepting the facial nerve fibers as they cross the zygomatic arch)

tested by holding the eyelids open with a small swab onto a holder and asking the patient to close his eyelids. If slightest action is observed then injection may be repeated to obtain adequate akinesia.

c. *Atkinson block:* The needle enters through a skin wheal at the inferior border of the zygoma just inferior to the lateral orbital rim. The path of the needle is along the inferior edge of the zygomatic bone and then superiorly across the zygomatic arch, ending at the top of the ear. Three to four ml of the anesthetic is injected as the needle is advanced (**Figures 14.4 and 14.5**).

d. *Spaeth block:* The Spaeth block avoids the inconsistencies of the O'Brien block as well as the postoperative discomfort caused by going through the parotid gland and entering the temporomandibular joint. An injection is made into the back of the mandibulbar condyle just below the ear, catching the facial nerve before it divides (**Figure 14.6**). To locate the landmarks, the fingers are placed along the posterior border of the mandible as superiorly as possible. The needle is placed just anterior to the most superior finger. Bone should be reached shortly. If not, the needle is withdrawn and the position rechecked before a second attempt is made. After the bone is reached, the needle is pulled back slightly and suction is placed on the syringe to make sure that a vessel has not been punctured; 5 ml of anesthetic is then injected. Although rarely required, the needle can be redirected superiorly towards the outer canthus for 1.5 inches and an additional 5 ml is injected. After 30 seconds, nearly complete facial palsy should be evident.

e. *Nadbath block:* An injection is made into the cavity between the mastoid process and the posterior border of the mandibular ramus. The skin is pierced, and a skin wheal is made 1 or 2 mm anterior to the mastoid process and inferior to the external auditory canal. A 12 mm, 26-gauge needle is used, with the injection of anesthetic extending from the skin wheal, passing through a taut

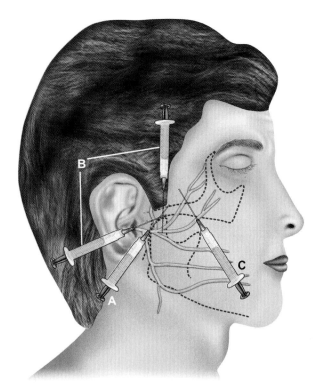

FIGURE 14.5: Diagrammatic presentation of O'Brien and Atkinson techniques. (A) Classic O'Brien technique; (B) Modified O'Brien technique; (C) Atkinson technique

membrane midway, to the full depth of the needle; 3 ml is injected (**Figure 14.7**).

The Nadbath block ensures ease of performance, and there are few complaints relating to the original injection or subsequent pain in the jaw area. The most common side effect is a bitter taste as the parotid gland secretes

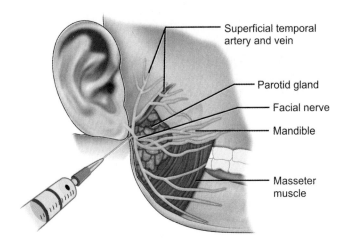

FIGURE 14.6: Spaeth block (facial nerve is blocked where it crosses the posterior edge of the mandible)

the anesthetic. Other problems reported are dysphonia, swallowing difficulty, and respiratory distress. Judging from the fact that these complications are seen predominantly in very thin patients and most certainly are secondary to the diffusion of anesthetic to the jugular foramen, 1 cm deeper than the stylomastoid foramen, the length of the needle—i.e. the depth of injection—is critical.

Preexisting unilateral oropharyngeal or vocal cord dysfunction is a definite contraindication, for bilateral vocal cord paralysis could result. The nadbath block should never be done bilaterally. If, after a unilateral Nadbath block, dysphonia or difficulty with swallowing or respiration occurs, lateral positioning will allow the paralyzed vocal cord to fall out of the way, clearing the airway.

Proper administration of local anesthesia requires knowledge of orbital anatomy, various anesthetic techniques, and the properties of the drugs used. Prompt recognition of side effects and complications following injection results in the best possible patient care.

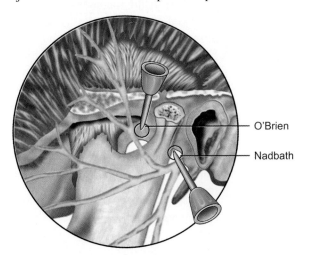

FIGURE 14.7: Needle positions for O'Brien and Nadbath ocular akinesia (*Courtesy:* Ciba Geigy Clinical Symposia)

f. *Retro-ocular (retrobulbar) injection:* Anesthesia and akinesia of the eye are achieved by injecting a local anesthetic solution into the retrobulbar space within the muscle cone (**Figure 14.8**).

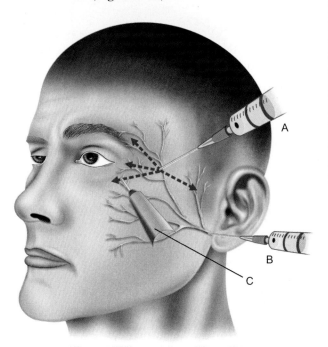

FIGURE 14.8: Local anesthesia techniques. (A) Van Lint's akinesia (dotted arrows); (B) Nadbath facial nerve block; (C) Retrobulbar needle position

In this method, patient is asked to look upwards and to the opposite side. A 3.5 cm in length 23 gauge sharp edge round tipped needle is inserted in the quadrant between the inferior and the lateral rectus muscles and directed posteriorly until the resistance of orbital septum is encountered. After it has penetrated the orbit, the needle is directed towards the apex of the orbit, and advanced until it meets the resistance of the intermuscular septum. When this structure is penetrated, the needle tip is in the retrobulbar space. About 3-4 ml of local anesthetic mixture solution is injected taking care, to minimize the needle movement to prevent possible vessels' lacerations. Following the injection the globe should be intermittently compressed for several minutes for distributing the anesthetic solution and to ensure hemostasis. A properly placed retrobulbar injection is effective within seconds. It blocks all extraocular muscles except superior oblique muscle, affects the ciliary ganglion and anesthetize the entire globe (**Figure 14.9**).

Gills-Loyd Modified Retrobulbar Block

Before the anesthetic is administered, the patient's vision is checked and the A scan examined. Then, prior to the first injection, 2 drops of proparacaine 0.5% are given topically. The eyes are either fixed in primary gaze or directed slightly superiorly, avoiding the superonasal position. With sharp 27 gauge needle, enter is effected at

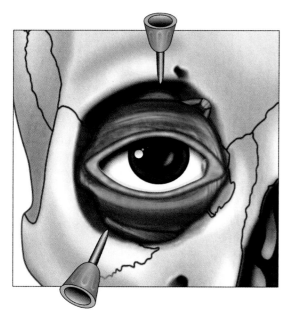

FIGURE 14.9: Needle positions for retrobulbar and peribulbar anesthesia (frontal view) (*Courtesy:* Ciba Geigy Clinical Symposia)

LE 4:00, RE 8:00, 5 mm medial to the lateral canthus. The needle is inserted parallel to the optic nerve. A preretrobulbar injection of 1.5 ml of pH adjusted xylocaine is administered subconjunctivally. After 30 seconds, a 5 ml retrobulbar injection of pH adjusted bupivacaine and hyaluronidase is injected with a 25 gauge, 1¼ inch needle. After 8 to 9 minutes, the eye is checked for akinesia. A 1 to 3 ml supplemental injection of full strength anesthetic is given as needed to complete the block. 1.0 ml bolus is administered subdermally into the inferolateral lid to anesthetize the distal branches of the seventh cranial nerve; this technique does not require a total seventh nerve block. Next 0.5 ml of cefazole is injected subconjunctivally, and gentle eye compression is administered for 30 to 60 minutes with a Super-Pinky Decompressor prior to surgery.

COMPLICATIONS OF RETROBULBAR INJECTION

A number of complications can occur as a result of retrobulbar injection, among them are retrobulbar hemorrhage, perforation of the globe, retinal vascular obstruction, and subarachnoid injection.

RETROBULBAR HEMORRHAGE

Retrobulbar hemorrhage probably occurs in 1 to 5% of the cases. It seems to occur less frequently if a blunt tipped needle is used, but this has not been demonstrated in any controlled study.

Retrobulbar bleeding may occur at a number of sites. The four vortex veins leave the globe approximately 4 mm posterior to the equator and could well be subjected to the shearing forces of an inserted needle, as could the central retinal or ophthalmic vein. An arterial source of bleeding

must be postulated to explain severe hemorrhages that produce the rapid onset of proptosis, hemorrhage, chemosis, and immobility of the globe. The posterior ciliary arteries supplying the choroid, the central retinal artery, and other ophthalmic artery branches are all subject to damage. Even the ophthalmic artery can be reached in the area of the optic foramen with a 1½ inch needle.

Most instances of retrobulbar hemorrhage resolve without complication, but should a complication arise, particularly during elective surgery, it is prudent to postpone the operation for at least 3 to 4 weeks and then consider general anesthesia if the patient can tolerate it.

Even when general anesthesia is employed, severe positive pressure can develop in an open eye if the operation is performed within several days after the hemorrhage.

Vision may be permanently decreased following a retrobular hemorrhage. This probably occurs as a result of closure of the central retinal artery or damage to the smaller vessels that supply the retrobulbar optic nerve.

If examination reveals that the central retinal artery has closed because of increased intraorbital and intraocular pressures, a lateral canthotomy should be performed. Other possible therapeutic modalities include anterior chamber paracentesis and orbital decompression. Prior to decompression of the orbit, computed tomographic scanning of the region should be undertaken to help localize the blood and rule out the possibility of bleeding within the optic nerve sheath, which also might have to be decompressed.

PERFORATION OF THE GLOBE

This is another sight-threatening complication of ophthalmic surgery with retrobulbar anesthesia. Highly myopic eyes are particularly suscepticle to this complication because of their long axial lengths. General anesthesia should be considered as an alternative in such eyes.

The scleral perforation should be repaired as soon as possible. Cryopexy or laser treatment of the break(s) may suffice, although vitreous traction that develops along the needle tract through the vitreous gel is better negated by a scleral buckling procedure. If the fundus view is obscured by vitreous hemorrhage, a pars plana vitrectomy is warranted to visualize the break(s). Although double scleral perforations probably have a worse prognosis than the single variant, the latter also can be devastating. I have seen one case in which the retina in the posterior pole was partially aspirated through the needle following a scleral perforation anterior to the equator.

Inadvertent injection of lidocaine into the vitreous cavity appears to be tolerated by the globe. However, it can cause an extreme elevation of the intraocular pressure and rapid opacification of the cornea.

RETINAL VASCULAR OBSTRUCTION

Retinal vascular obstruction has been reported after retrobulbar anesthesia. The most common types are central retinal artery obstruction and combined central retinal artery-central retinal vein obstructions. Central retinal artery obstruction seems to occur more commonly in conjunction with diseases that affect the retinal vasculature, such as diabetes mellitus and sickling hemoglobinopathies. Nevertheless, it also can be seen in people with good health. Fortunately, the condition more often than not reverses spontaneously and the central retinal artery reperfuses within several hours. The causes are uncertain, but spasm of the artery, direct trauma to the vessel from the needle, and external compression by blood or an injected solution are possible mechanisms that could cause obstruction. Ophthalmic artery obstruction also can be induced, possibly by injection and subsequent compression within the optic foramen.

Therapy is directed towards relieving the obstruction and keeping the retina viable. Anterior chamber paracentesis may help, the aim being to lower the intraocular pressure and decrease the resistance to blood through the central retinal artery. Although paracentesis widens vessels narrowed by artery obstruction, fluorescein angiography shows that the filling occurs in a retrograde fashion, via the retinal veins. Hence its value is questionable.

Combined obstruction of the central retinal artery central retinal vein is a much more serious complication. Ophthalmoscopically, a cheery-red spot is seen, as well as numerous intraretinal hemorrhages and dilated retinal veins. The mechanisms of obstruction include direct trauma to the central retinal vessels from the needle or compression from blood or fluid injected into the nerve sheath. Blood within a dilated optic nerve sheath has been demonstrated in these cases.

The visual prognosis of these eyes is generally grim. Computed tomography of the retrobulbar optic nerve may be used to determine whether a nerve sheath hemorrhage is present. If an optic nerve sheath hematoma is discovered, decompression of the nerve sheath may be of limited benefit.

Neovascularization of the iris may develop after combined central retinal artery-central retinal vein obstruction. If the anterior chamber angle is not yet closed by a fibrovascular membrane, aggressive, full scatter panretinal photocoagulation treatment should be administered in an attempt to prevent neovascular glaucoma.

Injecting with the eye in the primary position may help prevent this complication. In contrast, injecting with the eye looking up and in, places the optic nerve and central retinal vessels more in the pathway of the needle and thus probably should be avoided.

Multiple emboli with the retinal arterial system have caused vascular obstruction following retrobulbar corticosteroid injection. No therapy is available for this visually devastating complication which likely results from injection into the central retinal or ophthalmic artery. In theory, the use of a needle shorter than 1½ inches may help to prevent the complication, as can having the patient gaze in the primary position during the injection.

SUBARACHNOID INJECTION

Among the most recently recognized complications of retrobulbar anesthesia, inadvertent injection into the subarachnoid space may be the most serious. The subarachnoid space extends around the retrobulbar optic nerve up to the globe and can be violated with a retrobulbar needle at any point along its course.

Optic atrophy and blindness have also been reported following retrobulbar blocks but they are fortunately rare. Due to these potential complications retro-ocular injection is out of favor with eye surgeons worldwide.

PERIBULBAR (PERIOCULAR) TECHNIQUE

Since the exit of retrobulbar akinesia, peribulbar akinesia is considered a safe and effective technique of local anesthesia for cataract surgery. It is method of choice with eye surgeons for giving local anesthesia to cataract. As the name indicates, peribulbar anesthesia is a technique in which a local anesthetic is injected into peribulbar space and is not aimed at blocking a particular nerve.

TECHNIQUE

Periocular anesthesia is administered at two sites: lower temporal quadrant and nasal to caruncle **(Figure 14.10).**

The required local anesthetics are lidocaine 1% and bupivacaine 0.75% with hyaluronidase. Bupivacaine is preferred as it is a longer acting anesthetic agent which can provide prolonged anesthesia and analgesia.

In the first stage, injection of 0.5 cc of 1% lidocaine with a 26 G needle is done under the skin at about 1 cm away from the lateral canthus in the lower lid, along the orbital rim. The same needle is passed deeper to inject 0.5 cc of lidocaine into the orbicularis muscle and 1.0 cc into the muscle sheath. A second injection is done in the similar fashion in the upper eyelid just below the supraorbital notch. Pressure is applied at both for a minute using gauze pieces.

In the second stage, combination of 6.0 ml of 0.75% bupivacaine, 3 ml of 1% lidocaine and 0.25 cc of hyaluronidase is filled into a 10 ml disposable syringe fitted with a 1-1/4 inch 23 G hypodermic needle. The needle is first introduced deep into the orbit through the anesthetized site in the lower eyelid. One ml is injected just beneath the orbicularis muscle and then the needle is advanced up to the equator of the globe to inject 2 to 3 ml of the solution. The same procedure is followed in the upper nasal quadrant through the preanesthetized site to inject 1ml and another 1 ml may be injected around superior orbital fissure, by deeper penetration.

At the end of the procedure, fullness of the lids is noted due to the volume of the injected. Firm pressure with the flat of the hand is applied over the globe and is maintained for a minute. Then, before surgery, any pressure device as per the

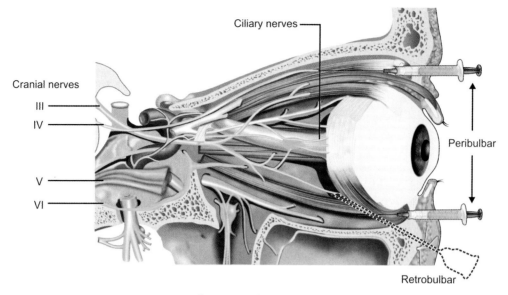

FIGURE 14.10: Needle positions for peribulbar and retrobulbar akinesia (*Courtesy:* Ciba Geigy Clinical Symposia)

surgeon's choice like Honan's balloon, super pinky ball, balance weight or simple pad-bandage is applied for 20 to 30 minutes, to achieve the desired response of hypotony.

The efficacy of the anesthesia is evaluated after about 10 minutes of injection and if inadequate, 2 to 4 ml more can be injected. In case of persistent inferior or lateral movement injection lower temporal quadrant and in case of persistent movements upwards of nasally, the upper quadrant could be infiltrated in the same fashion.

Hyaluronidase is essential as it helps in the spread of the drug. Otherwise, there are chances of the eye being proptosed due to high orbital pressure induced by the large quantity of the fluid injected.

Single injection of 5 to 6 ml of anesthetic mixture injected from any site posterior to equator of the globe also achieves same results. For convenience, however, it may be done through lower lid the junction of lateral and middle one-third, along the floor of the orbit.

Adequacy of akinesia is determined by the absence of ocular movements in all directions.

This technique is certainly better than retro-ocular technique and has least complications.

ADVANTAGES

The advantages reported are:
- The injection is done outside the muscle cone and so, the inherent complications of passing the needle into the muscle cone is completely eliminated.
- It does not enter the retrobulbar space and thereby avoids retrobulbar hemorrhage, injury to optic nerve and entry of anesthetic agents into subarachnoid space and other complications like respiratory arrest.
- Since the needle is constantly kept parallel to the bony orbit, it avoids injury to globe and entry of anesthetic agents into the eyeball.

- It causes less pain on injection.
- The procedure is easier and can be performed without causing damage to vital structures.
- It does not reduce vision on table.
- No facial block is required.

DRAWBACK

The possible drawbacks of this procedure are:
- Chemosis of conjunctiva
- Delayed onset of anesthetic effect
- Potential risk of orbital hemorrhage. Though it occurs rarely, the magnitude of the problem is comparable to retrobulbar hemorrhage and necessitates postponement of surgery.

MECHANISM

The exact mechanism is not known but this procedure may best be described as 'infiltration anesthesia' where nerve endings in all tissues in the area of injection get anesthetized.

Peribulbar anesthesia is a safe and reliable technique for achieving akinesia and anesthesia of the globe. In case of inadequate anesthesia, repeat injections in the similar manner can be safely used to achieve the purpose.

SUPERIOR RECTUS INJECTION

The induction of temporary paralysis of the superior rectus muscle is essential for any intra-ocular operation where the surgical field is upper half of the eye. This injection also affects the action of levator palpebrae superioris.

In this injection, patient is asked to look down. The upper lid is retracted and 2.5 cm long needle is passed into Tenon's capsule at the temporal edge of the superior rectus muscle. The needle is directed posteromedially and about

1 ml of anesthetic mixture of 2% xylocaine is injected around the muscle belly behind the equator. This injection can also be made through the skin of the upper orbital sulcus.

TENON'S CAPSULE INJECTION

The injection of anesthetic mixture can be given into Tenon's capsule around the upper half of the eyeball and into the belly of superior rectus muscle. It is considered safer than the retro-ocular injection across the postganglionic fibers of the ciliary body and may be effective in inducing extraocular muscle akinesia.

PARABULBAR (FLUSH) AKINESIA

Parabulbar (flush) administration is a new route for local anesthesia which is highly useful, safe, effective and technically easier **(Figures 14.11 and 14.12).** This method consists of a limbal sub-tenon administration of retrobulbar anesthesia using a blunt irrigating cannula. This technique can be used for anterior and posterior segment surgery.

TOPICAL ANESTHESIA

Since the advent of retrobulbar and peribulbar techniques in the early part of this century, both procedures are mainstay of local anesthesia for intraocular surgery till today. They do carry the risk of perforation of globe, optic nerve and the inadvertent injection of anesthetic at wrong places.

These accidents are mainly due to:
- Carelessness on the part of ophthalmologist who considers the procedures lightly and occurs more often with senior eye surgeons.

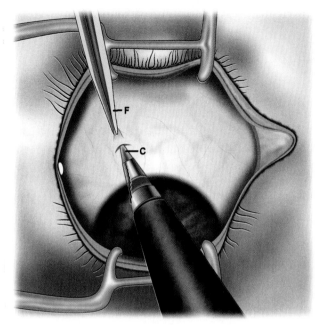

FIGURE 14.12: Parabulbar (flush) local anesthesia (surgeon view). C: Conjunctiva, F: Forceps

- Using long needles for these techniques endangers the perforation of globe, piercing the optic nerve and entering crowded retrobulbar space and even touching the intracranial space on forceful injection of copious amounts.
- Anesthetics given through local injection with little knowledge of anatomy of this area.
- Retrobulbar hemorrhage with its adverse effects on nerve and globe is very common complication of this technique.
- Injury caused by perforation of globe can lead to hole formation, retinal detachment, vitreous hemorrhage and central and branch vein occlusions.

To overcome all these practical difficulties, use of topical anesthesia in intraocular surgery has been widely suggested and used at an International ophthalmic level. Topical anesthesia meaning topical application of 4% xylocaine or 0.5-0.75% proparacaine one drop 3-4 times at regular intervals in the eye has become increasingly popular and accepted. In present day high-tech intraocular surgery—especially phaco surgery—topical anesthesia is the anesthesia of choice with the eye surgeons worldwide.

INDICATIONS TO USE TOPICAL ANESTHESIA

- Its indications in intraocular surgery are mainly when performing phacoemulsification and IOL implantation through a clear corneal tunnel and corneoscleral incisions.
- Topical anesthesia is ideally suited for small incision and stitchless cataract surgery. However, it is not a advocated to perform standard/ manual extracapsular cataract extraction and IOL implantation.

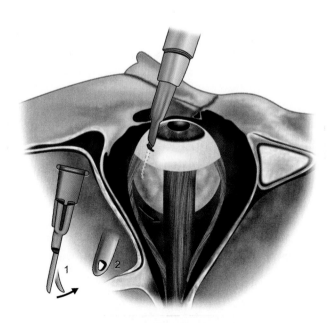

FIGURE 14.11: Parabulbar (flush) local anesthesia (cross-section view). 1: Direction of the needle, 2: Blunt needle

- Proper selection of patient is of great importance in this technique. It is important to have a patient who will comply with the instructions given during surgery.
- Patients who are noncooperative, hard of hearing, with language problem and anxious patients are poor candidates for surgery under topical anesthesia. Capsulorhexis requires the maximum cooperation of the patient.
- Intraocular surgery likely to be problematic in patients with rigid small pupils responding poorly to dilating drops and eyes with lenticular subluxation and high grade nuclear sclerosis are relative contraindications for topical anesthesia.
- Eye surgeon operating with topical anesthesia should be proficient and experienced at phacoemulsification.
- This procedure requires the use of foldable IOL either as a silicone lens or an acrylic lens. This is essential because corneal tunnel suture lens incision cannot be larger than 3.5 mm. Otherwise, corneal complications may arise and the incision would not be self-sealing.

HOW TO ACHIEVE SURFACE ANESTHESIA FOR INTRAOCULAR SURGERY

Generally, 3 applications of 4% xylocaine or 0.4% benoxinate HCl or 0.5-0.75% proparacaine 10 minutes apart starting 30 minutes before surgery are recommended. A drop is thereafter instilled prior to the incision. 1 cc of 4% xylocaine or 0.4% benoxinate HCI or 0.5-0.75 proparacaine (from fresh vial) is drawn into sterile disposable syringe and OT staff person is asked to instil a few drops of the same prior to cauterization of bleeders and if required during surgery, conjunctival anesthesia is used (pinpoint and mini pinpoint surface anesthesia).

Apart from giving topical anesthesia one has to give systemic analgesia. Besides it, surgeon should have a commanding hypnotic voice (vocal local anesthesia).

- Most surgeons doing corneal tunnel incision under topical anesthesia prefer to do it from temporal side.

CAN ONE CONVERT HALF WAY THROUGH SURGERY UNDER TOPICAL ANESTHESIA

Intraoperative conversion from topical to peribulbar anesthesia can definitely be achieved if surgical situation warrants it. Since corneal tunnel incision is sutureless and self-healing, a peribulbar injection can safely be given during the surgery.

ADVANTAGES OF TOPICAL ANESTHESIA

- Phacoemulsification experts feel that use of topical anesthesia with a clear corneal tunnel self-healing incision is a significant advancement in intraocular surgery. With topical anesthesia, visual recovery is immediate.
- It prevents the well-known complications of retrobulbar and peribulbar injections as mentioned in the early part of this chapter.
- It lessens the time of operating room use, thereby lowering costs.
- There is no immediate postoperative ptosis as seen in retrobulbar or peribulbar and Van Lint, O' Brien infiltrations last for 6 to 8 hour due to temporary akinesia of the lids.
- With topical anesthesia photon laser intraocular surgery can be OPD procedure.
- In practice, we have seen the anxiety of patients to peribulbar and retrobulbar injections prior to surgery. With topical anesthesia this problem is over and patient compliance will be better during intraoperative period.
- The need of qualified anesthesiologist is over in operation theater during the operation as a number of ophthalmologists have been seen to prefer anesthesiologist by their side for local anesthesia (retrobulbar and peribulbar anesthesia).
- No risk of postponement of intraocular surgery as seen in cases of retrobulbar hemorrhage.
  Again its main advantage is that it provides for immediate postoperative visual recovery.

DISADVANTAGES OF TOPICAL ANESTHESIA

- Only a highly experienced surgeon can operate with topical anesthesia. The eye can move which makes the operation more difficult. If the eye movement occurs when capsulorrhexis is being done, an undesirable capsular tear may take place leading to failure of this important step of the operation.
- The chances of intraoperative complications with topical anesthesia can be high if the surgeon is not highly skilled. If such complications arise surgeon should be ready to convert to other methods of local anesthesia during the intraoperative stage, because topical anesthesia along may not be adequate to handle intraoperative complications. Surgeon should be of cool temperament who can handle such a situation without anxiety.
- Topical anesthesia is not indicated in all patients especially in anxious and stressed patients, people with hearing difficulties, children and very young patients.
- As in our country a large number of patients come from rural areas who are illiterate and poor, their compliance remains very poor and they do not respond adequately to the command during surgery with topical anesthesia.
- The presence of very opaque cataract is a contraindication to the use of topical anesthesia. This is because surgeon depends on the patient's ability to visually concentrate on the operating microscope light in order

to avoid eye movement during the operation. Patients, who are not able to fix the eyes, may lead to complications.

- Some patients may feel pain during surgery with topical anesthesia. One patient observed a lot more pain and felt as if a sword was being used to cut him up. The pain continued postoperatively for quite some time.
- In principle, adequate selection of patients is fundamental when considering the use of topical anesthesia.

In spite of these hurdles, topical anesthesia will be a safe and common technique for local anesthesia during intraocular surgery in the near future.

NO ANESTHESIA CATARACT SURGERY

This is the latest technique of cataract surgery in which no anesthesia is required (whether local or topical). Neither topical or intracameral anesthetics agents are used. This technique has been devised by Dr. Amar Agarwal (India) and has been acclaimed and accepted worldwide.

BIBLIOGRAPHY

1. Arora R, et al. Peribulbar anesthesia. J Cataract Ref Surg 1991; 17: 506-08.
2. Bloomberg L. Administration of periocular anesthesia. J Cataract Ref Surg 1986;12: 677-79.
3. Bloomberg L. Anterior peribulbar anesthesia. J Cataract Ref Surg 1991;17: 508-11.
4. Davis DB. Posterior peribulbar anesthesia. J Cataract Ref Surg 1986;12: 182-84.
5. Fichman RA. Topical anesthesia, Sanders DR, Slack 1993;1661-72.
6. Furuta M, et al. Limbal anesthesia for cataract surgery. Ophthalmic Surg 1990;21: 22-25.
7. Garg A. Topical anesthesia: Current trends in ophthalmology. New Delhi. Jaypee Brothers Medical Publishers (P) Ltd., 1997;1-5.
8. Hay A, et al. Needle perforation of the globe during retrobulbar and peribulbar injection. Ophthalmology 1991;98: 1017-24.
9. Kimble JA, et al. Globe perforation from peribulbar injection. Arch Ophthalmol 1987;105: 749.
10. Shriver PA, et al. Effectiveness of retrobulbar and peribulbar anesthesia. J Cataract Ref Surg 1992;18: 162-65.
11. Zahl K, et al. Ophthalmol Clin North Am. Philadelphia: WB Saunders, 1990.

CHAPTER 15

Ocular Anesthesia for Small Incision Cataract Surgery

Samuel Masket

INTRODUCTION

Traditional methods of local ocular anesthesia for cataract surgery have employed injection of anesthetics to the periorbital region. It is well recognized that regional infiltration can produce ocular anesthesia, ocular akinesia, orbicularis akinesia, and varying degrees of amaurosis. However, recent trends strongly indicate that only ocular anesthesia is necessary for routine small incision cataract surgery. The 1997 American Society of Cataract and Refractive Surgery member survey for the year 1996 suggests that roughly 15 percent of surgeons employ non-injection anesthesia (topical with or without intracameral agents) routinely.[1] Nevertheless, the great majority of surgeons continue to use anesthetic injections with some degree of risks, that include damage to the globe, optic nerve, and periocular structures, and central nervous system (CNS) toxicity including brainstem anesthesia, apnea, and death. Very rarely, the patient may sustain bilateral ocular anesthesia as a result of anesthetic spread through the cavernous sinus. Moreover, with anesthetic injection, there is the potential for cosmetic blemish of the lids and conjunctiva. *It is worth noting that patients often rate the quality of their cataract surgery by how the eye looks as well as how the eye sees during the early postoperative period.*

The risks of periorbital anesthetic injections are of some consequence, in that the overall occurrence rate for retrobulbar hemorrhage is in the vicinity of one percent of all cases, the likelihood increases with long needles and intraconal injection.[2] Furthermore, ocular penetration and optic nerve damage are not terribly rare. The risks of those maloccurrences increase in patients who are uncooperative for injection, those with high myopia, those with prior scleral buckling surgery, and when the injections are administered by non-ophthalmologists. Additionally, no needle types, injection sites, or injection styles are immune to the risk for damage to the globe or other orbital structures.[3-5]

Another issue regarding the blind passage of sharp needles into the orbit concerns those patients on anti-coagulant medications or those with naturally occurring coagulopathies. It should be obvious that these patients are at greater risk for periocular hemorrhage with needle injection, but often the medical necessity for anticoagulation dictates that patients remain on treatment during the perioperative period. Often, the systemic risk to cessation of anticoagulant treatment is greater than the risk of intraoperative bleeding. Indeed, the published guidelines for cataract surgery in the United Kingdom suggest that cataract surgery should proceed up to an INR (International Normalized Ratio) of 4.0 for patients taking Coumadin. It is evident that non-injection forms of local anesthesia are safer for anticoagulated patients.

Additional, consequences of periocular anesthetic include an inability of the patient to move the eye during and after surgery. While it was once considered essential that the eye be fully still for safe surgery, it is now recognized that purposeful eye movements, on command, can benefit the progress of surgery. As an example, in cases with narrow palpebral fissures, the eye can be moved to facilitate incisions, etc. A further consequence of regional anesthetic infiltration is amaurosis. As a result, the patient cannot see to fixate a target. However, with topical/intracameral anesthesia, the patient can be asked to follow a light source or other visual target to help fixate the globe in a satisfactory position for surgery.

Movement away from periocular injection toward topical methods of ocular anesthesia is natural, given the overall changes in small incision cataract surgery that have progressed to outpatient surgery with methods that allow for immediate ambulation, rapid return to a full lifestyle, and stable optical results of surgery within days.[6] The immediate use of the eye after cataract surgery is possible only with topical/intracameral methods and is in keeping with the concepts of modern surgery.

Topical anesthesia resurfaced in this decade as a useful tool after Fichman's suggestion regarding the use of tetracaine 0.5 percent applied to the eye as the only anesthetic for cataract surgery.[7] Other agents, such as bupivacaine and lidocaine have been popularized because of a reduced tendency to cause corneal epitheliopathy and to have a longer period of action as compared with tetracaine. However, patients are not universally comfortable with topical anesthesia as the only agent. Many surgeons employ small amounts of intravenous, oral, or sublingual sedation as an adjunct. However, in 1995 Gills suggested the routine use of intracameral non-preserved lidocaine in addition to topical anesthesia with or without systemic sedation,[8] although the concept had been mentioned earlier by Fichman who considered intraocular tetracaine for use in difficult case situations. Safety and efficacy of intracameral lidocaine has been further established by Koch[9] and Masket with Gokmen in separate studies.[10] In the latter investigation, approximately 40 percent of more than 300 patients receiving only topical anesthesia required intraoperative conversion to a deeper level of local anesthesia, whereas fewer than one percent of 300 cases receiving intracameral lidocaine had need for an additional local anesthetic method. In the same study, safety was measured by comparing the degree of corneal edema on the first postoperative day between the two groups, a reduced likelihood for corneal edema was associated with the use of intracameral nonpreserved lidocaine hydrochloride one percent, but this finding may be related to the use of chop style phacoemulsification for the latter group. Nevertheless, based upon the early post-operative appearance of the cornea, nonpreserved lidocaine is seemingly nontoxic although Koch reports reduced contrast sensitivity and visual acuity in the first few hours after surgery.

Other methods to provide ocular anesthesia for cataract surgery without the risks of blind pass, sharp needle orbital injection have evolved during the same era as the movement to topical anesthesia. Posterior sub-Tenon's infiltration employs a blunt cannula (**Figure 15.1**) to place local anesthesia directly in the retrobulbar space. A conjunctival button hole incision, performed under topical anesthesia, is necessary for the cannula to gain direct access to the sub-Tenon's space. This method was suggested as an alternative to sharp needle orbital injection,[11] and has been further popularized by Greenbaum as a primary method for cataract anesthesia. He coined the term "parabulbar" anesthesia to describe the concept.[12] Additionally, the method may be used for surgeons in transition to topical/intracameral anesthesia and is very useful to convert from topical methods in cases where complications occur, surgery is prolonged, or if the patient is otherwise in need of a deeper level of anesthesia. As long as the cataract incision is self-sealing, the parabulbar infiltration may be given at any time during the surgery. Varying with the nature of the agent used for infiltration, parabulbar anesthesia may provide complete ocular akinesia and amaurosis. Other alternatives include anterior subconjunctival injection given diffusely or only focally in the region of the incision, so-called "pin-point" anesthesia.[13]

It is evident that traditional ocular anesthesia for cataract surgery, utilizing sharp needles passed blindly through the skin of the lids or the conjunctiva engenders risks (**Table 15.1**) that are avoidable with topical/intracameral or other recently developed means for local anesthesia. However, in addition to the greater safety associated with newer anesthetic systems, topical and topical/intracameral methods avoid the need for patching and allow the patient the use of the eye immediately following surgery in the overwhelming majority of cases. Advantages, therefore, include safety, improved cosmesis, ability to use the eye immediately following surgery, and the ability to move and fixate the eye during surgery in response to the surgeon as an aid to the procedure (**Table 15.2**).

TABLE 15.1	Risk of injection anesthesia

- Damage to optic nerve
- Retrobulbar hemorrhage
- Ocular penetration/perforation
- Central nervous system anesthesia
- Apnea
- Unintended bilateral ocular anesthesia
- Damage to extraocular muscles/diplopia
- Esthetic blemish

TABLE 15.2	Advantages of topical/intracameral anesthesia

- Avoids pain, blemish and risk of injection anesthesia
- Allows immediate useful vision after surgery
- Eliminates need for patch after surgery
- Reduces anxiety and/or heavy sedation associated with injection anesthesia
- Compatible for patients on anticoagulants
- Patients can aid surgeon by moving eye for favorable exposure

Varying with the experience of the surgeon, certain conditions may contraindicate the use of topical/intracameral anesthesia (**Table 15.3**). Given the ability to move the eye, the patient can aid in the surgery or create significant obstacles, cataract surgery under topical/intracameral anesthesia is, by necessity, interactive. Poor patient co-operation is a relative contraindication, as is the inability of the surgeon and patient to adequately

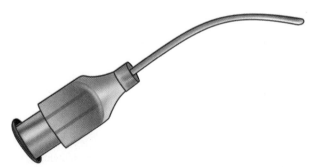

Masket Sub-Tenon Anesthesia Cannula

FIGURE 15.1: Blunted reusable cannula for sub-Tenon's (parabulbar) anesthesia. (*Courtesy* Rhein Medical, Tampa, Florida)

TABLE 15.3	Contraindications to topical/intracameral anesthesia

Relative
- Language barrier
- Anticipated difficult surgery
- Poorly co-operative patient

Absolute
- Total deafness
- Coarse nystagmus

communicate in the same language. Often, an interpreter or bilingual family member can be present in the operating theater in order to facilitate surgery without need for injection anesthesia. However, absolute congenital deafness with speaking difficulty is an absolute contraindication, since the patient may become disoriented under the surgical drapes and cannot be expected to communicate by the usual means of lip reading or sign language, patients of this nature often require general anesthesia. Ocular conditions may also act as relative or absolute contraindications, cataracts too dense to allow fixation on the microscope light, potentially complicated surgery (preoperative zonulysis, etc.), and nystagmus are common examples. Nevertheless, the huge majority of patients may safely experience small incision cataract surgery under topical/intracameral anesthetic with very limited sedation.

METHODS

The author prefers the use of lidocaine HCl 4.0 percent nonpreserved for topical anesthetic. It is long acting and nonmucogenic (previous experience with 0.75% bupivacaine HCl suggests that it causes undesired mucus production.) Intracameral anesthesia is achieved with unpreserved lidocaine HCl 1.0 percent. Some surgeons advocate diluting the intracameral agent with balanced salt solution (BSS) solution in order to raise the pH and reduce the mild discomfort associated with anterior chamber instillation.

1. Administer topical proparacaine HCl 0.4 percent to initiate anesthesia with little sting. Administer dilating agents (cyclopentylate or tropicamide and phenylephrine 2.5%), topical antibiotics, a topical non-steroidal anti-inflammatory drug (NSAID), and lidocaine HCl 4.0 percent four times at five minute intervals prior to surgery.

2. After the patient is brought into the theater, several drops of the 4.0 percent lidocaine are administered prior to the sterile "prep". The latter begins with instillation of two drops of half strength Betadine solution (not Betadine scrub) directly to the operative eye. At this time, very small amounts of intravenous sedation may be given, depending upon the mental and medical status of the patient, the anxiety of the surgeon, and the observations of the anesthetist or equivalent. The author generally asks that 0.5 to 1.0 mg of midazolam HCl be administered IV.

3. During the draping process communicate with the patient about the operative process. Tell them that they will feel slight pressure from the lid speculum and that they will need to fixate on the light of the microscope. Tell them that requests to look up, down, etc. should be achieved by moving the eye and not the head. Reassure them that they will feel no pain.

4. Begin surgery with the microscope light at low levels of illumination, sufficient only to perform a paracentesis. Place 0.2 cc of nonpreserved lidocaine HCl in the anterior chamber and follow that with the viscoelastic of choice. The anesthetic will be washed out as the viscoagent fills the chamber if the lip of the sideport is depressed as the viscoelastic is injected. Slowly increase the microscope light and perform the clear corneal incision. Continue with routine surgical procedure.

5. Generally, no further anesthesia is necessary. However, in situations with prolonged surgery or very sensitive patients, additional intracameral anesthetic may be administered for complaints of "pressure" or intraocular pain. For surface discomfort, the conjunctiva may be swabbed with a pledget of any sterile topical anesthetic, but care should be taken to avoid placing the agent near or in the incision if it contains preservatives. Additionally, small increments of intravenous sedation can be added as may be (rarely) necessary.

6. In the very unlikely case that the patient cannot tolerate the microscope light even at low illumination and continues to squeeze the lids against the speculum, additional doses of IV medicine could be given until the intracameral anesthetic is administered. In author's observations, once the eye has received the intracameral agent, all lid squeezing and signs of anxiety or discomfort abate rapidly. However, in extreme situations or should an operative complication occur that will significantly prolong surgery, one can stop surgery, given a self-sealing incision, pressurize the eye to normal, and administer deep sub-Tenon's local anesthetic with a blunt cannula (**Figure 15.1**) through a conjunctival buttonhole entry in the superior or inferior nasal quadrant.

Prior to incising the conjunctiva, a pledget of local anesthesia may be placed on the area for a few moments. The cannula should reach the retrobulbar space with ease if the buttonhole opening includes Tenon's capsule. Only 2.0 cc of local agent is necessary, given direct access to the muscle cone. Relative amaurosis will be achieved in a matter of seconds, and, with strong local agents, akinesia can be established in a few minutes.

REFERENCES

1. Leaming DV. Practice styles and preferences of ASCRS members: 1996 survey. J Cataract Refract Surg 1997;23: 527-35.
2. Cionni R, Osher R. Retrobulbar hemorrhage. Ophthalmology 1991;98: 1153-55.
3. Duker JS, Belmont JB, Benson WE, et al. Inadvertent globe perforation during retrobulbar and peribulbar anesthesia. Ophthalmology 1997;98: 519-26.
4. Hay A, Flynn HW Jr, Hoffman JI, et al. Needle penetration of the globe during retrobulbar and peribulbar injections. Ophthalmology 1991;98:1017-24.
5. Grizzard WS, Kirk NM, Pavan PR, et al. Perforating ocular injuries caused by anesthesia personnel. Ophthalmology 1991; 98: 1011-16.
6. Masket S, Tennen DG. Astigmatic stabilization of 3.0 mm temporal clear corneal cataract incisions. J Cataract Refract Surg 1996;22(10): 1451-55.

7. Fichman RA, Fine IH, Grabow HR. Clear-corneal Cataract Surgery and Topical Anesthesia Thorofare: Slack Inc. 1993.

8. Gills JP, Cherchio M, Raanan MG. Unpreserved lidocaine to control discomfort during cataract surgery using topical anesthesia. J Cataract Refract Surg 1997;23: 545-50.

9. Koch PS. Anterior chamber irrigation with unpreserved lidocaine 1% for anesthesia during cataract surgery. J Cataract Refract Surg 1997;23: 551-54.

10. Masket S, Gokmen F. Efficacy and apparent safety of intracameral lidocaine as a supplement to topical anesthesia. J Cataract Refract Surg 1998 (in print).

11. Stevens JD. A new local anaesthesia technique for cataract extraction by one quadrant sub-Tenon's infiltration. Br J Ophthalmol 1992;76: 670.

12. Greenbaum S. Anesthesia in cataract surgery. In Greenbaum S (Ed): Ocular Anesthesia, Philadelphia: WB Saunders, 1997; 1-55.

13. Fukasaku H, Marron JA. Pin-point anesthesia—a new approach to local ocular anesthesia. J Cataract Refract Surg 1994;20: 468.

Phaco Steps

CHAPTER 16

Preparing for the Transition to Phacoemulsification

L Samuel Boyd, Benjamin F Boyd, Cristela F Aleman

INTRODUCTION

The transition from planned extracapsular extraction to phacoemulsification fundamentally refers to the gradual change that the ophthalmic surgeon who already masters the planned extracapsular must undertake in order to dominate the new technique of phaco, which is equipment dependent. This transition should be progressive and atraumatic. This learning curve is achieved with effort, dedication and proper training to perform each phase of the transition well.

As proposed by those who taught the transition to phacoemulsification in the 1980s, it is imperative to have a plan that allows many opportunities to revert back to a more familiar technique when one feels uncomfortable. The original "Three Steps to Phaco," pioneered by William Maloney, MD; David Dilman, MD; and I Howard Fine, MD; allowed an entire generation of surgeons performing extracapsular cataract extraction to take on a different set of surgical skills in a predictable manner. A similar approach can be taken as bimanual phacoemulsification is adopted.

MAIN ELEMENTS OF PHACO MACHINES

In this chapter, the authors discuss the use of the phaco machine and the rationale behind it, the three elements of most phaco systems (irrigation, aspiration and ultrasonic energy), fluidics and phacodynamics, and the importance of understanding the surge phenomenon. The chapter also features information on the rationale behind high vacuum - low ultrasound power technology; the new technology of the peristaltic pump, particularly in the three main equipment sources available such as the Alcon's Legacy 2000, Allergan's Prestige (and the Sovereign) and Storz Millennium; and some useful information about the new phaco tips and their contribution toward a better operation.

SURGICAL TECHNIQUES IN THE TRANSITION

ANESTHESIA

During the transition, it is advisable that the surgeon utilize the type of anesthesia with which he/she feels more safe and in better control. It is unnecessary to add a new source of stress or immediate change at this stage of the procedure. Nevertheless, when the surgeon is in charge of the situation and masters the phaco technique, it is ideal to use topical anesthesia because of its ability to provide immediate visual recovery. The combined use of topical and intracameral anesthesia, intracameral anesthesia is more effective than topical anesthesia alone and should be tried before the surgeon attempts to operate using topical or intracameral anesthesia alone.

THE INCISION

Role of the Ancillary Incision

This is an important step. Although there are techniques to perform it with only one hand, phaco is fundamentally a two-handed procedure.

The ancillary incision is made before the main incision is performed. This incision serves as an entry for a second instrument, which is necessary for maneuvers to remove the nucleus. This wound is also utilized in irrigation of the anterior chamber (AC) with intracameral local anesthetic and for the insertion of viscoelastic before making the main incision and during several other steps of the operation. At the end of surgery, the ancillary incision also serves to inject fluid into AC to test for leaks in the wound.

The Main Incision

During the early stages of the transition, the surgeon should plan to start the operation as a phaco but learn how to convert to the planned extracapsular he or she is accustomed to do successfully if this becomes necessary. This will provide additional comfort and confidence. The surgeon may start with a small stepped limbal valvulated incision slightly larger than the phaco tip (**Figure 16.1**) even though he knows that he plans to convert to his usual planned extracapsular. It is not advisable to start the transition with a corneal incision because, upon enlarging it, the resulting astigmatism may be severe. The more anteriorly located the incision, the more astigmatism the patient may end up with. By starting the transition with a limbal incision, the surgeon will use the same area for the incision that he is accustomed to use in his planned extracapsular but will make the incision valvulated (stepped) and smaller than the usual extracapsular. The surgeon must master the technique of the small incision valve-like incision at the limbus, so that it can be part of his armamentarium in the future. Once the surgeon is certain that he will not need to convert from

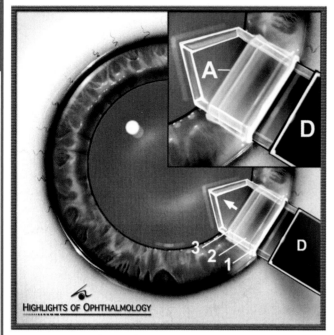

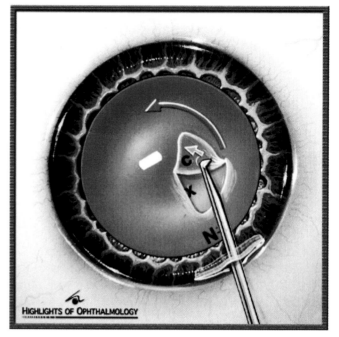

FIGURE 16.1: Final step of self-sealing, stepped, valvulated tunnel incision at the limbus performed with the diamond knife - surgeon's view. A diamond knife blade (D) enters the first incision (1), the second tunnel incision (2), and is then directed slightly oblique to the iris plane and advanced (arrow) into the anterior chamber. This forms the internal aspect of the incision into the chamber (A). This is the third sted (3) in the three-step self-sealing incision (*Source:* Highlights of Ophthalmology)

FIGURE 16.2: Continuous curvilinear anterior capsulorhexis with cystotome - step 1. Anterior capsulorhexis is one of the steps of phacoemulsification that is practically the same both for the surgeon beginning with the transition or the more advanced surgeon, with the exception that some advanced surgeons prefer to do a smaller capsulorhexis. The technique shown here is the initial step performed with the cystotome needle. In the transition, it is recommended that it should be continued with forceps. With an irrigating cystotome, the center of the anterior capsule is punctured creating a horizontal V-shaped tear. The tear is extended towards the periphery and continued circumferentially in the direction of the arrow. In the surgeon's transition stage, the cystotome is introduced through a 3.5 to 4.0 mm limbal incision. The initial puncture of the anterior capsule with the cystotome needle shown here as made in the mid periphery is the technique initially utilized by the pioneers of capsulorhexis and is shown here in this form for historical reasons. The present method has been modified to start the puncture in the center as a frontal incision. This leads to better results and facilitates the maneuver. C: Capsule, X: Cortex, N: Nucleus (*Source:* Highlights of Ophthalmology)

phaco to planned extracapsular and therefore will not need to enlarge the incision, he may choose to make a corneal incision if he wishes, but not before. This is what we refer to as a safe transition from a large to a small incision, a transition that must be undertaken step by step as the surgeon progresses in his learning curve.

Later, as he progresses and learns to master phacoemulsification, the surgeon is ready to make two significant changes in the technique: (1) Operate from an oblique position and make the incision in the upper right quadrant, temporally. (2) Perform a corneal incision instead of a limbal incision.

ANTERIOR CAPSULORHEXIS

This again is a vital step in the transition. Changing from the can opener capsulotomy to the anterior continuous circular capsulorhexis (CCC) is one of the fundamental steps in the transition **(Figures 16.2 to 16.4)**. The surgeon must learn first by practicing capsulorhexis on the skin of a grape or by using a very thin sheet of plastic wrap such as the one that covers some chocolate candies. Once the surgeon understands the concept of the technique and can do it in the laboratory, he or she may begin to use it for the patient.

The surgeon must keep in mind that the space needed to adequately maneuver the cystotome or the capsulorhexis forceps in order to do a proper continuous circular capsulorhexis is larger than the wound or paracentesis required to simply introduce a cystotome and perform a can opener capsulotomy.

It is highly recommended to make the capsulorhexis under sufficient viscoelastic. The latter should be injected into the AC as a first measure before trying the capsulorhexis. It is also fundamental not to begin with dense, hard cataracts where it is difficult to see the edge of the capsulorhexis. It is prudent to try performing this procedure over and over again in cataracts that are less dense until the surgeon is able to perform them in eyes with poor visualization of the edge of the capsule.

Since the surgeon, in the initial stages that are being discussed here, will most probably need to convert to extracapsular cataract extraction (ECCE), it is important that before he performs two relaxing incisions radially in the anterior capsule at 10 and 12 o'clock following the CCC, in order to facilitate the removal of the complete nucleus with a planned manual extracapsular extraction. If

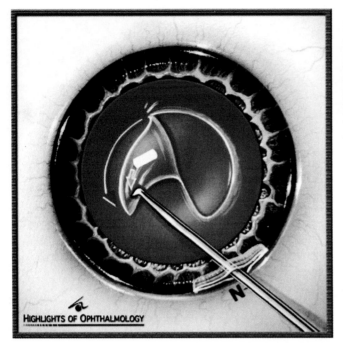

FIGURE 16.3: Continuous curvilinear anterior capsulorhexis with forceps- step 2. After having made the initial tear of the anterior capsule with an irrigating cystotome in the center of the anterior capsule, the tear is extended toward the periphery in a circular direction, this time utilizing forceps as shown in this figure. The tear is extended toward the periphery and continues circumferentially in a continuous manner for the remaining 180 degrees, as initially described by Gimbel. N: Incision (*Source:* Highlights of Ophthalmology)

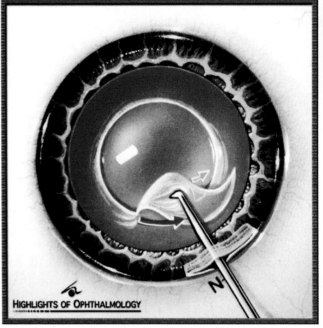

FIGURE 16.4: Continuous curvilinear anterior capsulorhexis with forceps - step 3. The flap of the capsule is flipped over on itself. The forceps engage the underside of the capsule. The tear is continued toward its radial segment. In the transition, beginning surgeons are encouraged to use forceps in order to perform the continuous circular capsulorhexis (CCC). Viscoelastic is essential in this maneuver. The correct size of the CCC is 5.5 mm to 6.0 mm. A larger CCC, would be undesirable because the nucleus may come out of the bag too quickly, forcing the surgeon to do emulsification in the anterior chamber which may lead to endothelial damage. For the early steps of the transition, when the surgeon may have to convert to extracapsular cataract extraction (ECCE), it is important to perform two relaxing incisions radially at 10 and 2 o'clock in the anterior capsule, in order to facilitate the removal of the complete nucleus in an ECCE if necessary. N: Incision (*Source:* Highlights of Ophthalmology)

these relaxing incisions in the anterior capsule are not done, the surgeon may confront serious problems in removing the nucleus.

STAINING OF THE ANTERIOR CAPSULE

Over the red reflex observed through the microscope, the anterior capsule and the border of the progressively performed continuous circular capsulorhexis can be very well visualized. This allows the completion of the circle under adequate visual control. On the other hand, when the surgeon is dealing with white, hypermature cataracts that have either been allowed to get into that advanced stage or have been produced by trauma, the details and border of the CCC cannot be well visualized because this white cataract interferes with fundus reflex. Consequently, the step-by-step progress in the performance of the CCC is not well visualized.

These important considerations have led to the development of a very effective technique to control the performance of the CCC in white cataracts. It consists in staining the anterior capsule of the lens in order to adequately visualize the details during the performance of the CCC (**Figure 16.5**).

Without the dye, it is nearly impossible to see the anterior capsule. These cataracts are risky. It is very difficult to distinguish the anterior capsule from the underlined cortex. This technique should be useful even when the surgeon is

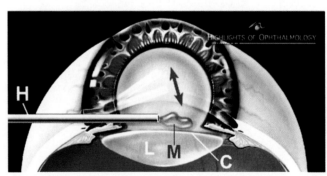

FIGURE 16.5: Staining the anterior capsule in dense cataracts to perform adequate CCC. White cataracts (L) present a problem because the red reflex is not present making the capsulorhexis quite difficult and risky. A viscoelastic is first injected into the anterior chamber immediately followed by the injection of a bubble of air, which partially displaces the viscoelastic from the anterior chamber. This leaves the corneal endothelium lubricated with the viscoelastic. A hydrodissection cannula (H) is introduced through the corneal incision over the anterior capsule (C) filled with a few drops of trypan blue to be instilled over the anterior capsule. M: Dye-Trypan blue (*Source:* Highlights of Ophthalmology)

in the capsulorhexis learning process, no matter the density of the cataract.

HYDRODISSECTION

Once the surgeon is able to perform a circular continuous capsulorhexis (CCC) without problems, he is ready to go into the next step, which is hydrodissection **(Figure 16.6)**. This step should not be undertaken before mastering the capsulorhexis. If not, tears in the anterior capsule may extend towards the equator when performing the injection with fluid to do the hydrodissection. The surgeon should have clearly in mind the anatomy of the crystalline lens and what he wants to achieve with hydrodissection. With this maneuver, by using waves of liquid, we wish to separate the anterior and posterior capsules from the cortex and the nucleus from the epinucleus. When this is achieved, the nucleus is liberated so that it will be free for the ensuing maneuvers of rotation, fracture and emulsification, all of which will come as the next steps in the procedure. As long as the surgeon is not sure that the nucleus has been freed of its attachments through the hydrodissection and will rotate easily, he should not proceed to try to rotate it mechanically because this may lead to rupture of the zonules. Also, if the nucleus is not separated from the cortex by hydrodissection **(Figure 16.7)**, the surgeon should not proceed to apply the phaco ultrasound to the nucleus because he or she may well meet with complications by extending the effects of ultrasound not only to the nucleus but peripherally to the cortex. This can lead to the feared rupture of the posterior capsule. Instead, the surgeon should decide to convert to an ECCE.

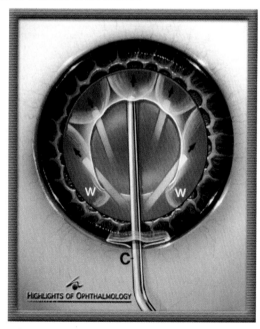

FIGURE 16.6: Hydrodissection of the lens capsule from the cortex during phacoemulsification—surgeon's view. Following circular curvilinear anterior capsulorhexis, a cannula (C) is inserted into the anterior chamber. The cannula tip is placed between the anterior capsule and the lens cortex at the various locations shown in the ghost views. Balanced salt solution is injected at these locations (arrows) to separate the capsule from the cortex. The resultant fluid waves (W) can be seen against the red reflex. These waves continue posteriorly to separate the posterior capsule from the cortex (*Source:* Highlights of Ophthalmology)

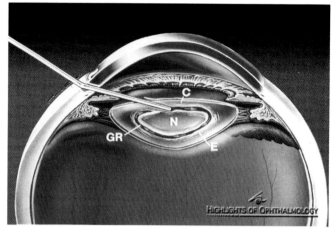

FIGURE 16.7: Hydrodissection—separation of nucleus and epinucleus and the cortex. In this stage, the cannula is advanced beneath the cortex (C) and the infusion with balanced salt solution is started in order to separate the nucleus (N) from the epinucleus (E). The pink arrows between these two structures, nucleus (N) and epinucleus (E), show the flow of fluid. The gold "ring" of fluid separating the nucleus from the epinucleus is here identified as (GR) (*Source:* Highlights of Ophthalmology)

THE MECHANISM OF THE PHACO MACHINE

OPTIMAL USE OF THE PHACO MACHINE

Several worldwide surgeons and teachers, describe the three main functions of the phaco machine: (1) irrigation, (2) aspiration, and (3) emulsification of the nucleus fragments **(Figure 16.8)**. Irrigation is done with the irrigation bottle, aspiration with the aspiration pump and emulsification with ultrasonic energy through the titanium needle present in the phaco tip of the handpiece. Many types of phaco tip shapes have been created to more efficiently handle nuclear extraction. A command pedal, which is controlled by the surgeon's foot, guides the machine into the following four positions: 0 (zero) which is at rest; position 1 for irrigation, position 2 for irrigation/aspiration; and position 3 for irrigation, aspiration and emulsification **(Figure 16.9)**.

The first function (irrigation) controlled by the foot pedal is provided by a bottle with balanced salt solution (BSS). The liquid flows by gravity. The amount of liquid that reaches the AC depends on the height of the bottle, the diameter of the tubing and the pressure already existing in the anterior chamber. The flow rate into the eye is determined by the balance of the pressure in the tubing - regulated by the height of the bottle, and the back pressure in the anterior chamber. When the two are equal, there is no flow. If there is leakage or aspiration of fluid from the anterior chamber, the pressure in anterior chamber (AC) drops, and fluid in the tubing flows into restore the pressure in the AC, and, indirectly thereby, the volume. The tubing is purposely made wide enough so that it impedes the flow of the BSS only slightly under normal rates of flow. It does limit maximum flow during AC collapse.

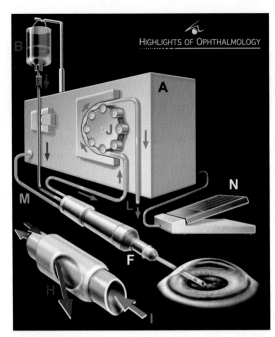

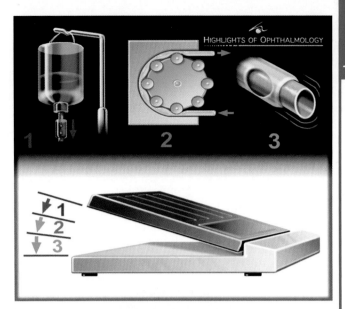

FIGURE 16.8: The principles of how the phaco machine works. This conceptual view shows the three main elements of most phaco systems. (1) The irrigation (red): Intraocular pressure is maintained and irrigation is provided by the bottle of balanced salt solution (B) connected via tubing to the phaco handpiece (F). It is controlled by the surgeon. Irrigation enters the eye via an infusion port (H) located on the outer sleeve of the bi-tube phaco probe. Height of the bottle above the eye is used to control the inflow pressure. (2) Aspiration (blue): (I) enters through the tip of the phaco probe, passes within the inner tube of the probe, travels through the aspiration tubing and is controlled by the surgeon by way of a variable speed pump (J). The peristaltic type pump is basically a motorized wheel exerting rotating external pressure on a portion of the flexible aspiration line, which physically forces fluid through the tubing. Varying the speed of the rotating pump controls the rate of aspiration. Aspirated fluid passes to a drain (L). (3) Ultrasonic energy (green) is provided to the probe tip via a connection (M) to the unit. All three of these main phaco functions are under control of the surgeon by way of a multi-control foot pedal (N) (*Source:* Highlights of Ophthalmology)

FIGURE 16.9: Basic phaco foot pedal functions. The foot pedal controls inflow, outflow and ultrasonic rates. With the foot pedal in the undepressed position, the inflow valve is closed, the outflow pump is stationary, and there is no ultrasonic energy being delivered to the phaco tip. With initial depression of the pedal (1), the irrigation line from the raised infusion bottle is opened. Further depression of the pedal (2), starts and gradually increases the flow rate of the **aspiration** pump to a maximum amount preset by the surgeon. Further depression of the pedal (3) turns on increasing ultrasonic power to the phaco tip for lens fragmentation (*Source:* Highlights of Ophthalmology)

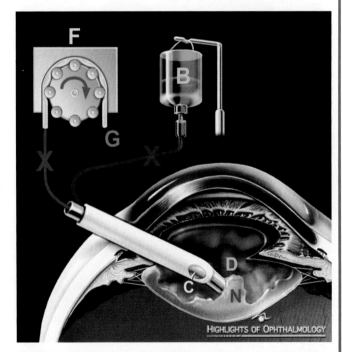

The second function, which is aspiration, is provided by a pump, which creates a difference in pressure between the aspiration line and the anterior chamber. The pumps may be a peristaltic pump, a venturi pump, a diaphragm pump, a rotary vane pump or a scroll pump. The peristaltic pump has become the most widely known and used. Many feel it is safer. Just like inflow, a base level of suction occurs whenever the pump is activated, depending on how hard the pump is working. When there is occlusion of the tip with the foot pedal in the aspiration position (position 2), the pump will continue to pump and create more and more suction until the material, which is provoking the occlusion is aspirated, or until the suction in the tubing reaches the maximum that the surgeon has preset on the control panel **(Figure 16.10)**. This latency period before reaching maximum suction level provides a greater security margin allowing the surgeon to take immediate action in case the tip grasps (and sucks in) the iris or the posterior capsule instead of grasping the lens mass. The reason for limiting

FIGURE 16.10: Fluid dynamics - balance of inflow and outflow during phacoemulsification - tip occluded with lens material - hydrostatic closed system. This view is a close-up complement of the fluid dynamics. When the tip of the phacoemulsification probe is occluded with nuclear material, the vacuum pressure rises to a level to which the machine is set, and the inflow and outflow rates go down. With the aspiration port occluded, no fluid can enter or exit the eye. F: Fluid movement, G: Gravity, B: Bottle, C: Phaco probe, D: Excavated nucleus, N: Nucleus (*Source:* Highlights of Ophthalmology)

the maximum suction pressure is to limit the rush of fluid out of the eye, the moment the fragment, which occluded the tip is aspirated. This provides the surgeon the opportunity to stop aspiration and avoid collapse of the anterior chamber.

The third function of the phaco machine is the production of ultrasonic vibrations leading to emulsification of the lens. It is carried out by a crystal transducer located in the handpiece, which transforms high-frequency electrical energy into high-frequency (ultrasonic) mechanical energy. The crystal drives the titanium tip of the phaco unit to oscillate in its anterior-posterior axis. It is precisely the anteroposterior oscillation of the phaco tip, which produces the emulsification **(Figure 16.11)**.

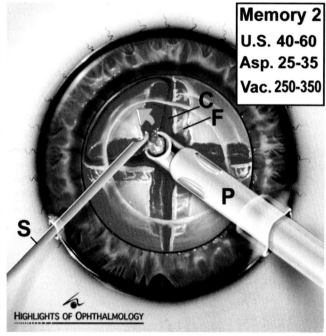

FIGURE 16.11: Emulsification of lens fragments. This surgeon's view shows the management of the lens quadrants. The apex of each of the four loose quadrants is lifted, the ultrasound phaco tip is embedded into the posterior edge of each and by means of aspiration the surgeon centralizes each quadrant for emulsification. C: Capsule, F: Nuclear piece, P: Phaco probe, S: Chopper (*Source:* Highlights of Ophthalmology)

PARAMETERS OF THE PHACO MACHINE

These parameters need to be set and reset depending on the type of cataract: soft, medium-hard, very hard; the stage of the operation; and also, importantly, the various situations which the surgeon must solve. These parameters are:

1. The amount of ultrasonic energy applied to the nuclear material for its emulsification. It is expressed as a percentage of the phaco machine's available power and it determines the turbulence, which is generated in the AC during surgery. It is ideal to use the least amount of power possible during the operation. This is possible by combining other functions of the machine and maneuvers within the nucleus to facilitate fracture and emulsification of the lens. The use of excess phaco energy may result

in damage to structures beyond the nucleus, such as the posterior capsule and the endothelium.

2. The aspiration flow rate measures the amount of liquid aspirated from the AC per unit of time. In practical terms, this determines the speed with which the lens material is sucked in into the phaco tip. This is synonymous with the power of "attraction" or suction of the lens fragments into the irrigation/aspiration handpiece. High maximum flow rates may result in collapse of the AC if the irrigation cannot keep up.

3. The third parameter measures the vacuum or negative pressure created in the aspiration line and actually determines the force with which the material is fixated onto the orifice in the phaco tip. This is known as fixation power or grasp and depends on the aspiration force. The higher the aspiration pressure, the more rapid the aspiration flow, and the less the amount of time it takes to obtain the maximum vacuum power. If the occlusion at the tip is broken or interrupted, due to the negative pressure in the aspiration line, fluid is rapidly sucked out of the eye. This may lead to collapse of the AC with risk of damage to the corneal endothelium as well as the posterior capsule. This is known as the surge phenomenon **(Figure 16.12)**.

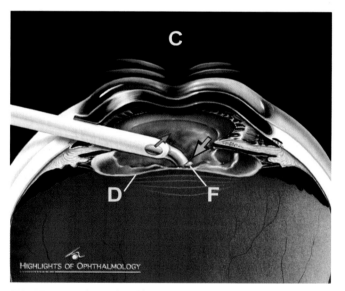

FIGURE 16.12: Physical problems caused by surge. During the surge phenomenon when a nuclear piece (F) is abruptly aspirated from the eye, the anterior chamber may collapse due to a sudden loss of intraocular fluid. The cornea (C) may cave in, resulting in possible endothelial cell damage if it comes near the phaco probe. The posterior capsule (D) may also be damaged from anterior displacement toward the instrument. The fluid outflow rate must be brought under control, and the inflow rate (small red arrow) and outflow rate (large blue arrow) are again equalized with the eye repressurized, to reestablish a balanced system with constant, controlled intraocular pressure is not maintained (*Source:* Highlights of Ophthalmology)

FLUID DYNAMICS DURING PHACO

Michael Blumenthal, MD, has made profound studies on this most important subject. Its understanding really makes a difference between success and failure in small incision cataract surgery, particularly in phacoemulsification. There are two factors specifically involved: (1) the amount of inflow and (2) the amount of outflow during any given period of the surgery. Fluid dynamics are responsible for the following intraocular conditions during surgery: (a) fluctuation in the AC depth; (b) turbulence; and (c) intraocular pressure.

Fluctuation in the AC depth is the consequence of the following conditions: the amount of outflow exceeds the amount of inflow in a given period. As a result, the AC is reduced in depth or collapses. When the amount of outflow is reduced below the amount of inflow, the AC depth is recovered. This phenomenon, when repeating itself, increases fluctuation. When fluctuation occurs abruptly, as in the sudden release of blockage of the phaco tip in aspiration, this is called "surge." The new machines are equipped with special sensors that prevent the possibility of this unpleasant event.

NUCLEUS REMOVAL AND APPLICATION OF PHACO

FRACTURE AND EMULSIFICATION

Fracture and emulsification is really when the surgeon begins to utilize the ultrasound energy in the phaco machine and apply it within the patient's eye. During the transition period, this is a step that should be preceded by a good number of hours of practice in the experimental laboratory until the surgeon is confident in the application of the ultrasound energy. It implies that he or she has been able to successfully perform all the previous steps over and over again in different patients. This experience will serve the surgeon as the requisite basis for success in the emulsification and removal of the nucleus in the present patient.

In removing the nucleus, the surgeon first attempts to divide the nucleus by fragmenting it into smaller portions that in due time will then be emulsified individually (**Figure 16.13**). If the fracture or division of the nucleus has been incomplete and has resulted in large pieces or incomplete fractures, the surgeon will not be able to perform the phacoemulsification successfully or he will need to use so much ultrasound energy that there may be endothelial damage. Present techniques of phacoemulsification are precisely geared to avoiding the use of large amounts of ultrasound energy.

There are different techniques for the fracture of the nucleus. In the end, the surgeon will decide which one he prefers or feels more secure with. Often, it depends on the type and maturity of the cataract. At this stage of the transition, when the surgeon is only beginning in his experience in fracturing and dividing the lens to apply the ultrasound, the most recommended procedure is to divide it into four quadrants, the well known "divide and conquer" first presented by Gimbel. Later, the surgeon will be able

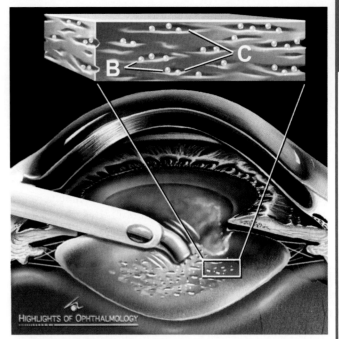

FIGURE 16.13: The role of cavitation in breaking the cataract inside the bag. There are two forces involved in emulsifying a cataract. One is the mechanical force of the ultrasound and other is the mechanism of cavitation. The magnified section of cataract presented here shows that as the phaco tip makes its tiny ultrasonic movements, the energy releases bubbles (B) inside the nucleus creating cavities (C). The build-up of bubbles inside the nucleus creates new hollow spaces (C) in the lens structure, the phenomenon of cavitation. This cavitation facilitates the break-up and destruction of the cataract (*Source: Highlights of Ophthalmology*)

to utilize other modern techniques which also use high vacuum and low phaco but which may be too difficult in the transition.

At this stage of division or fracturing of the lens in the transition, it is recommended that the surgeon use a discretely high amount of ultrasound, low or no vacuum, low aspiration and the conventional height of the bottle (65–72 cm).

The Divide and Conquer Technique

In the "divide and conquer" technique, the phacoemulsification instrument is used to create a deep tunnel in the center or the upper part of the nucleus. The nucleus is split into halves, sometimes fourths, and even occasionally into eighths. Splitting the nucleus is safer for the endothelium and easier to learn, especially for the less experienced ophthalmologist converting from planned extracapsular surgery to phacoemulsification. It is easier to keep smaller particles away from the endothelium without having to push them against the posterior capsule than it is to emulsify a large, cumbersome nucleus.

The nuclear fracturing techniques developed by Gimbel are in part possible because of the CCC (capsulorhexis) technique that Gimbel and Neuhann originated. The mechanical fracturing of the lens causes extra physical stress within the capsule, and that cannot be done without great risks of tears extending around posteriorly unless you have a proper CCC. There is almost an interdependence of these two methods. The fracturing techniques have not only provided more efficiency in phacoemulsification in routine cases; they have also made phacoemulsification in difficult cases safer and more feasible.

Gimbel clarifies that not only there are lamellar cleavage planes corresponding to the different zones of the lens, but also there are radial fault lines corresponding to the radial orientation of the fibers. Until the development of these nuclear fracturing techniques, we had not taken advantage of this construction. The lens fractures quite readily in radial or pie-shaped segments. To accomplish this radial fracturing, the surgeon must sculpt deeply into the center of the nucleus and push outwards. Sculpting is used to create a trench or trough in the nucleus. Then the surrounding part is divided into two hemisections. The separation must occur in the thickest area of the lens located at the center of the nucleus.

An additional consideration with these types of nuclear fractures is whether the segments should be left in place until all the fracturing is complete or whether they should be broken off and emulsified as soon as they are separated. With a lax capsule and particularly with a dense, or brunescent nucleus, Gimbel considers that it is safer to leave the segments in place to keep the posterior capsule protected. The segments are easier to fracture if they are held loosely in place by the rest of the already fractured segments still in the bag **(Figure 16.14)**.

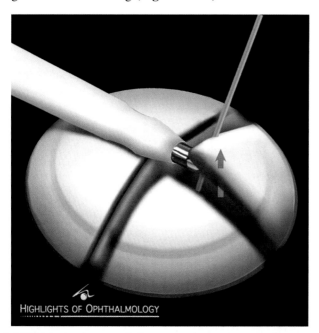

FIGURE 16.14: Phacoemulsification - slicing process. This cross section view shows the phacoemulsification probe removing the nucleus fragments within the capsular bag. Note the apex of one of the fragments created in the nucleus being lifted with the second instrument (arrow) and the ultrasound tip embedded into the posterior edge of each segment ready for emulsification. The epinucleus and cortex will then be removed during the phaco process. If we operate on a softer cataract, the freed fractured pieces are emulsified immediately (*Source:* Highlights of Ophthalmology)

EMULSIFICATION OF THE NUCLEAR FRAGMENTS

If the surgeon has been successful in the fragmentation of the nucleus, the next step is to emulsify the pieces of segments of the divided nucleus. He may do this with the linear continuous mode or with the pulse mode. The latter done during the transition provides more security for the surgeon and allows him to use less ultrasound which is the definite tendency at present.

The surgeon may later slowly begin to utilize other more specialized techniques known as the different "chop" techniques which we will discuss later. These techniques facilitate much more the emulsification of the segments or pieces of the fractured nucleus than the divide and conquer but they are a little more complex. During this step of emulsification of the nuclear fragments, the surgeon may deliver low ultrasound, high vacuum and a larger flow of aspiration, with a conventional height of the bottle of fluid.

ASPIRATION OF THE EPINUCLEUS

It is during this specific step that there is a higher incidence of rupture of the posterior capsule for the surgeon in the period of transition. This is due to his lack of familiarity with handling large fragments of epinucleus and cortex since in the planned extracapsular extraction he is accustomed to remove a large and complete nucleus that includes all the epinucleus and a significant amount of cortex. During the transition, the surgeon has to manage safely the irrigation/aspiration handpiece. Later, when he masters the technique, he may aspirate the epinucleus and cortex by maintaining the aspiration with the tip of the phaco handpiece. For this stage of the aspiration of the epinucleus, the surgeon will use very low or no ultrasound power, a moderate-to-high vacuum, and high flow of aspiration, with the bottle of fluid maintained at the conventional height.

ASPIRATION OF THE CORTEX

This step is closely related to the previous one. There can also be a larger incidence of posterior capsule rupture during this stage since the surgeon does not have the epinucleus as a barrier, which up to a few seconds before was protecting the posterior capsule. The surgeon should use a larger quantity of viscoelastic whenever required with the purpose of protecting the posterior capsule. During the transition period, he may help his maneuvers by using the Simcoe cannula with which the planned extracapsular surgeon usually feels safe. This cannula may be introduced through the ancillary incision. The Simcoe cannula has the disadvantage, though, that the aspiration hole or aperture is smaller than that of the irrigation/aspiration handpiece of the phaco machine. Consequently, the aspiration of the masses of cortex may become more difficult and slow. During this stage, the surgeon should use zero (0) phaco power, maximum vacuum and the highest flow of aspiration as compared with all the previously mentioned memories.

The fluid bottle is maintained at the conventional height. The aspiration of the cortex is also performed with the bimanual aspiration technique, which is very useful especially in the subincisional cortex aspiration process.

INTRAOCULAR LENS IMPLANTATION

ENLARGING THE INCISION AND IMPLANTING THE LENS

In order to accomplish this, if it is necessary the surgeon needs to extend the small incision. In extending the incision, the surgeon must maintain the valve-like, auto-sealing characteristics present in the original small incision. The preferred intraocular lens (IOL) implantation is performed as shown in **Figure 16.15**. After this stage has been mastered, the surgeon may then change to the implantation of the foldable lenses but this must be done only after the surgeon is completely satisfied with his phaco technique.

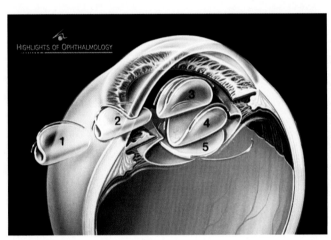

FIGURE 16.15: Concept of foldable intraocular lens implantation. This cross section view shows the movement of the foldable intraocular lens during insertion. Folding forceps removed for clarity. (1) Folded lens outside the eye. (2) Folded lens passing through small incision. (3) Folded lens placed posteriorly into the capsular bag through anterior capsule opening and then rotated 90 degrees. (4) Lens slowly unfolded in the bag. (5) Final unfolded position of lens within the capsular bag (*Source:* Highlights of Ophthalmology)

REMOVAL OF VISCOELASTIC

Throughout the different stages of this procedure, the presence of viscoelastic in the AC is always a measure to keep in mind in order to prevent or minimize damage to the surrounding structures during surgical maneuvers, particularly the corneal endothelium. When removing viscoelastic from the anterior chamber, the phaco machine must be in zero phaco or ultrasound, high vacuum, very low aspiration and the bottle of fluid should be significantly lower. After all the surgical steps have been accomplished, it is important, as we all know, to remove the viscoelastic in order to avoid a high intraocular pressure postoperatively, with subsequent corneal edema, blurred vision and pain during the first postoperative days.

Even though this measure of removing all the viscoelastic has been emphasized over and over again in lectures and published papers, there are still surgeons who are not fully aware of the importance of taking this step and the consequent complications.

Closure of the Wound

If a good incision has been made, valve-like, auto-sealing and waterproof, no suture will be absolutely necessary even in those cases where the wound has been extended to an arc of 5.2 mm for IOL implantation. As long as these two requisites are met, that is, extending the incision to 5.2 mm with a special knife blade of that size and maintaining a valve-like, auto-sealing incision, there is little danger of complications without sutures. Nevertheless, if the surgeon is not sure he has made a valvulated incision from the beginning, even a 3 mm incision with no sutures will leak. If so, to leave the patient without any sutures would be to take an unnecessary risk. It is more prudent to place two or three 10-0 nylon sutures in the wound and they may be removed early in the postoperative stage. This decision really depends on the ability of the surgeon to create a valve-like, self-sealing incision.

WHAT TO DO IF NECESSARY TO CONVERT

When the surgeon decides to convert from phaco to extracapsular, viscoelastic is placed in the anterior chamber. The incision is enlarged to one side and two or three sutures are placed (pre or post placed). The incision is completed to the other side and two or three more sutures are put in place (pre or post placed). The two superior sutures are placed at either end of the "valve incision," so that irrigation/aspiration (I & A) can be performed unhindered at that site. These two sutures are tied with a slipknot prior to I & A, and then loosened to place the IOL. The other sutures are tied and knots buried before I & A. At the end of the operation, an additional suture can be placed if the incision is not secure. To reduce risks, the surgeon may preplace the three 10-0 nylon sutures across a groove on each side, first before enlarging the incision.

RECOMMENDED READING

1. Seibel BS. Phacodynamics: Mastering the Tools and Techniques of the Phacoemulsification Surgery, 3rd edition, 1999.

BIBLIOGRAPHY

1. Barojas E. Importance of hydrodissection in phaco. Guest Expert. In: Boyd BF (Ed.). The Art and the Science of Cataract Surgery. Panama: Highlights of Ophthalmology; 2001.
2. Benchimol S, Carreño E. The transition from planned extracapsular surgery to phacoemulsification. Highlights of Ophthalmology. International English Edition, Vol 24, 1996; No 3.

3. Boyd BF. Preparing for the transition. In: Boyd BF (Ed.). The Art And Science of Cataract Surgery. Highlights of Ophthalmology; 2001. p. 93-132.

4. Carreño E. From can opener to capsulorhexis: the crucial step in the phaco transition. Course on How to shift successfully from manual ECCE to machine-assisted small incision cataract. AAO, Oct. 1999.

5. Carreño E. Hydrodissection and hydrodelineation. Guest Expert. In: Boyd BF (Ed.). The Art and the Science of Cataract Surgery of HIGHLIGHTS, 2001.

6. Centurion V. The transition to phaco: a step by step guide. Ocular Surgery News, Slack; 1999.

7. Drews RC. YAG laser demonstration of the anatomy of the lens nucleus. Ophthalmic Surgery. 1992;23:822-4.

8. Koch PS. Simplifying phacoemulsification safe and efficient methods for cataract surgery, 5th ed. Thorofare, NJ: Slack; 1997. p. 87-98.

9. Seibel SB. The fluidics and physics of phaco. In: Agarwal´s et al. Phacoemulsification, Laser Cataract Surgery and Foldable IOL. 2nd edition. New Delhi: Jaypee Brothers Medical Publishers; 2000. p. 45-54.

CHAPTER 17

Incisions

Luis W Lu, Alejandro Espaillat, Ana Claudia Arenas, Francisco Contreras-Campos

INTRODUCTION

Intracapsular cataract extraction, popular during the 1970s, generally utilized a large corneal incision performed superiorly, creating an against-the-rule astigmatism as a consequence. The switch to extracapsular cataract extraction (ECCE) with intraocular lens (IOL) implantation was a real improvement in the quality of vision, but did little to resolve the post-cataract astigmatic errors due to the large incisions needed to introduce the IOL. With the introduction of phacoemulsification and new foldable IOL designs, creating the correct small incision (**Figures 17.1 and 17.2**) became crucial to determine the successful outcome of the procedure and minimize the residual amount of astigmatism.

THE LIMBAL INCISION

In 1989, McFarland and Ernest introduced an incision architecture that allowed the phacoemulsification and intraocular lens implantation without the need of suturing. Besides lengthening the "scleral tunnel", as named by Girard and Hoffmann, this incision ended in a corneal entrance and a posterior lip, the so-called corneal lip, which acted as a one-way valve with self-sealing characteristics. Paul Koch described what he called the "incision funnel" indicating that there were certain characteristics of self-sealing incisions with respect to length and configuration,

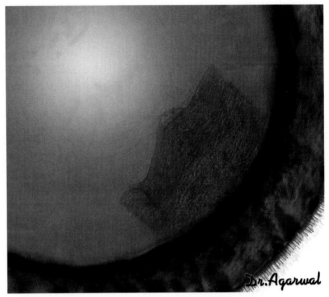

FIGURE 17.2: Illustration showing the clear corneal incision (*Courtesy:* Dr Agarwal's Eye Hospital, India)

that imparted self-sealability as well as astigmatism neutrality.

There are two aspect views of these incisions: sagittal and anteroposterior and three components: the external incision, the intratissue tunnel and the internal incision. From the sagittal aspect, limbal incisions can be made in one of the following configurations varying between single-plane, grooved beveled and triplane with a groove and a bevel.

The external component may also be in one of the following theoretical configurations: the single-step "stab" incision, as initially introduced by Howard Fine and the two-step grooved incision introduced by Charles Williamson, who felt that the wound should be larger on the outside than the inside, creating a trapezoid configuration.

The sagittal shape and the direction of the tunnel may also vary, but usually are made flat by blades advancing in a single plane. On the other hand, its anteroposterior configuration can be as a parallelogram.

The third component of these incisions, the internal opening, may have a single-plane "Stab" or biplane "Steeped" sagittal shape. The anteroposterior aspect of the wound incision could be made limbus-parallel, tangential or limbus antiparallel "corneal frown".

The limbal incision could be located superior, oblique or temporal. Superiorly located incisions, when not under the influence of sutures, are known to have an against-the-

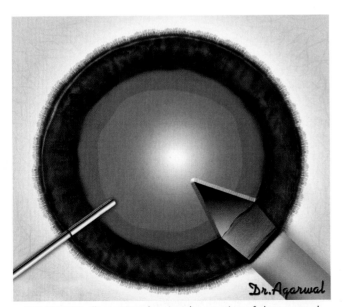

FIGURE 17.1: Illustration showing the creation of clear corneal incision (*Courtesy:* Dr Agarwal's Eye Hospital, India)

rule astigmatic effect. The oblique location, whether nasal or temporal, is advocated by some surgeons who prefer this site for ergonomic reasons as well as for greater wound stability. The temporal wound incision has been shown to be the most astigmatically neutral of these three locations, achieving stability almost immediately, and maintaining it for life.[1, 2]

The limbal incision is very simple to perform, making the maneuvers of entrance and instrumental manipulation easy for the surgeon. It is used primarily by the surgeon in transition to phacoemulsification from the classic ECCE. The technique usually starts with a conjunctival peritomy, followed by a perpendicular limbal incision made with a metal or diamond blade and an oblique entrance to the anterior chamber. The length of the incision could be as small as 2.5 mm initially to keep a close system and a deep anterior chamber during the phacoemulsification procedure, then it could be enlarged up to 6.0 mm, depending on the type of the IOL used.

Both limbal and clear corneal incisions heal by fibroblast response. The key is the timing of the healing process: seven days for vascular origin (limbal) and 60 days for avascular origin (corneal). Clear corneal incisions are also more subject to foreign body sensation than limbal incisions.[1, 2]

THE SCLERAL INCISION

The scleral pocket incision was developed to provide a self-sealing and an astigmatically neutral incision.[1,2] The incision size and configuration are determined by the surgeon's preference and the chosen style of intraocular lens. The options for incision configuration include, linear shape or tangential to the limbus, smile shape or concentric to the limbus, and frown shape or opposite of the limbal curvature. The frown configuration minimizes against-the-rule astigmatism and is reportedly the most astigmatically neutral of these incision.[3, 4] A potential disadvantage of the frown incision is the difficulty in enlarging it, if conversion to ECCE is necessary.

The technique usually follows the creation of a conjunctival flap with the base at the fornix and blunt dissection of the sub-Tenon's space with scissors. Mild cautery of the bleeding conjunctival and episcleral vessels is performed with high frequency bipolar diathermy. The globe is fixated and the scleral incision is then made in three steps. The first step is to mark the lateral limits of the scleral incision with calipers, followed by the creation of a vertical groove of a desired length and configuration, 40–50% scleral depth, using a microsurgical steel or diamond blade held perpendicular to the surface of the sclera. The second step is the creation of the scleral tunnel, with a rounded crescent blade, dissecting a lamellar flap anteriorly through the sclera, 1–2 mm into clear cornea. The dissection is carried forward to Descemet's membrane at the anterior edge of the vascular arcade. The last step is the advancement of the scleral tunnel incision, aiming the tip of the keratome toward the center of the lens, dimpling the Descemet's membrane of the cornea, before entering the anterior chamber creating a triplanar self-sealing incision.

The scleral tunnel must extend into the clear cornea to avoid the prolapse of the iris, damage to the structures of the chamber angle, fluid loss and a flat anterior chamber and to create a valve effect which will seal the wound at the end of the surgery. Some of the disadvantages of the scleral tunnel incisions are that it can surgically induce astigmatism, from the use of cautery to control bleeding conjunctival and episcleral vessels,[5, 6] presents a difficult access to the anterior chamber with limited movement of the surgical instruments and a difficult access to the lens nucleus, aspiration of the lens cortex and IOL manipulation.

THE CLEAR CORNEAL INCISIONS

The more advanced incision for phacoemulsification surgery is the clear cornea incision. The indications for clear corneal cataract surgery have expanded significantly since the last few years. Initially the indications were limited to those patients on anticoagulants, with blood dyscrasias, patients with cicatrizing diseases such as ocular pemphigoid or Stevens Johnson syndrome. However, the greatest advantage of the clear corneal incision has been the ability to do surgery with topical anesthesia. Another big advantage of clear corneal incisions is the tremendous safety with relative astigmatism neutrality, coupled with exceptional results.

This is a bloodless, self-sealing, sutureless and quick incision, best performed temporally, where the distance from the visual axis to the periphery is longer and accessibility to the eye is optimal. This temporal approach includes also better preservation of pre-existing corneal configuration and of the limbal zone at the 12 o'clock position in case of a future filtering surgery. It can also be used to reduce the patient's natural astigmatism by approximately 0.50 diopters in that meridian.[5, 6]

This type of incisions can be classified, after Fine, depending on:

LOCATION

- Corneal tunnel incision: entry posterior to limbus, exit at the cornea-scleral junction.
- Corneal tunnel incision: entry just posterior to the limbus, exit in clear cornea.
- Clear corneal tunnel incision: entry and exit in the clear cornea.

ARCHITECTURE

- Single plane no groove
- Shallow groove < 400 microns
- Deep groove > 400 microns.

SIZE AND PLANAR CONFIGURATION

- Single-plane incision 2.5 by 1.5 mm, rectangular tunnel
- Two-plane incision 2.5 by 1.5 mm rectangular tunnel.
- Three-plane incision 2.5 by 1.5 mm rectangular tunnel plus perpendicular arcuate component.

When making the incision, a decision must be made as whether to groove or not to groove, the external aspect to the incision. Non-grooved single-plane incisions utilize a 2.5–3.0 mm steel or diamond knife.[7] First the anterior chamber is filled with a viscoelastic agent through the paracentesis site, giving the eye stability prior to entry into the anterior chamber. The globe is then fixated with a fixation ring or forceps, to avoid creating conjunctival tears, hemorrhages or corneal abrasions. The uniplanar incision is made inserting the blade in-and-out through the cornea at the surgical limbus, 1 mm anterior to the limbal vessels in the plane of the cornea until the shoulders, which are 2 mm posterior to the point of the knife, touch the external edge of the incision. After the tip enters the anterior chamber, the initial plane of the knife is reestablished to cut through Descemet's in a straight line configuration.

A grooved, triplanar, self sealing, clear-cornea incision **(Figures 17.3A to C)** has three steps. The first step is the creation of an approximately 300 µm deep, perpendicular incision to the corneal surface, 1 mm anterior to the limbal vessels, using steel or preferably a calibrated diamond blade. The second step is the creation of a 1.75–2 mm stromal tunnel, parallel to the iris plane, dissecting the corneal stroma in a lamellar fashion.

The third and final step is to downward tilt the keratome blade 30 degrees toward the visual axis, in order to penetrate the anterior chamber.[8] The stability of the wound depends on the construction of the internal valve, the total width of the incision and the length of the tunnel.[9] Generally, the clear-corneal incision is limited to 4 mm or 5 mm in length in order to be self-sealing. The use of a foldable IOL that could be inserted through a 3–4 mm incision allows the surgeon to perform a purely corneal sutureless tunnel of 1.5–2.0 mm length, with minimal variation in the preexisting astigmatism.[10]

When properly created, the clear-cornea incision will seal by itself. This can be hastened by stromal hydration.[11] Stromal hydration is best accomplished by the injection of fluid via syringe attached to a 27-gauge cannula tightly against the lateral wall of the deeper layers of the incision causing immediate opacification. All properly created incisions usually seal after 1–2 min, when the stroma opposes properly.

In summary, one has to understand the rationale of clear corneal incisions:

- Excellent access to the anterior chamber for proper capsulorhexis performance, access to the cataract, and IOL placement
- Virtually bloodless incision
- Enables the formation of a self-sealing incision, resistant to deformation or leakage

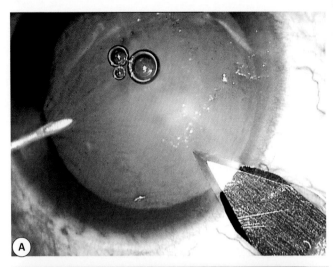
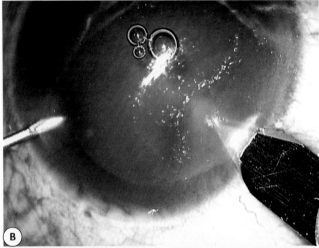
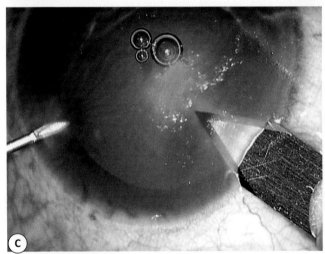

FIGURES 17.3A TO C: Steps in clear corneal incision
(*Courtesy:* Dr Agarwal's Eye Hospital, India)

- Variable incision architecture capable of eliminating pre-existing astigmatism
- Faster physical rehabilitation of the patient
- Being an anastigmatic incision, the refractive stability is almost perfect, enabling additional reading spectacles to be prescribed in a short period of time
- Faster healing with virtually no irritation and redness.

THE SIDE PORT INCISION

A side port incision is a small paracentesis **(Figures 17.4A and B)** limbal incision 1 mm wide, and 0.75 mm long, usually created 90 degrees away from the main incision, using a 15–30 degrees metal blade or a 1 mm diamond blade.

The side port incision should always be used during phacoemulsification because it provides an access route for the introduction of viscoelastic, saline, anesthetics and antibiotics to the anterior chamber. It can also be used to introduce additional instruments during the surgery to stabilize the globe, manipulate the lens nucleus, protect the posterior capsule, keep the iris in place and facilitate the removal of the lens cortex, as well as the insertion of the IOL.

The paracentesis incision is generally performed with the anterior chamber still closed or with the chamber open but previously filled with a viscoelastic agent. The incision is performed through the clear cornea, just in front of the limbal vessels, tangential to the iris. The external end of the incision is usually larger than the internal wound, to

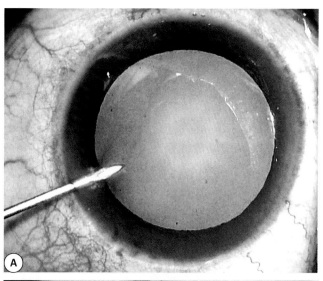

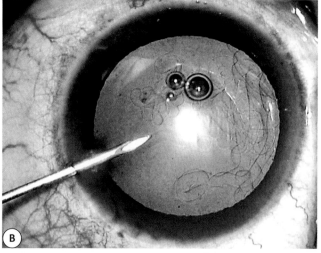

FIGURES 17.4A AND B: Steps in side port incision. Note a 26 G needle injects viscoelastic inside the eye and has also created the side port (*Courtesy:* Dr Agarwal's Eye Hospital, India)

facilitate the introduction of the surgical tools. When performed correctly, the paracentesis incision is self-sealing. It is very important to avoid creating a paracentesis that is too narrow, wide, superficial, deep, anterior or posterior, to facilitate the introduction of surgical instruments and prevent fluid leakage, iris prolapse and corneal folds.

RELAXING INCISIONS

Improved spherical and astigmatic outcomes are now well-recognized benefits of modern small-incision cataract surgery. The combination of limbal or corneal relaxing incisions with cataract surgery is fundamental to the current definition of "Refractive Cataract Surgery", which has come to represent a reality for cataract patients.

Over the past several years, great efforts have been made to study the astigmatic effects of various cataract incisions. By manipulating the size, location and shape of the incisions, surgeons could tailor the astigmatic outcome according to the patient's pre-existing astigmatism. If a patient has enough pre-existing astigmatism to warrant reduction, modern astigmatic keratotomy may then be conservatively added to arrive at the desired cylindrical outcome. Arcuate astigmatic relaxing incisions (RIs) have proven to be extremely safe and reliable[12] and have been used since the early 1970s to reduce high pre-existing astigmatism in cataract surgery.[13] The RIs can be made at the limbus (LRIs) or at the cornea (CRIs), depending on the amount of astigmatism. Although CRIs remain a powerful tool for correcting high astigmatism, they have a limited predictability and often may result in overcorrection particularly in patients with lower amounts of preoperative astigmatism. Most surgeons prefer to use LRIs to correct the preoperative astigmatism, because they are easy to perform, more comfortable for the patient, result in more regular corneal topographies with less corneal distortion, postoperative refractions are less variable, overcorrections are rare and are effective in patients with low to moderate astigmatism, usually three diopters or less.

To create a relaxing incision some surgeons advocate placing an orientation mark at the limbus at the 12 o'clock position before the patient is supine. The surgeon will then determine the amount and axis of the corneal cylinder through corneal topography. The refractive cylinder is usually not considered in phakic patients, because any lenticular astigmatism would be removed by the cataract surgery and cannot be included in the surgical plan. The LRIs are created using a diamond blade which incorporates a special preset 600 μm diamond microknife. The globe is fixated with a modified Fine-Thornton fixation ring and the diamond blade is placed in the steep axis at the limbus just anterior to the palisades of Vogt, creating an incision of an appropriate length by visually following the degree marks on the metal ring. The number and length of incisions are determined according to the various nomograms previously published.[12-15]

Astigmatic keratotomy, whether primary or associated with cataract surgery, is a simple, low-cost and effective procedure. Following surgery, these incisions appear to heal quickly and are nearly unidentifiable within several days leaving a long lasting effect on the patient's quantity and quality of vision.

Cataract surgery is a procedure which is in a constant evolution and undoubtedly will continue to improve in the future. In the mean time, following the previous suggestions will help surgeons achieve a successful outcome of a phacoemulsification cataract extraction.

REFERENCES

1. Fine HI. Architecture and construction of a self-sealing incision for cataract surgery. J Cataract Refract Surg. 1991;17 (Supp): 672-6.

2. Steinert RF, Brint SF, White SM, et al. Astigmatism after small incision cataract surgery. A prospective, randomized, multi-center comparison of 4 and 6.5 mm incisions. Ophthalmology 1991; 98: 417-24.

3. Singer JA. Frown incision for minimizing induced astigmatism after small incision cataract surgery with rigid optic intraocular lens implantation. J Cataract Refractive Surgery.1991; 17(Supp):677-88.

4. Koch PS. Mastering phacoemulsification: A simplified manual of strategies for the spring, crack and stop and chop technique. 4th edition. Thorofare NJ: Slack; 1994;19.

5. Long DA, Monica ML. A prospective evaluation of corneal curvature changes with 3.0 to 3.5 corneal tunnel phacoemulsi-fication. Ophthalmology 1996;103:226-32.

6. Leyland MD. Corneal curvature changes associated with corneal tunnel phacoemulsification. Ophthalmology. 1996;103: 867-88.

7. Fine IH. Self-sealing corneal tunnel incision for small-incision cataract surgery. Ocular Surgery News.1992.

8. Williamson CH. Cataract keratotomy surgery. In: Fine IH, Fichman RA, Grabow HB (Eds).Clear-Corneal Cataract Surgery and Topical Anesthesia. Thorofare, NJ: SLACK; 1993. pp. 87-93.

9. Buratto LL.Phacoemulsification: Principles and Techniques. 1st edition. Thorofare, NJ: Slack, 1998, 41.

10. Albert DM. Ophthalmic Surgery: Principles and Techniques.1st edition. Malden, MA: Blackwell Science; 1999;25(283):

11. Mackool RJ. Current Personal Phaco Procedure. In Fine IH (Ed): Clear-Corneal Lens Surgery. Thorofare, NJ: SLACK; 1999; 239-50.

12. Gills JP, Gayton JL. Reducing pre-existing astigmatism. In Gills JP, Fenzl R, Martin RG (Eds). Cataract Surgery: The State-of-the Art. Thorofare, NJ: SLACK Inc; 1998.

13. Troutman RC. Management of pre-existing corneal astigmatism. In: Emery JM, Paton D (Eds). Current Concepts in Cataract Surgery. St. Louis, Mo: CV Mosby, 1976.

14. Masket S, Tennen DG. Astigmatic stabilization of 3.0 mm temporal clear corneal cataract incisions. J Cataract Refract Surg. 1996; 22:1451-5.

15. Nichamin LD. Intraoperative astigmatism. In Ford JG, Karp CL (Eds). Cataract Surgery and Intraocular Lenses, a 21st Century Perspective. Ophth. Monographs 7, 2nd edition. AAO, LEO series; 2001.

Capsulorhexis

Tobias Neuhann

HISTORY

"Cataract surgery has been developed to its ultimate state and any improvements from this date will be insignificant," said one of the most renowned US ophthalmologists in 1962. Fortunately, this statement proved to be wrong throughout the four decades to follow until today and ophthalmological progress has continued to solve major problems and challenges, managing both a multitude of different anatomic conditions as well as of material characteristics and designs of ophthalmic implants and devices.

One of the major problems of the late 1970s and early 1980s was pupil capture of intraocular lenses due to sulcus implantation. This problem was seriously taken by the members of today's American Society of Cataract and Refractive Surgery (ASCRS). As result of this, discussion was favoring the idea of intraocular lens implantation into the capsular bag. The Simcoe loops (modified C-loop), a new design of that time, provided a considerable improvement in intracapsular centration compared to the generally used J-loops. However, the problem of decentration remained in 10–15%.

Analyzing this decentration showed that disregarding targeted and correct endocapsular implantation, tears of the anterior capsule originated, so that at least one loop luxated into the sulcus, thus mostly forming the precondition for later decentration. The Kelman Christmas-tree, also the Galand letterbox technique, as well as the most frequently applied can-opener technique produced jagged edges which formed a locus minoris resistentiae, so that the logical conclusion was to develop a method to open the capsular bag in such a way that only smooth edges were created. Based on mutual experiences and observations, author's brother Thomas F. Neuhann and author were the first to describe the reproducible method of capsulorhexis.[1]

At the same time and completely independent of their development, Dr Howard Gimbel worked on the same idea, produced the same result and called his new technique continuous tear capsulotomy. In the attempt to find the most suitable and precise term for the new technique and to take the original terminological approach of both inventors into account, Neuhann and Gimbel finally decided to call their mutual development "the continuous curvilinear capsulorhexis (CCC)".[2] It has become the standard technique for planned anterior as well as posterior capsular opening. Taking into account that two independent

developments had been made in the old as well as in the new-world and that this approach has remained the method of choice for opening all kinds of capsules. Until today, it shows that the CCC simply was the most logical conclusion summing up the experiences of the past **(Figure 18.1)**.[3,4]

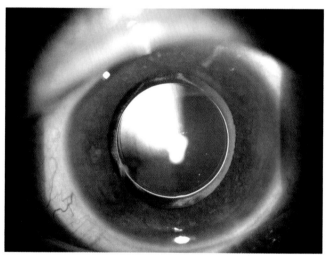

FIGURE 18.1: CCC with IOL in situ, a clinical picture (*Courtesy:* Dr Agarwal's Eye Hospital, India)

NEEDLE TECHNIQUE

Using the needle technique, first an initial puncture of the anterior capsule within the central area, to be removed, is required. This puncture is then extended in a curve-shaped manner to the targeted eccentric circle, to be described. Either pushing starts the circular tear or by pulling the central anterior capsule in either direction, while the flap to be created is gently lifted. The next step is to turn over the flap and apply the vectorial forces in tearing with the needle, in such a way that a more or less concentrically opening originates. Once the full circle is almost completed the end will automatically join the beginning of the curve *outside in* **(Figures 18.2 to 18.4)**.

Another option is to place the first puncture directly within the planned curvature and start the rhexis with a curved enlargement of this tiny hole. In this case, the tear is brought around on both sides, until the ends finally join together as already described above.[5]

The needle technique can be performed by using balanced salt solution (BSS) or viscoelastics. In addition the below factors are essential for the success of the needle capsulorhexis:

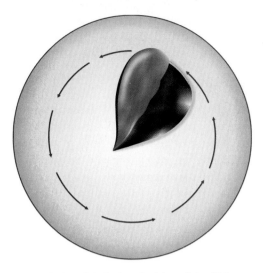

FIGURE 18.2: Basic principles of the CCC

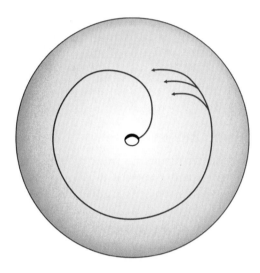

FIGURE 18.3: The right and safe way to perform the CCC

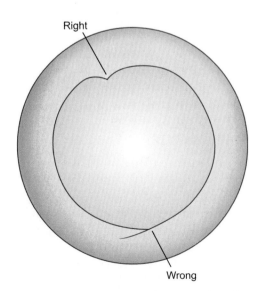

FIGURE 18.4: Right and wrong approach to close the CCC

NEEDLE

1. Although many different needles could theoretically be applied, only the 23-gauge needle is recommended. The lumen of this type of needle is just sufficient to produce a pressure exchange between the anterior chamber and the BSS irrigating bottle.

2. The metal of such a cannula offers just enough rigidity to provide the necessary resistance for difficult manipulations. Needles with higher gauge do not meet the described requirements and this alone may cause a CCC failure, even though this fact is unfortunately not generally known.

3. A higher, i.e. positive pressure in the anterior chamber, compared to the intracapsular pressure is mandatory. This becomes especially noticeable with intumescent lenses, where the lens protein is hydrated, resulting in a volume increase inside the capsular bag, which results in a considerable increase in the endocapsular pressure as a consequence. The necessary prerequisite for a successful capsulorhexis is a pressure of the anterior chamber that is greater than or equal to that inside the capsular bag. The pressure in the anterior chamber can be adjusted via the height of the infusion bottle.

4. The needle tip should be as sharp as possible, since a blunt needle will lead to stellate burst, which is more difficult to handle **(Figure 18.5)**.

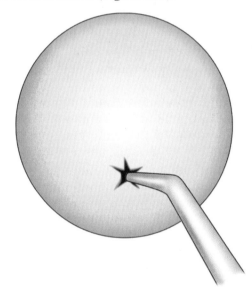

FIGURE 18.5: Stellate burst created by a blunt needle

FORCEPS TECHNIQUE

The principle of the forceps capsulorhexis exactly follows the principle of the needle technique. In addition to the known Utrata forceps, there are mini forceps that are similar in construction to the forceps developed for the posterior segment of the eye. The advantage of the mini forceps is that they can be inserted into the anterior chamber via a paracentesis, so that the incision is not exposed to needless strain **(Figure 18.6)**.[5]

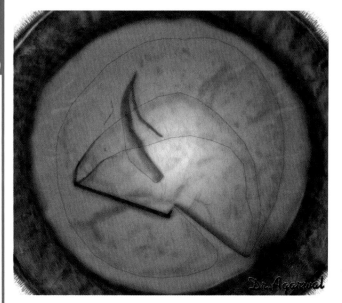

FIGURE 18.6: Rhexis completed (*Courtesy:* Dr Agarwal's Eye Hospital, India)

COMPARISON OF THE NEEDLE AND FORCEPS TECHNIQUES

The forceps technique is easier to learn. For this reason it is also the most frequently applied capsulorhexis technique. However, applying the forceps technique, the use of viscoelastics is mandatory.

The advantage of the needle technique is that it is economical, since it can be performed with application of BSS as well as viscoelastics and the cost of the needles is neglectable.

To point out the difference between the needle and the forceps technique, the following example might be appropriate: "to turn over a page of a book, one can take the sheet between two fingers and turn it from one side to the other (this is what one has to do with the forceps), or one can take a moistened finger, press the page a bit down and then turn it over (that is what one has to do with the needle, here the counter hold is the cortex)." With this in mind, the consequences appear quite clear cut. Author always uses a needle technique, the initial puncture peripheral or central, for the great majority of his cases. He uses forceps tchnique in those situations, where the needle so to say, lacks the other branch. This is mainly the case in the presence of a liquefied cortex or in cases, where a secondary enlargement of the capsulorhexis diameter is required.[5]

THE TWO-STEP NEEDLE TECHNIQUE

Today the two-step needle technique belongs to the past. Here, the capsule is first opened peripherally, with the needle below the incision and the incision is enlarged in a curve-shaped manner to the right and left, applying the sharp edges of the needle accordingly, so that a larger flap

is created. By bending the same needle now in such a way that the flap, which is transformed into an incision, is flipped around the tear is completed in a known way.[5]

CAPSULOSTRIPSIS

This technique was invented by F Rentsch and described by JH Greite at the 1995 ASCRS meeting. This approach is specifically designed for difficult cases, where the intracapsular pressure exceeds that of the anterior chamber. With this method a vitrector with infusion sleeve is used to create an irregular opening in the anterior capsule. Experience shows that a guillotine-type cutter is preferable to a rotating system. To prevent the capsule from tearing, extremely slow motion is essential. The resulting opening in the capsule is a jagged; however, the rounded, mouse-bite-like cuts of the vitrector tip, nevertheless produce a stable rim because of the favorable distribution of forces of this series of mini arcs.

This technique is rather time-consuming compared to conventional CCC performed by an experienced surgeon. On the other hand, it is easy to perform and provides a reliable alternative for hypermature or even milky cataracts without sufficient red reflex and other cases with difficult CCC, such as subluxated lenses or cataracts in children with elastic capsules.[6-8]

DIATHERMY CAPSULOTOMY

Another alternative method to create a circular and stable aperture of the anterior capsule that has been quite frequently discussed for some time is diathermy capsulotomy. In the attempt to create a circular rim in opening the capsule with this method, mostly bridges remain that have to be cut with microscissors. To perform this technique, the use of viscoelastics is required. The method is especially recommended for intumescent cataracts, but a number of surgeons find it easier to perform than the CCC in general.

However, even though the postoperative result may resemble that of a capsulorhexis, it should not be neglected that comparative studies demonstrated that the CCC is more stable and has a perfectly smooth edge in contrast to the diathermy opening, which is marked by multiple irregularities and offers less stability and less elasticity. Hence, the application of diathermy in routine cataract surgery cannot be recommended.[9-11]

CAPSULORHEXIS SIZE

The author prefers a capsulorhexis that is somewhat smaller than the optic diameter of the intraocular lens (IOL), to be implanted. The CCC provides enough stability and elasticity to allow intraocular manipulations, even with a smaller anterior aperture without any hazard. In fact, no study has ever been able to show that a larger CCC diameter relative to the IOL optic is more advantageous. Supporting this preference, comparative studies found that in addition, a slightly smaller capsulorhexis diameter seems to reduce the postoperative opacification of the posterior capsule.[12-14] When it comes to rhexis fixated IOL implantation, this type of IOL is completely excluded in the presence of an excessive rhexis diameter, for instance in case of damage of the posterior capsule, which is another reason why the rhexis size should be kept somewhat smaller than the lens optic. Furthermore, study results suggest that a smaller capsulorhexis size is likely to produce a smaller postoperative intraocular pressure (IOP) as well as better effectivity of sharp edges of some IOL designs.

DIFFICULT CASES

SMALL PUPIL

The fact that several different methods are available for intraoperative extension of a narrow pupil, capsulorhexis has become much easier to perform in such cases. The generally applied measures in such cases are:
• Removal of the pupillary membrane
• Bimanual stretching
• Removal of synechiae
• Iris hooks
• Pupil dilator.

To perform a capsulorhexis in the usual way, first the pupil is extended, using one of these methods. This is followed by creation of the CCC with needle or forceps.

PSEUDOEXFOLIATION SYNDROME, UVEITIS AND PIGMENTOSA

With these patients, often a thickened anterior capsule can be clinically observed, which is hard to tear. Another common finding in such cases is also a subluxated lens, which can only be diagnosed intraoperative. An important aspect of surgery in such patients is to strictly refrain from a rather small capsulorhexis, as the result of this might be an undesired shrinkage of the anterior capsule.

CAPSULES OF INFANTS, CHILDREN AND JUVENILES

Due to the high elasticity of the anterior capsule a smaller rhexis must be performed in such patients than is the case with adults. Here, it must be taken into account that the rhexis opening still enlarges by 0.5–1.0 mm after completion of the rhexis. Regarding pediatric posterior capsulorhexis, the necessity of an accompanying anterior vitrectomy is controversially discussed. Here, in a number of cases a self-sealing closure provided by the IOL could be successfully achieved.[15]

A new method to create a CCC in infantile and juvenile capsules was recently described by Nischal.[16] This new modification is called the two-incision push-pull capsulorhexis. Here, two stab incisions are made proximally and distally to the incision approximately 4.5–5.0 mm apart in the anterior capsule, thus outlining the diameter of the

planned capsulorhexis. One end of the distal edge of the proximal anterior capsule stab is grasped, using a fine capsulorhexis forceps and gently pushed toward the corresponding point of the distal stab incision and continued until halfway to the distal stab incision. A corresponding procedure is performed with the proximal edge of the distal anterior capsule stab incision, until half a CCC has been created. An analogous procedure is performed on the other side, resulted in a complete capsulorhexis opening.

This technique is specifically designed to meet the special conditions of the elastic pediatric capsule because the tearing forces are always directed to the pupillary center, thus resulting in a curvilinear tear. The technique can be applied for the anterior as well as posterior CCC.

CAPSULORHEXIS IN CALCIFIED CAPSULES OR ANTERIOR FLAPS

These cases mostly require a completely individual CCC, where an additional application of Ong or Vannas scissors or comparable tools are required.

POSTERIOR CAPSULORHEXIS

A series of indications, such as large-scale capsular fibroses, damage of the posterior capsule[17] or less frequent conditions, like persisting arteria hyaloidea as shown by Greite at the European Society of Cataract and Refractive Surgeons (ESCRS) 1990 meeting, may require a primary or secondary posterior capsulotomy. In the same way as the anterior CCC, the posterior capsulorhexis also offers the preservation of a stable capsule. First, the anterior capsulorhexis is performed using forceps or needle in the usual way and phacoemulsification or IOL explantation are carried out as preferred. The anterior segment is filled with viscoelastics to stabilize the posterior capsule. Then, the posterior capsule is first perforated only and viscoelastics are injected prior to further manipulations. This instillation of viscoelastics behind the capsule is vital to prevent a vitreous prolapse. The posterior CCC can then be carried out with needle or forceps in the same way as an anterior CCC. In some cases a successive vitrectomy may be necessary to prevent the vitreous from invading the capsular bag via the posterior opening. The remaining tire-like capsular residue provides a stable and secure site for intraocular lens fixation.[18] Gimbel, especially recommends a posterior capsulorhexis in pediatric cataract surgery, to avoid secondary membrane formation after cataract extraction.[19]

CAPSULORHEXIS IN THE PRESENCE OF A BROKEN POSTERIOR CAPSULE

If rupture of the posterior capsule occurs intraoperative (**Figures 18.7 and 18.8**) and cannot be transformed into a posterior CCC placement of the IOL in the ciliary sulcus with the known disadvantages of this fixation as listed below, seems to be the only option. To avoid this, rhexis fixation of the IOL is the possible solution. The author at

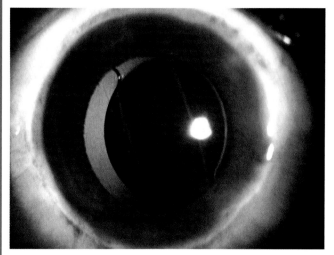

FIGURE 18.7: PC rupture and IOL in bag (*Courtesy:* Dr Agarwal's Eye Hospital, India)

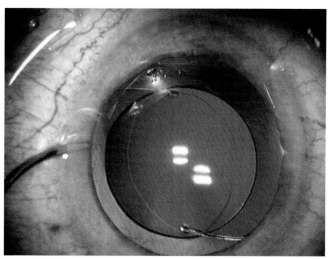

FIGURE 18.9: Rhexis fixation of an IOL; clinical picture

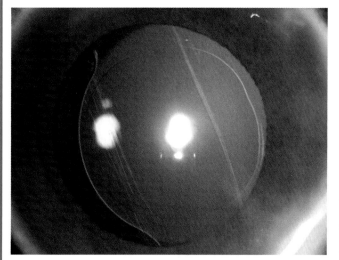

FIGURE 18.8: Magnified view of PC rupture and IOL in bag (*Courtesy:* Dr Agarwal's Eye Hospital, India)

the 1991 ASCRS film festival, first presented the applicable technique. The precondition for this method is an intact anterior capsulorhexis with a diameter that is smaller than that of the IOL optic. In rhexis fixation, the lens optic is manipulated behind the anterior capsulorhexis rim with a spatula, while the loops remain in the sulcus. This approach leaves the IOL optic securely positioned inside the capsule in a button-like manner (**Figure 18.9**). This method is also an option for pediatric surgery, where mostly a posterior capsulorhexis is performed as well as to prevent secondary cataract formation.[20,21] The only restriction using this method is the implied exclusion of plate-haptic IOLs.

The advantages of this technique are:
• No sunset or sunrise syndrome is possible.
• Rotation and decentration are excluded.
• The calculated lens power is effective because of the reliable location of the optic.
• Iris chafing cannot occur.
• Vitreous prolapse is prevented by stable endocapsular placement of the implant.

• Secondary cataract formation is avoided due to removal of the posterior capsule.

Howard Gimbel described a variation of this technique in the middle of the 1990s. In his modified approach, he used the opened posterior capsule as support/fixation location in infantile or juvenile lens implantation, thus trying to prevent a vitreous prolapse, calling this procedure capsular capture.[19]

ANTERIOR AND POSTERIOR CAPSULORHEXIS

MJ Tassignon works on that same topic to fixated IOLs on the capsulorhexis. Her technique is called "bag in the lens". The IOL has no haptics, but only a hinge of the IOL edge and is fixated, while clipping the two capsular leaves in this edge hinge. Further, clinical investigation is currently running to evaluate this very interesting IOL design and technique.

INSUFFICIENT RED REFLEX

In cases of an insufficient or completely missing red reflex due to mature or hypermature cataract, blue staining of the anterior capsule is now possible to increase the visibility for performance of the CCC. This method has become very fast, the most recommended technique in such cases.[22-26]

Another option to deal with this problem is capsulo-stripsis, instead of a capsulorhexis, as already described earlier in this chapter.

COMPLICATIONS AND PITFALLS

There are three major potential intraoperative problems an ophthalmic surgeon may find himself confronted with performing the CCC:

DISCONTINUITY OF THE CAPSULORHEXIS

To avoid this complication the capsulorhexis should never be completed from inside out, but also stellate bursts originating from initial puncturing attempts with a blunt needle may destroy an intact capsular margin in the course of surgery to form a discontinuity, which presents a most critical source for a radial tear down into the peripheral capsule. In the presence of such a discontinuity, the entity of mechanical forces inside the capsular bag concentrate on this weakest point and the only effective remedy is to repair the discontinuity immediately. If such a repair by transformation of the tear into a smooth edge is no longer possible, utmost care must be employed in the remaining intracapsular manipulations.

TEAR INTO THE ZONULA

If a tear has already reached a zonular fiber, a conventional repair of the capsulorhexis is too hazardous because it might result in further rupture right along the zonular fiber toward the equator. To cope with this critical situation two different approaches are available. One way is to follow the end of the respective zonula down to its origin, gently free it with the forceps and use this singled-out zonular fiber to tear a smooth edged curve, to unite with the otherwise intact capsulorhexis. The other and more risky approach is to firmly and briskly pull the flap toward the center.

INSUFFICIENT CAPSULORHEXIS SIZE

Realizing during the process of circular tearing that the capsulorhexis will be smaller than originally planned is not really an intraoperative problem. In such cases, all the surgeons have to direct the vector forces in such a way that the circle is not closed, but rather proceeds further into the periphery. With this kind of spiral shaped enlargement, the CCC diameter can be increased to the desired size. Once the capsulorhexis is large enough, the circle is closed in the usual way.

CAPTURED VISCOELASTICS

If the anterior capsular rim adheres to the anterior IOL surface after implantation, viscoelastics residues may be trapped behind the lens. Usually this problem does not occur, if the viscoelastics are carefully removed. If it does, mostly the lens blocks the passage for the viscoelastics into the anterior chamber and at the same time allows the aqueous to invade the area behind the implant, thus pushing the IOL against the cornea. In such a situation, an additional puncture of the peripheral anterior or in comparably narrow pupils, posterior capsule is required to provide for a release of the viscoelastics into the anterior chamber or the vitreous, respectively.

DISADVANTAGES OF THE CCC

As of the introduction of the CCC, a new problem was described over time, which is the capsular shrinkage syndrome or capsular phimosis.[27] This complication is not known in any other capsulotomy technique and solely relates to the CCC. The genuine pathomechanism could not be clarified until today. Clinically this problem can be observed, especially in patients suffering from pseudoexfoliation syndrome (PEX), uveitis, retinopathy pigmentosa or subluxation in combination with polymethylmethacrylate (PMMA) or silicone IOL implantation. All these diseases have a considerably reduced number of zonula fibers in common. The fact that up to now this complication has not been described in patients suffering from these diseases in context with an acrylic IOL implantation, allows the conclusion that a certain mechanical interaction of acrylic lens surface and capsule successfully prevent this problem, so that the acrylic IOL is presently the lens of choice in such cases. This however, is not valid for low-water acrylics.

A potential remedy to avoid the problem of capsular shrinkage is the insertion of a capsular tension ring.

DISCUSSION

The development of the capsulorhexis definitely introduced a new age in small incision cataract surgery (**Figures 18.10 to 18.16**). This applies both for the development of new phacoemulsification techniques as well as for the important role phacoemulsification plays in modern cataract surgery in general. In addition, the CCC has opened the gate for the development of a multitude of new and refined foldable IOLs and implantation devices because it was the first capsulotomy technique to offer a stable and reliable anterior capsular opening, so that today even a toric correction is possible with implantation of posterior chamber IOL.

While capsulorhexis as a principle is well established, its technical performance is being refined and advanced. In this context, author is stressing again that capsulorhexis in essence really is not a technical procedural detail, but a fundamental surgical principle. Its theory needs to be well understood, as only then its technical details emanate as a logical consequence. In other words, one should be convinced that this anterior capsular opening is what one wanted to have.

Also secondary surgery including intraocular lens exchange benefits from the specific properties of the capsulorhexis aperture. Intraocular manipulations in the anterior as well as posterior segment of the eye were belonging to the realm of phantasy only two decades ago, are feasible today. Now circular apertures at any required numbers and dimensions in both the anterior and the posterior capsule can be created securely and without taking the risk of tear originating from intraoperative manipulations. What is more, the structural integrity of the capsule is not only maintained throughout the course of surgery, but also postoperatively, thus forming the precondition for stable, safe and permanent IOL placement. From its invention 20 years ago, the CCC has managed to form a reliable basis for all new developments of the ophthalmic

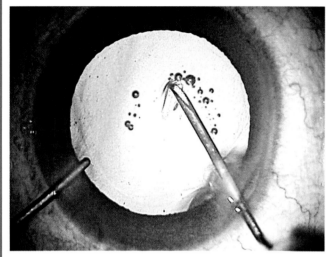

FIGURE 18.10

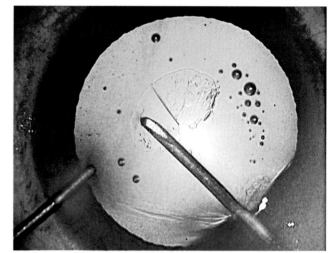

FIGURE 18.11

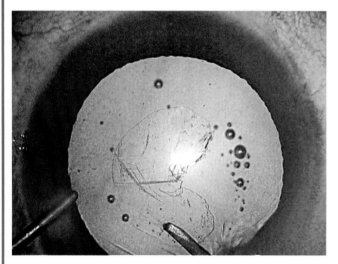

FIGURE 18.12

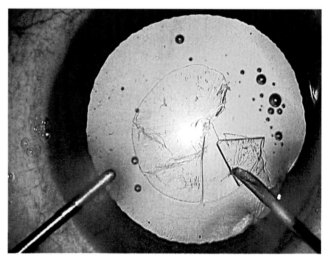

FIGURE 18.13

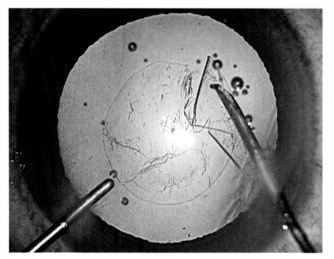

FIGURE 18.14

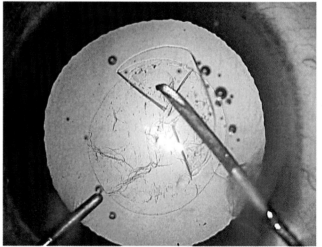

FIGURE 18.15

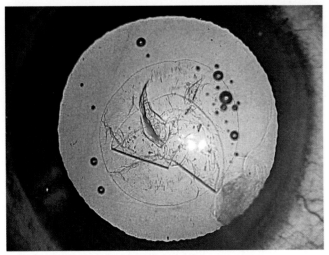

FIGURE 18.16

FIGURES 18.10 TO 18.16: Steps of capsulorhexis with a needle
(*Courtesy:* Dr Agarwal's Eye Hospital, India)

market and no comparable technique to open the capsular bag has been invented ever since. In this way, the CCC occupies its place as one of the important milestones of ophthalmology.

REFERENCES

1. Neuhann T. Theorie und Operationstechnik der Kapsulorhexis. Klin Monatsbl Augenheilkd. 1987;190:542-5.
2. Gimbel HV, Neuhann T. Continuous curvilinear capsulorhexis (letter). J Cataract Refract Surg. 1991;17:110-1.
3. Assia EI, Apple DJ, Barden A, et al. An experimental study comparing various anterior capsulectomy techniques. Arch Ophthalmol. 1991;109(5):642-7.
4. Krag S, Thim K, Corydon L, et al. Biomechanical aspects of the anterior capsulotomy. J Cataract Refract Surg. 1994;20(4): 410-6.
5. Neuhann T. Capsulorhexis, Phacoemulsification, Laser Cataract Surgery and Foldable IOLs. In: Agarwal S, Agarwal A, Sachdev MS, et al (Eds). New Delhi: Jaypee Brothers Medical Publishers (P) Ltd;1998. pp. 81-88.
6. Wilson ME, Bluestein EC, Wang XH, et al. Comparison of mechanized anterior capsulectomy and manual continuous capsulorhexis in pediatric eyes. J Cataract Refract Surg. 1994; 20(6):602-6.
7. Wilson ME, Saunders RA, Roberts EL, et al. Mechanized anterior capsulectomy as an alternative to manual capsulorhexis in children undergoing intraocular lens implantation. J Pediatr Ophthalmol Strabismus. 1996;33(4):237-40.
8. Andreo LK, Wilson ME, Apple DJ. Elastic properties and scanning electron microscopic appearance of manual continuous curvilinear capsulorhexis and vitrectorhexis in an animal model of pediatric cataract. J Cataract Refract Surg. 1999;25(4):534-9.
9. Morgan JE, Ellingham RB, Young RD, et al. The mechanical properties of the human lens capsule following capsulorhexis or radiofrequency diathermy capsulotomy. Arch Ophthalmol. 1996;114:1110-5.
10. Krag S, Thim K, Corydon L. Mechanical properties of diathermy capsulotomy versus capsulorhexis a biomechanical study. J Cataract Refract Surg. 1997;23(1):86-90.
11. Sugimoto Y, Kuho E, Tsuzuki S, et al. Histological observation of anterior capsular edges produced by continuous curvilinear and diathermy capsulorhexis. J Jpn Ophthalmol Soc. 1996;100(11):858-62.
12. Ravalico G, Tognetto D, Palomba M, et al: Capsulorhexis size and posterior capsule opacification. J Cataract Refract Surg. 1996;22(1):98-103.
13. Hollick EJ, Spalton DJ. Capsulorhexis size? Smaller seems better. J Cataract Refract Surg. 1997;2(5):12.
14. Cekic O, Batman C. Effect of capsulorhexis size on post-operative intraocular pressure. J Cataract Refract Surg. 1999; 25(3):416-9.
15. Gimbel HV, Chin PK, Ellant JP. Capsulorhexis. Ophthalmol Clin North Am.1995;8(3):441-5.
16. Nischal KK. Two-incision push-pull capsulorhexis for pediatric cataract surgery. J Cataract Refract Surg. 2002;28(4):593-5.
17. Galand A, Van Cauwenberge F, Moossavi J. Le capsulorhexis posterieur chez l´adulte. J Fr Ophtalmol. 1996;19(10):571-5.
18. Sandler G. Pediatric Ophthalmology, Benefits Seen to Posterior Capsulorhexis, Anterior Vitrectomy in Children. http://news.eyeworld.org/October/08 Kellan WZ. html.html.
19. Gimbel HV, DeBroff BM. Posterior capsulorhexis with optic capture—maintaining a clear visual axis after pediatric cataract surgery. J Cataract Refract Surg. 1994;20(6):658-64.
20. Behrendt S, Wetzel W. Vollständige Okklusion der Kapsulorhexisöffnung durch Vorderkapselschrumpfung. Ophthalmologe 1994;91(4):526-8.
21. Neuhann T. When posterior capsule tears, use capsulorhexis for IOL fixation. Phaco and Foldables. 1991;4(6):1-3.
22. Fritz WL. Fluorescein blue, light-assisted capsulorhexis for mature or hypermature cataract. J Cataract Refract Surg. 1998;24(1):19-20.
23. Nahra D, Castilla M. Fluorescein-stained capsulorhexis. J Cataract Refract Surg. 1998;24(9):1169-70.
24. Melles GR, de Waard PW, Pameijer JH, et al Färbung der Linsenkapsel mit Trypanblau zur Visualisierung der Kapsulorhexis bei Maturkataraktchirurgie. Klin Monatsbl Augenkeilkd. 1999;215(6):342-4.
25. Gotzaridis EV, Ayliffe WH. Fluorescein day improves visualization during capsulorhexis in mature cataracts. J Cataract Refract Surg. 1999;25(11):1423.
26. Nodarian M, Feys J, Sultan G, et al. Utilisation du bleu trypan pou la realisation du capsulorhexis dans la chirurgie de la cataracte blanche. J Fr Ophtalmol. 2001;24(3):274-6.
27. Sabbagh LB. Rhexis can hold IOL when posterior capsule breaks. Ocular Surgery News.1992;3(3):1-10.

CHAPTER 19

Divide and Conquer Nucleofractis Techniques

Howard V Gimbel, Ellen Anderson Penno

INTRODUCTION

Phacoemulsification, since its origin in the 1960s, has changed through the years and phacotechniques are still evolving. Besides the advantages of a smaller wound, phacoemulsification allows the removal of even dense brunescent nuclei through continuous curvilinear capsulorhexis (CCC) openings. In the early 1980s, as phacoemulsification was being applied to more and more denser nuclei, the author developed *in-situ* nuclear fracturing techniques which added to the safety and efficiency of phacoemulsification.[1-3] With the preservation of an intact capsular bag using CCC, fixation and centration of the intraocular lens (IOL) are ensured after safe and efficient in-the-bag phacoemulsification.[3]

The two-instrument nucleofractis technique was developed to facilitate subdivision of the nucleus into small pieces, so that they could be removed more efficiently through the phacoemulsification handpiece and thus through a small cataract incision. The term derives from the Latin *divide et impera* and nucleofractis comes from the prefix *nucleo* (nucleus) and the Greek suffix *fractis* (to fracture). Good nucleofractis skills can be learned by most ophthalmologists. Recent studies have demonstrated rates of vitreous loss by third-year resident surgeons learning nucleofractis techniques to be comparable to those found with standard extracapsular techniques.[4-6] Because the fracturing procedure in divide and conquer places a stretching force on the anterior capsular opening, can-opener-type capsulotomies are associated with an unacceptably high rate of peripheral capsular tears.

This led to the development of the CCC, which provides a strong tear-resistant border that maintains its integrity, despite the stretching forces produced with nucleofractis.[3,7,8]

The basic technique of nucleofractis is founded on the anatomic relationship of the lens fibers and the lenticular sutures. During embryologic development, lens fibers elongate and join, forming the two Y sutures, one anterior and one posterior. As more fibers are added, these sutures branch out into increasingly complex patterns.[9] These radially oriented sutures create potential cleavage planes that are susceptible to fracturing. The lens epithelial cells lay down concentric layers of nuclear tissue that become denser peripherally. These concentric layers resemble the lamellar organization of a tree-trunk or an onion. Radial and lamellar zones form cleavage planes within the lens nucleus and may be split by instruments and divided into smaller and more manageable pieces for phacoemulsification.

Divide and conquer nucleofractis (**Figures 19.1 to 19.17**) can be viewed as four basic steps: (i) sculpting until a thin posterior plate of nucleus remains, (ii) fracturing of the posterior plate and nuclear rim, (iii) breaking away a wedge-shaped section of nuclear material for emulsification and (iv) rotating the remaining nucleus for further fracturing and emulsification. All of the techniques described in this chapter represent variations on this theme. Which one is used depends on surgeon preference, density of the nucleus, degree of pupillary dilation and whether or not an intact CCC is present.

DOWN-SLOPE SCULPTING

Divide and conquer nucleofractis begins with sculpting until a thin posterior plate of nucleus remains. A variation from the traditional sculpting method involves nudging the lens inferiorly with the second instrument. With the lens nudged towards the 6 o'clock position, the surgeon can sculpt very deeply down the slope of the posterior curvature of the upper part of the capsule. This technique has thus been termed "down-slope sculpting".[10]

The author first began using this nudging maneuver in small pupil cases out of necessity because of limitations of pupil size and capsular opening. The technique was then extended to almost all cases. It was found that down-slope sculpting greatly enhanced the speed and efficiency of the nucleofractis techniques and has increased the safety, because the sculpting is parallel rather than somewhat perpendicular to the posterior capsule.

With traditional techniques, if the nucleus is broken through unexpectedly when sculpting a deep, long trench towards 6 o'clock, the tip is more perpendicular to the inferior portion of the posterior capsule because of its concavity and is directly perpendicular to the equatorial capsule. With down-slope sculpting, considerable nuclear material remains ahead of the tip at the end of each sculpting pass. Therefore, breaking through is unlikely with the "cushion" present. The risk of engaging the capsule is thus minimized.

Down-slope sculpting in the upper pole of the lens to just past the center reduces the chance of posterior capsule rupture with the phaco port. If the lens is nudged inferiorly by the second instrument and deep sculpting is done from just inside the continuous curvilinear capsulorhexis to the center of the lens, then the tip will travel parallel to the concave slope of the posterior aspect of the nucleus and the posterior capsule. Although the surgeon cannot visualize

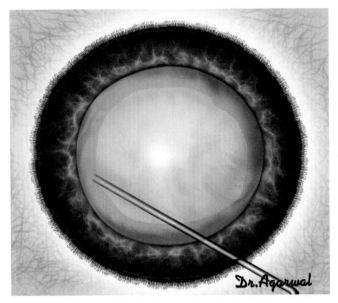

FIGURE 19.1: Hydroprocedures: Good hydroprocedures are also important for a successful divide and conquer procedure. Hydrodissection frees up the cortex from the capsular bag and makes cortical removal easy. More importantly, hydrodelineation delineates the nucleus from the epinucleus. This allows the nucleus to freely rotate within the capsular bag for maneuvers such as sculpting, etc. (*Courtesy:* Dr Agarwal's Eye Hospital, India)

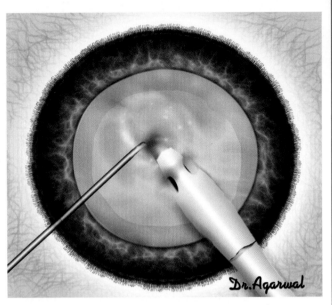

FIGURE 19.3: Sculpting: With the tip adequately exposed on the phaco probe, it is used to sculpt longitudinally along the nucleus. This creates a trench in the nucleus. It is useful to perform downslope trenching wherein the second instrument pushes the nucleus downwards so that trenching can be started above the center of the nucleus (*Courtesy:* Dr Agarwal's Eye Hospital, India)

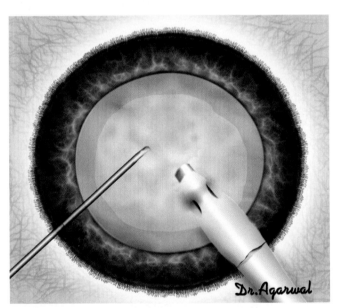

FIGURE 19.2: Sculpting (*Courtesy:* Dr Agarwal's Eye Hospital, India)

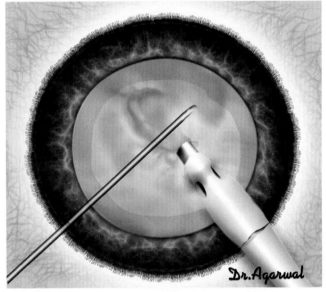

FIGURE 19.4: Nucleus rotation: Trenching thus started above the centre of the nucleus can be carried on in a downslope direction thus allowing deep sculpting in the central thickest portion of the nucleus. Once trenching is completed in the inferior direction, the nucleus is rotated 180 degrees so that the superior pole now comes to lie inferiorly (*Courtesy:* Dr Agarwal's Eye Hospital, India)

the tip when going "down-slope", the depth of the sculpting is determined by visualizing the depth of the groove and translucency of the remaining tissue.

Furthermore, with traditional sculpting techniques, the deepest part of the sculpting inevitably ends up inferior to the center of the lens. If the surgeon rotates the lens 90° after sculpting each quadrant, then the nuclear material deep in the center or posterior pole of the nucleus may still impede complete fracturing to the center and the sections will tend to hang together in the middle of the lens. However, with down-slope sculpting, complete and efficient fracturing and subsequent emulsification can be accomplished, by sculpting deeply and fracturing through the entire posterior plate of the nucleus.

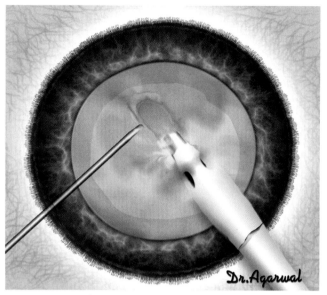

FIGURE 19.5: Sculpting: Sculpting is then carried on again in the inferior direction. The trench already created is extended in the opposite direction. It is important to follow the slope of the nucleus upwards now so as to avoid going through the nucleus and posterior capsule. This is especially important as the trench becomes more deep (*Courtesy:* Dr Agarwal's Eye Hospital, India)

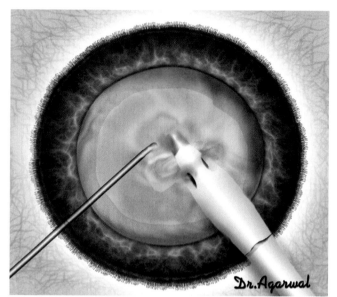

FIGURE 19.7: Trenching: Trenching is again started in a downward direction starting from the wall of the trench already created. Sculpting can be started at a deeper level this time as it is started from the depth of the previous groove. This creates a trench at right angles to the one already created (*Courtesy:* Dr Agarwal's Eye Hospital, India)

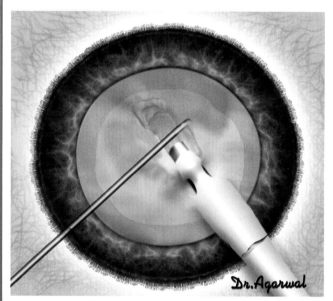

FIGURE 19.6: Nucleus rotation: The nucleus is thinned leaving only a thin posterior plate so that it can be easily cracked later. The nucleus is then rotated 90 degrees to bring the trench to lie horizontally (*Courtesy:* Dr Agarwal's Eye Hospital, India)

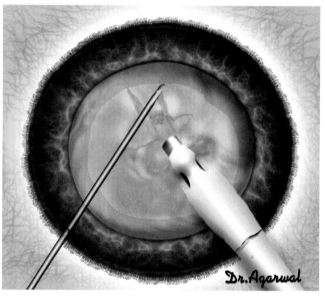

FIGURE 19.8: Nucleus rotation: The nucleus is then rotated 180 degrees and again sculpted downwards. This finally gives a cruciate trench which is equally deep along its length in all directions. The posterior plate should be thinned out along the cruciate trench to allow easy cracking (*Courtesy:* Dr Agarwal's Eye Hospital, India)

The surgeon must be cautious when the CCC is small to avoid tearing the edge of the anterior capsule superiorly with the tip or the sleeve of the phaco instrument. In the author's experience, small CCCs are most likely to occur in cases with poor visualization, such as when hypermature, white cataracts are present. Ordinarily, the risk is low because one is not sculpting much past the center when first beginning the trench.

Care must also be exercised in displacing the nucleus within the capsular bag, so that the whole bag is not displaced and the upper zonular ligaments are not unduly stretched and broken. Adequate hydrodissection is essential to allow inferior nucleus displacement, while minimizing stress to the upper zonular apparatus. Also, when tipping the handle of the phaco handpiece up to sculpt down towards the posterior pole, the surgeon must not push the tip posteriorly faster than the tip is chiselling its way through the lens material. The zonular ligaments may also be torn with such a maneuver. These risks are greatest in lenses with hard epinuclei and where the zonules are already weakened.

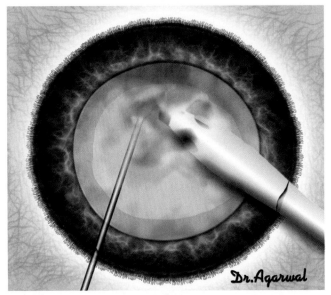

FIGURE 19.9: Cracking: The phaco tip and the second instrument are both placed deep within the trench created in preparation for cracking the thin posterior plate. It is important to place them both deep in the trench so that forces exerted are able to crack the posterior plate (*Courtesy:* Dr Agarwal's Eye Hospital, India)

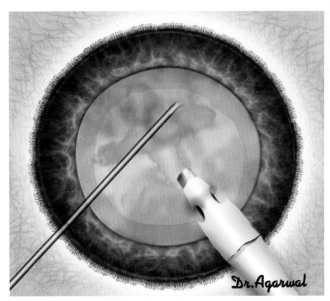

FIGURE 19.11: Nucleus rotation: If the posterior plate has not cracked along its entire extent or if the superior nuclear rim has not cracked, the nucleus is rotated 180 degrees using the second instrument and then cracked again (*Courtesy:* Dr Agarwal's Eye Hospital, India)

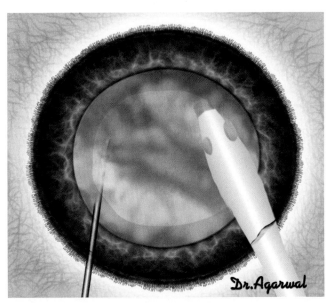

FIGURE 19.10: Cracking: Moving the two instruments thus placed opposite to each other cracks the thin posterior plate as well as the nuclear rim. The two instruments can be either moved outwards against their respective walls or in a cross-handed technique so that each instrument pushes the opposite wall (*Courtesy:* Dr Agarwal's Eye Hospital, India)

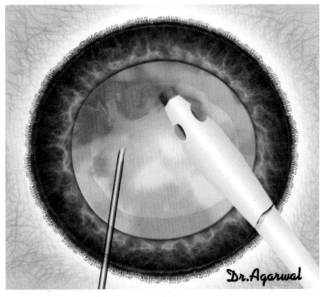

FIGURE 19.12: Cracking: The cracking is completed along its extent after having rotated the nucleus. It is important to separate any fibers in the posterior plate which might be still left between the two hemisections (*Courtesy:* Dr Agarwal's Eye Hospital, India)

Limiting sculpting to the superior part of the nucleus adds safety because of the reduced risk of contacting the posterior capsule and adds efficiency because of the rapidity with which the posterior pole of the nucleus is reached with the phaco tip. With instruments this deep in the nucleus, the fracturing can be effectively initiated and safely completed.

THE FRACTURE

The fundamental principle underlying nucleofractis is the creation of fractures within the nucleus to facilitate the removal of the cataract, through a small incision while causing the least possible trauma to the eye. If the nuclear rim is very hard or if the CCC is not intact, splitting the

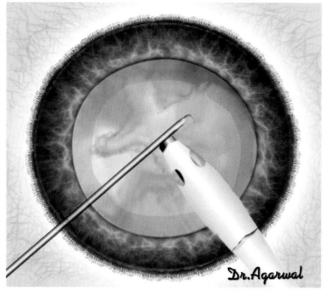

FIGURE 19.13: Nucleus rotation: The nucleus is now rotated 90 degrees for cracking along the second trench. While cracking, the two instruments should be moved only in a horizontal plane with no stress directed inferiorly to avoid stress on the zonules resulting in dialysis or subluxation (*Courtesy:* Dr Agarwal's Eye Hospital, India)

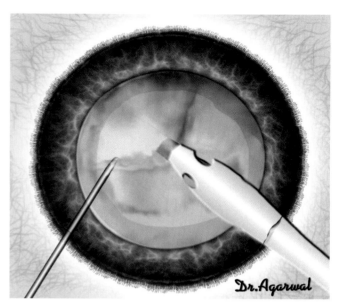

FIGURE 19.15: Quadrant removal: The phaco tip is embedded into the apex of the quadrant and brought out from the capsular bag. Each quadrant is similarly removed in turn for phacoemulsification (*Courtesy:* Dr Agarwal's Eye Hospital, India)

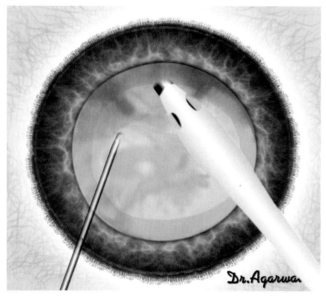

FIGURE 19.14: Cracking: Each hemisection of the nucleus is then cracked so that eventually the nucleus is divided into four quadrants, each of which is completely separated along the posterior plate as well as the nuclear rim (*Courtesy:* Dr Agarwal's Eye Hospital, India)

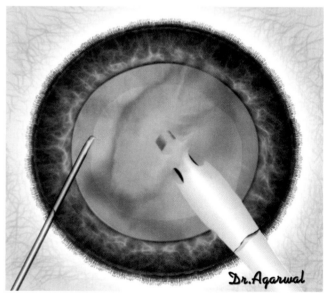

FIGURE 19.16: Quadrant removal: Once the quadrants are brought out, they are emulsified taking care to work deep in the anterior chamber at the iris plane. Dispersive viscoelastics should be used in case of dense nuclei (*Courtesy:* Dr Agarwal's Eye Hospital, India)

nucleus along a groove is achieved using a bimanual technique or a nuclear cracker. Regardless of the fracturing technique used, nucleofractis is facilitated by deep sculpting of the posterior pole of the lens nucleus. This will be discussed in more detail under "polar expenditions".

With the parallel instrument technique, a deep central groove is sculpted within the lens nucleus and the phaco probe is placed deep within the groove against the right-hand wall (for right-handed surgeons). A second instrument is placed in the groove against the other wall. The fracture is created by pushing the two walls away from each other.

Alternatively, with a cross-handed technique, each instrument is placed against the opposite wall of the groove. With both the parallel instrument and cross-handed techniques, placing the two instruments as deeply as possible within the groove provides the most efficient application of the cracking force.

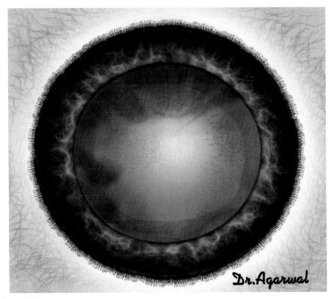

FIGURE 19.17: Quadrant removal: Once the first quadrant has been removed, subsequent quadrants are easier to bring out from the bag as they are no longer compactly arranged (*Courtesy:* Dr Agarwal's Eye Hospital, India)

As sculpting proceeds to deeper layers, the phaco tip is moved in a lateral sweeping motion. It is important to avoid occlusion of the tip during this procedure.

The lens is stabilized inferior to the groove with a second instrument through the paracentesis. After lateral sculpting is sufficiently deep, a horizontal fracture is created as described later in the "multi-directional divide and conquer" section of this chapter. Phaco sweep is a variation of down-slope sculpting which enhances visualization of the phaco tip and results in increased safety for the removal of central nuclear material.

In addition, the motion of the probe remains parallel to the posterior capsule, diminishing the risk of its inadvertent rupture.

CRATER DIVIDE AND CONQUER (CDC) TECHNIQUE

Divide and conquer nucleofractis phaco, described by the author was the first nucleofractis (two-instrument) cracking technique developed.[1, 12] It is still used for hard lenses and is now combined with the phaco chop for dense brunescent nuclei. The phaco chop technique will be discussed later in this chapter.

After adequate hydrodissection, a deep crater is sculpted into the center of the nucleus, leaving a dense peripheral rim that can later be fractured into multiple sections. The crater must include the posterior plate of the nucleus, otherwise, fracturing of the rim will be much more difficult. A shaving action is used to sculpt away the central nuclear material. When the central material is no longer accessible to the phaco probe, the lens should be rotated and additional central sculpting performed to enlarge and deepen the crater. The size of the central crater should be expanded for progressively denser nuclei. Enough of the dense material must be left in place, however, to allow the phaco probe and second instrument to engage the rim and fracture the lens into sections.

The surgeon uses experience as a guide to determine how deeply the central crater should be sculpted. The peripheral nuclear rim stretches the entire capsular bag and acts as a safety mechanism, to prevent the posterior capsule from suddenly moving anteriorly and being cut by the phacoprobe. For harder nuclei, small sections should be fractured from the rim. Rather than emulsify the sections as they are broken away, the sections should be left in place within the rim to maintain the circular rim and the tension on the capsule. Leaving the sections in place also facilitates rotation and the progressive fracturing of the remaining rim. It is sometimes advisable to initially remove one small section to allow space for fracturing the other segments of the remaining rim. If one small fragment is removed, the remaining segment can maintain capsular stretch and help to avoid rupture of the capsule. After the rim is fractured around the entirety of its circumference, each segment can

An alternative fracturing technique involves creating a full diameter groove, aligning the groove midway between the main incision and moving the two instruments away from each other deep within the trench. The density of the lens and the preference of the surgeon will dictate the appropriate fracturing techniques necessary to achieve consistent and predictable results in nucleofractis. All fracturing techniques currently used by the author, use the principles of deep sculpting followed by fracturing of the posterior plate of the nucleus and then the posterior rim. Once the initial fracture is achieved, rotation and additional fractures are used to break away wedge-shaped sections of the lens nucleus for emulsification.

PHACO SWEEP

Another variation on the theme of sculpting is a technique the author calls "phaco sweep".[11] In traditional sculpting techniques, the phaco tip is moved from the superior to the inferior portion of the nucleus to create a groove. By using the phaco tip in a lateral motion (nasal to temporal and back again), the central nucleus can be sculpted quickly and deeply, while maintaining constant visualization of the tip of the instrument. The author prefers to use a 30° Kelman tip to perform phaco sweep. With this tip, the removal of lens material is more efficient and easier to perform. However, this technique is also possible with standard straight tip phacoemulsification handpieces. The engineers at Alcon Surgical explain this difference on the basis of a three-dimensional propagation of the ultrasound wave front from the bent Kelman tip. Standard handpieces tend to direct their ultrasound power primarily in the forward direction, somewhat limiting their cutting efficiency for this technique.

then be brought to the center of the capsule for safe emulsification. One must be more cautious at this point because as more segments are removed, less lens material is available to expand the capsule, and the capsule will have a greater tendency to be aspirated into the phaco tip, especially if high aspiration flow rates are used.

TRENCH DIVIDE AND CONQUER (TDC) TECHNIQUE

Recognizing the efficiency of fracturing maneuvers during CDC, the author stopped sculpting the right side of soft lenses after making the central trench and instead made a central fracture.

Using the down-slope sculpting technique described earlier allows the phaco tip to remove more of the upper part of the nucleus during sculpting and to reach the posterior pole of the lens very early for effective fracturing. Then, the left side is divided by fracturing and also the right side. These variations were named "trench divide and conquer (TDC)" techniques.[10,13,14]

Using a 30° or 45° tip, the TDC technique begins with a shallow trench or trough sculpted slightly to the right of the center of the lens surface. The lens is stabilized with the spatula through the paracentesis. Then, nudging the loosened lens nucleus inferiorly with the second instrument, down-slope sculpting is performed very deeply to the posterior pole of the lens. Adequate hydrodissection is essential to down-slope sculpting because then the nucleus is not attached to the peripheral cortex and capsule and the nucleus can easily be displaced in the capsular bag.

Placing the instrument tips deep in the center of the lens, fracturing is accomplished by pushing towards the right with the phaco tip, as the cyclodialysis spatula is pushed to the left. This is accomplished in foot position two (irrigation/aspiration only and no ultrasound power). The lens usually splits from the center to the superior and inferior rim of the nucleus if the instruments are held deep in the center. If the split does not readily extend to the equator inferiorly or superiorly, moving the instruments away from the center can produce the mechanical advantage necessary to extend the fracture through the nuclear rim.

After this first crack has been obtained, the depth of the sculpted groove in the lens can be determined and the surgeon can gauge how much deeper sculpting should be continued to facilitate further fracturing.

In all but brunescent nuclei, usually three to five sculpting passes allow one to get deep enough into the lens to start fracturing.

Either before the first fracture or immediately afterward, the Down-slope technique may be used to sculpt the majority of the upper part of the lens. Keeping the probe deep in the tissue and close to the posterior cortex, the surgeon then burrows deeply into the left hemisection and

creates a second crack that intersects with the first, isolating a pie-shaped section of nucleus. In soft nuclei, this is usually performed about 60° from the first fracture, but in hard nuclei, the crack is shortened to about 30° away.

The isolated pie-shaped section can then either be emulsified or left in place as the next crack is made in a similar fashion. The remaining right section of nucleus is then maneuvered with the second instrument and brought to the midpupillary zone. A final split is made after impaling the tip with a short burst of ultrasound, pushing with the phaco tip towards the 6 o'clock position, while stabilizing the upper portion. The piece can then be fractured into halves or thirds and emulsified as they are fractured. Alternatively, the right hemisection may be rotated to the left side and fractured in a way similar to the first hemisection.

Rather than utilizing grooves to start the fractures, the surgeon simply needs to get the instruments deep into the center of the lens to fracture through the naturally occurring radial fault lines of the lens. Except in brunescent nuclei where notches are sculpted in the nuclear rim so that the spatula has a wall to push against, the principal advantage of the technique is that pregrooving the nucleus for subsequent fracturing is completely unnecessary.

MULTIDIRECTIONAL DIVIDE AND CONQUER (MDC) TECHNIQUE

Down-slope multidirectional nucleofractis is begun by debulking the superior part of the lens. The phaco sweep technique is initiated with small lateral movements of the phaco tip at the bottom of the previously formed groove. The Kelman tip works very well for this side-to-side movement, to create a deep groove horizontally. The phaco tip is then used to stabilize the upper portion while the spatula pushes inferiorly against the wall, creating a horizontal fracture.

This horizontal fracture is a combination of separation and shearing. The second instrument pushes towards 6 o'clock and the phaco tip pushes down and away, so that these opposing forces result in the splitting of the nucleus as the horizontal fracture.

Multidirectional nucleofractis occurs when the phaco tip is used to engage the inferior hemisection and multiple pie-shaped sections are fractured using the second instrument to stabilize the nucleus. The sections are brought into the central pupillary zone for safe emulsification.

The multidirectional fracturing is accomplished without rotating the lens. With the natural fault lines in the lens, this can be accomplished very easily without the chopping technique through the use of two-instrument separation. The fracturing is enhanced by not only separation but again by shearing (pushing down on one segment and away on the other) so that the separation is in two planes.

The superior hemisection is rotated inferiorly and emulsified in a similar fashion. Alternatively, the superior section is nudged inferiorly with the spatula and the phaco tip is burrowed into the bulk of the nucleus, which is fractured without rotation.

PHACO CHOP

Kunihiro Nagahara first introduced the phaco chop technique in 1993 at the annual meeting of the American Society of Cataract and Refractive Surgery (ASCRS) in Seattle, Washington. This technique also uses the lamellar structure of the nucleus to create radial fractures in the lens. The phacoemulsification probe is directed into the central core of the nucleus until occlusion of the port occurs. A modified lens hook is then inserted just beneath the anterior capsular leaflet at the 6 o'clock position, just adjacent to the phaco probe, but extending to the equator of the lens. The tip is drawn centrally from the equator of the lens towards the phaco tip. This chop must encompass at least half of the anteroposterior diameter of the lens. The two instruments can then be used in a standard bimanual technique to complete the fracture. The nucleus is rotated slightly after the first chop and the procedure is repeated until pie-shaped wedges are created throughout the lens. These wedges can then be aspirated into the center of the capsular bag for safe emulsification.

While the phaco chop technique can reduce phacoemulsification time significantly, this technique poses a persistent threat to anterior capsular integrity. Traversing the chopping instrument through the cortex towards the equator ensures that the anterior capsule remains anterior to the chopping instrument. The risk to capsular integrity with the phaco chop technique is greatest for surgeons with limited experience.

As discussed earlier, the author has incorporated this phaco chop technique into the crater divide and conquer method for dense brunescent nuclei.[15] It can be difficult to separate the nuclear rim in very hard lenses. In this modified technique, the central nucleus is sculpted away as described earlier (see "Crater Divide and Conquer" section). However, rather than fracture the remaining nucleus by traditional nucleofractis techniques, the chop maneuver is used to split and then separate the nuclear rim using shearing forces **(Figures 19.18A to C)**. Creating a central crater provides a space where rim segments can be easily maneuvered following the chop. Fracturing is thus made easier and zonular and capsular stress is reduced.

The use of the chop technique is safer in the presence of anterior capsular tears because stretching of the capsule is reduced. For soft and moderately soft nuclei, the chop technique does not offer sufficient added efficacy to offset the increased risk of capsular tears.

Steve Arshinoff presented his "slice and separate" modified phaco chop technique at the 1997 annual meeting of the American Society of Cataract and Refractive Surgery. This method is designed to be used for moderately dense nuclei. Dr Arshinoff describes impaling the nucleus and

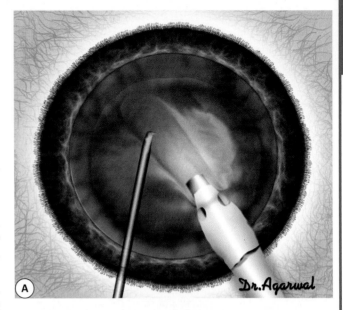

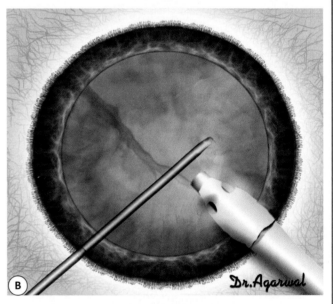

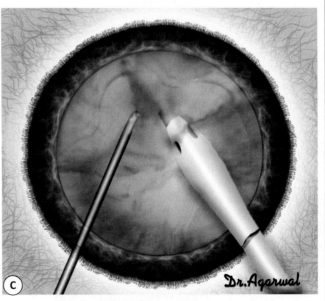

FIGURES 19.18A TO C: Stop and chop *(Courtesy: Dr Agarwal's Eye Hospital, India)*

using a phaco chopper to slice across the nuclear part of the lens from anterior to posterior, passing by the phaco tip. The nucleus is then rotated 15° to 20° and the same maneuver is repeated on the distal half. After the second slice, the segment is vacuumed out and the procedure is repeated—slice and vacuum—until the nucleus is removed. The slice maneuver is always started in the lens center and the posterior capsule remains protected by the remaining nuclear and cortical material. Dr. Arshinoff emphasizes the need for good hydrodissection for success in this technique and notes that the slice and separate technique is difficult to perform on very soft nuclei, due to difficulty in stabilizing the lens.

POLAR EXPEDITIONS

Regardless of the fracturing technique used—crater divide and conquer (CDC), trench divide and conquer (TDC) or multidirectional divide and conquer (MDC)—the key is to sculpt nuclear material away centrally, leaving a thin layer of epinuclear material. Deep sculpting to the posterior pole of the lens facilitates the fracturing of the nucleus because it provides for safe and efficient segmentation and removal of the nuclear segments by taking advantage of the natural fault lines of the lens. Deep sculpting also allows one to obtain the mechanical advantage required to effectively fracture through the entire lens. Sculpting should be deep enough to be right through the nucleus into the epinucleus. The bent Kelman tip facilitates this deep sculpting.

The expedition to the posterior pole can be accomplished with forward sculpting or phaco sweep lateral sculpting to thin the posterior plate, before fracturing is attempted.[16] Once a thin posterior plate is achieved, the segments fracture very easily with the two-handed technique. In a brunescent lens, the phaco chop instrument is used to fracture segments in the crater chop, so that the segments are smaller and more easily managed.

In trench divide and conquer (TDC) nucleofractis, polar sculpting is limited to a central trough or trench. This works best in a very soft nucleus where one has to maintain most of the nucleus which is firm enough to fracture. The nucleus is nudged slightly inferiorly and stabilized with the second instrument. Then the polar expedition for the posterior pole of the lens begins. The trench has to be wide enough to allow the phaco sleeve to get down into the nucleus. Once deep enough, the fracture is obtained with the two instruments. The segments are broken away, similar to the other nucleofractis techniques. Once the fracture is through the posterior plate of the lens, the fractured segments fracture completely without being tied together at the apices, and small segments are easier to manage than large segments. Only low-ultrasound power is necessary for these small nuclear segments to be emulsified.

In multidirectional divide and conquer, down-slope sculpting towards the posterior pole is used initially. The upper part of the nucleus is removed and then with phaco sweep, polar expedition involves sculpting of the posterior pole before the horizontal fracture. The lens is stabilized and nudged inferiorly and the sculpting is done with forward passes until one is deep in the lens. Then, phaco sweep is used to delicately sculpt through the deepest part of the nucleus to the epinucleus before the horizontal fracture is made.

THE SMALL PUPIL

The most important goal in small pupil cataract surgery is to limit serious surgical complications. Relatively complication-free surgery in small pupil casescan be achieved with phacoemulsification techniques. These techniques also help to attain other goals, such as the use of a small incision, the minimal use of pupil enlarging surgery and certain verification of in-the-bag placement of a posterior chamber intraocular lens. The placement verification, long-term stability and centration can be virtually assured by obtaining and maintaining a continuous curvilinear capsulorhexis opening in the anterior capsule.[17] The lens nucleus, even though dense and large, can be fractured into small segments and removed by emulsification through relatively small capsule openings, small pupil openings, small scleral incisions and small conjunctival incisions. These are important considerations in many glaucoma patients who have small pupils from long-term miotic therapy and who have had or may in the future require filtering surgery.

The author developed the down-slope sculpting method, as described earlier in this chapter, in small pupil cases to quickly reach the posterior pole of the nucleus for efficient fracturing. The lens is nudged inferiorly, using a second instrument and the phacotip sculpts down the concave posterior capsule towards the posterior pole as described earlier, parallel to the capsule as opposed to perpendicular to it. Once the pole is reached, the two-instruments are held deep in the center. The spatula pushes inferiorly while the phaco tip pushes superiorly to create a horizontal fracture. The two instruments are repositioned to create a vertical fracture. The fractured segments can remain in the bag to stabilize it or be removed piece by piece. The second instrument holds back segments, while other segments are emulsified in the center of the lens. As well, the spatula brings nuclear material to the phaco tip to be emulsified. The phaco tip itself, stays mainly in the center of the lens.

Small pupil cases demonstrate the distinct advantage of nucleofractis techniques in that the phaco tip does not have to be put under the iris or under the small openings in the capsule. As such, there is little risk of iris or capsule flowing unexpectedly with the lens material into the tip of the phaco port. One should use a lower flow when the pupil is small. This may reduce efficiency, but certainly increases safety. Again, epinuclear material is brought to the phaco port using the second instrument. The phaco port itself does not go searching for this material in a small pupil case.

INTUMESCENT LENS

The nucleus in an intumescent lens can be safely and efficiently fractured and phacoemulsified, using the down-slope sculpting technique.[18] In intumescent cases with primary, small capsulorhexis openings, the nucleus is nudged inferiorly with a second instrument. The upper portion of the nucleus is then sculpted using the down-slope sculpting technique. The nudging maneuver allows the phacotip to get very deep into the nucleus for subsequent fracturing. The phaco tip should be maintained centrally to avoid stress on either the small capsulorhexis rim or a can-opener margin. Mechanical stress to the ring of the can-opener with the use of the phaco handpiece or by a second instrument, should be avoided. This is another instance in which down-slope sculpting nucleofractis is advantageous for safe emulsification, because the phaco tip always stays in the center of the lens. The second instrument is used to rotate, maneuver and help fracture the nuclear rim.

The depth of the sculpting is quite easy to gauge in an intumescent lens due to the whiteness of the nucleus and the red reflex exposed during fracturing. In doing phaco-emulsification out near the periphery or up near the capsule in the epinucleus, a low flow and low vacuum should be used so that a sudden break-through with a high flow and high vacuum can be avoided. This will avoid engaging the equatorial capsule with the phaco tip. The intumescent lens is usually easy to fracture and quite often the lens will fracture spontaneously just with the attempt at rotation.

CAPSULAR TENSION RINGS

Since phacoemulsification and continuous curvilinear capsulorhexis were developed, it has become possible to remove a cataract through a small incision and implant an intraocular lens (IOL) into the capsular bag. The centration and stability of the IOL in-the-bag is critical for maintaining excellent visual outcome. In some situations, placing an IOL in the capsular bag may be insecure, as in the case of a traumatic cataract with broken or loose zonules. To manage this situation, many anterior segment surgeons (including the first author) prefer to use phacoemulsification if possible, even if the capsular bag cannot be used for IOL placement. A sutured posterior chamber IOL (PC-IOL) or an anterior chamber IOL (AC-IOL) may be placed after phacoemulsi-fication is completed. Sutured fixation of a PC-IOL significantly increases surgery time and axial tilt of the IOL often occurs postoperatively. Implantation of an AC-IOL may be associated with postoperative corneal pathology, chronic cystoid macular edema or secondary glaucoma.

In 1991, Hara et al introduced an equator ring for maintaining the circular contour of the capsular bag after cataract removal. Following their work, different types of rings of varied material were developed. Cionni and Osher reported on four cataract surgery cases with extensive zonular dialysis managed with endocapsular rings. The

results showed that the ring facilitated phacoemulsification and PC-IOL in-the-bag implantation. In January 1995, the author began using a polymethylmethacrylate (PMMA) capsular tension ring (Morcher GMBH, Germany) to manage patients with zonular dialysis requiring cataract surgery **(Figure 19.19)**.

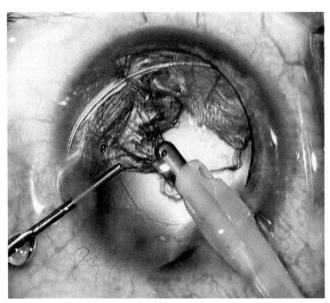

FIGURE 19.19: Capsular tension ring (*Courtesy: Dr Agarwal's Eye Hospital, India*)

A capsular tension ring may have potential benefits for cataract surgery patients with zonular dialysis—a capsular tension ring appears to enhance safety and efficacy during the phacoemulsification and PC-IOL implantation, it may help to avoid vitreous herniation, it maintains the circular contour of the capsular bag, it may reduce IOL decentration and it may inhibit lens epithelial cell proliferation on the posterior capsule by compression, which may reduce the incidence of secondary cataract.

Clinically, cataracts with loose zonules or broken zonules are commonly seen which present a challenge for surgeons when performing phacoemulsification and PC-IOL implantation. The capsular tension ring provides an alternative means to manage this situation.

CHALLENGES TO TOPICAL ANESTHESIA IN SMALL-INCISION CATARACT SURGERY

The use of topical anesthesia in cataract operations requires that surgeons learn new techniques and adapt to challenges not faced with the use of local or general anesthesia. The transition to topical anesthesia means that surgeons cannot use some of the techniques that have been entirely safe on the immobilized eye. Under topical anesthesia, one cannot rely on the patient's fixation or on voluntary immobilization of the eye and persistent ocular movements on a regular or irregular basis may occur. In some circumstances, the globe must be immobilized with a second instrument.

The author began using topical anesthesia for cataract surgery in 1993, specifically because of a case involving a very myopic eye with an axial length of 36.3 mm. In this case, it was felt that the risks of using peribulbar or even pin-point anesthesia were too high. The patient was relatively cooperative and communicative and fixated well. The author became convinced that topical anesthesia in long eyes adds an element of safety, reducing or eliminating the risks of the local anesthetic.

Topical anesthesia introduces new challenges to cataract surgery. A learning curve presents itself with changes in surgical technique and modifications must be made in reflex and habit that have evolved while doing surgery with peribulbar anesthesia surgery. Two-handed cataract extraction techniques are relatively advantageous in topical anesthesia cases, particularly because the second instrument—at almost 90° from the first—helps to stabilize the eye against unwanted movements in both the vertical and horizontal directions.

In general, the learning curve involves modifications to almost every stage of cataract surgery. The eye must be stable even before the paracentesis is done. If an eye is not very quiet, it is valuable to use a ring to stabilize the eye while making the paracentesis. Next, the eye needs to be stabilized with forceps during the incision. The surgeon cannot afford any sudden movements (particularly when using diamond knives) of an eye anesthetized only topically. Scleral incisions under topical anesthetic must be made with the eye stabilized with forceps (unlike clear corneal incision where the eye is stabilized by a ring), grasping and regrasping the sclera before continuing with dissection. Sometimes, with local anesthesia, when the incision is being made, the grasp on the sclera is released and reapplied in a different place when the blade is in the tunnel. In eyes under topical anesthesia, the author advocates that the blade be removed from the tunnel before the forceps are released and the sclera be grasped at another location before the blade is re-entered. One should never release the eye with the second instrument, unless the sharp instrument is taken away first, because if the eye moves unexpectedly with only the sharp instrument in the tunnel, the sclera could be inadvertently cut.

Some extremely nervous patients do not agree to topical anesthesia even after sedation. In patients with language barriers we now bring an interpreter or family member into the operating room. When faced with communication difficulties with extremely deaf or demented patients, we sometimes opt for a local anesthetic. However, nonverbal communication for instructions allows surgery to be done under topical anesthesia in many cases.

Topical anesthesia appears to be the growing trend in cataract surgery. It avoids the potential risks of damage to vessels, globe and nerves that exist when a needle is used. Surgeons who use topical anesthesia should already be experienced in phacoemulsification. A surgeon in the transi-

tion to phacoemulsification should probably not consider topical anesthesia until confident with phacoemulsification first. Initially, a surgeon should use topical anesthesia only on routine unchallenging cases. At the outset, surgeons should avoid using topical anesthesia on uncooperative patients or with patients who have difficulty in communicating. As one becomes more experienced and more confident, topical anesthesia can be used in more challenging cases. Cases in which local or general anesthesia is preferred will always exist and these include patients who are unable to co-operate, have extremely small pupils or very dense or subluxated lenses and those requiring more complex surgery or delicate dissection.

SUMMARY

Each of the nucleofractis techniques described in this chapter are variations of four basic steps: (i) sculpting to obtain a thin posterior plate of nucleus, (ii) fracturing the posterior plate and nuclear rim, (iii) breaking away wedge-shaped sections of nuclear material for emulsification and (iv) rotating the nucleus for further fracturing and emulsification. The techniques of continuous curvilinear capsulorhexis, down-slope sculpting, phaco sweep and polar expeditions are refinements which add efficacy and safety to the divide and conquer. The surgeon should be familiar with the variety of nucleofractis techniques described and be able to modify the surgical strategy, as dictated by specific patient characteristics and intraoperative events.

REFERENCES

1. Gimbel HV. Divide and conquer nucleofractis phacoemulsification—development and variations. J Cataract Refract Surg. 1991;17:281-91.
2. Gimbel HV, Ellant JP, Chin PK. Divide and conquer nucleofractis. Ophthalmol Clin North Am. 1995;8(3):457-69.
3. Gimbel HV, Neuhann T. Development, advantages, and methods of the continuous circular capsulorhexis technique. J Cataract Refract Surg. 1990;16:31-7.
4. Cruze OA, Wallace GW, Gay CA, et al. Visual results and complications of phacoemulsification with intraocular lens implantation performed by ophthalmology residents. Ophthalmology. 1992;99:448-52.
5. Noecker RJ, Allinson RW, Snyder RW. Resident phacoemulsification experience using the in situ nuclear fracture technique. Ophthalmology. 1994;25:215-21.
6. Pearson PA, Owen DG, Van Meter WS, et al. Vitreous loss rates in extracapsular cataract surgery by residents. Ophthalmology 1989;96:1225-7.
7. Gimbel HV, Neuhann T. Continuous curvilinear capsulorhexis (letter). J Cataract Refract Surg. 1991;17:110-1.
8. Neuhann T. Theorie und operationstechnik der kapsulorhexis. Klin Monatsble Augenheilkd. 1987;190:542-5.
9. Hogan M, Alvaradd J, Weddell J. Histology of the Human Eye. Philadelphia: WB Saunders; 1971.
10. Gimbel HV. Down slope sculpting. J Cataract Refract Surg. 1992;18:614-8.

11. Gimbel HV, Chin PK. Phaco sweep. J Cataract Refract Surg. 1995;21:493-6.

12. Gimbel HV. Divide and Conquer. (Video) Presented at the European Intraocular Implant Lens Council meeting; 1987.

13. Gimbel HV. CCC and nucleus fracturing. Ophthalmol Clin North Am. 1991;4:235.

14. Gimbel HV. Evolving techniques of cataract surgery—continuous curvilinear capsulorhexis, down-slope sculpting and nucleofractis. Semin Ophthalmol. 1992;7:193-207.

15. Gimbel HV. Nuclear phacoemulsification—alternative methods. In: Steinert RF (Ed). Cataract Surgery: Technique, Complications, and Management. Philadelphia: WB Saunders; 1995. pp. 148-81.

16. Gimbel HV, Austin A. 'Polar expedition' technique expedites phaco. Ocular Surgery News. 1997;15(9):27-32.

17. Gimbel HV. Nucleofractis phacoemulsification through a small pupil. Can J Ophthalmol. 1992;27(3):115-9.

18. Gimbel HV, Willerscheidt AB. What to do with limited view—the intumescent cataract. J Cataract Refract Surg. 1993;19:657-61.

CHAPTER 20

Stop and Chop Phacoemulsification

Amar Agarwal, Soosan Jacob

INTRODUCTION

Stop and chop phacoemulsification was first described by Paul Koch in 1994.[1] It is a technique that facilitates easier nucleus management by utilizing chop maneuvers. It is a useful technique for both experienced surgeons and even more so for those desiring to transition from divide and conquer to phaco chop.

Stop and chop involves sculpting of the nucleus along the center to create a groove (**Figure 20.1**) and to thin the posterior pole. This is followed by cracking the posterior plate into two halves (**Figure 20.2**). Once the nucleus is cracked into two pieces, the surgeon "stops" and proceeds further with "chop" maneuvers, hence the name "stop and chop". The cracked surface of the nucleus gives easier purchase of the hemisection by the phaco tip to chop it with the chopper (**Figure 20.3**). The nuclear rim is then chopped into multiple smaller fragments towards the central cracked groove which can be removed one by one (**Figure 20.4**).

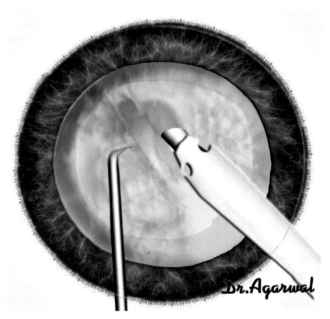

FIGURE 20. 2: The two instruments are inserted into the depth of the groove and moved apart to crack the nucleus

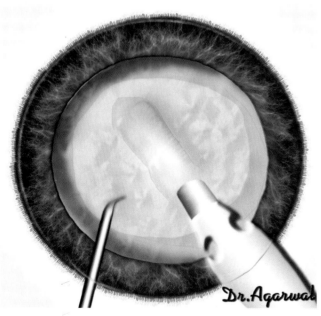

FIGURE 20. 1: A central groove is sculpted along the length of the nucleus till the red reflex is clearly seen

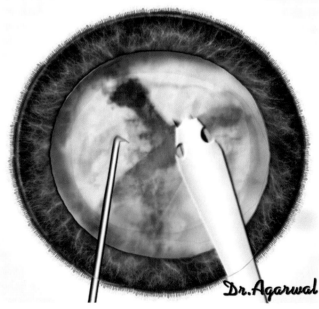

FIGURE 20. 3: The phaco tip is embedded into the hemi-nucleus and the chopper is used to chop the nucleus into two or three pieces

SURGICAL TECHNIQUE

PRELIMINARY STEPS

A continuous curvilinear capsulorhexis is created taking care to size it appropriately. Too small a rhexis can lead to capsular bag blow out on hydrodissection and too large a rhexis can lead to excessive nuclear mobility within the bag. A careful cortical cleaving hydrodissection[2] is performed to lyse capsule-cortical connections to facilitate easier cortex aspiration later on in the procedure. Hydrodelineation is performed to free the nucleus, to decrease its size

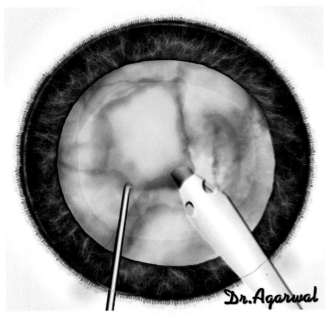

FIGURE 20. 4: The chopped fragments are removed one by one and emulsified in the iris plane

and to create a protective epinuclear shell. A Y-rod is then used to confirm rotational mobility of the nucleus. It is important that the nucleus should freely rotate before proceeding to the next step.

STOP AND CHOP

Using power based on the density of the nucleus, a central longitudinal trench is created with the phaco tip in continuous mode. It is deepened by making successive passes towards 6 'o clock till the red reflex is clearly visible. The trench is also widened enough to allow the phaco tip and sleeve access to successively deeper layers of the nucleus. At this stage, the vacuum used is low. The second instrument is used to avoid excessive nuclear movements while trenching. Power should be adjusted according to the grade of nuclear sclerosis. Using inadequate power at this stage leads to pushing of the nucleus instead of trenching and can result in unwanted stress on the zonules. Down-slope sculpting can be done to get a deep groove on the superior aspect as well. This is done by using the second instrument to push the lens downwards gently, while sculpting in a downward direction. This allows the surgeon better access to the upper part of the nucleus as well as allows safer and deeper access. Once the center of the nucleus has been crossed, the phaco tip follows the curve of the posterior capsule upwards instead. The nucleus is then rotated 180° and trenched in the opposite direction as well to get a trench of equal depth in both directions. Once the red reflex is seen equally well in both directions, the thinned out posterior plate can be cracked to divide the nucleus into two hemisections. This is done by inserting the phaco tip and the chopper into the depths of the groove and either moving them laterally apart or in a cross-handed manner so that both hands push in opposite directions. This

is a mechanical division of the nucleus and the tip is only placed within the nucleus without embedding. The nucleus can then again be rotated back 180° and cracked again, if the split has not extended through the entire length. This completely divides the nucleus into two hemi-sections. Once the nucleus is cracked into two, further trenching is "stopped" and the two hemi-nuclei are "chopped". The nucleus is rotated with the second instrument to make the groove lie perpendicular to the phaco tip. Using phaco power adjusted to the density of the nucleus and with pulse mode, the phaco tip is then embedded well into the depth of the crack at the junction of about one-third and two third of the hemi-nucleus. Once it is embedded, the foot-position is brought to two and it is held using vacuum alone. Vacuum levels are raised for this step, as higher vacuum is needed for holding the nucleus well. With the nucleus slightly pulled towards the surgeon, the chopper is embedded into the nucleus near the edge of the capsule and pulled towards the phaco tip. Once it reaches the phaco tip, it is moved laterally. This lateral movement chops and separates one-third of the nucleus from the remainder. This is again repeated so as to split the remaining two-third into two equal halves. Three nuclear fragments are thus obtained. These three fragments can then be removed in pulse phaco mode or, depending on surgeon discretion and nucleus density can be removed after the second hemi-nucleus is rotated downwards and also chopped into two or three.

FRAGMENT REMOVAL

The first fragment is caught with the phaco tip at its apex using a short burst of phaco and then holding with vacuum alone, it is manipulated out of the bag to be emulsified at the iris plane. Once the first fragment is removed, the other fragments are easier to remove as they no longer lie tightly packed together. All the nuclear fragments are emulsified in the iris plane. In case of dense cataracts, dispersive viscoelastics are used to protect the cornea.

COMPLICATIONS

Possible complications that can occur include the probe going through the posterior capsule while trenching in the deeper layers of the nucleus. This can be avoided to some extent by following the curve of the posterior capsule, i.e. downslope sculpting in the upper part of the nucleus and moving upslope again on crossing the center. Zonular dialysis may occur if sufficient energy is not used during trenching, as the nucleus ends up getting pushed rather than sculpted. The posterior plate may not crack as easily, especially in brown, leathery cataracts. In this case, the surgeon should ensure deep sculpting and insert the instruments well within the groove created before attempting cracking. Unless the split extends through and through, the pieces will not separate and an attempt to bring one fragment out will result in its coming out with the attached fragments. This can result in an overcrowding of the anterior chamber, endothelial touch of the fragment and inability to perform safe iris plane phacoemulsification.

Chopping needs to be performed carefully or can result in an accidental tearing of the capsulorhexis rim. This tear may extend around the equator of the capsule posteriorly, resulting in a posterior capsular tear and nucleus drop.

DISCUSSION

Stop and chop differs from Nagahara's phaco chop in requiring central sculpting which creates space for further manipulation of the nucleus. Once the nucleus is split into two, chopping techniques come into play. This helps in decreasing phacoemulsification time as well as permits easier removal of the nucleus, as compared to divide and conquer. It has also been shown to have an easier learning curve as well as a decreased incidence of accidental chopping of the rhexis in beginners, as compared to phaco chop. Hence, it is an easy transition technique for those surgeons who wish to learn phaco chop.

SUMMARY

Stop and Chop is an effective technique to master by all phaco surgeons. It can be utilized in difficult cases even by surgeons who routinely prefer chop, e.g. for brown cataracts where the initial trenching decreases the bulk of the nucleus and helps an easy first crack of the nucleus into two pieces.

CHAPTER 21

Phaco Chop Techniques

Uday Devgan

The most efficient technique of nucleus disassembly is a purely mechanical one where the nucleus can be chopped into segments within a few seconds. These smaller segments can then be easily removed with relatively little phaco energy. One can compare this to the divide and conquer technique where a tremendous amount of ultrasonic energy is required to create the grooves that are used to create the quadrants. A simple analogy is splitting of firewood: a grooving technique is similar to using a saw to cut through the piece of wood, whereas a chop technique is like using an axe to chop and split the firewood along the grain.

PHACO CHOP

The basic concept of chopping is holding the nucleus with the phaco probe while the chopping instrument splits it into pieces. The most common difficulty that beginning surgeons have in chopping techniques is failure to adequately fixating the nucleus, so that it can be chopped. If one is going to use a fork and knife to cut a piece of meat, one must first hold and immobilize the meat with the fork, so that the knife can do the cutting. Similarly, the phaco probe must achieve a high enough vacuum level to firmly fixate the nucleus so that the chopper can do the mechanical splitting of the cataract.

OCCLUSION

A high vacuum level is required to achieve the holding power that we desire for chopping. Depending on the phaco needle size that one is using, the vacuum level should be between 250 mm Hg and 400 mm Hg and if one is using a peristaltic fluid pump, it is to remember that total occlusion of the phaco tip is required to achieve the maximum preset vacuum level. With the vacuum setting high, one needs to bury the phaco tip into the nucleus using phaco power (foot pedal position 3), then once one has full occlusion of the tip, it is necessary to back off the pedal into position 2, so that the nucleus is being held by the high vacuum level. Now the cataract is well-fixated and one is ready to employ a chop technique.

HORIZONTAL CHOPPING

The original technique of chopping described by Nagahara is a horizontal chop. The phaco probe is embedded into the nucleus and the chopper is passed under the capsulorhexis and towards the lens equator. Once at the lens equator, the chopper is brought towards the phaco tip. It is the action of moving the chopper and the phaco tip together that does the chopping. When this is accomplished, the pieces need to be separated by pulling the two instruments apart. For most surgeons, this means bringing the chopper towards the left, while the phaco probe is pushed towards the right. A complete separation of the two pieces is required for complete mobilization of the halves and for further chopping into segments.

VERTICAL CHOPPING

In a nucleus with more density, vertical chopping is a very effective and safe technique. The phaco tip is embedded into the nucleus and a high vacuum level is used to fixate it. The chopper is then placed vertically, into the center of the nucleus, well within the confines of the capsulorhexis. Once the chopper and phaco tip are both fully buried in the center of the nucleus, the two instruments are pulled apart: The chopper to the left and the phaco probe to the right, thereby separating the two nuclear halves. These nuclear halves can then be further chopped into smaller segments and emulsified.

TILT AND CHOP

To minimize the stress on the capsular bag, which is particularly helpful in cases of pseudoexfoliation or trauma where there is zonular weakness, the nucleus can be tilted out of the capsular bag. A relatively large capsulorhexis of 5 mm or more, combined with hydrodissection or viscodissection, will aid in partially prolapsing the nucleus out of the capsular bag. With the nucleus tilted out of the capsular bag, it is very easy to place the chopper around the lens equator or even behind the nucleus. The chopper is brought towards the phaco tip and the two instruments are pulled apart to create the two nuclear halves. The tilt and chop technique is the author's preferred technique for very dense cataracts, where a significant amount of force is required to propagate the chop through the nucleus. By placing the chopper behind the nucleus, with the phaco probe in front of it, one is able to exert a high degree of chopping force, while being very gentle to the zonules and other intra-ocular structures.

SUMMARY

Chopping techniques are quickly becoming the preferred method for cataract surgery due to the efficiency and safety that they provide. While the technical skill required for chopping is higher, the great majority of ophthalmologists can master with practice.

CHAPTER 22

No Anesthesia Cataract Surgery with the Karate Chop Technique

Athiya Agarwal, Sunita Agarwal, Amar Agarwal

INTRODUCTION

On June 13th, 1998 at Ahmedabad, India, the first no anesthesia cataract surgery was done by the author (Amar Agarwal) at the Phako and Refractive Surgery conference. This was performed as a live surgery in front of 250 delegates. This has opened up various new concepts in cataract surgery.[1-4] In this surgery, the technique of karate chop was used.

For high refractive errors, clear lens extraction with phacoemulsification is a very good alternative. In such cases, if necessary, one can implant an IOL. This technique is very useful in hypermetropes, as LASIK does not give excellent results in such cases. *The most commonly done refractive surgery in the world is not PRK or LASIK, it is cataract surgery.* This is why this chapter will discuss phacoemulsification techniques for removal of cataract, as well as clear lens extraction.

NUCLEUS REMOVAL TECHNIQUES

Since the introduction of phacoemulsification as an alternative to standard cataract extraction technique, surgeons throughout the world have been attempting to make this new procedure safer and easier to perform, while assuring good visual outcome and patient recovery. The fundamental goal of Phaco is to remove the cataract with minimal disturbance to the eye, using least number of surgical manipulations. Each maneuver should be performed with minimal force and maximal efficiency should be obtained.

The latest generation Phaco procedures began with Dr. Howard Gimbel's "divide and conquer"nuclear fracture technique in which he simply split apart the nuclear rim. Since then, we have evolved through the various techniques namely four quadrant cracking, chip and flip, spring surgery, stop and chop and phaco chop.

Clear lens removal by phacoemulsification is a very good alternative to manage refractive errors. In these cases, as the nucleus is soft, one can use only *Phacoaspiration* to remove the nuclei, rather than use ultrasound power.

KARATE CHOP

Unlike the peripheral chopping of Nagahara or other stop and chop techniques, we have developed a safer technique called "Central Anterior Chopping" or "Karate Chop". In this method, the phaco tip is embedded by a single burst of power in the central safe zone and after lifting the nucleus a little bit (to lessen the pressure on the posterior capsule) the chopper is used to chop the nucleus. In soft nuclei, it is very difficult to chop the nucleus. In most cases, one can take it out in toto. But if the patient is about 40 years of age, then one might have to chop the nucleus. In such cases, we embed the phaco probe in the nucleus and then with the left hand cut the nucleus as if we are cutting a piece of cake. This movement should be done three times in the same place. This will chop the nucleus.

SOFT CATARACTS

In soft cataracts, the technique is a bit different. We embed the phaco tip and then cut the nucleus as if we are cutting a piece of cake. This should be done 2–3 times in the same area so that the cataract gets cut. It is very tough to chop a soft cataract, so this technique helps in splitting the cataract.

AGARWAL CHOPPER

We have devised our own chopper. The other choppers, which cut from the periphery, are blunt choppers. Our chopper is a sharp chopper. This is a 28 gauge chopper made by Gueder (Germany). It has a sharp cutting edge. It also has a sharp point. The advantage of such a chopper is that you can chop in the center and do not need to go to the periphery.

In this method, by going directly into the center of the nucleus without any sculpting ultrasound energy required is reduced. The chopper always remains within the rhexis margin and never goes underneath the anterior capsule. Hence, it is easy to work with even small pupils or glaucomatous eyes. Since we do not have to widen the pupil, there is little likelihood of tearing the sphincter and allowing prostaglandins to leak out and cause inflammation or cystoid macular edema. In this technique, we can easily go into even hard nuclei on the first attempt.

KARATE CHOP TECHNIQUE

INCISION

This chop is a modification of the Nagahara chop. The important feature is that we do not chop the periphery. A temporal clear corneal section is made. If the astigmatism is plus at 90 degrees then the incision is made superiorly.

First of all, a needle with viscoelastic is injected inside the eye in the area where the second site is made (**Figure 22.1**). This will distend the eye so that when one makes a clear corneal incision, the eye will be tense and one can create a good valve. Now one uses a straight rod to stabilize the eye with the left hand. With the right hand, one makes the clear corneal incision (**Figure 22.2**).

When the author started making the temporal incisions, he positioned himself temporally. The problem by this

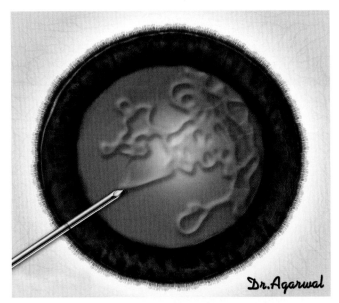

FIGURE 22.1: Eye with cataract. Needle with viscoelastic entering the eye to inject the viscoelastic. This is the most important step in no anesthesia cataract /clear lens surgery. This gives an entry into the eye through which a straight rod can be passed to stabilize the eye. The author notes that no forceps holds the eye

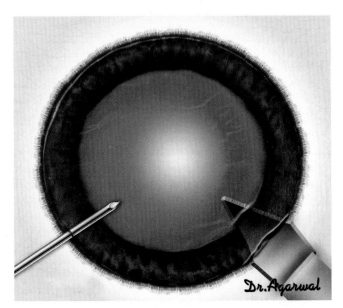

FIGURE 22.2: Clear corneal incision. The author observes the straight road inside the eye in the left hand. The right hand is performing the clear corneal incision. This is a temporal incision and the surgeon is sitting temporally

method is that, every time the microscope has to be turned which in turn would affect the cables connected to the video camera. Further, the theater staff would get disturbed between right eye and left eye. To solve this problem, we then decided on a different strategy. We have operating trolleys on wheels. The patient is wheeled inside the operation theater and for the right eye the trolley is placed slightly obliquely, so that the surgeon does not change his or her position. The surgeon stays at the 12 o'clock position. For the left eye, the trolley with the patient is rotated horizontally, so that the temporal portion of the left eye comes at 12 o'clock. This way the patient is moved and not the surgeon.

RHEXIS

Capsulorhexis is then performed through the same incision (**Figure 22.3**). While performing the rhexis, it is important to note that the rhexis is started from the center and the needle moved to the right and then downward. This is important because today concepts have changed of temporal and nasal. It is better to remember it as superior, inferior, right or left. If we would start the rhexis from the center and move it to the left, then the weakest point of the rhexis is generally where one finishes it. In other words, the point where one tends to lose the rhexis is near its completion. If one has done the rhexis from the center and moved to the left, then one might have an incomplete rhexis on the left hand side either inferiorly or superiorly. Now, the phaco probe is always moved down and to the left. So every stroke of the hand can extend the rhexis posteriorly, creating a posterior capsular rupture. Now, if we perform the rhexis from the center and move to the right and then push the flap inferiorly then if we have an incomplete rhexis near the end of the rhexis, it will be superiorly and to the right. Any incomplete rhexis can extend and create a posterior capsular tear. But in this case, the chances of survival are

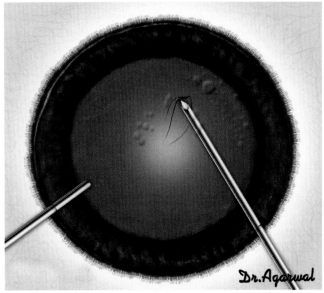

FIGURE 22.3: Rhexis being done with a needle

better. This is because we are moving the phaco probe down and to the left, but the rhexis is incomplete up and to the right.

If one is a left-handed person, one starts the rhexis from the center and move to the left and then down.

HYDRODISSECTION

Hydrodissection is then performed **(Figure 22.4)**. The author watches for the fluid wave to see that hydrodissection is complete. One does not perform hydrodelineation or test for rotation of the nucleus. Viscoelastic is then introduced before inserting the phaco probe.

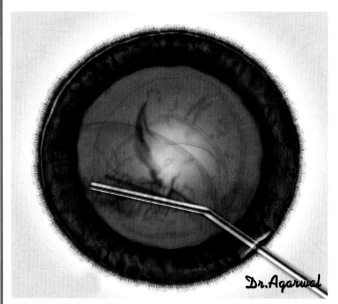

FIGURE 22.4: Hydrodissection

KARATE CHOP—TWO HALVES

The phaco probe is then inserted through the incision slightly superior to the center of the nucleus **(Figure 22.5)**. At that point, one applies ultrasound and sees that the phaco tip gets embedded in the nucleus **(Figure 22.6)**. The direction of the phaco probe should be obliquely downwards toward the vitreous and not horizontally towards the iris. Then only the nucleus will get embedded. The settings at this stage are 70% phaco power, 24 ml/minute flow rate and 101 mm Hg suction.

By the time the phaco tip gets embedded in the nucleus, the tip would have reached the middle of the nucleus. One does not turn the bevel of the phaco tip downwards when one does this step, as the embedding is better the other way. The author prefers a 15-degree tip but any tip can be used.

One should stop phaco ultrasound and bring his foot to position 2 so that only suction is being used. Then one should lift the nucleus. When the author requires to lift, it does not mean to lift a lot but just a little, so that when one applies pressure on the nucleus with the chopper, the direction of the pressure is downwards. If the capsule is a bit thin like in hypermature cataracts, one might rupture the posterior capsule and create a nucleus drop. So when

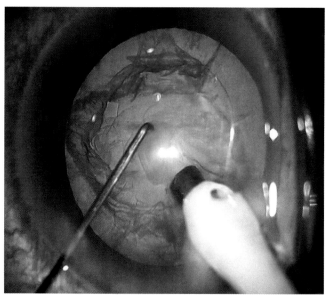

FIGURE 22.5: Phaco probe placed at the superior end of the rhexis

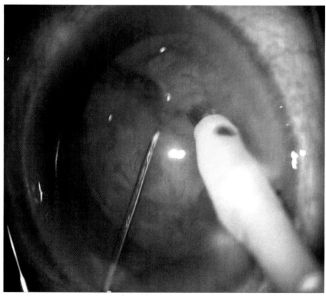

FIGURE 22.6: Phaco probe embedded in the nucleus. The author started from the superior end of the rhexis and notes it has got embedded in the middle of the nucleus. If the author had started in the middle then he would have embedded only inferiorly that is, at the edge of the rhexis and chopping would be difficult

the one lifts the nucleus, the pressure on the posterior capsule is lessened. Now, with the chopper one should cut the nucleus with a straight downward motion **(Figure 22.7)** and then move the chopper to the left when one reaches the center of the nucleus. In other words, one's left hand moves the chopper like a laterally reversed L.

One should *remember to not go to the periphery for chopping but to do it at the center.*

Once one has created a crack, one splits the nucleus till the center. Then one rotates the nucleus 180 degrees and crack again so to get two halves of the nucleus.

In brown cataracts, the nucleus will crack but sometimes in the center the nucleus will still be attached. One has to

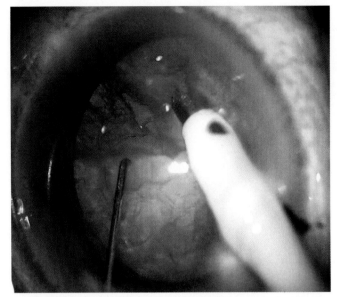

FIGURE 22.7: The left hand chops the nucleus and splits like a laterally reversed L, that is downwards and to the left

split the nucleus totally in two halves and should see the posterior capsule throughout.

KARATE CHOP—FURTHER CHOPPING

Now that two halves are obtained, one has a shelf to embed the probe. So, one has to place the probe with ultrasound into one-half of the nucleus **(Figure 22.8)**. One can pass the direction of the probe horizontally as now one has a shelf. The probe is embed, then pulled a little bit. This step is important so that one get the extra bit of space for chopping. This will prevent from chopping the rhexis margin. The force of the chopper is applied downwards. Then the chopper is moved to the left so that the nucleus

gets split. Again, one should see posterior capsule throughout so to know the nucleus is totally split. Then the probe is released, as the probe will still be embedded into the nucleus. Like this, one should create three quadrants in one-half of the nucleus. Then one makes another three halves with the second-half of the nucleus.

Thus, you now have six quadrants or pie-shaped fragments. The settings at this stage are 50% phaco power, 24 ml/minute flow rate and 101 mm Hg suction.

One needs to remember 5 words—Embed, Pull, Chop, Split and Release.

PULSE PHACO

Once all the pieces have been chopped, each piece have to be taken out one-by-one and in pulse phaco mode, one aspirates the pieces at the level of the iris. One should not work in the bag unless the cornea is preoperatively bad or the patient is very elder. The setting at this stage can be phaco power 50–30%, flow rate 24 ml and suction 101 mm Hg.

One needs to remember—It is better to have striate keratitis than posterior capsular rupture.

CORTICAL WASHING AND FOLDABLE IOL IMPLANTATION

The next step is to do cortical washing **(Figure 22.9)**. One should always try to remove the subincisional cortex first, as that is the most difficult. In **Figure 22.10**, it is to note the cortical aspiration complete and to note also the rhexis margins. It is also noted that everytime the left hand has the straight rod controlling the movements of the eye. If necessary, one should use a bimanual irrigation aspiration technique. Then it is necessary to inject viscoelastic and implant the foldable IOL. The author uses the plate haptic

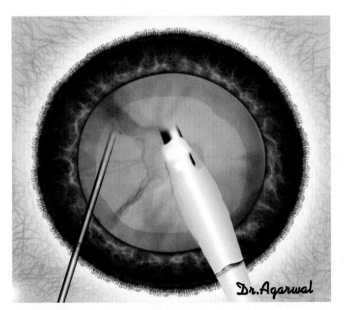

FIGURE 22.8: Phaco probe embedded in one-half of the nucleus. One needs to go horizontally and not vertically as a shelf of nucleus needs to be embedded. Chop and then the nucleus is chopped and split

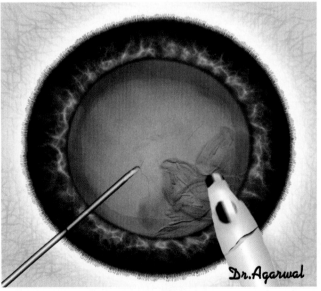

FIGURE 22.9: Cortical aspiration is completed. It is to note that straight rod in the left hand helps to control the movements of the eye

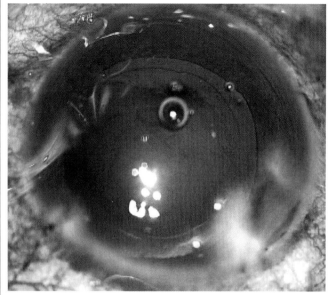

FIGURE 22.10: Eye distended with viscoelastic. Note the rhexis margins

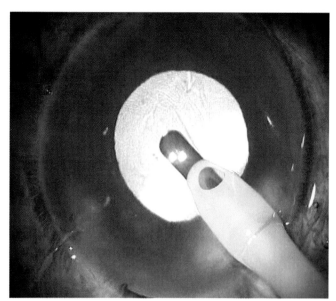

FIGURE 22.12: Foldable IOL in capsular bag. Viscoelastic removed with the irrigation aspiration probe

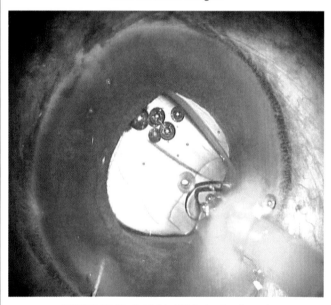

FIGURE 22.11: Foldable IOL being implanted

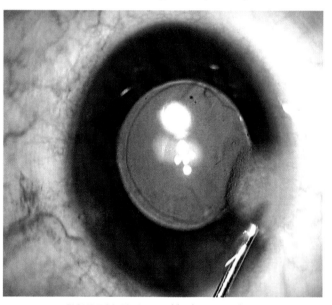

FIGURE 22.13: Stromal hydration is done and the case completed

foldable IOL **(Figure 22.11)** with large fenestration's generally as the author finds them superior. The viscoelastic needs to be taken out with the irrigation aspiration probe **(Figure 22.12)**.

STROMAL HYDRATION

At the end of the procedure, one should inject the BSS inside the lips of the clear corneal incision **(Figure 22.13)**. This will create a stromal hydration at the wound. This will create a whiteness, which will disappear after 4–5 hours. The advantage of this is that the wound gets sealed better.

NO PAD, S/C INJECTIONS

No subconjunctival injections or pad are put in the eye. The patient walks out of the theater and goes home. The patient is seen the next day and after a month glasses are prescribed.

NO ANESTHESIA CLEAR LENS EXTRACTION

In cases of clear lens removals, the same technique is followed. No anesthesia is used. If one is not good then it is advisable to use a parabulbar anesthesia (pin-point anesthesia) rather than a peribulbar block.

The reason is that in such cases, one could perforate the globe with the needle. Once the patient is draped, the syringe with viscoelastic is taken and the viscoelastic injected inside the eye using a 26 gauge needle. Then the temporal clear corneal incision is made. If the astigmatism is positive at 90 degrees then a superior incision is made.

The rhexis is then done using a needle. This is followed by hydrodissection. The phaco probe is passed into the eye and using phaco aspiration the soft nucleus is removed. One does not have to use ultrasound, as the nucleus in such cases is very soft. This is followed by cortical aspiration.

Depending on the biometry, a foldable IOL is implanted in the eye. If the patient has high myopia and an IOL is not required, then an IOL is not implanted. The authors have realized that chances of retinal detachment do not increase just because the eye is aphakic. The authors prefer to keep one eye emmetropic and the other slightly myopic to about 1 D to 1.5 D, so that the patient can see without glasses for distance and near with both eyes open.

Compared to LASIK, this is a very good alternative, as LASIK does not help much in hyperopes and in high myopes (powers above –15 D).

PHACODYNAMICS OF THE PHACO CHOP TECHNIQUE

We should take full advantage of the phaco machines capability, thereby decreasing physical manipulation of the intraocular tissues. In this phaco chop technique, we use a vacuum of 101 mm Hg, about 70% phaco power and the flow rate is 24 ml/minute.

In this phaco chop technique, the most important is the vacuum, which needs to be sufficient to stabilize the nucleus, while the chopper is splitting it. If the action of the chopper is dislodging, the vacuum seal on the phaco tip, it is said that the vacuum can be raised from 120 mm Hg to 200 mm Hg. After embedding the phaco needle with mild linear ultrasound power in foot switch position 3, it is important to raise the pedal back to foot switch position 2, while the vacuum builds up. This is because the purpose of ultrasound was to completely embed the aspiration port into the nucleus to obtain good vacuum seal. In foot switch 3, there is risk of adverse heat build up because the occluded tip prohibits any flow of cooling. Also, when manipulating the nucleus by pulling with the embedded tip, the vacuum seal is likely to be compromised by the vibrating needle if it is in foot switch position 3.

ADVANTAGES

The phacoemulsification procedure has been proved to be reasonably safe to the endothelium. As compared to the "divide and conquer" technique, this phaco karate chop technique eliminates the need for trenching, thereby producing significant reduction in phaco time and power consumed which in turn decreases endothelial cell damage. Even with increased density of cataract, there is a less pronounced increase in phaco time. Here we utilize the "Chop" to divide the nucleus by mechanical energy. It is safe and effective in nuclear handling during phaco-emulsification.

In conventional chop, the disadvantage is that the chopper is placed underneath the anterior capsule and then pulled towards the center. This can potentially damage the capsule and the zonules. In phaco chop, the author does not go under the rhexis, the vertical element of the chopper remains within the rhexis margin and it is visible at all stages. Hence, it is very easy to work with even small pupils

or glaucomatous eyes. The stress is taken by the impacted phaco tip and the chopper rather than transmitting it to the fragile capsule.

By going directly into the center of the nucleus with the phaco tip and not doing any sculpting, the author does not need as much ultrasound energy as is usually required. It is safe and easy to perform and there is no need to pass as much balanced salt solution (irrigating fluid) through the eye.

DISADVANTAGES

This technique demands continuous use of the left hand and hence requires practise to master it.

TOPICAL ANESTHESIA CATARACT/CLEAR LENS SURGERY

All cases done by the authors were previously done under topical anesthesia. Four percent xylocaine drops were instilled in the eye about 3 times 10–15 minutes before surgery. No intracameral anesthesia was used. It is not advisable to use xylocaine drops while operating. This can damage the epithelium and create more trouble in visualization. No stitches and no pad are applied. This is called the—*No injection, no stitch, no pad cataract surgery technique*. Now the authors have shifted all their cases, 100% to the no anesthesia technique.

NO ANESTHESIA CATARACT/CLEAR LENS SURGERY

The author has been wondering whether any topical anesthesia is required or not. So the patients were operated without any anesthesia. In these patients, no xylocaine drops were instilled. The patients did not have any pain. It is paradoxical because it is taught from the beginning that one should apply xylocaine. This is possible because one does not touch the conjunctiva or sclera. The author never uses any one-tooth forceps to stabilize the eye. Instead what is used is a straight rod which is passed inside the eye to stabilize it when rhexis is performed. The first step is very important. In this, the author first enters the eye with a needle having viscoelastic and inject the viscoelastic inside the eye. This is done in the area of the side port. Then, there is an opening in the eye through which a straight rod can be passed to stabilize the eye. The anterior chamber should be well maintained and the amount of ultrasound power used very less. If one tends to use the techniques like trenching, then the ultrasound power generated is high, which in turn generates heat. This causes pain to the patient. If these rules are followed, one can perform anesthesia cataract or clear lens extraction surgery. It is not necessary to do this, as there is no harm in instilling some drops of xylocaine in the eye. The point is that there is always a discussion about which anesthetic drop to use. It does not matter. The technique, which is performed, should not produce pain to the patient.

CONCLUSION

As in any other field, progress is inevitable in ophthalmology more so in refractive surgery. The author started to look on refractive surgery as a craft and should constantly try to improve the craft and become better everyday. By this, one will be able to provide good vision to more people than anyone dared dream a few decades ago. It also goes without saying that the author is and will be forever grateful to all his patients because without their faith, the author would never have had the courage to proceed.

Keeping this in mind, the author hopes and wishes that the effectiveness and the advantages of this "No Anesthesia Clear Lens Extraction Technique" be realized and practiced, thereby making the technique of phacoemulsification safer and easier providing good visual outcome and patient recovery.

REFERENCES

1. Agarwal S, Agarwal A, Sachdev MS, et al. Phacoemulsification, Laser Cataract Surgery and Foldable IOL's. 2nd edition. Delhi: Jaypee Brothers; 2000.
2. Agarwal A, Agarwal S, Agarwal A. No anesthesia cataract surgery with the karate chop technique. In: Agarwal A (Ed). Presbyopia: A Surgical Textbook; Slack Incoporated; 2002; 177–85.
3. Agarwal A, Agarwal S, Agarwal A. No anesthesia cataract and clear lens extraction with Karate chop; In: S Agarwal, A Agarwal, A Agarwal (Eds). Phako, Phakonit and Laser Phako: A quest for the Best; Highlights of Ophthalmology. Panama: Slack Inc; 2002; 113–20.
4. Agarwal A, Agarwal S, Agarwal A. No anesthesia Cataract and clear lens extraction with Karate chop; In: Martiz JR, Boyd BF, Agarwal AM (Eds). Lasik and beyond Lasik; Highlights of Ophthalmology. Slack Inc: Panama; 2001; 451–62.

CHAPTER 23

Supracapsular Phacoemulsification

Amar Agarwal, Soosan Jacob

INTRODUCTION

Supracapsular phacoemulsification comprise a variety of techniques which include Richard Lindstrom's tilt and tumble, Maloney's Supracapsular phaco, Pandit and Oetting's Pop and chop phaco, Can et al's Half moon supracapsular phacoemulsification. The most popular amongst these techniques is the Tilt and Tumble technique; therefore it will be described here. This utilizes hydrodissection to prolapse the nucleus out of the capsular bag. The prolapsed pole is then emulsified in the supracapsular plane. The inferior half of the nucleus is then rotated around to bring it to 6 o' clock position. This is then emulsified in turn. This is a good technique for soft nuclei and it is safer because of the supracapsular nature. However, it should be avoided in patients with borderline cornea, where phaco should be performed as far as possible from the corneal endothelium.

SURGICAL TECHNIQUE

PRELIMINARY STEPS

A moderate sized continuous curvilinear capsulorhexis is made. It should be large enough to allow the nucleus to prolapse out through the rhexis. A good cortical cleaving hydrodissection is done which helps later during cortex aspiration (**Figure 23.1**). The anterior capsule is lifted up and fluid is injected. Excessive and vigorous hydrodissection should be avoided.

NUCLEUS TILT AND TUMBLE

As the fluid is injected, the hydrostatic pressure within the bag increases and starts to lift up one pole of the nucleus out of the bag (**Figure 23.2**). The edge can be seen to tilt and lift up out of the capsular bag and at this point (**Figures 23.3 and 23.4**), hydrodissection is carried out very gently as excessive fluid trapped within the bag can lead to a capsular bag blow out. Unless this step is done very gently and carefully, an excessive build up of fluid can lead to a capsular bag blow out. Hydrodelineation decreases the size of the nucleus and therefore it allows an easier prolapse. It also makes phaco safer by decreasing the bulk of the nucleus that needs to be emulsified in the iris plane. Once hydrodelineation is performed, the remaining technique of tilting the nucleus remains the same. The inferior prolapsed half of the nucleus is emulsified in the iris plane, while supporting it with the second instrument. Once this is

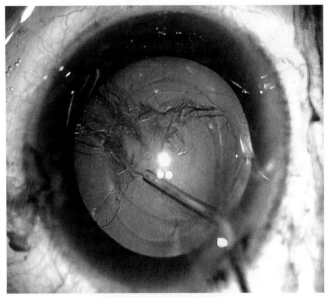

FIGURE 23.1: Cortical cleaving hydrodissection is done to facilitate cortex aspiration later in the surgery

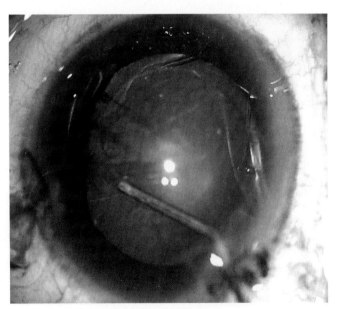

FIGURE 23.2: Hydrodelineation is done to gently build up hydrostatic pressure within the capsular bag

accomplished, the nucleus is tumbled upside down, so that the superior pole of the nucleus now faces up and this is also then emulsified in the iris plane (**Figure 23.5**).

After nuclear emulsification, cortex removal and intraocular lens (IOL) implantation are carried on, according to the surgeon's preferred technique.

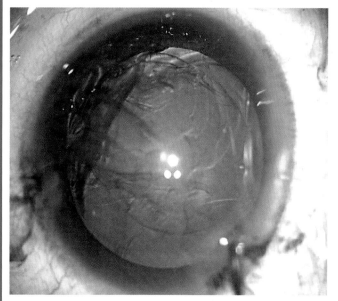

FIGURE 23.3: As the hydrostatic pressure builds up, the inferior pole of the nucleus prolapses out

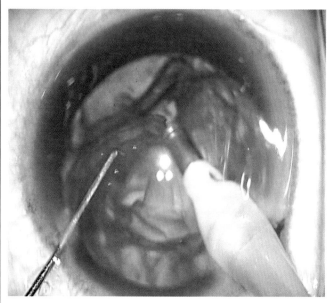

FIGURE 23.4: Once the inferior pole of the nucleus is prolapsed out, it is removed by phacoemulsification. The superior pole is then tumbled down and removed similarly

PHACO SETTINGS

Tilt and tumble generally works well for softer nuclei and hence the power used is usually low. For denser nuclei, higher power can be used. Vacuum and flow rate can be kept at medium settings.

GAS FORCED INFUSION

In our experience, nucleus removal becomes safer and easier with gas forced infusion or an air pump. This can be simply achieved by using the commonly available fish tank air pump. On connecting this to the bottle of balanced salt solution used for irrigation through a Millipore filter, pressurized air enters the irrigation bottle. This causes more fluid to enter the eye and thus maintains a deep anterior

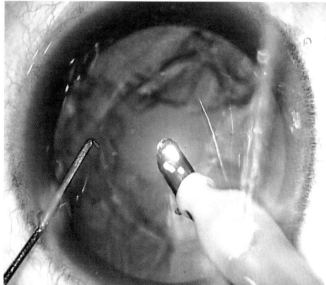

FIGURE 23.5: The nucleus is emulsified with the phaco tip

chamber and prevents surge. As air pump increases the fluid entering the eye, it deepens the anterior chamber and allows safer phacoemulsification. This is because it keeps the posterior capsule safely away from the nucleus during surgery, while at the same time also allowing nuclear emulsification at a safer distance from the endothelium.

COMPLICATIONS

A rhexis towards the slightly larger size allows easier prolapse of the nucleus. Too small a rhexis does not allow the pole to prolapse out; while at the same time it can lead to a capsular bag blow out because of excessive hydrostatic pressure within the bag. This can ultimately result in a nucleus drop and should therefore be avoided at all costs. Excessive and forceful hydroprocedures can also result in a similar blow out and should also be avoided. Small pupils can mechanically hinder prolapse of the nucleus into the anterior chamber. Pupil expansion techniques such as pupil expanders, iris hooks, Malyugin ring, etc. may be used in such a case. Most of the nucleus is emulsified supracap-sularly in this technique, therefore almost all the phaco energy is used in the anterior chamber. Patients with low endothelial count to begin with may therefore go for endothelial decompensation and this technique should be avoided in them. Harder nuclei are also associated with the problems of bigger bulk. Prolapsing these nuclei is more difficult as compared to soft nuclei. They also require more phaco energy to emulsify and hence a nucleofractis technique and quadrant removal may be a more preferred technique in such cases. Hydrodelineation should be done to decrease the size of the nucleus prolapsed, thereby decreasing the phaco energy used. Dispersive viscoelastics should also be used to coat the endothelial surface to protect the endothelium. The soft shell technique described by Steve Arshinoff can also be used to make the surgery more endothelium friendly.

DISCUSSION

Supracapsular phacoemulsification as proposed by Maloney et al. involves prolapsing the nucleus into the larger ciliary sulcus or supracapsular space where the nucleus can be more easily emulsified. This is safer although it does carry the risk of greater damage to the cornea and would be ideal for very soft nuclei. Pandit and Oetting's pop and chop phaco is also a type of supracapsular phacoemulsification where part of the nucleus is disassembled in the anterior chamber. This is done by chopping a fragment of the prolapsed pole of the nucleus and emulsifying it. Once this is done, it is manipulated back into the bag where the rest of it can be removed, using conventional chop techniques. This partial removal of the nucleus provides more space in the bag. Can et al. proposed a similar technique of half moon supracapsular phacoemulsification where the distal half of the nucleus is prolapsed out and then horizontally chopped from the equator to divide the nucleus into two pieces. These are then placed back into the bag either before or after removing a wedge of nucleus. The remaining nuclear disassembly is carried out in the conventional way.

SUMMARY

Supracapsular phacoemulsification technique refers to partial or complete removal of the nucleus in the supracapsular area. These are ideal for softer nuclei and should be used with caution in patients with borderline corneas.

CHAPTER 24

Hydrodissection and Hydrodelineation[1]

I Howard Fine, Richard S Hoffman, Mark Packer

HYDRODISSECTION

Hydrodissection of the nucleus in cataract surgery has traditionally been perceived as the injection of fluid into the cortical layer of the lens under the lens capsule to separate the lens nucleus from the cortex and capsule.[2] With increased use of continuous curvilinear capsulorhexis and phacoemulsification in cataract surgery, hydrodissection became a very important step to mobilize the nucleus within the capsule for disassembly and removal.[3-6] Following nuclear removal, cortical cleanup proceeded as a separate step, using an irrigation and aspiration handpiece.

CORTICAL CLEAVING HYDRODISSECTION

Fine first described cortical cleaving hydrodissection, which is a hydrodissection technique designed to cleave the cortex from the lens capsule and thus leave the cortex attached to the epinucleus.[7] Cortical cleaving hydrodissection usually eliminates the need for cortical cleanup as a separate step in cataract surgery, thereby eliminating the risk of capsular rupture during cortical cleanup.

A small capsulorhexis, 5–5.5 mm, optimizes the procedure. The large anterior capsular flap makes this type of hydrodissection easier to perform. The anterior capsular flap is elevated away from the cortical material with a 26 gauge blunt cannula (e.g. Katena Instruments No. K7-5150) prior to hydrodissection. The cannula maintains the anterior capsule in a tented-up position at the injection site near the lens equator. Irrigation prior to elevation of the anterior capsule should be avoided because it will result in transmission of a fluid wave circumferentially within the cortical layer, hydrating the cortex and creating a path of least resistance that will disallow later cortical cleaving hydrodissection. Once the cannula is properly placed and the anterior capsule is elevated, gentle, continuous irrigation results in a fluid wave that passes circumferentially in the zone just under the capsule, cleaving the cortex from the posterior capsule in most locations **(Figures 24.1A to C)**. When the fluid wave has passed around the posterior aspect of the lens, the entire lens bulges forward because the fluid is trapped by the firm equatorial cortical-capsular connections. The procedure creates, in effect, a temporary intraoperative version of capsular block syndrome, as seen by enlargement of the diameter of the capsulorhexis. At this point, if fluid injection is continued, a portion of the lens prolapses through the capsulorhexis. However, if prior to prolapse the capsule is decompressed by depressing the central portion of the lens with the side of the cannula in a way that forces fluid to come around the lens equator from behind, the cortical-capsular connections in the capsular fornix and under the anterior capsular flap are cleaved. The cleavage of cortex from the capsule equatorially and anteriorly allows fluid to exit from the capsular bag via the capsulorhexis, which constricts to its original sizeand mobilizes the lens in such a way that it can spin freely within the capsular bag. Repeating the hydrodissection and capsular decompression starting in the opposite distal quadrant may be helpful. Adequate hydrodissection at this point is demonstrable by the ease with which the nuclear-cortical complex can be rotated by the cannula.

HYDRODELINEATION

Hydrodelineation is a term first used by Anis to describe the act of separating an outer epinuclear shell or multiple shells from the central compact mass of inner nuclear material, the endonucleus, by the forceful irrigation of fluid (balanced salt solution) into the mass of the nucleus.[8]

The 26 gauge cannula is placed in the nucleus, off center to either side and directed at an angle downward and forward towards the central plane of the nucleus. When the nucleus starts to move, the endonucleus has been reached. It is not penetrated by the cannula. At this point, the cannula is directed tangentially to the endonucleus and a to-and-fro movement of the cannula is used to create a tract within the nucleus. The cannula is backed out of the tract approximately halfway and a gentle but steady pressure on the syringe allows fluid to enter the distal tract without resistance. Driven by the hydraulic force of the syringe, the fluid will find the path of least resistance, which is the junction between the endonucleus and the epinucleus and flow circumferentially in this contour. Most frequently, a circumferential golden ring will be seen outlining the cleavage between the epinucleus and the endonucleus **(Figures 24.2A and B)**. Sometimes the ring will appear as a dark circle rather than a golden ring.

Occasionally, an arc will result and surround approximately one quadrant of the endonucleus. In this instance, creating another tract the same depth as the first but ending at one end of the arc and injecting into the middle of the second tract, will extend that arc (usually another full quadrant). This procedure can be repeated until a golden or dark ring verifies circumferential division of the nucleus.

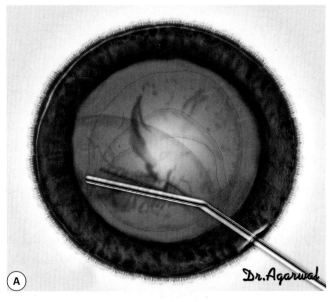

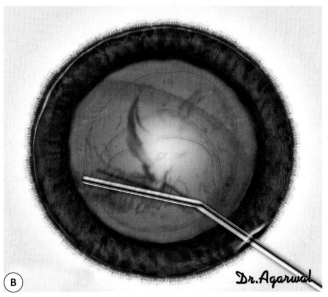

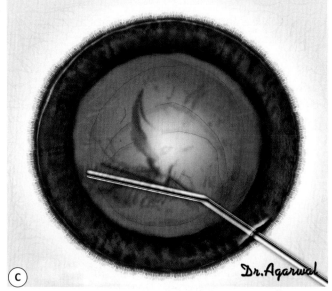

FIGURES 24.1A TO C: Illustration showing the steps of hydrodissection (*Courtesy:* Dr Agarwal's Eye Hospital, India)

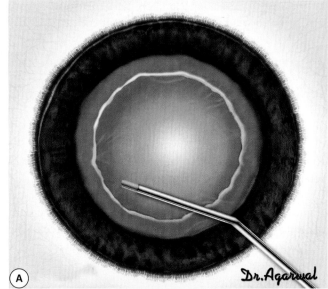

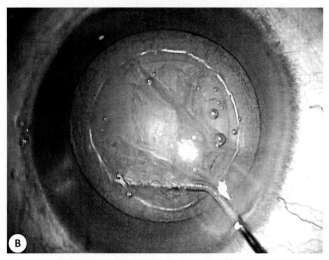

FIGURES 24.2A AND B: Golden ring (*Courtesy:* Dr Agarwal's Eye Hospital, India)

For very soft nuclei, the placement of the cannula allows creation of an epinuclear shell of any thickness. The cannula may pass through the entire nucleus if it is soft enough, so the placement of the tract and the location of the injection allow an epinuclear shell to be fashioned as desired. In very firm nuclei, one appears to be injecting into the cortex on the anterior surface of the nucleus and the golden ring will not be seen. However, a thin, hard epinuclear shell is achieved even in the most brunescent nuclei. That shell will offer the same protection as a thicker epinucleus in a softer cataract.

Hydrodelineation circumferentially divides the nucleus and has many advantages. Circumferential division reduces the volume of the central portion of nucleus removed by phacoemulsification by up to 50%. This allows less deep and less peripheral grooving and smaller, more easily mobilized quadrants after cracking or chopping. The epinucleus acts as a protective cushion within which all of the chopping, cracking and phacoemulsification forces can be confined. In addition, the epinucleus keeps the bag on stretch throughout the procedure, making it unlikely that a knuckle of capsule will come forward, occlude the phaco tip and rupture.

CORTICAL CLEAN-UP

Cortical clean-up is dramatically facilitated by cortical cleaving hydrodissection. After evacuation of all endonuclear material, the epinuclear rim is trimmed in each of the three quadrants, mobilizing cortex as well in the following way. As each quadrant of the epinuclear rim is rotated to the distal position in the capsule and trimmed, the cortex in the adjacent capsular fornix flows over the floor of the epinucleus and into the phaco tip. Then the floor is pushed back to keep the bag on stretch until three of the four quadrants of the epinuclear rim and forniceal cortex have been evacuated. It is important not to allow the epinucleus to flip too early, thus avoiding a large amount of residual cortex remaining after evacuation of the epinucleus.

The epinuclear rim of the fourth quadrant is then used as a handle to flip the epinucleus. As the remaining portion of the epinuclear floor and rim is evacuated from the eye, 70% of the time the entire cortex is evacuated with it.[9] Downsized phaco tips with their increased resistance to flow are less capable of mobilizing the cortex because of the decreased minisurge accompanying the clearance of the tip, when going from foot position two to foot position three in trimming of the epinucleus.

After the intraocular lens is inserted, these strands and any residual viscoelastic material are removed using the irrigation and aspiration tips, leaving a clean capsular bag.

If there is cortex still remaining following removal of all the nucleus and epinucleus, there are three options. The phacoemulsification handpiece can be left high in the anterior chamber while the second handpiece irrigates the cortex-filled capsular fornices. Often, this results in floating up of the cortical shell as a single piece and its exit through the phacoemulsification tip (in foot position two) because cortical cleaving hydrodissection has cleaved most of the cortical capsular adhesions.

Alternatively, if the surgeon wishes to complete cortical cleanup with the irrigation and aspiration handpieces before lens implantation, the residual cortex can almost always be mobilized as a separate and discrete shell (reminiscent of the epinucleus) and removed without ever turning the aspiration port down to face the posterior capsule.

The third option is to viscodissect the residual cortex by injecting the viscoelastic through the posterior cortex onto the posterior capsule. We prefer the dispersive viscoelastic device chondroitin sulfate-hyaluronate (Viscoat®, Alcon Laboratories, Fort Worth, Texas). The viscoelastic material spreads horizontally, elevating the posterior cortex and draping it over the anterior capsular flap. At the same time, the peripheral cortex is forced into the capsular fornix. The posterior capsule is then deepened with a cohesive viscoelastic device (e.g. Provisc®, Alcon

Laboratories, Fort Worth, Texas) and the IOL is implanted through the capsulorhexis, leaving the anterior extension of the residual cortex anterior to the IOL.

Removal of residual viscoelastic material accompanies mobilization and aspiration of residual cortex anterior to the IOL, which protects the posterior capsule, leaving a clean capsular bag.

TAKE HOME PEARLS

CORTICAL CLEAVING HYDRODISSECTION

- Is an easy and atraumatic procedure.
- Adds safety and reduces surgical time.
- Provides better for better cortical clean-up.

HYDRODELINEATION

- Circumferentially divides the nucleus.
- Provides a protective cushion.
- Reduces posterior capsule rupture during phacoemulsification.

CORE MESSAGE

CORTICAL CLEAVING HYDRODISSECTION

- Cleaves the connections between the cortex and the lens capsule.
- Facilitates mobilization and rotation of the lens within the capsule.
- Facilitates cortical clean-up.
- Adds safety to the procedure by reducing the incidence of capsule rupture occurring during cortical clean-up.

HYDRODELINEATION

- Divides the nucleus into an endonucleus and an epinuclear shell.
- Reduces the portion of the lens that has to be removed with ultrasound energy.
- Provides a cushion within which cracking and grooving are contained.
- Provides a protective cushion that keeps the capsule stretched and reduces the likelihood of capsule rupture during phacoemulsification.

SUMMARY

In summary, the lens can be divided into an epinuclear zone with most of the cortex attached and a more compact central nuclear mass. The central portion of the cataract can be removed by any endolenticular technique, after which the protective epinucleus is removed with all or most of the cortex attached. In most cases, irrigation and aspiration of the cortex as a separate step are not required, thereby eliminating that portion of the surgical procedure and its attendant risk of capsular disruption. Residual cortical cleanup may be accomplished in the presence of a posterior chamber IOL, which protects the posterior capsule by holding it remote from the aspiration port.

REFERENCES

1. This chapter has been previously published: Minimizing Incisions and Maximizing Outcomes in Cataract Surgery, 2010, pp. 135-139, "Hydrodissection and Hydrodelineation", IH Fine, R Hoffman, M Packer, Figs. 6.47-6.54. Used with kind permission of Springer Science+Business Media.
2. Faust KJ. Hydrodissection of soft nuclei. Am Intraocular Implant Soc J. 1984;10:75-7.
3. Davison JA. Bimodal capsular bag phacoemulsification: A serial cutting and suction ultrasonic nuclear dissection technique. J Cataract Refract Surg. 1989;15:272-82.
4. Sheperd JR. In situ fracture. J Cataract Refract Surg. 1990;16:436-40.
5. Gimbel HV. Divide and conquer nucleofractis phacoemulsification: Development and variations. J Cataract Refract Surg. 1991;17:281-91.
6. Fine IH. The chip and flip phacoemulsification technique. J Cataract Refract Surg. 1991;17:366-71.
7. Fine IH. Cortical cleaving hydrodissection. J Cataract Refract Surg. 1992;18(5):508-12.
8. Anis A. Understanding hydrodelineation: The term and related procedures. Ocular Surg News 1991;9:134-7.
9. Fine IH. The choo-choo chop and flip phacoemulsification technique. Operative Techniques in Cataract and Refractive Surgery. 1998;1(2):61-5.

MICS/Phakonit

History of Microincision Cataract Surgery (MICS): From Phakonit to Microphakonit

Amar Agarwal

INTRODUCTION

When Phakonit was started in 1998, the author did not realize it would become so popular so fast.

HOW IT ALL STARTED

The author is basically a vitreoretinal surgeon and used to do all his lensectomies with the phaco handpiece. The author did not have a fragmatome (an instrument to remove cataracts by vitreoretinal surgeons), so author used to remove the infusion sleeve and pass the phaco needle into the lens through the pars plana. Infusion would be through the infusion cannula which is connected in all vitrectomies. This way the author realized that he could remove the cataracts in patients in whom he had to continue with vitrectomy for proliferative vitreoretinopathy or any other posterior segment pathology.

He subsequently began to think about using this system for cataracts for the anterior segment surgeon. The problem was to have an irrigation system present inside the eye. On August 15th 1998, India's Independence day, the thought of taking a needle, bending it like a chopper and using that for irrigation and chopping occurred to the author (**Figure 25.1**). He also realized that there could be a corneal burn, so thought of irrigating the corneal wound from outside. With this idea in mind, the author went to the operation theater.

When the case began, he took out the infusion sleeve from the phaco handpiece and took a 20 gauge needle and connected it to the irrigation bottle. Then he took a needle holder and bent the needle in such a way that it could also be used for chopping. One can understand when we bend a needle like that it will obviously not come out very well. Another problem with using a needle was that as the needles have a bevel if one pulls out the needle a little bit, the bevel would be outside the eye and the chamber would collapse. For the incision the author used the microvitreoretinal blade (MVR blade) which vitreoretinal surgeons use for vitrectomies. This does not create a perfect valve as the diamond and saffire knives of today do but that was enough at that time (Later on the author designed his own irrigating choppers and knives).

When the author had finished the rhexis, he knew the hydrodissection was important and tricky. The reason was that the incision size was very less and so the amount of

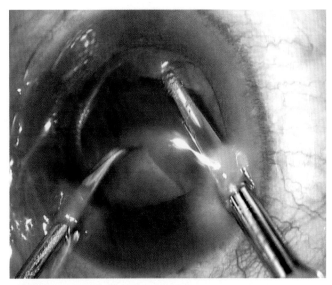

FIGURE 25.1: Phakonit done with a bent needle. The needle was bent like a chopper and the first case of Phakonit was done with this instrument. Later on instruments like the refined irrigating choppers were made

fluid escaping from the eye would not be much. So, the author was careful that he did not hydrodissect with a lot of fluid, otherwise he could get a dropped nucleus during hydrodissection.

When the surgery started, the author realized that he was having a lot of anterior chamber shallowing. Whenever he would start to remove the nucleus, the chamber would partially collapse. It was obvious that the amount of fluid entering the eye was not enough as compared to the amount exiting the eye. So the author stopped the surgery and shifted to an 18 gauge needle. To the author's surprise everything went well after that. He knew then that the amount of fluid was balanced with an 18 gauge needle. He could chop the hard cataract though not very well as compared to a chopper but he knew that with more refined instruments, this surgical technique would work. Once the surgery was complete, the author realized that this could be the next frontier in cataract surgery as the incision was reduced drastically.

TERMINOLOGY OF PHAKONIT

The author wanted to give a name to this surgical technique and started thinking of various names. Some names which came to the author's mind at that time were microphaco,

TABLE 25.1 Evolution of anesthetic techniques for cataract surgery

Technique	Year	Author
General anesthesia	1846	—
Topical cocaine	1881	Koller
Injectable cocaine	1884	Knapp
Orbicularis akinesia	1914	Van Lint, O'Briens Atkinson
Hyaluronidase	1948	Atkinson
Retrobulbar (4% cocaine)	1884	Knapp
Posterior peribulbar	1985	Davis and Mandel
Limbal	1990	Furata et al.
Anterior peribulbar	1991	Bloomberg
Pinpoint anesthesia	1992	Fukasawa
Topical	1992	Fichman
Topical plus intracameral	1995	Gills
No anesthesia	1998	Agarwal
Cryoanalgesia	1999	Gutierrez-Carmona
Xylocaine jelly	1999	Koch and Assia
Hypothesis, no anesthesia	2001	Pandey and Agarwal
Viscoanesthesia	2001	Werner, Pandey, Apple, et al

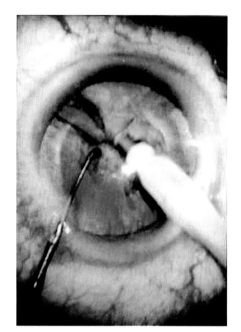

FIGURE 25.2: No anesthesia cataract surgery. Note the karate chop with the Agarwal chopper (Katena, USA)

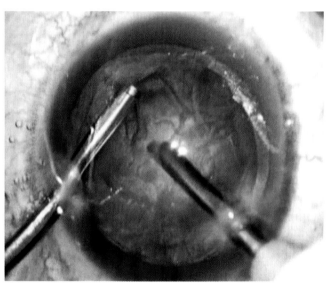

FIGURE 25.3: Phakonit being done with proper instruments. Note the bare phaco needle and an irrigating chopper in the left hand

miniphaco, etc. Then he thought of "phakonit" which was "phako with a needle incision technology". The reason he thought of this was because we did phaco using a needle (N) through an incision (I) and with the tip (T) of the phaco needle for the surgery. The author used in the phaco a "K" and not a "C" as he felt it looked better with a K and so termed it as "phakonit" and not "phaconit".

NO ANESTHESIA CATARACT SURGERY

On June 13th 1998, in Ahmedabad, India, the author had done the first live surgery of "no anesthesia cataract surgery" for a workshop organized by the Indian Intraocular Implant and Refractive Society. Later on a study was done by the author and his colleagues which was subsequently published in the journal of cataract and refractive surgery[1,2] (**Table 25.1 and Figure 25.2**).

FIRST LIVE SURGERY OF PHAKONIT

On August 22nd 1998, the first live surgery of Phakonit was done in Pune, India for the Indian Intraocular Implant and Refractive Society Conference. The author had to operate with just a needle and no refined instruments and under no anesthesia and so was under a lot of tension. Anyway, the surgery went off very well and there were about 350 ophthalmologists who watched the live surgery (**Figure 25.3**). In the ASCRS 99 conference in Seattle author and his colleagues did a live surgery in India which was telecast to USA of no anesthesia phakonit surgery.

PHAKONIT IN PHACOEMULSIFICATION BOOK

At that time author was writing his first book which was titled, Phacoemulsification, Laser Cataract Surgery and Foldable IOLs. The book was to be released in September 1998. He immediately contacted the publishers and informed them that he was sending a chapter titled "Phakonit" for the book and to please include it though it was quite late as the book was already in press. They agreed and that is how the Phakonit chapter came into publication in 1998 itself.[3-13]

PREVIOUS WORK DONE

Steve Shearing in 1985[14] published a paper on separating the infusion from the phaco handpiece. T Hara from Japan in

1987[15] also did the same. Author had not heard of any of this work when the concept of phakonit was started by him. Gradually as phakonit became more popular, work done by these early pioneers got appreciated more and more.

IRRIGATING CHOPPERS

Author subsequently worked with many companies to make the irrigating chopper and other instruments for Phakonit like the phakonit knives, etc. Various companies now have bimanual phaco instruments designed by various surgeons of the world.

AIR PUMP

One of the main problems in Phakonit was the fluidics. As explained earlier, the amount of fluid entering the eye was less as compared to the amount of fluid exiting the eye. Author's sister, Dr Sunita Agarwal understood this problem and started pushing air into the infusion bottle to get more pressurized fluid out of the bottle.[9] When it worked she then took an aquarium air pump and connected it to the infusion bottle via an IV set. This gave a constant supply of air into the infusion bottle and the amount of fluid coming out of the irrigating chopper was quite enough for them to move from an 18 gauge irrigating chopper to a 20 or 21 gauge irrigating chopper. This was the first time when pressurized fluid was used in anterior segment surgeries. This invention of air pump was made in 1999 and since then we have never looked back. They used the air pump not only in phakonit but in all our phaco cases. When we started microphakonit and moved to a 22 gauge irrigating chopper the air pump helped us tremendously. Bausch and Lomb in 2009 installed the air pump in their Stellaris machine to give a good control of the pressurized infusion system.

Arturo Perez-Arteaga from Mexico after reading on the air pump also used the Accurus vitrectomy machine which had an air pump for vitrectomies. He used this for Phakonit. Then others like Felipe Vejarano from Columbia also started and there was no looking back. Thus, the gas forced infusion could be external using an aquarium fish pump or internal in which the air pump is inbuilt inside the machine. In 2009 Bausch and Lomb fixed the air pump in their Stellaris MICS platform phaco machine.

THREE PORT PHAKONIT

Before the air pump, the author tried to solve the surge problem by fixing an anterior chamber maintainer. This was a three port phakonit,[2] but once the air pump invention was made, author realized that he did not need the anterior chamber maintainer. The usage of the anterior chamber maintainer made phakonit more cumbersome as three ports were made rather than two.

MICROINCISION CATARACT SURGERY

In 1999, P Crozafon reported the successful use of a sleeveless 21 gauge Teflon-coated tip for minimally invasive

bimanual phaco. In 1999, Hiroshi Tseunoka from Japan[16,17] studied the use of ultrasonic phacoemulsification and aspiration for lens extraction through a microincision. Jorge Alio from Spain[18] coined the term "microincision cataract surgery" (MICS). This meant cataract surgery being done through a 2.0 mm incision or less. This included laser cataract surgery (pioneering work done by Jack Dodick from USA) and ultrasound (phakonit). Randall Olson was the first to resurrect interest in the United States starting in the fall of 1999 and then to do studies published in peer review journals to answer the concerns of early critics.[19-22] He termed it microphaco. One problem in phakonit was that there would be a spray of fluid over the cornea whenever one would do phakonit. To solve this problem, one can use the hub of the infusion sleeve. There would be no infusion sleeve over the rest of the phaco needle but only be present over the base of the needle.[3] Using videos and a special vernier caliper sub 1 mm phakonit surgery was documented and demonstrated. In this, a 21 gauge irrigating chopper and a 0.8 mm phaco needle were used.[3]

MICS IOLS

Kristine Kreiner from Germany made an ultrasmall incision IOL[12] using a special copolymer as the lens material. The first lens was implanted by Kanellopoulos from Greece in 2000.[23] This was an Acrismart IOL (**Figures 25.4A to F**). The Thinoptx Company headed by Wayne Callahan made an ultrathin lens using the Fresnel principles.[8,10] Wayne and Scott Callahan began developing such a product using an inexpensive lathe, milling machine and blocking fixture. The first such lens was implanted by Jairo Hoyos from Spain. The second was implanted by Jorge Alio from Spain. They had heard of his work through Kenneth Hoffer (The first President of the ASCRS) and sent him some lenses and then he implanted the lens after Phakonit. The author also realized that it would be better to have a smaller optic lens and designed for Thinoptx a special 5 mm optic rollable IOL. They then made this special lens for me and we implanted five such lenses. These were the first 5 mm optic Thinoptx rollable IOL implanted. The first smaller sized rollable IOL was implanted on October 2nd 2001. These lenses could be rolled and hence the name "rollable IOL" was given rather than "foldable IOL" (**Figures 25.5A to D**).

MICROPHAKONIT; 700 MICRON CATARACT SURGERY

On May 21st 2005, for the first time the author used a 0.7 mm phaco needle tip with a 0.7 mm irrigating chopper to remove cataracts through the smallest incision possible as of now. He termed this as "microphakonit" to differentiate it from phakonit[24,25] (**Table 25.2**). When we wanted to go for a 0.7 mm phaco needle, the point which we wondered was whether the needle would be able to hold

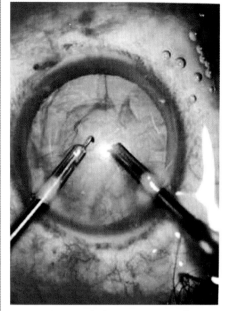

FIGURE 25.4A: Phakonit irrigating chopper and phako probe without the sleeve inside the eye

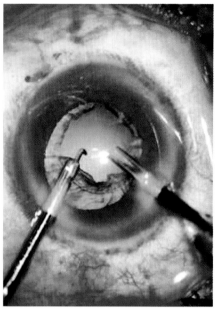

FIGURE 25.4B: Phakonit completed. Note the nucleus has been removed and there are no corneal burns

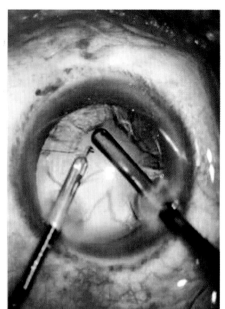

FIGURE 25.4C: Bimanual irrigation aspiration started

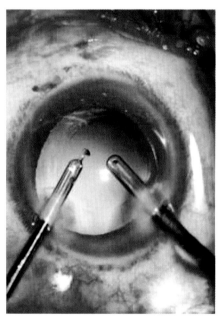

FIGURE 25.4D: Bimanual irrigation aspiration completed

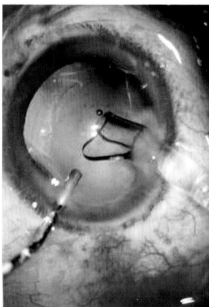

FIGURE 25.4E: The Acritec IOL being inserted

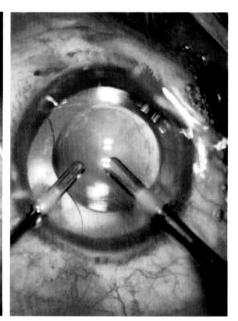

FIGURE 25.4F: Viscoelastic removed using bimanual irrigation aspiration probes

FIGURES 25.4A TO F: Phakonit with acritec IOL implantation

the energy of the ultrasound. We gave this problem to Larry Laks from MST, USA to work on. He then made this special 0.7 mm phaco needle **(Figure 25.6)**. As you will understand if we go smaller from a 0.9 mm phaco needle to a 0.7 mm phaco needle, the speed of the surgery would go down. This is because the amount of aspiration flow rate would be less. Bimanual irrigation aspiration is done with the bimanual irrigation aspiration instruments. These instruments are also designed by Microsurgical Technology (USA). The previous set we used was the 0.9 mm set. Now

with microphakonit we use the new 0.7 mm bimanual I/A set **(Figure 25.7)** so that after the nucleus removal we need not extend the incision **(Figure 25.8)**. Subsequently, Jorge Alio started 0.7 mm MICS and so also did others like Mark Packer, Robert Weinstock and many more.

BIMANUAL PHACO/BIAXIAL PHACO

Internationally, the name for phakonit became bimanual phaco. The idea was to separate it from coaxial phaco in which the irrigation is with the phaco handpiece. Then

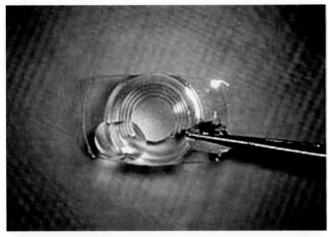

FIGURE 25.5A: Thinoptx rollable 5 mm IOL when removed from the bottle

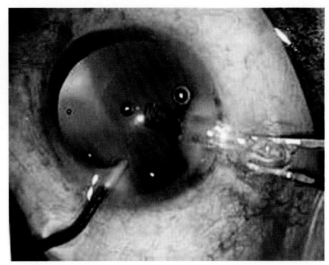

FIGURE 25.5B: The rollable IOL inserted through the incision

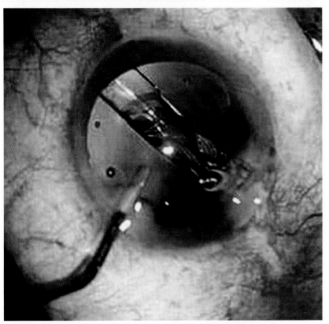

FIGURE 25.5C: Rollable IOL in the capsular bag

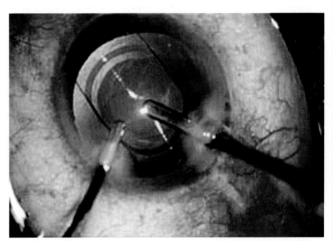

FIGURE 25.5D: Viscoelastic removed using bimanual irrigation aspiration probes

FIGURES 25.5A TO D: Phakonit with thinoptix 5 mm rollable IOL implantation

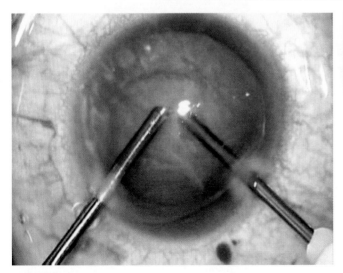

FIGURE 25.6: Microphakonit- 700 micron cataract surgery in a posterior polar cataract. 0.7 mm irrigating chopper and 0.7 mm phako tip without the sleeve are inside the eye. All instruments were made with the help of Larry Laks from MST, USA

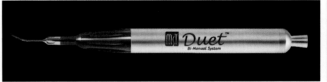

FIGURE 25.7: 700 micron bimanual irrigation aspiration set (MST, USA)

Steve Arshinoff coined the term "biaxial phaco" to make it more understandable and separate it from coaxial phaco.[26] Biaxial accurately describes what is being done in biaxial phaco, without referencing the size of the incision, which is likely to change with time, the number of surgeon's hands used for the procedure (or else the use of a chamber maintainer by a one handed surgeon would become bimanual surgery), or the size of the incision, which undoubtedly will decrease with time, irrespective of the axiality of the procedure.

TABLE 25.2	Evolution of techniques of cataract surgery	

Technique	Year	Author/Surgeon
Couching	800 BC	Susutra
ECCE* (Inferior incision)	1745	J Daviel
ECCE (Superior incision)	1860	Von Graefe
ICCE ** (tumbling)	1880	H Smith
ECCE with PC-IOL ***	1949	Sir H Ridley
ECCE with AC-IOL ****	1951	B Strampelli
Phacoemulsification	1967	CD Kelman
Foldable IOLs	1984	T Marrocco
CCC	1988	HV Gimbel and T Neuhann
Hydrodissection	1992	IH Fine
In-the-bag fixation	1992	DJ Apple/El Assia
Accommodating IOLs	1997	S Cummings /Kamman
Phakonit (Bimanual phaco)	1998	A Agarwal
Air pump to present surgery (gas forced infusion)	1999	S Agarwal
FAVIT Technique	1999	A Agarwal
MICS terminology	2000	J Alio
Microphaco terminology and using a 0.8 mm phaco needle	2000	R Olson
Eye enhanced cataract surgery	2000	SK Pandey/L Werner/ DJ Apple
Sealed Capsule irrigation	2001	Al Maloof
Factors for PCO Prevention	2002-2004	DJ Apple /L Werner/ SK Pandey
Microincisional coaxial phaco (MICP)	2005	Takayuki Akahoshi
Microphakonit cataract surgery with a 0.7 mm tip	2005	A Agarwal

*ECCE: Extracapsular cataract extraction
**ICCE: Intracapsular cataract extraction
*** PC IOL: Posterior chamber intraocular lens
**** ACIOL: Anterior chamber intraocular lens

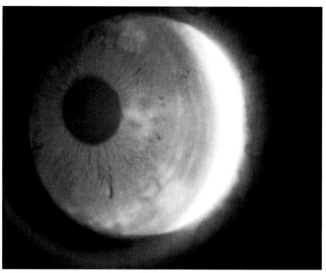

FIGURE 25.8: Corneal wounds after 700 micron cataract surgery. Note that in this high myopic patient an IOL was not implanted and so wound incisions are not extended

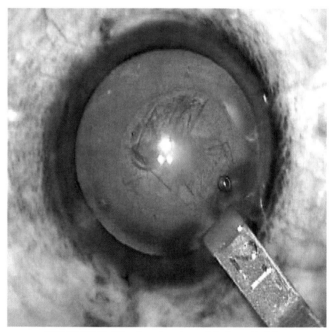

FIGURE 25.9: Microincisional coaxial phaco incision

MICROINCISIONAL COAXIAL PHACO

In 2005, Takayuki Akahoshi came out with a great concept. He designed with the help of Alcon, a nano sleeve, which was a thinner sleeve. The idea was to allow coaxial phaco through a sub 2 mm incision. Thus a new term was coined "MICP" which was microincisional coaxial phaco (**Figure 25.9**).

MICS-C-MICS AND B-MICS

The standard terminology, used for all the procedures is MICS. To differentiate MICP from bimanual phaco, the terminology used is C-MICS which is coaxial MICS and B-MICS which is biaxial MICS, respectively. In this book we will be using terminology of either coaxial or bimanual MICS.

SUMMARY

Today phakonit or MICS has taken the ophthalmologic world by storm. The only problem right now is to get more lenses into the market which will pass through sub 1 mm incisions and at the same time not reduce the quality of vision for the patients. These should also have an excellent injector system and should be user friendly. As one will notice that many surgeons and pioneers from different parts of the world have made bimanual MICS/coaxial MICS, reach their present status. We have come a long way in cataract surgery but still have a long way to go.

REFERENCES

1. Agarwal A, Agarwal S, Agarwal At. No anesthesia cataract surgery. In: Agarwal et al. (Eds). Textbook of Phacoemulsification, Laser Cataract Surgery and Foldable IOLs, 1st edition. New Delhi, India: Jaypee Brothers Medical Publishers; 1998. pp. 144-54.

2. Pandey S, Wener L, Agarwal A, et al. No-anesthesia clear corneal phacoemulsification versus topical and topical plus intracameral anesthesia: randomized clinical trial. J Cataract Refract Surg. 2001; 27(10):1643-50.

3. Agarwal A, Agarwal S, Agarwal At. Phakonit: A new technique of removing cataracts through a 0.9 mm incision. In: Agarwal et al (Eds). Textbook of Phacoemulsification, Laser Cataract Surgery and Foldable IOLs, 1st edition. New Delhi, India: Jaypee Brothers Medical Publishers; 1998. pp. 139-43.

4. Agarwal A, Agarwal S, Agarwal At. Phakonit and laser phakonit: Lens surgery through a 0.9 mm incision. In: Agarwal et al. (Eds). Textbook of Phacoemulsification, Laser Cataract Surgery and Foldable IOLs, 2nd edition. New Delhi, India: Jaypee Brothers Medical Publishers; 2000. pp. 204-16.

5. Agarwal A, Agarwal S, Agarwal At. Phakonit. In: Agarwal et al (Eds). Textbook of Phacoemulsification, Laser Cataract Surgery and Foldable IOLs, 3rd edition. New Delhi, India: Jaypee Brothers Medical Publishers; 2003. pp. 317-29.

6. Agarwal A, Agarwal S, Agarwal At. Phakonit and laser phakonit. In: Boyd/Agarwal et al. (Eds). Textbook of Lasik and Beyond Lasik. Panama: Highlights of Ophthalmology; 2000. pp. 463-8.

7. Agarwal A, Agarwal S, Agarwal At. Phakonit and laser phakonit-Cataract surgery through a 0.9 mm incision. In: Boyd/Agarwal et al. (Eds). Textbook of Phako, Phakonit and Laser Phako, Panama: Highlights of Ophthalmology; 2000. pp. 327-34.

8. Agarwal A, Agarwal S, Agarwal At. The phakonit thinoptx IOL. In: Agarwals (Ed). Textbook of Presbyopia. USA: Slack; 2002. pp. 187-94.

9. Agarwal A, Agarwal S, Agarwal At. Antichamber collapse. J Cataract Refract Surg. 2002; 28:1085.

10. Pandey S, Wener L, Agarwal A, et al. Phakonit: cataract removal through a sub 1.0 mm incision with implantation of the thinoptx rollable IOL. J Cataract Refract Surg. 2002; 28:1710.

11. Agarwal A, Agarwal S, Agarwal At. Phakonit: phacoemulsification through a 0.9 mm incision. J Cataract Refract Surg. 2001; 27:1548-52.

12. Agarwal A, Agarwal S, Agarwal At. Phakonit with an acritec IOL. J Cataract Refract Surg. 2003; 29:854-5.

13. Agarwal S, Agarwal A, Agarwal At. Phakonit with Acritec IOL. Panama: Highlights of Ophthalmology; 2000.

14. Shearing S, Relyea R, Loaiza A, et al. Routine phacoemulsification through a 1.0 mm non-sutured incision. Cataract. 1985; 6-8.

15. Hara T, Hara T. Clinical results of phacoemulsification and complete in the bag fixation. J Cataract Refract Surg. 1987; 13:279-86.

16. Tseunoka H, Shiba T, Takahashi Y. Feasibility of ultrasound cataract surgery with a 1.4 mm incision. J Cataract Refract Surg. 2001; 27:934-40.

17. Tseunoka H, Shiba T, Takahashi Y. Feasibility of ultrasound cataract surgery with a 1.4 mm incision-Clinical results. J Cataract Refract Surg. 2002; 28:81-6.

18. Jorge Alio. What does MICS require in Alios Textbook MICS. Panama: Highlights of Ophthalmology; 2004. pp. 1-4.

19. Soscia W, Howard JG, Olson RJ. Microphacoemulsification with Whitestar. A wound-temperature study. J Cataract Refract Surg. 2002; 28:1044-6.

20. Soscia W, Howard JG, Olson RJ. Bimanual phacoemulsification through two stab incisions. A wound-temperature study. J Cataract Refract Surg. 2002; 28:1039-43.

21. Randall Olson. Microphaco Chop in David Changs Textbook on Phaco Chop. Slack, USA; 2004. pp. 227-37.

22. David Chang. Bimanual Phaco Chop in David Changs Textbook on Phaco Chop. Slack, USA; 2004. pp. 239-50.

23. Kanellopoulos AJ. New laser system points way to ultrasmall incision cataract surgery. EuroTimes. 2000.

24. Agarwal A, Trivedi RH, Jacob S, et al. Microphakonit: 700 micron cataract surgery. Clinical Ophthalmology 2007; 1(3):323-5.

25. Agarwal A, Ashokkumar D, Jacob S. In vivo analysis of wound architecture in 700 microm microphakonit cataract surgery. J Cataract Refract Surg. 2008;34(9):1554-60.

26. Arshinoff Steve A. Biaxial phacoemulsification. Letter. J Cataract Refract Surg. 2005; 31:646.

CHAPTER 26

Wound Architecture in Microincision Cataract Surgery and In Vivo Analysis of 700 Micron Cataract Surgery

Dhivya Ashok Kumar, Amar Agarwal

INTRODUCTION

The advances in phacoemulsification techniques and phacomachines along with the invention of foldable intraocular lenses made the size of clear corneal incisions (CCI) less than 3 mm[1-13] possible. The smallest cataract incisions reported in 2005 using 700 micron cataract surgical instruments was termed as "microphakonit"[4-6] to differentiate it from 0.9 mm phakonit.[1-3,12,13] Recently there have been variable views on the risk of endophthalmitis[14,15] and cataract incisions. With the introduction of high speed anterior segment optical coherence tomography (OCT),[16-19] it is now possible to visualize the wound morphology.

ANTERIOR SEGMENT OPTICAL COHERENCE TOMOGRAPHY

Direct visualization of the wound can be achieved using anterior segment OCT. Postoperative wound morphology examination with the prototype anterior segment OCT (Carl Zeiss Meditec, Inc, Dublin, California, USA) Visante of 1310 nm wavelength has been done in a group of patients who underwent microphakonit procedure in our center. Corneal high resolution (10 mm × 3 mm) single scan mode was used. The axial resolution of the anterior segment OCT used is 18 microns and transverse resolution is 60 microns. This noncontact method of imaging provides micrometer scale cross-sectional images of the tissue.

WOUND EVALUATION

We looked for evidence of endothelial misalignment (gaping of the wound on the endothelial side), epithelial misalignment (gaping of the wound on the epithelial side), coaptation loss (loss of coaptation along the corneal stromal tunnel), stromal hydration and Descemet's status in the wound site. The images were bidimensional at a specific time and therefore did not take into account dynamic changes. The amount of stromal hydration was measured as the thickness of peripheral corneal thickness. Radial OCT scan, aligned more perpendicular to the width of the incision, was taken for analysis. The length of the corneal stromal tunnel from the epithelium to the endothelium was measured as incision length. Visante OCT analysis software system was used for measuring the endothelial misalignment, epithelial misalignment, coaptation loss, stromal hydration and incision length in millimeters. Angle of incision was defined as the angle of the incision line in the stroma to the corneal tangent. It was measured using hard copies of the images and a simple protractor.

There were 12 eyes of 11 patients included in the study. There were 24 clear corneal wounds studied which included the main port and the side port. Twelve eyes of eleven patients underwent phacoemulsification with 700 micron phaco tip (microphakonit) **(Figures 26.1A and B)**. Five out of twelve eyes had no IOL implantation (high myope with mean spherical equivalent of -20D±1.8) and seven eyes under-

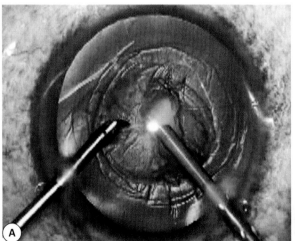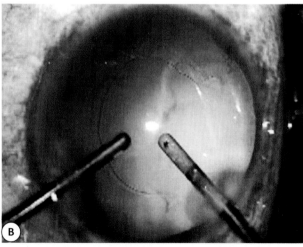

FIGURES 26.1A AND B: (A) Microphakonit performed with 700 micron phaco needle and 700 micron irrigating chopper (MST, USA) and (B) Bimanual irrigation aspiration done with 700 micron bimanual I/A set (MST, USA)

went foldable IOL implantation by extension of the main port of the microphakonit incision with a 2.8 mm keratome. The incisions were examined in the immediate postoperative period with mean duration of 30 minutes from the surgery, followed by day 1, day 3 and day 7 postoperative periods. Various parameters like endothelial alignment, epithelial alignment, coaptation loss, stromal hydration and Descemet detachment at the incision site were evaluated. Wound architecture changes of microphakonit compared with and without 2.8 mm keratome extension. Out of 24 clear corneal wounds, 17 were microphakonit without extension. On anterior segment OCT evaluation, 17.6% showed visible biplanar profile while 82.3% were straight or uniplanar. The mean incision length was 1.13 ± 0.1 mm. The mean angle of incision was 60.29 ± 11.4 degrees.

MICROPHAKONIT WITH NO WOUND EXTENSION

Endothelial Misalignment

As shown in **Table 26.1**, microphakonit wound in the postoperative period showed good endothelial alignment on an average by day 3 **(Figure 26.2)**. On comparing the correlation **(Table 26.2)** between the change in the endothelial alignment and stromal hydration from immediate postoperative time to day seven in microphakonit, there was no significant correlation seen. Similarly there was no significant correlation **(Table 26.2)** observed between the

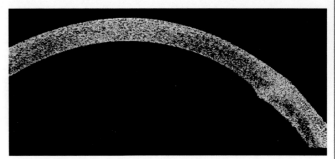

FIGURE 26.2: Anterior segment OCT cross-sectional image of the microphakonit wound showing good endothelial alignment on day 3

change in coaptation loss and the endothelial misalignment. No difference was seen in the amount of misalignment (p=0.265) between the temporal and superior incisions. There was a positive correlation (r=0.811, p=0.002) between the incision angle and endothelial misalignment **(Figure 26.3)**. No significant correlation was seen with the incision length (r=0.447, p=0.168) and endothelial misalignment.

Coaptation Loss

The mean coaptation loss seen in microphakonit was 0.03 ± 0.06 mm in the immediate postoperative period. Twelve (70.5%) out of the seventeen incisions showed no coaptation loss in the immediate postoperative period.

TABLE 26.1 Wound morphology in microphakonit without extension

Wound	EN Imm	D1	D3	D7	EP Imm	D1	D3	D7	CL Imm	D1	D3	D7	SH Imm	D1	D3	D7
1	0.17	0.16	0.1	0	0	0	0	0	0	0	0	0	0.9	0.75	0.7	0.67
2	0	0.05	0	0	0	0	0	0	0	0	0	0	0.82	0.82	0.8	0.7
3	0	0	0	0	0	0	0	0	0.2	0.1	0.1	0	1.6	0.9	0.9	0.72
4	0.3	0	0	0	0	0	0	0	0	0	0	0	1.02	0.9	0.87	0.81
5	0.1	0.16	0.13	0	0	0	0	0	0	0	0	0	1.2	1	1	0.72
6	0	0	0	0	0	0	0	0	0	0	0	0	1	0.9	0.85	0.75
7	0.1	0.2	0	0	0	0	0	0	0.1	0.1	0.1	0	1.4	1.4	1.2	0.7
8	0.05	0	0	0	0	0	0	0	0.1	0.1	0.1	0	1.2	1.2	1	0.65
9	0.2	0.16	0	0	0	0	0	0	0	0	0	0	0.9	0.9	0.8	0.6
10	0	0	0	0	0	0	0	0	0	0	0	0	0.9	0.77	0.7	0.67
11	0.01	0.01	0	0	0	0	0	0	0	0	0	0	0.9	0.9	0.85	0.8
12	0.07	0.07	0	0	0	0	0	0	0.1	0.1	0.1	0	1.5	1.5	1.3	0.7
13	0.09	0	0	0	0	0	0	0	0	0	0	0	0.8	0.8	0.7	0.7
14	0.2	0	0	0	0	0	0	0	0	0	0	0	1.05	0.8	0.8	0.8
15	0	0	0	0	0	0	0	0	0.09	0.09	0.09	0	1.2	1.2	1	0.83
16	0.16	0.16	0.1	0	0	0	0	0	0	0	0	0	1	1	1	0.82
17	0	0	0	0	0	0	0	0	0	0	0	0	1	0.9	0.9	0.76
Mean	0.085	0.057	0.019	0	0	0	0	0	0.035	0.029	0.029	0	1.082	0.979	0.904	0.729
SD	0.092	0.077	0.044	0	0	0	0	0	0.06	0.046	0.046	0	0.236	0.219	0.167	0.061

Keys: EN: Endothelial misalignment; EP: Epithelial misalignment; CL: Coaptation loss; SH: Stromal hydration; Imm: Immediate; D: Day; SD: Standard deviation

TABLE 26.2 Correlation analysis

	Immediate - Day1		Day1-Day3		Day3-Day7	
	r-value	p -value	r-value	p -value	r-value	p -value
EN - SH	0.098	0.707	-0.101	0.699	-0.162	0.534
EN - CL	-0.076	0.771	-0.187	0.471	-0.319	0.211
SH - CL	0.883	0	0.883	0	0.881	0
IOP - CL	-	-	-	-	-0.604	0.01
IOP - EN	-	-	-0.321	0.208	-0.347	0.172

Keys: EN: Endothelial misalignment; CL: Coaptation loss; SH: Stromal hydration; r: Pearson's correlation coefficient

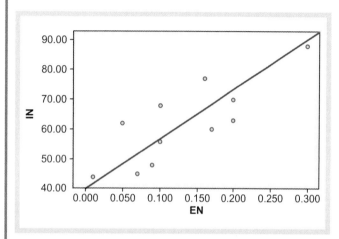

FIGURE 26.3: Scatter plot showing the correlation between endothelial misalignment and incision angle. EN—Endothelial misalignment, IN—Incision angle

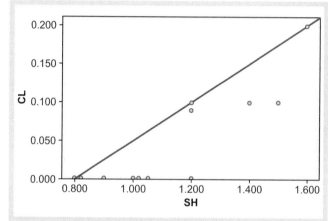

FIGURE 26.5: Scatter plot showing the positive correlation between change in stromal hydration and coaptation loss in the postoperative period. SH—Stromal hydration, CL—Coaptation loss

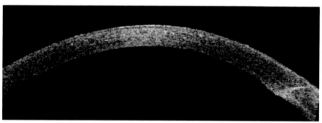

FIGURE 26.4: High resolution cross-sectional image of the anterior segment OCT showing dense apposition line in microphakonit wound

Dense wound apposition line was seen as early as day 1 (**Figure 26.4**) in all eyes with microphakonit. There was a significant positive correlation (**Figure 26.5**) seen between the change in stromal hydration and coaptation loss in the postoperative period (**Table 26.2**). The change in coaptation loss showed significant correlation with change in stromal hydration over the period (p <0.001) as shown in **Table 26.2**. There was no significant difference (p=0.338) between the superior and temporal incisions. There was no significant correlation noted between the endothelial misalignment and coaptation loss in the immediate postoperative period.

Stromal Hydration

The mean immediate postoperative stromal hydration in microphakonit wound was 1.08 ± 0.23 mm. The resolution

of stromal hydration was seen by the change in the peripheral corneal thickness. The mean peripheral corneal thickness on day 7 in microphakonit wound was 0.729 ± 0.06.

EPITHELIAL MISALIGNMENT

No epithelial misalignment was observed on immediate, day 1, 3 and 7 postoperative period. No fish mouthing was seen in any of the microphakonit incisions.

Descemet's Membrane

Localized subclinical Descemet's tear was noted in 1 out of 17 of the microphakonit wounds in anterior segment OCT.

MICROPHAKONIT WITH 2.8 MM WOUND EXTENSION

On comparison of microphakonit with 2.8 mm extension (**Table 26.3**) in the seven eyes which underwent IOL implantation, there was no significant difference in the mean early (30 minutes of surgery) endothelial misalignment (p=0.253) and coaptation loss (p=0.535) between the microphakonit with and without 2.8 mm extension. Twenty-nine point four percent of the seventeen microphakonit incisions had coaptation loss in the

TABLE 26.3	Microphakonit with 2.8 mm extension							
	Endothelial misalignment				**Coaptation loss**			
Wound	Imm	Day 1	Day 3	Day 7	Imm	Day 1	Day 3	Day 7
1	0	0	0	0	0.07	0.05	0	0
2	0	0	0	0	0.1	0.09	0.09	0.04
3	0.2	0.15	0	0	0	0	0	0
4	0.02	0	0	0	0	0	0	0
5	0.18	0.2	0.1	0.08	0.07	0.07	0.06	0.06
6	0.1	0.2	0.16	0.17	0	0	0	0
7	0.4	0.34	0.3	0.2	0	0	0	0
Mean	0.128	0.127	0.08	0.064	0.034	0.03	0.021	0.014
SD	0.145	0.132	0.116	0.088	0.043	0.039	0.037	0.025

Imm: Immediate; SD: Standard deviation

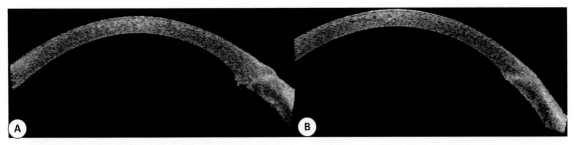

FIGURES 26.6A AND B: High resolution cross-sectional image taken in the anterior segment OCT showing wound healing over a period of time in microphakonit. Immediate postoperative (30 minutes from surgery) shows endothelial misalignment (A). Day 1 shows well formed apposition line with decrease in endothelial misalignment (B)

immediate 30 minutes postoperative period OCT while 42.8% of the 2.8 mm incisions showed immediate coaptation loss. There was no significant difference in the amount of stromal hydration between 2.8 mm and microphakonit incisions as measured from the peripheral corneal thickness on corneal side. One out of seven incisions of 2.8 mm extension had localized descemet detachment seen in OCT and localized subclinical Descemet's tear was noted in 1 out of 17 of the microphakonit wounds.

CORRELATION OF IOP WITH WOUND ARCHITECTURE

For each of the wound feature in the 17 microphakonit wounds, namely the endothelial misalignment and coaptation loss, the mean IOP of those with the feature was compared with the mean IOP of those without that feature. A two-tailed unpaired student "t test" was used with equal variance in the two groups. Out of 17 incisions of the microphakonit, there were both main port and side port of the same eye in five eyes (10 incisions) in microphakonit without extension. The effect of IOP was equal on both the wounds in the same eye. There was no significant difference between the mean IOP of the eyes with and without endothelial misalignment (p=0.557) or coaptation loss (p=0.237) in the 17 microphakonit wounds. On comparing the endothelial misalignment in the 17 microphakonit wounds according to day 1 IOP less than

10 mm Hg and more than 10 mm Hg, no significant difference was seen in the mean endothelial misalignment (p=0.857) and coaptation loss (p=0.291). There was a significant negative correlation between the change in IOP and coaptation loss from day 3 to day 7 but no correlation was observed with change in endothelial misalignment and IOP (**Table 26.2**).

ADVANTAGES OF MICROINCISION

Faster Wound Healing

In our series,[19] thick dense apposition line was seen in 88.2% of the eyes on day 3 and 100% on day 7 of microphakonit wounds. The wound healing seemed to be faster in microphakonit without extension (**Figure 26.6**) as 82.3% of the eyes had no endothelial gape on day 3 and 100% on day 7 (**Figure 26.7, Table 26.1**) as compared to 57.1% on day 3 and 57.1% on day 7 in 2.8 mm extended wounds. Similarly 70.5% and 100% of the 17 microphakonit wounds showed no coaptation loss (**Figure 26.7**) on day 3 and day 7, respectively; whereas 28.5% of the wounds in 2.8 mm size showed persistent coaptation loss even on day 7.

No Difference in Healing in Main or Side Port

On comparing the main port with side port incision in immediate postoperative period of the five eyes of microphakonit without IOL implantation, no significant difference in the wound morphology namely coaptation loss

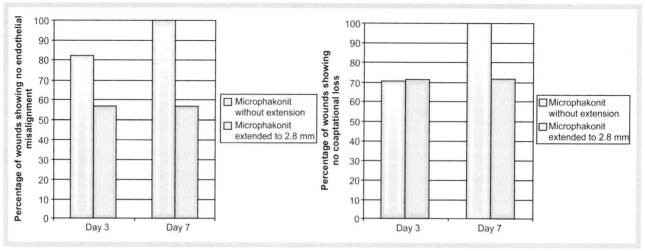

FIGURE 26.7: Graphical representation comparing wound healing in microphakonit wound with and without 2.8 mm extension

(p=0.374) and endothelial misalignment (p=0.146) was seen between the wounds with and without phaco needle. Similarly there was no significant difference noted in the wound healing between the incision which had the phaco tip and which didn't. The settings kept in all eyes were 50% ultrasound and pulse mode was used. There was no difference in wound morphology observed based on the settings of ultrasound used in the phaco tip.

Early Tight Closure at the Incision Site

One of the advantages that were seen with the microphakonit in this clear corneal wound morphology study by anterior segment OCT was the tight closure at the incision site in the immediate postoperative period **(Figure 26.8)** as compared to the incisions in which extension was made.

Less Fluid Ingress and Infection

Tight closure at the incision site in the immediate postoperative period decreases the chance of ingress of fluid

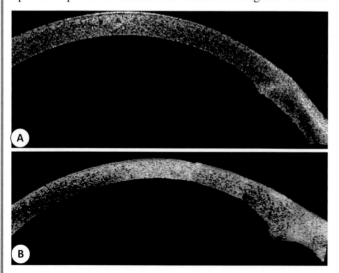

FIGURES 26.8A AND B: High resolution cross-sectional image of wound in the anterior segment OCT on day 1. Microphakonit without extension is shown in **A** and microphakonit with 2.8 mm extension is shown in **B**

and organisms from the ocular surface into the anterior chamber and would in turn decrease the chances of endophthalmitis.

Self Sealed/No Sutures

The incisions in microphakonit were also self sealed without any suture and no external wound gaping as early as day 1 which was seen as well formed tunnel in OCT. Moreover the incisions used for microphakonit[4-6] are so small and self-sealing that the chance of their opening as a result of lid or ocular movements is negligible. This makes the postoperative entry of periocular bacteria into the eye a remote possibility. Added to it is the early wound healing **(Figure 26.7)** seen in smaller incisions which further decreases the risk of entrance of microbes via the wound.

Lesser Postoperative Leak and Shallow Anterior Chamber

Microphakonit wounds have lesser postoperative leak and shallow anterior chamber and thereby lesser incidence of postoperative infection by its property of early wound apposition and healing.

No Change with IOP

There was no significant difference between the mean IOP of the eyes with and without endothelial misalignment (p=0.557) or coaptation loss (p=0.237). We also observed no significant difference in the endothelial misalignment and coaptation loss in the wounds less than 10 mm Hg and more than 10 mm Hg unlike Calladine et al.[17] study which showed more endothelial misalignment in higher IOP.

CONCLUSION

Though there are evidences[14,15] of postcataract endophthalmitis in clear corneal incisions, as of now there are no studies comparing the incidence of endophthalmitis between smaller (sub 1 mm) and larger clear corneal incisions. Corneal wound construction and design play a pivotal role in the prevention of postoperative inflammation and infection. With the appropriate use of aseptic methods, including careful draping, proper selection of anesthesia including the no anesthesia technique,[18] preoperative, intraoperative and postoperative chemoprophylaxis along with the selection of the most optimum clear corneal wound design and construction, the risks for postoperative infection should be low.

REFERENCES

1. Agarwal A, Agarwal S, Agarwal et al. Phakonit: phacoemulsification through a 0.9 mm incision. J Cataract Refract Surg. 2001;27:1548-52.
2. Pandey S, Wener L, Agarwal A, et al. Phakonit: cataract removal through a sub 1.0 mm incision with implantation of the Thinoptx rollable IOL. J Cataract Refract Surg. 2002; 28: 1710.
3. Agarwal A, Agarwal S, Agarwal et al. Phakonit with an acritec IOL. J Cataract Refract Surg. 2003;29:854-5.
4. Agarwal A, Trivedi R, Jacob S, et al. Microphakonit: 700 micron cataract surgery. Clinical Ophthalmology. 2007;1(3): 323-5.
5. Agarwal A, Jacob S, Sinha S, et al. Combating endophthalmitis with microphakonit and no-anesthesia technique. J Cataract Refract Surg. 2007;33(12):2009-11.
6. Agarwal A, Jacob S, Agarwal A. Combined microphakonit and 25-gauge transconjunctival sutureless vitrectomy. J Cataract Refract Surg. 2007; 33(11):1839-40.
7. Tsuneoka H, Shiba T, Takahashi Y. Feasibility of ultrasound cataract surgery with a 1.4 mm incision. J Cataract Refract Surg. 2001;27:934-40.
8. Tsuneoka H, Shiba T, Takahashi Y. Ultrasonic phacoemulsification using a 1.4 mm incision (clinical results). J Cataract Refract Surg. 2002;28:81-6.
9. Alio J, Rodriguez-Prats JL, Galal A, et al. Outcomes of microincision cataract surgery versus coaxial phacoemulsification. Ophthalmology. 2005;112(11):1997-2003.
10. Dosso AA, Cottet L, Burqener ND, et al. Outcomes of coaxial microincision cataract surgery versus conventional coaxial cataract surgery. J Cataract Refract Surg. 2008;34(2):284-8.
11. Agarwal A, Agarwal S, Agarwal A. Antichamber collapse. J Cataract Refract Surg. 2002;28:1085-6.
12. Agarwal A, Agarwal S, Agarwal At. Phakonit: A new technique of removing cataracts through a 0.9 mm incision. In: Agarwal A, Agarwal S, Agarwal A (Eds). Phacoemulsification, Laser Cataract Surgery and Foldable IOL'S, 1st edition. New Delhi: Jaypee Brothers Medical Publishers; 1998. pp. 139-43.
13. Agarwal A, Agarwal S, Agarwal At. Phakonit and laser phakonit: Lens surgery through a 0.9 mm incision. In: Agarwal A, Agarwal S, Agarwal A (Eds). Phacoemulsification, Laser Cataract Surgery and Foldable IOL'S, 2nd edition. New Delhi: Jaypee Brothers Medical Publishers; 2000. pp. 204-16.
14. Nakagi Y, Hayasaka S, Kadoi C, et al. Bacterial endophthalmitis after small-incision cataract surgery: effect of incision placement and intraocular lens type. J Cataract Refract Surg. 2003;29:20-6.
15. Colleaux KM, Hamilton WK. Effect of prophylactic antibiotics and incision type on the incidence of endophthalmitis after cataract surgery. Can J Ophthalmol. 2000; 35:373-8.
16. Izatt JA, Hee MR, Swanson EA, et al. Micrometer-scale resolution imaging of the anterior eye in vivo with optical coherence tomography. Arch Ophthalmol. 1994; 112:1584-9.
17. Calladine D, Packard R. Clear corneal incision architecture in the immediate postoperative period evaluated using optical coherence tomography. J Cataract Refract Surg. 2007; 33: 1429-35.
18. Pandey SK, Werner L, Apple DJ, et al. No-anesthesia clear corneal phacoemulsification versus topical and topical plus intracameral anaesthesia; randomized clinical trial. J Cataract Refract Surg. 2001;27:1643-50.
19. Agarwal A, Kumar DA, Jacob S, et al. In vivo analysis of wound architecture in 700 micron microphakonit surgery. J Cataract Refract Surg. 2008;34(9):1554-60.

CHAPTER 27

Phakonit

Amar Agarwal, Athiya Agarwal, Sunita Agarwal

HISTORY

On August 15th, 1998 the author (Amar Agarwal) performed the first 1 mm cataract surgery by a technique called Phakonit.[1,2] Since Charles Kelman started phacoemulsification, various new modalities have developed which have made this technique more refined. One problem still persists which is the size of the incision. The normal size of the incision is 3.2 mm. With time and more advances in phaco machines and phaco tips, this reduced to 2.8 mm and then to 2.6 mm. The author performed this technique for the first time in the world on August 15th, 1998. It was performed without any anesthesia. No anesthetic drops were instilled in the eye nor was any anesthetic given intracamerally. The first live surgery in the world of Phakonit was performed on August 22nd, 1998 at Pune, India by the author at the Phako and Refractive surgery conference. This was done in front of 350 ophthalmologists.[1,2] In 1999, a live surgery of Phakonit under no anesthesia was telecast live via satellite from India by the author to Seattle USA to the American Society of Cataract and Refractive Surgery (ASCRS) 1999 conference.

The problem with this technique was to find an intra-ocular lens (IOL), which would pass through such a small incision. Then on October 2nd, 2001 the author (Amar Agarwal) did the first case of a Phakonit Rollable IOL. This was done in his Chennai (India) hospital. The lens used was a special lens from Thinoptx. This was a Rollable IOL, which was implanted after a Phakonit procedure, and as it was a rolled IOL it was called the Thinoptx Rollable IOL. This lens uses the Fresnel principle and was designed by Wayne Callahan (USA). It is manufactured by the company Thinoptx. The first Rollable IOL was implanted by Jaino Hoyos (Spain). The author modified the lens to a 5 mm optic to make it pass through a smaller incision. The lens goes through a sub 1.5 mm incision.

PRINCIPLE

The problem in phacoemulsification is that we are not able to go below an incision of 3 mm. The reason is because of the infusion sleeve. The infusion sleeve takes up a lot of space. The titanium tip of the phaco handpiece has a diameter of 0.9 mm. This is surrounded by the infusion sleeve which allows fluid to pass into the eye. It also cools the handpiece tip so that a corneal burn does not occur.[3]

The authors separated the phaco tip from the infusion sleeve. In other words, the infusion sleeve was taken out.

The tip was passed inside the eye and as there was no infusion sleeve present the size of the incision was 1.2 mm. In the left hand, an irrigating chopper was held which had fluid passing inside the eye. The left hand was in the same position where the chopper is normally held; i.e. the side port incision. The assistant injects fluid (BSS) continuously at the site of the incision, to cool the phaco tip. Dr DP Prakash (India) used a 0.8 mm phaco needle with a 21 gauge irrigating chopper and demonstrated through a digital caliper the incision in this case would be a sub 1 mm incision.

TERMINOLOGY

The name "PHAKONIT" has been given because it shows phaco (PHAKO) being done with a needle (N) opening via an incision (I) and with the phako tip (T). It is also because it is phaco with a needle incision technology.

SYNONYMS

- Bimanual phaco
- Micro phaco
- Microincision cataract surgery.

TECHNIQUE OF PHAKONIT FOR CATARACTS

ANESTHESIA

All the cases done by the author have been done without any anesthesia, but the technique of phakonit can be done under any type of anesthesia also. In the cases done by the author no anesthetic drops were instilled in the eye, nor was any intracameral anesthetic injected inside the eye. The authors have analyzed that there is no difference between topical anesthesia cataract surgery and no anesthesia cataract surgery. They have stopped using anesthetic drops totally in all their hospitals.

INCISION

In the first step, a needle with viscoelastic is taken and pierced in the eye in the area where the side port has to be made. Then a special knife to create an incision is made (**Figure 27.1**). The viscoelastic is then injected inside the eye. This will distend the eye so that the clear corneal incision can be made. Now a temporal clear corneal incision

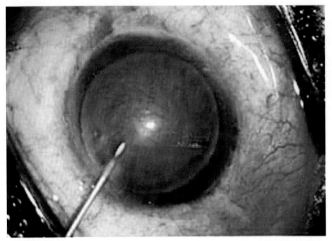

FIGURE 27.1: A 26 gauge needle with viscoelastic making an entry in the area where the side port is. This is for entry of the irrigating chopper

is made. The problem here is that the diamond knives are all 2.6 mm or larger. Since our aim is to make only a 1.2 mm opening, these diamond knives are not sufficient. So a special blade is used **(Figure 27.2)**. This creates an opening of 1.2 mm. When this incision is made, it should be done in such a fashion that a clear corneal valve is made. The authors have devised a keratome of 1.2 mm which they now use. This keratome creates a good valve. This keratome and other instruments for phakonit are made by microsurgical Technology (USA) and Gueder (Germany).

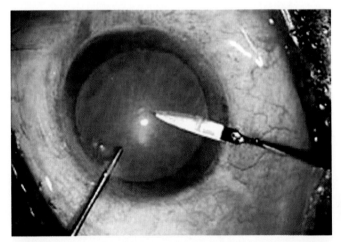

FIGURE 27.2: Clear corneal incision made with the keratome (1.2 mm). Note the left hand has a straight rod to stabilize the eye as the case is done without any anesthesia. These instruments are made by Microsurgical Technology (USA) and Gueder (Germany)

RHEXIS

The rhexis is then performed. This is done with a needle **(Figure 27.3)**. In the left hand, a straight rod is held to stabilize the eye. The advantage is that the movements of the eye can get controlled as one is working without any anesthesia.

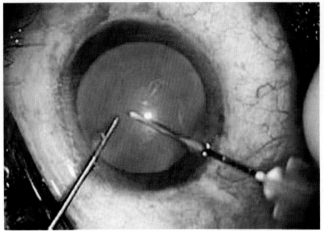

FIGURE 27.3: Rhexis started with a needle

HYDRODISSECTION

Hydrodissection is performed and the fluid wave passing under the nucleus is checked. One has to check for rotation of the nucleus.

PHAKONIT

After enlarging the side port a 20 gauge irrigating chopper connected to the infusion line of the phaco machine is introduced with foot pedal on position 1. The phaco probe is connected to the aspiration line and the phaco tip without an infusion sleeve is introduced through the incision **(Figure 27.4)**. Using the phaco tip with moderate ultrasound power, the center of the nucleus is directly embedded starting from the superior edge of rhexis with the phaco probe directed obliquely downwards towards the vitreous. The settings at this stage is 50% phaco power, flow rate 24 ml/min and 110 mm Hg vacuum. When nearly half of the center of nucleus is embedded, the foot pedal is moved to position 2, as it helps to hold the nucleus due to vacuum rise. To avoid undue pressure on the posterior capsule, the nucleus is lifted a bit and with the irrigating chopper in the left hand the nucleus chopped. This is done

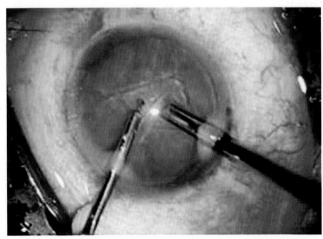

FIGURE 27.4: Phakonit irrigating chopper and phako probe without the sleeve inside the eye

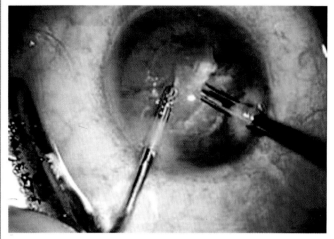

FIGURE 27.5: Phakonit started. Note the phako needle in the right hand and an irrigating chopper in the left hand. Phakonit being performed. Note the crack created by karate chopping. The assistant continuously irrigates the phaco probe area from outside to prevent corneal burns

with a straight downward motion from the inner edge of the rhexis to the center of the nucleus and then to the left in the form of an inverted L shape (**Figure 27.5**). Once the crack is created, the nucleus is split till the center. The nucleus is then rotated 180° and cracked again, so that the nucleus is completely split into two halves.

The nucleus is then rotated 90° and embedding done in one-half of the nucleus with the probe directed horizontally (**Figure 27.6**). With the previously described technique, three pie-shaped quadrants are created in one-half of the nucleus. Similarly, three pie-shaped fragments are created in the other half of the nucleus. With a short burst of energy at pulse mode, each pie-shaped fragment is lifted and brought at the level of iris, where it is further emulsified and aspirated sequentially in pulse mode. Thus, the whole nucleus is removed (**Figure 27.7**). It is to note in **Figure 27.7** that no corneal burns are present. Cortical wash-up is to be done with the bimanual irrigation aspiration technique (**Figures 27.8 and 27.9**). Many doctors like Jorge Alio

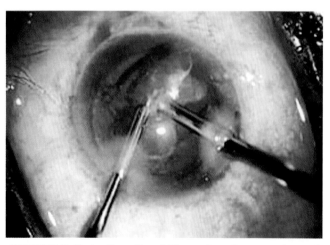

FIGURE 27.6: Phakonit continued. The nuclear pieces are chopped into smaller pie-shaped fragments

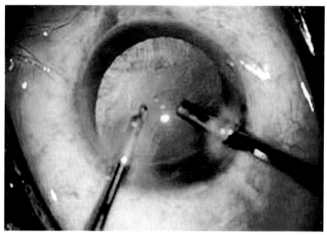

FIGURE 27.7: Phakonit completed. Note the nucleus has been removed and there are no corneal burns

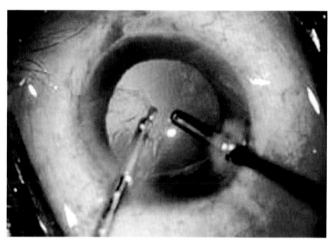

FIGURE 27.8: Bimanual irrigation aspiration started

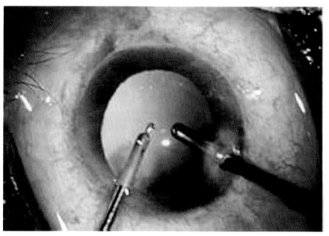

FIGURE 27.9: Bimanual irrigation aspiration completed

(Spain), Richard Packard (UK), F Vejanaro (Columbia), Randall Olson (USA) have devised their own instruments for Phakonit.

ANTICHAMBER COLLAPSER

One of the real bugbears in Phakonit when we started it was about the problem of destabilization of the anterior chamber during surgery. This was solved to a certain extent

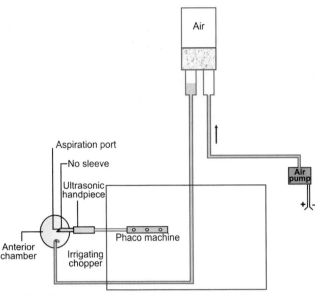

FIGURE 27.10: Anti-chamber collapser (air pump) in phakonit

by using an 18 gauge irrigating chopper. A development made by us (SA) was to use an anti-chamber collapser[4,5] which injects air into the infusion bottle (**Figure 27.10**). This pushes in more fluid into the eye, through the irrigating chopper and also prevents surge. Thus, we were not only able to use a 20 gauge on 21 gauge irrigating chopper but also solve the problem of destabilization of the anterior chamber during surgery. This increases the steady-state pressure of the eye making the anterior chamber deep and well maintained during the entire procedure. It even makes phacoemulsification a relatively safe procedure by reducing surge, even at high vacuum levels. Thus, this can be used not only in Phakonit but also in Phacoemulsification.

SURGE

When an occluded fragment is held by high vacuum and then abruptly aspirated, fluid rushes into the phaco tip to equilibrate the built up vacuum in the aspiration line, causing surge. This leads to shallowing or collapse of the anterior chamber. Different machines employ a variety of methods to combat surge. These include usage of non-complaint tubing,[4] small bore aspiration line tubing,[4] microflow tips,[4] aspiration bypass systems,[4] dual linear foot pedal control[4] and incorporation of sophisticated microprocessors[4] to sense the anterior chamber pressure fluctuations.

The surgeon dependent variables to counteract surge include good wound construction with minimal leakage[5] and selection of appropriate machine parameters, depending on the stage of the surgery.[5] An anterior chamber maintainer has also been described in literature to prevent surge but an extra side port makes it an inconvenient procedure. Another method to solve surge is to use more of phaco-aspiration and chop the nucleus into smaller pieces.

TECHNIQUE

A balanced salt solution (BSS) bottle is used (**Figure 27.10**). The bottle is kept at a height of about 65 centimeters above the operating field. The automated air pump, which is similar to the pump used in fish tanks to supply oxygen to the fish, is utilized to forcefully pump air into the irrigation bottle at a continuous rate. The air pump is connected to the BSS bottles through an IV set.

A millipore air filter is used between the air pump and the infusion bottle, so that the air pumped into the bottle is sterile. Sterile air is pumped into the infusion bottle, pressurizing it to force fluid into the anterior chamber, thereby neutralizing surge and maintaining a deep anterior chamber throughout the procedure.

DISCUSSION

Surge is defined as the volume of the fluid forced out of the eye into the aspiration line at the instant of occlusion break. When the phacoemulsification handpiece tip is occluded, flow is interrupted and vacuum builds up to its preset values. Additionally, the aspiration tubing may collapse in the presence of high vacuum levels. Emulsification of the occluding fragment clears the block and the fluid rushes into the aspiration line to neutralize the pressure difference created between the positive pressure in the anterior chamber and the negative pressure in the aspiration tubing. In addition, if the aspiration line tubing is not reinforced to prevent collapse (tubing compliance), the tubing constricted during occlusion then expands on occlusion break. These factors cause a rush of fluid from the anterior chamber into the phaco probe. The fluid in the anterior chamber is not replaced rapidly enough to prevent shallowing of the anterior chamber.

The maintenance of intraocular pressure (steady-state IOP) during the entire procedure depends on the equilibrium between the fluid inflow and outflow. In most phacoemulsification machines, fluid inflow is provided by gravitational flow of the fluid from the balanced salt solution (BSS) bottle through the tubing to the anterior chamber. This is determined by the bottle height relative to the patient's eye, the diameter of the tubing and most importantly by the outflow of fluid from the eye through the aspiration tube and leakage from the wounds.

The inflow volume can be increased by either increasing the bottle height or by enlarging the diameter of the inflow tube. The intraocular pressure increases by 10 mm Hg for every 15 centimeters increase in bottle height above the eye.[5] High steady-state intraocular pressure (IOP) increase phaco safety by raising the mean IOP level up and away from zero, i.e. by delaying surge related anterior chamber collapse. Air pump increases the amount of fluid inflow thus making the steady-state IOP high. This deepens the anterior chamber, increasing the surgical space available for maneuvering and thus prevents complications like posterior capsular tears and corneal endothelial damage. The phenomenon of surge is neutralized by rapid inflow of fluid at the time of occlusion break. The recovery to steady-state IOP is so prompt that no surge occurs and this enables the surgeon to remain in foot position 3 through the occlusion break. High vacuum phacoemulsification can be safely performed in hard brown cataracts using an air pump. Phacoemulsification under topical or no anesthesia[6] can be safely done, neutralizing the positive vitreous pressure occurring due to squeezing of the eyelids.

THINOPTX ROLLABLE IOL

Thinoptx the company that manufactures these lenses has patented technology that allows the manufacture of lenses with plus or minus 30 dioptre of correction on the thickness of 100 microns. The Thinoptx technology, developed by Wayne Callahan, Scott Callahan and Joe Callahan, is not limited to material choice but is achieved instead of an evolutionary optic and unprecedented nano-scale manufacturing process. The lens is made from off-the-shelf hydrophilic material, which is similar to several IOL materials already on the market. The key to the Thinoptx lens is the optic design and nano-precision manufacturing. The basic advantage of this lens is that they are ultra-thin lenses. Thinoptx has made a special lens for Phakonit which has a 5 mm optic.

LENS INSERTION TECHNIQUE

The lens is taken out from the bottle. The lens is then held with a forceps **(Figure 27.11)**. The lens is then placed in a bowl of BSS solution that is approximately body temperature. This makes the lens pliable. Once the lens is pliable, it is taken with the gloved hand holding it between the index finger and the thumb. The lens is then rolled in a rubbing motion. It is preferable to do this in the bowl of BSS, so that the lens remains rolled well.

The lens is then inserted through the incision carefully **(Figure 27.12)**. One can then move the lens into the capsular bag **(Figure 27.13)**. The natural warmth of the eye causes the lens to open gradually. Viscoelastic is then removed with the bimanual irrigation aspiration probes **(Figure 27.14)**. The tips of the footplates are extremely thin which allow the lens to be positioned with the footplates rolled to fit the eye.

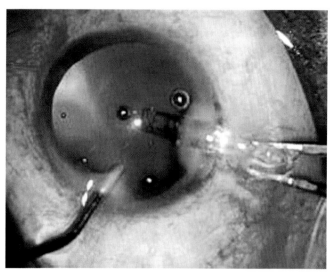

FIGURE 27.12: The rollable IOL inserted through the incision

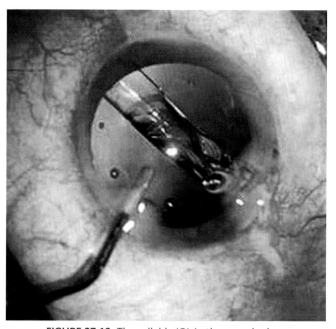

FIGURE 27.13: The rollable IOL in the capsular bag

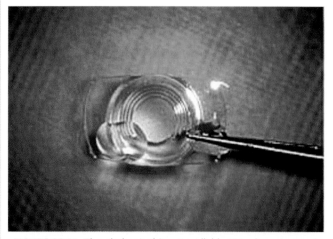

FIGURE 27.11: The phakonit thinoptx rollable IOL when removed from the bottle

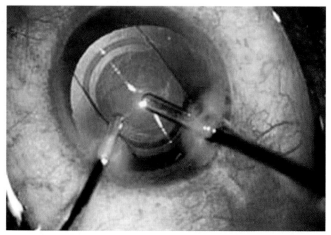

FIGURE 27.14: Viscoelastic removed using bimanual irrigation aspiration probes

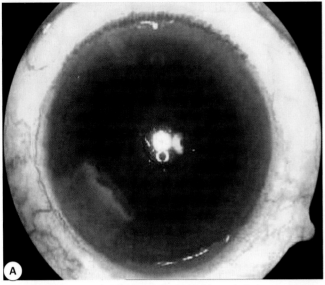 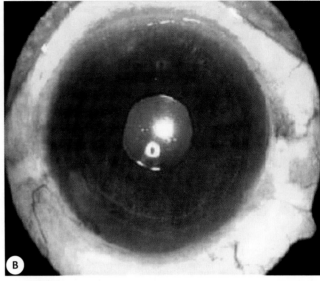

FIGURES 27.15A AND B: Phako foldable and phakonit thinoptx IOL. The figure on the left shows a case of phako with a foldable IOL and the figure on the right shows phakonit with a thinoptx rollable IOL

ROLLER

Thinoptx have devised a special injector to implant the Rollable IOL after Phakonit. The advantage of this roller is that it not only rolls the lens but also inserts the lens inside the eye.

TOPOGRAPHY

We also perfomed topography with the Orbscan to compare cases of phakonit and phaco and we found that the astigmatism in phakonit cases is much less compared to phaco **(Figures 27.15 to 27.18).** Stabilization of refraction is also faster with Phakonit compared to phaco surgery.

LASER PHAKONIT

Laser Phakonit uses laser energy (coupled with ultrasound energy in hard nuclei) to remove the nucleus. This technique was started first time in the world by the author (Sunita Agarwal). The laser machine used is the Paradigm Laser Photon. In these cases, two ports are used. One port has

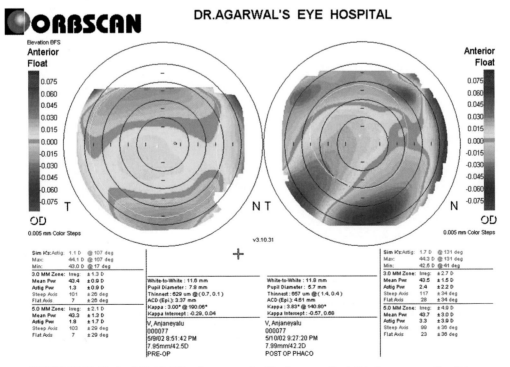

FIGURE 27.16: Phako foldable IOL orbscan results. The figure on the left is the preoperative Orbscan. The figure on the right is the one day postoperative Orbscan. Note the difference between the two Orbscan pictures. This is the site where the clear corneal temporal incision was made

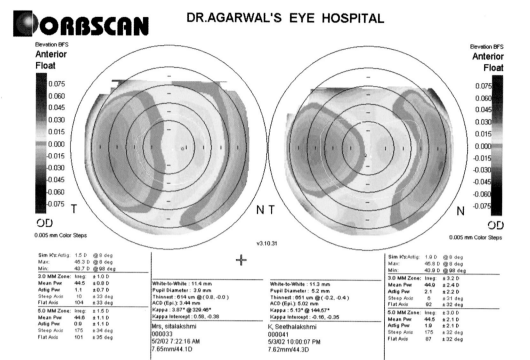

FIGURE 27.17: Phakonit thinoptx rollable IOL Orbscan results. The figure on the left is the preoperative Orbscan. The figure on the right is the one day postoperative Orbscan. Note the similarity between the two Orbscan pictures. This shows the minimal astigmatism created even on one day postoperative

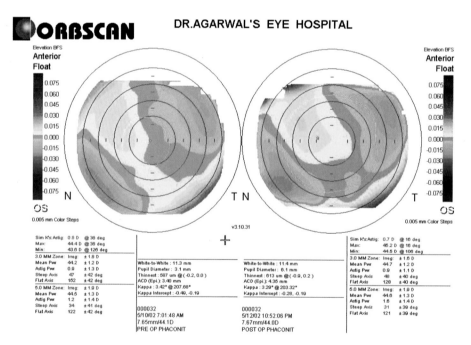

FIGURE 27.18: Phakonit thinoptx rollable IOL Orbscan results. The figure on the left is the preoperative Orbscan. The figure on the right is the one day postoperative Orbscan. Note the similarity between the two Orbscan pictures. This shows no astigmatism created even on one day postoperative. Do note the astigmatism preoperative is 0.8 D and postoperative on day one is 0.7 D

fluid (BSS) flowing through an irrigating chopper of 20 gauge and in the other hand is the phaco probe without a sleeve. In the center of the phaco probe is passed the laser probe. The diameter of the phaco probe is 900 microns. The laser probe reduces the orifice opening to 550 microns. Thus the nucleus can be removed through a very small opening.

THREE-PORT PHAKONIT

Another technique by which one can perform Phakonit is to use an anterior chamber maintainer. The author started this technique. He called it three-port phakonit. Just as a three port vitrectomy, here also there are three ports, hence the name Three-Port Phakonit.

There are pros and cons in every technique. The problem in three-port phakectomy is that it is too cumbersome. Surgeons prefer to have two ports only. Some surgeons prefer three ports, as an anterior chamber maintainer is present in the eye and thus the anterior chamber is always formed. At present, it is easier to perform Phakonit using a 20 gauge irrigating chopper with the anti-chamber collapser.

ANTERIOR CHAMBER (AC) STABILITY IN PHAKONIT

One of the real bugbears in Phakonit when we started it was about the problem of destabilization of the anterior chamber during surgery.[1-5] This was solved to a certain extent by using an 18 gauge irrigating chopper. Another solution would be to raise the bottle to the roof which is not very practical. The main problem in Phakonit was that the amount of fluid entering the eye through the irrigating chopper was not equal to the amount of fluid exiting the eye through the sleeveless phaco needle. With better methods as discussed below on AC stability, one can use a 21 gauge irrigating chopper.

SOLUTION

Different surgeons have tried different methods to solve this problem of anterior chamber stability. The various methods are:
• Air pump or Anti-chamber collapser
• Anterior Vented Gas Forced Infusion System (VGFI) of the Accurus Surgical System
• STAAR Surgical's disposable Cruise Control device
• Well designed irrigating choppers from Duet (Microsurgical Technology).

The anterior vented gas forced infusion system (AVGFI) of the Accurus Surgical System in the performance of phakonit

This was started by Arturo Pérez-Arteaga from Mexico.

The AVGFI is a system incorporated in the Accurus machine that creates a positive infusion pressure inside the eye; it was designed by the Alcon engineers to control the intraocular pressure (IOP) during the anterior and posterior segment surgery. It consist of an air pump and a regulator who are inside the machine; then the air is pushed inside the bottle of intraocular solution, and so the fluid is actively pushed inside the eye without raising or lowering the bottle. The control of the air pump is digitally integrated in the Accurus panel; it also can be controlled via the remote. Also the footswitch can be preset with the minimal and maximum of desired fluid inside the eye and go directly to this value with the simple touch of the footswitch. Arturo Pérez-Arteaga recommends to preset the infusion pump at 100–110 cm H_2O; it is enough strong irrigation force to perform a microincision phaco. This parameter is preset in the panel and also as the minimal irrigation force in the footswitch; then he recommends to preset the maximum irrigation force at 130–140 cm H_2O in the foot pedal, so if a surge exist during the procedure the surgeon can increase the irrigation force, by the simple touch of the footswitch to the right. With the AVGFI the surgeon has the capability to increase even more these values.

Cruise control:
The Cruise Control is a disposable, flow-restricting (0.3 mm internal diameter) device that is placed in between the phaco handpiece and the aspiration tubing of any phaco machine. The goal is very similar to that of the flare tip (Alcon): Combining a standard phaco tip opening with a narrower shaft to provide more grip with less surge. This has been popularized by David Chang (USA) for phakonit surgery. STAAR Surgical introduced this disposable Cruise Control device, which can be used with any phaco machine.

Duet system:
Larry Laks (USA) created the Duet system (Microsurgical Technology-MST). The advantage of this was a whole bimanual phaco set for Phakonit. The Duet system has phakonit knives also (**Figure 27.19**) handles on which various irrigating choppers can fit (**Figure 27.20**). The MST

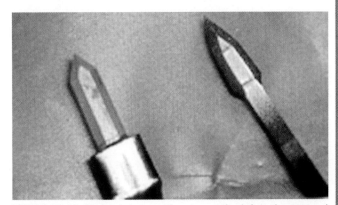

FIGURE 27.19: Phakonit knives. The one on the left is the Agarwal sapphire phakonit knife made by Huco (Switzerland). The one on the right is the one made by Microsurgical Technology

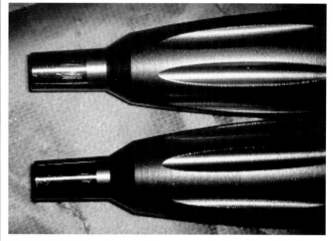

FIGURE 27.20: Duet system. These are the handles of the Duet system (Microsurgical Technology). The irrigating choppers and bimanual irrigation aspiration sets can be interchanged with the handles

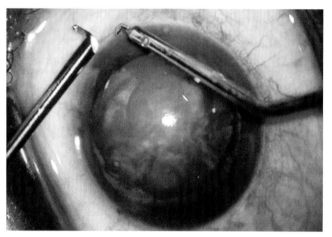

FIGURE 27.21: Two designs of irrigating choppers. The one on the left has a larger opening for fluid so that AC stability is more. This has been designed by Larry Laks (Microsurgical Technology). The one on the right has two openings on the sides (Gueder –Germany)

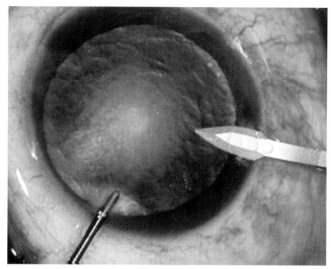

FIGURE 27.22: Clear corneal incision made with the microsurgical technology knife

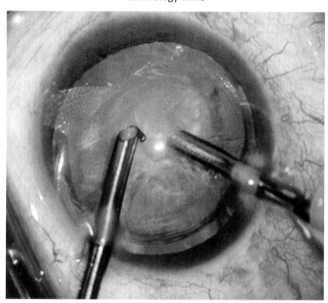

FIGURE 27.23: Phakonit being done with the Agarwal sharp irrigating chopper from Microsurgical Technology

20 gauge Duet irrigating choppers provide the best inflow of comparable devices. The MST shaft design gives an impressive inflow rate of 40 cc/min at 30 in of bottle height and is available with an assortment of interchangeable chopper tips. This whole design was created by Larry Laks. The idea was to have the opening in the irrigating choppers larger (**Figure 27.21**). The clear corneal incision can be created with the MST knife (**Figure 27.22**) and then Phakonit started using the Agarwal sharp MST irrigating chopper (**Figure 27.23**).

Once Phakonit is completed, the bimanual irrigation aspiration set from the Duet system is used (**Figure 27.24**) and the cortical aspiration completed (**Figure 27.25**).

SUMMARY

There are various problems, which are encountered, in any new technique and so also with Phakonit. With time, these

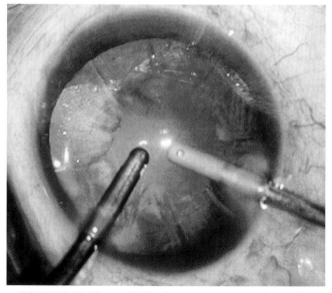

FIGURE 27.24: Bimanual irrigation aspiration started using the Duet system (MST)

TABLE 27.1 The differences between phako and phakonit

Feature	Coaxial phako	Bimanual phako (Phakonit)
Incision size	>3 mm	Sub 1.4 mm
Airpump	Non mandatory	Mandatory
Hand usage	Single handed phako possible	Two hands (Bimanual)
Non -dominant hand entry and exit	Last to enter and first to exit	First to enter and last to exit
Capsulorhexis	Needle or forceps	Better with needle
IOL	Foldable IOL	Rollable IOL
Astigmatism	Two unequal incision create astigmatism	Two equal ultra small incisions negate the induced astigmatism
Stability of refraction	Later than phakonit	Earlier than phako

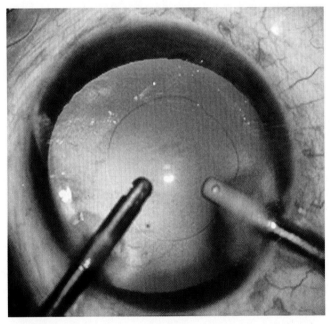

FIGURE 27.25: Bimanual irrigation aspiration completed

will have to be solved. The differences between phako and phakonit are shown in **Table 27.1**. The important point is that today we have broken the 1 mm barrier for cataract removals. This can be done easily by separating the phaco needle from the infusion sleeve. As the saying goes—

"We have miles to go before we can sleep".

REFERENCES

1. Agarwal S, Agarwal A, Sachdev MS, et al. Phacoemulsification. Laser Cataract Surgery and Foldable IOLs, 2nd edition. Delhi: Jaypee Brothers Medical Publisher(P) Ltd; 2000.
2. Boyd BF, Agarwal S, Agarwal A, et al. Lasik and Beyond Lasik; Highlights of Ophthalmology; 2000, Panama.
3. Ronge LJ. Clinical Update. Five Ways to avoid Phaco Burns; 1999.
4. Fishkind WJ. The Phaco Machine : How and why it acts and reacts? In: Agarwal's Four volume Textbook of Ophthalmology. Jaypee Brothers: New Delhi; 2000.
5. Seibel SB. The fluidics and physics of phaco. In: Agarwal's, et al. Phacoemulsification, Laser Cataract Surgery and Foldable IOLs, 2nd edition. Jaypee Brothers: New Delhi; 2000. pp.45-54.
6. Agarwal, et al. No anesthesia cataract surgery with karate chop. In: Agarwal's Phacoemulsification, Laser Cataract Surgery and Foldable IOLs 2nd edition. New Delhi Jaypee Brothers; 2000. pp. 217-26.

CHAPTER 28

No Anesthesia Sub 1 mm (700 micron) Microincision Cataract Surgery: Microphakonit

Athiya Agarwal, Soosan Jacob, Amar Agarwal

HISTORY

On August 15th, 1998 the author performed 1 mm cataract surgery by a technique called PHAKONIT[1-13] [Phacoemulsification (phako) being done with a Needle Incision Technology (NIT)]. Dr. Jorge Alio (Spain) coined the term MICS or Microincision cataract surgery[14] for all surgeries including laser cataract surgery and Phakonit. Dr. Randall Olson (USA) first used a 0.8 mm phaco needle and a 21 gauge irrigating chopper and called it Microphaco.[15-18] On May 21st, 2005, for the first time, a 0.7 mm phaco needle tip with a 0.7 mm irrigating chopper was used by the author to remove cataracts through the smallest incision possible as of now. This is called microphakonit.

MICROPHAKONIT (0.7 MM) NEEDLE TIP

When the author wanted to go for a 0.7 mm phaco needle, the point which he wondered was whether the needle would be able to hold the energy of the ultrasound. The author gave this problem to Larry Laks from MST, USA to work on. He then made this special 0.7 mm phaco needle. As one will understand, if one goes smaller from a 0.9 mm phaco needle to a 0.7 mm phaco needle, the speed of the surgery would go down. This is because the amount of aspiration flow rate would be less.

It was decided to solve this problem by working on the wall of the 0.7 mm phaco needle. There is a standard wall thickness for all phaco tips. If one says the outer diameter is a constant the resultant inner diameter is an area of the outer diameter minus the area of the wall.

The inner diameter will regulate the flow rate/ perceived efficiency (which can be good or bad, depending on how one looks at it). In order to increase the allowed aspiration flow rate from what a standard 0.7 mm tip would be, MST (Larry Laks) had the walls made thinner, thus increasing the inner diameter. This would allow a case to go speed wise, closer to what a 0.9mm tip would go (not exactly the same, but closer). With the gas forced infusion it would work very well. Finally, the author decided to go for a 30° tip to make it even better.

MICROPHAKONIT (0.7 MM) IRRIGATING CHOPPER

There are two designs of 20 gauge (0.9 mm) irrigating choppers which we designed **(Figure 28.1)** for phakonit when we used the 0.9 mm needle and irrigating chopper. One is the Agarwal irrigating chopper made by the MST (Microsurgical Technology) company. The opening for the fluid in this is end opening. This is incorporated in the Duet system. The other irrigating chopper is made by Geuder, Germany. This has two side openings. Depending on the convenience of the surgeon, the surgeon can decide which design of irrigating chopper they would like to use. There are advantages and disadvantages of both types of irrigating choppers. The end opening chopper has an advantage of more fluid coming out of the chopper. The disadvantage is that there is a gush of fluid which might push the nuclear pieces away. The advantage of the side opening irrigating chopper is that there is good control, as the nuclear pieces are not pushed away but the disadvantage is that the amount of fluid coming out of it is much less. That is why if one is using the side opening irrigating chopper, one should use an air pump or gas forced infusion.

The MST in their irrigating chopper increased flow by removing the flow restrictions incorporated in other irriga-

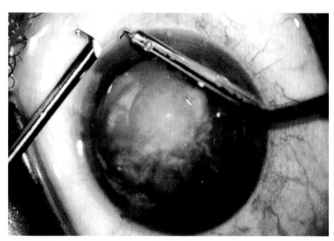

FIGURE 28.1: Two designs of Agarwal irrigating choppers. The one on the left has an end opening for fluid (microsurgical technology). The one on the right has two openings on the sides (Geuder – Germany)

ting choppers as a bi-product of their attachment method. They also had control of incisional outflow by having all the instruments to be of one size and created a matching knife of the proper size and geometry **(Figure 28.2)**.

When the author decided to go smaller to using a 0.7 mm irrigating chopper **(Figure 28.3)** he decided to go for an end-opening irrigating chopper. The reason is as the bore of the irrigating chopper was smaller, the amount of fluid coming out of it would be less and so an end-opening chopper would maintain the fluidics better. With gas forced infusion, the author thought he would be able to balance the entry and exit of fluid into the anterior chamber and that is what happened.

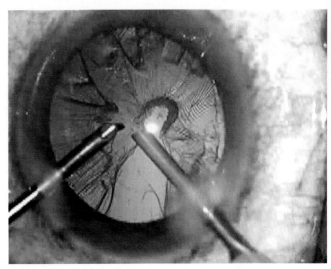

FIGURE 28.3: Microphakonit . 0.7 mm irrigating chopper and 0.7 mm phako tip without the sleeve inside the eye. All instruments are made by MST, USA. The assistant continuously irrigates the phaco probe area from outside to prevent corneal burns. Please note that the nucleus has been removed and there are no corneal burns

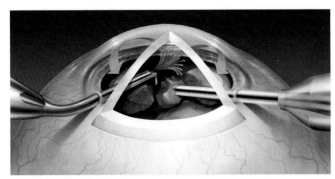

FIGURE 28.2: Phakonit. Notice the irrigating chopper with an end opening (*Courtesy:* Larry Laks, MST, USA)

The author measured the amount of fluid coming out of the various irrigating choppers with and without an air pump **(Table 28.1)**. He also measured the values using the simple aquarium air pump (external gas forced infusion) and the Accurus machine giving internal gas forced infusion.

The microphakonit irrigating chopper which the author has designed is basically a sharp chopper which has a sharp cutting edge and helps in karate chopping or quick chopping. It can chop any type of cataract. **Table 28.2** shows the differences between C-MICS which is Coaxial microincisional cataract surgery and B-MICS which is bimanual microincisional cataract surgery.

AIR PUMP AND GAS FORCED INFUSION

The main problem in phakonit the author had was the destabilization of the anterior chamber during surgery. He solved it to a certain extent by using an 18 gauge irrigating chopper. Then, Sunita Agarwal suggested the use of an antichamber collapser[19] which injects air into the infusion bottle. This pushes more fluid into the eye through the irrigating chopper and also prevents surge. Thus, the author was able to use a 20/21 gauge irrigating chopper as well as solve the problem of destabilization of the anterior chamber during surgery. Now with a 22 gauge (0.7 mm) irrigating chopper, it is extremely essential that gas forced infusion be used in the surgery. This is also called external gas forced infusion.

When the surgeon uses the air pump contained in the same phaco machine, it is called internal gas forced infusion (IFI). To solve the problem of infection, the author uses a millipore filter connected to the machine. The Stellaris machine made by Bausch and Lomb has an inbuilt air pump to give pressurized infusion. When the author is using a 0.7 mm irrigating chopper the problem is that the amount of fluid entering the eye is not enough. To solve this problem gas forced infusion is a must. The author presets the infusion pump at 100 mm Hg when he is operating microphakonit.

| TABLE 28.1 | Fluid exiting from various irrigating choppers (Values in ml/minute) |

Irrigating chopper	Without gas forced infusion	With gas forced infusion using the accurus machine at 50 mm Hg	With gas forced infusion using the accurus machine at 75 mm Hg	With gas forced infusion using the accurus machine at 100 mm Hg	Air pump with regulator at low	Air pump with regulator at high
0.9 mm Side opening	25	36	42	48	37	51
0.9 mm End opening	34	51	57	65	52	68
0.7 mm End opening	27	39	44	51	41	54

TABLE 28.2 Phaco vs phakonit

	Feature	Phaco (C-MICS)	Phakonit (B-MICS)
1.	Incision size	3 mm	Sub 1.4 mm
2.	Air pump	Not mandatory	Mandatory
3.	Hand usage	Single handed phaco possible	Two hands(bimanual)
4.	Non-dominant hand entry and exit	Last to enter and first to exit	First to enter and last to exit
5.	Capsulorhexis	Needle or forceps	Better with needle
6.	IOL	Foldable IOL	Rollable IOL
7.	Astigmatism	Two unequal incisions create astigmatism	Two equal ultrasmall incisions negate the induced astigmatism
8.	Stability of refraction	Later than phakonit	Earlier than phaco
9.	Iris prolapse- intraoperative	More chances	Less chances due to smaller incision

BIMANUAL 0.7 MM IRRIGATION ASPIRATION SYSTEM

Bimanual irrigation aspiration is done with the bimanual irrigation aspiration instruments. These instruments are also designed by Microsurgical Technology (USA). The previous set the author used was the 0.9 mm set. Now with microphakonit the author uses the new 0.7 mm bimanual I/A set **(Figures 28.4 and 28.5)**, so that after the nucleus removal he does not need to enlarge the incision.

DUET HANDLES

All these instruments of the 0.7 mm set fit onto the handles of the Duet system. So if a surgeon has already got the handles and is using it for phakonit they need to get only the tips and can use the same handles for microphakonit **(Figure 28.6)**.

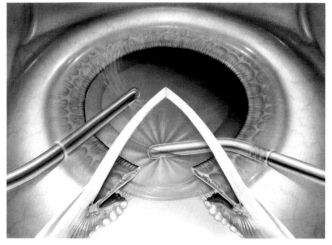

FIGURE 28.5: Soft tip I/A from MST, USA
(*Courtesy,* Larry Laks-MST, USA)

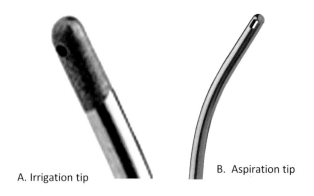

A. Irrigation tip   B. Aspiration tip

FIGURE 28.6: 700 micron irrigation aspiration tips
(*Courtesy,* Larry Laks-MST, USA)

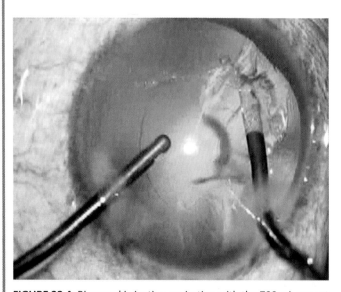

FIGURE 28.4: Bimanual irrigation aspiration with the 700 micron set

DIFFERENCES BETWEEN 0.9 MM AND 0.7 MM SETS IN CATARACT SURGERY

See **Table 28.3.**

TABLE 28.3 The differences between the two techniques and shows the differences between phakonit and microphakonit

Features	Phakonit	Microphakonit
Irrigating chopper	0.9 mm	0.7 mm
Phaco needle	0.9 mm	0.7 mm
Control in surgery	Good	Better control
Valve construction	Extremely important	Not very important as incision is much smaller
Iris prolapse	Can occur if valve is bad	Very rare
Intraoperative floppy iris syndrome	Can be managed	Much better to manage as incision is much smaller and there is better control
Hydrodissection	Can be done from both incisions	To be careful as very little space is there for escape of fluid
Air pump (gas forced infusion—GFI)	Can be done without it though better with it	Mandatory. 0.7 mm irrigating choppers even with higher end machines need GFI
Flow rate	Can keep any value	Do not keep it very high. 20-24 ml/min
Bimanual I/A	0.9 mm	0.7 mm

TECHNIQUE

INCISION

The incision is made with a keratome. This can be done using a sapphire knife or a stainless steel knife. One should be careful when one is making the incision, so that the incision is a slightly long, as one would be using gas forced infusion in microphakonit. Before making the incision, a needle with viscoelastic is taken and pierced in the eye in the area where the side port has to be made. The viscoelastic is then injected inside the eye. This will distend the eye, so that the clear corneal incision can be made easily. One should make one clear corneal incision between the lateral rectus and inferior rectus and the other between the lateral rectus and superior rectus. This way, one is able to control the movements of the eye during surgery.

RHEXIS

The rhexis is then performed of about 5–6 mm. This is done with a needle **(Figure 28.7)**. In the left hand a straight rod is held to stabilize the eye. This is the globe stabilization rod. The advantage of this is that the movements of the eye can get controlled if one is working without any anesthesia or under topical anesthesia. One can use a micro rhexis forceps also **(Figures 28.8 and 28.9)**.

HYDRODISSECTION

Hydrodissection is performed and the fluid wave passing under the nucleus checked. It is required to check for rotation of the nucleus. The advantage of microphakonit is that one can do hydrodissection from both incisions so that even the subincisional areas can get easily hydrodissected. The problem is as there is not a lot of escape of fluid, one should be careful in hydrodissection as if too much fluid is passed into the eye, one can get a complication.

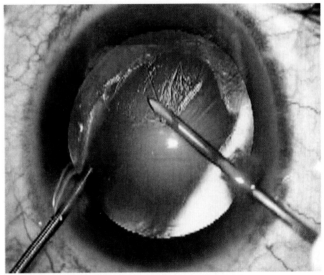

FIGURE 28.7: Rhexis done with a 26 gauge needle. This has viscoelastic in it so that if the chamber shallows one can inject viscoelastic inside the eye. Please note that the other hand has a globe stabilization rod (KATENA, USA)

MICROPHAKONIT

The 22 (0.7 mm) gauge irrigating chopper connected to the infusion line of the phaco machine is introduced with foot pedal on position 1. The phaco probe is connected to the aspiration line and the 0.7 mm phaco tip without an infusion sleeve is introduced through the clear corneal incision. Using the phaco tip with moderate ultrasound power, the center of the nucleus is directly embedded starting from the superior edge of rhexis with the phaco probe directed obliquely downwards towards the vitreous. The settings at this stage are 50% phaco power, flow rate 20 ml/min and 100–200 mm Hg vacuum. Using the karate chop technique, the nucleus is chopped. Thus the whole nucleus is removed. Cortical wash-up is then done with the bimanual irrigation

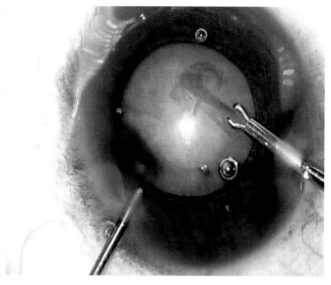

FIGURE 28.8: MST rhexis forceps used to perform the rhexis in a mature cataract. Please note the Trypan blue staining the anterior capsule

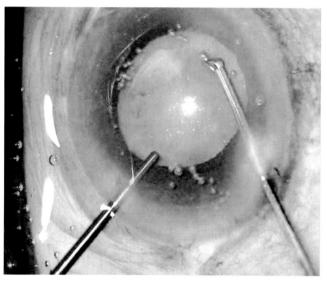

FIGURE 28.9: Twenty-five gauge micro rhexis MST forceps for sub 1 mm cataract surgery

aspiration (0.7 mm set) technique. During this whole procedure of microphakonit gas forced infusion is used.

SUMMARY

With microphakonit, a 0.7 mm set is used to remove the cataract. At present this is the smallest one can use for cataract surgery. With time one would be able to go smaller with better instruments and devices. The problem at present is the Intraocular lense (IOL). We have to get good quality IOLs going through sub 1 mm cataract surgical incisions, so that the real benefit of microphakonit can be given to the patient.

REFERENCES

1. Agarwal A, Agarwal S, Agarwal. No anesthesia Cataract surgery. In: Agarwal et al. Textbook Phacoemulsification, Laser Cataract Surgery and Foldable IOLs, 1st edition. India: Jaypee; 1998; 144-54.
2. Pandey S, Wener L, Agarwal A, et al. Apple D No anesthesia Cataract surgery; J Cataract and Refractive Surgery 2001; 28:1710-3.
3. Agarwal A, Agarwal S, Agarwal A. Phakonit: A new technique of removing cataracts through a 0.9 mm incision; In Agarwal et als. Textbook Phacoemulsification, Laser Cataract Surgery and Foldable IOLs, 1st edition; India Jaypee, 1998. p 139-43.
4. Agarwal A, Agarwal S, Agarwal A. Phakonit and laser phakonit: Lens surgery through a 0.9 mm incision; In: Agarwal et als. Textbook Phacoemulsification, Laser Cataract Surgery and Foldable IOLs, 2nd edition; India Jaypee, 2000;p 204-16.
5. Agarwal A, Agarwal S, Agarwal A. Phakonit; In: Agarwal et als. Textbook Phacoemulsification, Laser Cataract Surgery and Foldable IOLs, 3rd edition; India Jaypee, 2003;pp 317-29.
6. Agarwal A, Agarwal S, Agarwal A. Phakonit and laser phakonit; In: Boyd/Agarwal et al Textbook Lasik and Beyond Lasik, Highlights of Ophthalmology, Panama; 2000. pp. 463-8.
7. Agarwal A, Agarwal S, Agarwal A. Phakonit and laser phakonit-Cataract surgery through a 0.9 mm incision; In: Boyd/Agarwal et al Textbook Phako, Phakonit and Laser Phako, Higlights of Ophthalmology, Panama, 2000;pp. 327-34.
8. Agarwal A, Agarwal S, Agarwal A. The Phakonit Thinoptx IOL; In: Agarwals Textbook Presbyopia, Slack, USA; 2002. pp. 187-94.
9. Agarwal A, Agarwal S, Agarwal A. Antichamber collapser. J Cataract and Refractive Surgery. 2002;28:1085.
10. Pandey S, Wener L, Agarwal A, et al. Phakonit: Cataract removal through a sub 1.0 mm incision with implantation of the Thinoptx rollable IOL. J Cataract and Refractive Surgery. 2002;28:1710.
11. Agarwal A, Agarwal S, Agarwal A. Phakonit: phacoemulsification through a 0.9 mm incision. J Cataract and Refractive Surgery 2001;27:1548-52.
12. Agarwal A, Agarwal S, Agarwal A. Phakonit with an acritec IOL. J Cataract and Refractive Surgery 2003;29:854-5.
13. Agarwal S, Agarwal A, Agarwal A. Phakonit with Acritec IOL. Highlights of Ophthalmology; 2000.
14. Jorge Alio. What does MICS require in Alios Textbook MICS. Highlights of Ophthalmology 2004. pp. 1-4.
15. Soscia W, Howard JG, Olson RJ. Microphacoemulsification with Whitestar. A wound-temperature study. J Cataract and Refractive Surgery. 2002;28;1044-6.
16. Soscia W, Howard JG, Olson RJ. Bimanual phacoemulsification through two stab incisions. A wound-temperature study. J Cataract and Refractive Surgery. 2002;28:1039-43.
17. Randall Olson. Microphaco chop. In: David Changs Textbook on Phaco Chop. Slack, USA; 2004. pp. 227-37.
18. David Chang. Bimanual phaco chop. In David Changs Textbook on Phaco Chop. Slack, USA; 2004. pp. 239-50.
19. Agarwal A. Air pump in Agarwal's textbook on Bimanual phaco: Mastering the phakonit/MICS technique. Slack, USA; 2005.

CHAPTER 29

1.8 mm C-MICS with the Stellaris Vision Enhancement System

Terence M Devine

WHY COAXIAL MICROINCISION CATARACT SURGERY (C-MICS)?

Phacoemulsification techniques have evolved as improvements in technology and techniques allowed surgeons to use progressively smaller incisions. Compared to Kelman's original 3.5 mm procedure, achieving 2.8 mm capability seemed a major step forward to most of the surgeons, so that many still question the need to go smaller. However, the evidence that shows significant advantages to sub-2 mm surgery is mounting. This includes reduced inflammation,[1] corneal edema,[2] endothelial cell loss[3] and surgically induced astigmatism,[2,4] as well as improved corneal wound strength[5] and fluidics efficiency.[6]

Many surgeons therefore have adopted the Phakonit or biaxial/bimanual microincision cataract surgery (B-MICS) phaco techniques popularized by Dr Amar Agarwal, Dr Jorge Alio and others. A number of surgeons, however, found B-MICS more difficult or less efficient than their customary 2.8 mm cataract surgery and reverted to their previous technique. Others have embraced the new 1.8 mm coaxial MICS (C-MICS) procedure introduced with the Stellaris[TM] Vision Enhancement System for phacoemulsification **(Figure 29.1)**.[7]

In contrast to B-MICS, 1.8 mm C-MICS maintains the infusion sleeve to reduce leakage, improve chamber stability, protect the cornea from friction and stress, and maintain a water-tight seal. The nondominant hand is not "pinned" inside the eye to maintain infusion and smaller, more ergonomic side port instruments can be used. The 1.8 mm C-MICS procedure now offers the benefits of sub-2 mm surgery with little or no learning curve. It is compatible with any technique and surgeons can utilize their familiar fluidics settings. It offers improved visibility and maneuverability which benefits any case, but is particularly helpful with small pupils, IFIS cases, pseudoexfoliation or situations with disrupted zonules or capsule. The smaller incision is an obvious advantage for patients with previous radial keratotomy (RK) or corneal transplants because it allows the surgeon to work between the RK incisions or penetrating keratoplasty (PK) sutures. There is also early evidence that C-MICS may provide improved safety in terms of capsule tears. I performed the first 1.8 mm C-MICS cases with the Stellaris on October 30, 2006. In a computer based review of my cases through May 31, 2010, we found an incidence of 0.00014 unplanned anterior vitrectomies (1 out of 6846

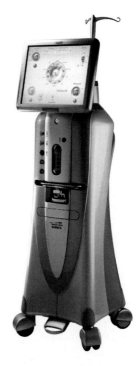

FIGURE 29.1: The Stellaris Vision Enhancement System designed for sub-2 mm coaxial and biaxial microincision cataract surgery (MICS)

cases). For these and other reasons, many surgeons have now adopted 1.8 mm C-MICS even if they plan to enlarge the incision for IOL insertion.

FLUIDICS CONTROL

In terms of fluidics, the principle for safety with the Stellaris is simple; inflow must always replace any outflow through the needle and any leakage through the incisions. The difficulty from an engineering perspective lies in the fact that the anterior chamber only contains approximately 0.3 ml or 6 drops of fluid. This means that if outflow exceeds inflow by six drops, the anterior chamber will collapse with potential damage to endothelium, capsule and other intraocular tissues. This inflow/outflow balance must be maintained at all times but becomes most critical in the situation of postocclusion surge.

Postocclusion surge occurs when an occluded phaco needle suddenly aspirates a piece of nucleus. The amount of fluid aspirated at that moment is related to several things:
- The internal diameter of the needle and aspiration tubing which determines the resistance to outflow.

- The tubing compliance or "stiffness": During occlusion, soft aspiration tubing will compress as vacuum rises and then rebound when occlusion breaks, adding to the volume of fluid drawn from the anterior chamber. The compliance of the pump and vacuum transducers may also influence surge.

- The "differential pressure" when the needle is occluded: The differential pressure is the difference between the positive intraocular pressure (IOP) related to bottle height and the negative pressure inside the needle determined by vacuum level generated by the pump. Higher vacuum can produce higher surge.

The volume of aspirated "surge" fluid must be immediately replaced by infusion or the chamber will collapse. This fluidics challenge becomes amplified for sub-2 mm phaco, because the smaller diameter infusion instruments for B-MICS or the smaller infusion sleeves for C-MICS deliver less fluid per second for any given bottle height.

To overcome this limitation, one alternative is to increase the bottle height to increase the potential infusion volume per second. The problem with this approach is that IOP is directly proportional to the bottle height and inversely proportional to the outflow. Therefore, whenever aspiration is stopped, either by tip occlusion or the surgeon returning to foot pedal position one, the IOP is solely determined by the bottle height. Balanced salt solution (BSS) produces approximately 0.73 mm Hg pressure per centimeter of bottle height. For example, with no outflow, a 150 cm bottle height would produce 110 mm Hg IOP (**Table 29.1**).

TABLE 29.1	Pressure of BSS in mm of Hg at the eye based on bottle height (cm) without any outflow from the eye

Bottle height	IOP
150	110
140	102
130	95
120	87.6
110	80.3
100	73
90	65.7
80	58.4
70	51.1

The magnitude of IOP is only part of the concern. As aspiration is restored, the IOP will decrease in proportion to the outflow rate. During surgery, the needle tip is continually alternating between states of occlusion and nonocclusion. This can create dramatic fluctuations in IOP which theoretically could produce stress or traction on macular capillaries, choroidal vessels, vitreous and other intraocular structures. The clinical significance of this has not yet been determined.

Another alternative for increasing the infusion potential for sub-2 mm phaco was popularized by Dr Amar Agarwal. He used an aquarium type air pump to pressurize the infusion bottle.[8] Subsequently, an automated infusion option called DigiFlow™ has been introduced for the Stellaris.

The DigiFlow technology pressurizes the infusion bottle with a digitally controlled air pump. It allows the surgeon to set the "actual" bottle height and then a precise amount of additional air pressure can be selected to achieve the desired "effective" bottle height. For example, a surgeon could set an "actual" bottle height of 100 cm and create an "effective" bottle height of 140 cm by adding an infusion pressure of 29.2 mm Hg (one cm of water equals 0.73 mm Hg; therefore providing 40 cm x 0.73 = 29.2 mm Hg additional pressure to obtain the effective height of 140 cm). This has a practical value to surgeons who desire bottle heights greater than their operating room ceiling permits. A possible additional value may be suggested from the results of the DigiFlow field observation evaluation (FOE) conducted by the manufacturer.[9]

The FOE included 55 surgeons from the USA, India and Spain. Of these, 76% reported improved chamber stability with DigiFlow compared to gravity feed for the same equivalent bottle heights.

One explanation for this is that with gravity feed, as fluid drains from the infusion bottle, a partial vacuum is created within. This must be equilibrated by air entering the bottle from its vent. This equilibration may be faster with pressurized infusion and could explain the clinical impression of improved chamber stability noted in the DigiFlow FOE.

CHAMBER STABILITY

In designing the Stellaris for fluidics safety with 1.8 mm C-MICS, the decision was made to engineer each component of the system to work synergistically to optimize chamber stability. The C-MICS needle and sleeve were designed as a balanced pair using computational fluid dynamics, computer-aided design (CAD) and FEA (finite element analysis) computer modeling. Various sizes and configurations were analyzed for their effects on intraocular pressure stability. The Stellaris global evaluation, involving 45 surgeons from 13 countries, looked specifically at the chamber stability with the MICS phaco needle. Of 811 cases, chamber stability was rated good or excellent in 803 (99%).

The Stellaris Attune™ handpiece was designed with a 50% larger infusion channel to deliver more BSS per second at any given bottle height. Stellaris tubing was created with a large diameter, high compliance (soft) infusion line and a smaller diameter, and low compliance (stiff) aspiration line. This combination optimizes the ability to deliver BSS, stabilize the chamber and minimize post-occlusion surge for vacuum settings up to 300 mm Hg.

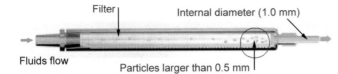

FIGURE 29.2: Stable Chamber tubing has a small internal diameter, low compliance tubing for aspiration which increases resistance to outflow and reduces the potential for chamber instability and postocclusion surge

For higher C-MICS, vacuum levels up to 600 mm Hg, Stable Chamber™ tubing was developed **(Figure 29.2)**. This incorporates a short section of flexible tubing connecting the hand piece to a filter, maintaining the natural flexibility and "feel" of "standard tubing". The tubing connecting the filter to the Stellaris console has low compliance (stiffer) and a smaller internal diameter which increases resistance to outflow and further reduces the potential for chamber instability and postocclusion surge. The filter captures nuclear fragments and prevents clogging of the smaller tubing.

The Stellaris pump technology was completely redesigned and now incorporates a Stable Chamber Fluidics Module™ which produces even more precise vacuum control than its predecessor, the Venturi pump. It is electric and therefore has the additional advantage of eliminating the need for external compressed gas.

The system uses two sensors to provide simultaneous feedback to the computer **(Figure 29.3).** One sensor directly monitors the speed of the pump while the other monitors vacuum at the aspiration cassette. The two sources of information are then processed by the computers PID (proportional-integral-differential) computer algorithms. PID algorithms are commonly used in jet aircraft control systems. In effect, the PID can compare the vacuum

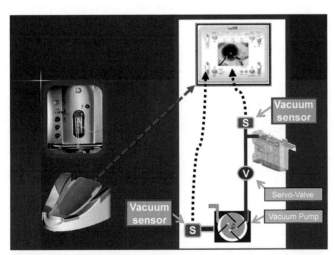

FIGURE 29.3: The Stellaris vacuum module system uses two sensors to provide simultaneous feedback to the system computer. One sensor directly monitors the speed of the vacuum pump while the other monitors vacuum at the aspiration cassette. The two sources of information are then processed by the computers PID (proportional-integral-differential) computer algorithms maintain reliable vacuum levels and minimize postocclusion surge

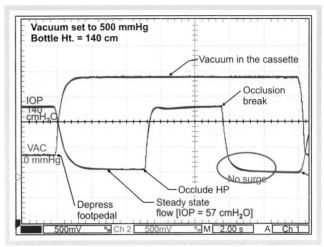

FIGURE 29.4: At occlusion break, IOP returns to baseline without postocclusion surge (red oval)

readings, updated every 5 milliseconds and analyze what has just occurred inside the cassette, what is happening now and in a sense anticipate what may happen next. It can then feed back to control the pump speed and also a servo valve that modulates vacuum and pressure to further reduce postocclusion surge **(Figure 29.4)**.

The effectiveness of this has been demonstrated by Dr Randy Olson who presented a study during the 2008 ASCRS meeting that showed the Stellaris, with a standard needle had 0.16 mm of posterior capsule deflection when measuring postocclusion surge in a cadaver eye.[10] This was less than one half the measured deflections for the Infiniti system (0.33 mm) at the same vacuum settings.

OPTIMIZING CUTTING EFFICIENCY

During phaco, as a surgeon steps down on the foot pedal to increase ultrasonic power, the actual effect is to increase the stroke or excursion of the needle. Stroke creates the major components of power; the acoustical wave, the mechanical impact of the tip (often referred to as the "jackhammer effect"), a fluid wave and cavitation.

The acoustical wave propagates away from the tip at a velocity of approximately 1500 meters per second at a frequency between 28.5 KHz and 40 KHz depending on the manufacturer. Its effect during phacoemulsification is poorly understood. It has, however, raised the question of why we can hear the handpiece during phaco if the frequency is "ultrasonic". The sound we hear is caused by spurious mechanical vibrations as well as some bubble dynamics. Cavitation may contribute to the sound but the handpiece remains audible even when tested in air with no cavitation.

The second component is the mechanical impact. As a phaco needle accelerates forward and strikes the nucleus, it can produce a cutting effect; sometimes referred to as the "jackhammer effect". This impact may also tend to "push" the nucleus away from the needle tip creating lens "chatter" unless it is balanced with adequate vacuum and flow.

The third component, the fluid wave, is also created by the forward acceleration of the needle. As it pushes fluid from its leading edges, it adds to the tendency to drive the nucleus away from the tip.

The fourth component of ultrasonic power is cavitation. As the phaco needle accelerates forward, it displaces fluid in front of it during what is called the "compression cycle". As the needle retreats, a low pressure area develops in front of the needle and cavitation bubbles begin to form during what is called the "expansion cycle". As the needle moves forward again, it compresses the newly formed cavitation bubble. Since diffusion of gas (or vapor) into or out of the bubble is related to the surface size, less gas can escape during compression and more gas can enter the bubble during expansion. Bubble growth during each expansion is, therefore, slightly larger than shrinkage during compression. A cavitation bubble therefore goes through a growth period of several cycles of expansion and contraction until it reaches a critical "resonant" size. Growing beyond this point, it can no longer absorb further energy and it implodes **(Figure 29.5)**. During implosion, the cavitation bubble creates an unusual environment as it releases its energy in the form of heat, pressure and "microjets" of fluid. The heat is in excess of 5500°C (9000°F), hotter than the surface of the sun. The pressure waves are in excess of 1000 atmospheres (equivalent to being at the bottom of the ocean) and the fluid microjets have been photographed emanating from the imploding bubble and impacting the nearest hard surface at velocities of approximately 400 kilometers per hour.[11]

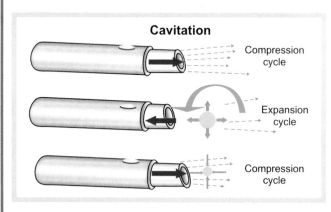

FIGURE 29.5: Cavitation in phacoemulsification is the formation of vapor bubbles when the pressure of the fluid in a small region of the anterior chamber falls below its vapor pressure. As the bubble is compressed, then expanded, it reaches a point where it can absorb no more energy and rapidly collapses, producing a high energy shock wave

This raises the question, "why doesn't cavitation damage the eye?" The heat, pressure and microjets from imploding cavitation bubbles occur in microscopic spaces in considerably less than a microsecond and have cooling rates above 10 billion°C per second. At any given time, therefore, the bulk of the liquid remains at the ambient temperature.[11]

Furthermore, with longitudinal (axial) phaco, studies have shown that cavitation is highly localized as a narrow beam of energy, less than 1 mm wide, directly in front of the tip. It should be noted that with torsional phaco, where the needle moves from side to side rather than forward and back, the cavitation bubbles are produced along the length of the needle shaft with little or no cavitation energy at the tip.[12] Possible effects of shaft cavitation in the incision should be considered if using torsional phaco without a sleeve for B-MICS.

Mark E Schafer, PhD, has used a hyperbaric chamber to study the relative cutting effects of the mechanical "jackhammer" energy and cavitation. He designed the experiment with a standard phaco handpiece and needle suspended by a solenoid above a fixed density resin block (approximately equivalent to a grade three nucleus). With the hyperbaric chamber at normal atmospheric pressure and active cavitation, 20% power could burrow 5 mm into the block in less than 5 seconds. With the hyperbaric chamber pressurized, cavitation was suppressed and at 20% power, there was no effective cutting. By increasing the power to 60% with cavitation still suppressed, he could achieve 5 mm of cutting in approximately 10 seconds but noted that it produced a "coring" effect and tended to clog the needle **(Figure 29.6)**.[13] These findings are consistent with the clinical recommendations of several Infiniti OZil™ (Alcon, Fort Worth, TX) surgeons who suggest blending torsional phaco with longitudinal to prevent clogging.[14,15]

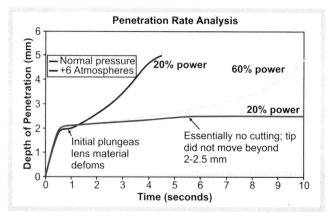

FIGURE 29.6: At normal pressure and 20% power, it takes 4–5 seconds for the tip to cut 5 mm into a resin block with a density similar to a 3+ cataract (blue line). When pressure is increased to the point where there is no cavitation (red line), there is virtually no cutting of the block. With power increased to 60%, the handpiece cut about 5 mm in about 10 seconds, at which point the needle was completely clogged with lens material

Based on this and other research, the current evidence suggests that the "jackhammer effect" initiates lens removal by cutting relatively large pieces of nucleus which are then emulsified by cavitational energy. The Stellaris Attune handpiece **(Figure 29.7)** was designed with a six crystal handpiece and a stroke length increased by 25% in order to optimize mechanical disintegration of the nucleus. It also optimizes cavitational emulsification by operating at a frequency of 28.5 KHz.

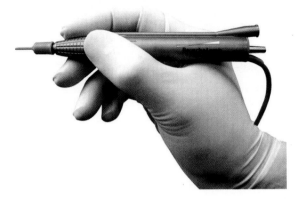

FIGURE 29.7: The Stellaris Attune handpiece has a 25% increased stroke length to improve mechanical cutting and operates at a frequency of 28.5 KHz to maximize the efficiency of cavitation in nuclear emulsification

The size and energy of cavitation bubbles are inversely proportional to the frequency creating them. At 28.5 KHz, the Attune handpiece produces cavitation bubbles of approximately 115 microns diameter as compared to 82 microns with a 40 KHz machine. This means that bubbles formed at 28.5 KHz produce 2.68 times greater energy than those occurring at 40 KHz to optimize cavitational disintegration of the nucleus.

CONTROLLING ULTRASOUND POWER

All major manufacturers have incorporated various "power modulation" options with different trade names into their equipment. The concept was pioneered by Anton Banko, the coinventor of phacoemulsification and founder of "Surgical Design Corporation". At the suggestion of Dr Jerre Freeman MD, he developed the first "Pulser Power™" (Surgical Design Corporation, Armonk, New York) which allowed surgeons to choose from 1 to 20 ultrasound (US) pulses per second as an alternative to continuous power. Each pulse had an equal "on" period (pulse duration) and "off" period (pulse interval) creating a 50% duty cycle. The concept was that the "off" period would allow for aspiration flow and lens material to approach the needle tip unopposed by the "jackhammer" mechanical effect or the fluid wave and improve followability. The "off" period would also provide a time for cooling. Since that original innovation, many refinements have been added allowing surgeon's choices in duty cycles; shorter "on" and "off" times ("micropulses") and a variety of foot pedal options to control them such as "burst", "multiburst", "fixed burst" and "pulse" mode.

Anton Banko's original predictions regarding followability have since been confirmed experimentally. Doctors Teruki Miyoshi MD and Hironori Yoshida MD published their work, "Ultra high-speed digital video images of vibrations of an ultrasonic tip and phacoemulsification"[16] which concluded that "using micropulse" (8 msec US "on" and 4 msec US "off"), "the study provided a visual demonstration of hyperfollowability. Hyperfollowability

means that once captured by an ultrasonic tip, nuclear fragments are emulsified and aspirated more efficiently (with micropulse) as if they were automatically rotating without drifting away from the tip".

An additional benefit of pulsing ultrasonic power was demonstrated by Mark E Schafer, PhD. He used acoustical methods to measure cavitation during continuous and pulsed power, and concluded: "more cavitation (cutting) energy is delivered with pulses than with continuous ultrasound at the same power (stroke)". This occurs because the "off" portion of the duty cycle allows more time for cavitation bubbles to form during their growth cycle.[12]

With this background, the Stellaris was designed with the "Attune Energy Management System" which allows "on" and "off" times as low as 2 milliseconds, pulse rates up to 250 pulses per second (PPS) and surgeon programmable duty cycles. It offers a variety of power modes including pulse, burst, multiburst, fixed burst and continuous power. It also offers a unique choice of traditional "square wave" pulses or "waveform" pulses **(Figure 29.8)**. These names derive from their appearance on oscilloscope tracings. With traditional square waves, the power spikes abruptly up to the selected power limit, plateaus for the selected "on" time and drops steeply back down to baseline.

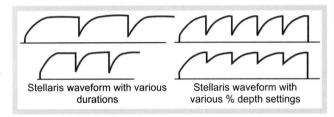

Stellaris waveform with various durations | Stellaris waveform with various % depth settings

FIGURE 29.8: The Stellaris advanced waveform allows the user to select variable waveform duration and depth. Such unique combination of duration and depth settings may produce better efficiency and followability

With "waveform" pulses, the power ramps up gradually over the course of the selected "on" time, reaches the selected power limit and then drops abruptly back down towards baseline, but not to zero power. The surgeon can select the percentage of the "drop" before power begins to ramp up again. Compared to square wave pulses, the potential advantages of "waveform" include less initial repulsive force as the power ramps up more slowly to improve followability and less total energy per pulse for identical power limits and duty cycles.

THERMAL EFFECTS AND CORNEAL WOUND BURN

The clinical significance of properly designed power modulation has become more evident with the increase in reports of corneal wound burn. In 2008, Dr Ismail Hamza presented his one year data at the ASCRS film festival including 400 cases performed with the OZil custom pulse mode.[17] He described a 3.5% incidence of wound burn out of 400 cases (14 cases of wound burn). Minimizing thermal effects during the phaco procedure becomes more important

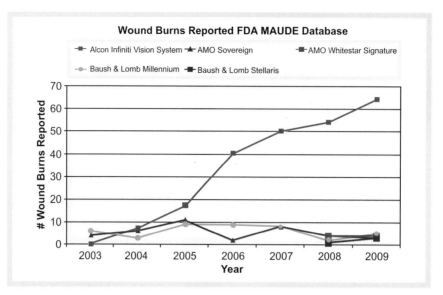

FIGURE 29.9: Total number of wound burns reported for the Infiniti, Millennium, Sovereign, Stellaris, and Signature phacoemulsification systems from 2003 through 2008. The Stellaris and Signature systems had a full year of data only for 2008

as the incision sizes decrease and incision leakage is minimized to optimize chamber stability.

The FDA "Manufacturer and User Facility Device Experience" (MAUDE) database includes surgeons' voluntary reports and machine manufacturer's reports of corneal wound burn in the United States.[18] A review of the database from 2003 to 2009 showed the number of corneal wound burns reported for the AMO Sovereign™ and Bausch + Lomb Millennium™ machines remained stable at less than 10 cases per year. Similarly low numbers were reported for the more recently introduced AMO Signature™ and B+L Stellaris (**Figure 29.9**). In contrast, the Alcon Infiniti reports of corneal wound burn have steadily increased from 2003 to 2009. One possible explanation for this could be the increased use of torsional phaco (OZil).

At the 2010 ASCRS meeting, Mikhail Boukhny, PhD presented a paper showing a "decrease in the percentage of corneal wound burns" since the introduction of OZil.[19] The potential flaw in their calculated percentage (# burns/ # procedures) derives from their use of FDA data for the number of reported burns and global pack sales for the total number of procedures. For this percentage to be accurate, all international cases of wound burn would need to be reported to the FDA with the same frequency as the US cases and all packs sold would have already been used in a procedure.

To investigate other possible explanations, experiments were conducted in 2008 and 2009 using an infrared camera to simultaneously measure the temperature of a phaco needle at its tip, shaft and hub while its aspiration port remained immersed in water with a constant flow rate of 30 ml/min (**Figure 29.10**).[20]

This study clearly demonstrated that with a straight needle operating in longitudinal motion, mechanical heat was generated in the hub well outside of the eye. The OZil needle, however, showed a substantial and rapid temperature rise in the needle shaft itself at approximately the position of the corneal incision. The authors hypothesized that torsional motion creates heat within the shaft because of internal metallic stress. This may lead to inaccurate assessments of energy available for thermal heating at the phaco incision site. The infiniti cumulative dispersive energy (CDE) calculation for energy appears to be based only upon the predicted frictional heat that would be created by the frequency of the torsional stroke. However, the heat from internal metallic stress rises rapidly with torsional amplitude is essentially at the wound location and adds to whatever frictional heat may exist.

The thermal profiles for the Stellaris, Infiniti OZil and AMO Sovereign have also been compared. The Stellaris had the lowest absolute temperature rise and was the most consistent in terms of cooling of the tip region.[21] These results appear to be consistent with recent clinical outcomes. In 2009, Dr Randall J Olson et al conducted a web based survey of ophthalmologists in the United States and Canada. His group worked through state and provincial societies and queried ophthalmologists three times regarding incidence of wound burn and type of machine used. He found the Stellaris had the lowest incidence followed by the signature with the Infiniti reporting the highest rate of burns (**Table 29.2**).[22] These studies suggest that current machine measures of energy during surgery are not only calculated differently by each manufacturer, but also are not considering all potential sources of heat, which may be misleading to the surgeon.

1.8 MM C-MICS FLUIDICS AND MACHINE SETTINGS

Another fluidics advance for the Stellaris is the wireless, bluetooth and dual linear foot pedal (**Figure 29.11**). It has

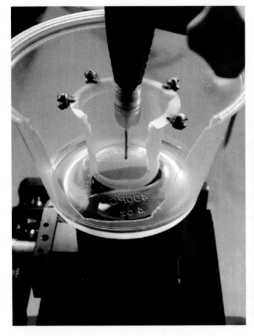

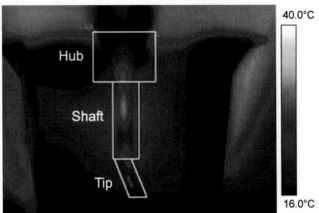

FIGURE 29.10: Phaco tip is immersed in fluid and irrigation is kept constant at 30 ml/min (right). An infrared camera simultaneously records thermal images at the tip, shaft, and hub of the phaco needle (left)

TABLE 29.2	Website based survey launched in Canada and the US in the summer of 2009 gathered information on wound burns including machine, power modulation, approach, OVD and incision size*		
Phaco Machine	**# Wound burns**	**# Surgeries**	**#Wound burns/ 1000 surgeries**
Infiniti	187	455,507	0.41
Signature	7	32,609	0.21
Stellaris	3	22,992	0.13

*From: Olson RJ, Chan C, Bradley M, Sorenson T. An analysis of wound burns in the United States and Canada. Poster presented at the ASCRS Symposium on Cataract, IOL and Refractive Surgery. Boston, MA; 2010.

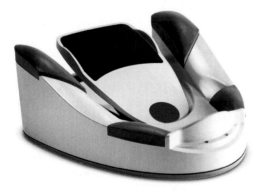

FIGURE 29.11: The dual linear foot pedal provides on-demand independent linear control of aspiration and phaco power that is customizable to each surgeon's technique and uses wireless connectivity for OR convenience

a variety of programmable options and can be used like a traditional phaco foot pedal in solely the up-down or pitch direction. In this case, the surgeon will program two or more, "low" and "high" phaco settings and manually switch between them on the panel. Most users, however, find a significant advantage in utilizing the dual linear function where power can be controlled in either the up and down "pitch" direction, or horizontally in the "yaw" direction. Vacuum can then be programmed to be controlled in the other direction.

Author's personal preference for both standard phaco and C-MICS is to control linear power in the pitch direction and vacuum in the horizontal or yaw direction. This dual linear movement actually creates "trilinear" control. For example, with C-MICS, using standard tubing, the author programmed linear vacuum between 50 and 300 mm Hg in the yaw direction. As he steps straight down in pitch to control linear power, he generated 50 mm Hg, the low end of his linear vacuum range. If he moves his foot pedal horizontally in yaw, he will linearly increase vacuum **(Figure 29.12)**. The farther he moves in yaw, the higher the vacuum will increase until he reaches the horizontal

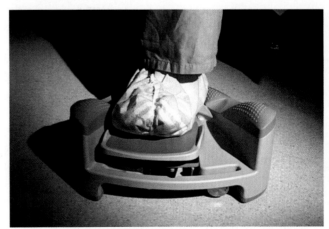

FIGURE 29.12: By programming linear vacuum in the yaw direction, vacuum/flow can be modified without changing power

limit of the footpedal and the upper limit of his selected vacuum range.

To understand "trilinear" control, we need to recognize that if the phaco needle tip is not occluded, stepping straight down on the foot pedal produces 50 mm Hg vacuum in the collection cassette. Inside the eye, however, the effect is to create approximately 20 cc/min of flow with the C-MICS needle (larger needles would create higher flow for the same vacuum level).

Moving the foot pedal horizontally in the yaw direction will linearly increase the vacuum in the cassette, but in the eye they were increasing the flow and followability. With the foot pedal at full excursion in yaw, they reached their maximum selected vacuum level (in this example 300 mm Hg). At that level, the flow inside the eye through the unoccluded C-MICS tip is approximately 45 cc/min. In other words, when the tip is not occluded, moving the foot pedal to the right increases the vacuum in the cassette, but inside the eye it is controlling the flow rate and providing linear "followability".

Once the tip is occluded with the nucleus, flow stops and vacuum migrates from the collection cassette to just inside the tip of the needle. Here, it now provides vacuum holding force for chopping and aspiration. Moving the foot pedal horizontally in the yaw position is now controlling the vacuum holding force between 50 and 300 mm Hg.

The difference between a standard foot pedal and a dual linear foot pedal can be compared to the difference between driving a car with cruise control and using the gas pedal. On a straight highway where conditions are stable, cruise control is convenient. On a winding mountain road, however, the driver will need to speed up or slow down to match the changing conditions.

In the eye, the dual linear foot pedal provides this "gas pedal-like" control of followability. One can use very low flow and followability when working close to iris or capsule, and precisely increase the followability as one starts to work more centrally in a safe position. This offers a level of safety and control not available with panel settings on a machine with a single function foot pedal. This trilinear function facilitates phacoemulsification with any case using any technique but is particularly valuable when dealing with small pupils, IFIS cases with floppy iris and cases with capsule tears or broken zonules.

For surgeons who prefer high vacuum techniques, 1.8 C-MICS can be safely performed up to 600 mm Hg with the Stable Chamber™ tubing. As previously described, Stable Chamber™ tubing incorporates a small internal diameter, low compliance tubing for aspiration. This increases resistance to outflow and reduces the potential for chamber instability and postocclusion surge. Increased resistance to outflow also means that for any given vacuum level there will be less flow and followability compared to standard tubing.

Each surgeon may have a different preference for followability rates, or how quickly or slowly material can be drawn to the phaco tip. My preference is 20 ml/min for sculpting or working close to capsule or iris and up to 45 cc/min to draw material to the tip when working centrally. With standard tubing the author achieved this flow range using a vacuum range of 50–300 mm Hg.

With Stable Chamber tubing, author can achieve that same flow range and followability by using a vacuum range of 200–600 mm Hg. With that setting, the "feel" for how slowly or quickly material is attracted to the tip is identical to the "feel" at the lower vacuum settings with standard tubing.

The advantage of using 600 mm Hg with Stable Chamber tubing only becomes apparent when the tip is occluded. At that time, flow stops and vacuum migrates to the tip, but instead of 300 mm Hg there is 600 mm Hg vacuum holding force to facilitate chopping or quadrant removal. Then, as the nucleus is aspirated, the eye is protected from high vacuum surge by the flow restriction of the Stable Chamber tubing.

1.8 MM C-MICS TECHNIQUE

In terms of technique, C-MICS is compatible with any chopping, divide and conquer, phaco flip or other variation a surgeon chooses. Early adopters often said the only "learning curve" involved was performing the "continuous curvilinear capsulorhexis" (CCC) through the smaller incision. Standard Utrata capsulorhexis forceps did not open widely enough and made this step difficult. There are now several designs available through STORZ Ophthalmics (St. Louis, MO) and other companies made specifically for C-MICS. There are also a variety of choices in diamond and disposable blades.

It should be stressed that proper incision size is important. The smaller infusion sleeves may be thinner and more easily crimped if the incision is too tight. Aside from crimping in the incision, they could also potentially crimp outside of the eye at the needle hub by "telescoping" as the surgeon advances the needle forward. This is not an issue with a true 1.8 mm incision but surgeons should not "experiment" with smaller incisions with this technology.

There are two final points regarding the sleeves. The sleeve is designed for the infusion to be directed laterally at approximately 30–40° through each of the infusion side ports. If the sleeve is positioned too far, back from the front "flair" of the needle, excess infusion will be directed forward reducing followability and pushing lens material away from the tip. The correct position is for the front edge of the sleeve to slightly overlap the wider front portion of the needle. Before entering the eye, the surgeon can verify this by engaging foot pedal position one (infusion) and observing that the majority of fluid is directed laterally.

The final point is that with the smaller incision and somewhat thinner sleeve, it is easier to insert using reverse flow through the needle. This can be programmed to be activated by moving the foot pedal to the left in yaw. The reverse flow immediately inflates and lubricates the corneal tunnel and pressurizes the anterior chamber before the sleeve is introduced.

In summary, the Stellaris was engineered to balance multiple technologies in order to optimize safety and efficiency for sub-2 mm C-MICS and B-MICS. This integrated design offers these same advantages for traditional 2.8 mm techniques and can readily be adapted to go below 1.8 mm for C-MICS, as lens technology and surgeon preferences evolve. At the time of this writing, the Stellaris is available either with anterior vitrectomy capability, or the newly released combined phaco and posterior segment Stellaris.

REFERENCES

1. McDonald JE. Comparison of postoperative flare/cells after microincision cataract surgery compared to small incision cataract surgery. Paper presented at the ASCRS Symposium on Cataract, IOL and Refractive Surgery. San Francisco, CA, USA; 2009 April 6.

2. Braga-Mele R. Is smaller truly better? An evaluation of phaco incision size and astigmatism. Paper presented at: AAO Annual Meeting. San Francisco; 2009.

3. Zafirakis P. Stellaris phaco platform versus Infinity torsional phaco mode. Paper presented at: ASCRS Annual Meeting. San Francisco; 2009.

4. Heng WJ. Surgically induced astigmatism in standard vs microincision coaxial phacoemulsification. Paper presented at the 11th Conference of the China Cataract Society in Xi'an, China; 2008.

5. Barrett GD. Minimizing astigmatism and improving wound security. Paper presented at: Asia-Pacific Academy of Ophthalmology; 2009.

6. Hunkeler JD. Comparison of BSS usage between Stellaris MICS and Infiniti Intrepid. Paper presented at: ASCRS Annual Meeting. Boston; 2010.

7. Mackool R. Point/Counterpoint: Can Bimanual phaco still deliver? CRST; 2002.

8. Agarwal A. Microincisional Cataract Surgery: The Art and Science. USA: Slack Inc; 2010.

9. Bausch + Lomb. Pressurized infusion field observation study #606; 2009.

10. Olson RJ. Comparison of fluidics of a new generation of phacoemulsification machines. Paper presented at the ASCRS Symposium on Cataract, IOL and Refractive Surgery, Chicago IL, USA; 2008, April 6.

11. Suslick KS. The chemical effects of ultrasound. Sci Am. 1989;260:80-6.

12. Schafer ME. In vitro and ex vivo measurements of cavitation from ultrasonic phacoemulsification systems. Paper presented at: ASCRS Annual Meeting: Washington DC; 2005, April 15-20.

13. Schafer ME. Quantifying the impact of cavitation in decreasing the use of ultrasonic energy during phacoemulsification. Paper presented at: ASCRS Annual Meeting. San Francisco, CA; 2006, March 17-22.

14. Lane SS. Paper presented at: ASCRS/Storm Eye Meeting; 2007.

15. Zacharias J. Ophthalmology Times; 2007, February 1.

16. Teruki Miyoshi, Hironori Yoshida. "Ultra-high-speed digital video images of vibrations of an ultrasonic tip and phacoemulsification". Journal of Cataract & Refractive Surgery. 2008;34(6):1024.

17. Hamza I. Wound burn in MICS with OZil Custom Pulse Mode. Video presented at: 2008 ASCRS Film Festival, Chicago, IL; 2008, April 4-9.

18. The FDA "Manufacturer and User Facility Device Experience" (MAUDE) database (http://www.acessdata.fda.gov/scripts/cdrh/cfdocs/cfMAUDE/Search.cfm.) accessed January 27, 2009 for 2003-2008. Updated 2/27/2010 to add 1/1/09 through 12/31/09.

19. Dimalanta RC, Boukhny M. Mechanism of temperature increase during longitudinal or torsional phacoemulsification. Boston: ASCRS; 2010.

20. Schafer ME, Devine TM. Analysis of thermal characteristics in alternative needle designs. Paper presented at: ASCRS Annual Meeting. San Francisco, CA; 2009.

21. Schafer ME. Thermal response of phacoemulsification tips in normal and occluded conditions. Paper presented at the Congress of the ESCRS. Barcelona, Spain; 2009, Sept. 15.

22. Olson RJ, Chan C, Bradley M, et al. An Analysis of Wound Burns in the United States and Canada. Poster presented at the ASCRS Symposium on Cataract, IOL and Refractive Surgery. Boston, MA; 2010.

CHAPTER 30

Microcoaxial Phacoemulsification

Vaishali Vasavada, Viraj A Vasavada, Abhay R Vasavada, Shetal M Raj

INTRODUCTION

Modern cataract surgery has undergone a series of remarkable technical refinements. Many of these advances have focused on technologies that involve a change in the type and size of the incision. Small incisions are associated with faster patient rehabilitation, improved prognosis for visual acuity and reduced surgically induced astigmatism.[1,2] These smaller incisions also increase wound stability, reduce ocular trauma and reduce the risk of iris prolapse. Currently, there are two popular small incision phacoemulsification techniques: bimanual phacoemulsification and coaxial MICS (microcoaxial phacoemulsification).

BIMANUAL MICROCOAXIAL PHACOEMULSIFICATION (MICS)

Bimanual MICS conventionally known as microincision cataract surgery (MICS) requires two incisions, each smaller than 1.5 mm, in order to perform emulsification. In this technique started by Amar Agarwal, the irrigation and aspiration are separated from each other,[3-5] and two paracentesis incisions ranging from 1.2 to 1.5 mm are made to accommodate the sleeveless phacoemulsificaiton tip and the irrigating chopper. This technique was introduced with the purpose of reducing the incision size; however, one of the major limitations of this technique is that the surgeon often has to enlarge the incision[5-7] or create a third incision[8,9] in order to implant an IOL of 6.0 mm optic. Alternatively, the surgeon would have to use an IOL that can be implanted without enlarging the incison.[10,11] The IOLs designed for implantation through the MICS incision are still evolving, and do not have a proven track record. The use of multifocal IOLs, aspherical IOLs and spherical IOLs with proven optic and edge designs and materials through microincisions in the bimanual technique still remains an issue.[5]

CONVENTIONAL COAXIAL PHACOEMULSIFICATION

Conventional coaxial phacoemulsification requires a 2.8–3.5 mm wide incision, so as to insert a phaco tip with a silicone sleeve through a single valvular incision for coaxial aspiration and irrigation.[12,13] This silicone sleeve acts to cool the tip, and it also seals and protects the incision from thermal injury when performing phacoemulsification.

MICROINCISIONAL COAXIAL PHACOEMULSIFICATION

A recent development in coaxial phacoemulsification facilitates IOL implantation through a 2.2 mm incision. This technique, which is referred to as microcoaxial phacoemulsification (MCP) or coaxial MICS requires an incision of 2.2 mm or less and accommodates a sleeved phaco tip. This allows aspiration and irrigation through the same incision coaxially and allows implantation of a full-sized IOL without enlarging the incision. This technique offers all the advantages of standard coaxial surgery with the added benefit of using a small incision. From a clinical perspective coaxial MICS technique involves minimal learning curve, it also provides favorable fluidics, a stable anterior chamber and excellent postoperative outcomes.[14,15]

THE MICROCOAXIAL INCISION

One of the most critical steps in contemporary cataract surgery is the creation of a clear corneal incision. Even with the adoption of small-incision cataract extraction techniques, wound integrity is a concern. There have been reports of increased incidence of endophthalmitis following inception of clear corneal incisions.[16] It has been suggested that poorly constructed and distorted wounds may increase the risk of postoperative endophthalmitis. Although smaller wounds would self-seal more easily, this is possible only if wound morphology and integrity are maintained. Small incision phacoemulsification techniques often use tight wound geometry, which may give rise to "oar locking" and lead to difficulties in intraocular manipulations. At times, such geometry adds stress to the incision, leading to wound distortion, corneal hydration and thermal injury.

It has been suggested that with phacoemulsification techniques employing clear corneal incisions, construction and integrity of the incision at the end of the surgery play a pivotal role in the reported increased rates of infection. It is therefore, crucial to have a square or near-square architecture of the incision and employ a surgical technique that minimizes incision distortion. Our previous randomized experimental study of rabbits eyes found that immediately after surgery, incisions used for sleeveless phacoemulsification had greater collagen damage on histomorphological and immunohistochemical analysis than the incisions used for sleeved tip phacoemulsification.[17] In another clinical study,[18] author found that ingress of trypan blue from the ocular surface into the anterior chamber was found to be less with microincision coaxial incisions, as compared to bimanual phacoemulsification.

With coaxial MICS, a single plane, temporal, clear corneal incision of 2.0–2.2 mm is created using a sharp trapezoidal keratome placed parallel to the dome of the cornea, making the internal entry in a single motion. It is of utmost importance to pay attention to the architecture and design of the incision. For a microcoaxial incision of 2.2 mm width, an internal entry of at least 1.5 mm is mandatory to ensure good self sealing nature of the wound **(Figure 30.1)**. More importantly, there should be minimal stress and distortion of the incision during intraocular manipulations.

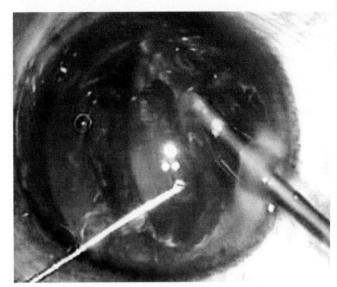

FIGURE 30.2: Microincisional coaxial phacoemulsification (*Courtesy:* Dr Agarwal's Eye Hospital, India)

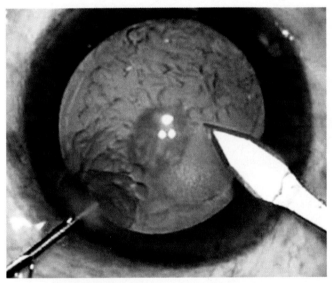

FIGURE 30.1: Single-plane clear corneal incision measuring 2.2 mm (*Courtesy:* Dr Agarwal's Eye Hospital, India)

SURGICAL TECHNIQUE AND INSTRUMENTATION

Surgery is performed using a conventional 0.9 mm phaco tip with specially modified smaller diameter sleeves, the "ultrasleeve" and the "nanosleeve". With coaxial MICS **(Figure 30.2)**, there is a reduction in fluid inflow into the eye by about 30%. This reduced inflow, in turn, restricts the limit to which the aspiration flow rate can be increased. The lower irrigation flow are compensated by thinner sleeve designs as well as innovations in ultrasound modulations, innovative phaco-tip designs, raising the bottle height and improved tubings/cassettes with superior fluid dynamics.

One of the merits of this technique is that surgeons can use their conventional instruments and techniques. It is not necessary to have expensive sideport capsulorhexis forceps or to use unfamiliar irrigating choppers. The technique of nucleus emulsification remains the same as in coaxial phacoemulsification. Our technique of choice is the step-by-step chop in situ and lateral separation technique,[19] as it allows division of nuclear fragments within the area of the capsulorhexis, with minimal stress to the zonules. Whatever the technique of nucleus division is, fragment removal should be confined to a posterior plane as far as possible **(Figures 30.3A and B)**, thereby minimizing damage to the corneal endothelium. Further, using lower fluidic parameters and progressively reducing them by adhering to the principles of slow motion technique[20] and step-down technique[21] allows the surgeon to perform fragment removal safely at the posterior plane **(Figure 30.4)**.

INTRAOCULAR LENS (IOL) IMPLANTATION

IOL implantation can be performed using a plunger type injection system and the appropriate cartridge with the wound assisted injection technique **(Figure 30.5)**. Even though the cartridge does not pass through the internal entry of the 2.0/2.2 mm incision, it suffices to place the cartridge at the outer edge of the incision and use the plunger to implant the lens into the eye. The key point is to provide counter force to the cartridge. Keeping a rigid ocular tension during implantation is another important point. Typically, there is an enlargement by about 1 mm following implantation of the IOL **(Figure 30.6)**. However, newer cartridges (e.g. D cartridge, Alcon) allow IOL implantation through these incisions **(Figure 30.7)**.

POWER MODULATIONS

With the advent of ultrasound power modulations, performing microcoaxial phacoemulsification (MCP) has become safer and more efficient. Several modulations of traditional ultrasound are now available, such as the pulse mode, burst

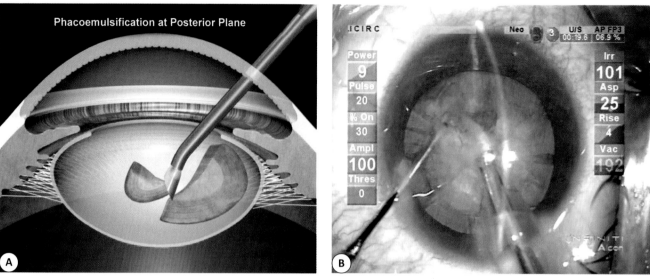

FIGURES 30.3A AND B: Schematic representation of nuclear fragment removal within the capsular bag (A). Fragment removal being performed at posterior plane, away from the corneal endothelium (B)

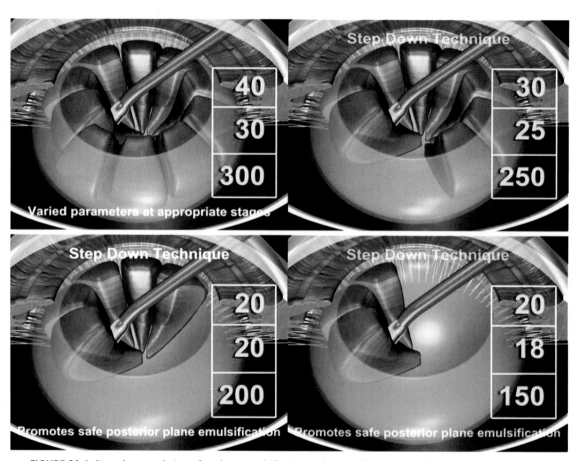

FIGURE 30.4: Step-down technique for phacoemulsification, wherein, the aspiration flow rate and vacuum are progressively reduced as more and more posterior capsule is exposed

mode, hyperpulse mode, Whitestaar® technology, ICE® technology and others. All these modulations allow interrupted use of ultrasound energy, thus minimizing heat induced damage to these small incisions, as well as making emulsification more efficient.

Newer ultrasound delivery modalities have come up, such as torsional ultrasound (Ozil™) and transverse ultrasound (Ellipse™), which allow ultrasound energy to be used much more efficiently. The torsional ultrasound (Ozil™) involves transverse oscillations of the phaco tip at a frequency of 32,000 Hz. This results in excellent followability with minimal repulsion of lens material, thereby allowing more efficient and faster emulsification. Combination of torsional ultrasound with MCP is extremely

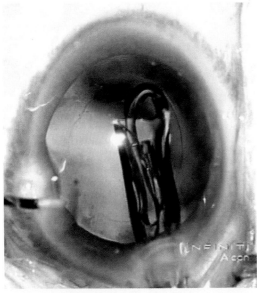

FIGURE 30.5: Wound assisted IOL implantation with the cartridge placed halfway in the corneal tunnel. Counterforce is provided by the second instrument

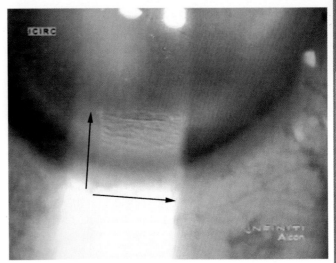

FIGURE 30.7: Micro-coaxial phaco incision

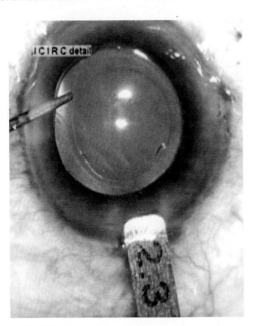

FIGURE 30.6: Incision enlargement by 0.1 mm following IOL implantation

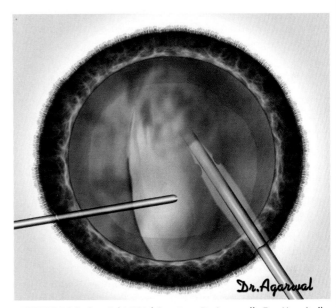

FIGURE 30.8: Coaxial MICS (*Courtesy:* Dr Agarwal's Eye Hospital)

beneficial, particularly in dense cataracts and other difficult scenarios.

COAXIAL MICS IN DIFFICULT SITUATIONS

Coaxial MICS (**Figure 30.8**) can be performed to emulsify cataracts in eyes with a compromised endothelium, small pupil and weak zonules, as well as those with posterior polar cataracts, subluxated cataracts and other difficult cataracts.

DENSE CATARACT AND COAXIAL MICS

Major concerns in dense cataract emulsification are corneal endothelial damage and woundsite thermal injury due to excessive dissipation of ultrasound energy, especially with smaller incisions. With coaxial MICS, there is some

reduction in irrigation and we need to have lower fluidic parameters to be more effective in order to perform posterior plane emulsification. Coaxial MICS in combination with torsional ultrasound is a boon for dense cataract emulsification; energy and aspiration work in harmony with OZil and microcoaxial because there is minimal to no repulsion of the lens substance; it stays at the tip. Using the Kelman tip with 45° bevel with torsional phaco through a 2.1 mm or 2.2 mm incision is the best combination to tackle dense cataracts. What is more striking, the incision at the end of phaco is undistorted, and there is no incisional hydration or stress seen. This will ensure clearer corneas on postoperative day one consistently.

MIOTIC PUPIL

A small pupil affects all steps of phacoemulsification, right from capsulorhexis to IOL insertion. Difficult maneuvering causes iris damage, sphincter tears, zonular dialysis, bleeding and so on. Poor exposure through a small pupil forces the surgeon to make a smaller rhexis, adding further to the difficulty and frequently leading to capsular dehiscence and nucleus drop the worst nightmare. The prolonged surgical time takes it toll thereafter. Corneal edema, uveitis, secondary glaucoma, cystoid macular edema, distorted pupil, the list is endless. All these lead to poor visual outcome, an unhappy patient and a frustrated surgeon.

PREOPERATIVE

A good surgeon should not wait unprepared to deal with the devil on the operating table.

A preoperative evaluation should include pupillary dynamics. Poor pupillary dilatation should be detected and noted down. Appropriate history is important for detecting any underlying etiology for the miotic pupil, may it be the use of miotics or long-standing diabetes. Any coexisting conditions like zonular weakness in pseudoexfoliation or synechiae in chronic uveitis should be detected preoperatively. The pupil should be dilated with a combination of cycloplegic, mydriatic and NSAID drops.

SPHINCTER SPARING TECHNIQUES

Pharmacological mydriasis alone may not be effective in cases with posterior synechiae, pupillary membrane or scarred pupils. Such pupils need intraoperative procedures. High molecular weight cohesive viscoelastics such as Healon-5 or Healon GV can be injected into the center of the pupil to mechanically dissect any synechiae and to stretch the sphincter. If this does not work, synechiolysis may be done with a blunt spatula passed through the side port incision. Viscomydriasis can then be repeated. Pupillary membranes can be stripped mechanically by the utrata forceps. Pure, preservative free adrenaline can be added to the irrigation bottle, after appropriate dilatation. Care should be taken in hypertensives and the irrigating solution should be immediately changed to an adrenaline free solution in case of a posterior capsular rupture.

SPHINCTER INVOLVING TECHNIQUES

Mini sphincterotomies less than 1 mm, and limited to the sphincter tissue can be made with either Vanass scissors or the vitreoretinal scissors. This gives adequate dilatation intraoperatively and maintains a functionally and esthetically normal pupil postoperatively. The disadvantage is that the incision is more difficult to create in the clock hour of the wound.

Dilatation can also be achieved by pupillary stretching using push-pull instruments. Under viscoelastic cover, two hooks are used in a slow, simultaneous and controlled fashion, to stretch the pupil in one or more axes. Bipronged, tripronged and quadripronged pupil stretchers are also very effective (**Figure 30.9**). The prongs should be maintained parallel to the iris plane and should not slip out into the pupil margin, especially on starting to depress the plunger to create the pupil stretch. The disadvantage of pupil stretch

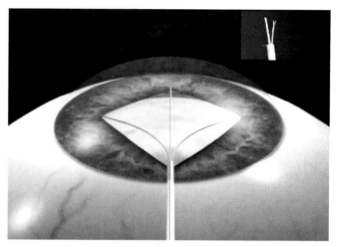

FIGURE 30.9: Tripronged pupil stretchers
(*Courtesy:* Dr Agarwal's Eye Hospital, India)

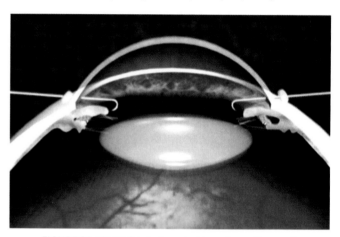

FIGURE 30.10: Iris hooks inserted to enlarge the pupil
(*Courtesy:* Dr Agarwal's Eye Hospital, India)

techniques is that the iris sometimes becomes flaccid and prolapses through the incision during surgery. Postoperatively, the pupil usually remains esthetically acceptable.

In very small pupils, commercially available iris hooks can be used to stretch the pupil (**Figure 30.10**). Gradual and optimal enlargement of the pupil to a size just adequate for the surgery should be attempted to avoid pupillary atony. The hooks should be placed parallel to the iris plane through small, short peripheral paracentesis. If not placed properly, they can pull the iris diaphragm forwards, resulting in chaffing and thermal damage during phacoemulsification of the nucleus.

The Malyugin ring made by microsurgical technology (MST, USA) is another great device to help surgery in small pupils (**Figures 30.11A to D**).

SUMMARY

In conclusion, this new era of microcoaxial surgery will enhance patient outcomes by minimizing surgically induced astigmatism, theoretically provide a potent barrier against postoperative infection, and encourage faster postoperative visual recovery.

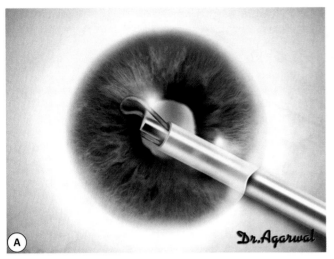
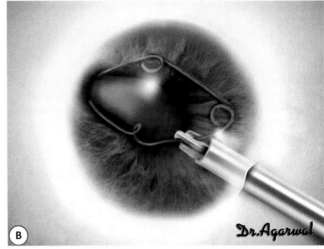
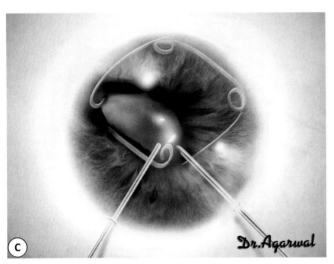
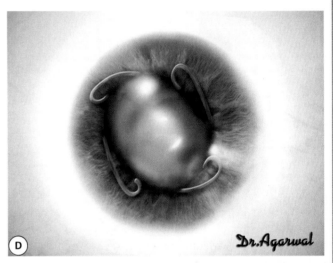

FIGURES 30.11A TO D: Steps of Malyugin ring for small puil phaco surgery (*Courtesy:* Dr Agarwal's Eye Hospital, India)

REFERENCES

1. Linebarger EJ, Hardten DR, Shah GK. Phacoemulsification and modern cataract surgery. Surv Ophthalmol. 1999;44(2):123-47.
2. Dick HB, Schwenn C, Krummenauer F, et al. Inflammation after sclerocorneal versus clear corneal tunnel phacoemulsification. Ophthalmology. 2000;107(2):241-7.
3. Alio JL, Rodriguez-Prats JL, Galal A, et al. Outcomes of micro-incision cataract surgery versus coaxial phacoemulsification. Ophthalmology 2005;112(11):1997-2003.
4. Alio JL, Rodriguez-Prats JL, Vianello A, et al. Visual outcome of microincision cataract surgery with implantation of an Acri.Smart lens. J Cataract Refract Surg. 2005;31(8):1549-56.
5. Dholakia SA, Vasavada AR. Intraoperative performance and longterm outcome of phacoemulsification in age-related cataract. Indian J Ophthalmol. 2004;52(4):311-7.
6. Dholakia SA, Vasavada AR, Singh R. Prospective evaluation of phacoemulsification in adults younger than 50 years. J Cataract Refract Surg. 2005;31(7):1327-33.
7. Tsuneoka H, Shiba T, Takahashi Y. Feasibility of ultrasound cataract surgery with a 1.4 mm incision. J Cataract Refract Surg. 2001;27:934-40.
8. Agarwal A, Agarwal A, Agarwal S, et al. Phakonit: phacoemulsification using a 1.4 mm incision: clinical results. J Cataract Refract Surg. 2001;27(6):1548-52.
9. Tsuneoka H, Shiba T, Takahashi Y. Ultrasonic phacoemulsification using a 1.4 mm incision: clinical results. J Cataract Refract Surg. 2002;28(1):81-6.
10. Donnenfeld ED, Olson RJ, Solomon R, et al. Efficacy and wound-temperature gradient of WhiteStar phacoemulsification through a 1.2 mm incision. J Cataract Refract Surg. 2003;29(6):1097-100.
11. Tsuneoka H, Hayama A, Takahama M. Ultrasmall-incision bimanual phacoemulsification and Acrysof SA30AL implantation through a 2.2 mm incision. J Cataract Refract Surg. 2003;29(6):1070-6.
12. Fine IH, Hoffman Rs, Packer M. Optimizing refractive lens exchange with bimanual microincision phacoemulsification. J Cataract Refract Surg. 2004;30(3):550-4.
13. Assaf A, El-Moatassem Kotb AM. Feasibility of bimanual micro-incision phacoemulsification in hard cataracts. Eye (Lond). 2007;21(6):807-11.
14. Vasavada V, Vasavada V, Raj SM, et al. Intraoperative performance and postoperative outcomes of microcoaxial phacoemulsification. Observational study. J Cataract Refract Surg. 2007;33(6):1019-24.
15. Osher RH. Microcoaxial phacoemulsification part 2: clinical study. J Cataract Refract Surg. 2007;33(3):408-12.
16. Taban M, Behrens A, Newcomb RL, et al. Acute endophthalmitis following cataract surgery: a systematic review of the literature. Arch Ophthalmol. 2005;123(5):613-20.

17. Johar SR, Vasavada AR, Praveen MR, et al. Histomorphological and immunofluorescence evaluation of bimanual and coaxial phacoemulsification in rabbits. J Cataract Refract Surg. 2008;34(4):670-6.

18. Praveen MR, Vasavada AR, Gajjar D, et al. Comparative quantification of ingress of trypan blue into the anterior chamber after microcoaxial, standard coaxial, and bimanual phacoemulsification: randomized clinical trial. J Cataract Refract Surg. 2008;34(6):1007-12.

19. Vasavada A, Singh R. Step-by-step chop in situ and separation of very dense cataracts. J Cataract Refract Surg. 1998:24(2): 156-9.

20. Osher RH. Slow motion phacoemulsification approach. J Cataract Refract Surg. 1993;19(5):667.

21. Vasavada AR, Raj S. Step-down technique. J Cataract Refract Surg. 2003;29(6):1077-9.

SECTION 5

PREMIUM IOLs

CHAPTER 31

Effect of the Shape Factor on the Quality of Images in Eyes Corrected with IOLs

I Pascual, A Beléndez, L Carretero, A Fimia, R Fuentes, C González, F Mateos, E Villegas

INTRODUCTION

In November, 1949 Dr Ridley implanted the first ever intraocular lens (IOL). As a result of the operation there was a refraction defect of –24 (+6) 30°. In order to analyze this result, we must consider the circumstances in which the surgical operation was carried out. Firstly, at that time the mechanical and optical properties of materials such as polymethyl methacrylate (PMMA) were not known as they are today. Secondly, the design of the lens was a copy of the crystalline lens, making implantation difficult, whereas modern lenses have a very different design. Thirdly, the surgical instruments that we have nowadays were not available then, e.g. at that time there were no surgical microscopes. In 1951, Dr Ridley presented the results of his operation at an ophthalmological congress in Oxford. The medical profession showed its disapproval and went as far as to say that such an operation should never have been performed. Nowadays, there are millions of people with implanted IOLs of different types, geometry, shape and size.

Enormous progress has been made in this field. Both the design of the lenses and surgical techniques have improved to such an extent that nowadays the operation takes only about 15 minutes and is carried out under local anesthetic with the patient sedated. This means that the patient is able to leave the hospital just a few hours after the operation, and the risks associated with a general anesthetic are avoided.

In this chapter, the latest advances made in the field of IOLs from a geometrical optics point of view are discussed, giving examples of how specific cases, mainly those involving high myopia, are being treated.[1]

Furthermore, we will analyze the image quality of pseudophakic eyes with IOLs in high myopia applying geometric optics [transverse spherical aberration (TA) and transverse chromatic aberration (TCA)], and wave optics [(polychromatic modulation transfer function (MTF)].[2,3]

GEOMETRY OF INTRAOCULAR LENSES

There are two basic aspects of an IOL. On the one hand, there is the optic zone, of which we need to consider the diameter, thickness, shape and radii of curvature. On the other hand, there are the haptics whose size, geometry and shape must be taken into account since they determine the zone where the lens will be implanted as well as the possible side effects of the lens being "off center" or inclined together with the possible effects of aberrations.

Figure 31.1 shows an example of an IOL that clearly demonstrates the way in which this type of lens has developed.

The design has become ever simpler, the lens lighter, and the haptics' configuration is such that they prove a minimum hindrance in the zone of union and to their insertion in the eye. This geometry prevents the lens from rotating, inclining or moving off center.

It should be emphasized that the geometry of the haptics is crucial when the lens is inserted, and contact with the cornea must be avoided at all times.

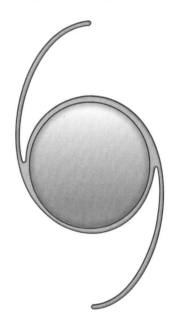

FIGURE 31.1: Intraocular lens (IOL) design

CLASSIFICATION OF INTRAOCULAR LENSES

Depending on the implant site, these lenses can be classified as: anterior chamber lenses, posterior chamber lenses and anterior chamber lenses for high myopia.

According to the optical way in which they work, they can be classified as: refractive monofocal lenses, refractive bifocal lenses, aspheric lenses and diffractive bifocal lenses. **Figure 31.2** shows the optical way in which a diffractive

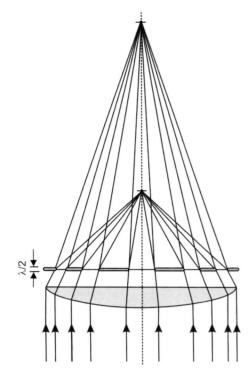

FIGURE 31.2: The way in which a diffractive bifocal intraocular lens (IOL) works

bifocal lens works. In theory, diffractive lenses show a large amount of chromatic aberration, however, this has not been demonstrated clinically.

FUNCTION

An important point to discuss is the need to implant IOLs as an alternative to other corrective systems. Corrective ophthalmic lenses have the disadvantages of variations in the size of the retinal image, restriction of the visual field and prismatic effects since they are usually very high power systems.

The use of contact lenses poses a problem when the eyes have undergone surgery, and there is a lack of tears. This is usually the case with elderly people who moreover have difficulty in putting the lenses every day.

In the case of intraocular lenses, no variations in the size of the image occur, and they also act as a barrier between the aqueous humor and the vitreous humor, thereby, maintaining the ocular structure. Nevertheless, we must not forget that a surgical operation is involved.

MATERIALS

The material to be used in an implant must be bio-compatible, have a high transmittance in the visible spectrum zone, and a refractive index that may be varied in order to control the geometry of the design.

Basically, PMMA is the material used, although in some cases (HEMA) is chosen for its high biocompatibility and the case with which it polymerizes.

POWER CALCULATION FORMULAS

Precision is very important in the power calculation of IOLs since normally, the objective is for the patient to have a specific postsurgical refraction, or even be emmetropic. The precision depends on three factors: (i) Biometric data (axial length, corneal power), (ii) Precision of the manufacturer's quality control of the IOLs' power, and (iii) The precision of the formulas used to calculate the required power. In a survey carried out in 1990,[5] 35% of the surgeons consulted stated that they believed the power calculation formula to be the most imprecise factor in the power calculation of IOLs.

There are two groups of calculation equations.[6] The first is made up of statistical type calculation equations based on the calculation of the linear regression of the numerical adjustment made. These empirical or regression formulas are a function of the axial length, corneal power and a specific constant for each type and brand of IOL. These equations are commonly used clinically due to the fact they are easy to use and are established on the majority of biometers. The most commonly used is the Sanders-Retzlaff-Kraff (SRK) which has been shown to be very accurate from a statistical point of view. However, in the case of high myopia, some calculation errors are seen using this equation.

The other group of equations correspond to the evaluation of the IOL implant power based on the principles of geometrical optics. These theoretical formulas are a function of the axial length, corneal power and desired depth of the anterior chamber. These equations do not produce errors, however, there are a great number of them, differing mainly in the approximations used in their development.

Possibly the most important parameter in IOL power calculation equations is the depth of the anterior chamber. There are innumerable models and statistical studies available to evaluate this parameter[7,8] and the one chosen depends on the individual surgeon and the surgical technique used.

Figure 31.3 shows just some of the different equations that exist together with a wide variety of terminologies used. It can therefore be said that these equations are personal and specific to the population studied in order to develop them. The most commonly used equation is the BK which gives excellent results. Nevertheless, most of these equations usually give rise to errors when the corneal power of axial length differs greatly from normal values. To be precise, high axial myopia needs to be given special treatment since many of the equations found in the literature give rise to significant errors. For example, the SRK-II[9] is a modified version of the SRK, and its parameters have been corrected so as to adapt it to the case of high myopia.

An alternative to optical-geometrical methods for power calculations is the use of the matrix method to obtain

Theoretical formulas

1. RD Binkhorst

$$D = \frac{1336\,(4r-a)}{(a-d)\,(4r-d)}$$

2. Colenbrander

$$F_L = \frac{N_1}{1-v-0.0005} - \frac{N_1}{\frac{N_1}{F_c} - v - 0.00005}$$

3. Eyodorov-Galin-Linsksz

$$D_p = \frac{n-aD_c}{(a-k)\left(1-\frac{k}{n}D_c\right)}$$

4. R. Binkhorst Extendida

$$D = \frac{1336(4R - \{4R - \{L+0.25 - 0.517\}\})}{\{(L+0.25 - 0.0517) - C\}\,(4R-C)}$$

5. Shammas

$$P = \frac{1336}{L-0.1-(L-23)-C-0.05} - \frac{1}{\frac{1.0125}{K} - \frac{C+0.05}{1336}}$$

Symbols used in the formulas:

	Keratometry Radius	Power	Thickness of the cornea plus depth of anterior chamber	axial length	power of the IOL
RD Binkhorst	r		d	a	D
Colenbrabder F_L		F_c	v	1	
F–G–L, D_p		D_c	k	a	

Regression formula

1. Formula SRK

$$D_p = A - 2.5\,A_1 - .9\,K$$

D_p = Implant power to obtain emmetropia
A = Constant
A_1 = Axial length in mm
K = Preoperative keratometry

FIGURE 31.3: Different equations used to calculate intraocular lens (IOL) power

accurate calculation equations for all types of eyes. In this way, we have obtained the following equation:[10]

$$P_7 = \frac{n_8(1-\delta_6 P_5)a - n_8 n_4 \delta_6 c - l'(aP_5 + n_4 c)}{l'(a - \delta_6 P_5 a - n_4 c \delta_6)} \quad (1)$$

where,

P_7 = power of the second surface of the IOL
n_8 = refractive index of vitreous humor
δ_6 = reduced thickness of the IOL
P_5 = power of first surface of the IOL
n_4 = refractive index of aqueous humor
l' = distance between the second surface of the IOL and the retina
a and c = coefficients related to the refraction and translation matrices used in the calculation.

Once P is calculated using Equation 1, we can find the IOL power P_L from the equation:

$$P_L = P_5 + P_7 - \delta_6 P_5 + P_7 \quad (2)$$

Moreover, the power of different types of lenses with different radii of curvature can be calculated, so that we can determine the shape factor of each lens in order to subsequently relate it to the quality of the image desired.

ABERRATIONS OF INTRAOCULAR LENSES

Just like any other type of lens, IOLs can have all kinds of chromatic and monochromatic aberrations. However, if the implanted IOL is correctly oriented with respect to the visual axis and has exactly the power necessary to focus near the fovea, the spherical aberration is the most important aberration to be considered and is the one that mostly affects the vision of the human eye.[11] For this reason, it is the aberration which has been studied most and the aim is to compensate for it at all times.

There are two possible IOL design principles—to minimize the spherical aberration of the whole eye[12] or to obtain the same spherical aberration as in phacic eye.[11]

With regard to the second criterion, Jalie[11] found that the IOL shape which most closely reproduces the average spherical aberration of the natural eye is planoconvex with the plane surface facing the cornea (convex plane, X = −1) for IOL powers ranging from + 15.94 to 17.98D.

However, Wang and Pomerantzeff[12] found that the shape factor which minimized spherical aberration of the whole eye was X = −0.52 (an unequal biconvex lens) for IOL powers—+19.4, +18.77, +19.17 and +19.61D.

On the other hand, Smith and Lu[13] found that for corneas with asphericities less negative than about −0.512, the spherical aberration of the eye as a whole is minimized with a planoconvex IOL with the curved surface facing the cornea (planoconvex, X = +1). Atchison's research[14] supports the use of a planoconvex IOL.

All these studies were carried out using general models of emmetropic theoretical eyes, except for the Atchison study[14] in which he also analyzed six ametropic eyes with refractive errors of approximately +10, +5, +2D (hypermetropia) and −2, −5, −10D (myopia). Nevertheless, in all cases the IOL power was positive. However, there do exist certain cases of highly myopic eyes in which when the image focal length of the cornea is less than the axial length of the eye, a negative IOL power is needed to achieve emmetropia.[1]

Some experimental studies[15,16] have been published on the optical quality modulation transfer function—(MTF) of the eyes implanted with IOLs by using a double-pass method. In these studies, the optical performance of different types of bifocal IOLs are compared with that of conventional monofocal IOLs. However, the optical performance of different types of monofocal IOLs are not compared.

Another recent study shows the use of MTF measurements to provide a standard test of minimum optical quality of positive intraocular lenses[17] using a water cell with plane entrance and exit windows. The results show that a meniscus-shaped lens gives an MTF that is significantly worse than the biconvex and planoconvex lenses.

Other studies show that in an emmetropic eye, diffraction and chromatic aberration are the factors that mostly affect image quality and therefore visual acuity.[18–22]

LN Thibos[20] designed a reduced model which predicts experimental values for chromatic aberration with a good degree of accuracy. However, this model is made up of only one refractive surface and cannot therefore be used to directly analyze the influence of any variation introduced in the eye on ocular chromatic aberration.

A real eye has aspheric surfaces, and the refractive indices of the ocular media depend on the wavelength. Furthermore, recent studies indicate that the human eye uses chromatic aberration to extract valuable directional information about "defocus" and to drive the accommodation response.[23]

For these reasons, it is of utmost importance to analyze diffraction and chromatic aberration together with spherical aberration in a theoretical pseudophakic eye model which more closely mimics a real eye.

In the pseudophakic eye, the total spherical aberration is the result of the contributions of the cornea and of the IOL. The amount of spherical aberration caused by the IOL depends mainly on the position of the object relative to the IOL and the shape of the lens.

We shall analyze the spherical aberrations of IOLs related to the shape of these lenses, taking into account at all times the eye which is nonaccommodated or focussed on infinity.

The schematic model of a pseudophakic eye used (Figure 31.4) is a centered system in which the cornea is represented by a single spherical diopter, the refraction index of the aqueous humor is the same as that of the vitreous humor (n) (schematic eye of Gullstrand-Emsley[24]), and the IOL is represented by a thin lens.

In order to study the spherical aberration of IOLs and the total spherical aberration of pseudophakic eyes, we have made use of Seidel's theory of aberrations, since this theory makes various premises, such as: the total aberrations of an optical system are the sum of the contributions of each surface, the aberrations of surfaces and of thin lenses can be expressed as simple equations, etc.

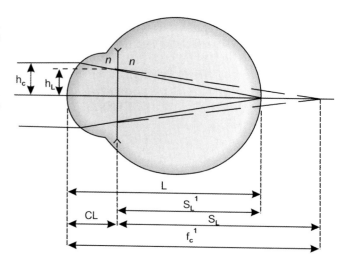

FIGURE 31.4: Schematic pseudophakic eye—corrected with an intraocular lens

Although nowadays, thanks to the facilities of modern computers, a finite pattern of rays can be widely used, a third order theory (Seidel's theory, or the primary aberration theory) can be of use in the preliminary design of any optical system without having to resort to a large number of data, since these simple third order theory equations give approximate values of the aberrations inherent in an optical system.

The use of Seidel's theory to study the spherical aberration of IOLs can be justified on the grounds that the majority of people who use IOLs have very small pupils and so the higher order aberrations are reduced to insignificant values.

SEIDEL'S THEORY: SPHERICAL ABERRATION

For a spherical diopter with radius of curvature r separating two mediums with refraction indexes n_1 and n_2, Seidel's spherical aberration or primary spherical aberration (S_{IS}) is given by the equation[25] where h is the height at which the light incides on the surface, and s′ is the distance to the Gaussian image.

$$S_{IS} = \frac{n_2(n_2 - n_1)h^4}{n_1^2} \left[\frac{1}{r} - \frac{1}{s^1} \right]^2 \left[\frac{n_2 - n_1}{r} + \frac{n_2}{s^2} \right] \tag{3}$$

Therefore, Seidel's spherical aberration of the cornea (S_{IC} can be calculated using the equation:

$$S_{IC} = \frac{h_c^4 P_c^3}{(n-1)^2 n^2} \tag{4}$$

The symbols used in this equation are defined in the Appendix.

Bearing in mind that we disregard the thickness of the IOL, Seidel's spherical aberration in this type of lens (S_{IL}) can be determined using the following equation for a thin lens.[25]

$$S_{IL} = \frac{h_L^4 P_L^3}{4n^2} \left[\frac{n_L^2}{(n_L - n)^2} + \frac{(n_L + 2n)n^2}{n_L(n_L - n)^2} X^2 + \frac{(3n_L + 2n)}{n_L} Y^2 + \frac{4n(n_L + n)}{n_L(n_L - n)} XY \right] \quad (5)$$

where,

$$Y = \frac{s_L' + s_L}{s_L' - s_L} \quad (6)$$

$$X = \frac{r_2 + r_1}{r_2 - r_1} \quad (7)$$

The symbols used in this equation are defined in the Appendix.

The power of the intraocular implant (P_L) can be calculated making use of Gauss' equation for a thin lens:

$$P_L = -\frac{n}{s_L} + \frac{n}{s_L'}$$

Since we have considered that the eye is focussed on infinity, the object distance (s_L) from the intraocular lens is (Fig. 59.4):

$$s_L = f_c' - CL \quad (8)$$

Our objective is for the eye to be emmetrope, therefore, the light beam will focus on the retina after having been refracted through the intraocular lens, so that **(Figure 31.4)**:

$$s_L' = L - CL \quad (9)$$

Therefore, the power P_L of the implant can be calculated by means of the equation:

$$P_L = \frac{(f_c' - L)n}{(f_c' - CL)(L - CL)} \quad (10)$$

If we take into consideration equations (8) and (9), equation (6) can be written as:

$$Y = \frac{L + f_c' - 2CL}{L - f_c'} \quad (11)$$

The symbols used in this equation are defined in the Appendix.

From equations (5), (10) and (11) we can see that Seidel's spherical aberration of an IOL depends on the position of the lens in the eye (CL), the corneal power (P_c), axial length of the eye (L) (all these data (CL, P_c and L) depend on the individual eye), and the shape factor.

From equation (5) we can see that, if the other variables (CL, P_c and L) are constant, S_{IL} is a function of the square of the shape factor and can therefore be simplified to:

$$S_{IL} = \frac{h_L^4 P_L^3}{4n^2} (AX^2 + BX + C) \quad (12)$$

where the parameter P_L is defined by equation 10 and,

$$A = \frac{(n_L + 2n)n^2}{n_L(n_L - n)^2} \quad (13)$$

$$B = \frac{4n(n_L + n)}{n_L(n_L - n)} Y \quad (14)$$

$$C = \frac{n_L^2}{(n_L - n)^2} + \frac{3n_L + 2n}{n_L} Y^2 \quad (15)$$

where the position factor Y is defined by equation (11).

Now we shall analyze the total Seidel's spherical aberration of the eye as a whole, which is the sum of Seidel's aberration of the cornea plus that of the IOL. Thus, if we add up the contributions of the cornea (S_{IC}) and of the IOL (S_{IL}) given by the equations (4) and (12), the total Seidel's spherical aberration for the eye as a whole is:

$$S_{IT} = h_c^4 [D + E(AX^2 + BX + C)] \quad (16)$$

where A,B and C are given by equations (13), (14) and (15), and:

$$D = \frac{n}{(n - 1)^2 f_c'^3} \quad (17)$$

$$E = \frac{P_L^3}{4n^2} \left(\frac{h_L}{h_C}\right)^4 \quad (18)$$

The relationship (h_L/h_c) depends on the individual parameters of the schematic eye and the position of the IOL in the eye **(Figure 31.4)**.

ANALYSIS OF SEIDEL'S SPHERICAL ABERRATION IN AN INTRAOCULAR LENS

Jalie[11] assumed that the spherical aberration of a pseudo-phakic eye should be the same as the spherical aberration of a phakic eye. In a phakic eye, most of the spherical aberration comes from the cornea and for this reason, it seems that the natural shape of the crystalline lens does not affect the value of the spherical aberration of the cornea. In other words, the crystalline lens itself is practically applanatic in the nonaccommodated state. The shape of an IOL should reproduce this situation.

If we consider equation (12), the value of X which is necessary to cancel out Seidel's spherical aberration in an intraocular lens (s_{IL}) is given by:

$$X = \frac{-B \pm \sqrt{B^2 - 4AC}}{2A} \quad (19)$$

The roots of this equation will be real numbers when:

$$\left(\frac{L + f_c' - 2CL}{L - f_c'}\right)^2 \geq \frac{n_L(n_L + 2n)}{n_L^2 - 2n_L n + n^2} \quad (20)$$

Therefore, Seidel's spherical aberration in an IOL (S_{IL}) will be cancelled out when the corneal power, axial length and position of the lens comply with equation (20), and the two shape factors that will cancel out S_{IL} are given by equation (19).

If Seidel's spherical aberration in an intraocular lens, S_{IL}, cannot be cancelled out because the corneal power, axial length and position of the lens do not comply with equation (20), it can at least be minimized (S_{ILmin}). Since equation (12) is square in terms of shape factor, S_{IL} as a function of X is a parabola with its vertex at (X_{Lmin}, S_{ILmin}). For a given position factor, the shape factor (X_{Lmin}) which minimizes Seidel's spherical aberration in an IOL is obtained taking derivatives of S_{IL} with respect to the shape factor X and equating to zero. In this way, we obtain:

$$X_{Lmin} = -2Y \frac{n_L^2 - n^2}{(n_L + 2n)n} \tag{21}$$

and the value of this minimum is:

$$S_{ILmin} = \frac{h_L^4 P_L^3}{4n^2} \left[\frac{n_L^2}{(n_L - n)^2} - \frac{n_L}{n_L + 2n} \right] Y^2 \tag{22}$$

ANALYSIS OF THE TOTAL SEIDEL'S SPHERICAL ABERRATION IN THE WHOLE EYE

In the previous section, we analyzed Seidel's spherical aberration in IOLs. In this way, the spherical aberration of a pseudophakic eye reproduces the spherical aberration of a phakic eye. However, instead of trying to reproduce the conditions of a phakic eye, we could try to improve them. Therefore, in this section we shall deduce what conditions are necessary to cancel out and minimize the total spherical aberration of the whole eye.

It can be seen that equation (16) is square in terms of the shape factor, and therefore, the value of X necessary to cancel out all of Seidel's spherical aberration is given by:

$$X = \frac{-B \pm \sqrt{B^2 - 4A\left(C + \dfrac{D}{E}\right)}}{2A} \tag{23}$$

The roots of this equation are real numbers if:

$$\left(\frac{L + f_c' - 2CL}{L - f_c'}\right)^2 \geq \frac{n_L + 2n}{n_L} + \left(\frac{n_L^2}{(n_L - n)^2} + \frac{D}{E}\right) \tag{24}$$

Therefore, the total Seidel's spherical aberration of the whole eye (S_{IT}) will be eliminated when the corneal power, axial length and position of the lens comply with equation (24), and the two shape factors which will cancel out S_{IT} are given by equation (23).

If the total Seidel's spherical aberration of the whole eye (S_{IT}) cannot be eliminated because the corneal power, axial length and position of the lens do not comply with equation (24), it can at least be minimized (S_{ITmin}). Since equation (16) is square in terms of shape factor, S_{IT} as a function of X is a parabola with its vertex at (X_{Tmin}, S_{ITmin}). The value

of the shape factor which minimizes the total Seidel's spherical aberration is obtained by taking derivatives of S_{IT} with respect to the shape factor X and equating to zero. Thus, we obtain:

$$X_{Tmin} = -2Y \frac{n_L^2 - n^2}{(n_L + 2n)n} \tag{25}$$

Therefore, the value of the shape factor which minimizes the total Seidel's spherical aberration is the same as that which minimizes the aberration of the IOL only.

If we substitute equation (25) in equation (16), we obtain the minimum value of the total Seidel's spherical aberration of the whole eye (S_{ITmin}):

$$S_{IT_m} = h_c^4 \left[D + E \left(\frac{n_L^2}{(n_L - n)^2} - \frac{n_L}{n_L + 2n} \right) Y^2 \right] \tag{26}$$

TRANSVERSE SPHERICAL ABERRATION (TA)

The eye is considered emmetropic for a wavelength of 555 nm (C,I,E maximum photopic luminous efficiency of mean observer). Using a computer program of rays tracing, we can calculate the retinal blur circle corresponding to this wavelength as function of the pupil diameter.[2,3]

CHROMATIC ABERRATION

The chromatic aberration on the retinal plane, or the transverse chromatic aberration (TCA), can be defined as the difference between the radii of the retinal blur circles corresponding to the limiting wavelengths, 430 and 680 nm[2,3]:

$$TCA = R_V - R_R$$

where R_V is the radius of the blur circle for lower wavelengths and R_R is the radius of the spot for higher wavelengths. The TCA will be positive if the green spot is greater than the red one and negative if the opposite occurs.

MODULATION TRANSFER FUNCTION (MTF)

The polychromatic MTF can be obtained using the point-spread function (PSF) taking into account spherical aberration and defocus coefficients.

The polychromatic PSF and MTF are computed by integration of their monochromatic counterparts through the visible spectrum (430–680 nm) sampled at 1 nm intervals. The monochromatic MTFs are weighted by the CIE photopic luminous efficiency function of the eye.

The monochromatic PSF is calculated taking into account the Stiles-Crawford effect.

$$PSF_\lambda = \frac{B}{\lambda^2} \left| \iint_\Sigma exp\left[i \frac{2\pi}{\lambda} w(\rho, \lambda) \right] \sqrt{A} \, J_0 \, (\alpha\rho) \, \rho \, d\rho \, d\theta \right|^2 \tag{27}$$

where,
B is a normalization term, and Σ is the exit pupil area
A is the Stiles-Crawford appodizing function

$0 < \rho < 1$ is the normalized radial coordinate in the exit pupil plane

θ is the angular coordinate in the exit pupil plane

α is given by the equation:

$$\alpha = \frac{\pi l d}{Z} \tag{28}$$

where l is the radial coordinate of the observation point, d is the distance between the planes of the exit pupil and the Gaussian image, and z the distance between the planes of the exit pupil and the plane where the PSF is calculated.

The rays entering the eye are not equally effective. In general, their efficiency decreases as they enter more eccentrically. For this reason, the Stiles-Crawford appodizing function, A, is assumed Gaussian[18]:

$$A = \exp(-0.05\, R_p^2\, \rho^2\, \ln 10) \tag{29}$$

where R_p is the exit pupil radius (in millimeters). $w(\rho,\lambda)$ is the aberration function for a rotationally symmetric system:

$$w(\rho, \lambda) = w_{20}(\lambda)\rho^2 + w_{40}(\lambda)\rho^4 + w_{60}(\lambda)\rho^6 \tag{30}$$

where w_{20} is the defocussing coefficient, w_{40} and w_{60} are the third and fifth spherical aberration coefficients respectively.

CALCULATION OF THE OPTIMUM BENGING FACTOR OF IOLS

The optical quality of the pseudophakic eyes can be calculated by means of the coefficient A^4.

$$A = \frac{1}{\lambda^o}\sqrt{2\int_0^1 w^2(\rho)\,\rho\,d\rho} \tag{31}$$

Where λ is the wavelength, $W(\rho)$ is the aberration function of a rotationally symmetric system:

$$W(\rho) = W_{20}\rho^2 + W_{40}\rho^4 + W_{60}\rho^6 + W_{80}\rho^8 + W_{100}\rho^{10} \tag{32}$$

where $0 < p < 1$ is the normalized radial coordinate in the exit pupil plane, W_{20} is the defocus coefficient, W_{40}, W_{60}, W_{80} and W_{100} are the third, fifth, seventh and ninth spherical aberration coefficients respectively.

The deformations [aberration function, $W(\rho)$] of an aberrated wavefront with respect to the reference sphere are related to the transverse spherical aberration in the observation plane[20] which in our study is placed at the Gaussian image point. Taking into account this relation, the coefficients W_{20}, W_{40}, W_{60}, W_{80} and W_{100} are calculated. W_{20} is negligible, due to the fact that the observation plane is the plane normal to the optical axis at the Gaussian image point (which is considered the retina), except for the IOLs with high spherical aberration because the spherical aberration of the pupil is important.

RESULTS

We applied this theoretical study to 12 theoretical cases of myopic pseudophakic eyes with different combinations of axial length (between 27 and 33 mm) and corneal power (between 42 and 48 D).

Table 31.1 shows the power of the IOL to be implanted so as to obtain emmetropia in these 12 cases. The IOL power range is between −9.80 D and +9.61 D.

TABLE 31.1	Calculation of the power of the intraocular lens to obtain emmetropia in 12 theoretical cases of pseudophakic eyes with different combinations of corneal power and axial length, using the schematic eye of Gullstrand-Emsley. All power in diopters

Pc/L	27	30	33
42	9.61	3.13	−2.02
44	7.05	0.57	4.48
46	4.46	0.02	7.17
48	1.83	4.64	9.80

Both the expression of Seidel's spherical aberration of an IOL (equation 12) and the expression of the total Seidel's spherical aberration (equation 16) depends on the height of incidence on the cornea (h_c). However, in this chapter we have not taken a specific height of incidence. Instead we have studied—S_{IL}/h_c^4 and S_{IT}/h_c^4 (S_{IL} and S_{IT} expressed in units of wavelength for a wavelength of 555 nm, and hc expressed in millimeters), From equations (19), (21), (23) and (25), we can see that the shape of the lens necessary to cancel out or minimize Seidel's spherical aberration does not depend on the height of incidence.

SEIDEL'S SPHERICAL ABERRATION IN AN IOL (S_{IL})

Figure 31.5 shows how S_{IL} varies as a function of the shape factor when $P_c = 46$ D and for all the axial lengths studied. For the other cases studied, the graphs show a similar parabolic shape.

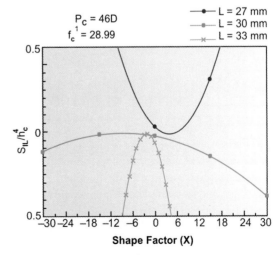

FIGURE 31.5: Variation of S_{IL}/h_c^4 as a function of the shape factor, when $P_c = 46$ D, and for all the axial lengths studied (27, 30, and 33 mm). S_{IL} is expressed in wavelength units when $\gamma = 555$ nm and h_c in millimeters

In general, it can be seen that when the IOL power increases in absolute value, the parabola is more closed indicating that Seidel's spherical aberration is more sensitive to variations in the shape factor. Therefore in the case of high IOL powers, the shape factor of the IOL should be carefully considered since it has a considerable effect on the spherical aberration.

In addition to analyzing Seidel's spherical aberration in the IOL as a function of the shape factor in these 12 cases of high myopia, we also studied the combinations of axial length and corneal power for which Seidel's spherical aberration in a thin IOL can be eliminated (equation 20). **Figure 31.6** represents the limits within which the axial length must fall, in cases of different corneal power, in order to eliminate Seidel's spherical aberration in an IOL. We have determined that in 8 of the 12 cases studied, it is possible to eliminate S_{IL} by choosing the appropriate shape factors (equation 19). The two shape factors are meniscuses with the convexity towards the cornea.

In the other 4 cases ($P_c = 42$ D and L= 27 mm, $P_c = 44$ D and L= 27 mm, $P_c = 46$ D and L= 33 mm and $P_c = 48$ D and L= 33 mm), S_{IL} could only be minimized and not eliminated.

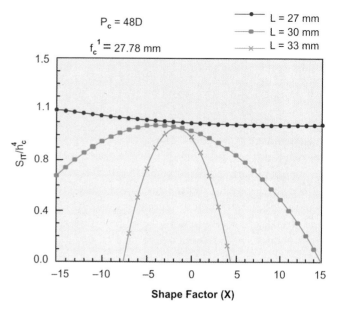

FIGURE 31.7: Variation of S_{IT}/h_c^4 as a function of the shape factor, when $P_c = 48$ D, and for all the axial lengths studied (27, 30, and 33 mm). S_{IT} is expressed in wavelength units when $\gamma = 555$ nm and h_c in millimeters

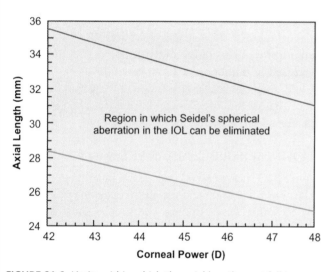

FIGURE 31.6: Limits within which the axial length must fall in cases of different corneal power in order to eliminate Seidel's spherical aberration in the IOL

TOTAL SEIDEL'S SPHERICAL ABERRATION OF THE WHOLE EYE (S_{IT})

Figure 31.7 shows how S_{IT} varies as a function of the shape factor when $P_c = 48$ D and for all the axial lengths studied. For the rest of the cases studied, the graphs present a parabolic shape and resemble that which would be obtained for S_{IL} as a function of the shape factor, since considering the contribution of the cornea modifies the position of the curves but does not affect their shape.

We have already reached the conclusion that S_{IT} can be eliminated when equation (24) is complied with, i.e. when the aberration of the IOL and that of the cornea have the same value but are of opposite signs. Of the 12 cases studied,

only in the 6 cases which required a negative power to obtain emmetropia can S_{IT} be eliminated by choosing the appropriate shape factors (equation 23). Of the two lenses which correspond to each case, one solution is a meniscus with a convex surface towards the retina, and the other is a meniscus convex towards the cornea. The meniscus which is convex towards the retina is called an inverted IOL lens,[26] and has several physiological advantages compared with the IOLs normally used—convex-plane, biconvex and plane-convex. For example, the risk of postoperative detachment of the retina is reduced, and the distance between the IOL and the iris is increased which means that the possibility of forming synechia is reduced. Consequently, these lenses are the ideal solution since they not only eliminate the spherical aberration, thereby, improving the image quality and also have physiological advantages.

For the 6 cases of corneal power and axial length that require a positive emmetropization power, it is not possible to eliminate S_{IT} completely, but it can be minimized. For each of these 6 cases, the two solutions which minimize S_{IT} are meniscuses which are convex towards the cornea. This means that from a physiological point of view these lenses are not ideal. In these 6 cases, we studied the S_{IT} which the most commonly used shapes present (convex-plane, biconvex, and plane-convex), and found that the flat-convex lens presents an aberration which is only slightly greater than the minimum value. This shape has always been considered to be the one that minimizes the spherical aberration. Possible meniscus lenses which are convex towards the retina were also studied. These lenses present a total Seidel's spherical aberration which is approximately twice that of the convex-plane lens aberration. However, the physiological advantages of these meniscus lenses should also be taken into account.

TRANSVERSE SPHERICAL ABERRATION, CHROMATIC ABERRATION AND MTF

The Seidel's spherical aberration, the transverse spherical aberration (TA), the transverse chromatic aberration (TCA), the modulation transfer function (MTF), and the coefficient A are very useful when applied to the design of IOLs. We use these parameters and functions to study the design of IOLs in myopic pseudophakic eyes with different combinations of axial length (between 27 and 33 mm) and corneal power (between 42 and 48 D).

Calculations of Seidel's spherical aberration were done employing a schematic model of a pseudophakic eye that (**Figure 31.4**) is a centered system in which the cornea is represented by a single spherical diopter, the refraction index of the aqueous humor is the same as that of the vitreous humor {(n) (schematic eye of Gullstrand-Emsley)},[24] and the IOL is represented by a thin lens.

The transverse spherical aberration, the chromatic aberration, the modulation transfer function and the coefficient A of the myopic pseudophakic eyes were studied using a modified version of the phakic theoretical eye used by Navarro et al,[27] replacing the crystalline lens by an IOL that corrects the highly myopic eye in the paraxial zone for a wavelength of 555 nm (CIE maximum photopic luminous efficiency of the mean observer).

We have studied 4 theoretical cases of pseudophakic eyes (IOL power = +10.8 D (Case A), +4.2 D (Case B), –3.2 D (Case C) and –8.4 D (Case D).

Figure 31.8 shows the transverse spherical aberration for the pseudophakic eyes studied at a 555 nm wavelength for 3, 5 and 8 mm pupil diameters. In cases of A, B and C, there is negative transverse spherical aberration (the image point moves nearer to the cornea as the radius of the pupil increases). In case D, the meniscus lens produces a positive transverse spherical aberration (the image point moves further from the cornea as the radius of the pupil increases), contrary to a planoconcave IOL. The TCA was calculated for the same cases than TA.

Taking into account spherical aberration, **Figure 31.9** shows the TCA for extreme wavelengths 430 and 680 nm. In the cases of A, B and C, the TCA difference between the meniscus IOL and the planoconvex or concave IOL is very small. For case D, the behavior for a negative planoconcave IOL (DC) is similar to cases A, B and C, but for a meniscus-shaped IOL (Dm), the evolution of the TCA as a function of pupil diameter is just the opposite due to the fact that the spherical aberration that is produced is positive.

Figures 31.10 and 31.11 show the polychromatic MTF for a positive IOL (case A) and for negative IOL (case D) respectively, for a pupilar diameter of 5 mm.

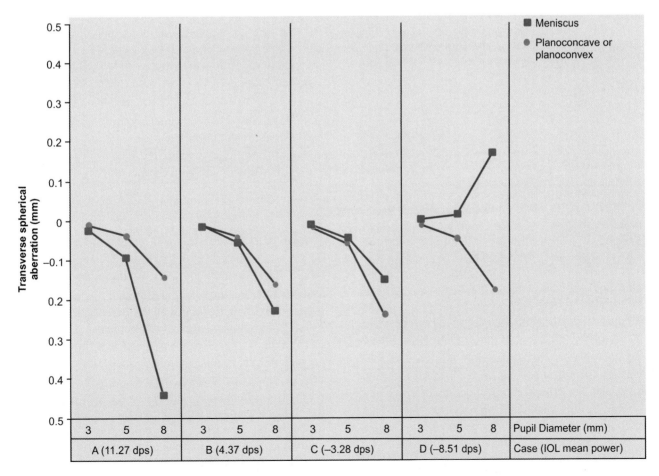

FIGURE 31.8: Transverse spherical aberration for each case of theoretical pseudophakic eyes with 3, 5 and 8 pupil diameters

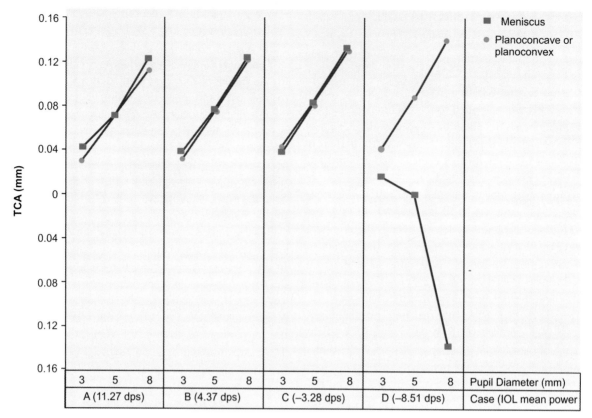

FIGURE 31.9: Chromatic difference of the blur circles (TCA) for each case of theoretical pseudophakic eyes with 3, 5 and 8 pupil diameters

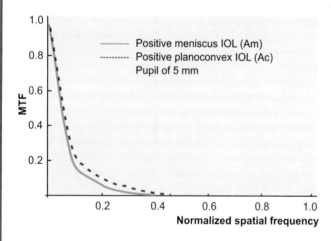

FIGURE 31.10: Polychromatic MTF for the pseudophakic eye A. Pupil diameter: 5 mm

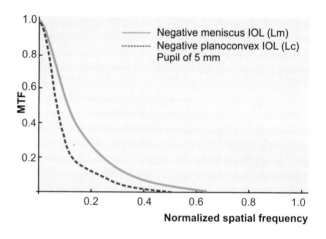

FIGURE 31.11: Polychromatic MTF for the pseudophakic eye D. Pupil diameter: 5 mm

DISCUSSION

The Seidel's aberration theory has proved to be very useful when applied to the design of IOLs. Studies have been done using this theory to determine how the shape of the lens affects the quality of the image.[12-14,26,28] All these studies were carried out using theoretical emmetropic eye models. However, in this chapter, theoretical myopic eyes were studied and for this reason, the results obtained regarding the most appropriate shape factors are different.

Considering all the findings, we can say that if we take into account the type of eye we wish to correct with an IOL, together with its dimensions and corneal power, we can find a lens whose shape factor is such that the spherical aberration of the lens is minimized or even eliminated. Therefore, we can conclude that if the lens used has the appropriate geometrical shape, it is possible to correct the eye by means of this IOL which, moreover, presents no spherical aberration. An analysis of the shape factors which appear indicates that the type of lens to be used in the case of high myopia should be shaped like a meniscus. It was also found that in certain cases and taking into consideration the position of the meniscus, not only the desired refractive effects but also extremely important physiological advantages were obtained.

Although it may be true that the theoretical variation of the spherical aberration is not very great when the shape factor is modified, when we analyze clinical cases of patients implanted with IOLs shaped like a meniscus, excellent results regarding the postsurgical visual sharpness were obtained. This was greater than expected in between 80 to 90% of the patients.[29]

For pseudophakic eyes with low myopia (IOL high positive power, case A), the planoconvex IOL is better than the meniscus IOL due to the fact that the planoconvex IOL gives less spherical aberration and TCA, and better polychromatic MTF for all the pupilar diameters.

For pseudophakic eyes with a medium myopia (IOL low power, cases B and C), the quality image given by TA, TCA and polychromatic MTF for meniscus and planoconvex concave IOLs is very similar. In these cases, it was better to implant a meniscus IOL due to the several physiological advantages it offers.

For pseudophakic eyes with very high myopia (IOL high negative power, case D), optically, the best IOL is the meniscus taking into account TA, TCA and polychromatic MTF. Furthermore, physiologically, it reduces the danger of postoperative retinal detachment which increases as myopia increases. These results agree with the results obtained using total Seidel's spherical aberration.

Taking into account A coefficient, in the case of a pseudophakic eye that is corrected with a positive IOL power, the planoconvex IOL ($X = +1$) gives the best optical quality. However, in the case of a pseudophakic eye, i.e. corrected with a negative IOL power, a meniscus with a specific bending factor gives the minimum A value and therefore the best image quality.

Considering all studies [Seidel's spherical aberration, transverse spherical aberration (TA), transverse chromatic aberration (TCA), polychromatic modulation transfer function (MTF); and A coefficient] in pseudophakic eyes, for positive IOLs lenses, the planoconvex IOL is the most adequate. This is in agreement with previous studies done by Smith and Lu[13] and Atchison.[14] However, for negative powers a meniscus IOL is the best, clinical study agrees with these results.[29]

Consequently, it is obvious that it is necessary to take the shape factor into account when calculating the power of IOLs, since it is then possible to choose the lens which, in addition to producing a minimum or no aberration, improves the quality of the final image.

APPENDIX

SIGN CONVENTIONS

1. The object is situated at the left of the optical system so that initially the light travels from left to right.
2. The radius of curvature r of a surface is positive if the center of curvature is to the right of its vertex.
3. The distance s of the object from (the vertex of) the surface is negative if the object is to the left of the surface.
4. The distance s' of an image from (the vertex of) a surface is positive if the image is to the right of the surface.
5. The height h of an object or h' of an image from the optical axis is positive if it is above the axis.

DEFINITION OF SYMBOLS

S_{IS}	Seidel spherical aberration of a spherical refracting surface
S_{IC}	Seidel spherical aberration of the cornea
S_{IL}	Seidel spherical aberration of an IOL
S_{ILmin}	Minimum Seidel spherical aberration of an IOL
S_{IT}	Total Seidel spherical aberration of the whole eye
S_{ITmin}	Minimum total Seidel aberration of the whole eye
h_c	Height above the optical axis at which the light incides on the cornea
p_c	Corneal power
f_c	Focal image distance from the cornea
n	Refraction index of aqueous humor and vitreous humor (taken here as 1.333333)
h_L	Height above the optical axis at which the light incides on the IOL
n_L	Refraction index of the IOL (taken here as 1.49)
P_L	IOL power
Y	Position factor of the IOL
X	Shape factor of the IOL
X_{Lmin}	Shape factor which minimizes Seidel's spherical aberration of an IOL
X_{Tmin}	Shape factor which minimizes the total Seidel's spherical aberration of the whole eye
$s_L, s_{L'}$	Gaussian distances of object and image from the IOL
r_1, r_2	Radii of curvature of the first and second surfaces of the IOL
CL	Position of the lens, distance from the cornea to the IOL (taken here as 3.6 mm)
L	Axial length of the eye.

REFERENCES

1. Gonzalez C, Pascual I, Bacete A, et al. Elimination and minimization of the spherical aberration of intraocular lenses in high myopia. Ophthal Physiol Opt. 1996;16: 19.
2. Villegas ER, Carretero L, Fimia A. Influence of chromatic aberration on image quality in pseudophakic eyes with high myopia: SPIE's BiOS 96. Ophthalmic Technologies. 1996; 2673: 125-34.
3. Villegas ER, Carretero L, Fimia A. Quality image in myopic pseudophakic eyes comparing two types of intraocular lenses. Biomedical Optics (In press).
4. Villegas ER, Carretero L, Fimia A. Optimum bending factor of intraocular lenses in pseudophakic eyes with high myopia. J Modern Optics. 1997;44: 941-52.
5. Leaming DV. Practice styles and preferences of ASCRS members-1989 survey. J Cataract Refract Surg. 1990;16: 624-32.

6. Retzlaff JA, Sanders DR, Kraff M. Lens Implant Power Calculation (3rd ed) Slack: New Jersey, 1990.

7. Holladay JT, Prager TC, Chandler TY, et al. A three-part system for refining intraocular lens power calculations. J Cataract Refract Surg. 1988;14: 17-24.

8. Retzlaff JA, Sanders DR, Kraff M. Development of the SRK/T intraocular lens implant power calculation formula. J Cataract Refract Surg. 1990;16: 333-40.

9. Sanders DR, Retzlaff JA, Kraff M. Comparison of the SRK II formula and other second generation formulas. J Cataract Refract Surg. 1988;14: 136-41.

10. Fimia A, Alio J, Pascual I, et al. New theoretical matrix formula for intraocular lens calculation using the optimal bending factor. J Cataract Refract Surg. 1993;19: 293-7.

11. Jalie M. The design of intraocular lenses. Br J Physiol Opt. 1978; 32: 1-21.

12. Wang GJ, Pomerantzeff O. Obtaining a high-quality retinal image with a biconvex intraocular lens. Am J Ophthal. 1982;94: 87-90.

13. Lu C, Smith G: The spherical aberration of intraocular lenses. Ophthal Physiol Opt. 1988;8: 287-94.

14. Atchison DA. Optical design of intraocular lenses: I. On-axis performance. Optom Vis Sci. 1989;66: 492-506.

15. Navarro R, Ferro M, Artal P, et al. Modulation transfer functions of eyes implanted with intraocular lenses. Appl Opt. 1993;32: 6359-67.

16. Artal P, Marcos S, Navarro R, et al. Through focus image quality of eyes implanted with monofocal and multifocal intraocular lenses. Opt Eng. 1995;34: 772-9.

17. Grossman LW, Faaland RW. Minimum resolution specification of intraocular lens implants using the modulation transfer function. Appl Opt. 1993;32: 3497-3503.

18. van Meeteren A. Calculations on the optical modulation transfer function of the human eye for white light. Opt Acta. 1974;21: 395-412.

19. Thibos LN, Bradley A, Zhang X. Effect of ocular chromatic aberration on monocular visual performance. Optom Vis Sci. 1991;68: 599-607.

20. Thibos LN, Ming Ye, Zhang X, et al. The chromatic eye—a new reduced-eye model of ocular chromatic aberration in humans. Appl Opt. 1992;31: 3594-3600.

21. Thibos LN, Bradley A, Still DL. Interferometric measurement of visual acuity and the effect of ocular chromatic aberration. Appl Opt. 1991;30: 2079-87.

22. Thibos LN. Calculation of the influence of lateral chromatic aberration on image quality across the visual field. J Opt Soc Am. 1987;A4:1673-80.

23. Kruger PB, et al. Chromatic aberration and ocular focus—Fincham revisited. Vision Research 1993;33: 1379-1411.

24. Bennett AG, Rabbetts RB. Clinical Visual Optics London: Butterworths, 1989.

25. Welford WT. Aberrations of Optical Systems Boston: Adam Hilger, 1986.

26. Lu C, Smith G. Optical Performance of the super-reversed intraocular lens. J Cataract Refract Surg. 1992;18: 293-300.

27. Navarro R, Santamaria J, Besco's J. Accommodation dependent model of the human eye with aspherics. J Opt Soc Am. 1985;A2: 1273-81.

28. Atchison DA. Optical design of intraocular lenses: II—off-axis performance. Optom Vis Sci. 1989;66: 579-90.

29. Bacete MA. Correccion de la ametropia post-afaquia en la miopia magna mediante lente intraocular con nuevas formas geométricas. Tesis doctoral. Universidad de Alicante, 1994.

CHAPTER 32

Materials for Intraocular Lenses

JM Legeais

POLYMETHYLMETHACRYLATE AND INTRAOCULAR LENSES

Polymethylmethacrylate (PMMA) is a polyacrylic derivative marketed under the brand names Plexiglas, Perspex, Diakon, Lucite, etc. The optical and organoleptic properties of PMMA have established it as the standard material for the manufacture of intraocular lenses (IOLs) **(Figure 32.1)**. It is amorphous, transparent and colorless. It has a refractive index of 1.49 to 1.50 and transmits 92% of the incident light. Chromophores can be incorporated into it and it is easily tinted. PMMA is rigid at room temperature. It has a vitreous transition temperature (i.e. the temperature at which it becomes flexible) of 105°C. It has a specific density of 1.19 gm/cm^3. PMMA is fairly water-repellent, has an angle of contact of 70° and a water absorption index of 0.25%.

It is insoluble in water and aliphatic hydrocarbons and stands up well to exposure to oils, fats, alkaline solutions and dilute acids. The manufacturing process for the optical part of the PMMA IOLs involves turning or molding. Leaves of PMMA are used in the manufacturing method that requires turning. The lenses are cut by rotating the slab of PMMA or by rotating the cutting tool. The thickness of the lens depends on the intended optical power and the edges are then polished until a satisfactory surface finish is obtained. Molding can be carried out by injection or by compression. In the injection method, the PMMA is heated to a temperature of 160 to 200°C until it melts and it is then injected into a mold with a compression pressure of about 140 kg/cm^2. The edges of the lens are polished after the mold has been opened. In the compression molding method, a steel mold is filled with PMMA and subjected to a pressure of 500 kg. It is then heated to a temperature of 20°C and the pressure raised to 2600 kg. The pressure is then brought back to normal and the mold is cooled by ventilation. Cast molding is a more recent method in which a mixture of methylmethacrylate monomer and a polymerization initiator are injected into the mold. This improves the reproducibility of the manufacturing process.

PMMA has to be sterilized at a low temperature, ethylene dioxide is therefore used to sterilize PMMA IOLs.

BIOCOMPATIBILITY AND PMMA

When a foreign material is introduced into a biological medium, the first phenomenon observed is the adsorption of macromolecules and particularly of proteins. Protein adsorption occurs rapidly and the layer deposited is of the order of 100 nm thick. This adsorption seems to result from acid/base and dipole/dipole interactions. These are directly related to the surface energy of the material, its chemical structure and the distribution of binding sites on the surface of the material. This layer of proteins mediates the chemical reactions that occur at the material-tissue interface over the next few minutes or hours.

Removing the natural lens and implanting the artificial IOL ruptures the blood/eye barrier. Adsorption of protein onto the implanted lens occurs immediately. Complement is then activated by the alternative pathway. Polymorpho-nuclear cells and monocytes are attracted, giving rise to macrophages and giant cells, and the IOL becomes the focus of a reaction to a foreign body. Kochounian et al used the Western blot method to identify the proteins adsorbed onto the surface of PMMA IOLs that had been incubated for 3 hours in rabbit plasma (*in vitro*) or implanted for 48 hours in the capsule of rabbits (*in vivo*). The protein layer consisted of at least 6 different proteins: albumin, complement fraction C$_3$, IgG, fibrinogen/fibrin, fibronectin and transferrin. The main proteins adsorbed *in vitro* were albumin IgG, fibronectin and fibrinogen. The dominant types adsorbed *in vivo* were fibronectin and fibrinogen.

Studies have also demonstrated the effect of surface properties on cell adhesion. These studies covered several factors, such as the free energy of the interface (FEI), the surface energy (SE) and the angle of contact (AC). If the

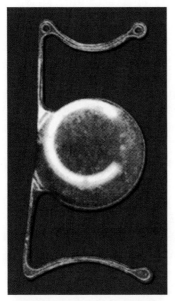

FIGURE 32.1: Anterior chamber lens (PMMA). Kellman IOL

FEI is used as the assessment criterion, the most hydrophilic materials, with a low FEI (< 5 ergs/cm^2) and the most water-repellent materials, which have a high FEI (> 40 ergs/cm^2) resulted in much lower cell adhesion than does PMMA. The intermediate FEI values (5 to 40 ergs/cm^2) of a PMMA make it favorable to cell adhesion and cell proliferation. The same conclusions were reached from a study of the SE and AC. The more hydrophilic (higher SE and lower AC), or more water-repellent (lower SE and higher AC) a material, the greater will be the adhesion of cells to its surface. The study of Tamada and Ikada showed that the adhesion and proliferation of rat fibroblasts is greatest on substrates with an AC of about 70° (the angle of contact of PMMA). Reich et al have developed a system for measuring the adhesive force between a material and the corneal endothelium of the rabbit and showed that these forces of adhesion were greater for PMMA.

The surface properties affect the opacification of the posterior capsule (OPC). Pathogenic aspects of OPC include the formation of Elschnig pearls, from equatorial epithelial cells that proliferate along the posterior capsule, and capsular fibrosis, due to anterior cuboid epithelial cells that undergo fibrous metaplasia. The epithelial cells of the lens require a surface on which to proliferate and the surface properties of the implanted lens determine the degree of postoperative OPC. Epithelial cells from rabbits, cattle, pigs and humans adhere *in vitro* less well to IOLs that are more hydrophilic or more hydrophobic than PMMA. However, no direct relationship was found *in vivo* between the surface properties and the degree of postoperative OPC.

PMMA IOL AND SURFACE PROPERTIES

The surface properties of a polymer can be altered by various methods, known collectively as surface treatment. These treatments make it possible to modify the surface energy of the polymer (hydrophilic-hydrophobic balance) by three methods:

1. Treatment of the surface proper
2. Coating with a deposit
3. Grafting by the attachment of new molecules.

TREATING OF THE SURFACE ITSELF

Various methods can be used to modify the surface of the polymer. The main ones are:

- Chemical techniques (chemical oxidation—exposure to ozone)
- Flaming
- Electromagnetic radiation (bombardment with ionizing radiation, bombardment with light rays; low-pressure cold plasma: crown discharges).

They are intended to create new chemical functions on the surface of the backing, which are then used to graft molecules or to alter some characteristics or the surface, such as roughness, hardness or slipperiness, without grafting molecules. The thickness treated is of the order of a few nanometers. Examples of the use of this method in ophthalmology tend to be linked to placing functional groups on the backing.

COATING WITH A DEPOSIT

Another polymer (deposit) with the desired properties is deposited on the backing to form a layer, which may reach a thickness of about 10 microns. The method usually is that known as the "soaking method", in which the backing is soaked in a solution of the deposit. The deposit is not made to adhere by chemical means and the two materials can have very different mechanical properties.

Teflon-coated Lenses

Polymethylmethacrylate intraocular lenses can be coated with a layer of a transparent fluorocarbon, Teflon AF. This is the first transparent, amorphous Teflon, which can be dissolved in fluoridized solvents (liquid fluorocarbons). This property means that it can be applied in very thin layers to substrates, rendering them entirely hydrophobic. The main steps in this process are:

- Soaking the PMMA lenses in a solution of Teflon AF in C8F18 for 3 seconds.
- Drying the lenses under vacuum at 37°C until the C8F18 has evaporated.

Teflon-coated lenses have been implanted in animals after phacoemulsification. No synechiae was observed between the iris and these implants over a follow-up period of 3 months. A significantly smaller number of cell deposits were found on the IOLs coated with Teflon than with those that were not. Another study, using a model of endothelial contact, demonstrated that the trauma induced by the implantation of Teflon-coated lenses was reduced, with less adhesion of the endothelial cells to their surface.

GRAFTING ON NEW MOLECULES

This method is used to bind one or more molecules (ligands) to the surface of a polymer (backing) by a covalent bond. The ligand is selected on the basis of specific new properties that the backing is required to have to make it more suitable for its final purpose. The grafting process includes the placing of functional groups on the backing and the binding of the ligand to them.

HEPARIN SURFACE-MODIFIED LENSES

The surface of PMMA lenses is heparin surface-modified by attaching heparin via covalent bonds in a series of chemical reactions.

- The lens surface is treated with sulfuric acid and potassium permanganate to create carbonyl and sulfate groups.
- They are then incubated with polyethyleneamine, a polymer that contains high levels of amines. This polymer reacts strongly with the surface of the treated lenses.

- The heparin is partially depolymerized with nitrous acid. The resulting molecular fragments have terminal aldehydes.
- The molecules containing aldehyde groups react with the primary amines to form bases, which can be reduced to form secondary amines. In this way, the fragments of aldehydes of the partially degraded heparin are coupled to the amine groups on the surface of the PMMA IOLs. Stable covalent bonds are then obtained by reduction with sodium cyanoborohydride. Larsson et al showed that the concentration of heparin on the surface of the lenses, obtained by this process was 0.6 mg/cm^2. It was found to have very satisfactory chemical stability.

Several studies have demonstrated the greater anti-adhesive effect of heparin surface-modified lenses compared to untreated PMMA IOLs.

Pekna et al showed that the grafting of heparin reduces complement activation by PMMA IOLs. In a model of endothelial injury using the rabbit cornea, heparin surface-modified lenses caused significantly fewer lesions and there was less adhesion of the endothelial cells to these lenses. Versura and Caramazza cultured human fibroblasts, monocytes and platelets on 4 types of IOLs: PMMA; heparin surface-modified PMMA, hydrogen and plasma-treated PMMA lenses. Electron microscopy identified reduced cell adhesion to heparin surface-modified IOLs and hydrogel lenses. A similar finding was reported by Joo and Kim for various cell models. Activation of the granulocytes by heparin surface-modified IOLs (assessed by the production of superoxide anions by exposed cells) was also reduced. Power et al followed by Cortina et al have demonstrated *in vitro* reduced adhesion of human epithelial cells to heparin surface-modified IOLs compared to PMMA IOLs. Power also compared the behavior of hydrogel IOLs, which had degrees of cell adhesion similar to those of heparin surface-modified lenses. Milazzo et al used organotypic cultures of chick embryo corneas and demonstrated that the surface of heparin surface-modified lenses is less propitious for cell adhesion and migration than the surface of unmodified PMMA lenses.

The antiadhesive property of heparin surface-modified IOLs seems to extend to bacteria, such as *Streptococcus epidermidis*, *Staphylococcus aureus* and *Pseudomonas aeruginosa*.

Rabbits were implanted with a heparin surface-modified or control artificial IOL and the number of leukocytes in the anterior chamber one day later was significantly lower in rabbits given heparin surface-modified lenses. The same thing was found in a similar type of study in which uveitis had been induced. The fibrinous reaction on heparin surface-modified IOLs was significantly less marked than that on PMMA intraocular lenses that had been implanted in monkeys for 4, 8 and 18 weeks. Larsson et al have shown that the concentration of heparin grafted to the surface of the PMMA IOLs by covalent bonding remained stable for 2 years after implantation in the anterior chamber of the rabbit.

These experimental findings have been confirmed in human studies. In a prospective study carried out by Borgioli et al 260 patients were given a heparin surface-modified lens and 264 a control lens. The number of patients presenting with cell deposits and posterior synechiae was reported to be lower in the group that had received heparin surface-modified lenses after 3 months and one year. In a group of 54 patients who had undergone surgery for cataract with phacoemulsification, Shah and Spalton found that there were fewer giant cells (counted by reflection microscopy) on the heparin surface-modified lens during the first year after surgery. Amon and Menapace, in a study involving 50 patients, found that 8% of the patients had giant cells on the lenses (mean follow-up time of 16 months versus one-third of cases after the implantation of conventional PMMA lenses. Zetterström carried out a study involving 40 patients with exfoliation syndrome. Two years later, the incidence of pigment and cell deposits was lower in the group of patients who were given a heparin surface-modified lens, opacification of the posterior capsule was also less marked in this group. Percival and Pai implanted heparin surface-modified lenses in 36 patients with a history of chronic uveitis. Cell deposits were found on only 16.6% of the lenses versus 22% in patients who also had a history of uveitis but had been given conventional lenses. Linn et al studied a group of patients with diabetes, glaucoma or chronic uveitis, found that the inflammatory reaction was less severe in the patients who were given heparin surface-modified lenses.

Damage to the heparin surface-modified surface has been caused by an Nd:YAG laser and by surgical instruments. The clinical consequences of this damage are not known.

SURFACE PASSIVATED INTRAOCULAR LENSES

Gupta and Van Osdel developed surface passivated IOLs in 1987. According to their patent, the process by which these lenses are produced consists of three steps, which are as follows:

1. PMMA intraocular lenses are subjected to surface treatment (or functionalization) consisting of exposure to ozone. This results in oxidation of the outer surfaces of the lenses.
2. The intraocular lenses are then exposed to a moist atmosphere, such as air, leading to hydrolysis of the outer, oxidized surfaces and the formation of hydroxyl groups.
3. The treated intraocular lenses are then soaked in a solution containing fluorocarbon (CF2) x, where x is between 6 and 12 and the binding agents. As a result, a layer of fluorocarbons is chemically bound to the outer layer of the lenses and reduces their energy. However, according to the marketing literature issued by Ioptex-Allergan, the purpose of the lens surface-passivation process is to lower the energy and reduce the irregularity of the surface. Many studies have given disappointing results. Koch et al did not find any significant difference

between the surface energy of surface-passivated lenses and unprocessed PMMA lenses. In this same study, ESCA (Electron Spectroscopy for Chemical Analysis) and SIMS (Static Secondary Ion Mass Spectroscopy) identified the presence of fluoride ions on the surface of only 1 of the 5 IOLs tested. Kochounian et al have shown that the passivated lenses activate the complement cascade, generating the same levels of C3a and C5a fractions as the conventional PMMA lenses. In a human study, Umezawa and Shimizu did not find any significant difference between the postoperative flare (measured using a laser flare cell meter) in the patients who had received surface-passivated and unprocessed PMMA lenses. However, using a model of endothelial contact in the cat, Balyeat et al have shown that passivated IOLs are associated with less epithelial injury and less adhesion of endothelial cells to their surface than unprocessed PMMA intraocular lenses.

INTRAOCULAR LENSES TREATED WITH COLD PLASMA CF4

Another PMMA IOL was developed in 1990. These lenses are fluoridated by cold plasma treatment. The term "plasma" is used in physics to describe an ionized and electrically neutral gas. It can be produced artificially by confining the gas to a closed, high-frequency electromagnetic field under low pressure (1 mbar). The gas is placed in an unpolymerizable or polymerizable reactor. The gas used may be CF4 CF3H or CF3Cl, which contain a single carbon atom. It produces a chemical change in the surface of the polymer by substituting atoms of fluorine or CF2 or CF3 groups for hydrogen atoms. The thickness affected is no more than 0.01 mm.

The findings of the study of PMMA IOLs treated with CF4 plasma carried out by Eloy et al were as follows: ESCA of their surfaces detected the grafting of the fluorine and the *de novo* appearance of carbon-containing functions, particularly CF, CF2 and CF3; measurement of the angle of contact with water showed that the surface energy of the treated lenses was lower than that of the processed lenses; the adhesion of human granulocytes to the surface of treated IOLs was reduced after incubation. The granulocytes in contact with the treated IOLs were less active, and this was reflected by the rate of superoxide production by these cells.

Despite the excellent optical and physicochemical properties of PMMA, it is not totally inert. Surface treatment of PMMAs improves their acceptability. According to the literature, heparin surface-modified IOLs are more effective, particularly in high-risk patients. However, the data for surface-passivated IOLs is disappointing, because no significant difference between treated and untreated PMMA IOLs has been demonstrated *in vivo*. The efficacy of cold plasma CF4-treated IOLs *in vivo* remains debatable.

SILICONE FOR IOL

The use of soft intraocular lenses (IOLs) for cataract surgery has been growing since the 1980s **(Figures 32.2 and 32.3)**. These lenses can be folded and inserted through small incisions, and may cause less postoperative astigmatism and allow quicker visual rehabilitation. The advantage of using small incisions has been demonstrated on several occasions by Oshika et al. The extent of the inflammatory reaction in the anterior chamber depends on the length of the incision and the differences remain statistically significant for one month after surgery. Postoperative astigmatism was found to be directly related to the length of the incision in most studies, except in that carried out by Neumann et al.

The first silicone soft IOL was used in 1984. This new generation of IOLs was accompanied by the development of various types of silicone materials with increasing refractive indices and types of IOLs that have been influenced by advances in surgical techniques. Capsulorhexis, for instance, was developed long after IOL of this type were first implanted.

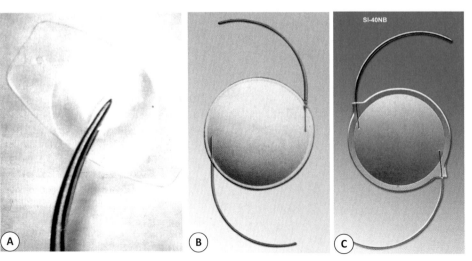

FIGURES 32.2A TO C: Silicone IOL

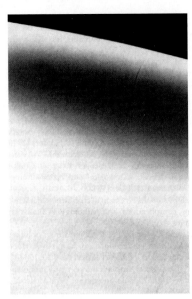

FIGURE 32.3: Silicone optic IOL observation by SEM (scanning electron microscopy)

The first elastomer used in the manufacture of the optical part of the soft IOLs was polydimethylsiloxane ($-Si(CH_2)3O-)n$. The main drawback of this material is its low refractive index (1.412 at 25°C), which makes it necessary to produce relatively thick lenses to achieve a given refractive index. These thick lenses are more difficult to fold. A second generation of silicone elastomers was then developed using a copolymer of diphenyl- and dimethylsiloxane, which has a refractive index of 1.464 ($-CH_3Si(C_6H_5)O-)n$. Silicones with even higher refractive indices have been developed, but have proved to be mechanically unsuitable for use as soft IOLs. Intraocular lenses made of various types of polydimethylsiloxane and polydimethyl-diphenylsiloxane materials have been exhaustively assessed and subjected to numerous tests. They have been shown to be very resistant to artificial aging in tests including exposure to ultraviolet light equivalent to 20 years of exposure under normal conditions of use. According to the study carried out by Kborz et al polydimethylsiloxane and PMMA IOLs seem to have equivalent optical qualities.

MOLDING FLASH AND SILICONE IOL

The most commonly used method for manufacturing silicone intraocular lenses is injection molding. This method often results in surface irregularities at the junction of the two sides of the lens, which take the form of a rough line visible all around the edges of the lens. This defect is known as molding flash, and it has been clearly identified by scanning electron microscopy. This defect can impair the biocompatibility of the lens. Newman et al have reported the case of a patient fitted with an early Staar silicone intraocular lens in the ciliary sulcus. The onset of glaucoma made it necessary to carry out explantation. Scanning electron microscopy identified severe molding flash all round the edge of the lens.

The quality of the lenses available has gradually improved, and routine assessment of this defect by various teams has shown that the quality of the finish of most IOLs is acceptable. In 1992, Tsai et al assessed the most commonly used IOLs, and although they found that the surface was smooth and regular and the finish acceptable, most of the lenses had molding flash. Similarly, in 1996, Omar et al compared these silicone IOLs with single-piece PMMA IOLs, which these authors, like many others, consider to set the standard for their quality of finish. Scanning electron microscopic examinations revealed that most of the silicone lenses had molding flash plus some irregularities at the optic loop junctions.

Investigation of the effects of folding these lenses sometimes detected surface changes, but these were usually temporary. So, although Brady et al have reported finding creases on the anterior surface of polydimethylsiloxane immediately after folding, these were no longer detectable by scanning electron microscopic examination ten minutes later.

The effects of the Nd:YAG laser have also been investigated by Newland et al who examined 17 silicone IOLs under the scanning electron microscope after standardized Nd:YAG exposure. The mean depth of the surface damage caused to these lenses was 143 (13.4 µm). According to the authors, these regions looked darker when viewed under a slit lamp, and looked very much like pigment deposits.

BIOCOMPATIBILITY AND SILICONE IOL

Silicone intraocular lenses were first used in 1984 by Mazzocco. Several studies of cell adhesion have subsequently been carried out both *in vivo* and *in vitro* and have shown that their safety is similar to that of IOLs made of PMMA.

Mondino et al incubated PMMA and silicone IOLs in serum. Using radioimmunological techniques, they demonstrated that the PMMA lenses activated the alternative complement pathway, whereas the silicone ones did not.

In vitro studies using cell models to evaluate the adhesion and toxicity of these materials have demonstrated better outcomes than those for standard PMMA.

Joo and Kim compared the adhesion of cells (platelets, human granulocytes, macrophage-like RAW 264.7 and rat fibrosarcoma L 929) to PMMA, heparin surface-modified PMMA, silicone and hydrogel. Less cell adhesion was found with the heparin surface-modified and hydrogel IOLs. There was slightly less cell adhesion to the silicone lenses than to the untreated PMMA lenses. In the same study, the authors evaluated granulocyte activation and measured the production of superoxide anions. Heparin surface-modified lenses and silicone lenses produced degrees of granulocyte activation intermediate between those found for PMMA and hydrogel IOLs.

In vitro animal studies carried out by Menapace et al, Kulnig et al found no differences between the numbers or types of cells deposited on PMMA and silicone IOLs.

According to these authors, the prevalence of cell deposits was not directly linked to the nature of the polymer, but depended on the severity of the postoperative inflammatory reactions. Several methods have been proposed to avoid between-animal differences, which could impair the validity of the data.

Okada et al developed a model for comparing the cell populations on PMMA and silicone IOLs. This system eliminates between-animal differences due to the surgical trauma or the postoperative inflammatory reaction. They coated half of the PMMA IOLs with polydimethylsiloxane and implanted them in albino rabbits. Examinations carried out 1, 2 and 3 weeks after surgery using a reflecting microscope found significantly fewer cells on the surfaces of the lenses coated with silicone. Similar conclusions were drawn from the study carried out by Cook et al, who implanted silicone-coated or PMMA-coated posterior chamber lenses (PCLs) in rabbits.

Carlson et al used fluorophotometric and histological methods to evaluate the inflammatory response in brown rabbits after phacoemulsification and the implantation of intraocular PMMA, silicone and hydrogel lenses. All 3 types of IOLs showed good biocompatibility during a 16-week follow-up. The only difference identified was the occurrence of nongranulomatous, chronic inflammation of the conjunctiva in the limbus of those rabbits which had been given a soft lens, although the authors did not identify any clinically significant repercussions.

No signs of toxicity were detected after implanting silicone PCLs in monkeys or cats. Both studies found that the cell loads deposited on the silicone lenses were significantly lighter than those on the PMMA lenses.

Endothelial contact models confirmed this tendency towards lower cell adhesion to Herzog et al demonstrated that the silicone IOLs caused less trauma of the endothelial cells.

Bacterial adhesion to this type of material is also an important factor. This is particularly relevant because cultures of the aqueous humor were positive for 29 to 43% of the patients who had undergone surgery for cataract. Cusamo et al cultivated coagulase-negative staphylococci on PMMA, silicone and hydrogel intraocular lenses. Bacterial growth was greatest on the silicone lenses, least on the PMMA and intermediate on the hydrogel IOLs. An increase in the incidence of endophthalmia after the implantation of soft lenses has not been confirmed, except in a context of suspected bacteriological risk arising from the use of polypropylene loops. The first clinical trials demonstrated good biocompatibility of silicone IOLs. The complications associated with them consisted essentially of decentering, which sometimes called for surgical repair. These problems are linked to the geometry of the lens and the operating technique, rather than to the materials of which they are made. The earliest silicone IOLs were initially implanted in the ciliary sulcus. The first silicone IOL was designed by Mazzocco. The first implantations

of these lenses into the capsular bag did not yet use the capsulorhexis technique, and the incidence of decentering was very high. Once capsulorhexis had been introduced by Neuhann and Gimbel, the shapes of the silicone IOLs were soon changed to make them more suitable for implantation in the capsular bag. At present, some authors believe that this decentering is primarily attributable to shortcomings in the capsulotomy technique, and that the shape and material is a secondary factor.

Silicone IOLs can be arbitrarily divided into three main groups: single-piece or "spindle" or "boat-shaped" lenses, three-piece lenses with polypropylene loops and lenses with PMMA loops.

The implantation of silicone IOLs of all three types calls for regular capsulorhexis and an intact posterior chamber. The nature of the single-piece and of the attached loops affect the risk of decentering and secondary lens deformity. Single-piece IOLs have no real anchor within the capsular bag. Secondary symphysis of the anterior chamber to the posterior chamber holds the loops in place. Fibrosis and contraction of the capsular bag can also lead to decentering and horizontal distortion of the lens. This seems to be particularly true of silicone single-piece IOLs and those with polypropylene loops, in which the forces brought to bear by the capsular bag on the loops are more readily transmitted to the ocular part of the lens. Polypropylene is very flexible and has a tendency to lose its "memory", becoming permanently distorted during implantation. A few cases of pupillary capture have been reported involving silicone IOLs with polypropylene loops. The flexibility of polypropylene seems to facilitate the forward shift of the lens during contraction of the capsular bag, particularly if the loops have no anterior angulation.

Studies have demonstrated that silicone lenses are not statistically significantly more often decentered than PMMA lenses: Blotnick et al examined seven eyes obtained postmortem 6 weeks to 13 months after surgery for cataract during which a 3-piece silicone intraocular lens (AMO SI-18NB/silicone lens, polypropylene loops) had been implanted. This IOL was the first 3-piece lens to come onto the market, hence the importance of this study. Macroscopic examination showed that the lenses were all located in the capsular bags, with minimal decentering except in two cases, in which significant decentering was associated with radial tearing of the capsulorhexis and secondary contraction of the capsular bag. Histological examination did not reveal any inflammatory reaction of the iris, ciliary body capsular bag or anterior chamber. An FDA report on this IOL investigated the behavior of these lenses in 500 patients over a period of 3 years. The clinical safety and visual acuity were similar to those of the PMMA IOLs. The complication rate after 3 years did not seem to be directly related to the lens type.

Auffarth et al studied the anchoring and centering of single-piece silicone IOLs (boat-shaped) and 3-piece lenses in 30 cadaver eyes. The mean displacement from the center observed for single-piece lenses was 0.26 (0.13 mm), while that for 3-piece lenses was 0.37 (0.31 mm) this difference was not statistically significant. The difference between them and PMMA single-piece or 3-piece IOLs was also not significant.

In another group of 100 explanted silicone IOLs (63 three-piece lenses with polypropylene loops and 37 boat-shaped lenses) Auffarth et al once again found no difference between these lenses and the PMMA IOLs with regard to the reasons for explantation (42% decentering, 27.7% inflammation). The authors think that the long-term clinical prognosis depends mainly on the quality of the surgery and above all on the anchoring of the lens in the capsular bag.

Disk-shaped silicone IOLs were produced at the same time as these boat-shaped IOLs and the three-piece lenses with separate loops. Some people thought that this shape would have the theoretical advantage of ensuring better centering. In a study of 35 eyes, Duncker et al found that 25 percent were located at least 1 mm off center, and decided to stop using this type of lens (FK-1 and Adatomed 90-D).

Other authors recommend the use of 3-piece silicone lenses with PMMA loops, which are stiffer than polypropylene loops and less sensitive to the forces exerted by the capsular bag. Egan et al monitored 100 patients for 4 months fitted with an AMO SI-40NB IOL. They found that this IOL provided excellent centering during surgery and after 4 months.

SURFACE MODIFICATION

Like PMMA IOLs, silicone lenses can also be surface-modified to alter their characteristics. Hettlich et al exposed polydimethylsiloxane lenses to oxygen plasma, which made their surfaces less water-repellant (the contact angle fell from 121.86 to 96.5°). They intended to evaluate the impact of these surface modifications on the foreign-body reaction induced by the IOL. The only difference observed was the significantly lower incidence of posterior synechiae in the rabbits that had been given a surface-modified lens. Similarly, several attempts were made to carry out surface-modification using heparin.

DISCOLORATION AND CAPSULAR OPACIFICATION OF SILICONE IOL

Miauskas was the first to report secondary discoloration of silicone lenses. In 1991, he reported 15 cases monitored for between 15 and 60 months after being implanted. The presence or absence of UV-blocks did not seem to affect the discoloration, as this occurred both in the IOLs manufactured by the Staar Surgical Co., which do not contain a UV block, and those manufactured by Iolab Co., which do. In the most severe instances (the surface of the lenses turned brown), there was an associated loss of contrast. Milauskas has subsequently identified another 9 cases involving these two types of lens. This discoloration

was attributed to the presence of impurities, which could account for the granular, brownish appearance under the slit lamp. The manufacturing process of these lenses has since been modified by adding an extra filtration of the silicone to remove all traces of impurity. In 1991, Watt also reported a case of brown discoloration of the center of a silicone lens (AMO Model S-18NGB) 6 weeks after surgery. In view of the location of the discoloration and the short interval since surgery, the author thought that this abnormality might already have been present when the IOL was implanted. In 1992, Koch and Heit reported two similar cases involving the same model of IOL. Allergan Medical Optics researchers have suggested that the brownish haze at the center of the lenses could have been due to diffusion of the light due to water vapor in the silicone immersed in an aqueous medium. This was attributed to defective polymerization or to the incomplete elimination of fractions of unpolymerized silicone. Kershner suggested that eyedrops may have affected the silicone. In 1992, Chapman et al investigated the possible interactions with compounds used before or after surgery. They found that none of the materials tested (PMMA, silicone and hydrogel) could have acted as a reservoir of these drugs (pilocarpine, gentamicin, dexamethasone, norepinephrine/noradrenaline) as the adsorption and desorption of these drugs was insufficient by any of the routes used (topical, subconjunctival and intravenous). It is unlikely that interactions of this type could contribute to the discoloration of silicone IOLs. No case has been recorded or reported in the literature since 1993.

The incidence of opacification of the anterior and posterior chamber after implantation of silicone IOLs has undergone considerable investigation. Fibrosis and opacification following surgery for cataract appears to be less frequent in the anterior chamber than in the posterior chamber. These effects are generally linked to a severe postoperative inflammatory reaction, promoted by capsular pseudoexfoliation or small-incision capsulorhexis. They can severely hinder the detailed examination of the fundus, taking retinographs and laser or surgical treatment of the retina. They may be combined with contraction of the capsular bag and lead to subsequent tilting or even folding of the lens. The material and shape of the lens may produce combined or independent effects. Auer and Gonvers studied two groups of 17 patients. Opacification of the anterior chamber occurred much more often when the lens was a single-piece silicone lens with flat loops (Staar® AA4203) (70%) rather than a PMMA lens (18%). It was suggested that this might have been due to the greater area in contact with the anterior chamber, which could have facilitated the proliferation of epithelial cells in the anterior chamber. Fibrosis and opacification of the posterior chamber appears to occur less frequently with single-piece silicone lenses with flat loops, because of the small area of contact between the IOL and the posterior chamber. Watts and Pearce demonstrated that a disk lens could act as a mechanical barrier, inhibiting the opacification of the posterior chamber. However, this was not observed in the study carried out by Duncker, in which 33% of the eyes displayed opacification of the posterior chamber after a mean follow-up time of 20.5 months.

The clinical results obtained with silicone IOLs are similar to those obtained with PMMA lenses. There is a considerable follow-up time, as the first implantations were carried out in 1984. Improvements in the manufacturing process have made it possible to solve the problems of lens discoloration which occurred in the early 1990s. But it is still possible to improve the surface finish of these lenses, as most of the models available have surplus material at the loop/lens junctions (molding flash). However, a recent circular from the DASS [French Social Security Authority] recommends avoiding the use of this type of material if there is silicone in the posterior segment, or if there is a risk of a slipped retina, because the adsorption of silicone to the surface of these lenses is irreversible.

SOFT ACRYLIC IOL

Silicone elastomers are some of the most frequently used materials in the manufacture of soft IOLs. Other materials are also used, including hydrogels and acrylics. The term "hydrogel IOLs" is generally taken to mean polyhydroxy-ethylmethacrylate (PHEMA) IOLs. In fact, the term encompasses a large group of polymers, of which PHEMA is just one. These materials all have a moisture content of at least 20 percent.

Soft "acrylic" IOLs are somewhat arbitrarily divided into groups. However, they all belong to the same group of chemicals, which includes stiff, hydrophobic poly-methylmethacrylate (PMMA) and soft hydrophilic hydro-gels, such as PHEMA. This large group of materials consists of monomers of esters of acrylic and methacrylic acids.

One important characteristic of the acrylics or acrylates is their vitreous transition temperature (VTT). This is the temperature at which the material undergoes a phase change and softens. The VTT of PMMA is 110°C. This means that it is stiff at room temperature, but becomes flexible from 110°C. Methacrylate monomers have much higher VTT values than acrylates. A polymer with an intermediate VTT can be obtained by selecting an appropriate combination of acrylates and methacrylates. For example, a copolymer containing 50% methacrylate (VTT = 10°C) and 50% methylmethacrylate (VTT = 105°C) would have a VTT of about 55°C. The materials used in the manufacture of soft IOLs, usually known as "acrylics", are copolymers synthesized from combinations of acrylics or acrylates. These ingredients are carefully selected to produce soft acrylic IOLs with high refractive indices and a VTT around room temperature while still having the optical properties of PMMA. These copolymers have a three-dimensional molecular structure, which enables them to retain a memory

of shape. In view of the large number of possible combinations, the various copolymers synthesized have differing refractive indices, moisture contents, folding and unfolding properties and surface properties. These materials can be synthesized by copolymerization using 0.5 to 2.0% of a cross-linking agent, such as ethyleneglycol dimethacrylate (EGDMA). PHEMA is synthesized from the monomers 2-hydroxyethylmethacrylate (HEMA) and HEGDMA.

The hydrophilicity of these materials, like that of PHEMA, is linked to the inclusion of an (OH) group which enables them to absorb water into the polymer mesh. This mesh is rigid when dry, but becomes soft in an aqueous medium. The molecules of water have a plasticizing effect which renders the material flexible.

HYDROGEL INTRAOCULAR LENSES

PHEMA is the hydrogel most commonly used in the manufacture of IOLs. It contains 38% water. The earliest models were single-piece IOLs, with a biconvex lens and flanged flat loops. Their rear surface has a continuous convex arc of curvature, giving it a "taco-like" appearance.

These materials are highly hydrophilic, which theoretically gives them the advantage of having a lower cell adhesion capacity than PMMA. The endothelial trauma caused by PMMA IOLs and hydrogel IOLs as a result of *in vitro* contact with the endothelium is nearly 20 times greater (3.6% of an endothelial area of 0.25 mm^2 for the hydrogels versus 62% for untreated PMMA IOLs and 27 to 57% for PMMA IOLs coated with a 1% solution of sodium hyaluronate Healon®). Reich et al have shown that the cell adhesion force is about 7 times lower than that of PMMA [0.09 (0.02 g/cm^2 or hydrogel vs. 0.66) (0.11 g/cm^2 for PMMA and 0.19) (0.05 gm/cm^2 for the Healon®-coated PMMA)]. Similarly, Power et al, who compared the *in vitro* adhesion of human lenticular epithelial cells to PMMA, heparin surface-treated PMMA and hydrogel, also demonstrated lower cell adhesion to the hydrogels. This has been confirmed for porcine, and bovine lenticular epithelial cells, as well as for human fibroblasts, monocytes and platelets. Bacterial adhesion to these IOLs remains controversial. Cusumano et al cultured coagulase-negative staphylococci on PMMA, silicone and hydrogel IOLs. Bacterial growth was greatest on the silicone lenses, least on the PMMA lenses and intermediate on the hydrogel lenses. In contrast, Ng et al demonstrated that the *in-vitro* adhesion of *S. epidermidis* to PMMA was 20 times greater than to hydrogel (p < 0.001). These results are confirmed by those of a study carried out by Hogt et al, who showed that the adhesion of *S. epidermidis* decreases as the HEMA content of the materials increases, and is therefore related to its hydrophilicity. This discrepancy between the findings of Cusumano et al and Ng et al is attributable to their use of differing methods, particularly involving different strains and concentrations of bacteria and the methods used to count the bacteria adhering to the materials. These materials cause little inflammatory reaction. Packard et al showed that implanting hydrogel IOLs in the rabbit for 2 months did not trigger any significant inflammatory reactions. Similarly, Amon and Menapace and Ravalico et al studied the cell deposits on PMMA and PHEMA IOLs and found that there was little cell reaction on the latter. Giant cells induced by foreign bodies were detected on only 9% of the PHEMA IOLs.

Hydrogel IOLs seem to be more resistant to the Nd:YAG laser than those made of PMMA or silicone. This has been demonstrated in several studies, including the *in vitro* study of Keates et al and a human study after discission of the posterior chamber. Skelnik et al compared hydrogel and PMMA IOLs immersed in a culture medium and exposed to an Nd:YAG laser and found that the PMMA lenses were always more severely damaged.

Despite their advantage in terms of biocompatibility, the earliest hydrogel IOLs had two drawbacks essentially linked to their design. The first posterior-chamber intraocular lens (PCL) made of poly-HEMA was developed and designed by Barrett, the IOGEL PC-12 model (Alcon). This was first implanted in 1983 in Perth, Australia. IOLs made of hydrogels with a higher water content than PHEMA, and hydrogel iris-supported IOLs had already been used in the 1970s. The PC-12 measured 6 mm wide and 12 mm long, and was intended for implantation in the sulcus or the capsular bag. This lens was often too long or too short, depending on whether it was implanted in the sulcus or the capsular bag, which is sometimes associated with a high degree of pigment dispersal. The design of the IOL was therefore modified to make it more suitable for implantation in the capsular bag. A second model, 1103, has a total length of 11.3 mm. The loops were shorter, and therefore less likely to be squashed once the IOL was positioned in the capsular bag. At the time, this single-piece lens was considered to be one of the best single-piece IOLs.

A more recent model, 1003, is supplied with a half-disk 6.5 mm wide and 10.3 mm long. It has a larger optical zone than the models mentioned above, which makes the center of the lens thicker. This IOL is smaller than the other models, and severe decentering has resulted from attempts to implant it in the capsular bag. Its wider and thicker optical zone resulted in more frequent contact between the iris and the anterior chamber, increasing the risk of fibrosis and iridocapsular synechia.

Many studies have shown that the visual acuity obtained with hydrogel IOLs is as good as that of PMMA IOLs. The only study in which the results for PMMA IOLs were significantly better than those for hydrogel IOLs (Alcon, Iogel PC-1103) was that of Lowe and Easty who investigated the sensitivity to contrast. This was not confirmed in the study of Weghaupt et al. They measured the contrast sensitivity of patients who had a PMMA implant in one eye and a hydrogel (Alcon, Iogel PC-1103) in the other. They did not find any significant difference.

Posterior chamber opacification (PCO) appears to be increased. Several studies have shown that the incidence of PCO is lower for PHEMA IOLs. Conflicting data have been obtained. Menapace evaluated the incidences of PCO and capsulotomy associated with PHEMA IOLs (PC-12, 1103, 1003) and found that 75% of these patients had impaired visual acuity and concomitant PCO over a period of 3 years. Theoretically, the posterior convexity of these lenses should prevent the migration of epithelial cells to lenses implanted in the capsular bag. However, the taco-style single-piece structure of these IOLs made it impossible to fuse the anterior and posterior chambers. A space developed behind the lens in 1/3 to 1/2 cases, within which there were numerous Elschnig pearls. According to the author, lens design was not the only factor responsible for this, and the properties of PHEMA were also implicated. The presence of Elschnig pearls in the capsular bag could have resulted in an osmotic pressure differential because fluid and nutrients pass through the IOL, which explains why Elschnig pearls filled the space behind the lens.

Levy et al have abandoned the use of hydrogel IOLs after the occurrence of two cases of this backward displacement of the IOLs into the vitreous humor during posterior capsulotomy using an Nd:YAG laser. The authors think that the lack of adhesion of the PHEMA to eye tissues and the design of these IOLs are responsible for these complications. This tendency has not been observed in any other study. The displacements reported by Levy et al led the FDA (Food and Drug Administration) to prohibit their use from September 1989.

Given the risk of backward displacement of the implant during YAG laser capsulotomy, Menapace and Yalon have recommended surgical aspiration of the Elschnig pearls if PCO occurs and substituting a PMMA IOL for the hydrogel IOL. The authors pointed out that it is easy to explant the soft and non-adhesive IOL and insert the PMMA lens because the anterior and posterior chambers are not attached.

The use of hydrogel IOLs has dwindled in the light of these incidents of decentering, backward displacement and pigment dispersal. The taco-style single-piece design is no longer considered suitable for hydrogel IOLs due to the symphysis of the anterior and posterior chambers. Barrett has recently produced a new design of PHEMA IOL intended to improve their attachment, eliminating the risk of backward displacement after YAG laser capsulotomy. The actual lens had a diameter of 6 mm and forms a continuous entity with the "C"-shaped loops. This design makes it possible to fuse the anterior and posterior chambers between the loops. The fixing and centering performance of these new IOLs obtained by Barrett in a group of 67 patients was excellent. Similar results were also obtained in Condon's study of 20 patients followed up for 6 months. However, Percival and Jafree reported one case of decentering caused by incomplete fusion of the bottom of the anterior and posterior capsules.

Another drawback often attributed to hydrogel IOLs is the fact that they do not incorporate UV filters. Despite this, the PC-12 model was monitored for 5 years after being implanted in 125 eyes and compared to a group of patients implanted with a PMMA PCL. The incidence of macular disease in these 2 groups were similar, despite the lack of incorporated UV-blocking chromophores in the hydrogel. Subsequently, Chirila was able to produce hydrogel IOLs containing melanin, which absorbs UV. These IOLs are currently undergoing experimental evaluation.

Bucher et al recently, reported a case of a PHEMA implant totally opacified by white deposits. Histological and physical examination showed that these deposits were due to calcification. These calcifications occurred even in patients without hypercalcemia. The authors suggested that the calcium was derived from residual lens fragments and the phosphorus from a solution of phosphated thymoxamine used preoperatively to induce miosis. This suggests that phosphated solutions should not be used with a PHEMA IOL.

SOFT ACRYLIC IOLs

The copolymers used in the manufacture of the soft acrylic IOLs discussed here are 3D chains synthesized from an ester of acrylic acid and an ester of methyacrylate acid (AcrySof®/Acrylens®) or from two esters of methacrylate acid (Memorylens®). A primer and a UV filter were included in their composition.

They have higher refractive indices than the PCLs. Despite being soft, they still have many of the advantages of PMMA, including its excellent optical characteristics. As a result of the three-dimensional arrangement of their chains, these lenses return to their initial shape and size after being inserted into the eye. They unfold more slowly than soft silicone IOLs. Only slight pressure is required to alter their shape. The forceps may often leave an imprint while they are being folded, but this disappears within a few minutes. However, their surface is fragile, and folding and insertion maneuvers can leave permanent marks. Soft acrylic IOLs are growing in popularity, and in Japan they are now preferred to silicone IOLs.

HYDROPHILIC SOFT ACRYLIC IOLs

Memory Lens®

Two models are currently supplied: the U780A, with an optical diameter of 7 mm and a total diameter of 14 mm, and the U940 A, with an optical diameter of 6 mm and a total diameter of 13 mm. Both models have a three-piece design with C-shaped polypropylene loops.

In the initial clinical trials, the Memory Lens had to be folded before being inserted. To do this it had to be attached to a folding device and heated in a heat exchanger supplied by the manufacturer. The heated IOL was folded and then cooled in a second chamber of the heat exchanger. These are complicated operations, and damage was sometimes caused at this stage. Prefolded IOLs are now available. These have to be kept at 8°C before use. Once implanted,

they slowly unfold (10 to 15 minutes) under the influence of body heat, and the folds have all disappeared by the day after the operation. The polypropylene loops on the prefolded IOL reach their normal position in the capsular bag as soon as they have been implanted. The hydrophilicity of the MemoryLens means that, unlike "hydrophobic" soft acrylic IOLs, its surfaces show no tendency to stick to each other or to the surgical instruments.

Pötzsch and Lötzsch implanted and compared 36 Memory Lens and 36 PMMA IOLs over a period of 4 years. The results for visual acuity, inflammatory reactions and opacification of the posterior chamber in the two groups were similar. There was less postoperative astigmatism in the MemoryLens group, and this IOL was also found to be more resistant to the YAG laser. This was confirmed by Johnson and Henderson, in a study in which MemoryLens and PMMA IOLs immersed in sterile physiological solution were exposed to the Nd:YAG laser. The MemoryLens IOLs suffered less damage.

Other hydrophilic soft acrylic IOLs are available in Europe, including the Hydroview® (Storz: 3 piece, PMMA loops, 18% water content, refractive index: 1.47) and the EasAcryl® (Chiron Vision: single-piece, 26% water content, refractive index 1.46). Akreos Disc® and First®, from the Chauvin group. The Haptibag® from Holtech and the ACR 6D® from Corneal are some of the best known of these. Clinical trials involving these IOLs are in progress.

HYDROPHOBIC SOFT ACRYLIC IOLs

The choice of material is controlled to some extent by patents (Allergan and Neslé/Alcon) which prevent the use of hydrophobic materials.

AcrySof was the first of the hydrophobic soft acrylic lenses to come onto the market. The MA60BM model has an optical diameter of 6 mm and a total diameter of 13 mm. The C-shaped loops are made of PMMA and have an anterior angle of 10°. The folding and unfolding of AcrySof depends on temperature. They are more flexible at higher temperatures which makes them easier to fold. Shugar has described a method for facilitating the implantation of AcrySof lenses without damaging them that is based on this characteristic. The IOLs are heated and coated with viscoelastic before being folded. It is advisable to handle AcrySofs using folding and insertion instruments and grasping them by the edges. The folding axis recommended by Shugar[48] corresponds to 6 O'clock to 12 O'clock, but Oh and Oh maintain that folding along the 4 O'clock to 10 O'clock axis makes it easier to handle the loops. Miller et al used the Staar 1-MTC-45 injection system to implant AcrySofs MA30BA through 2.8 mm incisions. This is not recommended, because this system has been specially designed for Staar silicone IOLs. However, the results of Miller et al show that a similar system for AcrySofs would make it easier to insert them through very small incisions, with less risk of damaging the optical part. A specific injector is now available. Several studies have reported creases or even cracks on the lens itself, all of which were produced during the folding and insertion maneuvers. Milazzo et al have shown that the marks produced on AcrySofs during folding are still visible under a slit lamp after a follow-up time of 17.75 (1.89 months, but have no impact on the visual recovery of the patients. Oshika and Shiokawa have shown that the procedures generally used for folding acrylic lenses do not affect their optical performance. In their study, damage to the material with deterioration of its optical properties was seen only after harsh treatment.

Shugar et al implanted 2 AcrySofs (1 in the capsular bag and 1 in the sulcus) in patients presenting with severe preoperative hypermetropia. The authors think that the AcrySof is appropriate for these multiple implantations because of its high refractive index, which makes it possible to produce thinner and flatter IOLs than with PMMA or silicone. AcrySof has a refractive index of 1.55 (37°C–550 nm), which is higher than that of any of the other materials used for IOLs. A 24D AcrySof lens is 0.3 mm thick. The fact that the AcrySof is flatter reduces the space between the two implanted lenses to a minimum. Where there is a space, lenticular epithelial cells can proliferate in it, leading to the formation of Elschnig pearls.

If the AcrySof IOL has to be explanted during or after surgery, it can be cut using Vannas scissors and the two halves removed as demonstrated by Koo et al. A special instrument has had to be devised to cut silicone IOLs. Neuhann has proposed an alternative method of intraocular folding for removing acrylic lenses without enlarging the incision. This preserves the advantages of small incisions.

Kohnen et al studied visual function in patients implanted with PMMA PCLs (n = 19), silicone (n = 20) and AcrySofs (n = 16). The outcome in terms of visual acuity was excellent in all three groups. However, significantly better results were obtained with regard to glare and contrast sensitivity with the PMMA lenses and AcrySofs. Oshika et al implanted AcrySofs in 64 patients who were monitored for 2 years. The intensity of postoperative "flare" was measured using a flare cell meter and was significantly higher in these patients than in those who had been given a PMMA or silicone lens. As a result of a burst capsule, one AcrySof was implanted in the ciliary sulcus with no adverse effect. Seven patients underwent YAG laser capsulotomy and the damage to the AcrySof lenses caused by this procedure was similar to but less severe than that incurred by the PMMA lenses. In the same study, the authors observed that AcrySof tended to stick to the forceps while it was being freed from the capsular bag. Sometimes the surfaces that came into contact with each other during folding stuck together. It was often necessary to introduce a second instrument through a lateral working incision to free the lens completely.

There have been some recent reports of glistening in the AcrySof lenses, which was first seen one week after surgery. In the study of Dhaliwal et al 17 of the 56 patients investigated displayed some glistening. Nine out of 10 patients with a silicone IOL in the other eye exhibited a loss of contrast sensitivity due to glistening in the eye fitted with the AcrySof. There was never any reduction of visual acuity and the glistening decreased with time in many of the patients. According to Alcon, this phenomenon is linked to hydration of the IOLs. Water vacuoles form in the lens and are visible as a result of the difference in the refractive indices of the polymer and of water. Placing AcrySof in BSS® at body temperature for 48 to 72 hours produced the same surface appearance. Other complications with the AcrySofs reported by Omar et al consisted of 9 cases of distention of the capsular bag. This distention was not specific to this type of IOL and had already been reported for hydrogel IOLs.

Sensar® IOL consists of a reticulated hydrophobic acrylic polymer that is now in the market in France. It has a lower refractive index than PMMA (1.47 versus 1.49) and a low melting point (13°C). This lower refractive index has the drawback of making it necessary to have a thicker lens for a given number of diopters, but it does cause less glare and reflection. An injection system is also provided.

The AcryLens (model ACR360) is a three-piece IOL with an optical diameter of 6 mm and a total diameter of 13.65 mm. C-shaped polypropylene loops have a forward angulation of 5°. Sanchez and Artaria implanted an AcryLens in each of 50 patients and monitored them for 12 months. The clinical outcomes were very similar to those obtained with other foldable IOLs. Two of these patients had preoperative complications (a radial tear of the capsulorhexis in one case and a burst posterior chamber in the other). Despite this, the AcryLens® was successfully implanted in the ciliary sulcus (as the AcrySof had been). This is an advantage over the spindle-shaped lenses, for instance, which cannot be implanted in the sulcus as they require a regular capsulorhexis and an intact capsular bag. Sanchez and Artaria also found the same tendency to stick to the surgical instruments as had been seen with AcrySof. The marks visible immediately after inserting these lenses were still visible by slit-lamp throughout the follow-up period. According to the authors, an injection system would simplify the insertion of these IOLs into the eye by preventing them from sticking to surgical instruments and protecting their fragile optical surfaces.

Surface Quality

Kohnen et al used scanning electron microscopy to analyze the quality of the surface of several acrylic, hydrogel and soft acrylic IOLs before and after folding. All the IOLs had smooth, uniform optical surfaces of excellent quality, in particular in the case of those containing HEMA (PHEMA, MemoryLens and Hydroview lenses). In the case of the Hydroview, the scan showed perfect fusion between the acrylic polymer (the optical part) and the PMMA (loops). There was no sign of the molding flash which is often associated with silicone IOLs, and the finish of the edges of all the lenses was thought to be generally of good quality. The AcryLens ACR360 had some fine irregularities on the polypropylene loops. Small gaps were found at the lens/loop junctions in the AcrySof MA60BM (PMMA loops) and the MemoryLens U940A (propylene loops). Minute linear defects were found in both hydrophobic acrylic IOLs (AcryLens ACR360 and AcrySof MA60BM) that had been folded for 1 minute. They were visible under very high magnification in the areas that had been gripped by the forceps. This confirmed the findings of other authors concerning the greater fragility of these lenses.

The main chemical constituents of the materials currently available for the manufacture of IOLs fall into just two groups: acrylate/methacrylate polymers and silicone elastomers. PMMA, hydrogel, PHEMA and the various copolymers used for the manufacture of soft acrylic IOLs all actually belong to the same group. It is the different chemical groups attached to the main chain of the standard polymer which produce the differing properties observed. Soft acrylic IOLs are becoming increasingly popular, and in some countries they are the most frequently used soft IOLs. Acrylic copolymers, in addition to those mentioned here, are also currently under investigation.

BIBLIOGRAPHY

1. Absolom DR, Thomson C, Hawthorn LA, et al. Kinetics of cell adhesion to polymer surfaces. J Biomed Mater Res. 1988;22: 215-29.
2. Allmer K, Hilborn J, Larsson PH, et al. Surface modification of polymers. V. Biomaterial applications. J Appl Polym Sci Pol Chem. 1990;28: 173-83.
3. Allmer K, Hult A, Ranby B. Surface modification of polymers. III. Grafting of stabilizers onto polymer films. J Appl Polym Sci Pol Chem. 1989;27: 3405-17.
4. Amon M, Menapace R. Cellular invasion on hydrogel and poly(methyl methacrylate) implants; in vivo study. J Cataract Refract Surg. 1991;17: 774-9.
5. Amon M, Menapace R. Evaluation of a one-piece poly (methyl methacrylate) intraocular lens with a 7 mm biconvex optic and a total diameter of 10 mm. J Cataract Refract Surg. 1993;19: 16-21.
6. Amon M, Menapace R. Long-term results and biocompatibility of heparin-surface-modified intraocular lenses. J Cataract Refract Surg. 1993;19: 258-62.
7. Anderson C, Koch DD, Gree G, et al. Alcon AcrySofTM acrylic intraocular lens. In Martin RG, Gills JP, Sanders DR (Eds): Foldable Intraocular Lenses. Thorofare: NJ Slack. 1993;161-77.
8. Apple DJ, Mamalis N, Loftfield K, et al. Complications of intraocular lenses. A historical and histopathological review. Surv Ophthalmol. 1984;29: 1-54.
9. Apple DJ, Mamalis N, Olson RJ, et al. Intraocular lenses: evolution designs, complications, and pathology. Williams and Williams: Baltimore; 1989; 429.
10. Arciola CR, Caramazza R, Pizzoferrato A. In vitro adhesion of Staphylococcus epidermidis on heparin-surface-modified intraocular lenses. J Cataract Refract Surg. 1994;20: 158-61.
11. Auer C, Gonvers M. Implant intraoculaire monobloc en silicone et fibrose de la capsule antérieure. Klin Monatsbl Augenheilkd. 1995;206: 293-5.
12. Auffarth GU, McCabe C, Wilcox M, et al. Centration and fixation of silicone intraocular lenses: Clinicopathological findings in human autopsy eyes. J Cataract Refract Surg. 1996; 22: 1281-5.
13. Auffarth GU, Wilcox M, Sims JCR, et al. Analysis of 100 explanted one-piece and three-piece silicone intraocular lenses. Ophthalmol. 1995;102: 1144-50.
14. Babizhayev MA, Chumayevskii NA. Tinting effect of ultraviolet radiation on intraocular lenses of polymethyl methacrylate. Biomed Mater Eng. 1994;4: 1-16.
15. Baldeschi L, Rizzo S, Nardi M. Damage of foldable intraocular lenses by incorrect folder forceps. Am J Ophthalmol. 1997;124: 245-7.
16. Balyeat HD, Nordquist RE, Lerner MP, et al. Comparison of endothelial damage produced by control and surface modified poly(methyl methacrylate) intraocular lenses. J Cataract Refract Surg. 1989;15: 491-4.
17. Barrett G, Constable IJ. Corneal endothelial loss with new intraocular lenses. Am J Ophthalmol. 1984;98: 157-65.
18. Barrett GD, Beasley H, Lorenzetti OJ, et al. Multicenter trial of an intraocular hydrogel lens implant. J Cataract Refract Surg. 1987;13: 621-6.
19. Barrett GD, Constable IJ, Stewart AD. Clinical results of hydrogel lens implantation. J Cataract Refract Surg. 1986;12: 623-31.
20. Barrett GD. A new hydrogel intraocular lens design. J Cataract Refract Surg. 1994;20: 18-25.
21. Barrett GD. The evolution of hydrogel implants. Dev Ophthalmol. 1991;22: 70-1.
22. Bechetoille A, Legeay G, Legeais V, et al. Dispositif à usage ophtalmologique formé d'un substrat polymérique comportant des groupements fluorés en surface, et procédé d'obtention. Brevet d'invention No. FR 51035 A, déposé le 21/11/90, Paris.
23. Blotnick CA, Powers TP, Newland T, et al. Pathology of silicone intraocular lenses in human eyes obtained postmortem. J Cataract Refract Surg. 1995;21: 447-52.
24. Borgioli M, Coster DJ, Fan RFT, et al. Effect of heparin surface modification of polymethylmethacrylate intraocular lenses on signs of postoperative inflammation after extracapsular cataract extraction. Ophthalmol. 1992;99: 1248-54.
25. Bourne WM, Kaufman HE. Endothelial damage associated with intraocular lenses. Am J Ophthalmol. 1976;81: 482-5.
26. Boyd W, Peiffer RL, Siegal G, et al. Fibronectin as a component of pseudophakic acellular membranes. J Cataract Refract Surg. 1992;18: 180-83.
27. Brady DG, Giamporcaro JE, Steinert RF. Effect of folding instruments on silicone intraocular lenses. J Cataract Refract Surg. 1994;20: 310-15.
28. Brinen JS, Greenhouse S, Pinatti L. ESCA and SIMS studies of plasma treatments of intraocular lenses. Surf Interface Anal. 1991;17: 63-70.
29. Brint SF, Ostrick DM, Bryan JE. Keratometric cylinder and visual performance following phacoemulsification and implantation with silicone small-incision poly(methyl methacrylate) intraocular lenses. J Cataract Refract Surg. 1991;17: 32-6.
30. Bronner A, Baikoff G, Charleux J, e t al. La correction de l'aphakie, Masson et Cie éditeurs, Paris, 1983;287-9.
31. Bucci FA, Lindstrom Rl. Total pupillary capture with a foldable silicone intraocular lens. Ophthalmic Surg. 1991;22: 414-5.
32. Buchen SY, Richards SC, Solomon KD, et al. Evaluation of the biocompatibility and fixation of a new silicone intraocular lens in the feline model. J Cataract Refract Surg. 1989;15: 545-53.
33. Bucher PJM, Buchi ER, Daicker BC. Dystrophic calcification of an implanted hydroxyethylmethacrylate intraocular lens. Arch Ophthalmol. 1995;113: 1431-5.

34. Carlson KH, Cameron JD, Lindstrom RL. Assessment of the blood-aqueous barrier by fluorophotometry following poly(methyl methacrylate), silicone, and hydrogel lens implantation in rabbit eyes. J Cataract Refract Surg. 1993;19: 9-15.

35. Carlson KH, Johnson DW. Cracking of acrylic intraocular lenses during capsular bag insertion. Ophthalmic Surg Lasers. 1995;26: 572-3.

36. Champetier G, Monnerie L. Introduction à la chimie macro-moléculaire, Masson et Cie éditeurs, Paris, 1969; 505-06.

37. Chapman JM, Cheeks L, Green K. Drug interaction with intraocular lenses of different materials. J Cataract Refract Surg. 1992;18: 456-9.

38. Chasset R, Legeay G, Touraine JC, et al. Fluoration du polyéthylène par plasma froid: mouillabilité, indice d'oxygène, coefficient de frottement. Eur Polym. 1988;24: 1049-55.

39. Chen TT. Clinical experience with soft intraocular lens implantation. J Cataract Refract Surg. 1987;13: 50-53.

40. Chirila TV, Vijayasekaran S, Constable IJ, et al. Melanin-containing hydrogel intraocular lenses: a histopathological study in animal eyes. J Biomater App. 1995;9: 262-74.

41. Chirila TV. Melanized poly (HEMA) hydrogels: basic research and potential use. J Biomater App. 1993;8: 106-45.

42. Christ FR, Buchen SY, Deacon J, et al. Biomaterials used for intraocular lenses. In Wise DL, Trantolo DJ, Altobelli DE et al (Eds): Encyclopedic Handbook of Biomaterials and Bioengineering. Part B. applications Marcel Dekker, InC. New York, 1995;2: 1261-1313.

43. Christ FR, Buchen SY, Fencil A, et al. A comparative evaluation of the biostability of a poly (ether urethane) in the intraocular, intramuscular, and subcutaneous environments. J Biomed Mater Res. 1992;26: 607-29.

44. Christ FR, Fencil DA, Van Gent S, et al. Evaluation of the chemical, optical, and mechanical properties of elastomeric intraocular lens materials and their clinical significance. J Cataract Refract Surg. 1989;15: 176-84.

45. Cobo LM, Ohsawa E, Chandler D, et al. Pathogenesis of capsular opacification after extracapsular cataract extraction; an animal model. Ophthalmol. 1984;91: 857-63.

46. Condon PI. Initial results with the IOGEL 1000 IOL. Eur J Implant Refract Surg. 1994;6: 176.

47. Cook CS, Peiffer RL, Jr, Mazzocco TR. Clinical and pathologic evaluation of a flexible silicone posterior chamber lens design in a rabbit model. J Cataract Refract Surg. 1986;12: 130-34.

48. Cortina P, Gomez-Lechon MJ, Navea A, et al. In vitro test of intraocular lens biocompatibility. Cataract Refract Surg. 1995;21: 112-3.

49. Crawford JB, Faulkner GD. Pathology report on the foldable silicone posterior chamber lens. J Cataract Refract Surg. 1986;12: 297-300.

50. Cumming JS, Ophth FC. Surgical complications and visual acuity results in 536 cases of plate haptic silicone lens implantation. J Cataract Refract Surg. 1993;19: 275-7.

51. Cumming JS. Postoperative complications and uncorrected acuities after implantation of plate haptic silicone and three-piece silicone intraocular lenses. J Cataract Refract Surg. 1993;19: 263-74.

52. Cunanan CM, Tarbaux NM, Knight PM: Surface properties of intraocular lens materials and their influence on in vitro cell adhesion. J Cataract Refract Surg. 1991;17: 767-73.

53. Cusumano A, Busin M, Spitznas M: Bacterial growth is significantly enhanced on foldable intraocular lenses. Arch Ophthalmol. 1994;112: 1015-6.

54. Davison JA. Capsular bag distension after endophacoemulsi-fication and posterior chamber intraocular lens implantation. J Cataract Refract Surg. 1990;16: 99-108.

55. Davison JA. Capsule contraction syndrome. J Cataract Refract Surg. 1993;19: 582-9.

56. Davison JA. Modified insertion technique for the SI-18NB intraocular lens. J Cataract Refract Surg. 1991;17: 849-53.

57. deGottrau P, Chevalley G, Dosso A, et al. Les implants pliables dans la chirurgie de la cataracte à la Clinique Ophtalmologique de Genève. Klin Monastsbl Augenheilkd. 1995;206: 296-9.

58. Dhaliwal DK, Mamalis N, Olson RJ, et al. Visual significance of glistenings seen inthe AcrySof intraocular lens. J Cataract Refract Surg. 1996;22: 452-7.

59. Dick B, Jacobi KW, Kohnen T. Alterations of heparin coating on intraocular lenses caused by implantation instruments. Klin Monatsbl Augenheilkd. 1995;206: 460-66.

60. Dickey JB, Thompson KD, Jay WM: Anterior chamber aspirate cultures after uncomplicated cataract surgery. Am J Ophthalmol. 1991;112: 278-82.

61. Duncker GIW, Westphalen S, Behrendt S. Complications of silicone discs intraocular lenses. J Cataract Refract Surg. 1995;21: 562-6.

62. Egan CA, Kottos PJ, Francis IC, et al. Prospective study of the SI-40NB foldable silicone intraocular lens. J Cataract Refract Surg. 1996;22: 1272-6.

63. Elias HG. MacromoleculeS. Synthesis, Materials and Technology Plenum PresS. New York. 1984;2: 926-7.

64. Eloy R, Parrat D, Due TM, et al. In vitro evaluation of inflammatory cell response after CF4 plasma surface modification of poly(methyl methacrylate) intraocular lenses. J Cataract Refract Surg. 1993;19: 364-70.

65. Fagerholm P, Koul S, Trocmé S. Corneal endothelial protection by heparin and sodium hyaluronate surface coating of PMMA intraocular lenses. Acta Ophthalmol. 1987;65: 110-14.

66. Faulkner GD. Early experience with STAARTM silicone elastic lens implants. J Cataract Refract Surg. 1986;12: 36-9.

67. Faulkner GD. Folding and inserting silicone intraocular lens implants. J Cataract Refract Surg. 1987;13: 678-81.

68. Fishkind WJ. ORC MemoryLensTM: A thermoplastic IOL. In Martin RG, Gills JP, Sanders DR (Eds): Foldable Intraocular Lenses SlacK. Thorofare, 1993;161-77.

69. Fogle JA, Blaydes JE, Fritz KJ, et al. Clinicopathologic observations of a silicone posterior chamber lens in a primate model. J Cataract Refract Surg. 1986;12: 281-4.

70. Francese JE, Pham L, Christ FR. Accelerated hydrolytic and ultraviolet aging studies on SI-18NB and Si20NB silicone lenses. J Cataract Refract Surg. 1992;18: 402-05.

71. Gimbel HV, Neuhann T. Development, advantages, and methods of the continuous circular capsulorhexis technique. J Cataract Refract Surg. 1990;16: 31-7.

72. Gupta A, van Osdel RL. Surface passivated intraocular lens. U.S. Patent No. 4,655,770. Ioptex, InC. California. 1987; 91702.

73. Hansen SO, Tetz MR, Solomon KD, et al. Decentration of flexible loop posterior chamber intraocular lenses in a series of 222 postmortem eyes. Ophthalmol. 1988;95: 344-9.

74. Herzog WR, Peiffer RL, Hill C. Comparison of the effect polymethylmethacrylate and silicone intraocular lenses on rabbit corneal endothelium in vitro. J Cataract Refract Surg. 1987;13: 397-400.

75. Hettlich HJ, Kaufmann R, Harmeyer H, et al. In vitro and in vivo evaluation of a hydrophilized silicone intraocular lens. J Cataract Refract Surg. 1992;18: 140-46.

76. Hettlich HJ, Kaufmann R, Otterbach F, et al. Plasma-induced surface modifications on silicone intraocular lenses; chemical analysis and in vitro characterization. Biomaterials. 1991;12: 521-4.

77. Hoffman AS. Ionizing radiation and gas plasma (or glow) discharge treatments for preparation of novel polymeric biomaterials. In Dusek K (Ed): Advances in Polymer Science Springer-VerlaG. Berlin, 1984;57: 142-57.

78. Hogt AH, Dankert J, Feijen J. Adhesion of coagulase-negative staphylococci to methacrylate polymers and copolymers. J Biomed Mater Res. 1986;20: 533-45.

79. Holladay JT, Ting AC, Koester CJ, et al. Silicone intraocular lens resolution in air and in water. J Cataract Refract Surg. 1988;14: 657-9.

80. Holladay JT, Van Gent S, Ting AC, et al. Silicone intraocular lens power vs temperature. Am J Ophthalmol. 1989;107: 428-9.

81. Humphry RC, Ball SP, Brammall JE, et al. Lens epithelial cells adhere less to HEMA than to PMMA intraocular lenses. Eye. 1991;5: 66-9.

82. Ichijima H, Kobayashi H, Ikada Y. In vitro evaluation of biocompatibility of surface-modified poly(methyl methacrylate) plate rabbit lens epithelial cells. J Cataract Refract Surg. 1992;18: 395-401.

83. Inoue H, Kohama S. Surface photografting of hydrophilic vinyl monomers onto diethyldithiocarbamated polydimethylsiloxane. J Appl Polym Sci. 1984;29: 877-89.

84. Janssen S. Biocompatibility and IOL. Bull Soc belge Ophtalmol. 1992;245: 103-07.

85. Johnson SH, Henderson C. Neodymium: YAG laser damage to VU-absorbing poly (mythyl methacrylate) and UV-absorbinb MMA-HEMA-EGDMA polymer intraocular lens materials. J Cataract Refract Surg. 1991;17: 604-07.

86. Joo CK, Kim JH. Compatibility of intraocular lenses with blood and connective tissue cells measured by cellular deposition and inflammatory response in vitro. J Cataract Refract Surg. 1992;18: 240-46.

87. Kaufman HE, Katz J, Valenti J, et al. Corneal endothelium damage with intraocular lenseS. contact adhesion between surgical materials and tissue. Science. 1977;198: 525-27.

88. Keates RH, Erdey RA, Ringel DM, et al. Seventy-six consecutive cases of IOGEL intraocular lens implants. J Cataract Refract Surg. 1990;16: 47-50.

89. Keates RH, Sall KN, Kreter JK. Effect of the Nd:YAG laser on polymethylmethacrylate, HEMA copolymer, and silicone intraocular materials. J Cataract Refract Surg. 1987;13: 401-09.

90. Kershner RM: In reply tO. Milauskas AT. Silicone intraocular lens implant discoloration in human. Arch Ophthalmol. 1991;109: 913-14.

91. Knight PM: In reply tO. What RH. Discoloration of a silicone intraocular lens 6 weeks after surgery. Arch Ophthalmol. 1991;109: 1494-5.

92. Knorz MC, Lang A, Hsia TC, et al. Comparison of the optical and visual quality of poly(methyl methacrylate) and silicone intraocular lenses. J Cataract Refract Surg. 1993;19: 766-71.

93. Koch DD, Heit LE. Discoloration of silicone intraocular lenses. Arch Ophthalmol. 1992;110: 319-20.

94. Koch DD, Samuelson SW, Dimonie V. Surface analysis of surface-passivated intraocular lenses. J Cataract Refract Surg. 1991;17: 131-8.

95. Koch HR. Lens bisector for silicone intraocular lens removal. J Cataract Refract Surg. 1996;22: 1379-80.

96. Kochounian HH, Kovacs SA, Sy J, et al. Identification of intraocular lens-adsorbed proteins in mammalian in vitro and in vivo systems. Arch Ophthalmol. 1994;112: 395-401.

97. Kochounian HH, Maxwell WA, Gupta A. Complement activation by surface modified poly(methyl methacrylate) intraocular lenses. J Cataract Refract Surg. 1991;17: 139-41.

98. Kohnen S, Ferrer A, Brauweiler P. Visual function in pseudophakic eyes with poly (methyl methacrylate), silicone, and acrylic intraocular lenses. J Cataract Refract Surg. 1996;22: 1303-07.

99. Kohnen T, Jacobi KW, Dick B. Effects of Nd:YAG microexplosions on heparin-coated PMMA intraocular lenses. Ophthalmol. 1995;92: 293-6.

100. Kohnen T, Magdowski G, Koch DD. Scanning electron microscopic analysis of foldable acrylic and hydrogel intraocular lenses. J Cataract Refract Surg. 1996;22: 1342-50.

101. Kohnen T. The variety of foldable intraocular lens materials. J Cataract Refract Surg. 1996;22: 1255-8.

102. Koo EY, Lindsey PS, Soukiasian SH. Bisecting a foldable acrylic intraocular lens for explantation. J Cataract Refract Surg. 1996;22: 1381-2.

103. Korinek P. Nouvelle génération de polymères fluorés. Matériaux et Techniques. 1991;2: 1-3.

104. Kulnig W, Menapace R, Skorpik C, et al. Tissue reaction after silicone and poly(methyl methacrylate) intraocular lens implantatioN. a light and electron microscopy study in a rabbit model. J Cataract Refract Surg. 1989;15: 510-18.

105. Kulnig W, Skorpik C. Optical resolution of foldable intraocular lenses. J Cataract Refract Surg. 1990;16: 211-6.

106. Larm O, Larsson R, Olsson P. A new non-thrombogenic surface prepared by selective covalent binding of heparin via a modified reducing terminal residue. Biomat Med Dev Art Org. 1983;11: 161-73.

107. Larsson R, Selén G, Björklund H, et al. Intraocular PMMA lenses modified with surface-immobilized hepariN. evaluation of biocompatibility in vitro and in vivo. Biomaterials. 1989;10: 511-6.

108. Larsson R, Selén G, Formgren B, et al. Long-term stability of heparin-surface-modified intraocular lenses in vivo. J Cataract Refract Surg. 1992;18: 247-51.

109. Legeais JM, Hallegot P, Chabala J, et al. Trifluorothymidine localization in the rabbit cornea by secondary ion mass spectrometry imaging microanalysis. Cur Eye Res. 1989;8: 971-3.

110. Legeais JM, Legeay G, Werner LP, et al. Teflon AF pour implant intraoculaire. Brevet d'invention INSERM No. FR 9604267, déposé le 04/04/96Paris.

111. Legeais JM, Renard G. La microanalyse en Ophthalmologie. J Fr Ophtalmol. 1991;14: 415-21.

112. Legeais JM, Werner LP, Legeay G, et al. In vivo studies—A fluorocarbon polymer for intraocular lenses. J Cataract Refract Surg. 1998;24: 371-9.

113. Lerman S. Assessing the biostability of intraocular lenses. Lens Eye Toxicity Res. 1992;9: 395-410.

114. Levy JH, Pisacano AM, Anello RD. Displacement of bag-placed hydrogel lenses into vitreous following neodymium: YAG laser capsulotomy. J Cataract Refract Surg. 1990;16: 563-6.

115. Levy JH, Pisacano AM: Initial clinical studies with silicone intraocular implants. J Cataract Refract Surg. 1988;14: 294-8.

116. Liesegang TJ, Bourne WM, Ilstrup DM: Short and long term endothelial cell loss associated with cataract extraction and intraocular lens implantation. Am J Ophthalmol. 1984;97: 32-9.

117. Lin CL, Shieh G, Chou JC, et al. Heparin-surface-modified intraocular lens implantation in patients with glaucoma, diabetes, or uveitis. J Cataract Refract Surg. 1994;20: 550-53.

118. Lindstrom RL. Foldable intraocular lenses. In Steinert RF (Ed): Cataract SurgerY. Technique, Complications and Management WB SaunderS. Philadelphia, 1995;279-94.

119. Lowe KJ, Easty DL. A comparison of 141 polymacon (IOGEL) and 140 poly(methyl methacrylate) intraocular lens implants. Br J Ophthalmol. 1992;76: 88-90.

120. Lundgren B, Holst A, Tärnholm A, et al. Cellular reaction following cataract surgery with implantation of the heparin-surface-modified intraocular lens in rabbits with experimental uveitis. J Cataract Refract Surg. 1992;18: 602-06.

121. Lundgren B, Ocklind A, Holst A, et al. Inflammatory response in the rabbit eye after intraocular implantation with poly(methyl methacrylate) and heparin surface modified intraocular lenses. J Cataract Refract Surg. 1992;18: 65-70.

122. Lundgren B, Selén G, Spangberg M, et al. Fibrinous reaction on implanted intraocular lenses. A comparison of conventional PMMA and heparin surface modified lenses. J Cataract Refract Surg. 1992;18: 236-9.

123. Mackool RJ. Ioptex AcrylensTM acrylic IOL. In Martin RG, Gills JP, Sanders DR (Eds): Foldable Intraocular Lenses. ThorofarE. NJ Slack. 1993;191-7.

124. Marcus DM, Azar D, Boerner C, et al. Pupillary capture of a flexible silicone posterior chamber intraocular lens (letter). Arch Ophthalmol. 1992;110: 609.

125. Martin RG, Sanders DR, van Der Karr MA, et al. Effect of small incision intraocular lens surgery on postoperative inflammation and astigmatism; a study of the AMO SI-18NB small incision lens. J Cataract Refract Surg. 1992;18: 51-7.

126. Martin RG, Sanders DR. Visual, astigmatic, and inflammatory results with the Staar AA-4203 single-piece foldable IOL. a randomized, prospective study. Ophthalmic Surg. 1992;23: 770-75.

127. Mazzocco TR. Early clinical experience with elastic lens implants. Trans Ophthalmol Soc UK. 1985;104: 578-79.

128. Menapace R, Amon M, Radax U. Evaluation of 200 consecutive IOGEl 1103 capsular-bag lenses implanted through a small incision. J Cataract Refract Surg. 1992;18: 252-64.

129. Menapace R, Juchem M, Skorpik C, et al. Clinicopathologic findings after in-the-bag implantation of open-loop polymethylmethacrylate and silicone lenses in the rabbit eye. J Cataract Refract Surg. 1987;13: 630-34.

130. Menapace R, Papapanos P, Radax U, et al. Evaluation of 100 consecutive IOGEL 1003 foldable bag-style lenses implanted through a self-sealing tunnel incision. J Cataract Refract Surg. 1994;20: 432-9.

131. Menapace R, Skorpik C, Wedrich A. Evaluation of 150 consecutive cases of polyHEMA posterior chamber lenses implanted in the bag using a small-incision technique. J Cataract Refract Surg. 1990;16: 567-77.

132. Menapace R, Skorpik Ch, Juchem M, et al. Evaluation of the first 60 cases of polyHEMA posterior chamber lenses implanted in the sulcus. J Cataract Refract Surg. 1989;15: 264-71.

133. Menapace R, Yalon M: Exchange of IOGEL hydrogel one-piece foldable intraocular lens for bag-fixated J-loop poly (methyl methacrylate) intraocular lens. J Cataract Refract Surg. 1993;19: 425-30.

134. Menapace R. Posterior capsule opacification and capsulotomy rates with taco-style hydrogel intraocular lenses. J Cataract Refract Surg. 1996;22: 1318-30.

135. Milauskas AT. Capsular bag fixation of one-piece silicone lenses. J Cataract Refract Surg. 1990;16: 583-6.

136. Milauskas AT. In reply tO. Watt RH. Discoloration of a silicone intraocular lens 6 weeks after surgery. Arch Ophthalmol. 1991;109: 1495.

137. Milauskas AT. Posterior capsule opacification after silicone lens implantation and its management. J Cataract Refract Surg. 1987;13: 644-8.

138. Milauskas AT. Silicone intraocular lens implant discoloration in humans. Arch Ophthalmol . 1991;109: 913-5.

139. Milazzo S, Sigot-Luizard MF, Borhan M, et al. In vitro organotypic culture method to evaluate the biocompatibility of heparin-surface-modified intraocular lenses. J Cataract Refract Surg. 1994;20: 638-42.

140. Milazzo S, Turut P, Blin H. Alterations to the AcrySof intraocular lens during folding. J Cataract Refract Surg. 1996; 22: 1351-4.

141. Miller KM, Grusha YO, Ching ECP. Injecting the Alcon MA30BA lens through a STAAR 1-MTC-45 cartridge. J Cataract Refract Surg. 1996;22: 1132-3.

142. Mondino BJ, Nagata S, Glovsky MM: Activation of the alternative complement pathway by intraocular lenses. Invest Ophthalmol Vis Sci. 1985;26: 905-08.

143. Mondino BJ, Rajacich GM, Summer H. Comparison of complement activation by silicone intraocular lenses and polymethylmethacrylate intraocular lenses with polypropylene loops. Arch Ophthalmol. 1987;105: 989-90.

144. Neuhann T. Theorie and Operationstechnic der Kapsulorhexis. Klin Monatsbl Augenheilkd. 1987;190: 542-5.

145. Neuhann TH. Intraocular folding of an acrylic lens for explantation through a small incision cataract wound. J Cataract Refract Surg. 1996;22: 1383-6.

146. Neumann AC, Cobb B. Advantages and limitations of current soft intraocular lenses. J Cataract Refract Surg. 1989;15: 257-63.

147. Neumann AC, McCarty GR, Osher RH. Complications associated with STAAR silicone implants. J Cataract Refract Surg. 1987;13: 653-6.

148. Neumann AC, McCarty GR, Sanders DR, et al. Small incisions to control astigmatism during cataract surgery. J Cataract Refract Surg. 1989;15: 78-84.

149. Newland TJ, Auffarth GU, Wesendahl TA, et al. Neodymium: YAG laser damage on silicone intraocular lenses. A comparison of lesions on explanted lenses and experimentally produced lesions. J Cataract Refract Surg. 1994;20: 527-33.

150. Newman DA, McIntyre DJ, Apple DJ, et al. Pathologic findings of an explanted silicone intraocular lens. J Cataract Refract Surg. 1986;12: 292-7.

151. Ng EWM, Barrett GD, Bowman R. In vitro bacterial adherence to hydrogel and poly(methyl methacrylate) intraocular lenses. J Cataract Refract Surg. 1996;22: 1331-5.

152. Nishi O, Nishi K. Intraocular lens encapsulation by shrinkage of the capsulorhexis opening. J Cataract Refract Surg. 1993;19: 544-5.

153. Noble BA, Hayward JM, Huber C. Secondary evaluation of hydrogel lens implants. Eye. 1990;4: 450-55.

154. Obstbaum SA. Development of foldable IOL materials (editorial). J Cataract Refract Surg. 1995;21: 233.

155. Obstbaum SA. The Binkhorst Medal Lecture—Biologic relationship between poly (methyl methacrylate) intraocular lenses and uveal tissue. J Cataract Refract Surg. 1992;18: 219-31.

156. Oh KT, Oh KT. Simplified insertion technique for the SI-26NB intraocular lens. J Cataract Refract Surg. 1992;18: 619-22.

157. Oh KT. Optimal folding axis for acrylic intraocular lenses. J Cataract Refract Surg. 1996;22: 667-70.

158. Okada K, Funahashi M, Iseki K, et al. Comparing the cell population on different intraocular lens materials in one eye. J Cataract Refract Surg. 1993;19: 431-4.

159. Omar O, Eng CT, Chang A, et al. Capsular bag distension with an acrylic intraocular lens. J Cataract Refract Surg. 1996;22: 1365-67.

160. Omar O, Mamalis N, Veiga J, et al. Scanning electron microscopic characteristics of small-incision intraocular lenses. Ophthalmol. 1996;103: 1124-9.

161. Oshika T, Shiokawa Y. Effect of folding on the optical quality of soft acrylic intraocular lenses. J Cataract Refract Surg. 1996;22: 1351-4.

162. Oshika T, Suzuki Y, Kizaki H, et al. Two-year clinical study of a soft acrylic intraocular lens. J Cataract Refract Surg. 1996;22: 104-09.

163. Oshika T, Yoshimura K, Miyata N. Postsurgical inflammation after phacoemulsification and extracapsular extraction with soft or conventional intraocular lens implantation. J Cataract Refract Surg. 1992;18: 356-61.

164. Oshika T. Intraoperative complications of foldable IOL. 2. Soft acrylic IOL. Jpn J Clin Ophthalmol. 1995;49: 1614-15.

165. Packard R. European clinical results with the AcrySof IOL. Eur J Implant Refract Surg. 1994;6: 178-9.

166. Packard RBS, Garner A, Arnott EJ. Poly-HEMA as a material for intraocular lens implantatioN. a preliminary report. Br J Ophthalmol. 1981;65: 585-7.

167. Pekna M, Larsson R, Formgren B, et al. Complement activation by polymethylmethacrylate minimized by end-point heparin attachment. Biomaterials. 1993;14: 189-92.

168. Percival P. Capsular bag implantation of the hydrogel lens. J Cataract Refract Surg. 1987;13: 627-9.

169. Percival P. Prospective study comparing hydrogel with PMMA lens implants. Ophthalmic Surg. 1989;20: 255-61.

170. Percival SPB, Jafree AJ. Preliminary results with a new hydrogel intraocular lens. Eye. 1994;8: 672-5.

171. Percival SPB, Pai V. Heparin-modified lenses for eyes at risk for breakdown of the blood-aqueous barrier during cataract surgery. J Cataract Refract Surg. 1993;19: 760-65.

172. Percival SPB. Five-year follow-up of a prospective study comparing hydrogel with PMMA single piece lenses. Eur J Implant Refract Surg. 1994;6: 10-3.

173. Pfister DR. Stress fractures after folding an acrylic intraocular lens. Am J Ophthalmol. 1996;121: 572-4.

174. Philipson B, Fagerholm P, Calel B, et al. Heparin surface modified intraocular lenses. Three-month follow-up of a randomized, double-masked clinical trial. J Cataract Refract Surg. 1992;18: 71-8.

175. Portolés M, Refojo MF, Leong FL. Reduced bacterial adhesion to heparin-surface-modified intraocular lenses. J Cataract Refract Surg. 1993;19: 755-59.

176. Potzsch DK, Losch-Potzsch CM: Four-year follow-up of the MemoryLens. J Cataract Refract Surg. 1996;22: 1336-41.

177. Power WJ, Neylan D, Collum LMT. Adherence of human lens epithelial cells to conventional poly(methyl methacrylate), heparin-surface modified, and polyHema lenses. J Cataract Refract Surg. 1994;20: 440-45.

178. Ravalico G, Baccara F, Lovisato A, et al. Postoperative cellular reaction on various intraocular lens materials. Ophthalmol. 1997;104: 1084-91.

179. Redbrake C, Salla S, Becker J, et al. Immunological reactions against PMMA lens material? Graefe's Arch Clin Exp Ophthalmol. 1993;231: 238-41.

180. Reich S, Levy M, Meshorer A, et al. Intraocular-lens-endothelial interface. adhesive force measurements. J Biomed Mater Res. 1984;18: 737-44.

181. Ridley H. Intraocular acrylic lenses. Trans Ophthalmol Soc UK. 1951;71: 617-21.

182. Saika S, Kobata S, Yamanaka O, et al. Cellular fibronectin on intraocular lenses explanted from patients. Graefe's Arch Clin Exp Ophthalmol. 1993;231: 718-21.

183. Saika S, Tonoe O, Kanagawa R, et al. Immunohistochemical study of deposits on intraocular lenses explanted from human eyes. Jpn J Ophthalmol. 1991;35: 96-101.

184. Saika S, Uenoyama S, Kanagawa R, et al. Phagocytosis and fibronectin of cells observed on intraocular lenses. Jpn J Ophthalmol. 1992;36: 184-91.

185. Sanchez E, Artaria L. Evaluation of the first 50 ACR360 acrylic intraocular lens implantations. J Cataract Refract Surg. 1996;22: 1373-8.

186. Schrage NF, Reim M, Burchard WC, et al. Scanning electron microscopic and energy-dispersive X-ray analysis findings on two brand new intraocular lenses. Ophthalmic Res. 1992;24: 51-4.

187. Shan SM, Spalton DJ. Comparison of the postoperative inflammatory response in the normal eye with heparin-surface-modified and poly(methyl methacrylate) intraocular lenses. J Cataract Refract Surg. 1995;21: 579-85.

188. Shan SM, Spalton DJ. Natural history of cellular deposits on the anterior intraocular lens surface. J Cataract Refract Surg. 1995;21: 466-71.

189. Shephard JR. Induced astigmatism in small incision cataract surgery. J Cataract Refract Surg. 1989;15: 85-8.

190. Shepherd JR. Capsular opacification associated with silicone implants. J Cataract Refract Surg. 1989;15: 448-50.

191. Shepherd JR. Continous-tear capsulotomy and insertion of a silicone bag lens. J Cataract Refract Surg. 1989;15: 335-9.

192. Shugar JK, Lewis C, Lee A. Implantation of multiple foldable acrylic posterior chamber lenses in the capsular bag for high hyperopia. J Cataract Refract Surg. 1996;22: 1368-72.

193. Shugar JK. Implantation of AcrySof acrylic intraocular lenses. J Cataract Refract Surg. 1996;22: 1355-59.

194. Skelnik DL, Lindstrom RL, Allarakhia L, et al. Neodymium: YAG laser interaction with Alcon IOGEL intraocular lenses. an in vitro toxicity assay. J Cataract Refract Surg. 1987;13: 662-8.

195. Skorpik C, Menapace R, Gnad HD, et al. Evaluation of 50 silicone posterior chamber lens implantations. J Cataract Refract Surg. 1987;13: 640-43.

196. Smetana K, Sulc J, Krcoca Z, et al. Intraocular biocompatibility of hydroxyethyl methacrylate and methacrylic acid copolymer partially hydrolyzed poly (2-hydroxy-ethyl methacrylate). J Biomed Mater Res. 1987;21: 1247-53.

197. Spangberg M, Kihlström I, Björklund H, et al. Improved biocompatibility of intraocular lenses by heparin surface modificatioN. a 12-month implantation study in monkeys. J Cataract Refract Surg. 1990;16: 170-77.

198. Steinert RF, Bayliss B, Brint SF, et al. Long-term clinical results of AMO PhacoFlex model SI-18 intraocular lens implantation. J Cataract Refract Surg. 1995;21: 331-8.

199. Steinert RF, Brint SF, White SM, et al. Astigmatism after small incision cataract surgery; a prospective, randomized, multi-center comparison of 4- and 6.5-mm incisions. Ophthalmol. 1991;98: 417-23.

200. Stoy V. Intraocular Lenses. US Patent No. 4,731,079. Kingston TechnologieS. Dayton. 1988;935224.

201. Tamada Y, Ikada Y. Fibroblast growth on polymer surfaces and biosynthesis of collagen. J Biomed Mater Res. 1994;28: 783-89.

202. Tsai JC, Castaneda VE, Apple DJ, et al. Scanning electron microscopic study of modern silicone intraocular lenses. J Cataract Refract Surg. 1992;18: 232-5.

203. Umezawa S, Shimizu K. Biocompatibility of surface-modified intraocular lenses. J Cataract Refract Surg. 1993;19: 371-4.

204. Uyama Y, Ikada Y. Electrostatic properties of UV-irradiated and surface-grafted polymers. J Appll Polym Sci. 1990;41: 619-29.

205. Versura P, Caramazza R. Ultrastructure of cells cultured onto various intraocular lens materials. J Cataract Refract Surg. 1992;18: 58-64.

206. Vrabec MP, Syverud JC, Burgess CJ. Forceps-induced scratching of a foldable acrylic intraocular lens (letter). Arch Ophthalmol. 1996;114: 777.

207. Wasserman D, Apple DJ, Castaneda VE, et al. Anterior capsular tears and loop fixation of posterior chamber intraocular lenses. Ophthalmol. 1991;98: 425-31.

208. Watt RH. Discoloration of a silicone intraocular lens 6 weeks after surgery. Arch Ophthalmol. 1991;109: 1494.

209. Watts MT, Pearce JL. Implantation of a disc lens in the capsular bag. Ophthalmic Surg. 1988;19: 546-8.

210. Weghaupt H, Menapace R, Wedrich A. Functional vision with hydrogel versus PMMA lens implants. Graefe's Arch Clin Exp Ophthalmo. 1993;231: 449-52.

211. Werner LP, Legeais JM, Durand J, et al. Endothelial damage produced by uncoated and fluorocarbon-coated polymethyl-methacrylate intraocular lenses. J Cataract Refract Surg. 1997;23: 1013-9.

212. Werner LP, Legeais JM: Les matériaux pour implants intra-oculaires. Partie I. Les implants intraoculaires en polymé-thylmétacrylate et modifications de surface. J Fr Ophthalmol. 1998;21: 515-24.

213. Werner LP, Legeais JM: Les matériaux pour implants intraoculaires. Partie II. Les implants en silicone. J Fr Ophthalmol. 1999;22: 492-512.

214. Wolter JR. Cytopathology of intraocular lens implantation. Ophthalmol. 1985;92: 135-42.

215. Zeigler JM, Fearon FWG. Silicon-based polymer science. A comprehensive resource. American Chemical Society, Washington DC, 1990.

216. Zetterström C. Incidence of posterior capsule opacification in eyes with exfoliation syndrome and heparin-surface-modified intraocular lenses. J Cataract Refract Surg. 1993;19: 344-7.

217. Ziemba SL. In reply to. Milauskas AT. Silicone intraocular lens implant discoloration in humans. Arch Ophthalmol. 1991;109: 914-5.

CHAPTER 33

Premium IOLs

Amar Agarwal

INTRODUCTION

Premium IOLs form a very important part of cataract refractive surgery today. Hyperopia is a form of refractive error in which parallel rays of light are brought to focus at some distance behind the sentient layer of the retina, when the eye is at rest. The image formed is therefore made up of circles of diffusion of considerable size and consequently blurred.[1] The hyperopic eye is small, the anterior chamber shallow and is predisposed to angle closure glaucoma. Patients with hyperopia, depending on their age and magnitude of refractive error, are unable to see clearly both at distance and near. This problem aggravates, as they approach the presbyopic age. The increase in plus lenses leads to spherical aberrations.

ALTERNATE TREATMENTS

Various surgical procedures were developed over the years to correct hyperopia including keratophakia, hexagonal keratotomy, automated lamellar keratoplasty (ALK), thermal keratoplasty, photorefractive keratectomy(PRK) and laser in situ keratomileusis (LASIK).[2] Significant regression, poor predictability and instability have been the bugbears of hyperopic refractive surgeries. Hexagonal keratotomy was fraught with poor wound healing, corneal edema and irregular astigmatism.[3] Thermal keratoplasty causes regression to pre-treatment steepness of the central cornea.[2, 4] Fyodorov's radial thermokeratoplasty causes damage to corneal endothelium. Holmium:YAG laser thermokeratoplasty causes regression.[5,6] Lamellar procedures include keratophakia, cryolathe keratomileusis, epikeratophakia, ALK and excimer laser PRK and LASIK.[2] Keratophakia caused induced keratometric astigmatism.[7] Epikeraophakia led to regression and problems with the cryolathe.[8, 9] PRK for hyperopia used large optical zones with attendant adverse effects.[10] ALK has been found to be unpredictable and caused ectasia in a few cases. LASIK has been tried for hyperopia with better predictability, less regression, less corneal haze than PRK. Posterior chamber phakic IOLs have been tried to treat hyperopia. The results support short-term safety, efficacy and stability with surgical implantable contact lens.[11] Iris-claw lens has been used in phakic eyes, but observation with specular microscopy is mandatory.[12] Clear lens extraction with posterior chamber IOL implantation for hyperopia has been proposed as an alternative treatment.

SURGICAL PROCEDURE

The eye is prepared for surgery with cyclopentolate hydrochloride 1% and phenylephrine 5% eye drops, 1 drop every 10 minutes 1 hour before surgery.[13] Routine cleaning and draping of the eyes is done. The approach used is temporal clear corneal. If the axis is plus at 90 degrees then a superior incision is made. The anterior chamber is entered through the side port through clear cornea with a 26 G needle and viscoelastic Hydroxypropylmethyl cellulose 2% injected. A temporal clear corneal incision is made of 3.2 mm width with a sapphire knife. A continuous curvilinear capsulorhexis is made with a bent 26 G needle mounted on a viscoelastic syringe. Hydrodissection is then done. Nucleus is emulsified and the remaining cortex aspirated. Peripheral iridectomy is done if the angles are found to be occludable. One 10-0 nylon suture can be used to close the tunnel if there is shallowing of the anterior chamber. This can be removed after a week.

TIPS

- It is very essential that one uses the air pump as gas forced infusion helps deepen the anterior chamber. This will prevent endothelial damage.
- It is better to do these complex cases under a peribulbar block as once again the pressure might be high and if operating under a block the vitreous pressure will not be that high.
- Use a suture to close the wound if necessary.
- Do an iridectomy by using a vitrectomy probe.
- Be careful of biometry. Whatever the reading comes in a high hyperope implant an IOL at least 2 dioptres higher. If it comes okay postoperatively fine otherwise if it comes myopic, then when one is doing the other eye, one adjusts the IOL power accordingly to make the other eye emmetropic. This way patient will be able to read and see distance without glasses.

LENSES

Various lenses can be implanted in the eye. Alcon has their multifocal IOL which is a single-piece acrylic lens under the name ReStor (Figure 33.1). Pharmacia/Pfizer has also designed a diffractive multifocal IOL, the Ceeon 811E that has been combined with the wavefront adjusted optics of the Technis Z9000 with the expectation of improved quality

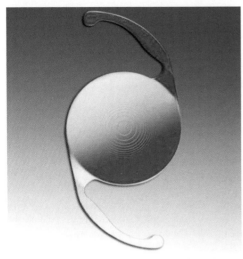

FIGURE 33.1: The Alcon ReStor multifocal IOL (*Courtesy* of Alcon Laboratories)

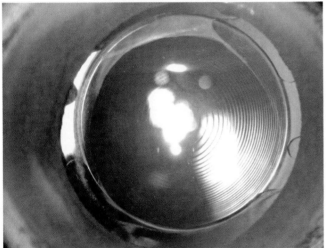

FIGURE 33.2: The Tecnis ZM001 multifocal IOL (*Courtesy:* Dr Agarwal's Eye Hospital, India)

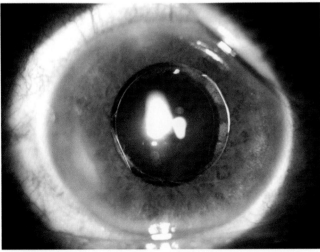

FIGURE 33.3: The Eyeonics Crystalens accommodating IOL (*Courtesy:* Dr Agarwal's Eye Hospital, India)

of vision in addition to multifocal optics **(Figure 33.2)**. The two accommodative IOLs that have received the most investigation to date are the Model AT-45 CrystaLens

(Figure 33.3) (Eyeonics, Aliso Viejo, California) and the 1 CU (Humanoptics, Mannheim, Germany). The new lens which is accommodating is the Synchrony IOL from AMO.

One of the most exciting technologies is the light adjustable lens (LAL) (Calhoun Vision, Pasadena, California). The LAL is designed to allow for postoperative refinements of lens power in situ. The current design of the LAL is a foldable three-piece IOL with a cross-linked silicone polymer matrix and a homogeneously embedded photosensitive macromer. The application of near-ultraviolet light to a portion of the lens optic results in polymerization of the photosensitive macromers and precise changes in lens power through a mechanism of macromer migration into polymerized regions and subsequent changes in lens thickness.

DISCUSSION

The refractive surgical correction of hyperopia has lagged far behind the advances that have occurred in the treatment of myopia and astigmatism. Clear lens extraction for the correction of high myopia is a concept known since at least 1800. After the invention of sterilization, clear lens extraction for myopia was done by Fukala and Vacher.[14]

The hyperopic eye with a smaller axial length, small anterior chamber and small corneal diameter is more vulnerable to intra-operative and post-operative complications. However, clear lens extraction with IOL implantation for hyperopia is considered to have same safety and efficacy as modern small incision cataract techniques, except in extremely hyperopic eyes like nanophthalmos. For presbyopic hyperopes, clear lens extraction with IOL implantation has a great appeal.[15]

There have been various studies of clear lens extraction for hyperopia in the last decade. In the study of Siganos et al using the SRK II formula for IOL power calculation, 100% of the eyes were within ± 1.0 D of emmetropia.[16] It was found to be a safe, effective procedure for the treatment of hyperopia from + 6.75 D to + 13.75 D. The SRK II formula proved superior to the SRK-T formula for IOL power calculation.[16] In the study of Lyle et al. 89% of the patients achieved 20/40 or better UCVA, all eyes had 20/25 or better BCVA. IOL power was calculated using Holladay formula, as it reduced the chance of postoperative residual hyperopia.[17] They found that this method was less accurate for hyperopia less than + 3.0 D.[17] Isfahani et al. reported the safety of clear lens extraction for the correction of hyperopia. They have reported a close association between achieved spherical equivalence and predicted spherical equivalence, using the Holladay Consultant formula for IOL power calculation. They have suggested that clear lensectomy is superior for the correction of moderate to high hyperopia in patients aged 35 or older. They reported postoperative malignant glaucoma in one nanophthalmic eye and recommended peripheral surgical iridectomies in all eyes with axial length less than 20 mm.[18]

In our study, 12 (60%) of the eyes achieved BCVA of more than 20/40. Clear lens extraction was done in amblyopic eyes also. Three patients achieved the intended refraction, whereas 16 (80%) eyes were within + 1.0 D of the intended refraction. We use the Holladay 2 formula for the IOL power calculation. The Holladay, Hoffer Q and SRK-T formulas are better than the older formulas for hyperopia. Hyperopic eyes with shallower anterior chambers are more prone to angle closure. All eyes in our series underwent gonioscopic evaluation preoperatively and surgical peripheral iridectomies were done in 5 eyes (25%) with occludable angles. We recommend preoperative gonioscopy in all patients who undergo clear lens extraction for hyperopia.

NANOPHTHALMOS

Such eyes are more prone to intraoperative and postoperative complications, like uveal effusion, retinal detachment, intraocular hemorrhage and malignant glaucoma. Foldable piggy-back IOLs may be required in such nanophthalmic eyes. Piggy-back IOLs in the bag have been associated with interlenticular pseudophakic opacification and a hyperopic shift.[19] Hence, one IOL must be placed in the bag and the other in the sulcus to avoid interlenticular pseudophakic opacification. In our study, the dioptric power of IOL ranged from +27 to +37 D. Eyes requiring more than +30 D were implanted with PMMA IOLs. The author did not implant Piggy-back IOLs in his series, as higher power IOLs are now available. However, PMMA IOL would require a larger incision thereby negating the advantages of a watertight environment which is particularly desirable in small eyes, especially nanophthalmic eyes.

SUMMARY

LASIK has been suggested as an alternative modality for hyperopia correction. But Ditzen and colleagues suggested preoperative corneal radius to be an important factor.[20] There was increased incidence of under-corrections and epithelial in-growth with hyperopia especially more than 6.0 D, due to problems with the suction ring and the microkeratome.[11] Regression and under-correction have been reported as major concern in LASIK for hyperopia. Goker et al. reported a regression and under-correction of more than 2.00 D in 12.9% eyes which underwent LASIK for hyperopia.[21] Lack of a special nomogram to achieve results comparable to LASIK for myopia was pointed out in study by Tabbara et al.[22] Postoperative glare is a common side-effect.[23] Dry eye, particularly in females, was reported after LASIK for hyperopia, which was associated with refractive regression.[24] Thus, choice of LASIK for correction of hyperopia should be made with caution.

Clear lens extraction with IOL implantation is a safe and effective procedure for the correction of hyperopia with minimal complications, especially in patients in the presbyopic age group. But care should be taken while doing surgery in nanophthalmic eyes. Further refinement is needed in the calculation of the IOL power in patients with hyperopia

REFERENCES

1. Abrams D. Hypermetropia. Duke-Elder's Practice of Refraction. 10th edition, B.I.Churchill Livingstone; 1997. p. 45.
2. Schallorn SC, Mcdonnell PJ. History and overview of refractive surgery. In: Krachmer JH, Mannis MJ, Holland EJ (Eds). Cornea. Mosby; 1997. pp. 1986-96.
3. Grandon SC, Sanders DR, Anello RD, et al. Clinical evaluation of hexagonal keratotomy for treatment of primary hyperopia. J Cataract Refract Surg. 1995;21(2):140-9.
4. Neumann AC, Sanders D, Raanan M, et al. Hyperopic Thermokeratoplasty: clinical evaluation. J Cataract Refract Surg. 1991;17(6):830-8.
5. Thomson VM, Seiler T, Durrie DS, et al. Holmium: YAG laser thermokeratoplasty for hyperopia and astigmatism: an overview. Refract Corneal Surg 1993;9(2):S134-7.
6. Nano HD, Muzzin S. Noncontact Holmium:YAG laser thermal keratoplasty for hyperopia. J Cataract Refract Surg. 1998; 24(6):751-7.
7. Villasenor RA. Keratophakia Long term results. Ophthalmology 1983;90(6):673-5.
8. Werblin TP, Blaydes JE. Epikeratophakia: existing limitations and future modifications. Aust J Ophthalmol 1983;11(3):201-7.
9. Ehrlich MI, Nordan LT. Epikeratophakia for the treatment of hyperopia. J Cataract Refract Surg. 1989;15(6):661-6.
10. Dausch D, Smecka Z, Klein R, et al. Excimer laser photorefractive keratectomy for hyperopia. J Cataract Refract Surg. 1997;23(2):169-76.
11. Sanders DR, Martin RG, Brown DC, et al. Posterior chamber phakic intraocular lenses for hyperopia. J Refract Surg. 1999;15(3):309-15.
12. Fechner PU, Singh D, Wulff K. Iris-claw lens in phakic eyes to correct hyperopia: Preliminary study. J Cataract Refract Surg. 1998;24(1):48-56.
13. Boyd B. IOL power calculation in standard and complex cases-Preparing for surgery. The art and science of cataract surgery.In: Boyd B (Ed). Highlights of Ophthalmology. Coral Gables; 2001. pp. 47-8.
14. Seiler T. Clear lens extraction in the 19th century - an early demonstration of premature dissemination. J Refract Surg. 1999;15(1):70-3.
15. Kohnen T. Advances in the surgical correction of hyperopia. From the Editor. J Cataract Refract Surg. 1998;24(1):1-2.
16. Siganos DS, Pallikaris IG. Clear lensectomy and intraocular lens implantation for hyperopia from +7 to +14 Diopters. J Refract Surg. 1998;14(2):105-13.
17. Lyle WA, Jin GJ. Clear lens extraction to correct hyperopia. J Cataract Refracr Surg. 1997;23(7):1051-6.
18. Isfahani AH, Rostamian K, Wallace D, et al. Clear lens extraction with intraocular lens implantation for hyperopia. J Refract Surg. 1999;15(5):316-23.
19. Shugar JK, Schwartz T. Interpseudophakos Elschnig's pearls associated with late hyperopic shift: a complication of piggy-back posterior chamber intraocular lens implantation. J Cataract and Refract Surg. 1999;25:863-7.
20. Ditzen K, Huschka H, Pieger S. Laser in situ keratimileusis for hyperopia. J Cataract Refract Surg. 1998;24(1):42-7.

21. Göker S , Er H, Kahvecioglu C. Laser in situ keratomileusis to correct hyperopia from +4.25D to +8.00D. J Refract Surg 1998; 14(1):26-30.

22. Tabbara KF, El-Sheikh, Islam SM. Laser in situ keratomileusis for the correction of hyperopia from +0.50 to +11.50D with the Keracor 117C laser. J Refract Surg. 2001;17(2): 123-8.

23. Procházková S, Kuchynka P, Novák P , et al. Treatment of intermediate hypermetropia using laser in situ keratomilieusis – retrospective study (1995-1999). Cesk Slov Oftalmol. 2001; 57(1):17-21.

24. Albeitz JM, Lenton LM, Mclean SG. Effect of laser in situ keratomileusis for hyperopia on tear film and ocular surface. J Refract Surg. 2002;18(2):113-23.

CHAPTER 34

Correction of Astigmatism with Toric IOL Implants—Practical Aspects

Christopher Khng

INTRODUCTION AND OVERVIEW

The increasing popularity of phacoemulsification and the reality of intraocular lens delivery through small incisions have led to improved predictability in the refractive outcomes of cataract surgery. This has spurred research into intraocular lenses that deal with the refractive aspects of cataract surgery and in particular the development of toric intraocular lens implants.

Astigmatism correction may be required in an estimated 15–29% of cataract cases.[1,2] This correction may be achieved by the use of toric IOLs, limbal relaxing incisions or astigmatic keratotomies, keratorefractive surgery or by the use of conductive keratoplasty (CK-A).

Toric IOL usage offers the advantages of same surgery convenience, efficacy, reproducibility and long-term stability. Currently, two popular methods for the correction of astigmatism during cataract surgery are toric IOL implants and limbal relaxing incisions (LRI).

CURRENT TORIC IOL MODELS

A few toric IOLs which are currently available include the Alcon Toric SN60T series 3-9 and the aspheric SN6AT series, the STAAR Toric, the Zeiss AT TORBI, and the Rayner T-Flex toric IOL, all of which are designed for capsular bag placement.

The Sulcoflex Toric (for sulcus placement) series from Rayner allows for touch up corrections in the event of unexpected astigmatism following cataract surgery.

PROBLEMS WITH TORIC IOLS

Toric IOLs have not always had a problem-free history. The silicone plate haptic STAAR Toric IOL (AA4203 TF and AA4203 TL) has been reported to rotate away from the axis of placement in the early postoperative period.[3,4] This problem of rotation has been overcome by the use of a tacky hydrophobic acrylic material in the Alcon AcrySof Toric IOL.[5] This tacky material results in increased adherence between the IOL and the capsular bag, reducing the likelihood of a postoperative misalignment.

Due to this problem with rotation, a few techniques have been introduced to reduce the likelihood of rotation with the STAAR Toric IOL. One method is to insert the lens back to front so that the lens alignment hash marks normally located on the front of the lens is now pressed against posterior capsule to reduce the risk of rotation. This causes a loss of about 0.25 D of spherical power with a slight hyperopic shift in refraction. Another approach to prevent postoperative rotation when using the STAAR Toric lens is to always choose the longer "TL" lens for a more snug fit.

The popularity of toric IOLs is the result of their relative ease of incorporation into a standard cataract routine. However, they may be more difficult to use correctly because of the necessity for careful attention to the choice of toric correction power and axis of orientation.

INDICATIONS FOR ASTIGMATISM CORRECTION WITH TORIC IOL

Modern phacoemulsification is now almost astigmatically neutral since incisions have gone down in size under 3 mm. Eyes in which the corneal astigmatism is at least 1 dioptre, and where the two major meridians of power are 90 degress apart (regular astigmatism) are candidates for implantation with the toric IOL. To ensure that the astigmatism is regular, corneal topography should ideally be obtained. If the surgeon does not have a topographer available to his disposal, one can be confident that the astigmatism is predominantly regular if the refractive cylinder corresponds to corneal cylinder and is correctable by spectacle lenses, leading to a good level of best corrected acuity.

TORIC IOL OR LIMBAL RELAXING INCISIONS (LRI)?

The two most common methods of correcting astigmatism at the time of cataract surgery are with toric IOLs or LRIs. Surgeons who are proficient with the technique of LRI may question the necessity of going to the extra expense of using a toric IOL, especially when the amount of astigmatism to be corrected is under 2 D. However, there are some clear advantages in the choice of a toric IOL.

No matter how precise the LRI, it is unlikely to equal the accuracy, precision of correction or optical quality of a toric IOL produced by modern manufacturing processes.

LRIs structurally damage and weaken the cornea and may adversely affect the integrity of the globe in case it is injured by blunt trauma. Toric IOLs do not physically weaken the eye.

The LRIs may induce a change in the spherical equivalent of the eye, especially if the incisions are longer, as needed for higher amounts of astigmatism. Incisions placed further from the limbus nearer the visual axis may also induce irregular astigmatism and higher order aberrations.

LRIs are based on a nomogram, which is how the average cornea behaves when incised. This therefore affects the predictability of the correction in non-average eyes.

The effect of the LRI may also be affected by healing of the incision over time, with possible loss of effect. Toric IOLs are not affected by any of these problems and therefore have better predictability and stability with time.

Incision gape caused by LRIs may be felt by patients as a foreign body sensation. The same incisions may also contribute to dry eye syndrome by transecting nerve fibers in the corneal nerve plexus as they enter from the long ciliary nerves, especially where the incisions are placed on the horizontal axis such as in correction of against-the-rule astigmatism.

Corneal perforations are uncommon with LRIs if on-axis pachymetry has been performed or the corneal thickness noted from an Orbscan or similar reading. However, the possibility of it occurring is always present.

ADVANTAGES OF TORIC IOL OVER LRI

• Predictability
• Stability
• Reduced likelihood of foreign body sensation
• Reduced risk of dry eye syndrome
• No corneal weakening—may be important in the event of severe blunt eye trauma
• Correction nearer to the nodal point of the eye
• Dangers of perforation for LRI.

DISADVANTAGES

• Added cost of IOL
• Not as straightforward to implant as standard IOL.

CALCULATION OF TORIC IOL POWER AND PLACEMENT AXIS

The important point to remember when implanting a toric IOL is that the spherical equivalent of the toric lens is identical to that of a spherical IOL of the same dioptric power. During selection of a toric IOL, biometry is done in the surgeon's usual preferred way and the IOL constant is input for the preferred toric IOL model. A printout is then obtained and the desired refractive error outcome chosen together with the corresponding lens implant (spherical equivalent) dioptric power. For example, when

a 20.0 D lens implant would normally be chosen for a –0.5 D refractive error based on biometry, a toric lens with a spherical equivalent of 20.0 D is required.

The next step is to determine the keratometric cylinder amount and axis. To simplify calculations, Alcon has come up with an easy-to-use website where the correct AcrySof Toric IOL model (e.g. SN60T5) is recommended together with an indication of the correct IOL placement axis.

To use this website, one first selects whether the spherical toric (SN60T series) or aspheric toric (SN6AT series) model is to be used. Then one enters data into the fields for the eye to be operated, flat K value and axis, steep K value and axis, the IOL spherical power to achieve the desired refractive error, the surgeon's surgically induced astigmatism and incision location. This generates an output (**Figure 34.1**) recommending the appropriate AcrySof Toric IOL model (e.g. SN60T5) and a diagram that can be brought into the operating room showing the axis of IOL placement and the incision location. The printout also generates a figure for the expected residual astigmatism amount and axis, which is useful to know. The Alcon Toric IOL calculator can be found at www.acrysoftoriccalculator.com.

If one chooses to do the IOL selection manually, then it is useful to remember that for the Alcon AcrySof Toric series of IOLs, the T3 corrects 1.0 D at the corneal plane, the T4 corrects 1.5 D, the T5 corrects 2.0 D and so on with an increase of 0.5 D with each higher T model till the T9 which corrects approximately 4.0 D.

One then looks at the patient's keratometry readings to determine the amount of corneal astigmatism by subtracting the corneal power of the flat axis (e.g. 43.25 D@13) from the power of the steep corneal axis (e.g. 44.75 D@103). This leads to the amount of the corneal astigmatism that should be corrected (e.g. 1.50 D). An IOL is chosen based on this power and the amount of expected residual cylinder that the surgeon will accept. In this example, the surgeon might consider the SN60T4 for correction of 1.50 D.

During surgery, the toric IOL flat axis (indicated by the three dots near each haptic insertion) (**Figure 34.2**) is then aligned to coincide with the steep corneal axis (103 in this example) to neutralize the astigmatism. It is extremely important that the surgeon does not make an error with the axis of placement or the resultant astigmatism will roughly be double what the eye started out with.

The K readings may be obtained by manual keratometer, auto-K or IOL-Master K.

SURGICAL TECHNIQUE FOR IMPLANTATION

CORNEAL REFERENCE MARKING

As the toric IOL is aligned relative to the corneal reference marks, care should be taken to ensure that they are placed correctly on the cardinal meridians. An accurate way to

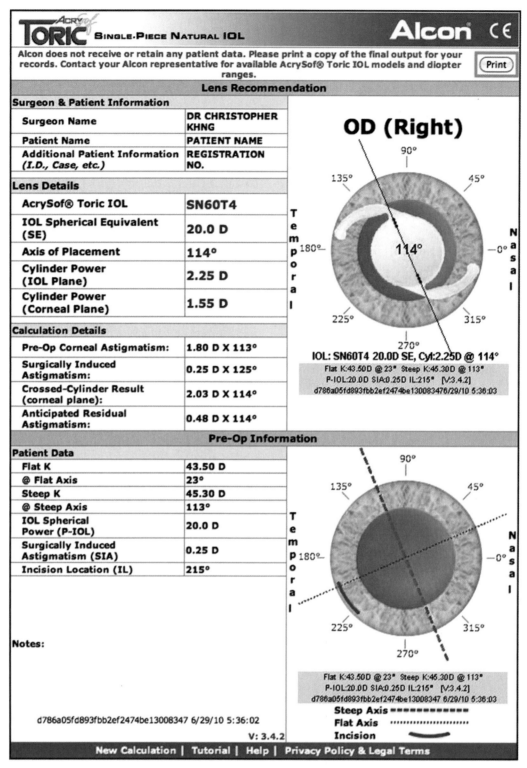

FIGURE 34.1: Printout from Alcon web calculator

mark either the horizontal or vertical axis is to mark the patient while seated upright at the slit lamp. The slit beam is narrowed and positioned to cut across the pupil center in the chosen axis. A fine tipped gentian violet marker pen is then used to dot where the slitbeam intersects with the limbus near each end of the beam.

A variety of reference marking instruments has been designed to help in achieving improved accuracy with the markings (**Figures 34.3 and 34.4**). All of these should be

used while the patient is seated upright, as it is suggested[6] that some eyes undergo appreciable amounts of cyclotorsion when changing from the upright to the recumbent position, thus partially invalidating the purpose of those markings.

In addition to the corneal reference markers, a variety of toric markers that help to indicate the axis that the IOL should be aligned with are readily available.

Blotchy ink marks should be avoided, as they reduce the accuracy of the marks. It might be better to use a fine point

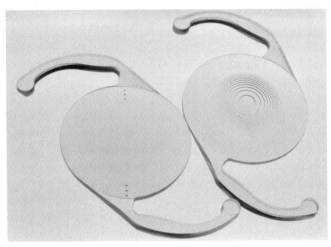

FIGURE 34.2: Alcon AcrySof Toric IOL (left) showing alignment dots

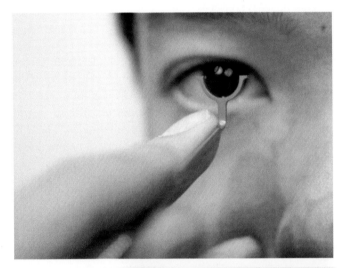

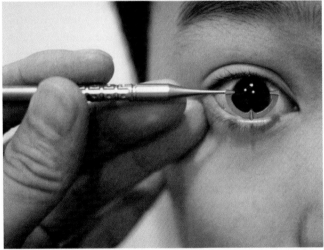

FIGURES 34.3 and 34.4: Corneal reference markers for marking cardinal meridians

remain visible long enough to be useful for alignment during IOL implantation.

Once the IOL alignment marks have been made on the cornea phacoemulsification may proceed as usual. Care should be taken to ensure that the capsulorhexis is centered, round and slightly smaller than the IOL optic so that the refractive outcome is predictable. ***Cortical cleanup*** should also be completed and ***polishing of the anterior and posterior capsules*** performed to minimize capsular bag shrinkage, which can adversely affect the refractive outcome.

The IOL can then be injected into the viscoelastic filled capsular bag. Once the IOL is fully unfolded, it is then rotated (counter clockwise) to be about 15 degrees short of the intended axis**.**

TWO-COMPARTMENT VISCOELASTIC REMOVAL TECHNIQUE TO PREVENT IOL ROTATION

A cohesive viscoelastic may be preferred over a dispersive so that complete viscoelastic removal may be more readily obtained. This should reduce the likelihood of retained dispersive material between IOL and posterior capsule at the end of surgery, which can prevent proper IOL seating and make a rotation more likely. Viscoelastic is first removed from behind the IOL and then from the front of the lens and the anterior chamber using IA. Once all viscoelastic has been cleared with the IA handpiece tip, the IOL is then rotated so that last 15 degrees (clockwise) to be on axis. Care has to be taken that the final alignment is only made when the eye is straight on and coaxial with the microscope view to avoid parallax errors when aligning the IOL. Usually one can avoid these errors by ensuring that the corneal reflex from the microscope light and the Purkinje reflexes off the IOL are all aligned, and the IOL plane is perpendicular to the axis of light travel. Sometimes this final alignment is more easily achieved by using the Sinskey hook to dial the IOL through the side port while the IA tip is in the main incision with the infusion on. Occasionally one will rotate too far in the clockwise direction and this will necessitate a further, almost 180 degrees to come on axis again. The AcrySof Toric will not permit easy counter clockwise rotation to correct an over rotation because of the tacky material and splaying open of the haptics when the IOL is rotated counter clockwise, increasing its adherence to the peripheral capsule. One possible way to avoid rotating another 180 degrees is to engage and pull in one of the haptics centrally with a Sinskey hook through the side port and then rotating the IOL counter clockwise while keeping the capsular bag fully distended with fluid pressure from the IA. This maneuver will generally allow about 15–25 degrees of backward rotation.

Once the lens is in proper alignment, the capsular bag is left slightly underinflated to allow it to "mold" to the posterior surface of the IOL to discourage inadvertent further rotation. The IOL is then gently tapped with the tip

like an inked tip of a Sinskey hook rather than a felt pen tip if possible. However, if using a pen, care has to be taken to ensure that the pen is held vertically enough so that only the extreme tip (and so the finest point) of the pen comes into contact with the cornea. The cornea should be left to dry out a bit before the corneal marks are made so that they

TABLE 34.1 Rotational misalignment effects

IOL rotational misalignment	10 deg	20 deg	30 deg	>30 deg
Loss of astigmatism effect	33%	66%	100% (but 90 degree axis change)	Adds astigmatism

of the IA or Rycroft cannula against the posterior capsule to gently "seat" it. Rotational misalignment of the IOL has a deleterious effect on the astigmatism correction, so care should be taken to prevent it **(Table 34.1)**.

During surgery, adequate pupil dilatation should be maintained to allow proper visualization of the alignment markings on the toric IOL. Pupil constriction, if desired, can be deferred to the last stage of the procedure after sealing the main and side port incisions. Deferring pupil constriction to the very end can alert the surgeon to inadvertent lens rotation resulting from shallowing of the chamber from improperly sealed incisions.

IMPORTANT SURGICAL POINTS

- CCC must be precise
- Total cortical cleanup
- Polishing anterior and posterior capsules
- 2-compartment removal of viscoelastic
- Avoid parallax errors during IOL alignment
- Make sure incisions sealed to prevent shallowing of chamber and lens movement and rotation.

MANAGING RESIDUAL ASTIGMATISM

If residual refractive astigmatism is present following toric IOL implantation, this amount may be left alone if it is not visually significant. If the astigmatism's magnitude is greater than anticipated, then an assessment of the amount of IOL rotation has to be made. If there is any malrotation, the decision of whether to go back into reposition the IOL depends on the amount of astigmatism, the patient's symptoms and level of visual acuity, the amount of angular misalignment, the toric power of the IOL and the patient's acceptance of other methods of visual correction such as toric contact lenses or glasses. One would be more inclined to surgically correct a malrotation if it is more than 10 degrees, the IOL is of a higher toric power, or the astigmatism magnitude is more than 0.75 D. If there is no significant IOL rotation and yet the astigmatism is of sufficient magnitude to bother the patient then it can be dealt with by excimer laser, touch up LRI, conductive keratoplasty (CK-A) or sulcus piggyback IOL (e.g. Rayner Sulcoflex Toric).

MANAGING TORIC IOL ROTATIONAL MISALIGNMENT

If a rotational misalignment has occurred which has required surgical correction, it may be prudent to wait for

a week before performing the correction. The one-week timing is chosen to allow easy capsular bag reopening and lens repositioning and to allow some capsular bag shrinkage to occur in order to minimize the probability of a malrotation occurring again. Some "malrotations" are the result of inaccurate corneal marking and intraoperative IOL alignment rather than subsequent rotation in the early postoperative period, so it is imperative that these are checked thoroughly the second time around. A cohesive viscoelastic is injected into the anterior chamber and used to open the capsular bag after the IOL alignment markings have been made. Once the capsular bag has been reopened, the IOL is rotated into alignment and care must be taken to observe that the same steps, as mentioned earlier to prevent inadvertent rotation, are followed.

SPECIAL SITUATIONS

- Very high corneal astigmatism
- Combining LRI with Toric IOL.

In patients with very high corneal cylinder, a toric IOL (of the maximum toric power, currently Alcon AcrySof SN60T9 correcting 4 D at the corneal plane) may be combined with astigmatic keratotomies or LRIs to reduce the amount of postoperative refractive cylinder. The AK or LRI may be done at the primary surgery or deferred to a later date as a staged procedure. It is important in such eyes for corneal topography to be done and a detailed slit-lamp examination to exclude keratoconus.

HOW DOES ONE CALCULATE RELATIVE AMOUNTS OF EACH CORRECTION?

If a combined "bioptic" approach is required, then usually the highest toric IOL power is used and the remaining power is what needs to be corrected by the second modality. For example, if a toric IOL and LRI are required to correct 5.5 D of corneal cylinder, the highest toric powered IOL (SN60T9) currently of 4 D (corneal plane) is chosen. This leaves 1.5 D of cylinder, which can then be corrected by LRI along the same axis as the toric IOL.

Keratorefractive surgery can be combined with toric IOL, either as touch up procedure or as planned procedures for higher amounts of astigmatism.

LASIK can be used following toric IOL implantation to effectively correct residual astigmatism. Alternatively, conductive keratoplasty-astigmatism (CK-A) may also be employed. It is important to remember that while using CK-A, the correct axis of correction is the *FLAT* axis, as CK *steepens* on the corrected axis as opposed to all the other techniques that flatten on the corrected axis.

COMBINING TORIC IOLS

In-the-bag, placement of a toric IOL may be combined with a sulcus-placed toric IOL. The Rayner Sulcoflex Toric is ideal for such a situation and has been designed for

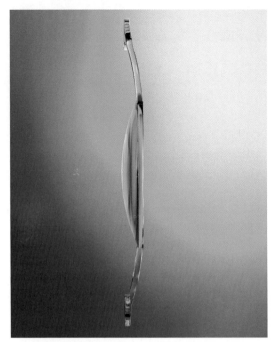

FIGURE 34.5: Profile view of Sulcoflex Toric

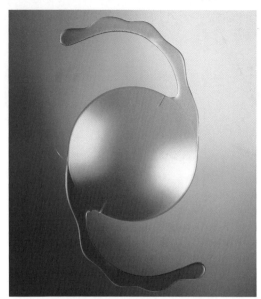

FIGURE 34.6: Rayner Sulcoflex Toric

placement in the sulcus. This IOL has been designed with a posterior concave surface to avoid contact with the primary IOL and capsular bag and an anterior convex surface, and is extremely thin to fit into the ciliary sulcus **(Figure 34.5)**. The optic size is 6.5 mm and overall length is 13.5 mm **(Figure 34.6).** It can be implanted with an injector system through a 2.8 mm incision. This sulcus placed IOL lends itself well also to "touch-up" astigmatism correction for residual amounts of cylinder.

In conclusion, toric IOLs are an excellent option for the correction of astigmatism when spectacle independence is desired. They require little extra effort on the part of the surgeon, but can provide a high degree of patient satisfaction.

REFERENCES

1. Hoffer KJ. Biometry of 7,500 cataractous eyes. Am J Ophthalmol. 1980;90:360-8; correction:890.
2. Grabow HB. Intraocular correction of refractive errors. In: Kershner RM (Ed). Refractive Keratotomy for Cataract Surgery and the Correction of Astigmatism. Thorofare, NJ: Slack, Inc; 1994. pp. 79-115.
3. Sun XY, Vicary D, Montgomery P, et al. Toric intraocular lenses for correcting astigmatism in 130 eyes. Ophthalmology. 2000;107:1776-81.
4. Ruhswurm I, Scholz U, Zehetmayer M, et al. Astigmatism correction with foldable toric intraocular lens in cataract patients. J Cataract Refract Surg. 2000;26:1022-7.
5. Chang DF. Comparative rotational stability of single-piece open-loop acrylic and plate-haptic silicone toric intraocular lenses. J Cataract Refract Surg. 2008;34:1842-7.
6. Smith EM, Talamo JH, Assil KK, et al. Comparison of astigmatic axis in the seated and supine positions. J Refract Corneal Surg. 1994;10:615-20.

CHAPTER 35

The Multifocal Intraocular Lens

I Howard Fine, Richard S Hoffman, Mark Packer

Multifocal intraocular lens technology offers patients substantial benefits. The elimination of a presbyopic condition and restoration of normal vision by simulating accommodation greatly enhances the quality of life for most patients. The only multifocal intraocular lens (IOL) available for general use in the US is the AMO® Array® (Allergan Surgical Products; Irvine, California). The advantages of astigmatically neutral clear corneal cataract surgery have allowed for increased utilization of multifocal technology in both cataract and clear lens replacement surgery. Careful attention to patient selection, preoperative biometry and lens power calculations, in addition to meticulous surgical technique and will allow surgeons to offer multifocal technology to their patients with great success.

LENS DESIGN

The principle of any multifocal design is to create multiple image points behind the lens. The goal of these lenses is to enable less reduction in visual acuity for a given amount of defocus by improving the depth of field. The AMO Array is a zonal progressive intraocular lens with five concentric zones on the anterior surface. Zones 1, 3 and 5 are distance dominant zones while zones 2 and 4 are near dominant. The lens has an aspherical component and thus each zone repeats the entire refractive sequence corresponding to distance, intermediate, and near foci. This results in vision over a range of distances. The lens uses 100 percent of the incoming available light and is weighted for optimum light distribution. With typical pupil sizes, approximately half of the light is distributed for distance, one-third for near vision, and the remainder for intermediate vision. The lens utilizes continuous surface construction and consequently there is no loss of light through defraction and no degradation of image quality as a result of surface discontinuities. The lens has a foldable silicone optic that is 6.0 mm in diameter with haptics made of polymethylmethacrylate and a haptic diameter of 13 mm. The lens can be inserted through a clear corneal or scleral tunnel incision that is 2.8 mm wide, utilizing the Unfolder® injector system manufactured by AMO (Allergan Surgical Products; Irvine, California).

CLINICAL RESULTS

The efficacy of multifocal technology has been documented in many clinical studies. Early studies of the one-piece AMO Array documented a larger percentage of patients who were able to read J2 print after undergoing multifocal lens implantation compared to patients with monofocal implants.[1-3] Clinical trials comparing multifocal lens implantation compared to monofocal lens implantation in the same patient also revealed improved intermediate and near vision in the multifocal eye compared to the monofocal eye.[4,5]

Many studies have evaluated both the objective and subjective qualities of contrast sensitivity, stereoacuity, glare disability, and photic phenomena following implantation of multifocal IOLs. Refractive multifocal IOLs, such as the Array, were found to be superior to diffractive multifocal IOLs by demonstrating better contrast sensitivity and less glare disability.[6] The Array does produce a small amount of contrast sensitivity loss equivalent to the loss of one line of visual acuity at the 11 percent contrast level using Regan contrast sensitivity charts.[2] This loss of contrast sensitivity at low levels is only present when the Array is placed monocularly and has not been demonstrated with bilateral placement and binocular testing.[7] In addition to relatively normal contrast sensitivity, good random-dot stereopsis and less distance and near aniseikonia were present in bilaterally placed patients compared to unilateral implants.[8]

One of the potential drawbacks of the Array lens has been the potential for an appreciation of halos around point sources of light at night in the early weeks and months following surgery.[9] Most patients will learn to disregard these halos with time and bilateral implantation appears to improve these subjective symptoms. Concerns about the visual function of patients at night have been allayed by a driving simulation study in which bilateral Array multifocal patients performed only slightly worse than patients with bilateral monofocal IOLs. The results indicated no consistent difference in driving performance and safety between the two groups.[10] In a study by Javitt et al, 41 percent of bilateral Array subjects were found to never require spectacles compared to 11.7 percent of monofocal controls. Overall, subjects with bilateral Array IOLs reported better overall vision, less limitation in visual function, and less use of spectacles than monofocal controls.[11]

PATIENT SELECTION

Our utilization of the Array multifocal IOL over the past two and one-half years has been extensive. We have utilized this device in approximately 30 percent of our cataract patients and in the majority of our clear lens replacement refractive surgery patients. As a result of our experience, we have developed specific guidelines with respect to the selection of candidates and surgical strategies that enhance outcomes with this IOL.

AMO recommends using the Array multifocal IOL for bilateral cataract patients whose surgery is uncomplicated and whose personality is such that they are not likely to fixate on the presence of minor visual aberrations such as halos around lights. There is obviously a broad range of patients who would be acceptable candidates. Relative or absolute contraindications include the presence of ocular pathologies, other than cataracts, that may degrade image formation or may be associated with less than adequate visual function postoperatively despite visual improvement following surgery. Pre-existing ocular pathologies which are frequently looked upon as contraindications include age-related macular degeneration, uncontrolled diabetes or diabetic retinopathy, uncontrolled glaucoma, recurrent inflammatory eye disease, retinal detachment risk, and corneal disease or previous refractive surgery in the form of radial keratotomy, photorefractive keratectomy, or laser assisted *in situ* keratomileusis.

We avoid the utilization of these lenses in patients who complain excessively, are highly introspective and fussy, or obsess over body image and symptoms. We are conservative when evaluating patients with occupations that include frequent night driving and occupations that put high demands on vision and near work such as engineers and architects. Such patients need to demonstrate a strong desire for relative spectacle independence in order to be considered for Array implantation.

In our practice, we have reduced patient selection to a very rapid process. Once we determine that someone is a candidate for either cataract extraction or clear lens replacement, we ask the patient two questions. The first question is, "If we could put an implant in your eye that would allow you to see both distance and near without glasses, under most circumstances, would that be an advantage?" Approximately 50 percent of our patients say "no" in one way or another. Those negative responses may include, "I don't mind wearing glasses", "My grandchildren wouldn't recognize me without glasses", "I look terrible without glasses", or "I've worn glasses all my life". These patients receive monofocal IOLs. For the 50 percent who say it would be an advantage, we ask a second question: "If the lens is associated with halos around lights at night, would it still be an advantage?" Approximately 60 percent of this group of patients say that they do not think they would be bothered by these symptoms and they receive a multifocal IOL.

There are special circumstances in which implantation of a multifocal IOL should be strongly considered. Alzheimer's patients frequently lose or misplace their spectacles and thus they might benefit from the full range of view that a multifocal IOL provides without spectacles. Patients with arthritis of the neck or other conditions with limited range of motion of the neck may benefit from a multifocal IOL rather than multifocal spectacles which require changes in head position. Patients with a monocular cataract who have successfully worn monovision contact lenses should be considered possible candidates for monocular implantation. The same is true for certain occupations such as photographers who want to alternate focusing through the camera without spectacles and adjust imaging parameters on the camera without placing spectacles on – in these patients the focusing eye could have a monofocal IOL and the non-dominant eye a multifocal. We almost always use the Array in traumatic cataracts in young adults in order to facilitate binocularity at near, especially if the fellow eye has no refractive error or is corrected by contact lenses.

Prior to implanting an Array, we inform all candidates of the lens statistics to ensure that they understand that spectacle independence is not guaranteed. Approximately 41 percent of the patients implanted with bilateral Array IOLs will never need to wear glasses, 50 percent wear glasses on a limited basis such as driving at night or during prolonged reading, 12 percent will always need to wear glasses for near work, and approximately 8 percent will need to wear spectacles on a full-time basis for distance and near correction.[11] In addition, 15 percent of patients were found to have difficulty with halos at night and 11 percent had difficulty with glare compared to 6 percent and 1 percent respectively in monofocal patients.

PREOPERATIVE MEASUREMENTS

The most important assessment for successful multifocal lens use, other then patient selection, involves precise preoperative measurements of axial length in addition to accurate lens power calculations. There are some practitioners who feel that immersion biometry is necessary for accurate axial length determination. However, in our practice we have found applanation techniques in combination with the Holladay 2 formula and the Holladay II back calculation to yield accurate and consistent results with greater patient convenience and less technician time. We are currently experimenting with the Zeiss IOLMaster™ for non-contact optical measurements. The IOLMaster™ is a combined biometry instrument for the measurement of axial length, corneal curvature, and anterior chamber depth. The axial length measurement is based on an interference-optical method termed partial coherence interferometry. Measurements are claimed to be compatible with acoustic immersion measurements and accurate to within 30 microns. This new technology offers the possibility of extremely accurate and efficient measurements with minimal patient inconvenience.

When determining lens power calculations, the Holladay 2 formula takes into account disparities in anterior segment and axial lengths by adding the white-to-white corneal diameter and lens thickness into the formula. Addition of these variables helps predict the exact position of the IOL in the eye and has improved refractive predictability. As a final check in the lens power assessment, we will also use the SRK T and the SRK II formulas and, for eyes with less than 22 mm in axial length, the Hoffer Q formula for comparative purposes.

SURGICAL TECHNIQUE

The multifocal Array works best when the final postoperative refraction has less than one diopter of astigmatism. It is, thus, very important that incision construction be appropriate with respect to size and location. We favor a clear corneal incision at the temporal periphery that is 3 mm or less in width and 2 mm long.[12] Each surgeon should be aware of his or her usual amount of surgically-induced astigmatism by vector analysis. The surgeon must also be able to utilize one of the many modalities for addressing preoperative astigmatism. Although we have utilized both T and arcuate keratotomies at the 7 mm optical zone, we are currently favoring limbal relaxing incisions[13,14] utilizing a Force blade (Mastel Precision Surgical Instruments; Rapid City, South Dakota) and a Nichamin nomogram.

In preparation for phacoemulsification, the capsulorhexis must be round in shape and sized so that there is a small margin of anterior capsule overlapping the optic circumferentially. This is important in order to guarantee in-the-bag placement of the IOL and prevent anterior/ posterior alterations in location which would affect the final refractive status. Hydrodelineation and cortical cleaving hydrodissection are very important in all patients because they facilitate lens disassembly and complete cortical cleanup.[15] Complete and fastidious cortical cleanup will hopefully reduce the incidence of posterior capsule opacification whose presence, even in very small amounts, will inordinately degrade the visual acuity in Array patients. It is because of this phenomena that patients implanted with Array lenses will require YAG laser posterior capsulotomies earlier than patients with monofocal IOLs.

Minimally invasive surgery is very important. Techniques that produce effective phacoemulsification times of less than 20 seconds and average phacoemulsification powers of 10 percent or less are highly advantageous and can best be achieved with power modulations (burst mode or 2 pulses per second) rather than continuous phacoemulsification modes.[16]

COMPLICATIONS MANAGEMENT

When intraoperative complications develop they must be handled precisely and appropriately. In situations in which the first eye has already had an Array implanted,

complications management must be directed toward finding any possible way of implanting an Array in the second eye. Under most circumstances, capsule rupture will still allow for implantation of an Array as long as there is an intact capsulorhexis. Under these circumstances, the lens haptics are implanted in the sulcus and the optic is prolasped posteriorly through the anterior capsulorhexis. This is facilitated by a capsulorhexis that is slightly smaller than the diameter of the optic in order to capture the optic in essentially an "in-the-bag" location. If full sulcus implantation is utilized then appropriate change in the IOL power will need to be made in order to compensate for the more anterior location of the IOL within the eye. When vitreous loss occurs, a meticulous vitrectomy with clearing of all vitreous strands must be performed.

It is important to avoid iris trauma since the pupil size and shape may impact the visual function of a multifocal IOL postoperatively. If the pupil is less than 2.5 mm, there may be an impairment of near visual acuity due to the location of the rings serving near visual acuity. For patients with small postoperative pupil diameters affecting near vision, we have had success utilizing the Argon laser to perform a mydriatic pupilloplasty.[17]

POSTOPERATIVE COURSE

If glasses are required after surgery, the spherical correction should be determined by over-plusing the patient to a slight blur and gradually reducing the power until the best acuity is reached. Patients are able to focus through the near portions of their IOL and thus it is possible to over-minus a patient if care is not taken to push the plus power. When using this defocusing technique, it is critical to stop as soon as distance acuity is maximized to avoid over-minusing. The cylinder power should be the smallest amount that provides the best acuity. If add power is necessary, prescribe the full add power for the required working distance.

If patients are unduly bothered by photic phenomena such as halos and glare, these symptoms can be alleviated by various techniques. Weak pilocarpine at a concentration of 1/8 percent or weaker will constrict the pupil to a diameter that will usually lessen the severity of halos without significantly effecting near visual acuity. Another approach involves the use of over-minused spectacles in order to push the secondary focal point behind the retina and thus lessen the effect of image blur from multiple images in front of the retina. Polarized lenses have also been found to be helpful in reducing photic phenomena. Perhaps the most important technique is the implantation of bilateral Array lenses as close in time as possible in order to allow patients the ability to use the lenses together which appears to allow for improved binocular distance and near vision compared to monocular acuity. Finally, most patients report that halos improve or disappear with the passage of several weeks to months.

CONCLUSION

We have had a great deal of success with the Array multifocal IOL in patients undergoing cataract and refractive surgery. We recognize that multifocal technology is not for every patient but does offer substantial benefits over monofocal lenses. Appropriate patient screening, accurate biometry and lens power calculations, and meticulous surgical technique will allow surgeons to maximize their success with this lens. As with any new technology, there is a learning curve to its utilization and we believe that the information provided in this chapter will be helpful in mastering its use.

REFERENCES

1. Percival SPB, Setty SS. Prospectively randomized trial comparing the pseudoaccommodation of the AMO Array multifocal lens and a monofocal lens. J Cataract Refract Surg. 1993;19: 26-31.
2. Steinert RF, Post CT, Brint SF, et al. A progressive, randomized, double-masked comparison of a zonal-progressive multifocal intraocular lens and a monofocal intraocular lens. Ophthalmology. 1992;99: 853-61.
3. Negishi K, Nagamoto T, Hara E, et al. Clinical evaluation of a five-zone refractive multifocal intraocular lens. J Cataract Refract Surg. 1996;22: 110-15.
4. Vaquero-Ruano M, Encinas JL, Millan I, et al. AMO Array multifocal versus monofocal intraocular lenses: Long-term follow-up. J Cataract Refract Surg. 1998;24: 118-23.
5. Steinert RF, Aker BL, Trentacost DJ, et al. A prospective study of the AMO Array zonal-progressive multifocal silicone intraocular lens and a monofocal intraocular lens. Ophthalmology. 1999;106: 1243-55.
6. Pieh S, Weghaupt H, Skorpik C. Contrast sensitivity and glare disability with diffractive and refractive multifocal intraocular lenses. J Cataract Refract Surg. 1998;24: 659-62.
7. Arens B, Freudenthaler N, Quentin CD. Binocular function after bilateral implantation of monofocal and refractive multifocal intraocular lenses. J Cataract Refract Surg. 1999; 25: 399-404.
8. Haring G, Gronemeyer A, Hedderich J, de Decker W. Stereoacuity and aniseikonia after unilateral and bilateral implantation of the Array refractive multifocal intraocular lens. J Cataract Refract Surg. 1999;25: 1151-56.
9. Dick HB, Krummenauer F, Schwenn O, et al. Objective and subjective evaluation of photic phenomena after monofocal and multifocal intraocular lens implantation. Ophthalmology. 1999; 106: 1878-86.
10. Featherstone KA, Bloomfield JR, Lang AJ, et al. Driving simulation study: Bilateral Array multifocal versus bilateral AMO monofocal intraocular lenses. J Cataract Refract Surg. 1999; 25: 1254-62.
11. Javitt JC, Wang F, Trentacost DJ, et al. Outcomes of cataract extraction with multifocal intraocular lens implantation – Functional status and quality of life. Ophthalmology. 1997;104: 589-99.
12. Fine IH. Corneal tunnel incision with a temporal approach. In Fine IH, Fichman RA, Grabow HB (Eds). Clear-Corneal Cataract Surgery and Topical Anesthesia. Thorofare, NJ: Slack Inc, 1993; 5-26.
13. Gills JP, Gayton JL. Reducing pre-existing astigmatism. In Gills JP (Ed): Cataract Surgery: The State of the Art. Thorofare, NJ: Slack, Inc, 1998; 53-66.
14. Nichamin L. Refining Astigmatic Keratotomy During Cataract Surgery. Ocular Surgery News April 15, 1993.
15. Fine IH. Cortical cleaving hydrodissection. J Cataract Refract Surg. 1992;18: 508-12.
16. Fine IH. The choo-choo chop and flip phacoemulsification technique. Operative Techniques in Cataract and Refractive Surgery. 1998;1(2): 61-65.
17. Thomas JV. Pupilloplasty and photomydriasis. In: Belcher CD, Thomas JV, Simmons RJ (Eds). Photocoagulation in Glaucoma and Anterior Segment Disease. Baltimore, MD: Williams and Wilkins. 1984;150-57.

CHAPTER 36

Angle Kappa: The Angle to the Mystery of Multifocal IOLs

Gaurav Prakash, Soosan Jacob, Amar Agarwal

INTRODUCTION

Multifocal intraocular lens (IOL) implantation for the correction of ametropia aims for a good unaided visual acuity for both near and distance. This is done by creating multiple focal points, which focus for distance and near.[1-3] Two inherent designs of multifocal optics have been used to develop these IOLs: refractive and diffractive. Refractive IOLs have multiple concentric rings in them with varying powers. Diffractive IOLs work on the Huygens- Fresnel principle.[4-6] Both the lens designs have improved significantly from their earlier prototypes. These include aspheric optics, change in the size of rings and making the IOL dominant for distance or near, and modifying the anterior or posterior surface of the IOLs.[3,5] In spite of these modifications, the implantation of a multifocal IOL can have less than satisfactory visual acuity and quality along with more photic phenomenon like haloes and glare compared to monofocal IOLs. Researchers have noted these factors and some studies have analyzed the governing factors for patient satisfaction after implantation of multifocal IOLs.[7, 9-22] Causes associated with photic phenomena noted in previous studies have included IOL decentration, retained lens fragments, posterior capsular opacification, dry-eye syndrome, uncorrected visual acuity, use of spectacles for distance purposes, postoperative astigmatism and postoperative spherical equivalent.[10,22] However, none of the studies in published literature have evaluated the role of misalignment between the visual axis and the pupillary axis, or the angle kappa as a specific predictor for patient symptoms.[23-28]

ANGLE KAPPA

Angles of the eye have, of late received, a renewed interest secondary to the significant role they play in refractive surgery. Angle Kappa is the angle between the visual axis and the pupillary axis **(Figures 36.1A and B)**. It is clinically very important to the refractive surgeon as patients, especially hyperopic patients have a large angle kappa and the center of the pupil is thus no longer the point through which a fovea-centric ray of light passes. Thus any treatment that is performed centered on the pupil results in a decentered ablation. This effect is more pronounced with corrections for astigmatism and higher order aberrations if angle kappa is not compensated for.

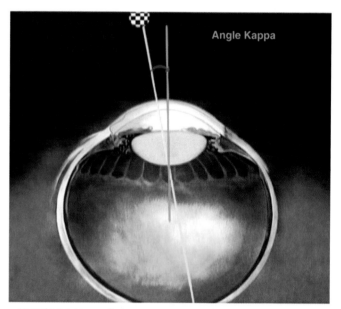

FIGURE 36.1A: Angle kappa is the angle between the visual axis and the pupillary axis

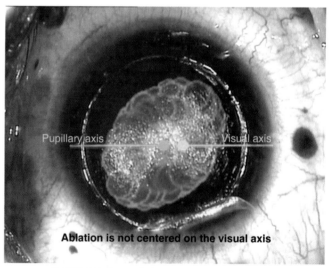

FIGURE 36.1B: Angle kappa in refractive surgery

ANGLE KAPPA AND MULTIFOCAL IOLS

WHAT ROLE DOES ANGLE KAPPA PLAY FOR THE CATARACT SURGEON?

We know that multifocal IOLs work by creating multiple focal points which focus for distance and near **(Figures 36.2A and B)**. We also know that patients with monofocal

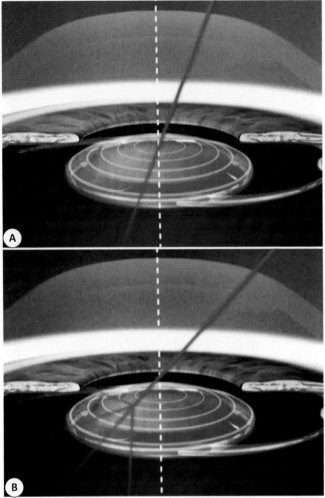

FIGURES 36.2A AND B: In eyes with small angle kappa, a fovea centric ray may pass through the central ring of the multifocal IOL (A); in eyes with large angle kappa, a fovea centric ray may hit on the edge of the ring causing edge glare effects and deterioration in quality of vision (B)

IOLs have traditionally been more satisfied with their visual outcome with regard to postoperative blurry vision, haloes, glare and decreased contrast sensitivity. Multifocal IOLs have been associated with these symptoms despite uneventful surgery with the IOL well centered in the bag. Many factors have been proposed for these phenomena, the most important being a decrease in the intensity of light falling on the retina due to splitting up of incident light into multiple focal points and due to superimposition of the defocused image onto the focused image. Irrespective of these factors being common to all patients, all patients are not equally affected by the symptoms. One of the factors proposed to account for this difference in symptoms is varying degrees of neuroadaptation. Other factors include IOL decentration, retained lens fragments, posterior capsular opacification, poor ocular surface and postoperative residual refractive error. The newer model multifocal IOLs have lesser symptoms associated with them.

A lesser studied entity is the angle kappa. Angle kappa is the distance between the center of the pupil and the light reflex. The vertex normal or the light reflex is near the visual axis at the corneal plane. Angle Kappa can be measured with the synoptophore or using the Orbscan II. The average angle kappa is about ±5 degrees. Effect of angle kappa on multifocal IOLs has been evaluated previously by attempting iridoplasty to make the pupil concentric to the center of the IOL. This could theoretically increase the effect of higher order aberrations because of an increase in the pupil size.

MULTIFOCAL GLUED IOL

Just as the corneal intercept of the visual axis is used for centration of ablation in LASIK, we attempted to use the angle kappa measurement as an intraoperative guide to center a multifocal IOL. We marked the visual axis using the coaxially sighted light reflex. We then marked the pupillary center and centered a multifocal IOL using the glued IOL technique (**Figures 36.3A to C**). We marked the visual axis and the pupillary center on the cornea.

Despite the inability to ensure perfect accuracy, we did observe promising results with this technique.

There are certain situations where, despite best attempts, a centered multifocal IOL in the bag may not be possible in a patient who is desirous of a multifocal. In such a patient, it is possible to perform a glued IOL and to adjust the centration by adjusting the location of the scleral flaps, sclerotomies and the degree of tuck of individual haptics. In other situations, such as microspherophakia, the preferred practice is to do a lensectomy and implant a glued IOL, which if multifocal needs to be centered on its rings. It would also be ideal to combine this with ray optics and to be able to center the IOL ideally so that the light ray passes from fixation through the centre of the rings to the fovea.

In the event of a posterior capsular rent, it is not advisable to place a multifocal IOL in the sulcus for fear of postoperative decentration. If in the bag multifocal IOL is not possible, a glued multifocal IOL may be preferable as the IOL is very stable with no postoperative decentration of the IOL occurring from its intraoperative positioning. In all these complicated situations and more importantly in the routine multifocal IOL patients, it is important to take the angle kappa into consideration for IOL centration. Future advances might also include IOL customization to match the angle kappa of the patients, though postoperative capsular contraction and IOL rotation would be challenges to be overcome.

ANGLE KAPPA AND MULTIFOCAL IOL

We also studied angle kappa in relation to visual satisfaction in multifocal patients and found photic phenomena to have an association with angle kappa. Multifocal IOLs work on either a refractive or a diffractive principle and have either multifocal zones or steps. In an eye with a small angle kappa, the ray of light would be able to pass through the IOL center without disturbance; but in an eye with a large

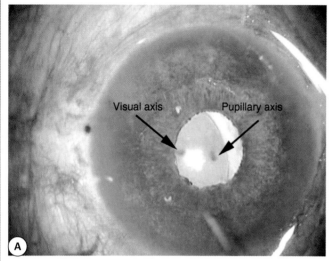

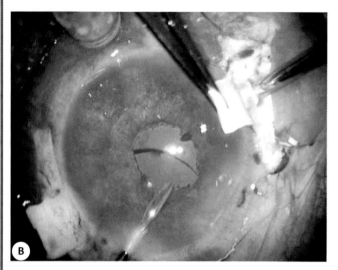

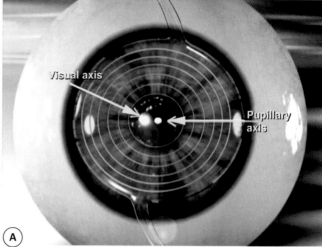

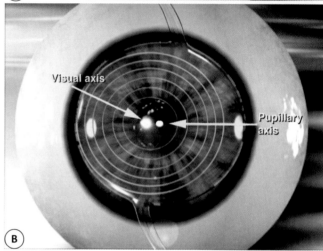

FIGURES 36.4A AND B: Figure A shows a multifocal IOL which is centered on the pupillary axis but not on the visual axis in an eye with large angle kappa; Figure B shows possible future customization of multifocal IOLs to allow centration of rings on the visual axis

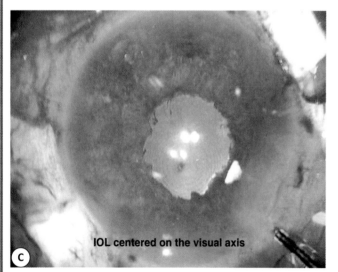

FIGURES 36.3A TO C: A glued multifocal IOL being done in an aphakic eye in an attempt to center the rings on the visual axis. Figure A shows the pupillary axis and the visual axis marked preoperatively; Figure B shows multifocal glued IOL and Figure C shows the multifocal IOL rings centered on the pupillary axis after a glued IOL procedure which allows adjustment of the rings by adjusting the flaps, sclerotomies and the degree of tuck of individual haptics

angle kappa, a fovea centric ray might hit on the edge of the ring, thus giving rise to edge glare effects, etc. **(Figures 36.4A and B).** This might be severe enough for having to explant such an IOL and replace it with a different IOL. A monofocal IOL in an eye with a large angle kappa would not cause as much visual disturbance as a decentered multifocal IOL because of the lack of steps or rings on its surface.

DISCUSSION

Multifocal IOL designs have come a long way since the earlier prototypes. At the cost of mild reduction in contrast sensitivity, many patients are satisfied with these newer models.[3,5,6,8] Neuroadaptation may also play a major role in some cases and hence enough time should be provided before drawing a conclusion on the severity of photic phenomenon.[6]

Improved patient compliance noticed with these newer IOLs was seen in our study too. The distance and near visual outcome was satisfactory with the multifocal IOL implantation in our study. We found that in cases having dissatisfaction, uncorrected postoperative visual acuity was the most important factor for patient satisfaction. This is intuitive because low intensity photic symptoms would happen in certain conditions, like around light sources or in night time driving; however, the effect of poor UCVA stays for the patient in all waking hours. Other than these factors, there was no effect of any other factor in the final resolution acuity satisfaction for distance or near. We did not find that cylindrical power had an effect, independent of UCVA in the patient dissatisfaction. Walkow and Klemen had similar finding with UCVA in a questionnaire based study on diffractive IOL, however they found cylindrical power to be an additionally important independent predictor of dissatisfaction.[22] The reason for this difference can be in our exclusion of high cylinders from the preoperative data and the low postoperative cylinders. We do agree that both high cylinders and on same lines induced higher order aberration (acquired aberropia) may have an impact on the final satisfaction of the patients.[23,24] We did not perform a wavefront analysis in our patients. A study correlating visual symptoms, angle kappa (and therefore coma aberration, which may be linked) and other higher order aberrations may provide further information on the same.[25-27]

Both the photic phenomenon evaluated in the study, i.e. haloes and glare, were found to have an association with angle kappa, which represents the angle between the visual axis and the pupillary axis. Even though many patients with high angle kappa were also asymptomatic, the strength of association was statistically significant, suggesting that angle kappa values may be considered in preoperative decision making in cases of multifocal IOL implantation. The reason for this association needs to be evaluated in detail, with simulation methods perhaps like ray tracing to confirm whether edge effect from the anterior IOL surface's rings may be responsible for the same. A higher angle kappa means that the actual misalignment between the anatomical center of the pupil-IOL complex (through which a foveacentric ray should pass ideally) and the visual axis may be large enough to misalign the ray on to a ring edge **(Figures 36.5A and B)**.

It may be noted that most self-reporting questionnaires are biased by the expectation levels and the mindset of the patient itself, and therefore, in spite of a scale based on objective parameters, the subjective perception of a symptom may vary from one patient to another.

It needs to be seen if the lens can be customized to match the kappa angle of the patient. Due to multiple variable factors including capsular contraction and IOL rotation, it seems unlikely that a multifocal IOL intentionally decentered towards the visual axis would stay in the same position in the postoperative period. However, the situation can be different in a case of a glued IOL for aphakia.[28] In cases with glued multifocal IOL where the IOL is being

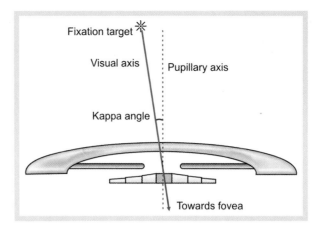

FIGURE 36.5A: Schematic ray diagram showing the incident ray passing through the central area in an eye with small angle kappa

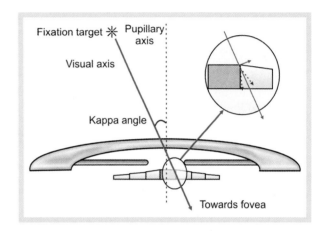

FIGURE 36.5B: Schematic ray diagram showing the incident ray passing through the ring edge area in an eye with large angle kappa

placed without capsular support, one of the haptics may be pulled furthermore to position the central ring of IOL under the visual axis before tucking the haptic to fixate the IOL. A feasibility study for the same with glued IOL is currently undergoing in our institution and the results may throw more light on this evolving concept.

The perception of photic phenomenon is multifactorial as evaluated in previous studies.[10,22] Our study suggests that there may be an additional role of misalignment between the visual and pupillary axis in the occurrence of photic phenomenon after multifocal IOL implantation. Further studies will be required to analyze the effect of the same on induced higher order aberrations and contrast sensitivity after multifocal IOL implantation.

CONCLUSION

To conclude, we propose that it is important to focus more research on the association between angle kappa and multifocal IOLs. It may be important to consider angle kappa for all prospective multifocal IOL patients and to avoid multifocal implantation in patients with large angle kappa till the time, advances make accurate centering of IOLs possible.

REFERENCES

1. Bellucci R. Multifocal intraocular lenses. Curr Opin Ophthalmol. 2005;16:33-7.

2. Lane SS, Morris M, Nordan L, et al. Multifocal Intraocular lenses. Ophthalmol Clin North Am. 2006;19:89-105.

3. Buznego C, Trattler WB. Presbyopia-correcting intraocular lenses. Curr Opin Ophthalmol. 2009;20:13-8.

4. Jay JL, Chakrabarti HS, Morrison JD. Quality of vision through diffractive bifocal intraocular lens. Br J Ophthalmol. 1991;75: 359-66.

5. Cillino S, Casuccio A, Di Pace F, et al. One-year outcomes with new-generation multifocal intraocular lenses. Ophthalmology. 2008;115(9):1508-16.

6. Palomino Bautista C, Carmona González D, Castillo Gómez A, et al. Evolution of visual performance in 250 eyes implanted with the Tecnis ZM900 multifocal IOL. Eur J Ophthalmol. 2009;19(5):762-8.

7. Häring G, Dick HB, Krummenauer F, et al. Subjective photic phenomena with refractive multifocal and monofocal intraocular lenses. Results of a multicenter questionnaire. J Cataract Refract Surg. 2001;27(2):245-9.

8. Leyland M, Zinicola E. Multifocal versus monofocal intraocular lenses in cataract surgery: a systematic review. Ophthalmology. 2003;110:1789-98.

9. Dick HB, Krummenauer F, Schwenn O, et al. Objective and subjective evaluation of photic phenomena after monofocal and multifocal intraocular lens implantation. Ophthalmology. 1999;106(10):1878-86.

10. Woodward MA, Randleman JB, Stulting RD. Dissatisfaction after multifocal intraocular lens implantation. J Cataract Refract Surg. 2009;35(6):992-7.

11. Pepose JS. Maximizing satisfaction with presbyopia-correcting intraocular lenses: the missing links. Am J Ophthalmol. 2008;146(5):641-8.

12. Kohnen T, Kook D, Auffarth GU, Derhartunian V. [Use of multifocal intraocular lenses and criteria for patient selection]. Ophthalmologe. 2008;105(6):527-32.

13. Chang DF. Prospective functional and clinical comparison of bilateral ReZoom and ReSTOR intraocular lenses in patients 70 years or younger. J Cataract Refract Surg. 2008;34(6):934-41.

14. Blaylock JF, Si Z, Aitchison S, et al. Visual function and change in quality of life after bilateral refractive lens exchange with the ReSTOR multifocal intraocular lens. J Refract Surg. 2008;24(3):265-73.

15. Chiam PJ, Chan JH, Haider SI, et al. Functional vision with bilateral ReZoom and ReSTOR intraocular lenses 6 months after cataract surgery. J Cataract Refract Surg. 2007;33(12): 2057-61.

16. Alfonso JF, Fernández-Vega L, Baamonde MB, et al. Prospective visual evaluation of apodized diffractive intraocular lenses. J Cataract Refract Surg. 2007;33(7):1235-43.

17. Mester U, Hunold W, Wesendahl T, et al. Functional outcomes after implantation of Tecnis ZM900 and Array SA40 multifocal intraocular lenses. J Cataract Refract Surg. 2007;33(6):1033-40.

18. Pepose JS, Qazi MA, Davies J, et al. Visual performance of patients with bilateral vs combination Crystalens, ReZoom, and ReSTOR intraocular lens implants. Am J Ophthalmol. 2007;144(3):347-57.

19. Chiam PJ, Chan JH, Aggarwal RK, et al. ReSTOR intraocular lens implantation in cataract surgery: quality of vision. J Cataract Refract Surg. 2006;32(9):1459-63.

20. Sen HN, Sarikkola AU, Uusitalo RJ, et al. Quality of vision after AMO Array multifocal intraocular lens implantation. J Cataract Refract Surg. 2004;30(12):2483-93.

21. Hunkeler JD, Coffman TM, Paugh J, et al. Characterization of visual phenomena with the Array multifocal intraocular lens. J Cataract Refract Surg. 2002;28(7):1195-204.

22. Walkow L, Klemen UM. Patient satisfaction after implantation of diffractive designed multifocal intraocular lenses in dependence on objective parameters. Graefes Arch Clin Exp Ophthalmol. 2001;239(9):683-7

23. Agarwal A, Prakash G, Jacob S, et al. Can uncompensated higher order aberration profile, or aberropia be responsible for subnormal best corrected vision and pseudo-amblyopia. Med Hypotheses. 2009;72(5):574-7.

24. Agarwal A, Jacob S, Agarwal A. Aberropia: a new refractive entity. J Cataract Refract Surg. 2007;33(11):1835-6.

25. Espinosa J, Mas D, Kasprzak HT. Corneal primary aberrations compensation by oblique light incidence. J Biomed Opt. 2009;14(4):044003.

26. Lu F, Wu J, Shen Y, et al. On the compensation of horizontal coma aberrations in young human eyes. Ophthalmic Physiol Opt. 2008;28(3):277-82.

27. Tabernero J, Benito A, Alcón E, et al. Mechanism of compensation of aberrations in the human eye. J Opt Soc Am A Opt Image Sci Vis. 2007;24(10):3274-83.

28. Agarwal A, Kumar DA, Jacob S, et al. Fibrin glue-assisted sutureless posterior chamber intraocular lens implantation in eyes with deficient posterior capsules. J Cataract Refract Surg. 2008;34(9):1433-8.

CHAPTER 37

Refractive Cataract Surgery

Pandelis A Papadopoulos

With the current advances in small incision cataract surgery and intraocular lens (IOL) technology, there is an increasing demand for the ophthalmic surgeon to perform "*refractive*" cataract surgery. The goal is to choose a surgical strategy that permits the correction of the patient's total refractive error in *one* operation. In the past, this was accomplished by choosing the appropriate combination of wound construction, placement and closure, as well as using techniques of incisional keratotomy. In recent years, multifocal, pseudoaccomodative and toric IOLs have enriched the surgeon's armamentarium and they play a significant role towards less spectacle dependency. In some cases piggyback or negative-power IOLs will also help the surgeon in correcting high refractive errors in cataract patients.

BIOMETRY

Precise axial length measurement is very important in refractive cataract surgery. Inaccurate ultrasound biometry or IOL miscalculation can lead to refractive errors that will destroy the final surgical outcome and can cause patient dissatisfaction. Measurement of axial length constitutes the largest source of error in IOL power calculation.[1] An error of 0.1 mm in axial length can cause an error of 0.3 D in IOL power. Measurement accuracy is considered satisfactory if there is no more fluctuation than 0.15 mm in the same eye and 0.3 mm between the fellow eyes.

ULTRASOUND BIOMETRY

Several methods were tested to improve the accuracy of axial length measurement. Among these, *Immersion A-Scan technique* is reported to be the most accurate and reproducible.[2,3] There seems to be no statistically significant difference between hand-held and slit-lamp attached A-probe measurements.[4] Manual rather automated A-scan measurements are indicated in eyes with asteroid hyalosis.[5] Falsely short axial length measurements may be obtained using automated A-scan biometry, leading to significant errors.

Falsely longer axial length measurements may occur if:[6]
a. A drop of fluid or methylcellulose increases the distance between the probe and the corneal surface in applanation biometry.
b. The probe is not aligned with the optical axis.

c. Low gain is used, that can lead to confusion of retinal and scleral peaks.
d. Higher than indicated ultrasound velocity is used.
e. A posterior staphyloma exists. In these cases *B-Mode-Guided Vector-A-Mode Biometry* can help to determine the position of the fovea.[7]
f. The eye is filled with silicone oil.
g. The eye has a scleral buckle after retinal detachment surgery.

Falsely shorter axial length measurements may occur if:
a. Pressure is applied on the cornea in applanation biometry. This error does not occur in immersion biometry.
b. The probe is not aligned with the optical axis.
c. Membranes or opacities (asteroid hyalosis) in vitreous exist.
d. A retinal detachment is present.
e. An IOL is present.
f. The choroid is thickened.
g. Lower than indicated ultrasound velocity is used.

Frequent evaluation of the surgical outcomes and personalizing of A-constants can further reduce the postoperative refractive error. Flowers, McLeod et al studied the use of personalized formula constants and concluded that they can significantly reduce the mean absolute predictive error for the SRK II, SRK/T, and Holladay formulas.[8]

Husain, Kohnen et al found that the Computerized Videokeratography-derived (CVK) corneal curvature values to be slightly less accurate than standard keratometry in predicting IOL power.[9] However, CVK provides important corneal curvature data for IOL calculations in patients with abnormal or surgically altered corneal surfaces.

The accuracy of IOL power calculation remains a major problem in very long and very short eyes. The accuracy of the newer generation theoretical intraocular lens power calculation formulas and of the empirical SRK I and II formulas was evaluated in a series of 500 IOL implantations including a series of unusually long and short eyes.[10] The prediction error of the theoretical formulas was found to be largely unaffected by the variation in axial length and corneal power, while the prediction of the SRK I formula was less accurate in the short and long eyes. The prediction of the SRK II formula was more accurate than the SRK I in that no systematic offset error with axial length could be demonstrated. However, because of a relatively larger scatter in the long eyes and a significant bias with the corneal power, the absolute error of the SRK II formula was higher than that of the theoretical formulas in the long eyes. The higher accuracy of the newer generation theoretical formulas was attributed to their improved prediction of the pseudophakic anterior chamber depth.

The following guidelines can help the surgeon to reduce the errors of axial length measurements and IOL power calculations:

a. Usage of theoretical formulas if the axial length is shorter than 22 mm or longer than 25 mm.
b. Repetition of measurements if there is an AXL difference of more than 0.3 mm between the eyes.
c. Multiple measurements if axial length is shorter than 22 mm or longer than 25 mm.
d. Multiple measurements if the corneal curvature is less than 40 D or more than 47 D.
e. Repetition of measurements if the astigmatic cylinder power difference is more than 1 D between the fellow eyes.
f. Repetition of measurements if the refractive cylinder differs significantly from keratometric cylinder.
g. Repetition of measurements if the axial length is incompatible with the refraction of the eye. (e.g. long axial length in a hyperopic eye).
h. Repetition of measurements in patients with poor fixation or poor co-operation.
i. Usage of B-Mode guided Vector A-Mode biometry in eyes with posterior staphyloma and age related macular degeneration.
j. Calculation of Personalized A-constant for each IOL type used.
k. Frequent analysis of refractive outcomes in order to localize the sources of error

An important issue that ophthalmologists will encounter more often in the near future is the IOL power calculation in eyes with previous refractive surgery. Significant calculation errors can occur due to wrong estimation of corneal power, that is caused by the change in the anterior and posterior corneal surface and due to incorrect estimation of the effective lens position. Many formulae were proposed by several authors (Awwad, Camellin, Calossi, Diehl, Feiz, Ferrara, Latkany, Masket, Rosa, Savini, Shammas, Seitz, Speicher and others). According to a recent study, when corneal power is known, the Seitz/Speicher method (with or without Savini adjustment) seems the best solution to obtain an accurate IOL power prediction. Otherwise, the Masket method may be the most reliable option.[11] Tang and Huang published an intraocular lens power calculation formula based on optical coherence tomography (OCT), that would not be biased by previous laser vision correction. Posterior corneal curvature was computed by combining IOLMaster keratometry with OCT corneal thickness mapping in order to avoid the calculation errors inherent in conventional IOL formulae.[12] Thus, patient data, prior to refractive surgery will not be necessary.

OPTICAL BIOMETRY

In recent years, non-invasive optical biometry methods based on the principle of partial coherence interferometry (PCI) have been developed.[14] The advantage of PCI is that this non-contact method neither requires local anesthesia nor represents a risk of infection.[14] In addition, the method precludes an additional source of error in AL (axial length) measurement caused by the indentation of the cornea. Moreover, pupil dilation is unnecessary in optical biometry using PCI, which has a high longitudinal and transversal resolution. In various publications, the accuracy is reported to be between 5 and 30 μm.[15,16] The main drawback of optical biometry is its limited usability in cases of fixation problems or advanced cataract.[13,16] In US biometry, the AL is determined by measuring the reflection of the anterior surface of the cornea and the limiting membrane.

The IOLMaster[TM] (Carl Zeiss) is the first commercially available instrument using optical biometry. It was introduced in Germany in September 1999 and was approved by the US Food and Drug Administration in March 2000. It is able to measure also the corneal curvature, the anterior chamber depth and the corneal diameter (white-to-white). The software of the instruments includes various IOL calculation formulas (Haigis, SRK/T, SRK II, Hoffer, etc). The IOLMaster measures the distance from the anterior surface of the cornea to the pigmented epithelium. Due to this difference, the IOLMaster measurements are on average 0.23 mm longer for the same eye.[17] A different A-constant should be used when the AL is measured by the IOLMaster. Several study groups have compared axial length and corneal radius measurements taken with the IOLMaster with those taken using traditional US systems and with keratometry measurements. The IOLMaster provides axial length measurements comparable to those by the immersion method.[18] The resulting correction factors were integrated in the software of the IOLMaster so that the IOL calculation formulas use customized constants. Updated optical A-constants of older and newer IOLs can be downloaded from the ULIB (User Group for Laser Interference Biometry) web site, found at URL: www.augenklinik.uni-wuerzburg.de/eulib/.

Recently, a new optical biometry device, the Haag Streit Lenstar 900 R, that utilizes Optical Low-Coherence Reflectometry (OLCR) with a dual scanning system in which the reflection from a reference beam is used to calculate distances within the eye, was introduced . According to a recent study, the mean differences in IOL power calculations were not statistically significant between the two devices.[19]

IOLS FOR THE CORRECTION OF PRESBYOPIA

MONOVISION WITH MONOFOCAL IOLS

Monovision is a means of presbyopic correction in which one eye is corrected for distance vision and the other eye for near vision. In clinical practice, the dominant eye is commonly corrected for distance. This practice is based on the assumption that it is easier to suppress blur in the non-dominant eye than in the dominant eye. Monovision limitations in refractive cataract surgery have not been clearly defined in the current ophthalmic literature, although the monovision success rate with contact lens correction is high. Ideally, the patient with monovision should be able to see clearly at all distances. The binocular clear vision range should be continuous and equal to the sum of the monocular clear ranges without interference from blurred images in one eye. However, input from the dominant eye produces a greater response to a given stimulus. Success and patient satisfaction in monovision patients were significantly influenced by the magnitude of ocular dominance.[20] In monovision, the postoperative target refraction may range from -1.5 to -2.75 D, depending from the intended working distance. Any reduction in intermediate vision created by the choice of full distance and near correction was well tolerated and accepted by highly motivated patients.[20,21]

MULTIFOCAL IOLS

Multifocal IOLs provide patients with an accomodative capacity, allowing multiple focal distances independent of ciliary body function and capsular mechanics.[22] This pseudoaccommodation results in full distance visual acuity and increased depth of focus including sufficient near visual acuity. Controversy exists over the quality of vision offered by these lenses. These IOLs have simultaneous multiple focal areas and therefore, multiple light distribution, which causes less light at every focal point and can also produce halos around light sources in the dark.

The AMO Array™ **(Figure 37.1)** was the first widely studied small-incision foldable multifocal IOL.[24-26] It has a five-zone refractive, progressive, aspheric configuration designed to provide true multifocality through a wide depth of focus and good visual acuity and contrast sensitivity for

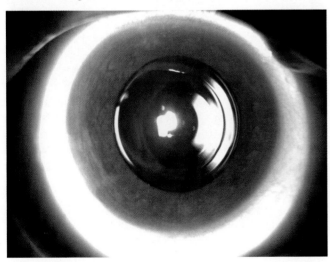

FIGURE 37.1: Multifocal IOL (*Courtesy:* Dr Agarwal's Eye Hospital, India)

distance, which results from the lens preponderant distance correction (50% for distance, 37% for near, 13% for intermediate).

According to study by Vaquero-Ruano et al, contrast sensitivity was found to be decreased at low contrasts with this IOL.[27] The most important subjectively reported optical side effects disappeared after the first 2 months. At 18 months 6% of the cases reported ghosting and 4% reported glare. In the same study, 28% of the patients could read J1+ without spherical addition, however the other 72% required a mean near addition of only 1.03 D. This could be explained by the 35% light distribution of the near area in the far preponderance design of the lens and the low refractive power. In another study by Papadopoulos et al, 37.5% of the patients could read J1 without correction at 3 months.[28]

A different concept of multifocality employs a diffractive design. Diffraction creates multifocality through constructive and destructive interference of incoming rays of light. An earlier multifocal IOL by 3 M employed a diffractive design. It encountered difficulty in acceptance, not because of its optical design, but rather, due to poor production quality and the relatively large incision size required for its implantation. Alcon introduced in 2005 a new diffractive multifocal IOL based on the 6 mm foldable three-piece AcrySof acrylic IOL, the Restor IOL. The diffractive region of this lens is confined to the center, so that the periphery of the lens is identical to a monofocal acrylic IOL. The inspiration behind this approach comes from the realization that during near work the synkinetic reflex of accommodation, convergence, and miosis implies a relatively smaller pupil size. Putting multifocal optics beyond the 3 mm zone creates no advantage for the patient and diminishes optical quality. In fact, bench studies performed by Alcon show an advantage in modulation transfer function for this central diffractive design, especially with a small pupil at near and a large pupil at distance.[23] The Restor IOL, that had initially a +4.0 D near add, has now also a +3.0 D add, which seems to be preferred by many surgeons and patients for its superior intermediate vision.[29] It is available with an aspheric optic.

Several IOL manufacturers offer now a wide choice of multifocal IOLs. The Acri.Tec (Now Zeiss) Acritwin™ IOLs were refractive/diffractive aspheric IOLs implanted bilaterally. One eye received the 447 D IOL with 70% of the light intensity in the distance focus, while in the accompanying eye, the IOL type 443 D with 30% of the light intensity in the distance focus has to be implanted. The Acri.Tec company (now owned by Carl Zeiss Meditec), has introduced the first multifocal MICS (Microincision Cataract Surgery) IOL, the Acri.Smart (Now AT Lisa) 366 D MICS, that could be implanted through a sub 2 mm incision. AMO (Abbott Medical Optics) has two multifocal IOL models: Tecnis and Rezoom, that have a diffractive and refractive design, respectively. Tecnis has a one-piece, hydrophobic aspheric optic that provided enhanced near

VA, reading acuity per speed, depth of focus, and spectacle independence compared with a monofocal IOL in a study of Packer et al.[30] Rezoom seems to function better in intermediate distances.[31] Rayner has also a multifocal, hydrophilic, acrylic one-piece IOL, the Rayner M-Flex, that is based on refractive aspheric optic technology and has 4 or 5 annular zones providing either +3 or +4 of additional refractive power for near.

Bilateral multifocal IOL implantation is reported to give the best multifocal effect. Forty percent of the multifocal group were able to do without spectacles, compared to 11% of the monofocal group. Careful selection of appropriate candidates is important for a satisfactory outcome. Accurate biometry is essential. Glare and ghosting were reported during night driving. Postoperative automated refractometry can be misleading, because of the variable refractive power in the central zone.[28] Absolute and relative contraindications for multifocal IOL implantation are summarized in **Table 37.1.**

TABLE 37.1	Contraindications for multifocal IOL implantation

Ocular and systemic diseases (loss of contrast sensitivity)
- Foveal impairment (e.g. maculopathy, diabetic retinopathy, retinal detachment surgery with macular involvement)
- Optic nerve anomalies, as in glaucoma, optic neuropathy
- Corneal disorders (e.g. dystrophy, scar leukoma, tear film dysfunction)
- Vitreous opacities
- Amblyopia
- Multiple sclerosis, Parkinson's, diabetes (with and without retinopathy)

Other conditions
- Astigmatism >1.00 diopter (applies to non-toric multifocal IOLs)
- Miosis <2.0 mm
- Age >85 years

Factors compromising multifocal function (preoperative or surgically induced)
- Biometric error
- Astigmatism >1.00 diopter (applies to non-toric multifocal IOLs)
- Abnormal pupil
- IOL tilt and decentration
- Capsular opacity
- Previous corneal refractive surgery

The effect of astigmatism on visual acuity in eyes with a diffractive multifocal intraocular lens was published by Hayashi et al. According to the authors, the presence of astigmatism in eyes with a diffractive multifocal IOL compromised all distance visual acuities, suggesting the need to correct astigmatism of greater than 1.00 D.[32] The introduction of toric multifocal IOLs by several IOL manufacturers, may solve this problem and extend the armamentarium of the refractive surgeon without compromising the optical quality of the cornea with invasive procedures.

ACCOMMODATIVE IOLS

Another approach to the correction of presbyopia has been introduced in the last few years with the so-called "accommodative" IOLs. True pseudophakic accommodation could be achieved by an anterior shift of the IOL optic during ciliary muscle contraction. In an eye of usual dimensions, an anterior shift of 600 μm of the IOL corresponds to an accommodative effect of 1 diopter current IOLs are too rigid to change position significantly during ciliary body contraction, so attempts have been concentrated mainly on more flexible accommodative IOL designs. A thin flexible hinge at the haptic-optic junction is common to all current models. Initially, two such IOLs [(1CU, HumanOptics, & AT-45, Eyeonics (Now Bausch & Lomb) Crystalens **(Figure 37.2)**] were, commercially available. Unfortunately, single or multi-center studies by independent researchers has shown that near-point accommodation did not induce significant movement of the so-called accommodating IOLs. In a study conducted by the author, 78% of the eyes implanted with the 1CU IOL had a visual acuity of 1.0 uncorrected for distance, but only 11% had J2 uncorrected for near. The overall satisfaction rate for near vision was very low. All patients required reading glasses.[33] The AT-45 model was reported to provide mean distance-corrected near visual acuity (DCNVA) of J5 at one month and six months. From one month on, the DCNVA was J3 or better in more than 60% of eyes.[34] The B&L Crystalens IOL had several modifications in its design. The latest version, Crystalens HD, was reported by Alio et al, to restore distance visual function after cataract surgery and improve near vision. The optical quality with this single-optic accommodating IOL was similar to that with a small-incision monofocal IOL.[35]

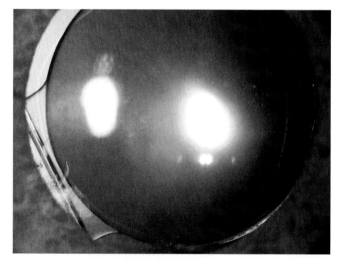

FIGURE 37.2: Accommodating IOL (*Courtesy:* Dr Agarwal's Eye Hospital, India)

A dual-optic lens design is currently in clinical trials. The Visiogen Synchrony Dual Optic IOL, a one-piece, silicone lens, consisting of a high plus-powered (front) optic attached by flexible bridges to a low minus-powered (back) optic, fits within the capsular bag. In a non-accommodated state, the distance between the two optics is shorter than in an accommodative state, when the bag slackens and the compressible haptics push the plus-powered optic forward. The first results are promising. In a recent study, the dual-optic accommodating IOL provided stable or improved reading ability over a two year period.[36]

Another interesting IOL design, NuLens (NuLens Ltd), according to Alio et al can provide near visual acuity improvement without compromising distance visual acuity. The accommodation mechanism of this IOL can produce an ocular power variation of 10.00 D.[37] This IOL has a semi-liquid silicone soft gel material in the center. The contraction and relaxation of the ciliary processes create movement of a piston into the soft silicone material. As a result of the movement of the capsular diaphragm, the material is displaced through an aperture in the piston, creating a bulge that gives the lens an increase in power.

Lenstec has developed the Tetraflex™ accommodating IOL, an acrylic, square-edged, one-piece microincision lens with equiconvex optics. According to the manufacturing company, the specially designed haptics and a 5 degree anterior angulation allow the lens to move forward during the accommodating process. The optic acts like a sail in the wind, catching the wave of the vitreous. Tetraflex is currently undergoing a US FDA Clinical Trial. Seventy-five percent of the Tetraflex patients reported near spectacle wear, either never or only occasionally for small print and/or dim light (21% never) compared with 46% of control patients (P<.001) (9% never).[38]

PIGGYBACK IOLS

Piggyback IOLs (Polypseudophakia) can provide appropriate pseudophakic optical correction for patients requiring very high IOL powers.[39,40] Since, primary polypseudophakia is considered for highly hyperopic eyes with small anterior segments, using thin, high-index optics allows two lenses to fit well into the capsular bag and remain optically stable. Acrylic IOLs with high refractive index are currently preferred as they offer several advantages.[41,42] The material's high index of refraction (usually 1,54), allows the biconvex optics to have flatter surfaces than plate-haptic silicone lenses, which by their design, have more steeply curved surfaces in view of their lower index of refraction (usually 1,41). Alignment of the optical zones of the two plate lenses could be tenuous as the capsular bag contracts around silicone optics postoperatively. Therefore, optical stability is more likely to be achieved with piggyback acrylic IOLs than with silicone or other lens materials.

With the first IOL, placing the loops within the bag can be achieved by any commonly practiced method. However, when placing the second set of loops, additional viscoelastic must be added to the bag and the loops presented in longitudinal fashion rather than having them open posteriorly over the first IOL. This will avoid displacing the first IOL from the bag or entwining the loops of the two IOLs. The question whether the loops of the two lenses should be left parallel or perpendicular to each other still remains unanswered. Negative-power IOLs are used in a piggyback fashion to correct high myopia. Fortunately, many IOL manufacturers have today a very large range of dioptric powers from -10 D up to +40 D.

Humanoptics and Rayner, have introduced IOLs that can be implanted in the sulcus to correct presbyopia or residual astigmatism in conjunction with a standard IOL, the Add-on and Sulcoflex, respectively. Combined implantation of an Add-on diffractive sulcus IOL and a monofocal capsular bag IOL was reported to be safe and effective in improving far and near visual acuity in cataract surgery. Preliminary visual acuity results were similar to those in eyes with a single 1-piece diffractive multifocal IOL.[43]

CONTROL OF ASTIGMATISM

An important goal in refractive cataract surgery is to control, and in some patients, to reduce corneal astigmatism. Several options for modulating astigmatism are available, including modifying incision placement, length, and construction; astigmatic keratotomy; limbal and corneal relaxing incisions (LRIs and CRIs) and toric intraocular lens (IOL) implantation.

The surgeon's major goal in managing astigmatism intraoperatively should be to preserve preoperative corneal asphericity, reduce a small amount of pre-existing astigmatism, or reduce high preoperative astigmatism without shifting the meridian. If the fellow eye is similar in astigmatic power and meridian, surgical astigmatic correction may not be indicated.

The temporal clear corneal, beveled single-plane or hinge incisions with a width of less than 3.3 mm retain the preoperative corneal cylinder within +-0.5 D of astigmatism. The astigmatically neutral incision allows the surgeon to perform predictable incisional keratotomy for the correction of preoperative astigmatism.

LIMBAL RELAXING INCISIONS AND ARCUATE KERATOTOMIES

The potential advantages of limbal relaxing incisions are preservation of the optical qualities of the cornea, less risk of inducing postoperative glare, less discomfort and more rapid recovery of vision.

They are placed at the limbus and can be made according to a modified Gills nomogram **(Table 37.2)**, based on preoperative corneal astigmatism as determined with standard keratometry and computerized videokeratography. The location of the steep axis is determined on the corneal topographic map and then the location relative to any significant landmark on the conjunctiva or limbus is noted. If a clear landmark is not evident preoperatively, the 6 and 12 o'clock semimeridians are marked with a 25 g needle in the corneal epithilium with patient sitting upright. Alternatively, a marking pen can be used to mark these

TABLE 37.2 Modified Gills nomogram to correct astigmatism with cataract surgery

Astigmatism (D)	Incision type	Length (mm)	Optical zone
1	One LRI	6.0	At limbus
1-2	Two LRIs	6.0	At limbus
2-3	Two LRIs	8.0	At limbus
> 3	Two LRIs + CRIs as indicated 3 months postoperatively	Lindstrom Surgical Nomogram for astigmatism	7-8 mm at cornea

TABLE 37.3 Nomogram for correction of astigmatism during cataract surgery (Budak, Friedman, Koch)

Astigmatism (D)	Incisions (mm)
<0.5	3.5 mm clear corneal temporal
With-the-rule	
0.5-1.25	3.5 mm superior limbal or 3.5 mm clear corneal temporal plus LRIs
=>1.50	3.5 mm clear corneal temporal plus LRIs (+ − CRIs at 3 months) or 3.5 mm superior limbal plus LRIs or 6.0 mm superior scleral
Against-the-rule	
0.5-1.25	3.5 mm clear corneal temporal
1.5-1.75	3.5 mm clear corneal temporal plus LRIs (+ − CRIs at 3 months)
>2.00	3.5 mm clear corneal temporal plus LRIs plus CRIs at 3 months
Oblique	
0.5-1.25	3.5 mm clear corneal on steeper meridian
1.5-1.75	3.5 mm clear corneal on steeper meridian plus LRIs (+ − CRIs at 3 months)
>2.00	3.5 mm clear corneal on steeper meridian plus LRIs plus CRIs at 3 months

semimeridians. A guarded diamond knife is set to at a depth of 600 μm. The incisions can be made before or after cataract surgery. Some surgeons prefer to perform the incisions at the conclusion of the surgery in the event that a complication occurs, altering the astigmatic strategy.

According to a study by Budak, Friedman and Koch, patients achieved a mean reduction in astigmatism of 1,47 D at 1 month postoperatively.[44] The mean with the wound (WTW) change was -0,70+-0,44D. Preoperative astigmatism was greater than 1,50D in 83,3% of the eyes preoperatively, compared with 25% postoperatively. No overcorrections were observed. None of the patients reported postoperative distortion in vision, glare or discomfort. Based on their early results the authors suggested a surgical nomogram for the correction of astigmatism during cataract surgery (**Table 37.3**).

In a similar approach Nichamin and Dillman developed a nomogram for clear corneal phaco and arcuate keratotomies[45] (**Table 37.4**). As seen in the nomogram, patients who are relatively spherical receive only a single-plane, beveled temporal incision placed just inside the vascular arcade. For those patients with modest pre-existing against the rule astigmatism, rather than enlarging the temporal incision, a peripheral nasal arcuate relaxing incision is placed according to the age-adjusted nomogram. If higher levels of astigmatism are present, a temporal limbal arcuate incision is placed so that it encompasses the posterior entry of clear corneal incision.

For pre-existing with-the-rule astigmatism the surgeon has two choices: utilize a superior clear corneal phaco incision, with or without arcuate limbal corneal incisions over the steep vertical axis, or retain the neutral temporal clear corneal phaco incision and place intralimbal arcs along the steep vertical axis. Although this latter approach may involve a greater number of incisions, it has the advantages of working temporally and the movement around the operating table is avoided.

After verifying the steep meridian with intraoperative keratoscopy or other method, the appropriate degree of arc is marked on the corneal surface. The incisions are placed

TABLE 37.4 Nomogram for clear-corneal phaco and astigmatic keratotomy (AK) surgery (Nichamin, Dillman, Maloney)

Astigmatic status—*Spherical*: (+0.75 × 90's + 0.50 × 180')

Incision Design—Neutral temporal clear corneal incision—TCC (3.2 mm or less single plane)

Astigmatic status—*Against-the-rule*: Steep axis (0 to 30°/150 to 180°): Intraoperative keratoscopy determines exact incision location

Incision design—Neutral TCC along with the following peripheral arcuate incisions

	Age:	30-50 years	51-70 years	71-85 years	>85 years
Preop cylinder		Degrees of	arc to be incised		
+0.75 to +1.50	Nasal limbal arc	50°	45°	30°	——
+1.75 to +2.50	Paired arcuate incisions	60°	50°	45°	30°
+2.75 to +3.50	Paired arcuate incisions	90°	75°	50°	45°
+3.75 to +4.50	Paired arcuate incisions	Reduce OZ (i.e. 7.0 mm)	90°	75°	60°

'TCC incision followed by nasal and temporal peripheral arcuate incisions
The temporal arc approximates the posterior border of the TCC

Astigmatic status—*With-the-rule*: Steep axis (45° to 145°): Intraoperative keratoscopy determines exact incision location

Incision design—Neutral TCC along with the following peripheral arcuate incisions

	Age:	30-50 years	51-70 years	71-85 years	>85 years
Preop cylinder		Degrees of	arc to be incised		
+1.0 to +1.75	Paired limbal arcs on steep axis	40°	35°	30°	—
+2.00 to +2.75	Paired limbal arcs on steep axis	60°	50°	45°	30°
+3.00 to +3.75	Paired limbal arcs on steep axis	75°	60°	50°	40°

Or

Incision design—superior clear cornea (SCC) with the following peripheral arcuate incisions

	Age:	30-50 years	51-70 years	71-85 years	>85 years
Preop cylinder		Degrees of	arc to be incised		
+1.5 to +2.00		SCC alone	SCC alone	SCC alone	—
+2.00 to +2.75	Inferior limbal arc	45°	30°	SCC alone	SCC alone
+3.00 to +3.75	*paired arcuate incisions	60°	45°	30°	SCC alone

*SCC incision followed by superior and inferior peripheral arcuate incisions. The superior arc approximates the posterior border of the SCC

just inside the limbus, taking care to keep the blade's footplates parallel to the corneal surface.

Arcuate keratotomy at a later date can be an alternative for the reduction of pre-existing or induced astigmatism. The number of incisions, the size of the optical zone and the arc length of the incision can be determined with reference to various nomograms.[46-48] The Thornton Nomogram for the correction of astigmatism is shown in **Table 37.5**. However, surgical outcomes in pseudophakic eyes with history of ocular surgery can be different from those with intact eyes.[49] The predictability of astigmatic keratotomy after cataract surgery has been addressed in very few published papers[50,51] and needs further evaluation with larger studies.

A more convenient way to perform more precise arcuate keratotomies is the Terry-Schanzlin Astigmatome (Oasis). It consists of an alignment speculum attached to a syringe to create suction and preset-depth single or double blades. Blade depth and Optical Zone (OZ) are preset to provide consistent depth and reproducibility. Preset depth options are 500, 550, 600, 650 and 700 μ for arcuate cuts at 8 mm. Pachymetry is required to determine corneal depth.

TABLE 37.5 Thornton nomogram for astigmatic keratotomy

Assumes cuts 98% deep (almost to Descemet's membrane) along the full length of the incision.

Age: For every year below age 30 add 1/2% to the astigmatic error. For every year above age 30 subtract 1/2%.

Sex: In premenopausal women (under age 40) subtract three years from actual age.

IOP: For every mm IOP below 12 add 2% to the astigmatic error. For every mm IOP above 15, subtract 2%.

Add or subtract the sum of the modifiers (%) from the actual amount of cylinder for the "Theoretical Cylinder".

Cylinder corrected by paired arcuate transverse incisions

Chord length of one pair arcuate transverse incisions

Theoretical cylinder	Degrees arc
0.50 D	20
0.75 D	23
1.00 D	25
1.25 D	28
1.50 D	32
1.75 D	35
2.00 D	38
2.25 D	42
2.50 D	45

Chord length of two pairs arcuate transverse incisions

Theoretical cylinder	Degrees arc
2.00 D	23
2.25 D	27
2.50 D	31
2.75 D	35
3.00 D	39
3.25 D	43
3.50 D	47
3.75 D	50

Chord length of three pairs arcuate transverse incisions

Theoretical cylinder	Degrees arc
3.25 D	22
3.50 D	26
3.75 D	30
4.00 D	35
4.25 D	40
4.50 D	45
4.75 D	50
5.00 D	54

Smaller OZ (5.5 to 7.5 mm)
−0.50 D to 1.00 D more

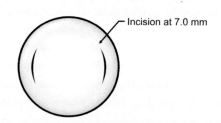

Incision at 7.0 mm

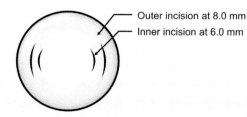

Outer incision at 8.0 mm
Inner incision at 6.0 mm

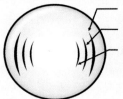

Outer incision just outside the 8 mm
Middle incision at the 7 mm
Inner incision inside 6 mm

Measurements should be taken centrally and at the location of the incisions. The double-blade design is commonly used for the treatment of regular astigmatism where two simultaneous arcs are desired exactly 180° apart. A single-blade variation is available for non-orthogonal and asymmetric corrections.

In the near future, it will be possible to perform LRIs and arcuate keratotomies before surgery with a femtosecond laser, that will also prepare the main and stub incisions with high precision.

TORIC IOLS

The advantages of toric IOLs versus astigmatic keratotomy are the facts that there is no additional intervention during surgery, no interference with corneal curvature and high predictability.[38] A potential problem is obtaining and maintaining the correct axis.

The STAAR Toric[TM] IOL was the first foldable single-piece, plate-haptic silicone injectable IOL, available commercially. It incorporates a cylindrical correction on the anterior surface of a spherical optic thereby producing a toric or spherocylindrical refracting element. The lens is available in a complete range of spherical powers with cylindrical adds of 2.0 and 3.5 D. The 2.0 D toric IOL is intended for use in cataract patients with 1.5 D to 2.25 D of preexisting corneal astigmatism. The 3.5 D Toric IOL is intended for use in cataract patients with 2.25 D to 3.5 D of preexisting astigmatism.[52] This toric IOL is indicated in cataract patients who will have a regular corneal astigmatism of 1.5 to 3.5 D. On corneal topography these patients will exhibit symmetrical bow-tie or wedge-type patterns. On keratometry, they will have regular mires with the steep and flat corneal meridians at approximately 90 degrees apart. The steep meridian of the spherocylindrical optic is orientated along the short axis of the IOL, so that the axis of the cylindrical correction lies along the long axis of the IOL which is indicated by the two markings at the haptic-optic junction. When used in conjunction with astigmatically neutral cataract surgery, these markings are simply aligned with the steep corneal meridian in order to maximize the effect of the cylindrical correction afforded by the lens.

The manufacturer of this IOL has developed software using the SRK/T formula to determine the IOL power and alignment axis. In addition, the probable postoperative astigmatism is displayed for misalignment up to 10 degrees. If the axis of the lens is within 10 degrees from the post-operative steep meridian it can be left uncorrected, but if it is greater than that postoperative realignment is indicated. At 30 degrees misalignment, the toric correction is lost. Beyond that the cylindrical correction may be increased.

Of the eyes implanted with the 3.5 D toric IOL, 42% had postoperative cylinder less than 0.5 D while 25% of the torics and 85% of the controls had greater than 1.5 D. Four of 175 IOLs in the FDA Study had to be re-aligned within one week after the surgery.[53]

Another toric IOL, the Humanoptics Torica (former Dr.Schmidt Microsil Toric), is available in a wider dioptric range, from -3.0 D to +30.0 D and from 2.0 D to 12.0 D for sphere and cylinder, respectively. This IOL has large serrated PMMA haptics that prevent IOL rotation. The same manufacturer has toric IOLs for sulcus fixation with 6.0 or 7.0 mm optic.

A few years ago, Alcon introduced the Acrysof Toric IOL, that was based on the familiar hydrophobic Acrylic Acrysof IOL platform. This IOL made toric IOLs popular to many ophthalmic surgeons, offering a wide choice of astigmatism correction up to 6 cylindrical diopters. The lens is reported to be fairly stable. In a study, mean axis rotation at one year was less than 4 degrees.[54] The results of another study by Kwartz and Edwards, showed a mean rotation of 3.3 degrees for up to 24 months postoperatively.[55] In our study, the Acrysof Toric Lens had a mean rotation of 4.2 degrees in six months.[56] The calculation of the IOL power and axis is made very easily on Internet at www.acrysoftoriccalculator.com.

In the past,patients with astigmatism higher than 1.0 Diopter were no good candidates for multifocal IOLs. Very recently, several companies (Alcon, Zeiss, Rayner) introduced toric multifocal IOLs, that are capable to correct all refractive errors and further reduce the dependency on glasses or contact lenses.

The evolution and the refinement of all the current and future techniques will allow the cataract surgeon to correct the refractive error of any patient with high precision in a single operation. The true refractive cataract surgery has become a reality in the beginning of the 21st Century.

REFERENCES

1. Olsen T. Sources of error in intraocular lens power calculation. J Cataract Refract Surg. 1992;18(2):125-9.
2. Giers U, Epple C. Comparison of A-scan device accuracy. J Cataract Refract Surg. 1990;16(2):235-42.
3. Olsen T, Nielsen PJ. Immersion versus contact technique in the measurement of axial length by ultrasound. Acta Ophthalmol (Copenh) (Denmark). 1989:67(1):101-2.
4. Whelehan IM, Heyworth P, Tabandeh H, McGuigan S, Foss AJ. A comparison of slit-lamp supported versus hand-held biometry. Eye. 1996;10(Pt 4):514-6.
5. Allison KL, Price J, Odin L. Asteroid hyalosis and axial length measurement using automated biometry. J Cataract Refract Surg. 1991;17(2):181-6.
6. Panidou I, Topouzidis H, Reptsis A, Alexandrou K, Zisiadis K. Biometric errors in IOL Power Calculation. Proceedings of the 31st Panhellenic. Ophthalmological Congress. 1998; 38-41.
7. Berges O, Puech M, et al. B-Mode-Guided Vector-A-Mode Versus A-Mode Biometry To Determine Axial Length and IOL Power. J Cataract Refract Surg. 1998;24:529-35.
8. Flowers CW, McLeod SD, McDonnell PJ, Irvine JA, Smith RE. Evaluation of intraocular lens power calculation formulas in the triple procedure. J Cataract Refract Surg. 1996;22(1): 116-22.

9. Husain SE, Kohnen T, Maturi R, Er H, Koch DD. Computerized videokeratography and keratometry in determining intraocular lens calculations. J Cataract Refract Surg. 1996; 22(3):362-6.

10. Olsen T, Thim K, Corydon L. Accuracy of the newer generation intraocular lens power calculation formulas in long and short eyes. J Cataract Refract Surg. 1991;17(2):187-93.

11. Savini G, Hoffer KJ, Carbonelli M, Barboni P. Intraocular lens power calculation after myopic excimer laser surgery: clinical comparison of published methods. J Cataract Refract Surg. 2010;36(9):1455-65.

12. Tang M, Li Y, Huang D. An intraocular lens power calculation formula based on optical coherence tomography: a pilot study. J Refract Surg. 2010;26(6):430-7.

13. Hitzenberger CK. Optical measurement of the axial eye length by laser Doppler interferometry. Invest Ophthalmol Vis Sci. 1991;32:616-24.

14. Drexler W, Findl Ï, Menapace R, et al. Partial coherence interferometry: a novel approach to biometry in cataract surgery. Am J Ophthalmol. l998;126:524-34.

15. Hitzenberger CK, Drexler W, Dolezal C, et al. Measurement of the axial length of cataract eyes by laser Doppler interferometry. Invest Ophthalmol Vis Sci 1993;34:1886-1893.

16. Kuck Ç, Makabe R. Vergleichende axiale Biometrie des Auges. Fortschr Ophthalmol. l985;82:91-3.

17. Papadopoulos, PA, Tyligadi A, et al. Accuracy of IOL calculations in Optical Biometry, Paper presented at 36th Panhellenic Congress Of Ophthalmology, Crete. 2003.

18. Findl Ï, Drexler W, Menapace R, et al. Teilkoharenz- Laser-interferometrie: eine neue hochprazise Biometrie Methode zur Verbesserung der Refraktion nach Kataraktchirurgie. Klin Monatsbl Augenheilkd 1998;212:29.

19. Rabsilber TM, Jepsen C, Auffarth GU, Holzer MP. Intraocular lens power calculation: clinical comparison of 2 optical biometrydevices. J Cataract Refract Surg 2010;36(2):230-4.

20. Handa T, Mukuno K, Uozato H, Niida T, Shoji N, Minei R, Nitta M, Shimizu K.Ocular dominance and patient satisfaction after monovision induced by intraocular lens implantation. J Cataract Refract Surg. 2004;30(4):769-74.

21. Greenbaum S, Monovision pseudophakia. J Cataract Refract Surg. 2002;28(8):1439-43.

22. I. Howard Fine, MD, Mark Packer, MD, Richard S. Hoffman. MD New lens technologies progress for correction of presbyopia. Ophthalmology Times. 2003.

23. Kriechbaum K, Findl O, Koeppl C, Menapace R, Drexler W. Stimulus-driven versus pilocarpine-induced biometric changes in pseudophakic eyes. Ophthalmology. 2005;112(3):453-9.

24. Fine IH. Design and Early Clinical Studies of the AMO Array multifocal IOL. In: Maxwell A, Nordan LT (Eds). Current Concepts on multifocal Intraocular Lenses. Thorofare, NJ, Slack Inc. 1991;105-15.

25. Percival SP, Setty SS. Prospectively randomized trial comparing the pseudoaccommodation of the AMO Array multifocal lens and a monofocal lens. JCRS 1993;19:26-31.

26. Jacobi PC, Konen W. Effect of age and astigmatism on the AMO Array multifocal intraocular lens. JCRS. 1995;121:556-61.

27. Vaquero-Ruano M, Encinas JL, et al: AMO Array Multifocal versus Monofocal Intraocular Lens: Long-term Follow-up, JCRS 1998;24:118-23.

28. Papadopoulos PA, Katsavavakis D, Kotsiras I. Early Results with the Foldable Multifocal IOL AMO Array SA40. Paper presented at the 31st Panhellenic Ophthalmological Meeting. 1998.

29. Alfonso JF, Fernández-Vega L, Puchades C, Montés-Micó R. Intermediate visual function with different multifocal intraocular lens models. J Cataract Refract Surg. 2010; 36(5):733-9.

30. Packer M, Chu YR, Waltz KL, Donnenfeld ED, Wallace RB 3rd, Featherstone K, Smith P, Bentow SS, Tarantino N. Evaluation of the aspheric tecnis multifocal intraocular lens: one-year results from the first cohort of the food and drug administration clinical trial. Am J Ophthalmol. 2010;149(4): 577-84.

31. Mesci C, Erbil HH, Olgun A, Yaylali SA. Visual performances with monofocal, accommodating, and multifocal intraocular lenses in patients with unilateral cataract. Am J Ophthalmol. 2010;150(5):609-18.

32. Hayashi K, Manabe S, Yoshida M, Hayashi H. Effect of astigmatism on visual acuity in eyes with a diffractive multifocal intraocular lens J Cataract Refract Surg. 2010;36(8):1323-9.

33. P.A.Papadopoulos, Sp.Georgaras. First Results with the Accomodative 1CU IOL, Presented at the 16th International Meeting of the HSIOIRS. Athens 2002.

34. Hantera MM, Hamed AM, Fekry Y, Shoheib EA. Initial experience with an accommodating intraocular lens: controlled prospective study. J Cataract Refract Surg. 2010;36(7): 1167-72.

35. Alió JL, Piñero DP, Plaza-Puche AB. Visual outcomes and optical performance with a monofocal intraocular lens and a new-generation single-optic accommodating intraocular lens. J Cataract Refract Surg. 2010;36(10):1656-64.

36. Bohórquez V, Alarcon R. Long-term reading performance in patients with bilateral dual-optic accommodating intraocular lenses. J Cataract Refract Surg. 2010;36(11):1880-6.

37. Alió JL, Ben-nun j, Rodríguez-Prats JL, Plaza AB. Visual and accommodative outcomes 1 year after implantation of an accommodating intraocular lens based on a new concept. J Cataract Refract Surg. 2009;35(10):1671-8.

38. Sanders DR, Sanders ML. Tetraflex Presbyopic IOL Study Group. US FDA clinical trial of the Tetraflex potentially accommodating IOL: comparison to concurrent age-matched monofocal controls. J Refract Surg. 2010;26(10):723-30.

39. Gayton JL. Implanting two Posterior Chamber Intraocular Lenses in Nanophthalmos, Ocular Surgery News. 1994;64-5.

40. Holladay J, Gills, et al. Achieving Emmetropia in Extremely Short Eyes with Two Piggyback Posterior Chamber Intraocular Lenses. Ophthalmology. 1996;103:1118-23.

41. Masket S. Piggyback Intraocular Lens Implantation, JCRS 1998;24:569-70.

42. Shugar JK, Lewis C, Lee A. Implantation of multiple foldable acrylic posterior chamber lenses in the capsular bag for high hyperopia. JCRS 1996;22:1368-72.

43. Gerten G, Kermani O, Schmiedt K, Farvili E, Foerster A, Oberheide U. Dual intraocular lens implantation: Monofocal lens in the bag and additional diffractive multifocal lens in the sulcus. J Cataract Refract Surg. 2009;35:2136–43.

44. Budak K, Friedman N, Koch D. Limbal Relaxing Incisions with Cataract Surgery. J Cataract Refract Surg. 1998;24:503-08.

45. Nichamin L, Dillman D, Maloney WF. Peripheral arcuate astigmatic keratotomy partners with clear corneal phaco surgery. Ocular Surgery News. 1997;17:15.

46. Lindstrom RL. The Surgical Correction of Astigmatism:A clinician's Perspective. Refr Corneal Surg 1990;6:441-54.

47. Thornton SP. Astigmatic Keratotomy: A review of Basic Concepts with Case Reports. JCRS 1990;16:430-35.

48. Thornton SP. Astigmatic Keratotomy in:Radial and Astigmatic Keratotomy. Slack Inc, NJ. 1994.

49. Georgaras S, Tsingos V, Papadopoulos PA. Correction of Postoperative Astigmatism. Proceedings of the 31st Panhellenic Ophthalmological Congress. 1998;214-21.

50. Guell JL, Manero F, Muller A. Transverse Keratotomy to Correct High Corneal Astigmatism After Cataract Surgery. JCRS 1996;22:331-6.

51. Oshika T, Shimazaki J, et al. Arcuate Keratotomy to Treat Corneal Astigmatism After Cataract Surgery. Ophthalmology. 1998;105:2012-6.

52. STAAR TORICTM IOL User's Guide, Staar Surgical, Monrovia, CA 1996.

53. Sanders D: Preliminary Results of the FDA Trial for the STAAR TORICTM IOL, XVth ESCRS Congress, Prague 1997.

54. Holland E, Lane S, Horn JD, Ernest P, Arleo R, Miller KM. The AcrySof Toric intraocular lens in subjects with cataracts and corneal astigmatism: a randomized, subject-masked, parallel-group, 1-year study. Ophthalmology. 2010;117(11): 2104-11.

55. Kwartz J, Edwards K. Evaluation of the long-term rotational stability of single-piece, acrylic intraocular lenses. Br J Ophthalmol. 2010;94(8):1003-6.

56. Papadopoulos P.A. "Toric IOLs in the Correction of Preoperative Astigmatism", Presented at the 22nd International Congress of HSIOIRS, Athens. 2008.

CHAPTER 38

Minimally Invasive Cataract Surgery and MICS IOLs: Our Experience, Our Technique, Our Outcomes

Jorge L Alio, P Klonowski

THE MODERN EVOLUTION OF CATARACT SURGERY

Cataract surgery is one of the most frequently performed surgeries and millions of the eyes are operated each year in the entire world. The first modern cataract surgery was done by Sir Harold Ridley in 1949 with the implantation of the first polymethyl methacrylate (PMMA) intraocular lens. The incision was longer than 10 mm, the intraocular lens was not perfect, and the surgery was complicated.

The spectacular progress of the cataract surgery technique in the 80s and 90s of the 20th century leaded to diminish the surgical trauma and percentage of the complications connected to the maneuvers and energy delivered into the eye. The technical progress made possible to think about diminish the incision seize. The idea to make the cataract surgery bimanually without phaco-tip sleeve was started in the end of the 80s. This method was described by Shearing in 1985, but the idea of diversification of the liquid was the main step to develop new surgical techniques, new surgical tools and new surgical possibilities.

Better visual outcome, aggressiveness surgery, separated infusion, minimal phaco power, new surgical tools and fluidics management evoke new idea of surgery microincision cataract surgery (MICS).

In 2001 Jorge Alio registered the concept of MICS as the surgery performed through incisions of 1.8 mm or less. Understanding this global concept implies that it is not only about achieving a smaller incision size but also about making a global transformation of the sugical procedure towards minimal aggressiveness.

Separated fluidics high volume of the liquids and high vacuum become also in the new tool. Especially in the case of the soft cataracts lens opacities classification system (LOCS) one or two the use of the ultrasound can be diminished or practically eliminated. The high vacuum and infusion chopper use permits the masses breaking and aspirating without US power. The phacoemulsification of the harder grade of the cataract needs to be supported by minimal doses of the US energy. Nowadays, the small doses of the ultrasound power and MICS concept can eliminate the phaco-tip overheating and the thermal injury of the cornea. These ideas diminish surgical trauma and improve cataract surgery refractive result.

The complications with MICS can occur during learning curve. Transition to MICS needs to understand the principles of MICS ideas and technique. In the first time of transition the problems with fluidics, anterior chamber stability and wound integrity can occur.[1,2]

MAIN CONCEPTS IN MICS

Incision

Diminishing of incision is the most interesting and important parameter of the modern surgery. Following the minimization idea smaller incision means lower wound dimension, less eye traumatism and faster healing.

Small wound construction satisfies the principles of the self sealing incision. The wound closing is more efficient and the leakage is no observed in short period of postoperative time. The watertight construction of the wound diminishes the iris prolapse complications. Faster wound healing reduces possibility of the bacterial infection. The reduction of the surgically induced astigmatism (SIA) by the small incision becomes more important advantage in the field of cataract and refractive lens surgery.[3]

Reduction of the cataract surgery incision leads to:
- Corneal tissue damage reduction
- Faster recovery of the wound
- Higher stability of the eye during surgery
- Easier capsulorhexis, hydrodissection performance
- Diminishing of the postoperative complications
- Wound leakage
- Risk of endophthalmitis
- SIA
- Improves optical quality of the cornea.

The idea of the small incision leads to progress in the instruments adaptation, machine construction and software programming. The small incision demand new technology of the foldable lenses. In the future probably, it will make the incision smaller.[2-4]

Fluidics

The fluid management is essential in MICS. The proper setup of machine with the balanced values protects the eye and helps the surgeon to pass through the all stages of the surgery without complications.

The fluid inflow should be balanced by outflow, but the balance should be corrected, based on the sufficient eye ball tension. The pressure of the infusion should make the infusion larger than the outflow of the liquid. This difference between inflow and outflow keeps the proper anatomy of the anterior segment of the eye and become the powerful tool in the breaking of the cataract masses. During the occlusion under high pressure in the phaco aspiration tip can break the masses without using of ultrasound power. At this moment fluidics become powerful tool in the process of the surgery. The MICS fluidics is more efficient than in the micro coaxial surgery. The gas forced infusion (GFI) support is obligatory in the MICS surgery. The continuous flow of the infusion liquid is supported by the gas which is delivered with the pressure to the infusion bottle. The GFI helps to stabilize and maintain the inflow of the liquid on the high level. This keeps the anterior chamber constant and permits to cool the tip. It equilibrates intraocular pressure (IOP) during the whole surgery. It is very important to keep IOP stable in the case of the severe retinal degenerations, proliferative vitreoretinopathy (PVR), neovascularizations and vascular diseases. Deregulation of the pressure can lead to accommodative convergence (AC) collapse and intrasurgical hypotony of the eye like in the standard coaxial phacoemulsification.

Some of the platforms such Accurus or Millennium are supported by internal pump. Infinity platform needs to be supported by external air pump connected with the air filter.

Other fluid problem is the postocclusion time and problems connected to the high vacuum and insufficient inflow. This dangerous circumstance can happen when occluded mass is aspirated suddenly by the tip and the pressure of the AC suddenly decreases. Some phaco machines have software to prevent the surge. Advanced medical optics (AMO) sovereign has virtual model of AC and in the moment of occlusion the pump decrease the vacuum. The use of the flow restrictors can also solve the problem. The restrictor can be connected to the aspiration tube. Small filters restrict the flow and surge does not exceed the limit values. The possibility of the AC collapse and rupture of the posterior capsule is practically eliminated (**Figure 38.1**).[5]

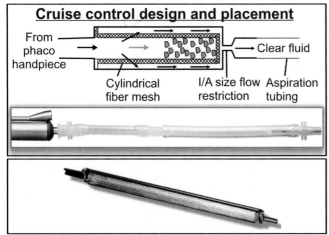

FIGURE 38.1: Cruise control™ system (STAAR surgical company MONROVIA, CA USA) and stable chamber system (Bausch and Lomb Company Rochester, NY, USA)

Power Modulation

Varying the power modulation during phacoemulsification can be saved and efficient method to improve the efficacy of cataract surgery. Pulsing ultrasound can dramatically diminish energy delivered into the eye. Changing on/off times and shortening the time of pulse one can achieve better result in cataract mass emulsification, corneal wound and endothelial cell protection. It is very important that very short power modulation like hyperpulse and ultrapulse can dramatically decrease possibility of wound burn during MICS surgery. During the on-time cycle the cornea is heating but during the off-time cycle phaco-tip and cornea are cooling. Also, short pulse energy seems to be more effective because it produces more cavitational energy than continuous power. The use of torsional phaco can additionally diminish the delivered energy. With the use of torsional phaco practically, one can eliminate the longitudinal ultrasound power or use it only in minimal way with the hard cataract. The active use of power modulation seems to change MICS to more efficient surgery.[5,6]

MICROINCISION CATARACT SURGERY (MICS) INSTRUMENTS

The MICS is bimanual procedure. Two incisions with the same diameter allow using the same instruments by the both wounds. This advantage is very helpful to clean the anterior and posterior capsule, remove cortical and nuclear fragments. The access to all regions of the anterior segment is ideal. The construction of the instrument permits to perfect maneuvers and liquid steam direction protects the posterior capsule integrity and endothelium stability.

MICS 18G

To perform MICS surgery one can use two types of the instruments depending on the incision size preferred by the surgeon. One can use tools for standard MICS (18 G instruments) and Micro MICS (22 G instruments).

To perform standard MICS 18 G surgery the author needs instruments specially designed for 1.5 mm incision. To make incision, the calibrated knife is necessary. The Alio´s MICS knife (Katena Inc, Denville, NJ, the USA) has trapezoid shape 1.25 mm/1.4 mm/2.0 mm which is necessary to make incision of the desired shape and dimensions. The other opportunity is the diamond knife with the same proportions (**Figures 38.2 and 38.3**).

The shape and dimension of the knives permit to make incision which is perfectly adapted to the MICS phaco tip

FIGURE 38.2: Alio´s MICS metal knife (Katena Inc, Denville, NJ, USA)

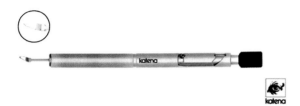

FIGURE 38.3: Alio´s MICS diamond knife
(Katena Inc, Denville, NJ, CUSA)

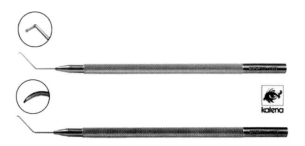

FIGURE 38.5: Alio-rosen MICS phaco prechopper and Alio Scimitar prechopper microincision cataract surgery (Katena Inc, Denville, NJ, USA)

of 0.9 mm. The incision is watertight, keep the anterior chamber stable and permit perfectly the maneuvering in the anterior chamber. The borders of the incision are perfectly adapted to close without suturing. The small amount of the fluid during hydration ascertain in incision closing.

Continuous curvilinear capsulorhexis (CCC) is essential in the each type of the phaco surgery. To make the capsulorhexis through the 1.25 mm incision, the micro forceps is obligatory. Alio´s MICS capsulorhexis forceps (Katena Inc, Denville, NJ, USA) is 23 G tool. This instrument is perfectly perpetrated to do tearing of the anterior capsule by the pointed catch which is situated at the end of the forceps. The CCC is easy with this thin and delicate forceps **(Figure 38.4)**.

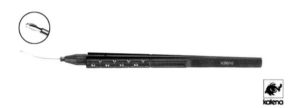

FIGURE 38.4: Alio's MICS capsulorhexis forceps (Katena Inc, Denville, NJ, USA)

During each capsulorhexis, the maintaining of the stable anterior chamber is essential. The disproportion between incision and tool can make conduct to the ophthalmic viscosurgical device (OVD), leakage during the CCC and tearing the capsule outside. With the 1.25 mm incision and 23 G instrument practically it does not happen.

Hydrodissection and hydrodelineation is the next stage of the surgery which permits to separate the lens from the capsule and divide the lens layers. This maneuver can be done by each type of the cannula prefer by surgeon but the washout of the OVD from the AC before is essential. The small incision and high density of the OVD can block the incision and lead to the increase the pressure in the anterior chamber and be dangerous for the stability of the posterior capsule.

Prechopping can facilitate the surgery. This stage of the surgery based on the mechanical division of the lens by the two prechoppers. This simple maneuver can be done by Alio-Rosen MICS phaco prechopper (Katena Inc, Denville, NJ, USA) or by Alio-Scimitar MICS prechoppers (Katena Inc, Denville, NJ, USA) **(Figure 38.5)**.

The shape of Scimitar prechopper is designed to perform and facilitate the 700 microns surgery. Scimitar prechopper has a curved tip with a blunt end and a sharp inferior edge. The choppers are crossed by situating symmetrically opposite oneself. Now, cutting movements are being made by gently crossing prechoppers. The cut will be made from the perimeter to the center of the nuclei. Internal edge has a sharp edge that facilitates the incisions of the lens masses. When the cut is made, two dividing hemispheres are made. The nucleus is then rotated about 90º and then for the second time prechopping is repeated as described.

Next stage of the surgery is phacoemulsification of the cataract lens. The MICS permits to do surgery bimanually. One port is for the irrigating chopper and the second is for the aspiration phaco tip without the silicon sleeve. The MICS gives opportunity to perform phacoemulsification from both sides, by right and left hand any time at all stages of surgery. It depends on corneal astigmatism, surgeon preferences and intraoperative conditions.

For the standard MICS surgery, the author uses two types of the irrigating choppers: Alio's original fingernail MICS irrigating hydromanipulator and Alio's MICS Irrigating Stinger (Katena Inc, Denville, NJ, USA) **(Figures 38.6 and 38.7)**.

First irrigating hydromanipulator fingernail helps to remove rather soft cataracts. There is irrigation hole on the bottom lower side of the tool. The diameter of the hole is 1 mm. It has also very thin walls to increase internal diameter of instrument. This irrigation cannula is assuring infusion in borders 72 cc/min. A large infusion directed to the bottom assures the excellent flow of liquids and also a fast and effective chilling phacoemulsification tip. An outstanding stability of the anterior chamber is assured

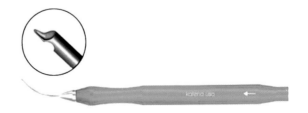

FIGURE 38.6: Alio's original fingernail MICS irrigating hydromanipulator (Katena Inc, Denville, NJ, USA). Not in use now

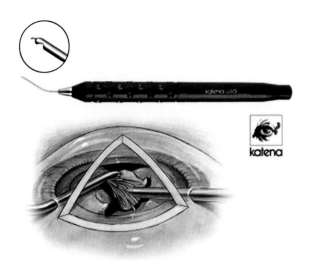

FIGURE 38.7: Alio's MICS irrigating stinger
(Katena Inc, Denville, NJ, USA)

through the function infusion and directs the liquid to the lens masses at the bag back, independently from high vacuum sets of phacoemulsification machine. The strength of the stream permits the bag to be held in a safe distance from the phacoemulsification tip and at the same time enables convenient manipulations of tools and lens masses. Additionally, this stream can clean the back bag from remaining cortical cells. A very fertile directed stream to the back bag is provided with the preservation of cells endothelium corneas before mechanical and thermal damage. The irrigation hole can be found situated on the side of the irrigating probe or on top and this can result in the turbulences in the anterior chamber. This effect can damage the endothelium cells and stabilities of the anterior chamber.

The tool which allows the removal of harder cataracts is Alio's MICS Irrigating Stinger. This tool has a 19 G diameter and it is equipped with a tip at the end which is angled downwards. This tool is useful to chop off segments or dividing masses of the nucleus in the phacoemulsification tip.

For removing remains of cortical masses is serving Alio's MICS aspiration handpiece (Katena Inc, Denville, NJ, the USA) **(Figure 38.8).**

There is a tool especially designed for delicate and safe manipulations within the anterior chamber. It has a diameter

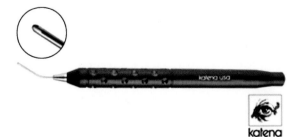

FIGURE 38.8: Alio's MICS aspiration handpiece
(Katena Inc, Denville, NJ, USA)

of 18 G. The cylindrical shape allows this tool to gently manipulate within the surgical wound. At the same time, the port diameter of 0.3 mm assures the stability of the hydrodynamic of liquid within the anterior chamber. This handpiece allows to remove remained masses from the bag and the full comfort of polishing the bag back.[7]

MICS 22 G

The Alio Stinger irrigating chopper duet system (Redmond, Washington, USA) is the 22 G inferior opening instrument. It has one hole on the inferior side of the cannula and provides the infusion stream directly backward, forcing cataract fragments to levitate towards the phaco tip pointed to masses and posterior capsule. This also allows maintaining anterior chamber deep and holding the capsule far from the phaco-tip. The fluid infusion with GFI is sufficient for 0.7 mm MICS demand. The end of the Stinger is equipped with a pointed tip which is angled downwards. It enables to break masses with ease and provide them to aspiration hole [7] **(Figure 38.9).**

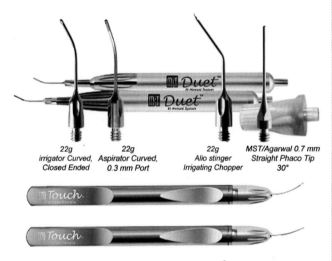

| 22g irrigator Curved, Closed Ended | 22g Aspirator Curved, 0.3 mm Port | 22g Alio stinger Irrigating Chopper | MST/Agarwal 0.7 mm Straight Phaco Tip 30° |

FIGURE 38.9: The 0.7 mm (22G) duet® system Alio stinger irrigating chopper

Microincision Cataract Surgery (MICS) Phacoemulsification Platforms

The MICS surgery can be made with the help of practically each type of the phaco platforms supported by venturi pump. This type of the pump is very powerful and effective in the vacuum construction. The surgery on venturi pump machine is the high vacuum and constant vacuum surgery. The vacuum about 550 mm Hg is very easy to achieve in few milliseconds in all of this types of machines. Other types of the pumps like peristaltic are not such effective.

In the case of soft cataracts having placed under pressure on 500–550 mm Hg, the author can only use Alio's MICS hydromanipulator irrigating fingernail. This makes it possible to divide and aspirate fragment masses of the lens without using ultrasound or using ultrasound in the minimum way. The torsional phacoemulsification with the oscillatory, mechanically moving tip can be helpful. Ultrasound energy can be eliminated. The Kelman Tip and Infinity System (Alcon Laboratories, Inc.) equipped with OZil energy are preferred. In the case of hard cataracts, when total occlusion tip is not causing aspiration of masses Stinger Alio's MICS irrigating chopper would be more useful. This headpiece has a narrow edge at the end which divides the masses and allows easy aspiration of the phacoemulsification tip. The fragmented elements of the hard cataracts are now easily aspirated using the high under pressure and in rare moments using of the ultrasound energy. Usually MICS is performed with up to 4% ultrasound power and fewer than 10 seconds of real phacoemulsification time.

Alcon Accurus 600: This device functions very well in MICS. Accurus device has the exerted inflow, high rate of the under pressure, advanced steering pump and very efficiently in reacting. This device is very useful for the MICS surgery. In the **Table 38.1** the author offers settings for cataract grade 3 (LOCS 3).

TABLE 38.1 Accurus 600 alcon settings for 19 G MICS

Quadrant	Phacoemulsification power	20%
	Vacuum	300 mm Hg
	Irrigation	90
	Mode burst	30 ms

Alcon infinity: This is a device with a highly efficient pump and good software which is effective in practice. The torsional phaco is the system which perfectly complement need to diminish the surgical trauma during cataract surgery. This lateral movement system of the phacoemulsification tip practically eliminates the US energy. For infinity most useful settings are shown in **Table 38.2.**

Bausch and Lomb millennium: The millennium is also adapted to lead the operation in the MICS mode. This highly efficient device has the software which reduces the power of ultrasound used for a surgery. It has modes: pulse, single burst, fixed burst, multiple burst, millennium updated by the mode pulsed pulselets for creating the model of cycle 250 milliseconds "on-time". It is a cut which considerable reduces the energy. In **Table 38.3** are shown standard settings for MICS.

AMO sovereign whitestar: The WhiteStar device is working well in mode of ultrapulse around 6 milliseconds on and 12 milliseconds off. For this device a height of the bottle is 90 cm, aspiration flow rate 26 ml/min, vaccum for nuclear emulsification 400 mm Hg, and for epinucleus 200 mm Hg.

Microincision Cataract Surgery (MICS) Intraocular Lenses

The MICS cataract surgery develops postoperative astigmatism in the minimal way. For up to 80% of MICS

TABLE 38.2 Infinity alcon settings for 19 G MICS

Chop	Phacoemulsification power	0
	Dynamic rise	0
	Vacuum	150
	Irrigation	110
	Torsional amplitude	Limit 40
		On: 20
		Off: 40
	Aspiration rate	15
Quadrant	Phacoemulsification power	0
	Dynamic rise	2
	Vacuum	500
	Irrigation	110
	Torsional amplitude	Limit 80
		On: 20
		Off: 40
	Aspiration rate	30
Epi	Phacoemulsification power	0
	Vacuum	28
	Irrigation	110
	Torsional amplitude	Limit 30
		On: 20
		Off: 40
	Aspiration rate	28

Note: For 21 G MICS forced air infusion with air pump is necessary

TABLE 38.3 Millennium Bausch and Lomb settings for 19 G MICS

Sculpture	Bottle height	100 cm
	Maximum bottle infusion	40 mm Hg
	Fixed vacuum	200 mm Hg
	Fixed U/S	10%
	Duration	20 ms
	Duty cycle	60%
Quadrant	Bottle height	100 cm
	Maximum bottle infusion	40 mm Hg
	Fixed vacuum	470 mm Hg
	Fixed U/S	10%
	Duration	20 ms
	Duty cycle	60%
I/A	Bottle height	80 cm
	Maximum bottle infusion	40 mm Hg
	Maximum vacuum	550 mm Hg

Note: For 21 G MICS forced air infusion with air pump is necessary

patients, the corneal astigmatism is less than 0.5 D. Only the 25% of coaxial cataract surgery patients have astigmatism less than 0.5 D. The MICS is the useful method to do a cataract surgery with refractive surgery. The MICS caused the foldable lenses evolution and now they can be implanted through 1.5 mm incision or less **(Table 38.4)**. The lenses should fulfil the high technology. Most of them are made of hydrophilic acrylic biomaterial. But only some

TABLE 38.4   **Microincision IOLs**

No	Name of the lens	Company
1	Zeiss - Acri.Tec MICS IOLs Family	Zeiss - Acri.Tec, Berlin, Germany
2	Akreos AO microincision MI60	Bausch and Lomb, Rochester, New York, USA
3	IOLtech MICS lens	IOLtech, La Rochelle, France and Carl Zeiss Meditec, Stuttgard, Germany
4	TetraFlex KH-3500 and ZR-1000	Lenstec, St Petersburg, Florida, USA
5	MicroSlim, Slimflex IOL	**PhysIOL, Liège, Belgium**
6	CareFlex IOL	W20 Medizintechnik AG, Bruchal, Germany
7	AcriFlex MICS 46CSE IOL	Acrimed GmbH, Berlin, Germany
8	Hoya Y-60H	*Hoya Corporation*, Tokyo, *Japan*
9	Miniflex IOL	Mediphacos Ltda, Minas Gerais, Brasil

of them can be used to MICS incision. Compression during injecting can damage the lens. The lens ruptures can occur. Decompression can also be a matter of damage of the lens. For MICS IOL, it should fulfil the following requirements. The IOL should be implantable through a sub-2 mm incision. After unfolding the IOL should not have any structural, mechanical changes or optical alteration or deformation. Haptics of the lens should defend from decantation. The structure of the lens should protect from posterior capsule opacifications (PCO). Some of the lenses can have a problem with PCO but precise cleaning of the capsule can prevent the epithelium proliferation.[8] Lenses should not induce halos, glare, night-vision phenomenon, aberrations or scattering. Microincision IOLs are described in **Table 38.4**.

Acri.Tec MICS's lenses: One can use Acri.LISA for multifocals implantation **(Figure 38.10)**. For toric implants and for cases with more than 3 D of astigmatism, one can use the toric Acri.Tec IOL, marking the axis of the implantation at the slit-lamp prior to surgery. Acri.Smart 48 S and Acri.Smart 46 S are the lenses with the optical diameter 5.5 mm and 6 mm. It is biconvex, equiconvex, nonangled lenses with hydrophobic surface. They can be

implanted on both sides. Acri.Smart 48 S IOLs water content of 25% in its fully hydrated state Acri.Smart lenses are designed with square truncated edges. The edge thickness corresponds to standard designed IOLs and is in the range 0.25–0.27 mm. The lens is made from acrylic material, a copolymer of hydroxyethylmethacrylate and ethoxymethacrylate with an ultraviolet absorber. The optic power of this lens range from 0.00 D to 32.00 D. Acri.Smart glide system with Acri.Glide cartridge is used to implant lens. Acri.Smart 48 S are the lenses which can be injected through 1.5 mm incision or smaller. They are very easy to apply. After injection, the lens unfold very quickly and with the control. It has no tendency to decentration or to tilt. The adhesion between posterior capsule and lens is perfect.[9] Wehner et al. investigation seems to confirm the stability of the Acri.Smart 46 S lens. There was no decentration, rotation of this lens during 19 months observation after MICS surgery. No unwanted complications occurred.[10]

CLINICAL RESULTS

Forty-five eyes with cataract grade 2, 3, 4 (LOCS III) were operated by MICS. The incision size was 1.46 mm (1.4–1.9). After 6 months after operation, 98.9% of the patients had best-corrected distance visual acuity (BCDVA) 20/25 (0.7 decimal value) or better and 71.3% of the patients had distance UCDVA 20/32 (0.6 decimal value) or better. The safety index for distance vision of the procedure was 2.5 and the efficacy index of the procedure was 1.8.

Ninety percent of the patients had a near BCNVA of 20/25 (0.8 decimal value). Sixty percent of the patients had a near UCNVA of 20/32 (0.6 decimal value) or better. The mean add for near was +1.5 D or less in 70% of cases and was +2.0 D in 26% of cases. The safety index for near vision of the procedure was 1.4 and the efficacy index of the procedure was 0.9. It can indicate that Acri.Smart has a pseudoaccommodative ability. In this study none of the lenses showed any change in position, decentration, tilt, PCO.[11]

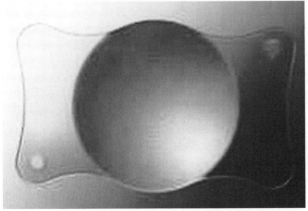

FIGURE 38.10: Acri.LISA 366D multifocal IOL (Zeiss-Acri.Tec, Berlin, Germany)

Akreos AO MI60 microincision is a hydrophilic acrylic with 26% hydration rate. Optic measures 6 mm and has a 360° posterior ridge barrier to prevent PCO. Haptics geometry consists of four-point support system, haptics angled at about 10°. Akreos has an aspherical optic. Akreos MI60 is an aspheric lens, it reduces the aberrations and improves contrast sensitivity.

Akreos AO MI60 can be implanted with a 1.8 Viscoglide cartridge and Viscoject Lens Injection System (Medicel AG, Widnau, Switzerland). This type of lenses has no tendency to decentration or PCO **(Figure 38.11)**.

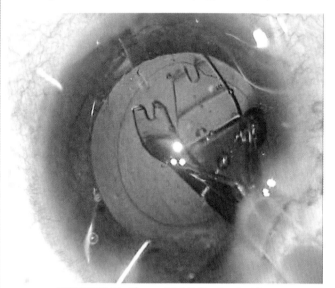

FIGURE 38.11: Akreos AO MI 60 microincision (Bausch & Lomb, Rochester, New York, USA)

IOLtech MICS lens (IOLtech, La Rochelle, France; and Carl Zeiss Meditec, Stuttgard, Germany) is biconvex. The total diameter is 12.0 mm and the optic diameter is 5.5 mm. The angulation is 13° between haptics and optics. This is the hydrophilic acrylic and monobloc lens. This lens has a square edge. The diopters range from +10.5 D to +25.5 D. The lens can be implanted with disposable injector and microincision cartridge. This lens shows pseudoaccommodative effect **(Figure 38.12)**.

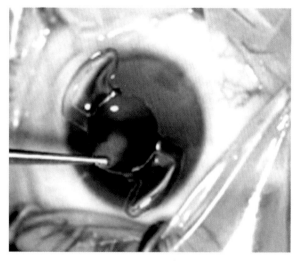

FIGURE 38.12: IOLtech MICS lens

Verges et al. (ESCRS congress, Portugal 2005, London 2006) showed data of 48 patients who underwent MICS surgery and implantation of IOLtech MICS lens through 1.8 mm incision. After 1 year follow-up, 92% of the patients reported UCDVA 20/25 and 96% BCDVA more than 20/25. Sixty-five percent of the patients achieved near visual acuity J 3 with distant correction and 98% of the patients J 5. Only two patients needed neodymium yttrium aluminium garnet (NdYAG) capsulotomy.

TetraFlex KH-3500 and ZR-1000 (Lenstec, St. Petersburg, Florida, USA) is the accommodating MICS IOL-lens. It is made from hydroxyethylmethacrylate (HEMA), consist of 26% water and the material is highly flexible. The lens is 11.5 mm of total length and 5.75 mm optic length with square edges. It is one-piece lens. The lens is available in powers from +5 D to +36 D. The TetraFlex KH-3,500 uses injector with 1.8 mm cartridge **(Figure 38.13)**.

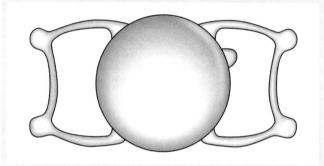

FIGURE 38.13: Tetraflex KH-3500

Chitkara, at the ESCRS winter refractive surgery meeting 2004, reported that the mean accommodation achieved binocularly was 3.42 D. Moreover, 89% of the patients achieved J 3 or better unaided binocular near vision at 6 months and 100% achieved J 5 or better.

ZR-1000 is the new one-piece lens from Lenstec. The length of this lens is 11.0 mm. The diameter of the optic is 5.5 mm and is made in square edge technology. The optic type is equiconvex and the haptic is plate. The angulation is 0°. This lens is made of 26% water content acrylic. The diopters of lens range from +10.0 D to +30.0 D. No clinical data is available for this lens **(Figure 38.14)**.

MicroSlim and SlimFlex MICS IOLs (PhysIOL, Liège, Belgium) is a hydrophilic acrylic lens with biconvex optics. Optic diameter is 6.15 mm, and overall diameter is 10.75 mm. The angulation is 5°. The power of the lens range is from +10.0 D to +30.0 D. This lens can be injected using Viscoject™ injector and 1.8 Viscoglide cartridge (Medicel, Widnau, Switzerland). No clinical data is available for this lens **(Figure 38.15)**.

Vryghem et al. presented on Congress of the ESCRS 2006 his experience in SlimFlex IOL implantation through 1.5 mm incision. The group of 50 patients underwent bilateral MICS with lens implantation. After 6 weeks mean

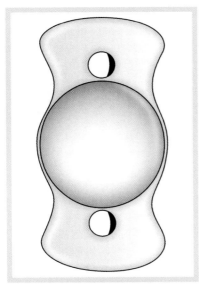

FIGURE 38.14: ZR-1000 IOL

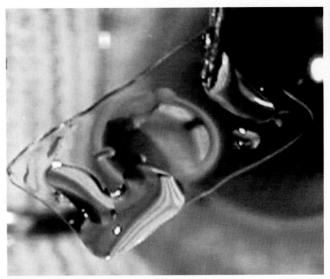

FIGURE 38.16: Acriflex MICS 46CSE IOL

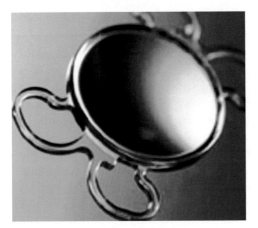

FIGURE 38.15: Microslim IOL

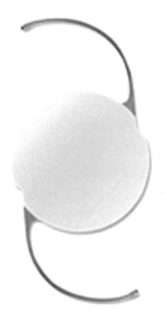

FIGURE 38.17: Hoya Y-60H MICS IOL

BCVA was 1.04. Less than 1% of the patients complained about halos or glare, and 3% of lenses resulted in small damage of the optic or haptics. No clinical data is available for this lens.

CareFlex IOL (W20 Medizintechnik AG, Bruchal, Germany) is a 26% hydrophilic acrylate, one-piece lens. Optic size is 5.8 mm, overall length is 10.5 mm and the haptic angulation is 0°. The optic design is a biconvex. The recommended anterior chamber depth is 5.1 mm. The lens is available from +10.0 D to +30.0 D. No clinical data is available for this lens.

AcriFlex MICS 46CSE IOL (Acrimed GmbH, Berlin, Germany) is made of 25% acrylic hydrophilic. The superficial is hydrophobic. The lens diameter is 11.0 mm and optic diameter is 6.0 mm. This is a monobloque type lens with perforated haptics. The angulation is 0°. The optic is biconvex with sharp edges. The lens is available from +15 D to +27 D. The clinical data is not available for this lens **(Figure 38.16)**.

Hoya Y-60H (Hoya Corporation, Tokyo, Japan) is a quite new lens for micro-surgery. This is hydrophobic foldable lens. The clinical data is not available, but Tsuneoka described possibility of implantation of this lens through 1.7 mm incision. He used Hoya F-1 cartridge to inject the lens[12] **(Figure 38.17)**.

Miniflex IOL (Mediphacos Ltda, Minas Gerais, Brasil) is also new MICS surgery lens and can be implanted through 1.8 mm incision. The material is Flexacryl® Hybrid Acrylic which brings together hydrophobic and hydrophilic monomers. The optics is aberration neutral. The lens can be implanted through 1.8 mm incision using a docking technique. The lens was presented on ESCRS 2008 in Berlin by Carlos Verges **(Figure 38.18)**.

Finally, we can conclude that MICS IOLs are not only the normal classic IOLs which are adapted to MICS incision. These lenses are the other type of intraocular IOLs. New technique and new idea of the construction lead to create thin and stable MICS IOL with the optical quality as good as standard intraocular IOLs.[8-13]

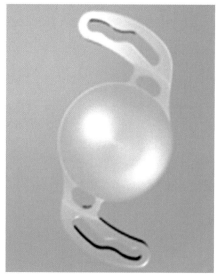

FIGURE 38.18: Miniflex IOL

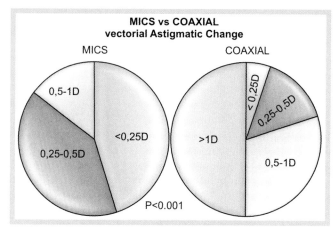

FIGURE 38.19: Comparison of MICS and coaxial vectorial astigmatic change

MICS IOL characterizes:
- Thin optic and haptic
- Perfect characteristic of kompresyjnosci
- Very good optical quality
- Long-term stability after implantation.

MICROINCISION CATARACT SURGERY (MICS) OUTCOMES

Astigmatism Control with MICS

Among the major advantages of MICS, the diminution of surgical trauma is resulting in reduction of surgically induced astigmatism (SIA), aberrations and improvement of the optical quality of the cornea after surgery.

Degraded optical quality of the cornea after incisional cataract surgery would limit the performance of the pseudophakic eye. Thus, it is important not to increase or to induce astigmatism and/or corneal aberrations after cataract surgery. Even with MICS, one could achieve reduction of the astigmatism and higher order corneal aberrations.

The optical quality of the cornea plays an important role in recovery of visual function after cataract surgery, and this is determined by combination of corneal and internal aberrations generated by the IOL and those induced by the surgery. These corneal refractive changes are attributed to the location and size of the corneal incision. The smaller incision, lower aberrations means better optical quality.

The author has described the improved control on corneal surgically induced astigmatism with MICS, when compared to conventional 3 mm phacoemulsification. A great advantage of MICS is the reduction of SIA and that the microincisions do not produce an increase in astigmatism **(Figure 38.19).**

The shorter is the incision, the less will be the corneal astigmatism, as it was estimated that the magnitude of the SIA studied by vector analysis is around 0.44 diopters and 0.88 diopters, rising as the size of the incision increases. This is considered important because today cataract surgery is considered more and more a refractive procedure.

Also, small incision surgery (3.5 mm incision without suture) does not systematically degrade the optical quality of the anterior corneal surface. However, it introduces changes in some aberrations, especially in no rotationally symmetric terms such as astigmatism, coma and trefoil. Therefore, one has to expect better results and lesser changes with sub 2 mm incision (MICS). This is supported by the finding that the corneal incision of less than 2 mm had no impact on corneal curvature, going hand in hand with the modern concept of making cataract surgery a refractive procedure, by controlling and even decreasing astigmatism and higher-order astigmatism (HOA) by using MICS, which is the state of the art.[14] The author can say that MICS sub 2 mm incision effectively decreases the induction or changes in corneal HOA during cataract surgery.

Corneal Aberration with MICS

Nowadays cataract surgery is not only a removal of a opaque lens, but also it is a part of refractive surgery. The author can obtain precisely IOL power calculation can reduce residual astigmatism and he does surgery without SIA and finally the author improves the corneal optical quality after cataract surgery. The final visual function is determined by the aberrations produced by the implanted intraocular lens and corneal aberrations changed by the postsurgical incisions. The smaller incision means lower aberrations and the better optical quality.[15,16]

Authors Elkady and Alio in prospective cumulative interventional nonrandomized, noncomparative study of 25 eyes of 25 patients, show that after the MICS incision smaller than 1.8 mm there was no statistical difference in corneal power, corneal astigmatism before and three months of follow-up after surgery.[17]

The root mean square (RMS) value of the total corneal aberrations decreased slightly after MICS (mean 2.15 ±

2.51 µm preoperatively, 1.87 ± 1.87 µm at 1 month and 1.96 ± 2.01 µm at 3 months); there was no statistically significant difference between the two follow-up visits (both p=1.00, Bonferroni). Analysis of individual Zernike terms showed a mean astigmatism of 0.85 ± 0.74 µm preoperatively, 0.65 ± 0.44 µm at 1 month, and 0.69 ± 0.46 µm at 3 months and a mean spherical aberration of 0.11 ± 0.25 µm, 0.09 ± 0.25 µm, and 0.19 ± 0.13 µm, respectively. Coma decreased (mean 0.45 ± 0.40 µm preoperatively, 0.39 ± 0.36 µm at 1 month, and 0.42 ± 0.44 µm at 3 months, respectively); there was no statistically significant difference between the two follow-up visits (both P = 1.00, Bonferroni). The mean HOA was 0.47 ± 0.26 µm preoperatively, 0.59 ± 0.32 µm at 1 month, and 0.54 ± 0.25 µm at 3 months; there was no statistically significant difference between the two follow-up visits (both p > .47, Bonferroni) **(Figure 38.20)**.

All aberration values, except HOA, decreased slightly, with no statistically significant differences between the follow-up visits. All aberration values were stable for three months after surgery, indicating that successful MICS depends on preventing induction of HOAs as well as a surgically neutral and stable procedure. Successful MICS gives visual quality equal to that in persons of the same age without pathology and leads to good patient satisfaction.[16,17]

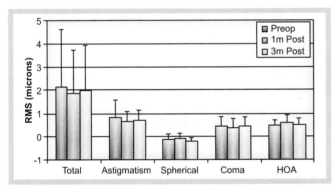

FIGURE 38.20: Corneal aberrations (Seidel coefficients) with a 6.0 mm aperture diameter over time (Preop = preoperative; m = month; HOA = higher-order astigmatism)

Clinical Efficacy of MICS

Advantages of MICS in the field of the refractive result as astigmatism control and aberration neutrality are supported by many papers of the various authors as described above, but the author should evaluate the other area of the MICS surgical technique. For each cataract surgeon very important is to compare available surgical techniques in the field of surgical technology and clinical efficacy. Seven years of MICS was an opportunity to evaluate this technique by many authors.

Relatively fast method to compare is evaluation of the surgical machine parameters settings. The Alio et al. comparing study of the MICS and coaxial phacoemulsification shows large difference between amounts of energy delivered into the eye. The effective phacoemulsification time (EPT) of the MICS was more than four times lower

than in the coaxial group and the astigmatism was almost three times lower than in the coaxial group. This means that intraocular injury connected with the phacoemulsification should be lower in the MICS group.[14] Also Kurz et al. indicate in publication important decrease of phacoemulsification time in MICS group comparing to coaxial surgery.[18] The Kahraman study shows decrease of phacoemulsificacion time in the MICS group compared to coaxial group (p=0.001).[19] Also, Tanaka study shows lower ultrasonic output in the bimanual group than in the coaxial group. Tanaka correlates it with better efficiency of nuclear treatment, including nuclear compliance, crushing and flexor hinge in the case of bimanual procedure.[20] The other studies did not show difference in the total surgery time between MICS and coaxial phaco.[14,21] The other study described by Crema et al. shows the total US time was lower in the coaxial phacoemulsification group than in the MICS group; the means were 0.50 minutes +/- 0.33 (SD) and 0.82 +/- 0.39 minutes, respectively. The mean US power was similar between groups (mean 10.1% +/- 3.76% and 10.0% +/- 4.0%, respectively).[22] Nowadays, one can compare also MICS and Micro-coaxial phaco. Cavallini study of MICS shows shorter total surgery time (p=0.04) and lower balanced salt solution (BSS) consumption (p=0.004) of the MICS group.[23]

The phacoemulsification process always affects on the corneal endothelial cells. Wilczynski et al. comparison study of the endothelial cell density shows that there is no difference in the MICS group and Micro Coaxial group in the lost of the endothelium.[24] Also Kahraman et al. study evaluates the endothelial cell loss in the MICS and Coaxial group but the results show the minimal difference between both groups. There were no statistically significant differences between preoperative and postoperative anterior chamber flare or endothelial cell loss.[19] No significant differences in corneal endothelial cell loss or endothelial morphology were found between MICS and standard incision techniques in the Mencucci et al study.[21] Morphology of the cells was not different in the MICS and coaxial group in the study of Mencucci or Kahraman.[19-21] The comparative study of the Crema et al. indicates lower cell lost in the coaxial group. The mean central corneal endothelial cell loss at 3 months was 4.66% +/- 6.10% in the coaxial phacoemulsification group and 4.45% +/- 5.06% in the MICS group and at one year, 6.00% +/- 6.72% and 8.82% +/- 7.39%, respectively. Postoperative inflammation in the anterior chamber evaluated by laser flare photometry was the same in MICS and coaxial groups in various studies.[14-19] Also Wylegala et al. in the article about corneal thickness after coaxial phacoemulsification or MICS indicate the difference in the postsurgery corneal edema. Micro-incision cataract surgery reduces risk of corneal edema when compared to standard coaxial phacoemulsification.[25]

The wound integrity and the self selling properties of the MICS and coaxial incisions are currently one of the most important agents in the endophthalmitis prophylaxis.

Irreversible changes may affect the cornea. Every incision of the cornea evokes the change of corneal curvature. The study of Kaufmann et al. confirms that MICS incision offers astigmatic neutrality in the cataract surgery and it supports the idea of MICS as the refractive procedure.[26] In the author's study, it is proven that MICS and microphaco provided similarly good incision quality and optically neutral incisions. The MICS incision respected corneal prolateness more, with less corneal edema in the short-term and less induced corneal aberrations in the long-term.[27] In the other studies, Tong et al support the perfect MICS optical result. Cataract surgery-related changes in corneal wavefront aberrations were dependent on incision size. The MICS technique had advantages over the small incision cataract surgery (SICS) in minimizing the destructive effect of the large incision size on the optical quality of the cornea.[15,28] Denoyer et al compared MICS with conventional coaxial surgery. This study shows that MICS could improve the optical performances of the pseudophakic eye reducing in three months surgically induced corneal higher-order aberrations. The postoperative root mean square of 3–6 was lower in MICS group 0.705 ± 0.285 µm versus 0.956 ± 0.236 µm in coaxial group and it was significantly different ($p < 0.001$) and the root mean square for the 3–6 order ocular aberration was lower in MICS 0.308 ± 0.122 µm versus coaxial group 0.488 ± 0.172 µm with significant difference ($P = 0.002$).[29] The latest publication of Saeed et al. show the smooth but significant difference between MICS and standard coaxial phacoemulsification in terms of uncorrected visual acuity recorded 1 hour and 2 weeks postoperatively. Nine eyes (18%) and one eye (2%) achieved a UCVA of C 6/12 at 1 hour, following MICS and coaxial phacoemulsification (CAP), respectively, and this difference was statistically significant ($p = 0.02$). The authors conclude that mean UCVA at 1 hour and at 2 weeks following cataract surgery was not significantly different between eyes undergoing MICS and CAP. However, a greater proportion of patients achieved a UCVA of C 6/12 following MICS when compared with CAP.[30] This result support other MICS investigations, smaller corneal complications, better incision leads to faster recovery and superior refractive result.[30] Astigmatic neutrality in biaxial microincision cataract surgery confirms Kaufmann et al article. His investigation, comparing keratometry of the surgical and non-surgical eye, shows the astigmatic neutrality of the sub-2 mm cataract surgery. The difference between groups was not statistically significant.[31] Wilczynski et al. article also confirm this result.[32]

Combining MICS and limbal relaxing incisions (LRI) cataract surgery can achieve superior refractive result. Ouchi et al. compare results of MICS and LRI-MICS groups. Statistically significant difference between both groups in UCVA is not surprising, but conclusion is very important. Limbal relaxing incision with bimanual MICS is an easy-to-follow combined surgery to correct pre-existing astigmatism with predictable accuracy. It confirms that MICS is SIA-neutral procedure.[33]

Quality of vision also depends on the quality of the lens implanted in the eye. Greater compression of the lens in the cartridge was a challenge for the MICS lens, but the results of comparative studies of standard lenses and MICS lenses were exceptionally good for MICS lens. There is no single method of assessing the surgical safety. The author can only take into account data from the publication but also important is the opinion of surgeons. Most of them are very much satisfied because of stable intraocular environment during lens removal, especially in patients with high myopia who are the greater risk of retinal detachment (RD) after lens extraction.[34] Practically MICS surgery can be performed under the stable anatomical conditions with the permanent use of the irrigating chopper.[35] The author can conclude as Muller et al. in the article about MICS that the advantages of MICS are less corneal astigmatism and fewer corneal surface irregularities, with favorable implications for visual quality and early rehabilitation. In the effort toward smaller incisions, special interest should be given to wound integrity, especially regarding the risk of endophthalmitis but tissue laceration can occur and smaller incisions are superior only if they cause less trauma.[36,37] However, bimanual MICS seems to be superior over the other surgical techniques because of the better refractive result, better fluidics, greater manual control and lower surgical time.[38] The author has found this technique to be simple and safe.

CONCLUSION

The MICS is a well-established surgical technique for cataract removal. The MICS offers distinctive advantages in terms of eliminating surgically induced astigmatism and reducing the changes in the aberration pattern of the cornea to the minimum. The MICS is the technique that best matches the concept of premium IOLs, as the control and correction of astigmatism and corneal aberrations seems to be mandatory at this moment in modern cataract surgery. Proven evidence exists to state that MICS is the best surgical option today for cataract removal; both biaxial and coaxial sub 2 mm incision. Micro-MICS (sub 1 mm surgery) is a feasible surgery, with the same standards and advantages of MICS, but IOL technology should be further developed, in order to use these sub 1 mm incisions for IOL implantation, something not feasible today. Future evolution on IOL technology and new surgical tools will make MICS the gold standard of cataract surgery, as biaxial technique, separating irrigation and aspiration functions, once new energies allow the nucleus to be softened and the cataract to be aspirated injecting a lens refilling substance. Biaxiality and sub 1 mm, even punctual surgery, are pending further development in the coming years.

REFERENCES

1. Alió JL, Rodriguez-Prats JL, Klonowski P, et al. MICS: Cirugia de la catarata por microincision. In: Lorente R, Mendicute J (Eds). Cirugia del cristalino (Tomo I). Sociedad de Española. Macline SL. 2008. pp. 539-44.

2. Alio JL, Rodriguez-Prats JL, Galal A. Micro-incision cataract surgery. Highlights of Ophthalmology International, Miami, 2004.

3. Wehner W. Microincision intraocular lens with plate haptic design. Evaluation of rotational stability and centering of a microincision intraocular lens with plate haptic design in 12-19 months of follow-up. Ophthalmologe. 2007;104(5):396-8.

4. Saeed A, O'Connor J, Cunnife G, et al. Uncorrected visual acuity in the immediate postoperative period following uncomplicated cataract surgery: bimanual microincision cataract surgery versus standard coaxial phacoemulsification. Int Ophthalmol. 2009;29(5):393-400.

5. Kaufmann C, Krishnan A, Landers J, et al, Astigmatic neutrality in biaxial microincision cataract surgery. J Cataract Refract Surg. 2009;35(9):1555-62.

6. Alio JL, Klonowski P, Rodriguez Prats JL. MICS instrumentation. In: Alio JL, Fine IH (Eds). Minimizing Incisions and Maximizing Outcomes in Cataract Surgery. Springer; 2010. pp. 25-37.

7. Alió JL, Klonowski P, Rodriguez-Prats JL,et al. MICS Microincision cataract surgery. In: Cavallini GM, Perez Arteaga A, Malyugin B (Eds). Instant Clinical Diagnosis in Ophthalmology. Lens Diseases. New Delhi: Jaypee Brothers Medical Publishers (p) Ltd; 2008. pp. 155-85.

8. Tanaka T, Koshika S, Usui M. Cataract surgery using the bimanual phacoemulsification technique with an Accurus system and Mackool microphaco tip. J Cataract Refract Surg. 2007;33(10):1770-4.

9. Alio JL, Klonowski P. MICS intraocular lenses. In: Alio JL, Fine IH (Eds). Minimizing Incisions and Maximizing Outcomes in Cataract Surgery. Springer; 2010. pp. 209-20.

10. Crema AS, Walsh A, Yamane Y, et al. Comparative study of coaxial phacoemulsification and microincision cataract surgery. One-year follow-up. J Cataract Refract Surg. 2007;33(6):1014-8.

11. Alió JL, El Kady B, Klonowski P. Acri.Lisa with MICS. In: Goes FJ (Ed). Multifocal IOLs. New Delhi: Jaypee Brothers Medical Publishers (p) Ltd; 2009. pp. 201-10.

12. Tsuneoka H. Implantation of a new Hoya-IOL, Y-60H, through a 1.7 mm corneal incision. In: Packer M. (Ed) Mastering the Techniques of Advanced Phaco Surgery. New Delhi: Jaypee Brothers Medical Publishers (p) Ltd; 2008. pp. 209-13.

13. Cavallini GM, Campi L, Masini C, et al. Bimanual Microphacoemulsification versus coaxial miniphacoemulsification: prospective study. J Cataract Refract Surg. 2007;33(3):387-92.

14. Alió JL, Klonowski P, El Kady B. Micro incisional lens surgery In: Kohnen T, Koch DD (Eds). Essentials in Ophthalmology. Cataract and Refractive Surgery. Springer; 2009. pp.11-24.

15. Tong N, He JC, Lu F, et al. Changes in corneal wavefront aberrations in microincision and small-incision cataract surgery. J Cataract Refract Surg. 2008;34(12):2085-90.

16. Weikert MP. Update on bimanual microincisional cataract surgery. Current Opinion in Ophthalmology. 2006;17(1):62-7.

17. Alió JL, Klonowski P, Rodriguez-Prats JL, et al. Microincisional cataract surgery (MICS). In: Garg A. et al. (Eds) Mastering the Techniques of Advanced Phaco Surgery. New Delhi: Jaypee Brothers Medical Publishers (p) Ltd; 2008. pp. 121-36.

18. Alió JL, Rodriguez-Prats JL, Vianello A, et al. Visual outcome of microincision cataract surgery with implantation of an Acri.Smart lens. J Cataract Refract Surg. 2005;31(8):1549-56.

19. Mencucci R, Ponchietti C, Virgili G, et al. Corneal endothelial damage after cataract surgery: Microincision versus standard technique. J Cataract Refract Surg. 2006;32(8):1351-4.

20. Wilczynski M, Supady E, Loba P, et al. Comparison of early corneal endothelial cell loss after coaxial phacoemulsification through 1.8 mm microincision and bimanual phacoemulsification through 1.7 mm microincision. J Cataract Refract Surg. 2009;35(9):1570-4.

21. Denoyer A, Denoyer L, Marotte D, et al. Intraindividual comparative study of corneal and ocular wavefront aberrations after biaxial microincision versus coaxial small-incision cataract surgery. Br J Ophthalmol. 2008;92(12):1679-84.

22. Kaufmann C, Krishnan A, Landers J, et al. Astigmatic neutrality in biaxial microincision cataract surgery. J Cataract Refract Surg. 2009;35(9):1555-62.

23. Kurz S, Krummenauer F, Gabriel P, et al. Biaxial microincision versus coaxial small-incision clear cornea cataract surgery. Ophthalmology. 2006;113(10):1818-26.

24. Kahraman G, Amon M, Franz C, et al. Intraindividual comparison of surgical trauma after bimanual microincision and conventional small-incision coaxial phacoemulsification. J Cataract Refract Surg. 2007;33(4):618-22.

25. Tong N, He JC, Lu F, et al. Changes in corneal wavefront aberrations in microincision and small-incision cataract surgery. J Cataract Refract Surg. 2008;34(12):2085-90.
    Alio JL, Agarwal A, Klonowski P. 0.7mm microincision cataract surgery. In: Alio JL, Fine IH (Eds). Minimizing Incisions and Maximizing Outcomes in Cataract Surgery. Springer; 2010. pp. 13-25.

26. Elkady B, Piñero D, Alió JL. Corneal incision quality: microincision cataract surgery versus microcoaxial phacoemulsification. J Cataract Refract Surg. 2009;35(3):466-74.

27. Alió JL, Rodriguez-Prats JL, Galal A, et al. Outcomes of microincision cataract surgery versus coaxial phacoemulsification. Ophthalmology. 2005;112(11):1997-2003.

28. Wilczynski M, Supady E, Loba P, et al. Comparison of surgically induced astigmatism after coaxial phacoemulsification through 1.8 mm microincision and bimanual phacoemulsification through 1.7 mm microincision. J Cataract Refract Surg. 2009;35(9):1563-9.

29. Ouchi M, Kinoshita S. Prospective randomized trial of limbal relaxing incisions combined with microincision cataract surgery. J Refract Surg. 2009;26:1-6.

30. Wylegała E, Rebkowska-Juraszek M, Dobrowolski D, et al. Influence of 3.0 mm incision coaxial phacoemulsification and microincision cataract surgery (MICS) on corneal thickness. Klin Oczna. 2009;111(7-9):207-11.

31. Müller M, Kohnen T. Incisions for biaxial and coaxial microincision cataract surgery. Ophthalmologe. 2010;107(2):108-15.

32. Müller M, Kohnen T. Incisions for biaxial and coaxial microincision cataract surgery. Ophthalmologe. 2010;107(2):108-15.

33. Sallet G. Viscoless microincision cataract surgery. Clin Ophthalmol. 2008;2(4):717-21.

34. Nochez Y, Favard A, Majzoub S, et al. Measurement of corneal aberrations for customization of intraocular lens asphericity: impact on quality of vision after micro-incision cataract surgery. Br J Ophthalmol doi:10.1136/bjo.2009.167775.

35. Cleary G, Spalton DJ, Hancox J, et al. Randomized intraindividual comparison of posterior capsule opacification between a microincision intraocular lens and a conventional intraocular lens. J Cataract Refract Surg. 2009;35(2): 265-72.

36. Paul T, Braga-Mele R. Bimanual microincisional phacoemulsification: the future of cataract surgery? Curr Opin Ophthalmol. 2005;16(1):2-7.

37. Fine IH, Hoffman RS, Packer M. Optimizing refractive lens exchange with bimanual microincision phacoemulsification. J Cataract Refract Surg. 2004;30(3):550-4.

38. Elkady B, Alió JL, Ortiz D, et al. Corneal aberrations after microincision cataract surgery. J Cataract Refract Surg. 2008;34(1):40-5.

CHAPTER 39

Functional Vision, Wavefront Sensing and Cataract Surgery

Mark Packer, I Howard Fine, Richard S Hoffman

INTRODUCTION

While the achievement of 20/20 visual acuity remains a laudable target for any cataract or refractive surgeon, the goal of high quality vision increasingly reflects our understanding of the visual system as a whole. In fact, Snellen acuity represents only a small portion of functional vision. A comparison of vision and hearing highlights the limitations of standard visual acuity tests: the auditory equivalent of a standard high-contrast Snellen eye chart would be a hearing test with only one high level of loudness for all sound frequencies. Today, contrast sensitivity testing is emerging as a more comprehensive measure of vision that will probably replace Snellen letter acuity testing, just as audiometric testing replaced the "click" and spoken-word tests used prior to the 1940s **(Figure 39.1)**.[1]

Engineers understand that Fourier analysis allows the representation of any visual object as a composite of sine waves of various frequencies, amplitudes and orientations. In fact, visual processing in the human nervous system works like Fourier analysis in reverse, with functionally independent neural channels filtering images to create what we see.[2] Thus, sine wave gratings are the building blocks of vision, just as pure tones are the building blocks of audition.

Ophthalmologists realize that patients may complain about haziness, glare and poor night vision despite 20/20 Snellen acuity. Contrast sensitivity testing has the ability to detect differences in functional vision when Snellen visual acuity measurements cannot.[3] For example, a patient

with loss of low frequency contrast sensitivity may be able to read 20/20 but be unable to see a truck in the fog. While blur due to refractive error alone affects only the higher spatial frequencies, scatter of light due to corneal or lenticular opacities causes loss at all frequencies. Glaucoma and other optic neuropathies generally produce loss in the middle and low frequencies. Contrast sensitivity testing thus offers critical information to help explain patients' complaints.

Numerous studies have demonstrated the relationship of contrast sensitivity and visual performance. From driving difficulty[4] and crash involvement,[5] to falls[6] and postural stability in the elderly,[7] to activities of daily living and visual impairment,[8] to the performance of pilots in aircraft simulators,[9] contrast sensitivity has consistently been found to provide a high correlation with visual performance.

Unfortunately, contrast sensitivity declines with age even in the absence of ocular pathology such as cataract, glaucoma or macular degeneration **(Figure 39.2)**. The pathogenesis of this decline in vision likely involves changes in the spherical aberration of the crystalline lens.

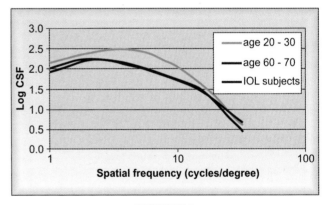

FIGURE 39.2

SPHERICAL ABERRATION

Spherical aberration is a property of spherical lenses. A spherical lens does not refract all parallel rays of incoming light to a single secondary focal point. The lens bends peripheral rays more strongly so that these rays cross the optical axis in front of the paraxial rays. As the aperture of the lens increases the average focal point moves towards the lens, so that a larger pupil produces greater spherical aberration.

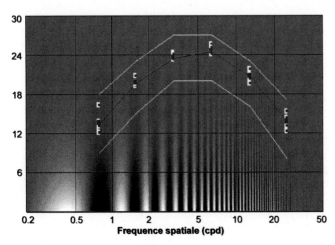

FIGURE 39.1

Spherical aberration of the cornea changes little with age. However, total wave-front aberration of the eye increases more than threefold between 20 and 70 years of age.[10] Wave-front aberration measurements combined with data from corneal topography demonstrates that the optical characteristics of the youthful crystalline lens compensate for aberrations in the cornea, reducing total aberration in younger people (**Figures 39.3 to 39.5**). Unfortunately, the aging lens no longer compensates so well, as both the magnitude and the sign of its spherical aberration change significantly (**Figure 39.6**).[11] Thus, a loss of balance between corneal and lenticular spherical aberration causes the degradation of optical quality in the aging eye (**Figures 39.7 to 39.9**).

It has been documented that the sine wave grating contrast sensitivity of a pseudophakic patient is no better than that of a phakic patient of a similar age who has no cataract. When a 65-year-old patient with cataracts has the cataracts removed and is implanted with IOLs the resulting visual outcome is no better than the visual quality of a 65-year-old without cataracts (**Figure 39.2**). The fact that the visual quality of the IOL patients is no better than that of their same-age counterparts may seem surprising because

an IOL is optically superior to the natural crystalline lens. However, this paradox is explained when one realizes that the intraocular implant has positive spherical aberration like the aged lens. It is not the optical quality of the intraocular lens in isolation that creates the image, but the optical

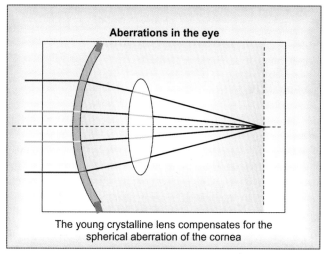

The young crystalline lens compensates for the spherical aberration of the cornea

FIGURE 39.5

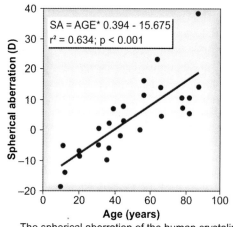

$$SA = AGE* 0.394 - 15.675$$
$$r^2 = 0.634; p < 0.001$$

The spherical aberration of the human crystaline lens increases with age (Glasser)

FIGURE 39.6

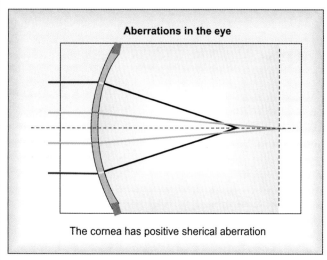

The cornea has positive sherical aberration

FIGURE 39.3

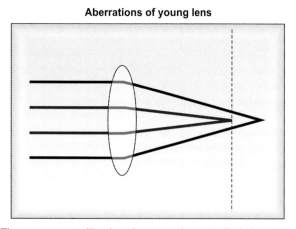

The young crystalline lens has negative spherical aberration

FIGURE 39.4

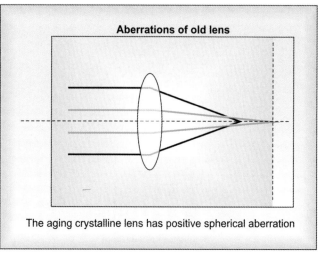

The aging crystalline lens has positive spherical aberration

FIGURE 39.7

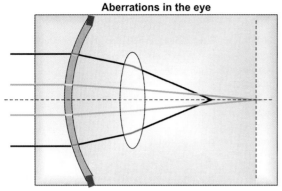

Aberrations in the eye

Old crystalline lens increases total spherical aberration of the eye

FIGURE 39.8

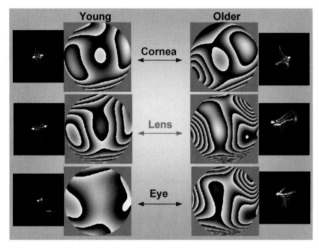

FIGURE 39.9

quality of the intraocular lens in conjunction with the cornea.

The spherical aberration of a manufactured spherical intraocular lens is in no better balance with the cornea than the spherical aberration of the aging crystalline lens **(Figure 39.10)**. Aberrations cause incoming light that would otherwise be focused to a point to be blurred, which in turn causes a reduction in visual quality. This reduction in

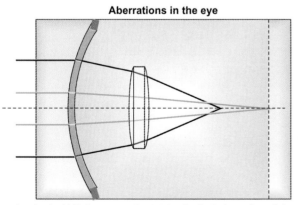

Aberrations in the eye

A spherical IOL increases the total spherical aberration of the eye

FIGURE 39.10

quality is more severe under low luminance conditions because ocular aberrations increase when the pupil size gets larger.

TECNIS IOL

The Tecnis Z9000 intraocular lens (Pharmacia), currently undergoing FDA-monitored clinical trials in the United States, has been designed with a modified prolate anterior surface to compensate for the spherical aberration of the cornea **(Figure 39.11)**. The Tecnis Z9000 shares basic design features with the CeeOn Edge 911 (Pharmacia), including a 6 mm biconvex square-edge silicone optic and angulated cap C polyvinylidene fluoride (PVDF) haptics. The essential new feature of the Tecnis IOL, the modified prolate anterior surface, acts like the youthful crystalline lens and compensates for corneal spherical aberration. The exciting new concept of the Z9000 is the potential for restoration of youthful optical quality and improvement of functional vision. Theoretical calculations and optical bench measurements support the hypothesis of improved contrast sensitivity with the Tecnis IOL **(Figure 39.12)**.

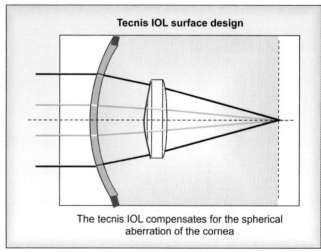

Tecnis IOL surface design

The tecnis IOL compensates for the spherical aberration of the cornea

FIGURE 39.11

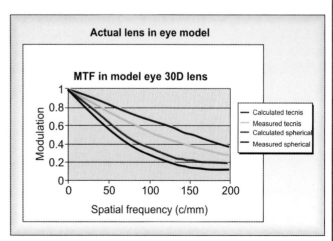

Actual lens in eye model

FIGURE 39.12

A study performed by Ulrich Mester, MD, of Salzabach, Germany, and reported at the American Society of Cataract and Refractive Surgery Symposium in Philadelphia (June 1-5, 2002), has compared the quality of vision obtained with the Tecnis IOL and a spherical acrylic IOL (Acrysof, Alcon Surgical). A total of 45 patients were enrolled and randomized to receive the Tecnis IOL in one eye and the SI 40 in the fellow eye. The average photopic contrast sensitivity values demonstrated a statistically significant advantage for the Tecnis IOL at all spatial frequencies. The contrast sensitivity curves showed an even greater difference under mesopic conditions.

SUMMARY

As advances in technology allow cataract and refractive surgeons to address higher order optical aberrations, the measurement of functional vision becomes increasingly critical as a gauge of our progress. Sine wave contrast sensitivity testing assumes a prominent place in our evaluation of surgical modalities because it reflects functional vision, correlates with visual performance and provides a key to understanding optical and visual processing of images. The Tecnis Z9000 study represents a first step towards the integration of wave-front technology and lens-based surgery.

REFERENCES

1. Ginsburg AP. The Evaluation of Contact Lenses and Refractive Surgery Using Contrast Sensitivity, in Contact Lenses: Update 2. Grune and Stratton, Inc, 1987;56.5.
2. Spillman L, Wooten DR (Eds).Visual Form Perception Based on Biological Filtering, in Sensory Experience, Adaptation and Perception. Hillsdale, NJ. Lawrence Erlbaum Associates, 1984.
3. Evans DW, Ginsburg AP. Contrast sensitivity predicts age-related differences in highway sign discriminability. Human Factors. 1985;27(12): 637.
4. McGwin G Jr, Chapman V, Owsley C. Visual risk factors for driving difficulty among older drivers. Accid Anal Prev. 2000; 32(6): 735-44.
5. Owsley C, Stalvey BT, Wells J et al: Visual risk factors for crash involvement in older drivers with cataract. Arch Ophthalmol. 2001; 119(6): 881-87.
6. Lord SR, Dayhew J: Visual risk factors for falls in older people. J Am Geriatr Soc. 2001;49(5): 508-15.
7. Lord SR, Menz HB: Visual contributions to postural stability in older adults. Gerontology. 2000;46(6): 306-10.
8. Rubin GS, Bandeen-Roche K, Huang GH et al: The association of multiple visual impairments with self-reported visual disability: SEE project. Invest Ophthalmol. Vis Sci 2001;42(1): 64-72.
9. Ginsburg AP, Evans DW, Sekule R et al: Contrast sensitivity predicts pilots' performance in aircraft simulators. Am J Optom Physiol Opt. 1982;59(1): 105-09.
10. Artal P, Berrio E, Guirao A et al: Contribution of the cor-nea and internal surfaces to the change of ocular aberrations with age. J Opt Soc Am A Opt Image Sci Vis. 2002;19(1): 137-43.
11. Glasser A, Campbell MC: Presbyopia and the optical changes in the human crystalline lens with age. Vision Res. 1998;38(2): 209-29.

CHAPTER 40

The Light Adjustable Lens

Richard S Hoffman, I Howard Fine, Mark Packer

Despite the introduction of more accurate intraocular lens (IOL) formulas and biometry instrumentation, cataract and refractive lens surgery have yet to achieve the ophthalmologist's ideal of perfect emmetropia in all cases.[1-5] This limitation stems from occasional inaccuracies in keratometry and axial length measurements, an inability to accurately assess the final position of the pseudophakic implant in a fibrosing capsular bag, and the difficulty of completely eliminating pre-existing astigmatism despite the use of limbal relaxing incisions and toric IOLs.[6,7] A new lens technology offers the hope of taking ophthalmologists one step closer to achieving emmetropia in all cases and also perhaps further improving the final result by addressing higher order aberrations.

THE IDEAL PSEUDOPHAKIC LENS

A pseudophakic lens that could be noninvasively adjusted or fine-tuned following implantation would allow for extreme accuracy in the final refractive outcome. Ideally, this lens would have the ability to be precisely adjusted using a non-toxic external light source and allow for several diopters of myopic, hyperopic, or astigmatic correction should a postoperative refractive surprise occur. Micron precision adjustment would allow for the possibility of modifying not only the lower order aberrations of sphere and cylinder but also higher order optical aberrations such as coma and spherical aberration. The lens should be stable following adjustment and composed of a safe biocompatible material. In addition, a foldable lens that could be inserted through a 2.5-3.0 mm clear corneal incision would insure control of surgically induced astigmatism.[8] Finally, if possible, an injectable flexible polymer design that could be injected through a 1 mm incision would further reduce any surgically induced astigmatism or higher order corneal aberrations and conceivably, depending on its final elasticity, could return accommodative ability to the lens/ciliary body apparatus.

LIGHT ADJUSTABLE LENS

This ideal lens technology is no longer science fiction and is currently being developed by Calhoun Vision (Pasadena, Ca). It is termed the light adjustable lens (LAL) **(Figure 40.1)**. The current design of the LAL is a foldable three-piece IOL with a cross-linked photosensitive silicone polymer matrix, a homogeneously embedded photosensitive

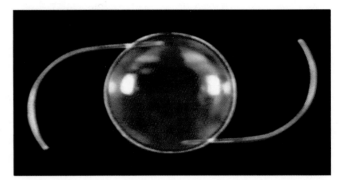

FIGURE 40.1: Calhoun Vision, Light Adjustable Lens (LAL) (*Courtesy of Calhoun Vision, Inc.*)

macromer, and a photoinitiator. The application of near-ultraviolet light to a portion of the lens optic results in disassociation of the photoinitiator to form reactive radicals that initiate polymerization of the photosensitive macromers within the irradiated region of the silicone matrix. Polymerization itself does not result in changes in lens power, however, it does create a concentration gradient within the lens resulting in the migration of non-irradiated macromers into the region that is now devoid of macromer as a result of polymerization. Equilibration from migration of the macromers into the irradiated area causes swelling within that region of the lens with an associated change in the radius of curvature and power. Once the desired power change is achieved, irradiation of the entire lens to polymerize all remaining macromer "locks-in" the adjustment so that no further power changes can occur.[9]

MODULATING REFRACTIVE POWER

The treatment of residual postoperative sphere and cylinder is fairly straightforward. In a patient whose postoperative refraction reveals residual hyperopia, power will need to be added to the LAL in order to achieve emmetropia **(Figure 40.2)**. Once postoperative refractive stability has been reached (2-4 weeks), irradiation of the central portion of the lens with the Light Delivery Device **(Figure 40.3)** polymerizes macromer in this region. Over the next 12-15 hours, macromer in the peripheral portion of the lens will diffuse centrally down the concentration gradient in order to achieve concentration equilibrium with the central lens which has been depleted of macromers due to their polymerization. This migration results in swelling of the central portion of the lens with an increase in the radius of curvature and an associated increase in the power of the

Adding Power to the LAL

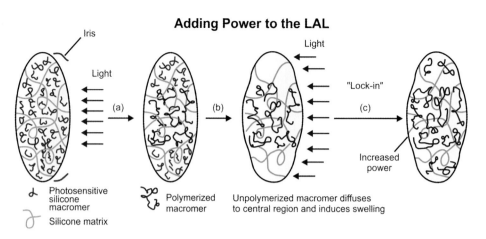

FIGURE 40.2: Cross-sectional schematic illustration of mechanism for treating hyperopic correction. (a) Selective irradiation of central portion of lens polymerizes macromer, creating a chemical gradient between irradiated and non-irradiated regions; (b) In order to re-establish equilibrium, macromer from the peripheral lens diffuses into the central irradiated region leading to swelling of the central zone; (c) Irradiation of the entire lens polymerizes the remaining macromer and "locks-in" the new lens shape (*Courtesy* of Calhoun Vision, Inc.)

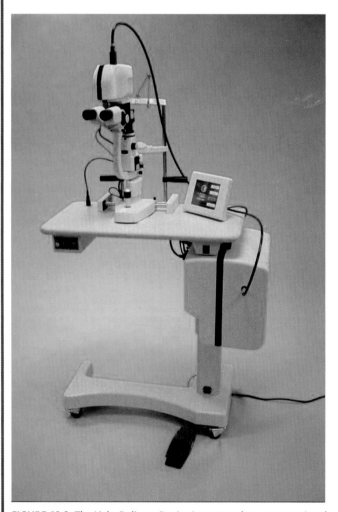

FIGURE 40.3: The Light Delivery Device is mounted on a conventional slit lamp. The refractive error and desired refractive outcome are entered on the color console and irradiation is activated using either a foot pedal or the joystick (*Courtesy* of Calhoun Vision, Inc.)

LAL. With variation in the duration and power of light exposure, differing amounts of hyperopia can be corrected. One day or more after this adjustment, the entire lens is treated to lock-in the fine adjustment. Since outdoor ultraviolet light can affect the LAL, patients wear sunglasses to eliminate UV exposure until the final lock-in is performed. Once final polymerization and lock-in is executed, no further UV protection is necessary.

In a patient with a myopic postoperative result following primary surgery, power will need to be reduced from the LAL in order to achieve emmetropia **(Figure 40.4)**. In this scenario, irradiation of the peripheral portion of the lens in a doughnut configuration will result in polymerization of macromers in this region with a resultant diffusion of central lens macromers into the peripheral irradiated portion of the lens. This creates swelling of the peripheral annulus of the lens with a concomitant increase in the radius of curvature and a decrease in lens power **(Figures 40.5A and B)**. Similarly, astigmatism can be treated by irradiating the LAL along the appropriate meridian in order to create a toric change in the radius of curvature of the lens and thus increase power ninety degrees from the treated meridian.

ANIMAL STUDIES

Nick Mamalis, MD, from the Moran Eye Center, University of Utah, has been instrumental in documenting some of the early data regarding the efficacy and accuracy of LAL adjustment in animal studies. In his pilot study, five rabbits underwent cataract surgery and LAL implantation followed by irradiation to correct 0.75 D of hyperopia. Each lens was then explanted and its power change analyzed. The mean power change was extremely close to the target correction

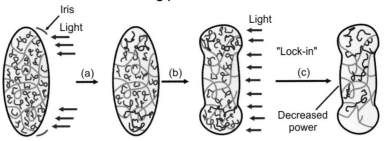

Reducing power from the LAL

FIGURE 40.4: Cross-sectional schematic illustration of mechanism for treating myopic correction. (a) Selective irradiation of peripheral portion of lens polymerizes macromer, creating a chemical gradient between irradiated and non-irradiated regions; (b) Macromer from the central zone diffuses peripherally leading to swelling of the peripheral lens; (c) Irradiation of the entire lens polymerizes the remaining macromer and "locks-in" the new lens shape with less power (*Courtesy* of Calhoun Vision, Inc.)

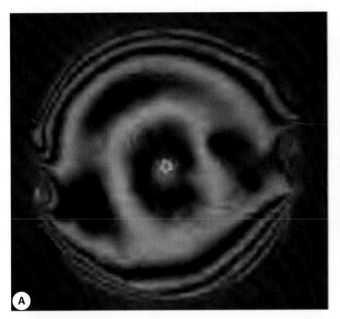

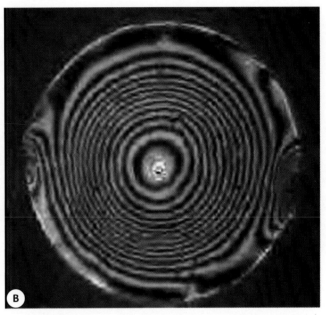

FIGURES 40.5A AND B: (A) Fizeau interference fringes of a LAL immersed in a water cell maintained at 35°C before irradiation. (B) Fizeau interference fringes of the same lens 24 hours following myopic peripheral irradiation. Note approximately 14 fringes of wavefront curvature added to the lens corresponding to approximately 1.5 D of myopic correction (*Courtesy* of Calhoun Vision, Inc.)

at 0.71 ± 0.05 D **(Figure 40.6A).** Four additional rabbits underwent LAL implantation and treatment to treat -1.00 D of myopia. These eyes also demonstrated precise adjustments averaging -1.02 ± 0.09 D of power reduction **(Figure 40.6B).**

In addition to these animal tests documenting the accuracy and reproducibility of LAL adjustments, Calhoun Vision has also performed extensive animal testing demonstrating biocompatibility and safety. Toxicology testing has revealed that no leaching of the macromers embedded in the cross-linked silicone matrix occurs despite experimental transection of the IOL.

RESOLUTION

Although, the ultimate determination of an IOL's effect on the quality of vision can best be determined by contrast

sensitivity testing after human implantation, the resolution efficiency of a lens can be determined utilizing optical bench studies. To monitor the resolution efficiency of the LAL after irradiation, the lens was evaluated on a collimation bench utilizing a standard 1951 US Air Force resolution target. **Figure 40.7A** demonstrates the quality of the resolution target through the LAL in air prior to irradiation. **Figure 40.7B** reveals the imaged target 24 hours following treatment of the LAL for -1.58 D of myopia. **Figure 40.7C** reveals the image through a +20 D AMO SI40 for comparison. Inspection of the images reveals that the resolution efficiency of the LAL is not compromised following irradiation.[9]

REFRACTIVE LENS EXCHANGE

Perhaps one of greatest possible uses of a LAL is as a platform for refractive surgery. The concept of exchanging

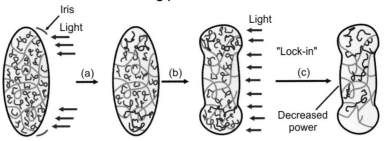

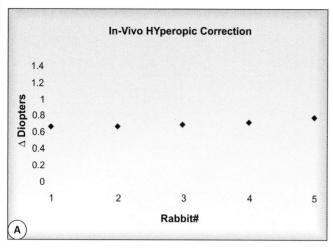

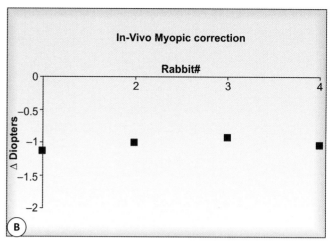

FIGURES 40.6A AND B: (A) *In vivo* hyperopic correction in five rabbit eyes. Target correction was 0.75 D and the mean result was 0.71 ± 0.05 D (B) *In vivo* myopic correction in four rabbit eyes. Target correction was -1.0 D and the mean result was -1.02 ± 0.09 D (*Courtesy* of Nick Mamalis, MD)

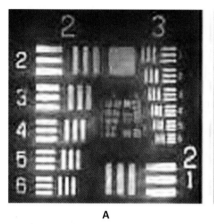
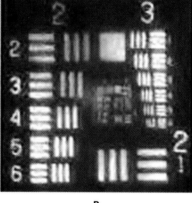
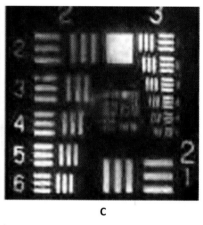

FIGURES 40.7A TO C: US Air Force resolution target imaged in air though a (A) LAL prior to irradiation; (B) LAL 24 hours following -1.58 D of treatment, and (C) 20 D AMO SI40 silicone IOL (*Courtesy* of Calhoun Vision, Inc.)

the human crystalline lens with a pseudophakic IOL as a form of refractive surgery is gaining popularity in the ophthalmic community. This stems from several problems inherent in excimer laser corneal refractive surgery including the limitations of large myopic and hyperopic corrections, the need to address presbyopia, and progressive lenticular changes that eventually will interfere with any optical corrections made in the cornea.

Currently acceptable methods of performing refractive lens exchange incorporate multifocal lenses as a means of maximizing the final refractive result.[10] Multifocal IOLs allow the presbyopic patient considering refractive surgery to address their distance refractive error in addition to their near visual needs without resorting to monovision with monofocal lens implants. In patients whose night-time visual demands preclude the use of multifocal technology, monofocal IOLs can still be used with the understanding that monovision or reading glasses will be necessary to deliver functional vision at all ranges.

The LAL is an ideal implant for refractive lens exchanges since emmetropia can be fine-tuned following insertion. In addition, Calhoun Vision has demonstrated *in vitro*, an ability

to irradiate multifocal optics of any near add onto any portion of the LAL **(Figures 40.8A to C).** Theoretically, a patient undergoing a refractive lens exchange could have their lens adjusted for emmetropia and then have multifocality introduced to determine if they were tolerant to multifocal optics. If intolerant, the multifocality could be reversed and a trial of monovision could be induced. Once the desired refractive status was achieved, the LAL could then be locked-in permanently. This would allow patients the option of experimenting with different refractive optics and deciding *in situ* which was best for them.

Until now, the potential drawbacks of refractive lens exchange have included the risk of endophthalmitis, retinal detachment, and the inability to guarantee emmetropia in these highly demanding patients.[11,12] Hopes of reducing or eliminating the risks of endophthalmitis are now being encouraged by the introduction of newer fourth generation fluoroquinolone antibiotics while the issue of lens power accuracy can now be potentially solved with the adjustment capabilities of the LAL.[13]

Retinal detachment following cataract and refractive lens surgery is more common in high myopes but can occur in

Multifocality after initial correction

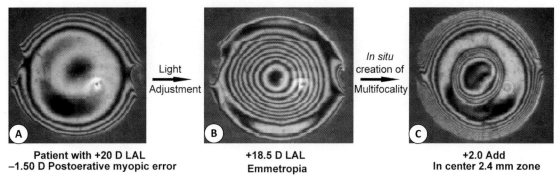

Light
Adjustment →

In situ
creation of
Multifocality →

(A) **Patient with +20 D LAL
−1.50 D Postoerative myopic error**

(B) **+18.5 D LAL
Emmetropia**

(C) **+2.0 Add
In center 2.4 mm zone**

FIGURES 40.8A TO C: A laser interferogram (A) demonstrates a 20 D LAL *in vitro*. If a -1.50 D postoperative error resulted, the lens could be irradiated to reduce the power and achieve emmetropia (B). This could then be followed by creation of a +2.0 D add power in the central zone of the lens (C) in order to yield a multifocal optic. (*Courtesy* of Calhoun Vision, Inc.)

any patient. Detachments usually occur secondary to tears from posterior vitreous detachments that develop by removing the space occupying crystalline lens and replacing it with a thin pseudophakic IOL. Calhoun Vision's research of an injectable silicone polymer with the same light adjustable properties as the LAL offer the possibility of reducing the risk of retinal detachment following lens surgery **(Figure 40.9)**. By reinflating the capsular bag with an adjustable polymer, vitreous detachment and subsequent retinal detachment risk would theoretically lessen. In addition, an injectable polymer would allow for the possibility of utilizing advanced phacoemulsification techniques through microincisions of 1.0 mm and implanting an adjustable lens material through these same minute incisions.

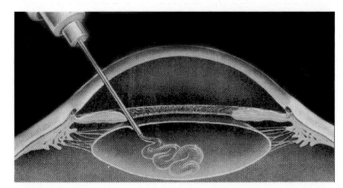

FIGURE 40.9: A soft and injectable light adjustable silicone polymer could be injected into the capsular bag and then irradiated postoperatively to achieve emmetropia. Refilling of the capsular bag would eliminate the creation of potential space behind the capsular bag and theoretically, decrease the incidence of vitreous detachment. A soft pliable material could also potentially allow for the return of accommodation. (Courtesy of Calhoun Vision, Inc.)

HIGHER ORDER ABERRATIONS

One of the hottest topics in the field of refractive surgery today is the concept of correcting higher order aberrations within the eye. The elimination of higher order optical aberrations would theoretically allow the possibility of achieving vision previously unattainable through glasses, contact lenses, or traditional excimer laser refractive surgery.[14]

One of the major limitations of addressing higher order aberrations with corneal ablations lies in the fact that higher order aberrations such as spherical aberration tend to remain constant within the cornea throughout life while aberration in the crystalline lens tends to change as a patient ages.[15-17] Thus, any attempt to perfect the human visual system with wavefront guided ablations to the cornea will be sabatoged at a later date by increasing positive spherical aberration in the naturally aging crystalline lens. If the higher order aberrations within the cornea are indeed stable throughout life, a better approach for creating an aberration-free optical system that endures as a patient ages would be the removal of the crystalline lens and replacement with an implant that could be adjusted using wavefront technology to eliminate higher order optical aberrations within the eye.

Calhoun Vision claims the ability to adjust the LAL with micron precision. If true, wavefront guided treatments could be irradiated onto the lens essentially negating any aberrations introduced into the optical system by the cornea. Spherical aberration has been successfully corrected on a LAL **(Figure 40.10)** and additional research investigating the treatment of other higher order aberrations is underway. In collaboration with Carl Zeiss Meditec, Calhoun Vision is developing a Digital Light Delivery Device (DLDD) that holds the promise of irradiating precise complex patterns onto the LAL as a means of correcting higher order aberrations **(Figure 40.11)**.

The core of the DLDD is a complex digital mirror device composed of a chip containing thousands of tiny aluminized silicone mirrors. The chip can be programmed in such a way that an inverse gray scale image of a patient's mathematically modeled wavefront pattern can be generated **(Figure 40.12)**. The gray scale image is generated by rapid fluctuations of the tiny mirrors within the chip and this image can then be irradiated directly onto the LAL

Correction of spherical aberration

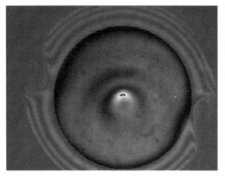

Before irradiation

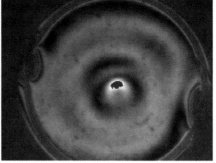

24 hours post irradiation

FIGURE 40.10: Irradiation of an annular ring at the edges of the LAL corrects spherical aberration. Note that two fringes from the interferometry pattern in the lens periphery are removed corresponding to 0.5 D of correction (*Courtesy* of Calhoun Vision, Inc.)

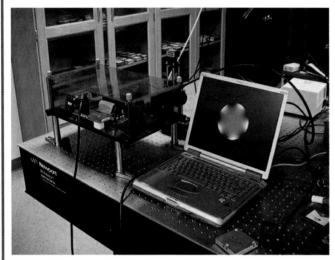

FIGURE 40.11: Digital Light Delivery Device (DLDD) (*Courtesy* of Calhoun Vision, Inc.)

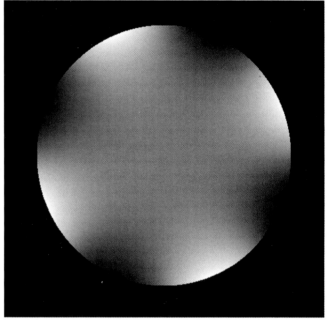

FIGURE 40.12: A tetrafoil spatial intensity pattern is represented digitally. This pattern can be directly transferred to a LAL or an inverse pattern could likewise be irradiated to the LAL to correct this aberration (*Courtesy* of Calhoun Vision, Inc.)

(Figures 40.13A and B). By creating an inverse or conjugate wavefront pattern, higher order treatments can be transferred to the LAL effectively neutralizing the eye's higher order aberrations. Ultimately, wavefront guided adjustments to the LAL could result in enhanced visual function that remains stable. Since aberrations in the cornea do not change with age and potential progressive crystalline lens aberrations are eliminated with lensectomy, wavefront treatments to the LAL should not change with time and should produce a stable aberration-free optical system throughout the patient's lifetime.

FINAL COMMENTS

Cataract surgery has come a long way since the time of intracapsular extraction and large incision extracapsular surgery. Incremental advancements in phacoemulsification technology have allowed ophthalmologists to offer their patients the safest and most rapidly visually rehabilitative cataract surgery ever. Emphasis now has shifted to

improving intraocular lens technology. Research into newer multifocal and accommodative IOLs will be instrumental in allowing ophthalmologists to provide not only state of the art cataract surgery but also offer refractive lens exchanges to their refractive surgery patients as a means of treating distance refractive errors and the presbyopic condition.

Current limitations in cataract and refractive lens surgery stem from the inability to guarantee emmetropia in even the most experienced hands. The light adjustable lens offers an incredible opportunity for ophthalmologists to deliver excellent postoperative visual acuities and in addition to many other options. IOLs will now have the potential of being fine-tuned following surgery to provide not only emmetropia but also multifocality and higher order

Creation of Tetrafoil wavefront correction

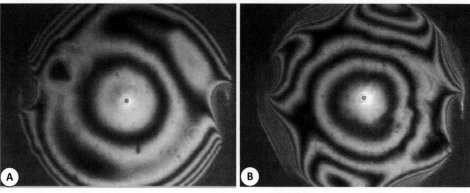

Before irradiation   Post tetrafoil wavefront irradiation

FIGURES 40.13A AND B: (A) LAL interferometry pattern before and after irradiation with DLDD to create tetrafoil wavefront. (B) 3-D representation of tetrafoil wavefront created in LAL (*Courtesy* of Calhoun Vision, Inc.)

aberration free corrections if the patient desires. The early reversible nature of the LAL prior to the final "lock-in" will allow patients the opportunity to experience monovision, multifocality, and wavefront guided treatments and then decide if that refractive status is acceptable.

The LAL is truly one of the great revolutions in modern cataract and lens surgery. Clinical trials in the United States should begin in 2003.

REFERENCES

1. Brandser R, Haaskjold E, Drolsum L. Accuracy of IOL calculation in cataract surgery. Acta Ophthalmol Scan. 1997;75: 162-65.
2. Drexler W, Findl O, Menapace R, et al. Partial coherence interferometry: a novel approach to biometry in cataract surgery. Am J Ophthalmol. 1998;126: 524-34.
3. Giers U, Epple C. Comparison of A-scan device accuracy. J Cataract Refract Surg. 1990;16: 235-42.
4. Watson A, Armstrong R. Contact or immersion technique for axial length measurements? Aust NZ J Ophthalmol. 1999;27: 49-51.
5. Packer M, Fine IH, Hoffman RS, et al. Immersion A-scan compared with partial coherence interferometry. Outcomes Analysis. J Cataract Refract Surg. 2002;28: 239-42.
6. Olsen T. Sources of error in intraocular lens power calculation. J Cataract Refract Surg. 1992;18: 125-29.
7. Pierro L, Modorati G, Brancato R. Clinical variability in keratometry, ultrasound biometry measurements, and emmetropic intraocular-lens power calculation. J Cataract Refract Surg. 1991;17: 91-94.
8. Masket S, Tennen DG. Astigmatic stabilization of 3.0 mm temporal clear corneal cataract incisions. J Cataract Refract Surg. 1996;22: 1451-55.
9. Schwiegerling JT, Schwartz DM, Sandstedt CA et al: Light-adjustable intraocular lenses. Review of Refractive Surgery; Newtown Square, Jobson Publishing, LLC, 2002.
10. Packer M, Fine IH, Hoffman RS: Refractive lens exchange with the Array multifocal lens. J Cataract Refract Surg. 2002;28: 421-24.
11. Rodriguez A, Gutierrez E, Alvira G. Complications of clear lens extraction in axial myopia. Arch Ophthalmol. 1987;105:1522-23.
12. Ripandelli G, Billi B, Fedeli R et al: Retinal detachment after clear lens extraction in 41 eyes with axial myopia. Retina. 1996;16: 3-6.
13. Mather R, Karenchak LM, Romanowski EG, et al. Fourth generation fluoroquinolones: new weapons in the arsenal of ophthalmic antibiotics. Am J Ophthalmol. 2002;133: 463-66.
14. Macrae SM, Krueger RR, Applegate RA. Customized corneal ablation. The quest for supervision. Thorofare, NJ, Slack Inc, 2001.
15. Guirao A, Redondo M, Artal P. Optical aberrations of the human cornea as a function of age. J Opt Soc Am A Opt Image Sci Vis. 2000;17: 1697-1702.
16. Oshika T, Klyce SD, Applegate RA, et al. Changes in corneal wavefront aberrations with aging. Invest Ophthalmol Vis Sci. 1999;40: 1351-55.
17. Artal P, Berrio E, Guirao A, et al. Contribution of the cornea and internal surfaces to the change of ocular aberrations with age. J Opt Soc Am A Opt Image Sci Vis. 2002;19: 137-43.

Difficult Cases

CHAPTER 41

Posterior Polar Cataract

Abhay R Vasavada, Shetal M Raj

INTRODUCTION

Posterior polar cataract (PPC) is a clinically distinctive entity consisting of a dense white, well demarcated, disk-shaped opacity, located in the posterior cortex or subcapsular region **(Figure 41.1).** Two types of PPC have been described in literature: stationary and progressive.[1] The stationary type consists of concentric rings around the central plaque opacity that looks like a bull's eye **(Figure 41.2).** This type is compatible with good vision. Normally the patient seeks help in the third or the fourth decade of life. The common symptom is intolerance to light. Glare is most severe when the source of light is close to the object

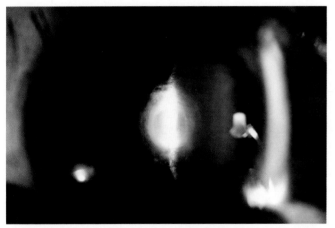

FIGURE 41.1: Posterior polar cataract (PPC) characterized by dense white, well demarcated, disk-shaped opacity

of vision. In the progressive type, changes take place in the posterior cortex in the form of radiating rider opacities **(Figure 41.3).** Patients with progressive opacity become more symptomatic as the peripheral extensions enlarge.

The inheritance pattern of this cataract is reported to be autosomal dominant.[2-7] Osher and colleagues had mentioned a positive family history for congenital cataracts in 55% (12/22) patients.[8] The gene for PPC has been linked with the haptoglobin locus on chromosome 16.[9] A recent study reported that mutations in the PITX3 gene in humans result in posterior polar cataracts and variable anterior segment mesenchymal dysgenesis (ASMD).[10] Studies have indicated that a majority of these patients present with bilateral cataracts, the incidence being 80% in our earlier study,[11] and 70% in a study conducted by Gavris and colleagues.[12] There is no gender predilection in PPC. The polar opacity consists of abnormal lens fiber cells and an accumulation of extracellular materials.[13-15]

PPC presents a special challenge to the phacoemulsification surgeon as it is known to be predisposed to posterior-capsule dehiscence during surgery.[8,11] In 1990, Osher and co-authors reported a 26% (8/31 eyes) incidence of posterior capsule rupture (PCR) during surgery in eyes with PPC.[8] We have earlier reported 36% (9/25 eyes) in 1999,[11] while in 2003, Hayashi and co-authors,[16] and Lee and co-authors,[17] reported 7.1% (2/28 eyes) and 11% (4/36 eyes), respectively. Liu and co-authors reported 16.4 % (10/61 eyes).[18] A study by Gavris and colleagues in 2004 reported an incidence of 40% (4/10 eyes).[12] Author's study reports that the anteroposterior dimensions of the lens in eyes with

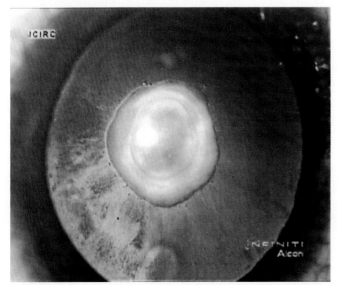

FIGURE 41.2: In the stationary type of PPC, concentric rings are seen around the central plaque opacity resembling bull's eye

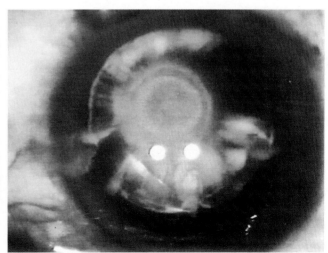

FIGURE 41.3: In the progressive type of PPC, changes take place in posterior cortex in the form of radiating rider opacities

posterior polar cataracts is significantly thinner compared to the posterior subcapsular cataracts (In press).

To prevent PCR, Osher and colleagues recommend slow-motion phacoemulsification with low aspiration flow rate, vacuum and infusion pressure.[8] Fine and co-authors avoid over pressurization of the anterior chamber with visco-dissection to mobilize epinucleus and cortex,[19] Allen and Wood also perform viscodissection,[20] and Lee and Lee prefer a lamda technique with dry aspiration.[17] We prefer inside-out delineation.[21] This technique, along with modern instrumentation, refined surgical strategies, better understanding of phacodynamics and cumulative surgical experience has enabled us to reduce PCR to 8% (2/25 eyes).[21]

DIAGNOSIS

The bull's eye appearance is pathognomonic of posterior polar cataracts **(Figure 41.1)**. However, this entity could be camouflaged under a dense nuclear sclerosis or a total white cataract. In our opinion, surgery should be delayed as far as possible and undertaken only if the patient finds it difficult to perform his routine activities. In our experience, the procedure should be governed by the following paradigm:

SURGERY

Counseling

During preoperative examination, the patient should be informed of the possibility of intraoperative PCR dropped nucleus, relatively longer operative time, secondary posterior segment intervention and likely delayed visual recovery. The need to perform Nd: YAG capsulotomy for residual plaque[8,11,16] and possibility of preexisting amblyopia especially in unilateral PPC should be envisaged at the preliminary stage.[16]

Anesthesia

Peribulbar anesthesia with oculopressure to soften the globe diminishes intraoperative posterior pressure.[8] With increasing experience, one may use topical anesthesia in a selective manner.

Surgical Technique

We prefer to use a closed chamber technique. The contours of the cornea and the globe should be maintained through the procedure.

Hayashi and co-authors perform either phacoemulsification, pars plana lensectomy or intracapsular cataract extraction depending on the size of opacity and density of nuclear sclerosis.[16]

Incision

A paracentesis is performed with 15 degrees ophthalmic knife (Alcon Surgical, Texas, USA). The aqueous is exchanged with Sodium Hyaluronate (Provisc, Alcon Laboratories, USA). A temporal corneal single plane valvular incision of 2.6 mm is performed. A cohesive viscoelastic in the AC prevents chamber collapse and forward movement of iris-lens diaphragm, during entry into the eye. Fine and co-authors caution against increasing the pressure in the AC.[19]

Capsulorhexis

The optimal size is approximately ≤5 mm. While a rhexis size of ≤ 4 mm could be detrimental in the event of necessity to prolapse the nucleus into the anterior chamber, a larger opening may not leave adequate support for a sulcus-fixated intraocular lens in case the PC is compromised.[11,19]

Hydro Procedures

Cortical-cleaving hydrodissection[22] can lead to hydraulic rupture and therefore should be avoided.[8,11] It would be logical to perform hydrodelineation to create a mechanical cushion of epinucleus.[11,16,20,23] Masket,[24] Hayashi and colleagues,[16] Allen and Wood,[20] Lee and Lee,[17] recommend hydrodelineation. In addition to hydrodelineation, Fine and co-authors also perform hydrodissection in multiple quadrants injecting tiny amounts of fluid gently, such that the fluid wave is not allowed to spread or extend across the posterior capsule.[19] The author and his colleagues propose "inside-out delineation" to precisely delineate the central core of nucleus.[21]

Inside-out delineation: A central trench is sculpted the slow motion technique (Infinity Phacoemulsifier, Alcon Laboratories, Texas, USA). In nuclear sclerosis ≤ grade 3 (grading system from grade 1 to 5),[25] preset parameters are: ultrasound energy (U/S) 30–60% (Supra-optimal power), vacuum 60 mm Hg, aspiration flow rate (AFR) 18 cc/min and bottle height (BH) 70 cm. Care should be taken not to mechanically rock the lens. Dispersive viscoelastic (Viscoat, Alcon Laboratories) is injected through the side-port before retracting the probe to avoid forward movement of iris-lens diaphragm. A specially designed right-angled cannula mounted on a 2 cc syringe filled with fluid, is introduced through the main incision and the tip is placed adjacent to the right wall of the trench at an appropriate depth, depending on the density of the cataract. It then penetrates the central lens substance and fluid is injected through the right wall of the trench **(Figure 41.4)**. Delineation is produced by the fluid traversing inside-out. A golden ring within the lens is evidence of successful delineation **(Figure 41.5)**. Fluid injection may be repeated in the left wall of the trench with another right-angled cannula **(Figure 41.6)**. The trench allows the surgeon to reach the central core of the nucleus. As fluid is injected at a desired depth, under direct vision, a desired thickness of epinucleus cushion can be achieved **(Figure 41.7)**. It provides a precise epinucleus bowl that acts as mechanical cushion to protect the posterior capsule during subsequent maneuvers.

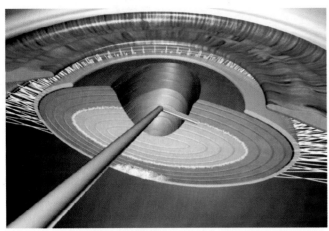

FIGURE 41.4: Sketch demonstrating technique of inside-out delineation. The cannula penetrates central lens substance and fluid is injected through right wall of the trench

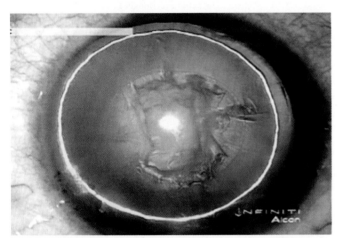

FIGURE 41.5: The golden ring indicates end point of inside-out delineation

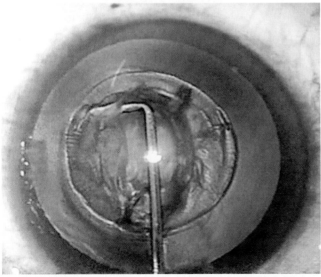

FIGURE 41.6: Fluid injection is repeated in the left wall of the trench with another right-angled cannula, if delineation is incomplete

With conventional hydrodelineation, the cannula is penetrated within the lens substance causing the fluid to traverse from outside to inside. It is sometimes difficult to introduce the cannula within a firm nucleus leading to

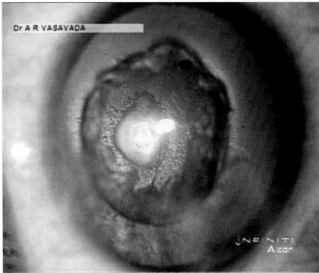

FIGURE 41.7: Mechanical cushion consisting of epinucleus; nucleus protects the posterior capsule

rocking and stress to the capsular bag and zonules. There is also a possibility of fluid being injected inadvertently in the subcapsular plane, leading to unwarranted hydro-dissection. Inside-Out delineation is easy to perform, provides superior control, reduces stress to zonules and precisely demarcates the central core of nucleus.

Rotation: An attempt to rotate the nucleus can lead to posterior capsule rupture and is therefore avoided.[11]

Division and fragment removal: All techniques are geared to facilitate the removal of nucleus within the cushion effect of the epinucleus. Bimanual cracking and division of the nucleus involve outward movements and can result in distortion of the capsular bag. In nuclear sclerosis ≥ 2 we use the step-by-step chop in situ and lateral separation technique[26] for chopping using U/S 40–50%, vacuum 150–250 mm Hg, AFR 18 cc/min and BH 70–90 cm. The resultant fragments are removed with stop, chop, chop and stuff technique.[27] In nuclear sclerosis < 2, the entire nucleus is aspirated within the epinucleus shell using AFR 16 cc/min and vacuum 100–120 mm Hg. **Figure 41.8** shows the capsular bag after the nucleus removal showing a central breach in the continuity of the epinucleus at the site of the posterior polar cataract. Traction of posterior lens fibers and posterior polar opacity during surgery are enough to break the weak posterior capsule. Thus the slow motion technique is recommended to reduce turbulence in the AC.[28] Collapse of the AC and forward bulge of the PC is prevented throughout the procedure by injecting viscoelastic before the instrument is withdrawn.[11,29]

Lee and co-authors use the lambda technique to sculpt the nucleus followed by cracking along both the arms and 21removal of central piece.[17]

Epinucleus removal: First only the peripheral lower half of epinucleus is stripped off using U/S 30%, vacuum 80–100 mm Hg, AFR 16 cc/minute and BH 80–90 cm. The

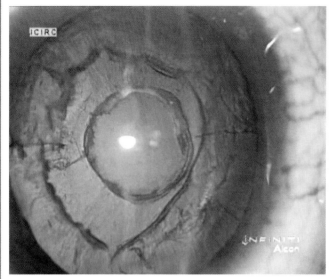

FIGURE 41.8: Capsular bag after nucleus removal showing a central breach in continuity of epinucleus at the site of PPC

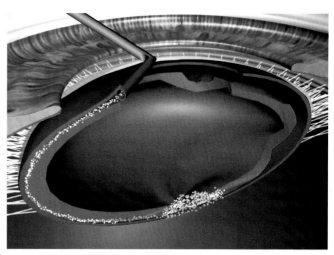

FIGURE 41.10: Sketch demonstrating the technique of injecting fluid in the subcapsular region to cleave the cortex from the capsule proximal to incision. The nucleus has been emulsified and the capsular bag is empty. Therefore, it is safe to hydrodissect at this stage

central area is attached to the left.[11,19,24] Then the peripheral upper epinucleus (subincisional epinucleus) is mobilized with a gentle focal and multiquadrant hydrodissection with a right angled cannula facing right and left **(Figures 41.9 and 41.10).** The fluid wave travels along the cleavage formed between the capsule and lower epinucleus that does not threaten the integrity of the posterior capsule. Also, it is safe to hydrodissect as the capsular bag is not fully occupied. Therefore, the hydraulic pressure built-up is not sufficient to rupture the posterior capsule. The entire epinucleus is then aspirated, finally detaching the central area.

Allen[20] and Fine[19] suggested viscodissection of the epinucleus performed by injecting viscoelastic (Healon 5 or GV and Viscoat respectively) under the capsular edge to mobilize the rim of epinucleus. It is removed with a

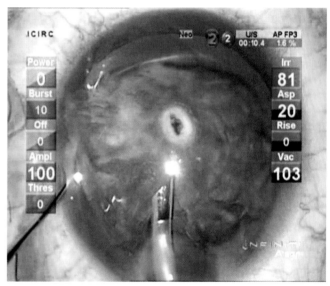

FIGURE 41.11: A pseudohole suggestive of a defect is observed in posterior cortex, but the posterior capsule remains intact

coaxial irrigation-aspiration (I/A) handpiece. Lee and colleagues perform manual dry aspiration with Simcoe cannula.[17]

Pseudohole: At times, the classical appearance suggestive of a defect is observed in the posterior cortex, but the posterior capsule remains intact. This is a "pseudohole" **(Figure 41.11).**

Cortex removal: Bimanual automated I/A, using AFR 20 cc/min and vacuum 400 mm Hg, optimizes control, ensures AC maintenance and aids in complete removal of the cortex.

Fine and colleagues using coaxial protect the PC with VES during cortex removal.[19]

Posterior capsule vacuum polishing: It is avoided even if the PC is not open because of its potential fragility.[8,11,16,19,24] The traction on an excessive adhered plaque to an otherwise

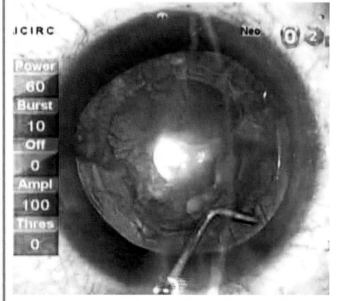

FIGURE 41.9: Removal of upper half of epinucleus using focal and multiquadrant hydrodissection

normal posterior capsule could eventually rupture the posterior capsule. Instead postoperative neodymium-yttrium-aluminum-garnet (Nd:YAG) laser posterior capsulotomy is preferable.

Posterior Capsule Dehiscence

If a defect is present in the PC, Viscoat is injected over the area of PC defect before the phaco or I/A probe is withdrawn from the eye,[29] and two-port limbal anterior vitrectomy is performed using cut rate 800 cuts/min, vacuum 300 mm Hg and AFR 25 cc/min. Once the AC is free from vitreous, the cortex is aspirated by bimanual I/A. A posterior capsulorhexis (PCCC) may be performed if the rupture is confined to a small central area **(Figure 41.12)**.

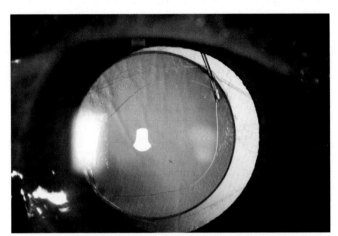

FIGURE 41.12: IOL capture to the rhexis in a case of a posterior capsular rupture

Intraocular Lens Implantation

In eyes with the PC defect, IOL is implanted in the bag, only if PCCC can be achieved. In eyes with a large posterior capsule defect, the IOL is placed over the anterior capsule in ciliary sulcus. Fine and colleagues have suggested capture of the optic through the anterior capsulorhexis.[19,30] We believe optic capture induces more inflammation.[31]

After intraocular-lens implantation, viscoelastic is removed by two-port vitrectomy rather than I/A as vitrectomy aspirates in a piecemeal and gradual manner and reduces the chances of rapid aspiration of vitreous.

We do not suture the main valvular incision, but suture paracentesis in eyes with posterior capsule defect. In these eyes, a periodic evaluation for retinal break, cystoid macular edema and raised intraocular pressure is necessary.

SURGICAL PEARLS

- Thorough counseling
- Avoid cortical-cleaving hydrodissection
- Inside-out delineation
- Closed chamber technique
- Slow motion technique for lens removal
- Focal and multiquadrant hydrodissection for cleavage of subincisional epinucleus.

KEY POINTS

- Posterior polar cataract (PPC) is a clinically distinctive entity consisting of a dense white, well demarcated, disk-shaped opacity located in the posterior cortex or subcapsular region. Two types of PPC have been described in literature: stationary and progressive.
- The inheritance pattern of this cataract is reported to be autosomal dominant.
- The bull's eye appearance is pathognomonic of posterior polar cataracts.
- Cortical-cleaving hydrodissection can lead to hydraulic rupture and should be avoided. It would be logical to perform hydrodelineation to create a mechanical cushion of epinucleus.
- At times the classical appearance suggestive of a defect is observed in the posterior cortex, but the posterior capsule remains intact. This is a "pseudohole".

REFERENCES

1. Duke-Elder S. Posterior polar cataract. System of Ophthalmology: Normal and Abnormal Development, Congenital Deformities. St Louis, MO: CV Mosby; 1964. pp. 723-6.
2. Tulloh CG. Hereditary posterior polar cataract with report of a pedigree. Br J Ophthalmol. 1955;39(6):374-9.
3. Tulloh CG. Hereditary posterior polar cataract. Br J Ophthalmol. 1956;40(9):566-7.
4. Nettleship E, Ogilvie FM. A peculiar form of hereditary congenital cataract. Trans Ophthalmol Soc UK. 1906;26:191-207.
5. Harman NB. New pedigree of cataract – posterior polar, anterior polar and microphthalmia, and lamellar. Trans Ophthalmol Soc UK. 1909;29:296-306.
6. Yamada K, Tomita HA, Kanazawa S, et al. Genetically distinct autosomal dominant posterior polar cataract in a four-generation Japanese family. Am J Ophthalmol. 2000;129(2):159-65.
7. Berry V, Francis P, Reddy MA, et al. Alpha-B crystallin gene (CRYAB) mutation causes dominant congenital posterior polar cataract in humans. Am J Hum Genet. 2001;69(5):1141-5.
8. Osher RH, Yu BC, Koch DD. Posterior polar cataracts: A predisposition to intraoperative posterior capsular rupture. Journal of Cataract and Refractive Surgery. 1990;16:157-62.
9. Maumenee IH. Classification of hereditary cataracts in children by linkage analysis. Ophthalmology. 1979;86:1554-8.
10. Addison PK, Berry V, Ionides AC, et al. Posterior polar cataract is the predominant consequence of a recurrent mutation in the PITX3 gene. Br J Ophthalmol. 2005;89(2):138-41.
11. Vasavada AR, Singh R. Phacoemulsification with posterior polar cataract. Journal of Cataract and Refractive Surgery. 1999;25:238-45.
12. Gavris M, Popa D, Caraus C, et al. Phacoemulsification in posterior polar cataract. Oftalmologia. 2004;48(4):36-40.
13. Eshaghian J, Streeten BW. Human posterior subcapsular cataract; an ultrastructural study of the posteriorly migrating cells. Arch Ophthalmol. 1980;98:134-43.
14. Eshagian J. Human posterior subcapsular cataracts. Trans Ophthalmol Soc UK. 1982;102:364-8.
15. Nagata M, Marsuura H, Fujinaga Y. Ultrastructure of posterior subcapsular cataract in human lens. Ophthalmic Res. 1986;18:180-4.

16. Hayashi K, Hayashi H, Nakao F, et al. Outcomes of surgery for posterior polar cataract. Journal of Cataract and Refractive Surgery. 2003;29:45-9.

17. Lee MW, Lee YC. Phacoemulsification of posterior polar cataracts—a surgical challenge. British Journal of Ophthalmology. 2003;87:1426-7.

18. Liu Y, Liu Y, Wu M, et al. Phacoemulsification in eyes with posterior polar cataract and foldable intraocular lens implantation. Yan Ke Xue Bao. 2003;19(2):92-4.

19. Fine IH, Packer M, Hoffman RS. Management of posterior polar cataract. Journal of Cataract and Refractive Surgery. 2003;29:16-9.

20. Allen D, Wood C. Minimizing risk to the capsule during surgery for posterior polar cataract. Journal of Cataract and Refractive Surgery. 2002; 28:742-4.

21. Vasavada AR, Raj SM. Inside-Out delineation. Journal of Cataract Refract Surgery. 2004;30:1167-9.

22. Fine IH. Cortico-cleaving hydrodissection. Journal of Cataract and Refractive Surgery. 1992;18:508-12.

23. Aziz Y Anis. Understanding hydrodelineation: the term and procedure. Doc Ophthalmol. 1994;87(2):123-37.

24. Masket S. Consultation Section. J Cataract Refract Surgery. 1997;23:819-24.

25. Emery JM, Little JH. Phacoemulsification and aspiration of cataracts, surgical technique, complications and results. St Louis, MO: CV Mosby; 1979. pp. 45-9.

26. Vasavada AR, Singh R. Step-by-step chop in situ and separation of very dense cataracts. J Cataract Refract Surgery. 1998;24:156-9.

27. Vasavada AR, Desai JP. Stop, chop, chop and stuff. J Cataract Refract Surgery. 1996;22:526-9.

28. Osher RH. Slow motion phacoemulsification approach (letter). J Cataract and Refract Surg. 1993;19(5):667.

29. Osher RH, Cionni R. In: Steinert RF (Ed). Cataract Surgery, Technique, Complications, Management, 2nd edition. Saunders; 2004. pp. 469-86.

30. Gimbel HV, DeBroff BM. Posterior capsulorhexis with optic capture: maintaining a clear visual axis after pediatric cataract surgery. J Cataract Refract Surg. 1994;20:658-64.

31. Vasavada AR, Trivedi R. Role of optic Capture in congenital cataract and IOL surgery in children. J Cataract Refract Surg. 2000;26:824-31.

CHAPTER 42

Phaco in Subluxated Cataracts

Athiya Agarwal

INTRODUCTION

The surgical management of cataract associated with zonular dialysis is a real challenge for the ophthalmic surgeon. Due to recent advances in equipment and instrumentation, better surgical techniques and understanding of the fluidics, the surgeon is able to perform relatively safe cataract surgery in the presence of compromised zonules. Implantation of a capsular tension ring can stabilize a loose lens and allow the surgeon to complete phacoemulsification and IOL implantation.

HISTORY

Insertion of a ring into the capsular bag fornix (equator) to support the zonular apparatus was first described by Hara and coauthors in 1991.[1] Hara et al. introduced the concept of "equator ring", "endocapsular ring" or "capsular tension ring". In 1993, the first capsular tension ring (CTR) for use in humans was designed.[2] In 1994, Nagamato and Bissen-Miyajima[3] suggested using an open PMMA ring to provide adaptability.

ADVANTAGES

This technique offers four main advantages:
- The capsular zonular anatomical barrier is partially reformed, so that vitreous herniation to the anterior chamber during surgery is reduced or even avoided.
- A taut capsular equator offers counter traction for all traction maneuvers, making them easier to perform and decreasing the risk of extending the zonular dialysis. The great advantage of using the capsular ring during the phacoemulsification rather than after, just to center the lens, is that it is a great deal safer. Any force that is transmitted to the capsule is not applied directly to the adjacent zonules, but rather distributed circumferentially to the entire zonular apparatus.
- The necessary capsular support for an in-the-bag centered implant is obtained.
- The capsular bag maintains its shape and do not collapse, which can lead to proliferation and migration of epithelial cells, development of capsular fibrosis syndrome and late IOP decentration.

DESIGNS AND DESCRIPTIONS

The capsular tension ring is made up of one-piece polymethyl methacrylate (PMMA) and is available in different sizes depending on their use in patients with emmetropia, low or high myopia. An injector is also present for loading the ring. The original capsular tension ring, with characteristic eyelets on both ends, is marketed by Morcher company in cooperation with Dr Mitchel Morcher. Meanwhile, various similar products are being marketed (e.g. by ophtec physiol, corneal, IOL tech, Acrimed, Rayner, Hanita, Lens Tec.). As a standard capsular tension ring, 12.0/10.0 mm diameter ring (Morcher type 14) and 13.0/11.0 mm diameter ring (ophtec 13/11) are most commonly used by surgeons. Morcher type 14 is used for normal axial length eyes, while types 14A and 14C are used for myopic eyes.

The modifications used by Morcher include two types of capsular tension rings with iris shields (Types L and G, with integrated iris shields of 60 and 90 degrees, respectively) and two types of capsular bending rings (CBRs) designed to prevent capsule opacification (types E and F). These modified versions incorporate fixation elements that allow the surgeon to suture the ring to the scleral wall, through the ciliary sulcus, without violating the capsular ring.[4]

SPECIAL DESIGNS FOR SUTURING IN SEVERE ZONULAR DEHISCENCE

In cases where severe or progressive zonular dehiscence is present, implantation of the capsular tension ring alone may not be adequate. This may lead to severe postoperative capsular bag shrinkage as well as IOL decentration and pseudophakodonesis.[5] Also complete luxation of the bag along with the capsular tension ring and the IOL cannot be excluded.

A modified design developed by Cionni with a fixation hook for severe or progressive cases of zonular deficiency[6] solves this problem. The hook is kept opposite to the meridian of decentration and is pulled peripherally using a transscleral fixation suture to counteract capsular bag decentration and tilt. In severe cases, two such rings or the two hooked model can be used. However the Cionni ring has its limitations like difficulty to implant if the capsulorhexis is small and in such cases the hook may even drag on the edge of the anterior capsule and as the fixation plane is anterior to the anterior capsule, it may lead to iris chafing leading to pigment dispersion and chronic uveitis.

An alternative is to fix the ring by guiding the needle of the scleral suture through the equator of the capsular bag, just inside the capsular tension ring.[7] This technique has to be completed as a one step procedure because the suture may cheese-wire through both capsules leaving along the equator.

Another alternative in cases of severe decentration is to make a small equatorial capsulorhexis through which a standard capsular tension ring can be inserted. A scleral suture can then be passed around the exposed capsular tension ring which is then used to center the lens before capsulorhexis.

INDICATIONS

The indications for use of capsular tension ring is in all cases of subluxation of lens (**Table 42.1**) ranging from the common ones like traumatic displacement (mechanical or surgical), Marfan's syndrome, pseudoexfoliation syndrome and hypermature cataract to the rare ones like aniridia and intraocular tumors.

APPLICATIONS

Zonular Dehiscence

The efficacy of the capsular tension ring in managing zonular dialysis has been demonstrated *in vitro*[8,9] depending on where the zonular defect presents. The capsular tension ring may be inserted at any stage of cataract procedure. By reestablishing the capsules contour, the capsular tension ring protects the capsular fornix from being aspirated, avoiding consecutive zonular dialysis extension, irrigation fluid running behind the capsular diaphragm with the posterior capsule bulging and vitreous prolapse into the anterior chamber with possible aspiration. With preexisting zonular defects, such as those caused by blunt trauma, the capsular tension ring is inserted before phacoemulsification is started.

Zonular Weakness

Ocular and systemic conditions may result in a zonular weakness that may be profound and progressive. Pseudoexfoliation syndrome with or without glaucoma and Marfan's syndrome are the most common causes. If zonular weakness is profound, the capsular tension ring is implanted before the cataract is emulsified and a 10-0 nylon anchoring suture may be temporarily threaded through the eyelets so as to remove the capsular tension ring if the zonules fail during surgery.

In pseudoexfoliation syndrome, the anterior capsule may contract excessively after in the bag IOL placement (capsular phimosis). This can be prevented by providing a locking mechanism that would prevent the eyelets from overlapping, suturing together the two eyelets together or by using two larger implants. This can be supplemented by meticulously polishing the anterior capsule leaf overlapping the implant.

In case of Marfan's syndrome, the zonules may be disintegrated or elongated while the remaining may be still functional, giving rise to lens decentration, which may be

TABLE 42.1	Etiology of subluxated lenses

A. *Isolated Ocular Abnormality*
- Simple ectopia lentis
- Simple microspherophakia
- Spontaneous, late subluxation of lens

B. *Associated with Other Ocular Abnormality*
- Aniridia
- Ectopia lentis et pupillae
- Uveal coloboma
- Cornea plana

C. *Assoicated with Heritable Systemic Syndromes*
- Marfan's syndrome
- Homocystinuria
- Weil Marchesani syndrome
- Ehlers-Danlos syndrome
- Reiger's syndrome
- Hyperlysinemia
- Sulfite oxidase deficiency
- Sturge-Weber syndrome
- Pflander's syndrome
- Crouzon's syndrome
- Sprengel's anomaly
- Oxycephaly

D. *Associated with Other Ocular Conditions*
- Mature or hypermature cataract
- Mechanical stretching of zonules
  - Buphthalmos
  - Staphylomas
  - Ectasias of globe
  - High myopia
  - Perforation of large central corneal ulcer
- Pull on zonules
  - Cyclytic inflammatory adhesions
  - Eales'disease
  - Persistent hyperplastic primary vitreous
  - Intraocular tumors
  - Retinal detachment
- Degeneration of zonules
  - Uveitis
  - Retinitis pigmentosa
  - Chalcosis
  - Prolonged silicone oil tamponade
  - High myopia
  - Hypermature cataract

E. *Traumatic Subluxation/Dislocation and Surgical Trauma*

progressive. In case of Weil-Marchesani syndrome, microspherophakia and zonular degeneration may occur. Secondary scleral suturing to remedy IOL decentration and tilt may be useful in such cases.[7]

Use of prolonged silicone oil tamponade may lead to progressive zonular atrophy and emulsified oil or oil bubble gaining access into the anterior chamber spontaneously or during the cataract surgery. In such cases, a large capsular tension ring should be implanted before phacoemulsification is done.

LENS COLOBOMA

A colobomatous lens (**Figure 42.1**) is due to defective or absent segment of zonules resulting in a notch in the lens.

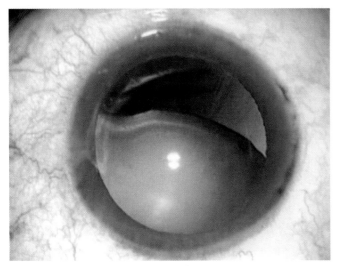

FIGURE 42.1: Lens coloboma

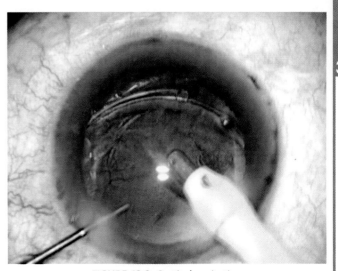

FIGURE 42.3: Cortical aspiration

It is a misnomer in that there is no actual lenticular substance missing. There is just a retraction of a crystalline area due to localized loss of tension on the lens capsule. Intact zonules are often seen in this area and therefore a localized area of defective ciliary body or zonules may lead to localized loss of traction on the lens capsule. It may occur along with a ciliary body coloboma. Lens coloboma is, therefore, more accurately referred to as "coloboma of the zonule and/or ciliary body".

Surgery in Lens Coloboma

Surgery is done using a capsular tension ring (CTR) which forms the capsular fornix **(Figures 42.2 to 42.4)**. The CTR which was first started by T Hara protects against capsular fornix aspiration, consecutive zonular dialysis, irrigation fluid flowing behind the capsule, vitreous herniating into the anterior chamber, IOL decentration and capsular phimosis. Minimal mydriasis or reactive miosis may be a problem. Conventional approaches to deal with normally positioned small pupils and cataract surgery may be used, such as mechanical stretching, iris retractors or multiple

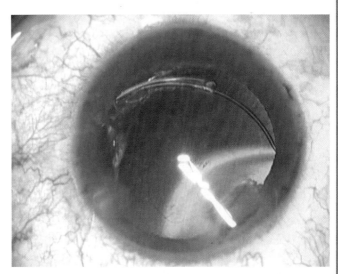

FIGURE 42.4: Cortex removed. Note the lens coloboma and endocapsular ring. At this stage, one can implant the foldable IOL comfortably

sphincterotomies. Vitreous loss may take place secondary to prolapse through the coloboma in the presence of an intact capsule. Giant retinal tears also occur with isolated lens coloboma. A large optic IOL is advisable for better visualization of the posterior segment, which is at greater risk of potential retinal detachment and also for optimal centration of the optic, relative to the ectopic pupil. Aberration free or aspheric IOLs may also be preferable in these eyes to decrease the effect of lens decentration on vision. A silicone IOL is not advised in case a complex retinal detachment occurs that requires the use of silicone oil.

SURGICAL TECHNIQUE

A case of subluxated lens, 3 months post surgery is shown in **Figure 42.5**.

Anesthesia

Both general and peribulbar anesthesia are suitable for creation of scleral windows and transscleral suturing of the

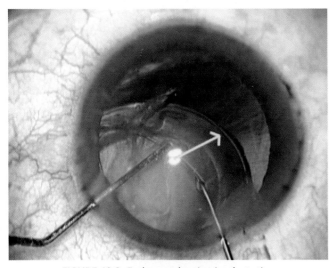

FIGURE 42.2: Endocapsular ring implantation

capsular ring or of the IOL, if necessary. Special mention is required about use of 1% intracameral lidocaine. There is a risk of its passage through the zones lacking zonular fibers and transitory loss of sight resulting from retinal toxicity as described in cases of capsular ruptures.[10]

Incisions

The first step is to make an incision in the eye which has a subluxated cataract. A needle with viscoelastic is injected inside the eye in the area where the second site is made. This will distend the eye, so that when you make a clear corneal incision, the eye will be tense and one can create a good valve. Now a straight rod is held to stabilize the eye with the left hand. With the right hand, the clear corneal incision is made.

Capsulorhexis

Commencing capsulorhexis is difficult because of capsular instability. It is better to begin the capsulorhexis in the area where the zonules are whole and the capsule offers sufficient resistance. If vitreous is present in the anterior chamber, the gel must be first isolated and vitrectomy should be performed, if required. After the vitreous has been removed from the anterior chamber, a viscoelastic, preferably dispersive, is inserted by first covering the zone. Capsulorhexis can be performed, after the zone of zonular dehiscence and iridocrystalline diaphragm have been stabilized. Trypan blue should not be used in such cases, as the trypan blue will go into the vitreous cavity through the zonular dehiscence and make the whole vitreous cavity blue. This will make visualization difficult in surgery. Completion of rhexis can be done using an intraocular rhexis forceps.

Hydrodissection-Hydrodelineation

Hydromaneuvers should be performed meticulously to ensure correct freeing of the lens nucleus. The hydrodissection cannula should be inserted in the direction of the zone of disinsertion rather than in the opposite direction, which would enlarge the disinsertion. Viscoelastic may be required to separate the nucleus and cortical material and also to separate the cortex from the lens capsule.

Implantation of Capsular Ring

Mostly capsular tension rings can be easily inserted in the capsular bag if it is well expanded with viscoelastic. The instruments used to implant a capsular tension ring include Kelman-McPherson type forceps special injectors (marketed by Ophtec and Geuder suitable for both Ophtec and Morcher CTRs and the one developed by Menapace and Nishi for use with CBR, Geuder Co.) and last but not the least, a guiding suture.

Phacoemulsification

Nuclear phacoemulsificaton can be performed using coaxial phaco or bimanual phaco/phakonit in the bag or out of the bag, depending on the surgeon's preference. In general, phacoemulsification in these situations may be considered a safe proposition if performed in a proper way.

Cortical Aspiration

When performing automated aspiration, movements of the tip should not be radial because of the risk of traction on the ring and the capsular bag.

Implantation of the Intraocular Lens

It is desirable to implant a larger diameter lens to minimize symptoms if lens decentration were to occur. The foldable lens is loaded and implanted in the capsular bag followed by viscoelastic removal. In either case, rotational maneuvers must be avoided or minimized.[11]

Cionni's Ring

If the lens continues to remain decentered after CTR insertion, a flexible nylon iris hook is used to engage the rhexis margin through a paracentesis opposite to the direction of subluxation. This gives capsular support till the end of surgery during which a transscleral fixation of one haptic of the IOL can be done for its centration.

When zonular dehiscence is large in extent or progressive in nature, capsular bag shrinkage resulting in IOL decentration and pseudophakodonesis may occur even after a successful surgery with capsular ring. Complete luxation of the bag and its contents has also been reported. For such cases, Cionni's modified design with a fixation hook is a good solution **(Figure 42.5)**. The hook is kept in the area of dialysis and is pulled peripherally using a transscleral fixation suture to counteract capsular bag

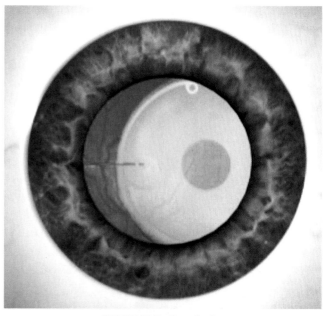

FIGURE 42.5: Cionni's ring

decentration and tilt. In severe cases, two such rings or the two hooked models can be used. If normal endocapsular ring is used, the ring and the IOLO might not be in the correct position (**Figure 42.6**). An alternative in cases of severe decentration (**Figure 42.7**) is to make a small equatorial capsulorhexis through which a standard capsular tension ring can be inserted. A scleral suture can then be passed around the exposed capsular tension ring which is then used to center the lens before capsulorhexis. Peribulbar anesthesia is suitable for creation of scleral windows and transscleral suturing of the capsular ring or of the IOL if necessary.

Ike Segments

Ike Ahmed designed the Ike segments which can be used for small segments.

Assia's Capsule Anchor

The capsular anchor (Hanita lenses, Kibbutz Hanita, Israel) is a novel device for the management of subluxation of the lens associated with moderate to severe zonular dehiscence or weakness. This was designed by Ehud Assia from Israel. It is a polymethyl methacrylate (PMMA) intraocular, uniplanar implant, inserted into the capsular bag after capsulorhexis is performed. An intact ACCC is a prerequisite for a safe use of the anchor. The two lateral arms of the device are inserted behind the anterior lens capsule whereas the central rod is placed in front of the capsule (**Figure 42.8**). A 10-0 or preferably 9-0 prolene suture is used to fixate the anchor to the scleral wall. The suture is either threaded through the hole in the base of the device or wraps around the neck of the anterior rod. A temporary safety suture can be used to prevent falling of the device during surgical procedures through the large zonular defect, especially if anterior vitrectomy was also performed. The anchor is usually inserted prior to removal of the lens material. Repositioning and stabilization of the lens capsule significantly facilitate phacoemulsification or aspiration of

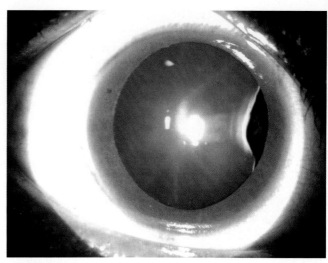

FIGURE 42.7: Lens coloboma

the lens material and implantation of a PC-IOL (**Figures 42.9A and B**).

Concept: The concept of the capsular anchor is different than that of the modified capsular rings. The later stabilize the capsular equator (the entire circumference, MCTR or partial circumference, CTS). The anchor clips a segment of the anterior capsule and supports only a limited portion of the lens equator. A conventional capsular tension ring can be used in conjunction with the anchor to reform the round contour of the capsular equator.

KEY POINTS WITH THE USE OF CAPSULAR TENSION RINGS

- Use a high viscosity viscoelastic.
- Make the incision at a meridian with no zonular dialysis, in order to avoid damage to zonular fibers with the movement of the phaco tip.
- Perform slow-motion phaco, with low flow rate, low vacuum and low infusion bottle height.

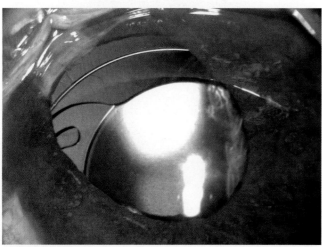

FIGURE 42.6: Endocapsular ring implanted without suturing to the sclera. Note that the ring and IOL are not in proper place

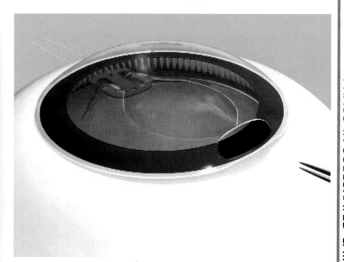

FIGURE 42.8: The capsular anchor. The two lateral arms are located behind the anterior capsule. The anterior central rod is placed in front of the capsule (*Courtesy:* Ehud Assia)

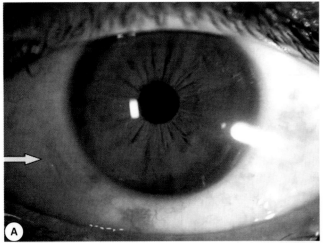

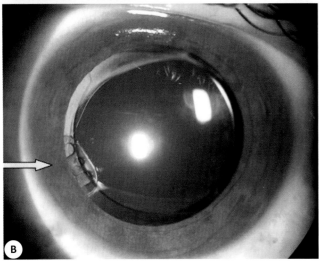

FIGURES 42.9A and B: Subluxated case, 3 months postoperatively. Nondilated pupil is round, suture is buried under the conjunctiva (arrow) (A). Dilated pupil, the anchor fixates the inferonasal anterior capsule to the scleral wall (arrow), PC-IOL is well centered (B) (*Courtesy:* Ehud Assia)

- Emulsification can be done in the bag when the nucleus is soft and in the anterior chamber if the nucleus is hard, thereby avoiding as much stress as possible to the already damaged zonular apparatus.
- Perform a careful two-port anterior vitrectomy with lax infusion bottle and low aspiration pressure when necessary.
- Try to place IOL haptics in the meridian of the zonular disinsertion.
- IOL stability must be checked at the end of the surgery, both in the frontal and sagittal plane in order to consider if suturing one haptic to the sulcus is necessary.[6]

Special Conditions

- *Coloboma shield for large sector iris defects or iridodialysis:* Tinted capsular tension ring with an integrated 60–90 degree sector shield designed by Rasch can be used to protect against glare and/or monocular diplopia (Morcher L and G). The capsular tension ring can be placed to cover sector iris defects and/or

coloboma. If more than 90 degrees of defect is present, then more than one capsular tension ring can be used.[4]

- *Multisegmented coloboma ring for aniridia:* This multisegmented ring designed by Rasch (Morcher type 50 C) is used in combination with the one of the same kind so that the interspaces of the first ring are covered by the sector shields of the second forming a contiguous artificial iris **(Figure 42.10).**

- *Anterior eye wall resection for uveal melanoma or other intraocular malignancy:* A combined use of a standard and coloboma capsular tension ring is advocated in cataract surgery after anterior eye wall resection for intraocular malignancy like uveal melanoma. Uveal tumors involving the anterior segment of the eye may need uveal resection resulting in large iris coloboma and zonular dehiscence. The crystalline lens may be cataractous or may become opaque after the surgery of the tumor requiring its removal sooner or later. For technical approach, intracapsular cataract extraction was considered previously, but the combined use of a standard and coloboma capsular tension ring may help preserve the capsular bag and cover the iris defects.

- *Along with primary posterior capsulorhexis for preexisting central capsule fibrosis or as a general preventive measure against capsule opacification:*[12] As the capsular tension ring is in place, vector forces during primary posterior capsulorhexis can be controlled in a better way as the ring stretches the posterior capsule, giving uniform radial vector forces. As the capsular tension ring is in place distortion in shape of the primary posterior capsulorhexis can be avoided and folds on the capsule caused by traction due to oversized and rigid lens loop can be prevented, which allows closer and

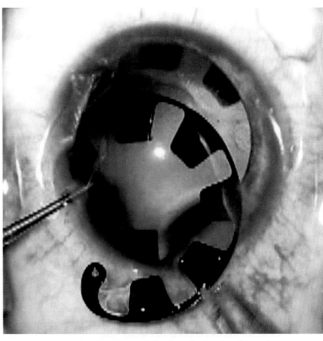

FIGURE 42.10: Aniridia rings being implanted

perfect apposition of the posterior capsule with the optic of the IOL, thereby preventing lens epithelial cells (LECs) from entering the retrolental space in the posterior capsulorhexis margin and thus preventing the secondary primary posterior capsulorhexis closure.

- *In combined cataract and vitreous surgery:* When the capsular tension ring is in place, the posterior capsule remains uniformly distended and a perfect peripheral view is possible. Also as the capsular tension ring is in place, silicone oil can be removed through the same phaco incision from the primary posterior capsulorhexis, which can be performed in a controlled manner with the capsular tension ring in place.

- *As a tool to measure capsular bag circumference:* The capsular tension ring *in vivo* can be visualized gonioscopically from a well-dilated pupil. The distance between the eyelets can be determined by adjusting the width of the slit beam of the slit lamp to fill in the space between the eyelets which can be read out on the slit lamp directly. This capsular bag biometry can be used for quantifying *in vivo* capsular bag circumference[13] and capsular bag shrinkage dynamics.[14]

- *For prevention of posterior capsular opacification:* Theoretically, the lesser is the space in between the optic lens and the posterior capsule, the lesser are the chances of lens epithelial cells from migrating behind the optic, i.e. no space, no cells. When the capsular bending ring is in place, this interspace is less common and if present, less in amount as compared to without a capsular bending ring. Also by keeping the anterior capsule away from the posterior capsule, myofibroblastic transdifferentiation of lens epithelial cells on the anterior capsule edge and back surface can be prevented. The capsular bending ring is an open, band shaped polymethyl methacrylate ring measuring 11 mm in diameter.

The ring is minimally polished to keep the edges sharp and rectangular, facilitating the creation of a sharp and discontinuous band in the equatorial capsule. A crooked islet is located at both the ring ends to prevent spearing of the capsular fornix and to facilitate manipulation during insertion. The capsular bending ring reduces anterior capsular fibrosis and shrinkage, as well as posterior capsular opacification. The ring may be useful in patients who are at high risk of developing eye complications from opacification that require Nd:YAG laser capsulotomy, in those expected to have vitreoretinal surgery and photocoagulation, and in cases of pediatric cataract.[15]

GLUED IOL

The latest technique for managing subluxated cataracts or colobomas is the use of the glued IOL. In this, a lensectomy vitrectomy is done and the lens is removed totally. Then a glued IOL is implanted. The advantage is that pseudo-exfoliations are progressive conditions and with glued IOL there is no problem (**Figures 42.11A and B**).

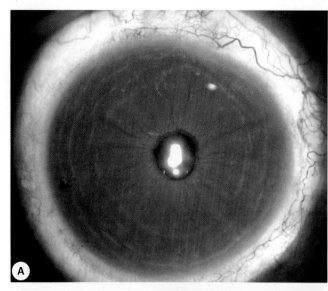

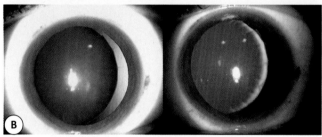

FIGURES 42.11 and B: Glued IOL; glued IOL done in right eye—one and a half year postoperatively (A); and subluxated cataract in left eye (B)

SUMMARY

Capsular tension rings or endocapsular rings have solved the problems of phaco in subluxated cataracts. They have made life much easier for the cataract surgeon.

REFERENCES

1. Hara T, Hara T, Yamada Y. "Equatorial ring" for maintenance of the completely circular contour of the capsular bag equator after cataract removal. Ophthalmic Surg. 1991;22:358-9.
2. Hara T, Hara T, Sakanishi K, et al. Efficacy of equator rings in a experimental rabbit study. Arch Ophthalmol. 1995;113:1060-5.
3. Nagamoto T, Bissen-Miyajima H. A ring to support the capsular bag after continuous curvilinear capsulorhexis. Cataract Refract Surg. 1994;20:417-20.
4. Menapace R, Findl O, Georgopoulos M, et al. The capsular tension ring: Designs, applications, and techniques. J Cataract Refract Surg. 2000;898-912.
5. Nishi O, Hishi K, Sakanishi K, et al. Explantation of endocapsular posterior chamber lens after spontaneous posterior dislocation. J Cataract Refract Surg. 1996;22:272-5.
6. Groessl SA, Anderson CJ. Capsular tension ring in a patient with Weill-Marchesani syndrome. J Cataract and Refract Surg. 1998;24:1164-5.
7. Fischel JD, Wishart MS. Spontaneous complete dislocation of the lens in pseudoexfoliation syndrome. Eur J Implant Refract Surg. 1995;7:31-3.
8. Sun R, Gimbel HV. In vitro evaluation of the efficacy of the capsular tension ring for managing zonular dialysis in cataract surgery. Ophthalmic Surg Lasers. 1998;29:502-5.

9. Gimbel HV, Sun R, Heston JP. Management of zonular dialysis in phacoemulsification and IOL implantation using the capsular tension ring. Ophthalmic Surg Lasers. 1997;28:273-81.

10. Gills J, Fenzl R. Intraocular lidnocaine causes transient loss of vision in small number of cases. Ocular Surgery News. 1996;14:26.

11. Agarwal Sunita, Agarwal Athiya, Sachdev S Mahipal, et al. Phacoemulsification, Laser Cataract Surgery and Foldable IOL's, 2nd edition. New Delhi, India: Jaypee Brothers; 2000.

12. Van Cauwenberge F, Rakic JM, et al. Complicated posterior capsulorhexis: etiology, management, and outcome. Br J Ophthalmol. 1997;81:195-8.

13. Vass C, Menapace R, Schametter K, et al. Prediction of pseudophacic capsular bag diameter on biometric variables. J Cataract Refract Surg. 1999;25:1376-81.

14. Strenn K, Menapace R, Vass C. Capsular bag shrinkage after implantation of an open loop silicone lens and a polymethyl methacrylate capsule tension ring. J Cataract Refract Surg. 1997;23:1543-7.

15. Nishi O, Nishi K, Menaopace R, et al. Capsular bending ring to prevent posterior capsule opacification: 2 year follow up. J Cataract Refract Surg. 2001;27:1359-65.

CHAPTER 43

Mature Cataracts

Amar Agarwal

INTRODUCTION

One of the biggest bugbears for a phaco surgeon is to perform a rhexis in a mature cataract **(Figures 43.1 and 43.2).** Once one performs rhexis in mature and hypermature cataracts, then phaco can be done in these cases and a foldable IOL implanted.

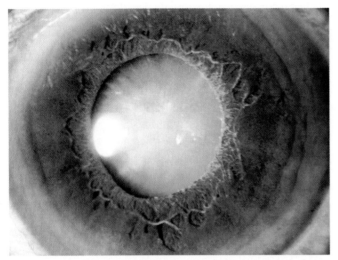

FIGURE 43.1: Mature cataract. It is difficult to visualize the rhexis in such cases, so we need to stain the anterior capsule with a dye

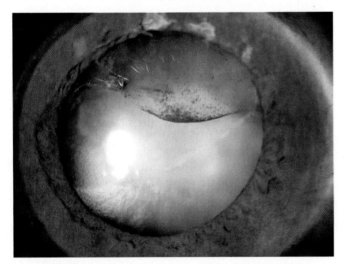

FIGURE 43.2: Mature cataract. Note that vitreous is there anterior to the cataract

RHEXIS IN MATURE CATARACTS

Various techniques are present which can help one perform rhexis in mature cataracts.

1. One should use a good operating microscope. If the operating microscope is good, one can faintly see the outline of the rhexis.
2. Use of an endoilluminator: While one is performing the rhexis with the right hand (dominant hand), (non-dominant hand) one can hold an endoilluminator in the left hand. By adjusting the endoilluminator in various positions, one can complete the rhexis as the edge of the rhexis can be seen.
3. Use of forceps: A forceps is easier to use than a needle especially in mature cataracts. One can use a good rhexis forceps to complete the rhexis.
4. Use of paraxial light.

With all these techniques, one is not very sure of completing a rhexis in all the cases. Many times if the rhexis is incomplete, one might have to convert to an extracapsular cataract extraction to prevent a posterior capsular rupture or nucleus drop.

TRYPAN BLUE

The solution to this problem is to have a dye, which stains the anterior capsule. This dye is trypan blue **(Figure 43.3).** Each ml contains 0.6 mg trypan blue, 1.9 mg of sodium mono-hydrogen orthophosphate, 0.3 mg of sodium di-hydrogen orthophosphate, 8.2 mg of sodium chloride, sodium hydroxide for adjusting the pH and water for injection. There are many other companies making this dye.

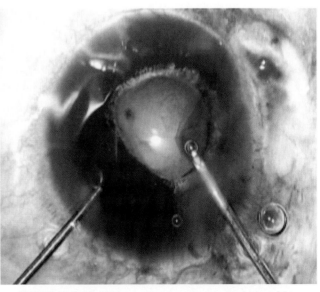

FIGURE 43.3: Rhexis in a mature cataract using trypan blue

INDOCYANINE GREEN (ICG)

ICG is available in the US. It comes as a lyophilized compound, which must first be dissolved in 0.5 cc of sterile diluent supplied by the manufacturer. It is then further diluted with 4.5 cc of BSS Plus (Alcon) immediately prior to use. This creates a 270 mOsm, 0.5% concentration. ICG creates a pale green staining of the capsule, which is gone by the conclusion of the case. One slight disadvantage is that the dye is lyophilized and larger particles often remain suspended in the mixture.

TECHNIQUE

We always tend to perform a temporal clear corneal incision. If the astigmatism is plus at 90 degrees, then the incision is made superiorly. Trypan blue can be injected under air or directly into the anterior chamber. Trypan blue is withdrawn from the vial into a syringe. This is then injected by a cannula into the anterior chamber between the air bubble and the lens capsule. It is kept like that for a minute or two for staining of the anterior capsule to occur. Next viscoelastic is injected into the anterior chamber to remove the air bubble and the trypan blue.

Now, rhexis is started with a needle. One can use a forceps also. We prefer to use a needle as it gives a better control on the size of the rhexis. Note that the left hand holding a rod stabilizing the eye while the rhexis is being performed. The rhexis is continued with the needle. Note the contrast between the capsule, which has been stained, and the cortex, which is not stained. The rhexis is continued and finally completed.

Hydrodissection is then done. One will not be able to see the fluid wave in such cases as the cataract is very dense. In such cases, a simple way is to see if the lens comes up anteriorly a little bit. This will indicate hydrodissection being completed. One can also test this by rotating the nucleus before starting phaco.

Then the phaco probe is inserted through the incision, slightly superior to the center of the nucleus. At that point, ultrasound should be applied and it should be checked whether the phaco tip gets embedded in the nucleus. The direction of the phaco probe should be obliquely downwards toward the vitreous and not horizontally towards the iris. Then only the nucleus will get embedded. The settings at this stage are: 80% phaco power, 24 ml/minute flow rate and 101 mm of Hg suction. By the time the phaco tip gets embedded in the nucleus, the tip would have reached the middle of the nucleus. Now with the chopper, the nucleus is cut with a straight downward motion and then the chopper is moved to the left when one reaches at the center of the nucleus. In other words, the left hand moves the chopper like an inverted L. One does not go to the periphery for chopping, but do it at the center. Once a crack is created, the nucleus is split till the center. Then the nucleus is rotated to 180 degrees and cracked again so that one can get two halves of the nucleus.

Now that one has two halves, a shelf is also present to embed the probe. So, now the probe should be placed with the ultrasound into one half of the nucleus and chop. Like this three quadrants are created in one half of the nucleus. Then another three halves are made with the second half of the nucleus. Thus, one can get six quadrants or pie-shaped fragments now.

Once all the pieces have been chopped, each piece is taken out one by one and in pulse phaco mode the pieces are aspirated at the level of the iris. One should not work in the bag unless the cornea is preoperatively bad or the patient is very elderly.

The next step is to do cortical washing. One must always try to remove the subincisional cortex first, as that is the most difficult. Note that everytime the left hand has the straight rod controlling the movements of the eye. If necessary, a bimanual irrigation aspiration technique can be used. Then inject viscoelastic and implant the IOL. At the end of the procedure, the BSS is injected inside the lips of the clear corneal incision. This will create a stromal hydration at the wound. This will create a whiteness, which will disappear after 4–5 hours. The advantage of this is that the wound gets sealed better.

ADVERSE EFFECTS

1. One is still not sure if extended contact of trypan blue with the corneal endothelium produces corneal damage. At present, no cases have been reported as the trypan blue is washed off with the viscoelastic and the BSS fluid.
2. Postsurgical inflammatory reactions and some bullous keratopathy have been known to occur after using vital staining agents.
3. Extreme care must be taken when using trypan blue on patients who are hypersensitive to any of its components.
4. During animal experiments, a teratogenic and/or mutagenic effect has been reported after repeated and/or high-dose intraperitoneal or intravenous injections with trypan blue. So, trypan blue should not be used in pregnant women.

SUMMARY

Trypan blue can make life much easier for the phaco surgeon especially in cases of mature and hypermature cataracts by staining the anterior capsule. Another dye is ICG, which is much costlier.

CHAPTER 44

Combined Cataract and Glaucoma Surgery

Amar Agarwal, Soosan Jacob

INTRODUCTION

Cataract is the foremost cause of blindness worldwide and continues to remain an important cause of visual impairment in the United States.[1-4] In the Baltimore Eye Survey, cataract was found to be the leading cause of blindness among the population over 40 years of age, and unoperated cataract was found to be four times more common among African Americans than Caucasian Americans.[3] The Salisbury Eye Evaluation Study (n=2,520) found that after refractive error, cataract was the leading cause of visual impairment in African Americans and Caucasian Americans.[4]

Cataract and glaucoma often co-exist in the elderly, especially so with the increasing longevity of the human race. It is especially important to be able to appropriately manage this patient sub-group in whom central vision is compromised due to cataract and peripheral vision due to the glaucoma.

SURGICAL OPTIONS

When a patient with cataract also has glaucoma, surgical options are cataract surgery alone, glaucoma surgery first followed later by cataract surgery, cataract surgery first followed later by glaucoma surgery or cataract surgery combined with filtering surgery. The decision is based on the degree of visual field damage, optic nerve head damage and retinal nerve fiber layer loss, the patient's response to medical or laser therapy, grade of cataract, and the surgeon's experience and personal preferences. The factors favoring a combined procedure are many. While cataract surgery with intraocular lens (IOL) implantation lowers intraocular pressure (IOP) by 2 mm Hg to 4 mm Hg in long-term studies,[5,6] a glaucoma procedure combined with cataract surgery lowers IOP more effectively (6–8 mm Hg).[7-9] Following either extracapsular cataract extraction (ECCE) or phacoemulsification, many of the glaucomatous eyes suffer an IOP spike to 30 mm Hg or more, which may lead onto anterior ischemic optic neuropathy or progressive glaucomatous damage. It is essential to avoid IOP spikes in eyes with severe optic disc damage and visual field loss close to fixation. Combining drainage surgery with cataract extraction can significantly reduce the frequency of these spikes. The disadvantages for performing filtration surgery first followed by cataract surgery 3–6 months after a mature bleb has formed, include delayed visual recovery, all attendant anesthetic as well as perioperative risks of having to undergo two intraocular surgical procedures, decreased cost efficiency and the possibility of inducing bleb failure.

In a patient who requires both cataract extraction and glaucoma surgery for IOP control, a combined surgery would be preferred. The advantages of a combined procedure (cataract extraction with IOL implantation and trabeculectomy) are avoiding the IOP rise that may occur following cataract surgery alone, rapid visual recovery, and long-term glaucoma control with a single operation. Phacoemulsification combined with trabeculectomy results in good IOP control as well as an improvement in the visual acuity.[7,10,11] The disadvantage of combined procedures is that they are technically slightly more difficult and time consuming.

In a patient for whom only glaucoma surgery is definitely indicated, the decision to combine it with a cataract extraction as well depends on the patient's age, visual acuity, visual requirements, grade of cataract, associated ocular comorbidity such as subluxated lens, pseudoexfoliation syndrome, etc. Trabeculectomy hastens the onset and progression of cataract which will make optic nerve head and field evaluation difficult and also result in an unhappy patient who then requires a second surgery for the cataract soon after. The second step cataract surgery may also result in failure of a previously functioning bleb, all of which lead to an extremely unhappy patient and a difficult situation for the surgeon. All of these factors favor a combined surgery for these patients.[12]

One may also consider combining glaucoma surgery in a patient who is going to undergo a cataract extraction depending on the IOP control, number of drugs required for IOP control and patient's intolerance or non-compliance with drugs.[12]

PREOPERATIVE PREPARATION

Apart from the usual preoperative preparations, it is extremely imperative to control the IOP prior to surgery to avoid choroidal effusion, choroidal hemorrhage or expulsive hemorrhage. Phacoemulsification is especially advantageous here, as it is a closed chamber procedure; nevertheless, IOP may suddenly drop to values close to zero even with phaco.[13] Preoperative control of IOP can be done with topical medications, systemic carbonic anhydrase inhibitors, oral glycerol or intravenous mannitol.

SURGICAL TECHNIQUES

Peripheral Iridectomy with Phacoemulsification

A simple peripheral iridectomy can be done with a vitrectomy probe at the time of phacoemulsification in some cases of angle closure glaucoma. Care should be taken that the iridectomy is in a position that is covered by the lids, in order to avoid intractable monocular diplopia for the patient.

Single Site Trabeculectomy with Phacoemulsification

Either a limbus based or fornix based conjunctival flap is created followed by a scleral flap which will be large enough to allow implantation of the IOL (**Figure 44.1**). Anterior chamber is entered under the scleral flap and phacoemulsification is performed as usual. After IOL implantation, sclerectomy and iridectomy are made and the scleral and conjunctival flaps are sutured.

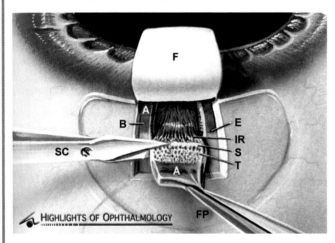

FIGURE 44.1: Trabeculectomy with Fornix Based Flap - Removing the Trabecular Window-Surgeon's View. This is a surgeon's view of the final incision to remove the trabecular window. It also reveals the surgeon's view of the structures most important to proper trabeculectomy. The trabeculectomy flap which is being excised has been hinged backwards exposing its deep surface to the surgeon's view. The Vannas scissors (SC), make the final cut just in front of the scleral spur (S), on the trabecular tissue which is here being reflected back with forceps (FP). The scleral spur is localized externally (E) by the junction of white sclera and gray band (B). Scleral flap (F). Clear cornea (A). Iris (I). Iris root (IR). Trabeculum (T). (*Courtesy:* Highlights of Ophthalmology, "Innovations in the Glaucomas - Etiology, Diagnosis and Management", English Edition, 2002, Editors: Benjamin F Boyd, MD, FACS; Maurice H Luntz, MD, FACS; Co-Editor: Samuel Boyd, MD)

Two Site Trabeculectomy with Phacoemulsification

Conjunctival and scleral flaps are made at the beginning of the surgery. Clear corneal phacoemulsification is then carried out in another quadrant. Filtering surgery is then completed at the end of the surgery (**Figures 44.2A and B**).

Trabeculectomy with Microphakonit

Here, 0.7 mm gauge phaco probe, irrigating chopper and I/A instruments are used for performing bimanual micro-incision cataract surgery (MICS). Trabeculectomy is performed as previously mentioned (**Figures 44.3A to C**).

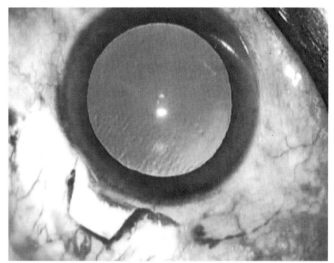

FIGURE 44.2A: Superficial scleral flap dissected out. Then phacoemulsification is done in another site and the IOL implanted

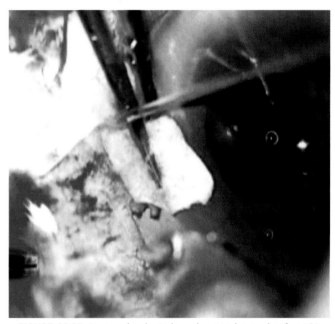

FIGURE 44.2B: Inner scleral window about to be made after IOL insertion

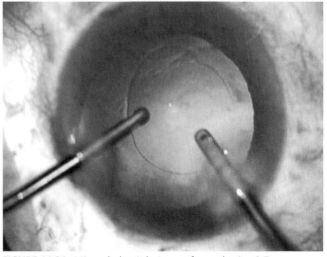

FIGURE 44.3A: Microphakonit being performed using 0.7 mm gauge instruments after making superficial scleral flap. Cortex has been removed with 0.7 mm gauge instruments in microphakonit

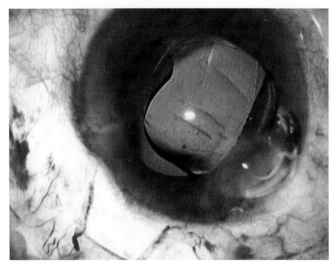

FIGURE 44.3B: IOL inserted after enlarging the microphakonit incision

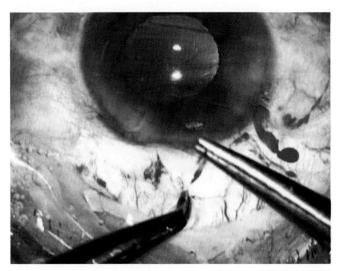

FIGURE 44.3C: The superficial scleral flap being sutured after taking the inner scleral punch and performing the iridectomy

Trabeculotomy with Phacoemulsification, Single Site and Two Site

In trabeculotomy,[14] a direct communication is created between the anterior chamber and the Schlemm's canal **(Figure 44.1)**. The conjunctival and scleral flaps are raised. In single site surgery, the scleral flap is then incised from its backside with a shallow incision, from which a sclerocorneal pocket is dissected with a keratome for the phaco probe. In two site surgery, the phacoemulsification is done from a different quadrant. Next, the Schlemm's canal is identified by its pigmentation and by the blood refluxed into the canal during phacoemulsification. In case of difficulty in identification because of too thick a remaining scleral bed, a second inner scleral flap is raised. Once the overlying sclera is thick enough, the Schlemm's canal can be easily identified. The scleral lamellae over Schlemm's canal are then incised parallel to the canal, taking care to avoid entering the anterior chamber. This can be facilitated by lifting the incised roof of Schlemm's canal

with a fine forceps and widening the incision after an initial puncture in the roof with fine Vannas scissors. A specially curved canalicular probe is then inserted into the Schlemm's canal, and the trabecular meshwork ruptured with a forward and inward motion. This is then repeated on the opposite side as well through the same entry site. The scleral flap and conjunctiva are closed in a water tight manner.

Non-Penetrating Glaucoma Surgery with Phacoemulsification

Viscocanalostomy and phacoemulsification: It is a non-perforating technique described by Stegman in 1991. It is aimed at avoiding fibrosis related bleb failure. It works by facilitating outflow of aqueous through the physiological pathway, viz. canal of Schlemm and the collector channels. This is done by creating a Descemetic window which is composed of the innermost layers of the trabecular meshwork and the Descemet's membrane.[15] Aqueous flows out through these layers and collects in an intrascleral space, through which it flows into the cut ends of the Schlemm's canal, which has been dilated previously by injecting high viscosity viscoelastic. It has also been postulated that there may be increased uveoscleral outflow after the surgery. The advantages of viscocanalostomy are: It is a non-penetrating procedure, postoperative complications such as hypotony, shallow anterior chamber, uveitis, endophthalmitis and cataract formation are avoided. Also the lack of external filtration avoids all bleb related complications, such as bleb failure due to scarring, blebitis, discomfort, etc.

Under retrobulbar or peribulbar anesthesia, a fornix-based conjunctival flap is made. As little cautery as possible is used to avoid damage to Schlemm's canal and the collector channels. An outer parabolic flap, sized 5 × 5 mm, approximately 200 μm thick, is then dissected, followe1d by an inner 4 × 4 mm scleral flap. One should be able to see the dark reflex from the underlying choroid after dissecting the inner flap. The cut is advanced towards the limbus and the Schlemm's canal is deroofed. The two openings of the canal remain patent at the lateral edges of the cut. The inner flap is then extended into the clear cornea by approximately 1 mm using blunt dissection with cotton tipped applicator. The inner scleral flap is then excised and the ostia of Schlemm's canal are cannulated with a specific cannula through which high-molecular-weight sodium hyaluronate (Healon GV®, Pharmacia & Upjohn, Sweden) is injected to distend it. This is done to prevent collapse and scarring in the early postoperative period. If adequate percolation is not seen through the Descemetic window, the juxtacanalicular meshwork along with the inner wall of the Schlemm's canal can be stripped with a fine forceps. The outer scleral flap is then tightly sutured and Healon GV® is injected beneath the flap, to prevent the intrascleral lake from collapsing and scarring in the early postoperative period. Two lateral stitches hold the conjunctiva in place. The conjunctiva is then closed. In case of perforation of the descemetic window, one can convert to a trabeculectomy. Viscocanalostomy can be combined with phacoemulsification,[15] using the same site or a different site. In single site, phacoemulsification is done via a superior scleral tunnel and a block of deep sclera is excised at the end and viscocanalostomy is completed as usual. In case of two site surgery, viscocanalostomy is done after phaco has been completed through the temporal approach. When viscocanalostomy is combined with phaco, aqueous leakage from the tunnel can be differentiated from a perforation of the Descemet's membrane, by drying the window surface with a sponge.

Deep sclerectomy and phacoemulsification: It is also a non-penetrating surgery, which differs from viscocanalostomy by producing subtenon filtration.

Under retrobulbar or peribulbar anesthesia, a 4 × 4 mm, 200-250 microns square superficial scleral flap is made followed by a deep scleral flap similar to that in viscocanalostomy. The dissection is extended anteriorly to deroof the Schlemm's canal and a descemetic window is created. The deep flap is excised and the superficial flap is closed less tightly to allow percolation into the subtenon space. The conjunctiva is then closed.[15]

Collagen or reticulated hyaluronic acid implants[15] can be inserted into the scleral lake for improving long-term filtration. These devices are slowly absorbed, thus maintaining the intrascleral lake and preventing its closure by fibrosis. A high molecular weight viscoelastic[15] (Healon5) may also be injected into the intrascleral lake to decrease wound healing. Deep sclerectomy can also be combined with the application of antimetabolites.[15] The hypotensive effect may also be increased even after surgery by perforating the descemetic window ab interno with a yttrium aluminium garnet (YAG) laser.

Deep sclerectomy can be combined with phacoemulsification just as in viscocanalostomy.

Laser sclerotomy with phacoemulsification: Here, the laser fiberoptic of the neodymium-doped yttrium aluminium garnet (Nd:YAG) laser is passed through the clear corneal incision and a short burst of laser is given directly opposite the planned site of sclerotomy.[16] The aiming beam is used as a guide and hence a goniolens is not required. When the aiming beam is seen around 1.5 mm from the limbus, a short burst of laser brings the laser fiberoptic out of the sclera and under the conjunctiva. The laser fiberoptic has a Helium Neon aiming beam and the diameter of the optic end is 380 microns. The fiberoptic is encased in a silicone sleeve. The remaining phacoemulsification is carried out as usual.

Seton procedure: This can be done in cases which do not respond to conventional surgeries **(Figure 44.4)**.

Antimetabolites

The use of antifibrotics (mitomycin-C,[17] and 5-fluoro-uracil[18]) to reduce the potential for bleb failure in combined phacotrabeculectomy is controversial. Mitomycin-C may

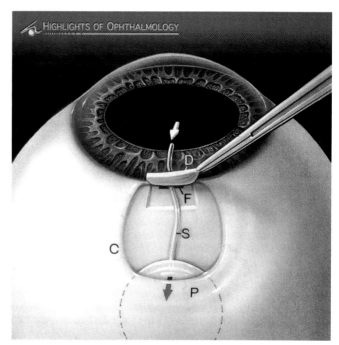

FIGURE 44.4: **Seton implantation procedure.** A fornix based conjunctival flap (C) is raised and the methylmethacrylate baseplate (P) of the Seton is pushed under the conjunctival flap posteriorly and sutured to the scleral surface. The implant has a biconcave shape with the inferior surface shaped to fit the sclera. A small 3 mm square half thickness lamellar scleral flap (D) is raised just as in a trabeculectomy. An incision (F) is made into the anterior chamber under this scleral flap and the long silicone tube (S) of the Seton is placed into the anterior chamber (the end of the silicone tube can be seen in the anterior chamber near the tip of the white arrow). Next, the scleral flap (D) is sutured down around the tube (S) of the Seton. Finally, the conjunctiva is sutured back in place. Aqueous then drains from the anterior chamber (white arrow) down through the tube (S) to the baseplate (P) (black arrow), where a bleb forms. (*Courtesy:* Highlights Of Ophthalmology, "Innovations in the Glaucomas - Etiology, Diagnosis and Management", English Edition, 2002, Editors: Benjamin F Boyd, MD, FACS; Maurice H Luntz, MD, FACS; Co-Editor: Samuel Boyd, MD)

result in lower long-term IOPs when used with combined procedures[9,17] but 5-fluorouracil does not seem to.[9,18] The potential vision-threatening complications of antimetabolites, such as bleb-related endophthalmitis,[19,20] hypotonic maculopathy[21,22] and late-onset bleb leaks[23] should be considered while deciding to use these agents.

Types of IOL

Friedrich et al. found that foldable silicone IOLs may induce late postoperative inflammatory membranes with pigment precipitates, especially after combined surgery.[24]

Complications

Postoperative uveitis or rise in IOP can usually be tackled with appropriate medications. Hyphema, if small usually resolves by itself. If very large, it may need to be evacuated.

Excessive filtration may occur leading onto choroidal detachment. When associated with a flat anterior chamber or other severe complications, it may require fluid drainage and bleb revision. Shallow anterior chamber may also be due to bleb leak. Hypotonic maculopathy may rarely be seen, especially in a young myopic patient. Other postoperative complications which may occur after routine phacoemulsification may occur in this setting too. Late postoperative complications include cystoid macular edema, capsular phimosis syndrome, IOL decentration, posterior capsular opacification, bleb failure, bleb related endophthalmitis, etc.

KEY-POINTS

- The summary of the evidence on IOP control with surgical treatment of coexisting cataract and glaucoma on long-term IOP re-control[25] states that there is good evidence that long-term IOP control is greater with combined procedures than with cataract extraction alone and fair evidence that trabeculectomy alone lowers long-term IOP more than combined ECCE and trabeculectomy. There is weak evidence that cataract extraction in glaucoma patients lowers IOP on average by 2 mm Hg to 4 mm Hg, trabeculectomy alone appears to lower IOP more than combined phaco and trabeculectomy, phaco and trabeculectomy lowers IOP by approximately 8 mm Hg in individuals followed-up for a mean of 1–2 years, ECCE and trabeculectomy lowers IOP by approximately 6–8 mm Hg in individuals followed-up for a mean of 1–2 years. The evidence was insufficient to determine the impact of cataract extraction on preexisting filtering blebs, to determine if other combined techniques (e.g. cyclodialysis and endolaser) work as well as cataract extraction and trabeculectomy and to determine if combined phaco and trabeculectomy lower IOP on the first postoperative day more than phaco alone.
- An Evidence-Based Practice Center sponsored by the Agency for Healthcare Research and Quality reviewed 131 studies on the treatment of adults with coexisting cataract and glaucoma, assessed the study quality and data, and reported it in evidence tables.[9] The investigators concluded that the findings that glaucoma surgery was associated with an increased risk of postoperative cataract and that a glaucoma procedure added to cataract surgery lowers IOP more than cataract surgery alone were strongly supported by the literature.
- The other findings that were found to be moderately supported by the literature[9] were that limbus and fornix-based conjunctival incisions provided the same degree of long-term IOP lowering in combined surgery; in combined surgery using phacoemulsification, the size of the cataract incision did not affect long-term IOP control; when used with combined procedures 5-fluorouracil was not beneficial in further lowering IOP, whereas mitomycin-C was efficacious in producing lower long-term IOPs when used with combined procedures.

- Findings weakly supported by literature[9] are that combined procedures resulted in lower IOP at 24 hours than cataract extraction alone; extracapsular cataract extraction (ECCE) alone appears to increase IOP at 24 hours; in the long-term, cataract surgery alone lowered IOP by 2–4 mm Hg, combined cataract and glaucoma surgery lowered IOP by 6–8 mm Hg, and the performance of a glaucoma procedure alone provided even greater long-term IOP lowering than combined cataract and glaucoma surgery; combined surgery in which the incisions for the cataract extraction and glaucoma procedure are separate, provided slightly lower long-term IOP than a one-site approach and that combined surgery in which phacoemulsification is used, provided slightly lower long-term IOP than nuclear expression.
- It is extremely imperative to control the IOP prior to surgery to avoid choroidal effusion, choroidal hemorrhage or expulsive hemorrhage.
- Newer techniques combining non-penetrating glaucoma surgery with phacoemulsification appear promising but long-term follow-up results have to be reported before they become widely practised.

References

1. Age-Related Eye Disease Study Research Group. A randomized, placebo-controlled clinical trial of high-dose supplementation with vitamins C and E and beta carotene for age-related cataract and vision loss: AREDS Report No. 9. Arch Ophthalmol. 2001;119(10):1439-52.
2. Sperduto RD, Hu TS, Milton RC, et al. The Linxian cataract studies. Two nutrition intervention trials. Arch Ophthalmol. 1993;111(9):1246–53.
3. Mares-Perlman JA, Klein BE, Klein R, et al. Relation between lens opacities and vitamin and mineral supplement use. Ophthalmology. 1994;101(2):315-25.
4. Leske MC, Wu SY, Connell AM, et al. Lens opacities, demographic factors and nutritional supplements in the Barbados Eye Study. Int J Epidemiol. 1997;26(6):1314-22.
5. Shingleton BJ, Gamell LS, O'Donoghue MW, et al. Long-term changes in intraocular pressure after clear corneal phacoemulsification: normal patients versus glaucoma suspect and glaucoma patients. J Cataract Refract Surg. 1999;25(7):885-90.
6. Tennen DG, Masket S. Short- and long-term effect of clear corneal incisions on intraocular pressure. J Cataract Refract Surg. 1996;22(5):568-70.
7. Wedrich A, Menapace R, Radax U, et al. Long-term results of combined trabeculectomy and small incision cataract surgery. J Cataract Refract Surg. 1995;21(1):49-54.
8. Gimbel HV, Meyer D, DeBroff BM, et al. Intraocular pressure response to combined phacoemulsification and trabeculotomy ab externo versus phacoemulsification alone in primary open-angle glaucoma. J Cataract Refract Surg. 1995;21(6):653-60.
9. Lau J, Ioannidis J, Balk E, et al. Evaluation of Technologies for Identifying Acute Cardiac Ischemia in Emergency Departments. Evidence Report/technology Assessment Number 26. (Prepared by the New England Medical Center Evidence-based Practice Center under Contract No. 290-97-0019) AHRQ Publication No. 01-E006, Rockville, MD: Agency for Healthcare Research and Quality. May 2001.

10. Wyse T, Meyer M, Ruderman JM, et al. Combined trabeculectomy and phacoemulsification: a one-site vs a two-site approach. Am J Ophthalmol. 1998;125(3):334-9.

11. Park HJ, Weitzman M, Caprioli J. Temporal corneal phacoemulsification combined with superior trabeculectomy. A retrospective case-control study. Arch Ophthalmol. 1997;115(3):318-23.

12. Guillermo L, Urcelay-Segura JL, Ortega-Usobiaga J, et al. Combined cataract extraction and filtering surgery. In: Agarawal S, Agarwal S, Agarwal A (Eds). Phacoemulsification. 3rd edition. pp. 596-608.

13. Burrato L, Zanini M. Phacoemulsification in glaucomatous eyes. In: Buratto L, Osher RH, Masket S (Eds). Cataract Surgery in Complicated Cases, NJ: Slack Inc; 2000.

14. Neuhann T, Ernest PH. Combined phacoemulsification with trabeculectomy. In: Buratto L, Osher RH, Masket S (Eds). Cataract Surgery in Complicated Cases, NJ: Slack Inc; 2000.

15. Obstbaum S, Zanini M. Combined cataract and glaucoma surgery. In: Buratto L, Osher RH, Masket S (Eds). Cataract Surgery in Complicated Cases, NJ: Slack Inc; 2000.

16. Sunita Agarwal, Sundaram, Asha B. Laser sclerotomy, laser phakonit and IOL implantation. In: Agarwal S, Agarwal A, Agarwal A (Eds). Phacoemulsification. 3rd edition. 2004. pp. 596-608.

17. Shin DH, Simone PA, Song MS, et al. Adjunctive subconjunctival mitomycin C in glaucoma triple procedure. Ophthalmology. 1995;102(10):1550-8.

18. Wong PC, Ruderman JM, Krupin T, et al. 5-Fluorouracil after primary combined filtration surgery. Am J Ophthalmol. 1994;117(2):149-54.

19. Higginbotham EJ, Stevens RK, Musch DC, et al. Bleb-related endophthalmitis after trabeculectomy with mitomycin C. Ophthalmology. 1996;103(4):650-6.

20. Greenfield DS, Suñer IJ, Miller MP, et al. Endophthalmitis after filtering surgery with mitomycin. Arch Ophthalmol. 1996;114(8):943-9.

21. Zacharia PT, Deppermann SR, Schuman JS. Ocular hypotony after trabeculectomy with mitomycin C. Am J Ophthalmol. 1993;116(3):314-26.

22. Costa VP, Wilson RP, Moster MR, et al. Hypotony maculopathy following the use of topical mitomycin C in glaucoma filtration surgery. Ophthalmic Surg. 1993;24(6):389-94.

23. Greenfield DS, Liebmann JM, Jee J, et al. Late-onset bleb leaks after glaucoma filtering surgery. Arch Ophthalmol. 1998;116(4):443-7.

24. Friedrich Y, Raniel Y, Lubovsky E, et al. Late pigmented-membrane formation on silicone intraocular lenses after phacoemulsification with or without trabeculectomy. J Cataract Refract Surg. 1999;25(9):1220-5.

25. Jampel HD, Lubomski LH, Friedman DS, et al. Treatment of Coexisting Cataract and Glaucoma. Baltimore: Evidence-Based practice center, Johns Hopkins University; 2000. Contract No. 290-097-0006, Task Order 3.

CHAPTER 45

Correcting Astigmatism Through the Use of Limbal Relaxing Incisions

Louis D "Skip" Nichamin

INTRODUCTION

In recent years, the concept of "refractive cataract surgery" has received increased attention from surgeons and the need for its adoption has recently been made more urgent by the increased availability of new presbyopia-correcting intraocular lenses. As such, the need to manage preexisting astigmatism has become a requisite aspect of modern phaco surgery. Experience with keratorefractive surgery has proven that astigmatism of as little as 0.75 diopters (D) may leave a patient symptomatic with blur vision, ghosting and halos. To fully embrace this notion of refractive cataract surgery, the dedicated surgeon must aspire to a level of accuracy that one would equate with corneal-based refractive surgery. The most popular approach to achieve this goal is through the use of corneal and specifically, limbal relaxing incisions (LRIs).

LIMBAL RELAXING INCISIONS

The modern era of cataract and astigmatism surgery began in the mid 1980s when several pioneering surgeons first suggested that astigmatic keratotomy might be combined with cataract and implant surgery.[1,2] Over time, other innovators began to recognize the benefit of moving these incisions out to a more peripheral, limbal location.[3-5] Indeed, experience has shown us that LRIs possess several advantages over astigmatic keratotomy incisions placed at a more central optical zone. These would include less of a tendency to cause a shift in the resultant cylinder axis and less likelihood of inducing irregular astigmatism. These incisions are easier to create and overall are simply more forgiving. Another important advantage gained by moving out to the limbus involves the "coupling ratio" which describes the amount of flattening that occurs in the incised meridian relative to the amount of steepening that results 90 degrees away; paired LRIs (when kept at or under 90 degrees of arc length) exhibit a very consistent 1:1 ratio and therefore, elicit little change in spheroequivalent, obviating the need to make any change in implant power.

THE PLAN

Perhaps the most challenging aspect of astigmatism surgery involves the determination of the quantity and exact location of the cylinder that is to be corrected, and thereby formulating a surgical plan. Unfortunately, preoperative measurements, such as refraction, keratometry and corneal topography, do not always correlate. Lenticular astigmatism may account for some of this disparity, particularly in cases where there is a wide variance between refraction and corneal measurements; however, some discrepancies are likely due to the inherent shortcomings of traditional measurements of astigmatism. Standard keratometry, for example, measures only two points in each meridian at a single optical zone of approximately 3 mm.

When confounding measurements do arise, one must assess the reliability of the particular measurement, possibly repeat particular studies and generally ignore outliers. Corneal readings are more heavily weighted than is the refractive cylinder, as the lens component will be removed, but some attention should be directed towards the habitual refraction (prior to cataract development) if it is available. When disparate readings do arise, for example, if topography shows 2 D of astigmatism and keratometry reveals only 1 D, it would be reasonable to correct for 1.5 D. Alternatively, if preoperative calculations vary widely, one may defer placing the relaxing incisions until a stable refraction postimplantation is obtained, and then correct the astigmatism. LRIs may be safely performed in the office in an appropriate treatment-room setting. Corneal topography is increasingly becoming the overall guiding measurement upon which the surgical plan is based. Topography is also helpful in detecting subtle corneal pathology such as keratoconus fruste which would likely negate the use of LRIs or subtle irregular astigmatism such as that caused by epithelial basement membrane dystrophy.

NOMOGRAMS

Once the amount of astigmatism to be corrected has been determined, a nomogram must be consulted to determine the appropriate arc length of the incisions. A number of popular nomograms are currently available.[6] Our nomogram of choice originated from the work of Dr Stephen Hollis and incorporates concepts taught by Spencer Thornton, MD, particularly his age modifiers.[7] As seen in **Table 45.1,** astigmatism is considered to be with-the-rule if the steep axis (plus cylinder) is between 45–135 degrees. Against-the-rule astigmatism is considered to fall between 0–44 and

TABLE 45.1 The "NAPA" nomogram: Nichamin age, a pachymetry-adjusted intralimbal arcuate astigmatic nomogram

With-the-rule (Steep Axis 45°-135°)						
Preop Cylinder (Diopters)	Paired Incisions in Degrees of Arc					
	20-30 years old	31-40 years old	41-50 years old	51-60 years old	61-70 years old	71-80 years old
0.75	40	35	35	30	30	
1.00	45	40	40	35	35	30
1.25	55	50	45	40	35	35
1.50	60	55	50	45	40	40
1.75	65	60	55	50	45	45
2.00	70	65	60	55	50	45
2.25	75	70	65	60	55	50
2.50	80	75	70	65	60	55
2.75	85	80	75	70	65	60
3.00	90	90	85	80	70	65
Against-the-rule (Steep Axis 0°-44°/136°-180°)						
Preop Cylinder (Diopters)	Paired Incisions in Degrees of Arc					
	20-30 years old	31-40 years old	41-50 years old	51-60 years old	61-70 years old	71-80 years old
0.75	45	40	40	35	35	30
1.00	50	45	45	40	40	35
1.25	55	55	50	45	40	35
1.50	60	60	55	50	45	40
1.75	65	65	60	55	50	45
2.00	70	70	65	60	55	50
2.25	75	75	70	65	60	55
2.50	80	80	75	70	65	60
2.75	85	85	80	75	70	65
3.00	90	90	85	80	75	70
Blade depth setting is at 90% of the thinnest pachymetry						

Source: Louis D "Skip" Nichamin, MD. The Laurel Eye Clinic, Brookville, PA

136–180 degrees. One aligns the patient's age with the amount of preoperative cylinder to be corrected and finds the suggested arc length that the paired incisions should subtend.

An empiric blade depth setting is commonly used when performing LRIs, typically at 600 microns. This would seem to be a reasonable practice when treating cataract patients; however, in the setting of refractive lens exchange surgery or when employing presbyopia-correcting IOLs, where ultimate precision is required, it is our preference to perform pachymetry and utilize adjusted blade depth settings. Pachymetry may be performed either preoperatively or at the time of surgery. Readings are taken over the entire arc length of the intended incision and an adjustable micrometer diamond blade is then set to approximately 90% of the thinnest reading obtained. Refinements to the blade depth setting as well as nomogram adjustments may be necessary depending upon individual surgeon technique, the instruments used and, in particular, the style of the blade **(Figures 45.1A and B)**. It should also be noted that in eyes that have previously undergone radial keratotomy, the length of the incisions should be reduced by approximately 50%, and in eyes that have undergone "significant" prior keratotomy surgery, it would be best to avoid additional incisional surgery and employ a toric IOL or laser technology instead.

SURGICAL TECHNIQUE

In most cases, the relaxing incisions are placed at the outset of surgery in order to minimize epithelial disruption **(Figures 45.2A to F)**. The one exception to this rule occurs when the phaco incision intersects or is encompassed within an LRI of greater than 40 degrees of arc; if it is extended

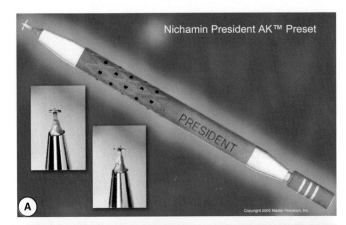

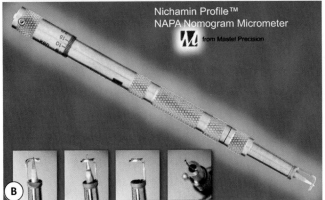

FIGURES 45.1A and B: Preset and adjustable micrometer (for use with the NAPA Nomogram) diamond knives by Mastel Precision. Similar designs are available from Storz instruments and other manufacturers

to its full arc length at the start of surgery, significant gaping and edema may result secondary to intraoperative wound manipulation. In this setting, the phaco incision is first made by creating a shortened LRI whose arc length corresponds to the width of the phaco and IOL incision. This amounts to a two-plane grooved phaco incision whose depth is either 600 microns or has been determined by pachymetry as described above. Just prior to IOL implantation, with a firm viscoelastic filled eye, the relaxing incision is extended to its full arc length as dictated by the nomogram. When an LRI is superimposed upon the phaco tunnel, the keratome entry is accomplished by pressing the bottom surface of the keratome blade downward upon the outer or posterior edge of the LRI. The keratome is then advanced into the LRI at an iris-parallel plane. This angulation will promote a dissection that takes place at mid-stromal depth which will help to assure adequate tunnel length and a self-sealing closure.

Proper centration of the incisions over the steep corneal meridian is of utmost importance. Increasing evidence supports the notion that significant cyclotorsion may occur when assuming a supine position.[8] As previously noted, an axis deviation of only 15 degrees may result in a 50% reduction of surgical effect.[9] This reduction in effect holds true for both relaxing incisions and toric IOLs. For this reason, most surgeons advocate placing an orientation mark at the 12:00 or 6:00 limbus while the patient is in an upright position. This is particularly important when employing injection anesthesia wherein unpredictable ocular rotation may occur. The author personally prefers placing multiple radial marks using a dedicated marking instrument to assure proper orientation. An additional measure that may be employed to help center the relaxing incisions is to identify the steep meridian (plus cylinder axis) intraoperatively by using some form of keratoscopy. The steep meridian over which the incisions are to be placed corresponds to the shorter axis of the reflected corneal mire. A simple hand-held device, such as the Maloney (Storz, Katena) or Nichamin (Mastel Precision) keratoscope, works well or a more robust and well-defined mire may be obtained through an elaborate microscope-mounted instrument such as the Mastel Ring of Light (Mastel Precision). Newer technology such as that offered by SMI, Inc (SG3000 Guidance System)[10] can be used to very accurately identify the steep meridian and intraoperative wavefront aberrometry (ORange) as developed by WaveTec[11] may help in titrating the length and effect of the relaxing incisions. Then, based off from the limbal reference mark (having been placed with the patient in the upright position) one then utilizes a Mendez Ring or similar degree gauge to find and mark the desired meridian over which the incisions are to be centered.

The LRI should be placed at the most peripheral extent of clear corneal tissue, just inside of the true surgical limbus. This holds true irrespective of the presence of pannus. If bleeding does occur, it may be ignored and will cease spontaneously. One must avoid placing the incisions further out at the true surgical limbus in that a significant reduction of effect will likely occur due to both increased tissue thickness and a variation in tissue composition; these incisions are therefore really intralimbal in nature. In creating the incision, it is important to hold the knife perpendicular to the corneal surface in order to achieve consistent depth and effect, and will help to avoid gaping of the incision. Good hand and wrist support is important, and the blade ought to be held as if one were throwing a dart such that the instrument may be rotated between thumb and index finger as it is being advanced, thus leading to smooth arcuate incisions. Typically, the right hand is used to create incisions on the right side of the globe and the left hand for incisions on the left side. In most cases it is more efficient to pull the blade toward oneself, as opposed to pushing it away.

COMPLICATIONS

LRIs have, without question, become a very safe and effective way of managing astigmatism at the time of cataract surgery. Nonetheless, as with any surgical technique, potential complications exist and several are listed in **Table 45.2**. Of these, the most likely to be encountered is the placement of incisions upon the wrong axis. When this occurs, it typically takes the form of a 90°

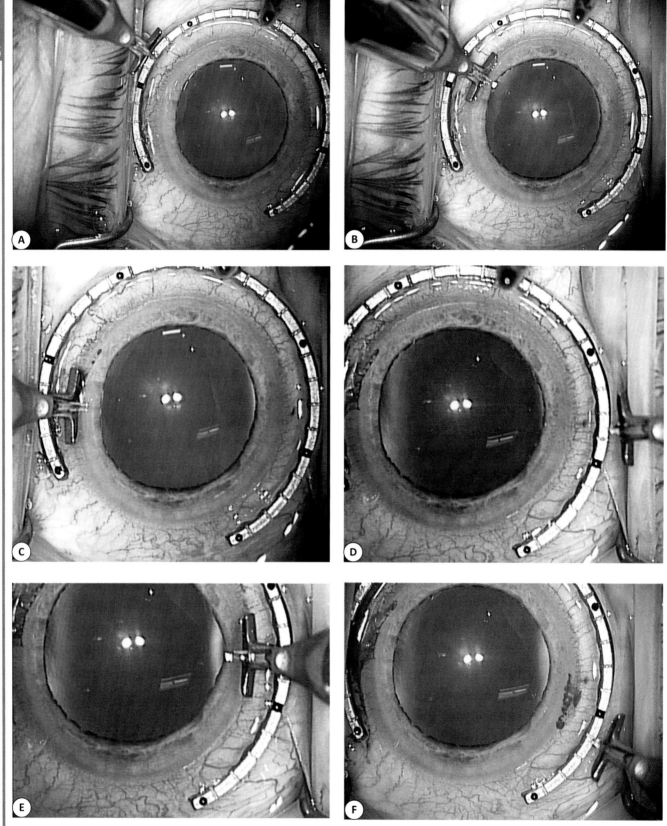

FIGURES 45.2A to F: A pair of limbal relaxing incisions, delineating 40° of arc is shown, placed over the steep 77° meridian. Note the faint 6 o'clock ink orientation mark in this right eye. Surgeon is seated temporally

TABLE 45.2 Potential problems associated with surgical techniques

- Infection
- Weakening of the globe
- Perforation
- Decreased corneal sensation
- Induced irregular astigmatism
- Misalignment/axis shift
- Wound gape and discomfort
- Operating upon the wrong (opposite) axis

error with positioning upon the opposite, flat meridian. This, of course, results in an increase and likely doubling of the patient's preexisting cylinder. Compulsive attention is required in this regard. The surgeon ought to consider employing safety checks to prevent this frustrating complication from occurring such as having a written plan that is brought into the OR and is kept visible and properly oriented. Incisions are always placed upon the plus (+) cylinder axis and opposite to the minus (–) cylinder axis.

Although very rare, corneal perforation is possible. This may be due to improper setting of the blade depth or as a result of a defect in the micrometer mechanism. This latter problem may arise after repeated autoclaving and many sterilization runs. Periodic inspection and calibration is therefore warranted, even with preset single-depth knives. When encountered, unlike radial microperforations, these circumferential perforations will rarely self-seal and will likely require placement of temporary sutures.

SUMMARY

Refinement of the refractive outcome may arguably be the solely most pressing challenge, faced by today's cataract surgeon. Along with the spherical error, preexisting astigmatism may now be safely and effectively reduced at the time of cataract surgery. Astigmatic relaxing incisions is the most common method used to accomplish this goal.

By moving these incisions out to an intralimbal location, the complications and difficulties associated with astigmatic keratotomy have been greatly reduced.

REFERENCES

1. Osher RH. Combining phacoemulsification with corneal relaxing incisions for reduction of preexisting astigmatism. Paper presented at the annual meeting of the American Intraocular Implant Society. Los Angeles; 1984.
2. Maloney WF. Refractive cataract replacement: a comprehensive approach to maximize the refractive benefits of cataract extraction. Paper presented at the annual meeting of the American Society of Cataract and Refractive Surgery. Los Angeles; 1986.
3. Budak K, Friedman NF, Koch DD. Limbal relaxing incisions with cataract surgery. J Cat Refract Surg. 1998;24(4)503-8.
4. Muller-Jensen K, Fischer P, Siepe U. Limbal relaxing incisions to correct astigmatism in clear corneal cataract surgery. J Refract Surg. 1999;15(5):586-9.
5. Nichamin LD. Changing approach to astigmatism management during phacoemulsification: peripheral arcuate astigmatic relaxing incisions. Paper presented at the annual meeting of the American Society of Cataract and Refractive Surgery. Boston; 2000.
6. Gills JP. A complete guide to astigmatism management. Thorofare: SLACK Inc; 2003.
7. Thornton SP. Radial and astigmatic keratotomy: the American system of precise, predictable refractive surgery. Thorofare: SLACK Inc; 1994.
8. Swami AU, Steinert RF, Osborne WE, et al. Rotational malposition during laser in situ keratomileusis. Am J Ophthal. 2002;133(4):561-2.
9. Abrams D. Ophthalmic optics and refraction. In: Duke-Elder SS (Ed). System of Ophthalmology. St Louis: Mosby; 1970. pp. 671-4.
10. Nuijts RM, Visser N. Assessment of cyclotorsion errors in marker-based toric IOL. Paper presented at the annual meeting of the American Society of Cataract and Refractive Surgery. Boston; 2010.
11. Packer M. Effect of intraoperative aberrometry on the rate of postoperative enhancement: retrospective study. J Cataract Refract Surg. 2010;36:747-55.

CHAPTER 46

Pediatric Cataract Surgery

Rupal H Trivedi, M Edward Wilson

INTRODUCTION

Cataracts remain one of the most important causes of treatable blindness in children. Over 2,00,000 children are blind from disorders of the lens, principally unoperated cataract, but also dense amblyopia following delayed surgery, complications of surgery or from associated ocular abnormalities.[1] Lens is responsible for 12% of anatomical abnormalities in children.[2] The prevalence of cataract in childhood has been estimated at 1 in 1,000 children.[1,3,4] The adjusted annual age-specific incidence of new diagnosis of cataract is reported to be highest in the first year of life.[5] Unilateral cataracts are reported to account for slightly over half of the cases.[6] Roughly one-third of childhood cataracts are inherited, one-third are associated with other diseases and the remaining one-third are idiopathic. Loss of vision in each of these cases of cataract is either preventable or treatable. While the number of children being blinded by cataract is numerically small when compared with blindness at other ages, the survivors may live for a long time and thus, the total years of blindness that can be prevented by treatment becomes very significant.

Aim of pediatric cataract surgery is to provide and maintain a clear visual axis and a focused retinal image. The successful management of cataracts in children has been an enigma to the practicing ophthalmologist for many decades. Dramatic improvements have occurred in outcomes during last few years due to advances in technology and microsurgical techniques. Best practices for the treatment of childhood cataract have now been established and are spreading to even more remote sites around the globe. Differences in pediatric and adult eyes demand a surgical approach that differs in many ways from the adult procedure (**Table 46.1**). The best surgical techniques for children continue to evolve because of cooperation and collaboration between pediatric ophthalmologists and adult cataract surgeons. This way, new adult-tested techniques can be selectively utilized for pediatric surgery.[7]

WHO SHOULD PERFORM PEDIATRIC CATARACT SURGERY: PEDIATRIC OPHTHALMOLOGIST OR ADULT CATARACT SURGEON?

As pediatric cataracts are relatively rare, many ophthalmologists lack surgical experience with this particular group of patients. The surgeon should have enough experience to feel comfortable with the specific difficulties of the

TABLE 46.1	Major differences between adult and pediatric cataract surgery

- Younger is the age at cataract surgery, higher will be the prevalence of PCO making primary posterior capsulectomy and vitrectomy is a rule rather than option for most younger children undergoing cataract surgery
- Increased inflammatory response
- A refractive state that is constantly changing due to growth of the eye makes difficult IOL power calculation
- Difficulty in documenting anatomic and refractive changes due to poor compliance
- Need of general anesthesia (for surgery as well as preoperative and postoperative examinations)
- A tendency to develop amblyopia
- Anatomical differences: Lack of hard nucleus, highly elastic anterior capsule, reduced scleral and corneal rigidity, poor preoperative pupillary dilation, enhanced posterior vitreous pressure

pediatric eye. In many locations, a pediatric ophthalmologist will gain surgical expertise from regional referrals. In other locations, an adult cataract surgeon with an interest in treating children will become the most experienced surgeon for these cases. Whoever performs pediatric cataract surgery must understand the importance of teamwork. Co-management among ophthalmologist works well in this setting. A pediatric ophthalmologist should generally be following these eyes for strabismus, amblyopia and other functionally related issues. The removal of the cataractous lens is only one aspect of the treatment regime. The ophthalmic physician examining the child and contemplating surgery should also assess his or her own commitment to the visual rehabilitation of the patient.

PREOPERATIVE CONSIDERATIONS

The preoperative evaluation of the patient with childhood cataract should include a search for an etiology, thorough careful history taking, detailed physical examination and necessary laboratory studies.

HISTORY

A cataract evaluation begins with a chief complaint from the parents (e.g. white spot in the pupil, visual inattentiveness, nystagmus, strabismus, smaller size of an eye, photophobia, ocular injury or family history of childhood cataract). At times, the evaluation is scheduled because of a referral from other physician who has identified the loss of the red reflex, indicating a possible lens opacity, or because the child has a systemic syndrome that has been known to be associated with cataracts. Specific information is gathered on age, birth weight, evidence of maternal infection (especially the TORCH infections), rash or febrile illness during pregnancy (may be suggestive of intrauterine infection), any other prenatal and perinatal history that may be pertinent (e.g. alcohol, tobacco, drug use, ionizing radiation during pregnancy), history of ocular trauma (unless cataract appears to be purely non-traumatic), age at onset of visual symptoms, ocular status on previous eye examinations (can be helpful in assessing visual prognosis after treatment), history of corticosteroid therapy (especially in posterior subcapsular cataract) and family history of cataract (especially in bilateral cataract).[8]

EXAMINATION

Assessment of Visual Function

The method of evaluating visual function will vary according to the age of the child and the level of cooperation. Documentation of the child's level of cooperation with the examination can be useful in interpreting the results and in making comparisons among the examinations over time.

Infant and preverbal child: The assessment strategy is to determine whether each eye can fixate on an object, maintain fixation and then follow the object into all directions. The assessment should be performed binocularly and then monocularly. This can be done by drawing the child's attention to the examiner's or family member face (infants <3 months) or a toy either hand-held or at 20 feet. The force with which the child objects to alternate occlusion of the eyes is useful to judge the relative vision in each eye. In an awake and alert child, if poor fixation and following are noted binocularly after 3–4 months of age, a significant visual loss is suspected.

For strabismic children, an assessment of binocular fixation pattern is performed in which the examiner determines the length of time that the nonpreferred eye can hold fixation. It can be reported as, "will not hold fixation with the nonpreferred eye, holds fixation briefly with nonpreferred eye or no fixation preference". With a straight-eyed child and those with small angle deviation, the base-down prism induced tropia fixation test can be used to separate the two eyes optically. The vertical prism (a 20 prism-diopter prism is used most commonly) is placed base down before one eye at a time for approximately 2 seconds and the fixation response is described. The results of the induced tropia test can be recorded as alternates or the preferred eye is the right/left and nonpreferred eye holds well, holds briefly or shows no hold.

Verbal child: Quantitative visual acuity (VA) assessment in cooperative verbal children can be assessed using optotype VA testing (identifying or matching symbols or letters), allowing quantification of VA on a Snellen or preferably, a logMAR scale. Distance VA should be determined monocularly whenever possible. The fellow eye

should be completely covered (with adhesive occluder to prevent peeking). In addition to VA, the testing distance, type of optotype, whether the optotype is presented a line at a time or isolated and cooperation level of the child should be documented in the medical record. Strabismic patients who develop amblyopia exhibit the "crowding phenomenon", whereby linear-optotype acuity is worse than single-optotype acuity. Thus, it is important not to rely on isolated letter VA tests in these children. Fusion and stereoacuity testing, at distance as well as near, may also be helpful when deciding how much visual dysfunction is present in a cataract patient. In children with posterior subcapsular cataracts (PSC) who complain of intolerable glare, but have good Snellen VA, glare testing should be performed to evaluate the need for surgery.[8]

Red reflex test: Although discussed under examination subsection, red reflex test is also a screening test, which should be a part of all infant evaluations in the newborn nursery, at 6 weeks of age and again at 6 months of age, consists of observing the red reflex from each eye with a direct ophthalmoscope with the +2 or +3 D lens focused on the child's pupil from 8 inches to 10 inches away.[9] This screening technique can be taught easily to primary care physicians or their nursing staff and if an abnormal red reflex is detected, urgent referral to an ophthalmologist can be made for more definitive diagnosis. The red reflex test can be used to detect the density and the extent of opacity in the visual axis. When both eyes are viewed simultaneously, potentially amblyogenic conditions, such as anisometropia, strabismus and asymmetric cataracts, can be identified. The most valuable test for determining the visual significance of cataract is analysis of the red reflex through the nondilated pupil with a retinoscope. Additional information can be obtained by further analysis following pupil dilation.

Ocular alignment and motility: Infants with profound bilateral dense cataracts develop nystagmus at approximately 3 months of age (at the time of development of fixation reflex). If manifest nystagmus develops, the visual prognosis will be worse. Ocular alignment is assessed by using the corneal light reflection, the binocular red reflex test and the cover test. Cover/uncover and alternate cover tests are performed in primary gaze at distance and at near. Accommodative targets are utilized when feasible. These tests require the patient's cooperation and interaction with the examiner in addition to sufficient vision to fixate on the target.

External Examination and Anterior Segment Evaluation

External examination of the eye with a suspected cataract usually consists of a penlight evaluation of eyelids, eyelashes, conjunctiva, sclera, cornea and iris.[8] Evidence of blepharitis, or any discharge or tearing should be evaluated and if applicable, treatment should be advised prior to the proposed surgery date. For pupil, size, shape,

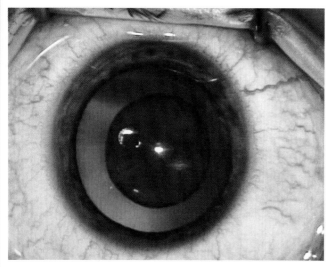

FIGURE 46.1: Lamellar cataract in a 10-year-old child

symmetry and reaction to light should be noted. Poorly dilating pupils may increase the risk of intraoperative difficulties and postoperative complications.

After dilation, a slit lamp evaluation should be carried out if the child is old enough to be cooperative. The morphology of the cataract may affect prognosis **(Figure 46.1)** and give a clue to the etiology. Unilateral PSC should prompt a careful search for evidence of trauma. Bilateral PSC may result from chronic uveitis, prolonged corticosteroid treatment for chronic disease, radiation treatment for malignancy or nonaccidental injury (child abuse). Children with juvenile idiopathic arthritis may have associated band-shaped keratopathy and posterior synechaie. Lens subluxation, iridodonesis and aniridia should be looked for. Total cataract involving the whole lens can occur in Down's syndrome, type 1 diabetes mellitus, in congenital rubella (where shaggy nuclear cataracts are more common) and posterior lentiglobus. In cases of unilateral cataract, examination of the fellow eye after pupil dilation is essential to rule out asymmetric bilateral findings. Anterior lenticonus is most often associated with Alport syndrome and should be investigated accordingly.[10] A sudden onset of total cataract may be an indication of unsuspected trauma, diabetic cataract[11] or preexisting ruptured anterior or posterior capsule.[12]

The ability of a child to cooperate for slit lamp examination is also an indirect indicator that child will likely cooperate for YAG-laser capsulotomy, if needed. In children above 5–6 years of age with intact posterior capsule and AcrySof[R] intraocular lens (IOL) implantation, visually significant posterior capsule opacification (PCO) is known to develop most often 18–24 months after the cataract surgery.[13,14] If a child in this age range seems to be cooperative for slit-lamp examination during the preoperative evaluation, the surgeon may decide to leave behind an intact posterior capsule (assuming high odds of getting child's cooperation for YAG if needed). Finally, a slit-lamp examination of both the parents, if possible, helps to establish the presence of familial cataracts. These findings can be subtle and the parents may not have been told that they have any pathology at all.

INDICATION FOR SURGERY

The measured VA or estimated fixation responses remained the single most significant indicator for surgery. For verbal children, cataract surgery is contemplated if Snellen VA is ≤ 20/50, or if the child is intolerant to glare or resistant to amblyopia therapy with gradually deteriorating visual function. Since a subjective VA cannot be obtained in infants with cataracts, greater reliance is placed on the morphology of the cataract, associated ocular findings and the visual behavior of the child.

The degree of visual impairment induced by opacity of the lens differs markedly depending on the location, size and density of the opacity. Posterior and central opacities tend to be more amblyogenic than anterior and peripheral ones. For central opacities, VA depends more on the density of the cataract than on its size. A cataract that blackens the retinoscopic reflex in an undilated pupil is considered visually significant. An asymmetry in the opacity of the lenses may lead to amblyopia. The presence of strabismus is an indication that the cataracts are longstanding and that early surgery, optical correction and treatment of amblyopia in the deviated eye may be indicated.

The decision to remove a partial cataract can be difficult. Nonverbal children add more difficulties to this decision. Individual judgment needs to make for partial cataract. The loss of accommodation after the cataract is removed that may negatively affect visual functioning more than the partial cataract was. Simple questions can help in determining the surgical need, the timing or urgency of surgery and the visual prognosis after cataract removal (e.g. Does your child appears to see well? Do your child's eyes look straight or do they seem to cross or drift or seem lazy? How long have you noticed a change in your child's visual function?). Frequently, even with poor vision, a child may be functioning reasonably well in a familiar environment. The child will be reluctant, however, to explore an unfamiliar area. Parents must be asked how well their child functions in a new environment as a useful indicator of vision.[8]

Timing of Surgery

Deciding on the appropriate timing of surgery is most critical during early infancy. In the case of a dense cataract diagnosed at birth, the surgeon can wait until 4–5 weeks of age. Avoiding surgery in the first 28–30 days of life decreases anesthesia-related complications and facilitates the surgical procedure, decreases postoperative inflammation with minimal or no reduction in visual prognosis. Waiting beyond this time, however, adversely affects visual outcome.[15-17] In the case of a bilateral cataract which is diagnosed at birth, it is important to keep the time interval to a minimum between the two eye surgeries. Birch and colleagues[16] reported visual outcome for dense bilateral cataract extracted by 31 weeks of age in a prospective study. Visual acuity outcome was assessed at ≥5 years of age. During weeks 0–14, mean VA decreased by one line with each 3 weeks' delay in surgery. From 14 weeks to 31 weeks, VA was independent of the subject's age at surgery, averaging 20/80. Despite the greater risk for secondary membrane formation and glaucoma in patients undergoing surgery at a very early age, better long-term VA outcomes were obtained with surgery performed during the patients' first 4 weeks of life.[16]

For older children with cataracts that developed after infancy, timing of surgery is not as crucial. Depending on age, laterality and density of cataract, surgery can often be decided based on convenience and other logistic issues. In eyes with penetrating trauma and cataract, primary repair of the corneal or scleral wound is usually preferred as the initial step. Cataract surgery with IOL implantation should be performed 1–4 weeks after repair.

If a partial cataract is being treated conservatively, it is important to carefully follow these children. Conservative treatment using mydriatics drops has not found widespread acceptance. Associated glare and loss of accommodation are the most common obstacles. Visual outcome has also been unimpressive.

Simultaneous Bilateral Cataract Surgery

Sequential cataract surgery, more popularly known as simultaneous bilateral cataract surgery (SBCS), remains controversial.[18] Almost every discussion on SBCS either starts or ends with a comment on the disagreement surrounding its use. The important question is not "can it be done?" but, more properly, "should it be done?" Even conservative surgeons, who vote against routine use of SBCS in children, are more likely to use this approach when anesthesia poses more than average risks or the patient lives far away and a visit for surgery on the second eye would be difficult.

Aphakic Rehabilitation

Intraocular lens implantation in children has the benefit of reducing dependency on compliance with other external optical devices (aphakic glasses and contact lens) and providing at least a partial optical correction. These are important advantages to the visual development in amblyopia-prone eyes. However, concerns about primary IOL implantation are the technical difficulties of implanting an IOL in the eyes of children, selecting an appropriate IOL power and higher risk of postoperative complications. A general consensus exists that IOL implantation is appropriate for children undergoing cataract surgery after their first birthday. In the USA, parents should be made aware that while IOL implantation has become the most common method used to correct aphakia in children overall, it is still considered "off label" by the Food and Drug Administration (FDA). A multicenter randomized clinical trial known as the infant aphakia treatment study (IATS) reported no statistically significant difference in grating VA at age 1 year between unilateral cataract patients in the IOL

and contact lens groups. Additional intraocular operations were performed more frequently in the IOL group. Until longer-term follow-up data are available, caution should be exercised when performing IOL implantation in children aged 6 months or younger given the higher incidence of adverse events and the absence of an improved short-term visual outcome compared with contact lens use. One of the caveats with IATS is that it provided contact lenses, spectacles and patches for participants at no charge. In addition, regular monitoring of their adherence to these treatments may have improved compliance. As a result, IATS visual outcomes may reflect efficacy (benefit under ideal conditions) rather than effectiveness (benefit under usual conditions).[19] In some locations, visual outcomes outside of a study environment may be better with an IOL if contact lens availability and compliance is anticipated to be poor.[19] On the other hand, when contact lenses are available and the parents are motivated to use them, aphakia may be ideal for unilateral cataract, allowing the IOL to be implanted at a later time when more eye growth has occurred. Patients with corneal diameter <9 mm or persistent fetal vasculature (PFV) causing stretching of the ciliary processes or tractional detachment of the retina were excluded from participation in IATS. Primary IOL implantation in these high risk eyes should be avoided.

Parental Counseling

The surgical team should be prepared for a quite lengthy discussion with parents and should be prepared to answer the following questions. What causes cataract in my child? How frequent is it? Is this cataract ready for removal? What will my child see after surgery? How often will my child need to visit the hospital after cataract surgery? Would you consider implanting an IOL for my child? Would you implant an IOL if this were your child? Useful web resources for parents: http://www.pgcfa.org/cataract.htm and http://www.ich.ucl.ac.uk/factsheets/families/F020023/ (information for families with cataract).

A coordinated plan of action can best be developed when the parents understand the reasons for, goals of, and the advantages and potential complications of cataract surgery. When properly informed preoperatively, the parents and the physician become partners with the common goal of doing what is best for the child. It is important to make decisions in partnership with the parents. Taking the extra time to help parents understand the implications of the cataracts their child has and the options for treatment will save time later and will promote better compliance with medications, glasses, contact lenses and occlusion therapy. The more they understand and accept the necessary steps, the better partner they will become in the battle for good visual function. Time spent establishing this partnership is not wasted, because a better informed family is much more likely to comply with the frequent follow-ups, medications, patching, glasses wear, etc. that are so essential to the eventual visual outcome.[8] Parents should be made aware that surgery is only one component of the treatment and successful visual outcome also depends on their ability to maintain adequate aphakic correction and follow through amblyopia therapy. A child operated for cataract requires regular scheduled care for the first decade of life and then every 1–2 years throughout the life. The changing refraction will require frequent follow-up examinations. Glaucoma is known to develop even years after cataract surgery in children. Parents need to understand that their child may need serial examinations under anesthesia (EUA) until the child is cooperative enough to get examined in the office. For eyes operated during early infancy, parents should be made aware that the first 6-month follow-up is very crucial. Despite performing primary posterior capsulectomy and vitrectomy, many of the infants who are implanted with an IOL develop secondary VAO from regrowth of lens cortex. This complication occurs most often in the first 6 months after implantation and the material can be easily aspirated with a return to the operating room. Earlier detection (and treatment if needed) can help to assure that the VAO does not worsen the long-term visual outcome. For eyes operated with an intact posterior capsule, parents should be made aware that the child is likely to require a secondary procedure for PCO. Parents, of the children with lens implants, are also made aware that glasses will likely still be needed postoperatively even when an IOL is implanted. In addition, glasses power may need to be changed frequently after surgery, because of the changing refraction that occurs with eye growth. Visual prognosis can be explained to the parent based on the preoperative evaluation (Table 46.2).[8,20] During preoperative visits, the physician can also ascertain the following factors: predicted level of compliance of child and family to postoperative correction of residual refractive error and to amblyopia therapy which helps in deciding whether to implant an IOL or not, and if implanting, how much residual refraction should be aim for while selecting an IOL power and the ease of developing a successful partnership with the child's parents or caretakers.

Laboratory Test

Exhaustive lists of possible laboratory investigations for a child with cataract can be found in several textbooks; however in an otherwise healthy child, most physicians do not advise extensive laboratory and genetic investigations.[8]

TABLE 46.2 Factors predicting poor visual prognosis

- Longer duration between onset of cataract and surgery
- Cataract: unilateral, dense, asymmetric bilateral
- Preoperative strabismus
- Preoperative nystagmus
- Severe preoperative visual impairment as per age appropriate standards
- Longer preoperative interocular axial length difference[20]
- Cataract associated with severe ocular anomalies or systemic problems

Children with unilateral cataracts do not usually receive any systemic work-up. For bilateral cataract patients, deciding on a list of laboratory investigations to detect the cause is usually based on the overall developmental health of the child, but may also be occasionally based on logistic issues, financial considerations, and parent's enthusiasm and willingness to spend time and efforts to do so. Developmental pediatricians and clinical geneticists are experts in selective investigation based on characteristics of the child. These specialists are invaluable and should be consulted when necessary. They will help the surgeon to choose laboratory investigations that are customized for each child and aimed at finding treatable systemic diseases that will require lifelong monitoring.

Based on history and examination, customized laboratory investigations can be advised. While recommending laboratory investigation, it is important to keep in the mind that the common causes of cataract in children include intrauterine infections, metabolic disorders and genetically transmitted syndromes. As compared to unilateral cataract, laboratory investigation of bilateral cases is more rewarding. After detailed evaluation, 86% of unilateral and 68% of bilateral cataract have no discernible cause.[21] Positive family history of childhood cataract or evidence of even a minor opacity of a similar type in one parent of sibling can confirm a diagnosis of hereditary cataract and make further studies unnecessary. Since cataracts can be the presenting sign of diabetes, children with acquired cataracts of unknown etiology should be questioned about classic symptoms of diabetes and evaluation for hyperglycemia should be performed.[11] If Lowe syndrome is suspected, the urine should be screened for amino acids. If there is a history of maternal rash, fever, flu-like symptoms or neonatal physical signs of intrauterine infection, then acute and convalescent TORCH titers should be obtained.

Preoperative Treatment

The surgeon may elect to prepare for surgery but the final decision on surgery may be delayed until the time of the EUA. As preoperative preparation of surgery, topical medications have been prescribed: antibiotic drop and the dilating drops (Peds combo, 2 ml 2% cyclopentalate, 0.5 ml 10% phenylephrine, 0.5 ml 1% tropicamide) given every 5 minutes (3 times). Dilating drops should be given for both eyes for dilated examination of both eyes.

Examination under Anesthesia

The author routinely performs EUA during the same session as the cataract surgery. However, performing EUA as a separate session is also an acceptable approach. Intraocular pressure (IOP) should be checked as soon as possible after induction of anesthesia. Although the tonopen is routinely used, if in doubt, we recheck IOP using the Perkin's applanation tonometer. In addition to high IOP, a difference of IOP between the two eyes is a cause for concern. The next step is to take keratometry measurements using a handheld device. The remaining examinations listed below can be performed in any order: examine the eye using the operating microscope, immersion A-scan ultrasound for globe axial length, horizontal corneal diameter, retinoscopy (if possible) and a retinal fundus examination. In the case of no view on fundus examination, a B-scan ultrasound examination is performed.

Calculation and Selection of IOL Power

Nihalani and Vanderveen recently reported that the predictive error was ≤ 0.5 D in 43% pediatric eyes and similar for all formulae.[22] Implantation of a fixed-power IOL into an eye that is still growing, makes it difficult to choose the IOL power to implant. IOL implantation at the calculated emmetropic power helps to fight amblyopia during childhood, but risks significant myopia at ocular maturity. Ideal IOL power should balance the best help to amblyopia management in childhood with the least possible refractive error in adulthood. With a growing eye, prone to develop a myopic shift of refraction after cataract removal, the surgeon faces the problem of deciding that which refraction should be the immediate postoperative aim.[23-26] We do not recommend the use of any published table alone for deciding IOL power. These tables are only meant to help as a starting point towards appropriate IOL power selection, which is a multifactorial decision customized for each child based on many variables like age, laterality (one eye or both), amblyopia status (dense or mild), likely compliance are shown in **Table 46.3**. It is noteworthy that we had selected less undercorrection than is typically advised to lessen late myopia (unpublished data). While implanting children with bilateral cataracts and no amblyopia, leaving hypermetropia is reasonable. However, in unilateral cataracts with dense amblyopia, less early dependence on glasses may help in the amblyopia treatment. The late myopia, even if marked, may be an acceptable trade for better visual outcome from amblyopia treatment. Refractive surgery or IOL exchange may be needed in these eyes at ocular maturity.

SURGICAL TECHNIQUE

The advances in surgical technique and technology have brought the pediatric cataract surgical technique closer to the adult procedure. One of the major challenges for pediatric cataract surgery has been the adaptation of techniques used for adult cataract surgery.[7]

Incision

Pediatric cataracts can be removed through a relatively small wound, as the lens has no hard nucleus. When an IOL is not being implanted, two paracentesis incisions are usually made in clear cornea near the limbus. These incisions should not be larger than necessary for the instruments being used. For instance, a microvitreoretinal (MVR) blade can be used that creates a 20-gauge opening for a 20-gauge vitrector/aspirator to enter the anterior chamber. A 20-gauge blunt tipped irrigating cannula can also be used through a separate MVR blade stab incision. If the instrument positions need to be reversed, the snug fit is maintained. For those using 23-gauge or 25-gauge instruments, the same principles apply. Anterior chamber stability is maintained by limiting wound leak and using a high irrigation setting. When a foldable IOL is being implanted, a tunnel incision is required. A corneal tunnel is preferred by some, since it leaves the conjunctiva undisturbed. Some prefer a scleral tunnel because it heals more transparently than a corneal tunnel. Author preferably uses a corneal tunnel near the limbus. Unlike adults, corneal incisions do not usually self-seal in children. Even in older children, suturing is recommended since postoperative eye rubbing is common. The incision can be sutured with 10/0 polyglactic acid (Vicryl) absorbable sutures. It takes 1–2 months for complete absorption. Corneal vascularization requiring suture removal is less frequent using Vicryl suture, as opposed to nonabsorbable suture (e.g. nylon). The use of nonabsorbable sutures occasionally calls for EUA for suture removal. It is better to use absorbable sutures rather than to subject the child to additional anesthesia. Locating the site of the tunnel according to the preexisting astigmatism (e.g. temporally in against-the-rule astigmatism) has not been studied as often in younger children. Mostly physicians prefer superior incision irrespective of preexisting astigmatism.

Anterior Capsulotomy

The anterior capsules in children are highly elastic and pose challenges in the creation of the capsulotomy.[27,28] While a manual continuous curvilinear capsulorhexis (CCC) is ideal,

TABLE 46.3	Expected postoperative residual refraction based on patient age at cataract surgery*	
Age at surgery	Residual refraction to minimize late myopia	Median residual refraction in our series
1st month	+ 12	+ 8.3
2–3 months	+ 9	+ 8.5
4–6 months	+ 8	+ 6.0
6–12 months	+ 7	+ 4.5
1–2 years	+ 6	+ 3.0
2–4 years	+ 5	+ 0.9
4–5 years	+ 4	+ 0.5
5–6 years	+ 3	+ 0.5
6–7 years	+ 2	+ 0.1
7–8 years	+1.5	+ 0.2
8–10 years	+ 1	+ 0.1
10–14 years	+ 0.5	0
>14 years	Plano	−0.1

*We do not recommend the use of any published table alone for deciding IOL power. These tables are only meant to help as a starting point towards appropriate IOL power selection, which is a multifactorial decision customized for each child based on many variables (especially age, laterality, amblyopia status, likely compliance with glasses and family history of myopia).

it is more difficult to perform in very young eyes. The vitrectorhexis is commonly used in the first 2 years of life.[27] Manual CCC is used most often in children, older than 2 years. While performing a manual CCC in a child, the following technical recommendations are offered.[29] Use of a highly viscous ophthalmic-viscosurgical-device (OVD) is recommended to flatten the anterior capsule. A slack anterior capsule will be easier to tear in a controlled fashion. The capsulorhexis edge must be regrasped frequently and begin with a smaller capsulotomy than desired. Due to the elasticity, the opening will be larger than it appears once the capsular flap is released. In order to control the turning of the CCC edge along a circular path, the tear must often be directed more towards the center of the pupil than would be necessary in an adult eye. Shearing is the term which is used when the capsule is torn by pulling in the direction of the tear. Ripping is the term used when the capsule is torn by pulling in a direction that is 90 degrees from the path of the tear, towards the center of the pupil. Pediatric CCC relies more on ripping than shearing. If the capsule begins to extend peripherally, it should be stopped before the edge is out of sight under the iris. The capsule edge should be regrasped and pull back against the path of the tear. This is called "pull-back" and can be used to recover a radial extension of the CCC. Converting to a vitrectorhexis or a radiofrequency diathermy, capsulotomy may also be warranted. Using a small incision capsulorhexis forceps that fits easily through a paracentesis will allow conversion to vitrector instruments when needed without leakage around the vitrector handpiece during use. Modifications of the manual anterior CCC technique have also been published and popularized, e.g. two-incision push-pull and four-incision technique.[30]

While a CCC using the techniques described above is a reasonable option beyond age 2, it will be more difficult when attempted on children younger than 2 years of age. The vitrectorhexis is an alternative anterior capsulotomy method that will be more consistently successful than manual CCC in the youngest patients. When creating a vitrectorhexis, the following surgical caveats are offered. A vitrector is used, supported by a Venturi pump, if possible. Peristaltic pump systems will not cut anterior capsule as easily. A bimanual technique with a separate infusion port is recommended. A snug fit of the instruments is maintained in the incisions through which they are placed. The anterior chamber of these soft eyes will collapse readily if leakage occurs around the instruments, making the vitrectorhexis more difficult to complete. A MVR blade can be used to enter the eye. The vitrector and a blunt-tip irrigating cannula fit snugly into the MVR openings. We use 20-gauge Grieshaber irrigation handpiece (Alcon). Disposable irrigation handpieces from Alcon-Grieshaber are now available as well. An anterior chamber maintainer can also be used if the surgeon prefers. It is not necessary to begin the capsulotomy with a bent-needle cystotome. Merely the vitrector is placed, with its cutting port

positioned posteriorly, in contact with the center of the intact anterior capsule. The cutter is turned on and the suction is increased using the foot pedal until the capsule is engaged and opened. A cutting rate of 150–300 cuts per minute and an aspiration, maximum of 150–250, is recommended. Adjustments may be needed for specific machines, especially those utilizing a peristaltic pump. With the cutting port facing down against the capsule, the capsule is engaged and the round capsular opening is enlarged in a spiral fashion to the desired shape and size. Care should be taken to avoid leaving any right-angle edges, which could predispose to radial tear formation. The completed vitrectorhexis should be slightly smaller than the size of the IOL optic being implanted.

A third option for creating an anterior capsulotomy in a child is available with the use of high frequency endodiathermy (Kloti radiofrequency endodiathermy). This instrument cuts capsule efficiently but results in an edge that tears easily, if stretched. The Fugo plasma blade has also been used to make an anterior capsulotomy. Our experience with the Fugo blade in children is in only a few cases, but the capsulotomy edge created in those cases was not very different clinically from that produced by the Kloti instrument mentioned above.[27,28]

Use of capsular dyes has started attracting pediatric cataract surgeons also. Visualization of the capsular flap is important to maintain control of any tears and to ensure that the edge is continuous. A report from the American Academy of Ophthalmology has concluded that "it is reasonable to consider the use of dye in cataract surgery in cases in which inadequate capsule visualization or inexperience with capsule visualization may compromise the outcome".[31] Both trypan blue and indocyanine green dyes provide excellent visualization of the anterior capsule flap during CCC. When injecting under air, the dye should be injected after the paracentesis, but prior to creating the main incision, to help with anterior chamber stability. Staining under air versus under OVD was reported to have similar efficacy and safety. In addition to better visualization, trypan blue has been reported to minimize epithelial cell proliferation in pediatric cataract surgery.[32] The staining affected the density and viability of LECs.

Hydrodissection

Hydrodissection has been thought to be less useful in children than in adults. However, one study has shown the intraoperative benefits of performing multiquadrant hydrodissection.[33] The potential benefits are: overall reduction in the operative time and a reduction in the amount of irrigating solution used to facilitate lens substance removal. A fluid wave can sometimes be generated in older children, but not reliably in infants and toddlers. Cortical material strips easily from the pediatric capsule even in the absence of hydrodissection if the proper technique is used. Attempts at hydrodelineation should be discouraged in children since it does not aid in lens removal and may lead to capsular rupture. Hydrodissection should not be done in children with posterior polar cataracts in children because of the fragility in the posterior capsule in these cases.

Lens Substance Aspiration (Phacoaspiration)

Thorough removal of lens substance is especially important for pediatric eyes. The best means of reducing the incidence of proliferative PCO is to remove as many of the lens epithelial cells as possible at the time of surgery. Since PCO is one of the most frequent postoperative complications in pediatric cataract surgery, meticulous removal of the lens substance is a crucial step in the management of pediatric cataracts.

The additional 0.5 ml of adrenaline to the infusion bottle (1:1000 for cardiac use) helps to maintain mydriasis and perhaps improves iris tissue tone and decreases iris floppiness. We reported a pediatric case of intraoperative floppy iris syndrome (IFIS) in one eye and no IFIS in the other eye as a result of the inadvertent absence of epinephrine in the irrigating fluid of the eye demonstrating signs of IFIS.[34] Use of intraoperative heparin has been reported in the literature, however need for heparin in modern pediatric cataract surgery is questionable.[35-37] The use of heparin should be avoided in eyes with a compromised blood-aqueous barrier (e.g. previous ocular surgery) as they are at high risk of developing postoperative hyphema.

Pediatric cataracts are soft but they may be "gummy". Phacoemulsification is not needed. Lens cortex and nucleus can be aspirated in every case with an irrigation/aspiration or vitrectomy handpiece. Bimanual approach using separate irrigation and aspiration helps to maintain the anterior chamber stability, decrease fluctuations of the anterior chamber and help for thorough removal of lens substance. When using the vitrector, bursts of cutting can be used intermittently to facilitate the aspiration of the more "gummy" cortex of young children. The advantage of using the vitrector is that it is possible to perform vitrectorhexis, irrigation/aspiration, posterior capsulectomy and vitrectomy—all with one instrument (the setting needs to be changed appropriately). This avoids extra manipulation and repeated entry into and exit from the eye. In older children, after a manual CCC, tapered 20-gauge or 23-gauge bimanual irrigation/aspiration hand pieces can be used.

Posterior Capsulectomy and Vitrectomy

In young children who undergo pediatric cataract surgery, PCO is rapid and virtually inevitable if the posterior capsule is left intact. PCO occurs much faster and is much more amblyogenic in younger children as compared with older children. The advent of vitreous suction cutting devices for removing the center of the posterior capsule and a portion of the anterior vitreous during the initial surgery in young children undergoing cataract surgery dramatically decreased the need for secondary surgery. A primary posterior capsulectomy and anterior vitrectomy during IOL implantation gives the best chance for maintaining a long-term clear visual axis in the pediatric patient (**Figure 46.4**). Secondary surgical (**Figure 46.3**) or neodymium-yttrium-aluminum-garnet (Nd: YAG) laser posterior capsulotomies are usually necessary in children when the posterior capsule is left intact. Larger amounts of laser energy are often needed as compared to adults and the posterior capsule opening may close, requiring repeated laser treatments or a secondary pars plana membranectomy.

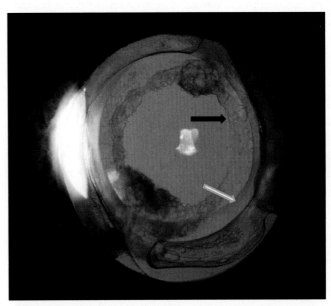

FIGURE 46.2: Clear visual axis after 5 years of cataract surgery with posterior capsulectomy and vitrectomy. Arrow shows edge of anterior and posterior capsulotomy

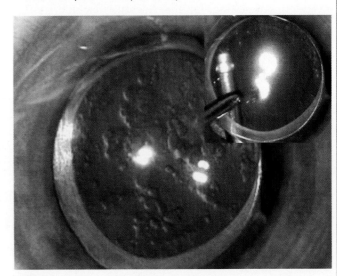

FIGURE 46.3: Surgical removal of posterior capsule opacification

As of today, primary posterior capsulectomy and anterior vitrectomy is common practice while managing younger children with cataract. An important question that remains is, "when the posterior capsule should be left intact?" We answer this question looking at several factors (age, association of posterior capsule plaque or defect, availability of YAG laser, expected cooperation of child approximately 12–24 months after cataract surgery for YAG). As a rough guideline, in children below 5 years of age, primary posterior capsulectomy and vitrectomy is the norm. In children who are 5–8 years of age, posterior capsulotomy can be performed without vitrectomy. In children above 8 years of age, posterior capsule can be left intact more often (**Figures 46.4A to F**). Even in children older than 8 years of age, posterior capsulectomy and vitrectomy is advisable if child deems to be noncooperative for YAG laser capsulotomy in the presence of dense plaque or preexisting posterior capsule defect, nonavailability of YAG and questionable follow-up. Anterior segment surgeons are often more accustomed to, and more comfortable with, a limbal (or anterior) approach. Our current strategy is to perform these procedures via the pars plana/plicata preferentially, whenever we intend to use a primary vitrectomy in pediatric eyes receiving IOL implantation. The size of the posterior capsule opening should be large enough to help in avoiding VAO, but small enough that sufficient peripheral capsular support remains for capsular fixation of an IOL. Even if the surgeon is not planning to implant an IOL in a specific eye, it is important to leave behind sufficient anterior and posterior capsular support (**Figures 46.5A to D**) at the time of cataract surgery to facilitate subsequent in-the-bag or sulcus-fixated IOL implantation (if needed). Ideally, the surgeon should aim for a central, circular opening in the posterior capsule about 1–1.5 mm smaller than the IOL optic. A Venturi vacuum pump system is advisable, as it cuts the capsule more easily than a peristaltic pump. Readers should follow the manufacturer's instruction manual for using a specific machine and setting. On the Accurus machine (Alcon Laboratories, Fort Worth, Texas), an irrigation rate of 30+ cc/min and a cutting rate of 600 cuts/min have been effective at our setting. When the pars plana/plicata approach is chosen, the IOL should be inserted into the capsular bag using OVD, while the posterior capsule is still intact. The OVD can be removed without fear of engaging vitreous, because removal precedes the posterior capsulectomy. While the irrigation cannula remains in the anterior chamber, a MVR blade is used to enter the pars plana/plicata 2–3 mm (2 mm in patients less than 1 year old, 2.5 mm in patients 1–4 years old, and 3 mm in patients over 4 years old) posterior to the limbus. The vitrector is then inserted through this incision and used to open the center of the posterior capsule. The endpoint for the vitrectomy is difficult to define. Sufficient vitreous should be removed centrally so that the LEC cannot use the vitreous face as a scaffold for VAO. Any vitreous that tracks forward past the plane of the posterior capsulectomy needs to be removed. VAO after primary posterior capsulectomy and vitrectomy is often blamed on an inadequate posterior capsule opening or an inadequate vitrectomy. These assertions have not been verified scientifically.

IOL Implantation

When an IOL is placed in a child's eye, in-the-bag implantation is strongly recommended. Care should be taken to avoid asymmetrical fixation with one haptic in the capsular bag and the other in the ciliary sulcus. This can lead to decentration of the IOL. In contrast to adults, dialing of an IOL into the capsular bag can be difficult in children. Often the IOL will dial out of the capsular bag rather than into it. This tendency can be blunted somewhat by the use of highly viscous OVDs. Foldable hydrophobic acrylic IOLs are used increasingly in children. The one-piece AcrySof® is suited for small soft eyes and can be inserted into the capsular bag with ease. When capsular fixation is not possible, sulcus placement of an IOL in a child is acceptable. To avoid decentration, a rigid PMMA IOLs

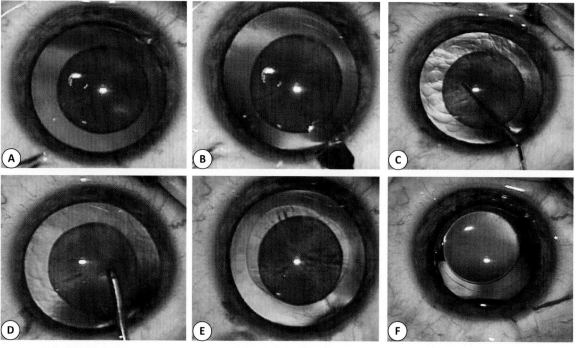

FIGURES 46.4A TO F: Cataract surgery with intraocular lens implantation (with intact posterior capsule)

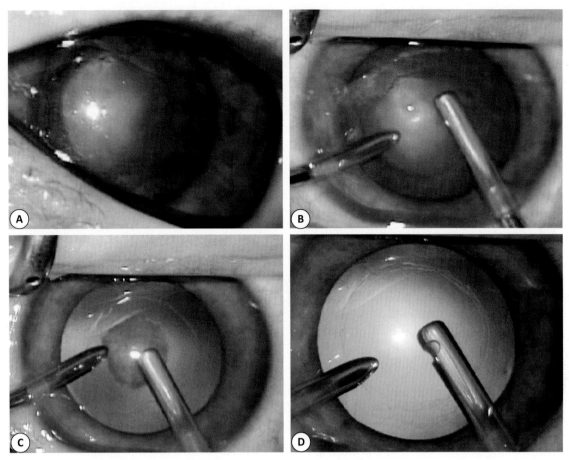

FIGURES 46.5A TO D: Cataract surgery (with posterior capsulectomy and vitrectomy)

should be considered or when a foldable lens (such as the 3-piece AcrySof® IOL) is used, optic capture through the anterior or combined anterior/posterior capsulorhexis should be attempted. Optic capture of an IOL maintained better IOL centration but was reported to predispose to an increased inflammatory response in one study.[38]

POSTOPERATIVE CONSIDERATIONS

Medications

Immediately at the end of surgery, a drop of dilute (5%) Povidone iodine is placed on the operative eye. An antibiotic steroid ointment and atropine ointment are placed on the eye. A patch and Fox shield are placed over the eye.[7] The shield is secured with 2 Tegaderm sheets instead of standard tape. The patch and shield should remain on the eye until the morning after surgery. With older children, the atropine ointment may be deleted. Babies who are left aphakic receive topical drops and Silsoft contact lens (usually a 7.5 base-curve and +32 D or +29 D power) at the end of surgery. The parents can then begin the drops right away. For older children (above age 6–7 years), the parents are allowed to remove the patch and shield 4–5 hours after the surgery and to begin the postoperative drops. The eye is still examined on the first postoperative day. Topical atropine (0.5% in children <1 year of age and 1% thereafter) is utilized once per day for 2–4 weeks in children

up to age 6 years. Topical steroid drop is used topically six times per day for 2 weeks and then 3–4 times per day for an additional 2 weeks. An antibiotic drop (the same bottle used preoperatively) is used for one week after surgery. Use of systemic steroids can be reserved for uveitis and some traumatic cases. However, some physicians prefer to use systemic steroids for all children.

Follow-up

A follow-up program of patching, monitoring of vision and therapy for amblyopia should be just as much as part of the treatment as the cataract surgery itself. Postoperative examinations can be scheduled at 1 week, 4 weeks, 3 months and 6 months, postoperatively. We also consider an yearly EUA in order to measure IOP, examine the peripheral retina, monitor eye growth using A-scan ultrasound and examine the position of the IOL and detect any secondary membrane or after-cataract formation. Once children become old enough and cooperative enough to undergo these examinations awake, the yearly EUA becomes unnecessary.

Correction of Residual Refractive Error

Uncorrected refractive error after pediatric cataract surgery can cause or worsen amblyopia. Even short intervals of uncorrected aphakia are potentially damaging to the prognosis in infants. When an IOL is implanted, residual hyperopia may be present. Correction of this residual hyperopia and any significant astigmatic error is necessary. Correction of refractive error itself helps as an optical treatment of amblyopia. Residual refractive error can be corrected after the wound stabilizes and the synthetic absorbable sutures dissolve. On the first postoperative day, these small soft eyes will not yield a reliable refraction by which this residual refractive error can be determined and marked temporary astigmatism will be seen initially. This resolves quickly over the first 2–4 weeks after surgery. If significant refractive error exists, glasses should be given at 2–4 weeks postoperatively. Defining a significant refractive error may vary among physicians and may vary according to the age of the patient. Any amount of hypermetropia, myopia greater than 3 D and astigmatism greater than 1.5 D, may be significant for aphakic/pseudophakic eyes. Lesser values of refractive error may warrant spectacle correction when strabismus or other risk factors are present.

During infancy: When a child is left aphakic, every effort should be made to minimize time intervals when the prescribed aphakic glasses or aphakic contact lenses are not worn. Nearly all infants will have residual refractive error after cataract and IOL surgery. The goal is to give contact lenses or glasses that over-correct the residual hyperopia by 2 diopters since the babies world is at near. Glasses for residual refractive error are often changed 1–2 times in the first year after surgery. At age 2 years and older, glasses or contact lenses are given without the 2 diopter overcorrection and a +3.00 diopter spectacle bifocal is added instead. Contact lenses should be considered as first-line optical treatment for unilateral aphakia in young children. One can fit these infants with a Silsoft silicone contact lens if possible. For children who are noncompliant with a contact lens, spectacle correction can be prescribed. If aphakia is unilateral, the spectacles are worn during patching, but usually removed when not patched. The Silsoft super-plus series is available in powers from +32 to +20 in 3 diopter increments. The aphakia series contains lens powers from +20 to +12 in one diopter increments. For power, needs less than +12.00, a daily wear contact lens is chosen. Since these daily wear lenses are more difficult to fit, we most often transition the babies into glasses as soon as the power needs are less than the minimum available in the Silsoft line. For bilateral surgeries, this transition is less troublesome. However, for unilateral pseudophakia, high residual refractive error requires a marked anisometropic glasses prescription. When dense amblyopia is present, the chance of achieving high-grade stereopsis is poor. In these patients marked anisometropic glasses are tolerated very well and may help achieve good VA.

After surgery in toddlers and preschool aged children: Unlike the infants, these children are prescribed their full cycloplegic refraction for distance and a +3.00 bifocal for near viewing as their first postoperative prescription. Toddlers are often much more active with near tasks and

school activities these days and bifocals should be added to the glasses from age 2 years on.

After surgery in school-aged and older children: When the pseudophakia is bilateral, bifocals (usually lineless progressive bifocals) are prescribed. However, with unilateral pseudophakia, the bifocal can be placed unilaterally, bilaterally or not at all. This is left up to the preference of the surgeon and the patient.

When young adulthood is near: Laser refractive surgery may likely be needed with this group of patients to minimize the use of glasses. IOL exchanges are also becoming more commonplace when the myopia is moderate to severe.

If compliance with glasses or contacts for the residual refractive error is poor, amblyopia may worsen or improve more slowly even when proper patching is being done. Accurate fitting and proper adjustment simplify the acceptance of spectacles. Straps may be useful in babies; cable temples and spring hinges are helpful in keeping glasses on active young children. Polycarbonate lenses have greater safety and are preferable for children. The children are sensitive to parental attitudes; if a parent believes the glasses detract from the child's appearance, compliance is likely to be poor. It may be helpful to suggest ways to give positive reinforcement suitable for the specific child. If positive reinforcement fails, the short-term use of an elbow extension with restraints may be useful to improve compliance.

Postoperative Complications

Posterior capsule opacification: Secondary PCO is one of the most common complications of pediatric cataract surgery; especially when the posterior capsule is left intact. PCO is generally delayed in eyes with a hydrophobic acrylic IOL as compared with a PMMA IOL.[14] VAO after acrylic implantation with an intact posterior capsule is more "proliferative" compared to the "fibrous" reaction commonly seen in conjunction with the PMMA IOLs. After a primary posterior capsulotomy and an anterior vitrectomy, VAO is rare in older children when an acrylic IOL has been used. When VAO does occur, it is usually in a baby operated in the first year-of-life. When infantile eyes are implanted with an IOL, VAO is common despite performing posterior capsulectomy and vitrectomy. Using hydrophobic acrylic IOLs, various articles have reported VAO averaging 44.0%, while ranging from 8.1% when all children under 2 years of age were reviewed, to 80% when all children operated below 6 months of age were included.[14] Secondary VAO in eyes implanted in infancy tends to occur within the first 6 months after cataract surgery. Thus, patients with longer follow-up will not likely change the incidence of VAO in infantile eyes. Eyes with associated ocular anomalies (e.g. anterior segment dysgenesis, iris hypoplasia, or persistent fetal vasculature) are at nine-fold higher risk for developing VAO as compared to eyes without associated ocular anomalies. In children older than 2 years of age at the time of cataract surgery, the secondary VAO rate after primary posterior capsulectomy and vitrectomy varies from 0% to 20.6% with an average of 5.1%.[14] In older children, some authors prefer to do only posterior capsulorhexis (without vitrectomy). The average rate of secondary intervention in these eyes is 13.8% (range 0–68%). With an intact posterior capsule, various articles have reported PCO ranging from 14.7% to 100% (average 25.1%, excluding eyes with 100% PCO in children younger than 4 years of age). With longer follow-up, even for older children, the average Nd:YAG laser capsulotomy rate may be higher than the 25.1% noted here. Stager and colleagues reported that 70% maintained a clear visual axis after a single Nd:YAG procedure, 84% after 2 Nd:YAG procedures, and 88% after 3 Nd:YAG procedures.[39] Surgical intervention to clear the visual axis was needed in 8%. The probability of maintaining a clear central visual axis after 24 months with a single Nd:YAG laser procedure was 35% in children <24 months of age and 74% in older children.

Deposits and synechiae: The incidence of deposits and synechiae was significantly higher in younger age groups (age at surgery less than 2 years of age) than in the older groups (P <0.04).[13] Younger age at the time of cataract surgery also increases the risk for synechiae formation.

Glaucoma: Congenital cataracts operated during first year of life are at higher risk for the development of glaucoma. Childhood cataracts that develop after infancy are usually not associated with microphthalmia, are almost always implanted with an IOL, and are at very low risk for the development of glaucoma. Since the eyes at highest risk for glaucoma are also the eyes most likely to be left aphakic, IOL implantation may falsely appear to be protective against glaucoma. However, The result of our study suggests that an IOL is not protective against the development of glaucoma.[40] For patients who underwent surgery during the first 4.5 months of their life, the glaucoma incidence was 24.4% in eyes with an IOL implant and 19% in aphakic eyes in our series (P = 0.55).[40] Recently published infant aphakia treatment study concurs with our results. This study reported that at one year after surgery, glaucoma had developed in 5% of eyes in the contact lens group and 12% of eyes in the IOL group (P=.32).[41] One (2%) eye in the contact lens group and 4 (7%) eyes in the IOL group required glaucoma surgery.

Retinal detachment: Although we have not analyzed our data for pseudophakic RD systematically, we do not recall seeing it in eyes with pediatric cataract in the absence of a predisposing etiology such as a history of RD, trauma or retinopathy of prematurity.

Functional Outcome

Visual outcome: The visual outcome in children is profoundly influenced by many extraneous factors. These include the age of the child at the occurrence of the lens opacity, the density of the opacity, the time elapsed between visual obscuration and reestablishment of a clear visual axis, associated ocular diseases or anomalies, the age of the child at surgery, the kind and success of aphakic optical correction used, the presence or absence of amblyopia and/or strabismus, and their therapeutic success or failure. We reported a median VA of 20/30, with median VA of unilateral and bilateral cases being 20/40 and 20/25, respectively.[42] Better VA was associated with bilateral cataract, older age at surgery, and normal interocular axial length difference. Amblyopia was the major cause of residual visual deficit. Birch and colleagues reported visual outcome for 37 infants with dense bilateral cataract extracted by 31 weeks of age in a prospective study.[16] Visual acuity outcome was assessed at ≥ 5 years of age. During weeks 0–14, mean VA decreased by 0ne line with each 3 weeks' delay in surgery. From 14 weeks to 31 weeks, VA was independent of the subject's age at surgery, averaging 20/80. Despite the greater risk for secondary membrane formation and glaucoma in patients undergoing surgery at a very early age, excellent long-term VA outcomes were obtained with surgery performed during the patients' first 4 weeks of life; no patient who had surgery on both eyes by 4 weeks of age had a VA outcome poorer than 20/60, and the mean VA was 20/40.

Strabismus: Children with cataracts may experience enough disruption in binocular fusion to lose proper ocular alignment. Strabismus occurs more often in aphakic/pseudophakic eyes of children compared to the general pediatric population. Earlier onset unilateral cataracts have the highest risk for strabismus and late-onset bilateral cataracts have the least risk. The patients with partial cataracts and relatively good preoperative VA tend to have less strabismus. While reviewing the literature in 2003, we noted that strabismus was present in 33.3% of patients preoperatively and in 78.1% of patients postoperatively.[17] Few preoperative strabismus cases resolved postoperatively, while some new strabismus cases were first diagnosed postoperatively. This new diagnosis of strabismus postoperatively may reflect the ongoing susceptibility of the infantile eye to amblyopia due to an uncorrected refractive error, the easier detection of strabismus in older children or the intensity of the occlusion prescribed.

Strabismus is a risk factor for the developing amblyopia, and amblyopia is a risk factor for developing strabismus. Occasionally, an intermittent strabismus will resolve as the VA improves. However, this is the exception rather than the rule. Strabismus associated with cataracts in children usually needs surgery. The surgery aids amblyopia treatment by achieving ocular alignment and possibly reducing suppression. Although strabismus surgery may promote amblyopia management in selected cases, it usually does not remove the need for amblyopia treatment. Conventional wisdom states that surgery should be performed after treating amblyopia.[43] The goal is to obtain the best possible VA in each eye before strabismus surgery because it promotes fusion and ultimately stable postoperative eye alignment; that said, strabismus correction can still be done during the treatment rather than at the completion of amblyopia treatment. Strabismus repair should be carried out in a timely manner and do not deferred indefinitely. Strabismus should be measured during several visits after cataract surgery. If the strabismus angle and pattern are stable, correction is planned at an elective time such as during a scheduled EUA. Strabismus repair can be done simultaneously with other intraocular surgery (e.g. surgical removal of visual axis opacification) if both surgeries are planned to be performed by the same surgeon or at the same institute. Combined surgery is considered at times, because of the difficulties of arranging surgery and to decrease number of anesthesia exposure. In patients undergoing simultaneous incision intraocular surgery and strabismus surgery, the muscle procedure should be done first to avoid disruption or opening of the cataract incision during extraocular muscle manipulation. For the same reason, it may be advisable to avoid using an adjustable suture during combined surgery. Pulling on the muscle during the adjustment could disturb the main incision.

Amblyopia management: The long-term visual outcome is often negatively affected by the development of amblyopia secondary to the cataract itself, or due to postoperative reopacification of the ocular media (**Table 46.4**). Most cataractous patients are predisposed to pattern deprivation, strabismus, and optical defocus types of amblyopia. Even when optically corrected, these eyes are focused at a fixed distance and continue to optical defocus promoting amblyopia if the fellow eye is normal. Although refractive correction alone can result in improved vision in aniso-metropic amblyopia, it is generally held that most postcataract cases will need amblyopia treatment. Amblyopia therapy requires a high level of effort. Noncompliance is a major hurdle. Adhesive skin patches should be used unless a skin allergy/irritation develops that is unresponsive to both local treatment with a skin emollient and a change in brand of patch, in which case a spectacle-mounted occluder should be prescribed.

There is no priori way to decide the intensity and duration of treatment that will maximize VA. Attempts to improve compliance with a specific regimen, followed by increasing the number of hours per day, are reasonable. Although not always effective, it may be helpful in children beyond infancy to begin by patching two per day, systematically increasing the percentage of occlusion as required to sustain improvement in visual acuity. A reward is the most effective strategy to encourage compliance. In infants, occlusion should be prescribed over the better eye for 1-hour/day per month of age until the child is 8-months old. The better eye should then be patched all hours the child is awake every-other-day, or one-half the child's waking hours every-day. If occlusion amblyopia develops,

TABLE 46.4	Results of the pediatric eye disease investigator group*

- For children of 3–7 years:
  • With severe amblyopia (20/100 to 20/400), prescribing six hours of daily patching produces an improvement in VA that is similar to the improvement produced by prescribing full-time daily patching.[44]
  • For moderate amblyopia (20/40 to 20/80), prescribing two hours of daily patching produces an improvement in VA similar to the improvement produced by prescribing six hours of daily patching.[45]
  • Refractive correction alone improves VA often and results in resolution of amblyopia in at least one-third of children with untreated anisometropic amblyopia.[46]
  • Following treatment with spectacles, two hours of daily patching combined with one hour of near-vision activities modestly improves moderate to severe amblyopia.[47]
  • Nearly one fourth of successfully-treated amblyopic children experience a recurrence within the first year off treatment. For patients treated with ≥ 6 hours of daily patching, the risk of recurrence is greater when patching is stopped abruptly, than when it is reduced to 2 hours per day before termination.[48]
- For patients of 7–12 years: Amblyopia treatment with near activities improves VA even if the amblyopia has been previously treated.[49]
- For patients of 13–18 years: Amblyopia treatment with near activities may improve VA when amblyopia has not been previously treated, but appears to be of little benefit if amblyopia was previously treated.[49]

*Not done for aphakic/pseudophakic eyes, however, until such studies for aphakic/pseudophakic eyes are performed, it may be reasonable to apply these principles for aphakic/pseudophakic eyes.

it is advisable to patch the opposite eye for a short period (e.g. 1 day/year-of-age), with frequent eye examinations.

The occlusion regimen may be modified or stopped if it is felt to be in the best interest of the child. It is advisable for parents to continue patching until vision is equalized or shows no improvement after three compliant cycles of patching. Once the ophthalmologist is convinced that maximal VA for that child has been gained, the treatment should be tapered or stopped. Children should be encouraged to engage in their normal activities during patching therapy. The parent should be told to have the child spend at least part of patching time each day performing eye-hand coordination activities at near such as crafts, coloring, tracing, cutting out shapes with scissors, completing workbook games (connect the dots, hidden pictures, and word finds), computer-generated or video games, computer/internet, reading or writing.

Early follow-up evaluation for children undergoing full-time patching should be spaced at an interval of 1 week for each year of life (e.g. every 2 weeks for a 2-year-old child).[43] The frequency of successive follow-up evaluations will depend on the age of the patient, severity of the amblyopia and intensity of occlusion therapy (high versus low percentage). Intervals may be adjusted based on the clinical response in an individual patient. The distance that the patient must travel for amblyopia treatment and the socioeconomic status of the parent should be considered when determining follow-up frequency. Less aggressive treatment and longer follow-up intervals are better than stopping therapy.

Infants who have developed nystagmus before surgery and children who have delays for such surgery may have amblyopia that is resistant even to aggressive occlusion treatment. Ideally, all amblyopia should be treated, although the difficulty of treatment for both the patients and the parent/caregivers should not be underestimated.[43] The difficulty in treatment should be weighed against the potential lifetime benefit of successful treatment.[43] The value of normal visual function and the effectiveness of treatment justify the difficulty and inconvenience of managing amblyopia in children. The pediatric eye disease investigator group has recently published several articles on amblyopia management for older children. Although not done for aphakic/pseudophakic eyes, until such studies for aphakic/pseudophakic eyes are performed, it may be reasonable to apply these principles for aphakic/pseudophakic eyes.[44-49]

SPECIAL SITUATION

Posterior Lentiglobus and/or Preexisting Posterior Capsule Defect

Posterior lentiglobus is a progressive well-circumscribed globular bulging of the posterior capsule of the lens. Early findings of posterior lentiglobus appear ophthalmoscopically as an "oil droplet in the central red reflex". During lens aspiration, the bulging of the posterior capsule helps to confirm the diagnosis of lentiglobus. Posterior lentiglobus increases the intraoperative challenges of cataract surgery in children because of the thin, floppy, and at times, ruptured posterior capsule. It is occasionally possible to convert a preexisting capsule rupture into a PCCC to better support the IOL and resist further tearing. However, sometimes the preexisting tear is very large and it is not possible to convert it into a round PCCC of desired size. When operating on an eye with lentiglobus, it is important to ensure that the opening is not extended into the posterior capsule. With posterior lentiglobus, low flow rate and low bottle height are recommended to reduce the possibility of an uncontrolled peripheral extension of the posterior capsule defect.

Vasavada and colleagues described a characteristic fish-tail sign in eyes with preexisting posterior capsule defect (when the globe was moved with forceps, the dots in the anterior vitreous moved with the degenerated vitreous).[12] Of 400 consecutive eyes that had undergone congenital cataract surgery, of which 27 eyes (20 children) had a confirmed preexisting posterior capsule defect. The visual axis remained clear in all the eyes and the IOL was well-centered in 24 eyes (88.88%).

Posterior Capsule Plaque

Posterior capsule plaque is commonly observed in eyes in congenital cataract. If a posterior capsule plaque is present, either the technique of plaque peeling (for small plaque) or vitrectorhexis (for large plaque) can be used depending on the extent of the plaque.

Secondary IOL Implantation

Eyes that are left aphakic are likely to require a secondary IOL implantation. Even if the surgeon is not planning to implant an IOL in a specific eye, it is important to leave behind sufficient anterior and posterior capsular support at the time of cataract surgery to facilitate subsequent in-the-bag or sulcus-fixated IOL implantation. The vast majority of children undergoing secondary IOL implantation have had a primary posterior capsulotomy and anterior vitrectomy. If adequate peripheral capsular support is present, the IOL is placed into the ciliary sulcus or in the reopened capsular bag.[50,51] Eyes operated for cataract surgery before their first birthday were more likely to received in-the-bag secondary IOL in our series.[51] Viscodissection and meticulous clearing of all posterior synechiae between the iris and the residual capsule is mandatory. The most common IOL used in secondary implantation is the three-piece AcrySof® IOL. It has a posterior angulation that helps to make it suitable for the sulcus. However, the haptics are soft and decentrations can occur, especially in eyes with large anterior segments and axial length measurements greater than 23 mm. Prolapsing the IOL optic through the fused anterior and posterior capsule remnants is very useful in preventing decentration and also eliminating the possibility of inadvertent pupillary capture. The Raynor C-flex IOL is a hydrophilic acrylic implant that can be used in the sulcus and is a very suitable alternative for secondary IOL implantation in children. When inadequate capsular support is present for sulcus fixation in a child, implantation of an IOL is not recommended unless every contact lens and spectacle option has been explored fully. Anterior chamber IOLs and scleral or iris-fixated posterior chamber IOLs are used in children when other viable options are absent but the long-term consequences of these placements are unknown. Anterior chamber IOLs should be of an open-loop flexible design and sized appropriately for the anterior chamber. Scleral-sutured IOLs are usually fixated with 10-0 prolene suture but concerns of biodegradation have surfaced as more late (5–15 years after surgery) IOL decentrations have been documented. A 10-0 polyester suture has now been tried. Many surgeons are now using 9-0 prolene and some are using 8.0 Gortex suture. Other suture materials are in design. Iris-fixation is also an alternative in children when inadequate capsule is present for sulcus or bag fixation. Iris fixation as in the "lobster-claw" style lenses (Verisyse™ Artisan) are utilized in some children as a phakic IOL for high myopia. Details on this IOL have been covered in another chapter.

Traumatic Cataract

Trauma is a common cause of unilateral cataract in children. At the time of presentation after the trauma to the eye, primary repair of a corneal or scleral wound may be needed along with a complete evaluation of damage to the intraocular structures (e.g. posterior capsule rupture, vitreous hemorrhage and retinal detachment). The authors prefer to defer cataract surgery and IOL implantation in traumatic cataract patients, even when anterior lens capsule has been ruptured. A delay of 1–4 weeks may be helpful to allow corneal healing and to reduce the inflammatory response. Longer delays are avoided in children within the amblyopic ages. Implantation of an IOL is preferred in the cases of traumatic cataracts with corneal injuries, because contact lenses may be difficult to fit. On the other hand, a rigid gas-permeable contact lens may be needed to help with control of astigmatism and, if worn, can also provide aphakic correction. For this reason, some surgeons are less likely to place an IOL primarily in these cases. Placement of the IOL in the capsular bag is preferred when capsular support is available. When stability of capsular bag is compromised, capsular tension ring can be used. Ciliary sulcus fixation of the IOL can also be done in absence of adequate capsular support for in-the-bag placement, but with a greater incidence of uveitis and pupillary capture.

Persistent Fetal Vasculature

The key to success in managing the child with PFV is early diagnosis and surgical intervention if needed. In cataract with associated blood vessel anomalies such as PFV, vitrectomy instrumentation is used to remove the posterior lens capsule, abnormal membrane, and anterior vitreous. Intraocular scissors and intraocular cautery are also used as needed. The rehabilitation of vision may be further facilitated using an IOL if PFV is not associated with stretched ciliary processes or tractional retinal detachment.

Retinopathy of Prematurity (ROP)

Cataract can be associated with ROP; however, occurrence of secondary cataract is more frequently reported.[52] Preventive measures play a significant role in minimizing the risk of cataract formation in eyes with ROP. Lambert and colleagues[53] reported a median interval of 3 weeks for diagnosis of cataract after laser photocoagulation. For cataract surgery in eyes with ROP, general principles of pediatric cataract surgery discussed in this chapter should be followed. These eyes are more often associated with fibrous changes in the anterior capsule. Lambert and colleagues recommended to defer cataract surgery if there are objective signs of anterior segment ischemia, because cataract surgery may accelerate the process of these eyes becoming phthisical.[53]

Aniridia

Cataracts develop in 50–85% of patients with familial aniridia, usually during the first two decades of life. Ectopia lentis has been reported in from 0% to 56% of patients with aniridia.[54] Literature has reported the thinning of the anterior capsule in association with congenital aniridia.[55] However, caution is needed as all aniridia eyes with a thin anterior capsule were from younger patients in this series compared with the control group. The younger the age, the thinner is the anterior capsule. It is not clear whether younger age or aniridia led to thinner capsules in this series. Aniridic eye may be associated with corneal vascularization and pannus, thick cornea, optic nerve hypoplasia, strabismus, nystagmus and glaucoma. Operating on a congenitally aniridic eye presents special challenges and implantation of an artificial iris device appears to be a reasonably effective method for reducing the subjective perception of glare resulting from the iris deficiency. The optical correction of aphakia in aniridic patients is difficult because concomitant corneal pannus may be a relative contraindication to contact lenses and nystagmus may exacerbate the optical aberration of aphakic spectacles. The lack of a normal iris presents difficulties in placement of an IOL.[56]

Retinoblastoma

Retinoblastoma is the most common intraocular malignancy of childhood. One of the treatment modalities used in this disease is external beam radiation therapy (EBRT). An expected side effect of EBRT for retinoblastoma is cataract formation, which impairs a child's visual development and an ophthalmologist's ability to examine the eye. While proceeding with the cataract surgery in eyes with retinoblastoma, it is prudent to get consultation with retinoblastoma specialist. It is important to weigh the expected benefit of visual rehabilitation against the risk of tumor recurrence and metastasis, and discuss it with the family before proceeding to cataract surgery. It is worthwhile to allow observation of at least 6–12 months after documented tumor regression before attempting for cataract removal. The clear corneal incision may reduce the risk of inadvertent conjunctival implantation of viable tumor cells and may allow for direct inspection of the incision site for tumor recurrence (unlike the limbal or scleral incision, which may be obscured by the overlying conjunctival flap). Presence of a posterior capsule opening theoretically increases the risk of dissemination of viable RB cells to the anterior chamber and extraocular extension through the incision site. If RB regression has been deemed stable for at least 6–12 months after cataract surgery, Nd-YAG laser posterior capsulotomy may be cautiously performed where required.[57] We prefer to avoid opening the posterior capsule, if the posterior capsule is not associated with plaque and age limits permits. However, more often these eyes are associated with posterior capsule plaque or defect.[58] In such case, it may become necessary to perform posterior capsulotomy. However, still, it is better to attempt manual posterior capsulorhexis (with an intake anterior vitreous face), to avoid vitreous phase disturbance and

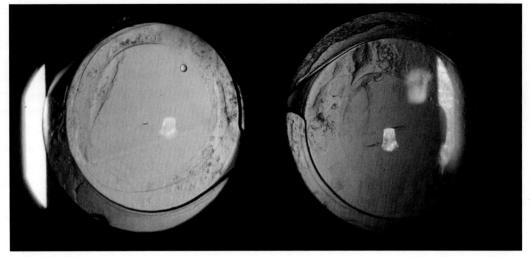

FIGURE 46.6: Four year follow-up of cataract surgery in a child with retinoblastoma (Both eyes were operated for cataract surgery with IOL implantation at 6 years of age with manual PCCC without vitrectomy)

subsequent vitrectomy (**Figure 46.6**). Cytolologic examination of vitrectomy fluid can provide direct intraoperative evidence of viable RB. Prompt enucleation and adjuvant chemotherapy with or without orbital radiotherapy may be considered in such situations. Close observation is warranted for several years to detect possible tumor recurrence and systemic metastasis. Tumor recurrence has been reported to range from 0% to 45% after various intraocular procedures. Even after a successful surgical outcome, the final VA depends on several factors.[59] In addition to clarity of the visual axis, other factors such as amblyopia, refractive error, macular tumors, radiation complications (keratopathy and/or retinopathy), optic atrophy or chronic retinal detachment can affect visual outcome.

Small Pupil

This topic will be covered in other chapter in this book.

Alport Syndrome

Anterior lenticonus is less common than the posterior lenticonus, and most often found in association with Alport's syndrome. It is a rare bilateral condition wherein the anterior surface of the lens protrudes to assume a conical form. Anterior capsule is thin in such eyes. Close follow-up is necessary in patients with anterior lenticonus. If signs of early lens capsule slitting, "cracking" or rupture are seen at the slit lamp, clear lens extraction can be considered to avoid an uncontrolled lens rupture and hydration.[10,60]

NEWER TECHNOLOGY

Triamcinolone

Intracameral triamcinolone (Kenalog) may have a potential benefit in the management of pediatric cataract.[61] Kenalog injection into the anterior chamber provides the anterior segment surgeon a means to localize and identify if any vitreous strands remaining in anterior chamber that otherwise might have gone unnoticed.

Sutureless Pars Plana Vitrectomy

Sutureless, pars plana vitrectomy through self-sealing sclerotomies has been reported in the literature.[62,63] No difference in the amount of visible vitreous incarceration between sutured and sutureless sclerotomies was reported, using ultrabiomicroscopy. However, wound leakage, extension, dehiscence, hemorrhage, vitreous and/or retinal incarceration, retinal tear and dialysis have been reported with this technique. Difficulty with the passage of instruments has also been observed when tunnel incisions are used.

Bag in the Lens

Tassignon and colleagues[64] reported the outcome of a surgical procedure they called "bag-in-the-lens" in eyes with pediatric cataract. In this technique, the anterior and posterior capsules are placed in the groove of a specially designed IOL after a capsulorhexis of the same size is created in both capsules. The authors reported a clear visual axis in all pediatric patients with an average follow-up of 17 months.

Sealed Capsule Irrigation

Perfect Capsule™ (Milvella Ltd) is a sterile single use ophthalmic instrument used to perform sealed irrigation of the capsular bag during cataract surgery in such a way that the irrigation fluid does not come in contact with the other ocular structures (**Figure 46.7**). A prospective case series comprising eyes of 12 children aged 1–12 years undergoing cataract surgery evaluated sealed irrigation of the lens capsular bag using 5-Fluorouracil (FU) (50 mg/ml). Results of the study found that the 5-FU sealed capsule irrigation system was effective in preventing the occurrence of PCO in 50% of the patients at 6 months. However, PCO was not severe enough in any of the eyes to warrant performing

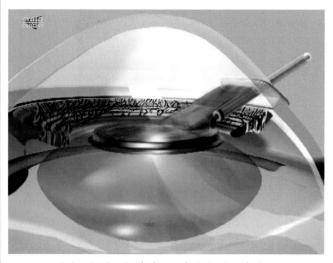

FIGURE 46.7: Sealed capsule irrigation device

a secondary procedure at 6 months postoperative period in any group (Viraj A Vasavada, Abhay R Vasavada, Sajani K Shah, Vaishali A Vasavada MS "Evaluation of PCO with 5-FU using sealed capsule irrigation in congenital cataract surgery and IOL implantation – Preliminary Results" presented at the Annual Symposium of ESCRS, 2009, Barcelona, Spain).

Multifocal and Accommodative IOL

Each of the multifocal IOLs represents a compromise based upon the simultaneous vision principle. Two or more images are formed on the retina at the same time, one image at near and the other at distance focus. The brain selects the image it wants to see. Some loss of contrast is inherent to simultaneous vision since the available light is split between the near focus and the distant focus. Uncorrected refractive error (cylinder of more than 1 diopter or the changes in sphere that occur with eye growth) may result in more significant blur because of the simultaneous vision concept. Alternating vision, which is provided by a monofocal IOL and bifocal glasses, results in only one object being in focus at a time and all incoming light, is directed to this focus. While the increased use of multifocal and accommodative IOLs for implantation during the teenage years is predictable, we would caution surgeons that these lenses may not be advantageous in growing or amblyopic eyes.[65] There is a growing interest in multifocal IOL implantation in children because they lose accommodation when a cataract is removed. Many have assumed that very little, if any, eye growth occurs in the second decade of life. Axial eye growth continues throughout the second decade of life, at least to age 20. Measurement data show variable growth throughout the second decade of life. Average axial growth was 0.53 mm.[65] With residual refractive error, especially the myopia that develops after eye growth, multifocality may (ironically) result in more spectacle dependence compared to a monofocal IOL with residual myopia. This deserves further study. The Crystalens accommodating IOL is engineered with a hinge designed to allow the optic to move back and forth in response to change of focus. It is unknown whether the fibrosis that often occurs throughout the pediatric lens capsule after surgery would influence the IOL movement. This IOL is not recommended when a primary posterior capsulectomy and anterior vitrectomy has been performed, which is necessary surgical steps for younger children undergoing cataract surgery.

Adjustable Power IOL

The ongoing development in adjustable IOL technology may prove very useful in the future of the surgical management of pediatric cataracts. The possibility of a lens that could be adjusted to counter the myopia induced by ocular growth is potentially exciting. An ideal pediatric adjustable IOL implant should be biocompatible, allow for safe repeatable adjustment procedures performed at any time after cataract surgery; and have an adequate refractive error adjustment range. As of today, this ideal adjustable IOL does not exist. However, the concept of such an IOL is being developed and after certain modifications, such an IOL may become available.[66]

SUMMARY

To summarize the given qualities and characteristics of children's eye, pediatric cataract surgery is technically challenging. Diligent preoperative and postoperative management is essential for satisfactory visual results. The timing of surgery is often crucial to prevent amblyopia. The surgeon must be cognizant of the many complications that may occur in pediatric cataract surgery and should be prepared to manage any that arise. The improvements in surgical technique and technology have improved the anatomical results obtained following pediatric cataract surgery. Adequate visual results, however, are still too often lacking.

CORE MESSAGES

- Pediatric cataract surgery itself is, but one-step among many, aimed at achieving normal visual function over a long lifespan.
- Cataract surgery is not the end of the journey; it is the beginning. Surgery is only one component of the treatment package for a child with cataract.
- Achieving better visual outcome requires a team approach that involves the patient, parents, ophthalmologist and other caregivers considering visual, economical, psychological and social issues.
- Lengthy discussions between the parents/caregivers and the surgeon are common. The outcome is often better when the parents/caregivers are informed and committed partners with the ophthalmic team.
- A cataract when reduced the VA to worse than or equal to 20/50, or blackens the retinoscopic reflex in undilated

pupil is likely visually significant enough to consider surgery. The most valuable test for determining the visual significance of cataract is analysis of the red reflex through the undilated pupil with a retinoscope.

- In the case of a dense cataract diagnosed at birth, surgeon can wait until 4 to 6 weeks of age. Waiting until this age decreases anesthesia-related complications and facilitate the surgical procedure. Waiting beyond this time, however, adversely affects visual outcome. In the case of a bilateral cataract, it is important to keep the time interval to a minimum between the two eye surgeries.

- For older children, timing of surgery can often be decided based on convenience and other logistic issues factoring in age, laterality and density of cataract.

- Even conservative surgeons, who vote against routine use of SBCS in children, are more likely to use this approach when anesthesia poses more than average risks or the patient lives far away and a visit for surgery on the second eye would be difficult.

- A general consensus exists that IOL implantation is appropriate for children undergoing cataract surgery after their first birthday. Until longer-term follow-up data are available, caution should be exercised when performing IOL implantation in children younger than 1 year.

- For IOL power selection, several nomograms based on age at surgery have been published. However, author does not recommend the use of any published table alone for deciding IOL power. Selection of an optimum power of IOL is multifactorial decision, customized to each child.

- Ideal IOL power should balance the best help to amblyopia management in childhood with the least possible refractive error in adulthood. The late myopia, even if marked, may be an acceptable trade for better visual outcome from amblyopia treatment.

- In an otherwise healthy child, most physicians do not advise extensive laboratory and genetic investigations. As compared to unilateral cataract, laboratory investigation of bilateral cases is more rewarding.

- Modifications of the manual CCC in older children and use of the vitrectorhexis in younger children (e.g. less than 2 years of age) can lead to successful anterior management in nearly every surgery.

- The surgeon should strictly adhere to the principles of a closed chamber technique. Proper wound construction and a tight-fit around the instruments helps assure chamber stability throughout irrigation and aspiration of cortex and nucleus.

- No phacoemulsification is needed. Phacoaspiration generally suffice the need to remove lens cortex.

- In young children who undergo pediatric cataract surgery, PCO is rapid and virtually inevitable if the posterior capsule is left intact. PCO occurs much faster and is much more amblyogenic in younger children as compared with older children. As a rough guideline, in children below 5 years of age, do primary posterior capsulectomy and vitrectomy. In children, 5–8 years of age, it is optional surgical step. In children above 8 years of age, an intact posterior capsule can be left more often.

- Even if the surgeon is not planning to implant an IOL in a specific eye, it is important to leave behind sufficient anterior and posterior capsular support at the time of cataract surgery to facilitate subsequent in-the-bag or sulcus-fixated IOL implantation.

- Suturing the wounds in children is the norm.

- In children beyond the infantile age group, combined posterior capsulectomy, vitrectomy and hydrophobic acrylic IOL implantation avoids the need for a secondary intervention in most eyes.

- In infant eyes, VAO is much more common when an IOL of any type is implanted compared with primary aphakia, even when a posterior capsulotomy and an anterior vitrectomy is performed.

- In pediatric eyes with an intact posterior capsule, PCO is almost inevitable. Nd:YAG capsulotomy can treat this complication but requires more energy and may need to be repeated.

- Single-piece acrylic IOLs have improved the intra-operative performance and helped to assure that proper capsular placement of the implant.

- Patients undergoing cataract surgery during early infancy are at higher risk for the development of glaucoma with or without an IOL implant.

- Amblyopia is major cause for poor visual outcome.

- Cataract operated children should be monitored and may need EUA during the higher risk years.

- Management of residual refractive error, amblyopia and strabismus need to be customized to the individual child based on measurements that can be a challenge to get and can change over time.

- Correction of residual refractive error can be aimed at mild myopia in children below 2 years of age. In children above 2 years of age, bifocal lenses can be prescribed (distance emmetropia, near +3 D).

- Despite the continuing threat of amblyopia, visual outcome after pediatric cataract surgery has improved over the last few years. We have refined surgical techniques and our understanding of the sensitive periods for developing and reversing of amblyopia has increased.

REFERENCES

1. Gilbert C. Worldwide causes of blindness in children. In: Wilson ME, Saunders RA, Trivedi RH (Eds). Pediatric Ophthalmology: Current Thought and A Practical Guide. Heidelberg, Germany: Springer; 2009. pp. 47-60.
2. Gilbert C, Foster A, Negrel AD, et al. Childhood blindness: a new form for recording causes of visual loss in children. Bulletin of the World Health Organization. 1993;71:485-90.
3. Foster A, Gilbert C, Rahi J. Epidemiology of cataract in childhood: a global perspective. J Cataract Refract Surg. 1997; 23 (Suppl 1):601-4.

4. Wilson ME, Trivedi RH. Visual impairment and blindness in children: Cataract. In: Johnson GJ, West SK (Eds). Epidemic Eye Disease. New York: Oxford University Press; 2010.

5. Rahi JS, Dezateux C. Measuring and interpreting the incidence of congenital ocular anomalies: lessons from a national study of congenital cataract in the UK. Invest Ophthalmol Vis Sci. 2001;42:1444-8.

6. Lim Z, Rubab S, Chan YH. Pediatric cataract: the Toronto experience-etiology. Am J Ophthalmol. 2010;149:887-92.

7. Wilson ME, Trivedi RH. Pediatric cataract surgery: operative and postoperative issues. In: Wilson ME, Saunders RA, Trivedi RH (Eds). Pediatric Ophthalmology: Current Thought and a Practical Guide. Heidelberg, Germany: Springer; 2009. pp. 326-43.

8. Trivedi RH, Wilson ME. Pediatric cataract: Preoperative issues and considerations. In: Wilson ME, Saunders RA, Trivedi RH (Eds). Pediatric Ophthalmology: Current Thought and a Practical Guide. Heidelberg, Germany: Springer; 2009. pp. 311-24.

9. American Academy of Pediatrics; Section on Ophthalmology; American Association for Pediatric Ophthalmology And Strabismus; American Academy of Ophthalmology; American Association of Certified Orthoptists. Red reflex examination in neonates, infants, and children. Pediatrics. 2008;122:1401-4.

10. Wilson ME, Trivedi RH, Biber JM, et al. Anterior capsule rupture and subsequent cataract formation in Alport syndrome. J AAPOS. 2006;10:182-3.

11. Wilson ME, Levin AV, Trivedi RH, et al. Cataract associated with type-1 diabetes mellitus in the pediatric population. J AAPOS. 2007;11:162-5.

12. Vasavada AR, Praveen MR, Dholakia SA, et al. Preexisting posterior capsule defect progressing to white mature cataract. J AAPOS. 2007;11:192-4.

13. Vasavada AR, Trivedi RH, Nath VC. Visual axis opacification after AcrySof intraocular lens implantation in children. J Cataract Refract Surg. 2004;30:1073-81.

14. Wilson ME, Trivedi RH, Buckley EG, et al. ASCRS white paper. Hydrophobic acrylic intraocular lenses in children. J Cataract Refract Surg. 2007;33:1966-73.

15. Birch EE, Stager DR. The critical period for surgical treatment of dense congenital unilateral cataract. Investigative Ophthalmology and Visual Science. 1996;37:1532-8.

16. Birch EE, Cheng C, Stager DR, Weakley DR, Stager DR, Sr. The critical period for surgical treatment of dense congenital bilateral cataracts. J AAPOS. 2009;13:67-71.

17. Wilson ME, Trivedi RH, Hoxie JP, et al. Treatment outcomes of congenital monocular cataracts: the effects of surgical timing and patching compliance. Journal of Pediatric Ophthalmology and Strabismus. 2003;40:323-9.

18. Nallasamy S, Davidson SL, Kuhn I, et al. Simultaneous bilateral intraocular surgery in children. J AAPOS. 2010;14:15-9.

19. Wilson ME, Trivedi RH. Multicenter randomized controlled clinical trial in pediatric cataract surgery: efficacy and effectiveness. Am J Ophthalmol. 2007;144:616-7.

20. Gochnauer AC, Trivedi RH, Hill EG, et al. Interocular axial length difference as a predictor of postoperative visual acuity after unilateral pediatric cataract extraction with primary IOL implantation. J AAPOS. 2010;14:20-4.

21. Johar SR, Savalia NK, Vasavada AR, et al. Epidemiology based etiological study of pediatric cataract in western India. Indian J Med Sci. 2004;58:115-21.

22. Nihalani BR, Vanderveen DK. Comparison of intraocular lens power calculation formulae in pediatric eyes. Ophthalmology. 2010;117:1493-9.

23. Trivedi RH, Wilson ME (Eds). Intraocular Lens Power Calculation for Children. New Delhi, India: Jaypee Brothers Medical Publishers; 2007. pp. 214-9.

24. Lambert SR. Ocular growth in early childhood: Implications for pediatric cataract surgery. Op Tech Cataract Refract Surg. 1998;1:159-64.

25. Plager DA, Kipfer H, Sprunger DT, et al. Refractive change in pediatric pseudophakia: 6-year follow-up. J Cataract Refract Surg. 2002;28:810-5.

26. Plager DA, Lipsky SN, Snyder SK, et al. Capsular management and refractive error in pediatric intraocular lenses. Ophthalmology. 1997;104:600-7.

27. Wilson ME. Anterior lens capsule management in pediatric cataract surgery. Trans Am Ophthalmol Soc. 2004;102:391-422.

28. Trivedi RH, Wilson ME, Bartholomew LR. Extensibility and scanning electron microscopy evaluation of 5 pediatric anterior capsulotomy techniques in a porcine model. J Cataract Refract Surg. 2006;32:1206-13.

29. Wilson ME, Trivedi RH, Bartholomew LR, et al. Comparison of anterior vitrectorhexis and continuous curvilinear capsulorhexis in pediatric cataract and intraocular lens implantation surgery: a 10-year analysis. J AAPOS. 2007;11:443-6.

30. Nischal KK. Two-incision push-pull capsulorhexis for pediatric cataract surgery. J Cataract Refract Surg. 2002;28:593-5.

31. Jacobs DS, Cox TA, Wagoner MD, et al. Capsule staining as an adjunct to cataract surgery: a report from the American Academy of Ophthalmology. Ophthalmology. 2006;113:707-13.

32. Nanavaty MA, Johar K, Sivasankaran MA, et al. Effect of trypan blue staining on the density and viability of lens epithelial cells in white cataract. J Cataract Refract Surg. 2006;32:1483-8.

33. Vasavada AR, Trivedi RH, Apple DJ, et al. Randomized, clinical trial of multiquadrant hydrodissection in pediatric cataract surgery. Am J Ophthalmol. 2003;135:84-8.

34. Wilson ME, Trivedi RH, Mistr S. Pediatric intraoperative floppy-iris syndrome. J Cataract Refract Surg. 2007;33:1325-7.

35. Bayramlar H, Totan Y, Borazan M. Heparin in the intraocular irrigating solution in pediatric cataract surgery. J Cataract Refract Surg. 2004;30:2163-9.

36. Dada T. Intracameral heparin in pediatric cataract surgery. J Cataract Refract Surg. 2003;29:1056.

37. Wilson ME, Trivedi RH. Low molecular-weight heparin in the intraocular irrigating solution in pediatric cataract and intraocular lens surgery. Am J Ophthalmol. 2006;141:537-8.

38. Vasavada AR, Trivedi RH. Role of optic capture in congenital cataract and intraocular lens surgery in children. J Cataract Refract Surg. 2000;26:824-31.

39. Stager DR, Wang X, Weakley DR, et al. The effectiveness of Nd:YAG laser capsulotomy for the treatment of posterior capsule opacification in children with acrylic intraocular lenses. J AAPOS. 2006;10:159-63.

40. Trivedi RH, Wilson ME, Golub RL. Incidence and risk factors for glaucoma after pediatric cataract surgery with and without intraocular lens implantation. J AAPOS. 2006;10:117-23.

41. Infant Aphakia Treatment Study Group, Lambert SR, Buckley EG, et al. A randomized clinical trial comparing contact lens with intraocular lens correction of monocular aphakia during infancy: grating acuity and adverse events at age 1 year. Arch Ophthalmol. 2010;128(7):810-8.

42. Ledoux DM, Trivedi RH, Wilson ME, et al. Pediatric cataract extraction with intraocular lens implantation: visual acuity outcome when measured at age four years and older. J AAPOS. 2007;11:218-24.

43. American Academy of Ophthalmology. Amblyopia, preferred practice pattern. San Francisco, CA, USA. American Academy of Ophthalmology; 2002.

44. Holmes JM, Kraker RT, Beck RW, et al. A randomized trial of prescribed patching regimens for treatment of severe amblyopia in children. Ophthalmology. 2003;110:2075-87.

45. Repka MX, Beck RW, Holmes JM, et al. A randomized trial of patching regimens for treatment of moderate amblyopia in children. Archives of Ophthalmology. 2003;121:603-11.

46. Cotter SA, Pediatric Eye Disease Investigator Group, Edwards AR, et al. Treatment of anisometropic amblyopia in children with refractive correction. Ophthalmology. 2006;113:895-903.

47. Wallace DK, Pediatric Eye Disease Investigator Group, Edwards AR, et al. A randomized trial to evaluate 2 hours of daily patching for strabismic and anisometropic amblyopia in children. Ophthalmology. 2006;113:904-12.

48. Holmes JM, Beck RW, Kraker RT, et al. Risk of amblyopia recurrence after cessation of treatment. Journal AAPOS. 2004;8:420-8.

49. Scheiman MM, Hertle RW, Beck RW, et al. Randomized trial of treatment of amblyopia in children aged 7 to 17 years. Archives of Ophthalmology. 2005;123:437-47.

50. Wilson ME, Englert JA, Greenwald MJ. In-the-bag secondary intraocular lens implantation in children. J AAPOS. 1999;3:350-5.

51. Trivedi RH, Wilson ME, Facciani J. Secondary intraocular lens implantation for pediatric aphakia. J AAPOS. 2005;9:346-52.

52. Anfuso T, Wilson ME. Nanophthalmos. In: Johnson SM (Ed). Cataract surgery in the glaucoma patients. Heidelberg, Germany: Springer; 2009. pp. 221-6.

53. Lambert SR, Capone A, Cingle KA, et al. Cataract and phthisis bulbi after laser photoablation for threshold retinopathy of prematurity. Am J Ophthalmol. 2000;129:585-91.

54. Nelson LB, Spaeth GL, Nowinski TS, et al. A review. Surv Ophthalmol. 1984;28:621-42.

55. Schneider S, Osher RH, Burk SE, et al. Thinning of the anterior capsule associated with congenital aniridia. J Cataract Refract Surg. 2003;29:523-5.

56. Trivedi RH, Wilson ME. Aniridia and cataracts. In: Wilson ME, Trivedi RH, Pandey SK (Eds). Pediatric Cataract Surgery: Techniques, Complications, and Management. Philadelphia: Lippincott, Williams & Wilkins; 2005. pp. 199-202.

57. Honavar SG, Shields CL, Shields JA, et al. Intraocular surgery after treatment of retinoblastoma. Arch Ophthalmol. 2001;119:1613-21.

58. Trivedi RH, Wilson ME. Cataract surgery in eyes treated for retinoblastoma. In: Wilson ME, Trivedi RH, Pandey SK (Eds). Pediatric Cataract Surgery: Techniques, Complications, and Management. Philadelphia: Lippincott, Williams & Wilkins; 2005. pp. 184-8.

59. Payne JF, Hutchinson AK, Hubbard GB, et al. Outcomes of cataract surgery following radiation treatment for retinoblastoma. J AAPOS. 2009;13:454-8.e3.

60. Trivedi RH, Wilson ME. Anterior lenticonus in Alport syndrome. In: Wilson ME, Trivedi RH, Pandey SK (Eds). Pediatric Cataract Surgery: Techniques, Complications, and Management. Philadelphia: Lippincott, Williams & Wilkins; 2005. pp. 194-8.

61. Shah SK, Vasavada V, Praveen MR, et al. Triamcinolone-assisted vitrectomy in pediatric cataract surgery. J Cataract Refract Surg. 2009;35:230-2.

62. You C, Wu X, Ying L, et al. Ultrasound biomicroscopy imaging of sclerotomy in children with cataract undergoing 25-gauge sutureless pars plana anterior vitrectomy. Eur J Ophthalmol. 2010;20:1053-8.

63. Lam DS, Chua JK, Leung AT, et al. Sutureless pars plana anterior vitrectomy through self-sealing sclerotomies in children. Arch Ophthalmol. 2000;118:850-1.

64. Tassignon MJ, De Veuster I, Godts D, et al. Bag-in-the-lens intraocular lens implantation in the pediatric eye. J Cataract Refract Surg. 2007;33:611-7.

65. Wilson ME, Trivedi RH, Burger BM. Eye growth in the second decade of life: implications for the implantation of a multifocal intraocular lens. Trans Am Ophthalmol Soc. 2009;107:120-4.

66. Nischal KK. Who needs a reversibly adjustable intraocular lens? Arch Ophthalmol. 2007;125:961-2.

CHAPTER 47

Small Pupil Phacoemulsification

Amar Agarwal, Soosan Jacob

INTRODUCTION

The pupil size has always played a very important role in performing any type of cataract surgery, be it an intracapsular cataract extraction, extracapsular cataract extraction, phacoemulsification, bimanual phacoemulsification or microphakonit.

A large sized, well-dilated pupil increases the ease of surgery dramatically, but unfortunately a miotic pupil (less than 4.0 mm), is a common bugbear that every surgeon faces at some time or the other. Miotic, non-dilating pupil **(Figure 47.1)** may be secondary to a variety of reasons **(Table 47.1)**. Phacoemulsification is especially difficult in these cases as it affects all steps right from capsulorhexis to emulsification of the nucleus, cortical removal and in-the-bag IOL insertion. The surgeon is forced to perform a small capsulorhexis, which further adds to the difficulty in performing surgery. A small pupil may cause damage to the patient's eye by emulsification of the iris or cause complications such as sphincter tears, intraoperative bleeding, zonular dialysis, posterior capsular rent or nucleus drop. Prolonged surgical time and increased maneuvering may result in postoperative complications such as striate keratopathy, uveitis, secondary glaucoma, floppy, torn or atrophic iris, irregular pupil, endophthalmitis, cystoid macular edema, etc, all resulting in a suboptimal surgical outcome and an unhappy patient. A study of 1,000 consecutive extracapsular cataract extractions showed that a small pupil was the most common factor associated with vitreous loss and capsular rupture.[1]

TABLE 47.1	Causes for miotic pupil

- Age related dilator atrophy
- Diabetes mellitus
- Synechiae
- Previous trauma
- Previous surgery
- Uveitis
- Iridoschisis
- Pseudoexfoliation syndrome
- Chronic miotic therapy
- Congenital
- Idiopathic
- Marfan's syndrome
- Chronic lues

A hypotonic, mid-dilated, irregular pupil postoperatively can also be esthetically bad, especially noticeable in light colored irides. Such a pupil can also have significant effect on the pupillary function leading onto iatrogenic glare dysfunction. Masket reported that an enlarged pupil can be responsible for postoperative glare disability in eyes that were anatomically normal except for having pseudophakia.[2] All these factors makes it mandatory, especially for a phaco surgeon to know how to tackle a miotic pupil.

There are a variety of techniques for the management of the small pupil, including iris hooks, iris rings, and pupillary stretching with or without the use of multiple half-width sphincterotomies.[3]

PREOPERATIVE EVALUATION

A dilated preoperative examination is mandatory for every patient, not just for assessing the posterior segment, but also to detect cases of suboptimal pupillary dilatation. Appropriate history is important for detecting any underlying etiology for the miotic pupil. One should check for intraoperative floppy iris syndrome and usage of tamsulosin (Flomax®, Boehringer-Ingelheim Pharmaceuticals, Inc., Ridgefield, CT) as suggested by David Chang. A careful slit-lamp examination is mandatory for detecting the cause as well as any associated complicating conditions that may co-exist, such as zonular weakness in a case of pseudoexfoliation. Proper planning of the surgical steps should be done preoperatively itself. Synechiolysis or membranectomy may be required in cases of chronic uveitis. For patients on chronic miotic therapy, these drugs

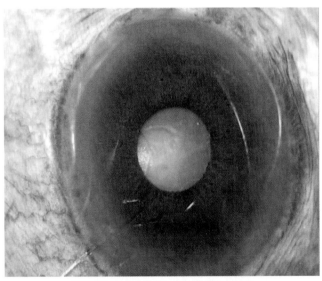

FIGURE 47.1: Miotic non-dilating pupil

should be stopped preoperatively and replaced if necessary with other suitable medications.

PHARMACOLOGICAL MYDRIASIS

The topical agents used preoperatively for dilating the patient's eye should include a cycloplegic, a mydriatic and a non-steroidal anti-inflammatory drug.[4]

CYCLOPLEGICS

The most commonly used cycloplegic agent is cyclopentolate hydrochloride 1%, which provides good cycloplegia and pupillary dilatation. The pupillary dilatation can last upto 36 hours. Tropicamide hydrochloride 1% is also a good pupillary dilator though shorter acting and with slightly lesser degree of cycloplegia. Atropine sulfate 1% is a longer lasting mydriatic and can be considered in cases of chronic uveitis, long standing diabetics, etc.

MYDRIATICS

Phenylephrine hydrochloride 2.5%, is a good pupil dilator, especially when combined with a cycloplegic. The 10% solution gives stronger dilatation, especially in resistant cases but the disadvantage is that it may increase the blood pressure in some patients and can also result in corneal punctate keratopathy. Mydricaine, a product which contains atropine, procaine and adrenaline can also be used as subconjunctival injections preoperatively.

NSAIDs

Non-steroidal anti-inflammatory drugs decrease the incidence of intraoperative constriction of the pupil. This is especially important in case of prolonged surgeries and surgery with increased intraoperative manipulation. Suprofen, diclofenac ketorolac, flurbiprofen, etc. are commonly used for this purpose.[5-10]

Pharmacological mydriasis may not be effective in all cases, especially in cases with posterior synechiae and scarred pupils. Such pupils have to be dealt appropriately during surgery to avoid a cascade of complications (**Table 47.2**).

TABLE 47.2	Methods for enlarging the pupil

Sphincter sparing techniques:
- Synechiolysis
- Pupillary membranectomy
- Viscomydriasis

Sphincter involving techniques:
- Mini sphincterotomies
- Pupil stretch
- Iris hooks
- Pupil ring expanders

INTRAOPERATIVE PROCEDURES NOT INVOLVING SPHINCTER

VISCOMYDRIASIS

A new ophthalmic viscosurgical device (OVD), 2.4% hyaluronate can be used for mechanically dilating the pupil in certain cases.[4,11] It is injected into the center of the pupil to mechanically dissect any synechiae and to stretch the sphincter. It should be completely removed at the end of the procedure to avoid postoperative intraocular pressure increase.

SYNECHIOLYSIS

A blunt spatula is passed through the side port incision after injecting viscoelastic into the eye.[4] A second side port incision may be required in case of extensive synechiae. This is followed by utilizing one of the other techniques to maintain the pupil in a dilated stage, e.g. viscomydriasis, iris hooks, pupil expanders, etc. A blunt rod can also be used to sweep any posterior synechiae free, without any stretch motions (**Figure 47.2**).

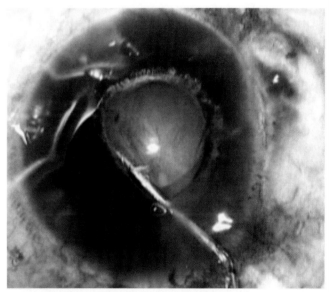

FIGURE 47.2: A blunt rod being used for synechiolysis

PUPILLARY MEMBRANECTOMY

Presence of pupillary membranes can result in small pupils. These membranes can be then taken care of with a combination of preoperative pharmacotherapy and intraoperative surgical removal by stripping the fine fibrin pupillary membrane using utrata forceps.

INTRAOPERATIVE PROCEDURES INVOLVING SPHINCTER

MINI-SPHINCTEROTOMIES

Mini-sphincterotomies[4,11] can be done with either Vannas scissors through the main port incision or with vitreoretinal scissors placed through the paracentesis. Very small partial cuts, no larger than 0.75 mm in radial length, are made limited to the sphincter tissue. As long as the incisions are kept very small, postoperatively the pupil should be normal both functionally and esthetically. The disadvantage is that regardless of the wound position, the incision is more difficult to create in the clock hour of the wound.

PUPIL STRETCH

Pupil stretch[12] can be done either using push-pull instruments or pronged instruments which stretch the pupillary sphincter. Pupillary stretching generally causes multiple fine partial sphincter tears. If combined with preplaced mini-sphincterotomies, the effect can be increased.[3] It generally results in a functionally and esthetically acceptable pupil postoperatively. The disadvantage is that the iris sometimes becomes flaccid and may either move into an undesirable location or may prolapse through the incision during surgery. Rarely, it may cause complications like hematoma or larger sphincter tears, pigment dispersion, postoperative uveitis, pressure spike and an abnormal and nonfunctional pupil postoperatively.

Bimanual Push-Pull Instruments

Using viscoelastic cover, two hooks are used in a slow, controlled fashion, to stretch the pupil in one or more axes.[2] One hook is used for pushing the pupillary margin and the other one for pulling. The push-pull should be done simultaneously, in a controlled manner, to avoid large sphincter tears. This technique usually achieves an adequately sized pupil for effective phacoemulsification. A two-handed, two-instrument bimanual stretch technique with an angled Kuglen hook and Lindstrom star nucleus rotator is very effective.

Pronged Instruments

Instruments available[12] are the Keuch two-pronged pupil stretcher (Katena) or the four-pronged pupil stretcher (Rhein Medical's Beehler pupil dilator). Postoperatively, the pupil continues to react normally. This technique, popularized by Luther Fry,[4] is an efficient and cost-effective method. The prongs (**Figure 47.3**) should be maintained parallel to the iris plane and should not slip out into the pupil margin, especially on starting to depress the plunger to create the pupil stretch.

IRIS HOOKS

Commercially available iris hooks (Grieshaber, Schaffhausen, Switzerland) have been originally used for posterior segment surgeries.[13] They can also be utilized for phacoemulsification[14] (**Figures 47.4 to 47.6**), but the disadvantage is that unless properly placed, they can pull the iris diaphragm forwards, resulting in chaffing and thermal damage during phacoemulsification.[15,16] To avoid this, the hooks should be placed parallel to the iris plane

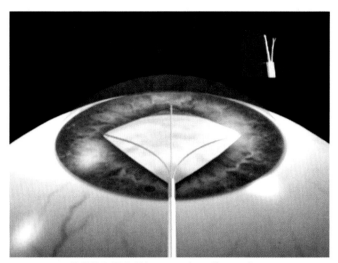

FIGURE 47.3: Tri-pronged pupil stretchers

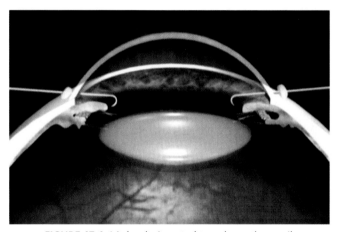

FIGURE 47.4: Iris hooks inserted to enlarge the pupil

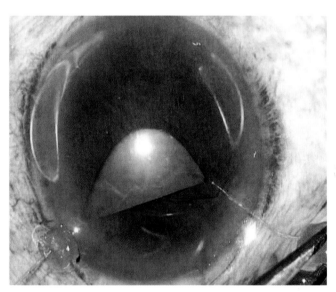

FIGURE 47.5: Iris hooks being placed

through small, short tract, peripheral paracenteses or by releasing the hooks after creating the capsulorhexis but before phacoemulsification. Gradual enlargement of the pupil should be done and one a pupil size just enough for the surgical procedure should be attempted for to avoid postoperative pupillary atony. The other disadvantage is that

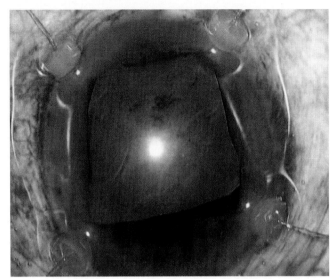

FIGURE 47.6: All four iris hooks in place

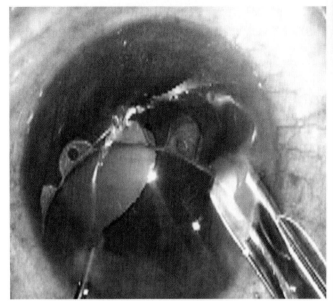

FIGURE 47.7: Perfect pupil device

it adds to the time and cost of surgery. Iris hooks have also been used in cases of zonular dialysis to stabilize the capsular bag by hooking it around the capsulorhexis margin.

IRIS RETAINER METHODS

Pupil Ring Expanders

They enlarge the pupil without sphincter damage. Here, incomplete pupil ring expanders are used to stretch the pupil.[17] They are inserted through the main port and manipulated into the pupil space. They can create the largest diameter pupil, creating a uniform expanding force approximately around 300° of the pupil. They thus have the least tendency for sphincter tears, as they do not produce point pressure on the pupillary margin. The disadvantages with these devices are that they are rigid, cumbersome and slightly difficult to insert into the eye through a small incision. They require manipulation to engage the sphincter. They may also hamper entry, exit and maneuvering of additional instruments through the incisions. It also adds to the time and cost of the surgery. The one-piece retaining rings are often difficult to position and even more difficult to remove.

Three expanders are the Grather, Siepser and Morcher[4] (**Table 47.2**). They are made of solid PMMA, silicone or expansible hydrogel material.

The Grather's pupil expander consists of a silicone ring with an indentation, which fits all along the edge of the pupil.[18] The iris fits like a tyre around the ring which is like an iron wheel. The disadvantage is that it can loosen easily with intraocular maneuvers.

Perfect Pupil Device™

This device is developed by John Milverton, MD, Sydney, Australia, and is a sterile, disposable, flexible polyurethane ring with an integrated arm (**Figure 47.7**) that allows easy insertion and removal.[11] It is inserted with a forceps or injected with an injector through the main port. The

integrated arm remains outside the eye to aid in easy removal. It can be inserted through an incision less than 100 microns. Because of the open ring design of the Perfect Pupil™, there is no interference with other instrumentation.

USE OF MALYUGIN RING FOR SMALL PUPIL PHACOEMULSIFICATION

The Malyugin ring (**Figure 47.8**) is a new device which has proved itself very useful for safe phacoemulsification in eyes with small, non-dilating pupils. The Malyugin ring is a square shaped, transitory implant with four circular scrolls that hold the iris at equidistant points with a gentle, stretching force. Insertion of the ring generally results in a pupillary diameter of about 6 mm, adequate for most phaco procedures. It keeps the iris sphincter from getting damaged during phaco procedures and allows the pupil to return to its normal size, shape and function at the end of the surgery.

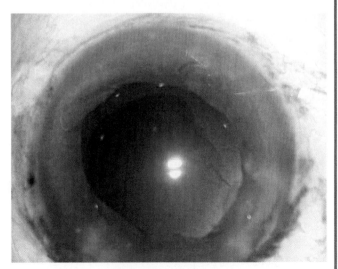

FIGURE 47.8: Malyugin ring

It has multiple advantages over the iris hooks. It is easier to implant and does not need multiple paracenteses wounds for insertion as it is introduced through the main port incision. Operating time is reduced and all risks associated with increased number of incisions are eliminated. It has no pointed ends and acts by producing a gentle, expansile force distributed over a wider area of contact with the pupil, thus causing lesser iris trauma. It may be especially useful in intraoperative floppy iris syndrome (IFIS) as there are lesser chances of iris prolapse as may occur in case of iris hooks through incorrectly sized paracenteses.

MODIFIED MALYUGIN RING IRIS EXPANSION TECHNIQUE

This technique is used in small-pupil cataract surgery with posterior capsule defects. Agarwal et al. modified the technique **(Figure 47.9)** for using the Malyugin ring for safe iris expansion in small-pupil cataract surgery in eyes with posterior capsule defects. This modification has two main advantages. First, while the ring is being injected, the chances of it dropping into the vitreous due to poor capsule support is reduced as it is well secured by the suture. Second, if a large posterior capsule defect occurs and the ring slips into the vitreous, it can be pulled back easily with the suture end. Thus, the surgeon can work effectively below the pupillary plane without fear of the ring slipping into the vitreous.

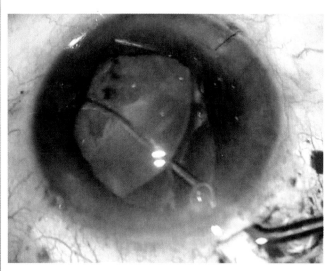

FIGURE 47.9: Agarwal's modification of the Malyugin ring in eyes with posterior capsular rupture

SURGICAL COMPLICATIONS

Bleeding may occur with these techniques.[4] It generally subsides on its own and any postoperative hyphema gets absorbed spontaneously. In case of significant bleeding intraoperatively, the intraocular pressure should be increased by elevating the bottle height, or by injecting a viscoelastic agent or air to the eye. In case of a major,

unresponsive bleed within the eye, one can add fibrin. Instrument-related damages that can occur include corneal endothelial damage,[4] iridodialysis, bleeding, iris pigment dispersion, etc. Postoperatively, the patient may have an atonic and distorted pupil. Large tears to the iris sphincter can result in latter. Pupillary dilatation should be done gradually to minimize sphincter tears and only the minimum amount of stretching that is required for the surgical steps should be done.[4] A forcibly, maximally dilated pupil can result in postoperative atonic pupil. Other postoperative complications which can be seen include uveitis, increased intraocular pressure, pigments on the IOL, etc. These can be avoided by careful, gentle instrumentation and as less manipulation as possible within the eye.

PHACOEMULSIFICATION PEARLS

- The experience of the surgeon and the nature of the cataract dictate the minimum pupil diameter for a case.
- Generally, if the pupil is large enough to perform an adequate capsulorhexis, it is large enough for the remainder of the surgical procedure.
- In cases with small pupil, the corneal incision must be made anteriorly to avoid the risk of iris prolapse with posterior corneal incisions.
- Capsular dyes such as indocyanine green (ICG) or trypan blue should be injected under the iris to aid in making the rhexis as well as to visualize the capsule as the pupil later enlarges.
- Hydrodissection should be gentle as an excessive fluid wave can cause iris prolapse.
- A retentive viscoelastic such as Healon5 should be used as it pressurizes the anterior chamber. As the intraocular pressure (IOP) increases, the viscoelastic remains in the eye and pushes down on the lens-iris diaphragm, thus mechanically enlarging the pupil. A cohesive type of viscoelastic is not as effective as it evacuates easily from the eye when IOP increases.
- Mini-sphincterotomies or the bimanual stretching technique of Luther Fry work well with fibrotic pupils such as those in patients on chronic miotic therapy. They are not as effective when the iris is elastic and floppy because the sphincter does not readily tear and the iris snaps back following stretching.
- A Sinskey or Kuglen hook can be inserted through the sideport incision to move the pupil away while doing capsulorhexis to achieve a larger sized rhexis.
- Sculpting is more difficult with small pupils as visualization is poor. The peripheral lens cannot be seen and the red reflex, which is required to visualize the depth of sculpting, is reduced by the smaller pupil diameter. These problems are overcome to a large extent using phaco chop techniques.
- For nucleus removal phaco chop, particularly vertical chop is the ideal technique in a miotic pupil, as it does not require a large pupil. Here, the phaco tip stays in

the center of the pupil for the majority of the time, and the chances of capturing the iris or capsular edge is much lesser. The second instrument can be used to move the pupil away to get a perfect position and then phaco chop can be performed.

- An injector is preferred over the folding forceps for inserting the IOL. The tip of the folder may catch the iris in the presence of iris prolapse or a flaccid iris and cause a dialysis. The injector tip immediately plugs the incision and there will be a net influx of viscoelastic instead.
- An injector separates the IOL from the surrounding tissues keeping it sterile. It also helps in exact positioning of the IOL which is an advantage in a small pupil or a flaccid iris.
- As long as the tip of the injector fits into the capsulorhexis, the IOL can be delivered into the bag without stretching or tearing the capsulorhexis.
- The second instrument or viscoelastic can be used to push the iris back and away from the bevel of the injector where it might otherwise be caught.
- For the trailing haptic, two instruments can be used: one to hold the iris and the other to dial in the trailing haptic.
- With plate haptic IOLs, anterior capsular contracture is greater and there is also more giant cell reaction, hence older silicone IOLs should be avoided in eyes that are likely to be inflamed.
- Latest generation silicone IOLs, such as clariflex (AMO), have no difference in long-term inflammatory profiles between hydrophobic acrylic and second generation silicone. The latest generation silicone achieved statistically significantly less inflammation than the AcrySof IOL in the long-term. The second generation and higher generation silicone IOLs are also more chemically pure and have a better overall design with a higher refractive index and thinner profile. Silicone IOLs also have a greater ease of implantation and reduced incision size as compared to acrylic IOLs.
- The Unfolder Emerald injector allows the surgeon to use a full size 6-mm optic acrylic IOL in a three-piece model through a 3-mm incision.
- A Lester hook (Katena Products, Inc.) can be used in the second hand to retract the pupil to re-tear and enlarge a small capsulorhexis.
- Irrespective of the method chosen for enlarging the pupil during phacoemulsification, the pupil should be constricted at the end of surgery with an intraocular miotic. If necessary, the pupil should be stroked with a blunt, gentle instrument to reduce its size. This prevents optic capture, capsular adhesion or other manner of pupillary deformity.

- Postoperatively, topical anti-inflammatory agents should be used to take care of the increased inflammatory activity secondary to increased maneuvering and longer and more difficult surgery.

REFERENCES

1. Guzek JP, Holm M, Cotter JB, et al. Risk factors for intraoperative complications in 1000 extracapsular cataract cases. Ophthalmology. 1987;94(5):461-6.
2. Masket S. Relationship between postoperative pupil size and disability glare. J Cataract Refract Surg. 1992;(18):506-7.
3. Fine IH. Phacoemulsification in the presence of a small pupil. In Steinert RF (Ed.). Cataract Surgery: Technique, Complications, & Management. Philadelphia: PA, WB Saunders; 1995. pp. 199-208.
4. Masket S. Cataract surgery complicated by the miotic pupil. In: Buratto L, Osher RH, Masket S (Eds). Cataract Surgery in Complicated Cases. Thorofare, NJ: Slack; 2000. pp. 131-7.
5. Thaller VT, Kulshrestha MK, Bell K. The effect of pre-operative topical flurbiprofen or diclofenac on pupil dilatation. Eye. 2000;14(Pt4):642-5.
6. Snyder RW, Siekert RW, Schwiegerling J, et al. Acular as a single agent for use as an antimiotic and anti-inflammatory in cataract surgery. J Cataract Refract Surg. 2000;26(8):1225-7.
7. Gupta VP, Dhaliwal U, Prasad N. Ketorolac tromethamine in the maintenance of intraoperative mydriasis. Ophthalmic Surg Lasers. 1997;28(9):731-8.
8. Solomon KD, Turkalj JW, Whiteside SB, et al. Topical 0.5% ketorolac vs 0.03% flurbiprofen for inhibition of miosis during cataract surgery. Arch Ophthalmol. 1997;115(9):1119-22.
9. Gimbel H, Van Westenbrugge J, Cheetham JK, et al. Intraocular availability and pupillary effect of flurbiprofen and indomethacin during cataract surgery. J Cataract Refract Surg. 1996;22(4):474-9.
10. Brown RM, Roberts CW. Preoperative and postoperative use of nonsteroidal antiinflammatory drugs in cataract surgery. Insight. 1996;21(1):13-6.
11. Kershner RM. Management of the small pupil for clear corneal cataract surgery. J Cataract Refract Surg. 2002;28(10):1826-31.
12. Shephard DM. The pupil stretch technique for miotic pupils in cataract surgery. Ophthalmic Surg. 1994;24:851-2.
13. De Juan Jr E, Hickingbotham D. Flexible iris retractors. Am J Ophthalmol. 1991;111:766-77.
14. Smith GT, Liu CSC. Flexible iris hooks for phacoemulsification in patients with iridoschisis. J Cataract Refract Surg. 2000;26:1277-80.
15. Nichamin LD. Enlarging the pupil for cataract extraction using flexible nylon iris retractors. J Cataract Refract Surg. 1993;19:793-6.
16. Masket S. Avoiding complications associated with iris retractor use in small pupil cataract extraction. J Cataract Refract Surg. 1996;22:168-71.
17. Graether JM. Graether pupil expander for managing the small pupil during surgery. J Cataract Refract Surg. 1996;22:530-5.
18. Benjamin Boyd. Phacoemulsification in small pupils. In The Art and Science of Cataract Surgery; Highlights of Ophthalmology. 2001.

CHAPTER 48

Intraoperative Floppy Iris Syndrome
David F Chang

In January 2005, John Campbell and the author reported and described a unique small pupil syndrome that we named intraoperative floppy iris syndrome (IFIS).[1-15] Besides a tendency for poor preoperative pupil dilation, severe IFIS exhibits a triad of intraoperative signs – iris billowing and floppiness, iris prolapse to the main and side port incisions and progressive intraoperative miosis **(Figure 48.1)**. Numerous studies have confirmed the initial suspicion that when such iris behavior is unexpected, the rate of cataract surgical complications is increased. Based upon parallel large retrospective (JC – 706 eyes) and prospective (DC – 900 eyes) clinical studies that had been conducted, the author identified a strong association of IFIS with either current or prior use of tamsulosin. This systemic alpha-1 antagonist is the most commonly prescribed medication for the symptomatic relief of benign prostatic hyperplasia (BPH). It is now universally recognized that other systemic alpha-1 antagonists, such as doxazosin, terazosin and alfuzosin are also associated with IFIS.

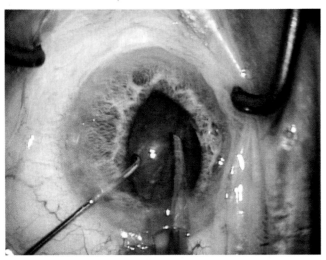

FIGURE 48.1: Patient on tamsulosin with iris billowing, intraoperative miosis and iris prolapse to the phaco and side port incisions

CLINICAL FEATURES

Although the author's original paper described a triad of signs, IFIS demonstrates a wide range of clinical severity. In a prospective study of 167 eyes in patients taking tamsulosin, the author classified IFIS as being mild (good dilation; some iris billowing without prolapse or constriction), moderate (iris billowing with some constriction of a moderately dilated pupil) or severe (classic triad and poor

preoperative dilation). Using this scale, the distribution of IFIS severity was - 10% no IFIS, 17% mild IFIS, 30% moderate IFIS and 43% severe IFIS. The tendency for iris prolapse often first appears during hydrodissection. Iris billowing may be seen when irrigation from the phaco tip is introduced, followed shortly thereafter by iris prolapse to both the incision and side port paracentesis. Progressive intraoperative pupil constriction may occur with or without accompanying iris prolapse. The combination of progressive miosis and iris floppiness increases the likelihood of iris aspirating the iris with the phaco tip.

When surgeons have not recognized or anticipated IFIS, the rate of reported intraoperative complications has been increased. Multiple retrospective studies have published higher rates of capsular rupture and vitreous loss. Complications of iris prolapse or aspiration include iridodialysis, iris sphincter damage, hyphema and significant iris stromal or transillumination defects. Such iris trauma can cause permanent pupil deformity with glare or photophobia. In 2009, a retrospective Canadian study of nearly 100,000 male cataract surgeries documented a doubling of the rate of serious postoperative complications including retinal detachment, retained nuclear fragments, and severe inflammation in tamsulosin patients.

One important caution with IFIS is that partial thickness sphincterotomies and manual pupil stretching are ineffective and can exacerbate iris billowing and prolapse. A medical history of systemic alpha-1 antagonist use should alert the cataract surgeon to anticipate IFIS and to consider alternative small pupil management strategies. Our multicenter, prospective study of 169 consecutive cataract surgeries in tamsulosin patients attained excellent outcomes with low surgical complications, by employing four specific operative techniques either alone or in combination. Using Healon5 viscomydriasis, iris retractors, preoperative topical atropine administration or pupil expansion rings, the incidence of posterior capsule rupture and vitreous loss was less than 1% in this clinical trial. However, because these were highly experienced cataract surgeons, this study may not be representative of the general surgical experience with IFIS. In a 2008 ASCRS membership survey, 95% of the respondents reported that tamsulosin increased the difficulty of cataract surgery and 77% believed that it also increased the risk of complications. Specifically, during the prior two years, IFIS had increased the rate of posterior capsular rupture for 52% of respondents and the rate of significant iris trauma for 23% of the respondents.

PHARMACOLOGY AND MECHANISM OF IFIS

Alpha-1 antagonists relax smooth muscle in the bladder neck and prostate. This permits more complete bladder emptying and thereby reduces the lower urinary tract symptoms of benign prostatic hyperplasia (BPH). There are at least three common human alpha-1 receptor subtypes - alpha-1A, alpha-1B and alpha-1D. Doxazosin, terazosin and alfuzosin are considered non-selective alpha-1 antagonists. Tamsulosin, however, is very selective for the alpha-1A receptor subtype, which predominates in the prostate as well as in the iris dilator smooth muscle. Because it theoretically should not block the vascular smooth muscle alpha-1D receptors, tamsulosin has a lower risk of causing postural hypotension. Although BPH is by far the most common indication, both men and women may take alpha-1 antagonists for other conditions. Tamsulosin is often briefly prescribed as an adjunctive medication to facilitate renal stone passage following shock wave lithotripsy. It may also be prescribed for urinary retention in women. Finally, alpha-1 antagonists, such as doxazosin, terazosin and prazosin have long been prescribed for systemic hypertension.

All alpha-1 antagonists may inhibit pupil dilation and cause IFIS. Several retrospective and prospective studies, however, suggest that the frequency and severity of IFIS is much higher with tamsulosin, as compared with non-selective alpha-1 antagonists. For example, the large retrospective Canadian study discussed earlier reported that tamsulosin significantly increased the rate of postoperative complications, but that non-selective alpha antagonists did not. A second Canadian retrospective study found that 86% of patients taking tamsulosin developed IFIS compared to only 15% of patients taking alfuzosin. These and other studies were supported by the 2008 ASCRS survey finding that 90% of respondents with sufficient experience believed that IFIS was more common with tamsulosin than with nonselective alpha-1 antagonists.

IFIS may also occur in patients without any history of alpha antagonist use.

In addition to confirming that IFIS was strongly correlated with alpha-1 antagonists, one prospective study found that IFIS was also associated with systemic hypertension in the absence of alpha blockers.

In the original publication, Campbell and the author hypothesized that IFIS was a manifestation of decreased iris dilator muscle tone and loss of intraoperative structural rigidity. Two separate slit lamp OCT studies have reported significant thinning of the mid-iris stromal thickness in tamsulosin patients when compared to control eyes. Another surprising but widespread finding is that IFIS can occur more than one year after tamsulosin has been discontinued. Ninety-five percent of ASCRS survey respondents have experienced IFIS in patients with only a prior history of alpha-1 antagonist use. Tamsulosin can even be recovered from aqueous samples taken 1-4 weeks after discontinuing the drug, suggesting that it has a very prolonged receptor binding time. The only large histopathologic study of

autopsy eyes from patients taking tamsulosin (26 eyes) showed atrophy of the iris dilator muscle, which could be consistent with a semi-permanent drug effect on iris morphology. Clearly, cataract surgical patients should be questioned about any prior alpha-1 antagonist use as well.

In conclusion, the mechanism of IFIS is not well understood. The stronger association with tamsulosin compared to nonselective alpha-1 antagonists and the occurrence of IFIS without any prior alpha blocker use suggest a more complex mechanism than that simply mediated by the alpha-1A receptor. The occurrence of IFIS long after tamsulosin cessation and the histopathologic findings further suggest a semi-permanent structural change occurring within the iris at some level. On the other hand, there are several anecdotal reports of IFIS occurring within 3–7 days of initiating tamsulosin treatment, meaning that chronicity is not necessary to cause this syndrome.

CLINICAL AND SURGICAL MANAGEMENT OF IFIS

PREOPERATIVE MANAGEMENT

The possibility of IFIS increases the importance of taking the patient's medication history prior to cataract surgery. A history of systemic alpha antagonists may not be elicited without direct questioning about current or prior use of prostate medication.

As discussed earlier, stopping tamsulosin preoperatively is of unpredictable and questionable value. With so many reported cases of IFIS occurring up to several years after the drug had been stopped, it is clear that ophthalmologists cannot rely solely upon drug cessation to prevent this condition. In the multicenter prospective trial mentioned earlier, tamsulosin was discontinued prior to surgery in 19% of patients, but did not result in any significant reduction in IFIS severity in this subgroup of eyes. In the 2008 ASCRS IFIS survey, 64% of respondents said that they never stop tamsulosin prior to surgery, compared to 11% who routinely do.

Preoperative atropine drops (e.g. 1% t.i.d. for 1-2 days preoperatively) can enhance cycloplegia as a means of preventing intraoperative miosis. However, the multicenter prospective tamsulosin study demonstrated that atropine, as a single strategy, is often ineffective for more severe cases of IFIS. In the ASCRS IFIS survey, 57% of respondents said that they never use topical atropine prior to surgery, compared to 19% who routinely do.

SURGICAL MANAGEMENT

The inter-individual variability in the severity of IFIS makes it difficult to determine whether one surgical strategy is superior to another. The severity of IFIS is likely to be greater in patients taking tamsulosin. Poor preoperative pupil dilation and billowing of the iris immediately following instillation of intracameral lidocaine are also predictive of greater IFIS severity. In contrast, if the pupil dilates well preoperatively, mild to moderate IFIS is more likely but the surgeon should still be prepared for iris prolapse and miosis. Patients taking nonselective alpha-1 antagonists or who have already discontinued these medications for several months are most likely to display mild to moderate IFIS.

Ideally, surgeons should be facile with several different approaches that may used alone or in combination to manage the iris in IFIS. In general, one should make a constructed shelved clear corneal incision, perform hydrodissection very gently, and consider reducing the irrigation and aspiration flow parameters if possible. Partial thickness sphincterotomies and mechanical pupil stretching are ineffective for IFIS and may worsen the iris prolapse and miosis.

Direct intracameral injection of alpha agonists, such as phenylephrine or epinephrine is a safe and simple pharmacologic strategy for IFIS. These alpha-1 agonists may further dilate the pupil **(Figures 48.2A and B)** and increase iris dilator muscle tone enough to reducing

billowing and the tendency for prolapse or sudden miosis. Preserved solutions should be avoided and one should dilute the 1:1000 commercial preparation in order to raise its acidic pH. American Regent and Cura Pharmaceuticals produce a bisulfite-free epinephrine solution. A 1:4000 epinephrine solution can be easily constituted by adding 0.2 ml of commercially available 1:1000 epinephrine to 0.6 ml of plain balanced salt solution or BSS Plus (Alcon) in a 3 ml disposable syringe. Because of the variable severity of IFIS, intracameral alpha agonists work well in some eyes but may have no detectable effect in others.

Although preferences for ophthalmic viscosurgical devices (OVD) vary widely, Healon 5 (Advanced Medical Optics) is a maximally cohesive single agent that is particularly well suited for viscomydriasis and for blocking the iris from prolapsing in IFIS **(Figure 48.3)**. Particularly, if mydriasis is insufficient after injecting an intracameral alpha agonist, Healon5 can be used to mechanically expand the pupil further. Viscomydriasis facilitates the capsulorhexis and combines with the epinephrine-induced iris rigidity to block iris prolapse. However, low flow and vacuum parameters (e.g. < 175–200 mm Hg; < 26 ml/min) should be used to avoid immediately aspirating Healon5 out of the eye. One should therefore not rely on this strategy if high vacuum and aspiration flow settings are desired for denser nuclei. In this situation, dispersive OVDs, such as DisCoVisc (Alcon) or Viscoat (Alcon) may persist longer within the anterior chamber. Finally, combining Healon5 with Viscoat has been advocated as a combination strategy whereby the Viscoat will better resist aspiration and delay the evacuation of Healon5.

The final category of strategies is the use of devices to mechanically expand and maintain the intraoperative pupil diameter. Disposable PMMA pupil expansion rings, such as the Morcher 5S Pupil Ring and the Milvella *Perfect Pupil,* have grooved contours and are threaded alongside the pupillary margin with dedicated metal injectors. Eagle Vision's Graether disposable silicone pupil expansion ring is inserted with a single use plastic injector. All of these

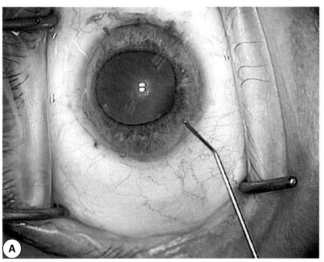

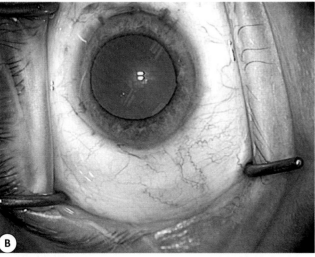

FIGURES 48.2A and B: Tamsulosin patient with pupil diameter before (A), and after (B) intracameral injection of 1:1000 unpreserved epinephrine mixture

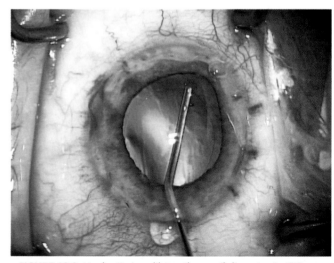

FIGURE 48.3: Healon5 viscodilates the pupil diameter in IFIS eye prior to IOL insertion

rings are relatively difficult to position if the pupil is less than 4 mm wide or if the anterior chamber is shallow. They will fail to engage the iris if the pupil diameter is larger than 7 mm.

Most surgeons find the Malyugin ring (Microsurgical technologies, Redmond WA) to be the easiest and fastest pupil expansion device to insert and remove. This is a 5-0 polypropylene single use device that is introduced with a disposable injector **(Figure 48.4)**. The way in which the iris drapes over the sides of the device creates a round 6 mm or 7 mm pupil diameter, depending on which of the two available sizes is used. The disposable injector tip fits through a 2.5 mm incision and is used to both place and extract the ring. Compared to bulkier and rigid plastic expansion rings, the thin profile of the Malyugin ring reduces the risk of accidental corneal or incisional trauma and does not impede instrument access to the cataract. The avoidance of multiple paracentesis sites, is advantageous in the presence of a bleb or pterygium, and avoids the problem of iris hooks being pushed against the lid speculum with a tight palpebral fissure. Finally, the smooth coils are very gentle on the pupil margin, and generally minimize iris sphincter damage.

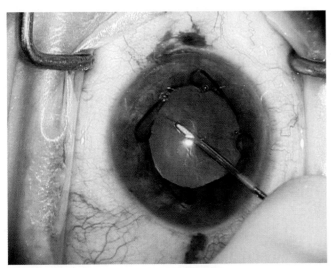

FIGURE 48.4: Malyugin ring (6 mm diameter) expands the pupil in an eye with IFIS

Iris retractors continue to be a popular mechanical strategy for managing IFIS. As described by Oetting and Omphroy, there are several advantages to placing the hooks in a diamond configuration **(Figure 48.5)**. The subincisional hook is placed through a separate paracentesis that is made just posterior to the temporal clear corneal phaco incision, so that it can pull the iris down and behind the phaco tip. This not only provides excellent access to subincisional cortex, but also avoids tenting the iris up in front of the phaco tip, such as occurs when the retractors are placed in a square configuration. Iris retractors may potentially overstretch a fibrotic pupil resulting in bleeding, sphincter tears and permanent mydriasis. This usually does not occur in IFIS because the pupil is so elastic that it readily springs

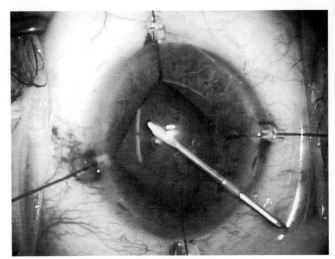

FIGURE 48.5: Reusable 4-0 Prolene iris retractors placed in a diamond configuration in IFIS patient

back to physiologic size despite being maximally stretched. Iris retractors therefore provide excellent surgical exposure for IFIS. Compared to 6-0 nylon disposable retractors (Alcon) 4-0 polypropylene retractors (Katena, FCI, Oasis) are stiffer and easier to manipulate. Reusable 4-0 polypropylene retractors can be repeatedly autoclaved in the manufacturer supplied storage case making them more cost effective than their disposable counterparts.

It is easier and safer to insert pupil expansion rings or iris retractors prior to creation of the capsulorhexis. If the pupil dilates poorly preoperatively (e.g. 3–5 mm diameter) or billows during injection of intracameral lidocaine, one should consider proceeding directly to mechanical devices because of the likelihood of severe IFIS. Both iris retractors and the Malyugin pupil expansion device provide reliable assurance that the pupil will be adequately large and cannot constrict intraoperatively. Mechanical devices also permit surgeons to use their preferred OVD, phaco technique and fluidic parameters. If the pupil dilates well preoperatively, but begins to constrict or prolapse after hydrodissection or during phaco, combining intracameral epinephrine and Healon5 can be an excellent rescue technique that may avoid the need to insert mechanical devices. If iris retractors are used, one should retract the pupil margin with a second instrument to avoid hooking the capsulorhexis margin with the retractors.

Eliciting a history of current or prior alpha-1 antagonist use should alert surgeons to anticipate IFIS and to employ these strategies either alone or in combination. Because of the variability in IFIS severity, many surgeons use a staged management approach. Pharmacologic measures alone may be sufficient for mild to moderate IFIS cases. Even if they fail to enlarge the pupil, intracameral alpha agonists can reduce or prevent iris billowing and prolapse by increasing iris dilator muscle tone. If the pupil diameter is still inadequate, viscomydriasis with Healon5 can further expand it for the capsulorhexis step. Finally, mechanical expansion devices assure the best surgical exposure for severe IFIS, and should be considered when other risk factors, such as weak zonules or a brunescent nucleus are present.

REFERENCES

1. Chang DF, Campbell JR. Intraoperative floppy iris syndrome associated with tamsulosin (Flomax). J Cataract Refract Surg. 2005;31:664-73.

2. Chang DF, Osher RH, Wang L, et al. Prospective multicenter evaluation of cataract surgery in patients taking tamsulosin (Flomax). Ophthalmology. 2007;114:957-64.

3. Chang DF, Braga Mele R, Mamalis N, et al. For the ASCRS Cataract Clinical Committee. ASCRS White Paper: Intraoperative Floppy Iris Syndrome – A Clinical Review. J Cataract Refract Surg. 2008;34:2153-62.

4. Chang DF, Braga-Mele R, Mamalis N, et al. For the ASCRS Cataract Clinical Committee. Clinical experience with intraoperative floppy-iris syndrome. Results of the 2008 ASCRS member survey. J Cataract Refract Surg. 2008;34:1201-9.

5. Bell CM, Hatch WV, Fischer HD, et al. Association between tamsulosin and serious ophthalmic adverse events in older men following cataract surgery. JAMA. 2009;301:1991-6.

6. Masket S, Belani S. Combined preoperative topical atropine sulfate 1% and intracameral nonpreserved epinephrine hydrochloride 1:4000 [corrected] for management of intraoperative floppy-iris syndrome. J Cataract Refract Surg. 2007;33:580-2.

7. Shugar JK. Intracameral Epinephrine for Prophylaxis of IFIS [letter]. J Cataract Refract Surg. 2006;32:1074-5.

8. Arshinoff SA. Modified SST-USST for tamsulosin-associated intraocular floppy iris syndrome. J Cataract Refract Surg. 2006;32: 559-61.

9. Manvikar S, Allen D. Cataract surgery management in patients taking tamsulosin. J Cataract Refract Surg. 2006; 32:1611-4.

10. Chang DF. Use of Malyugin pupil expansion device for intraoperative floppy iris syndrome: Results in 30 consecutive cases. J Cataract Refract Surg. 2008;34:835-41.

11. Schwinn DA, Afshari NA. Alpha (1)-Adrenergic receptor antagonists and the iris: new mechanistic insights into floppy iris syndrome. Surv Ophthalmol. 2006;51:501-12.

12. Cantrell MA, Bream-Rouwenhorst HR, Steffensmeier A, et al. Intraoperative Floppy Iris Syndrome Associated with {alpha}1-Adrenergic Receptor Antagonists. Ann Pharmacother. 2008;42:558-63.

13. Neff KD, Sandoval HP, Fernandez de Castro, LE, et al. Factors associated with intraoperative floppy iris syndrome. Ophthalmology. 2009;116:658-63.

14. Palea S, Chang DF, Rekik M, et al. Comparative effect of alfuzosin and tamsulosin on the contractile response of isolated rabbit prostatic and iris dilator smooth muscles. Possible model for intraoperative floppy iris syndrome. J Cataract Refract Surg. 2008;34:489-96.

15. Chang DF. Editorial. American Family Physician. Floppy Iris Syndrome: Why BPH can Complicate Cataract Surgery. 2009;79:1051-6.

CHAPTER 49

Phacoemulsification and Keratoplasty

Javier Mendicute, Yolanda Gallego, Aritz Bidaguren, Marta Ubeda, Cristina Irigoyen

INTRODUCTION

In certain circumstances, and despite the existence of a cataract, lens surgery may not be sufficient to achieve correct visual recovery. This is particularly true when associated with corneal pathology. In this kind of cases, the only way to restore the visual function is by associating cataract surgery with keratoplasty.

There are several classic ways of dealing with this problem: (1) Firstly, performing cataract or cornea surgery and subsequently implementing a keratoplasty or cataract surgery where necessary; (2) The simultaneous carrying out of both procedures (keratoplasty and cataract surgery); and (3) Triple procedures (keratoplasty, cataract surgery and intraocular lens implantation).

Given problems of infrastructure and the cornea donor requirements of keratoplasty, it used to be common practice to start by performing lens surgery; subsequently potentially considering a keratoplasty,[1-4] depending on the visual recovery achieved. Proceeding inversely was less common, i.e. first of all, performing a keratoplasty and subsequently cataract surgery where necessary. This latter option had the following drawbacks: Firstly, a new incision, either corneal or scleral, had to be made. This incision usually had to be long in the case of both intracapsular and extracapsular extraction; in the second place, endothelial damage to the transplanted cornea sometimes threatened its viability. It was also true that cataracts often developed following the keratoplasty, whether due to the surgical intervention itself or to the required postoperative medication.

Combined procedures were therefore considered. These first of all took the shape of double procedures combining intracapsular or extracapsular cataract extraction with keratoplasty. When the procedure implemented was intracapsular extraction, vitreous contact with the corneal endothelium was described as the cause of keratoplasty rejection, whether or not the anterior hyaloid was intact. Although vitreous-endothelium contact was avoided during extracapsular extraction, the potential appearance of secondary posterior capsule opacification, and the absence of Yag laser, meant that another surgical procedure was required to solve the problem at hand. In any case, double procedures were, at least in theory, highly attractive.

With the modern development of extracapsular lens extraction, plus introduction of the intraocular lens and Yag laser, triple procedures seemed to offer the best possible surgical option: an operation, an incision, three procedures (keratoplasty, extracapsular extraction and intraocular lens

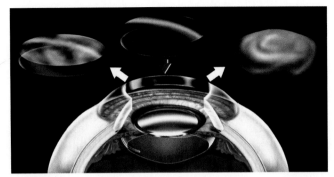

FIGURE 49.1: Triple procedure: keratoplasty, extracapsular cataract extraction and intraocular lens implantation

TABLE 49.1	Triple procedure with extracapsular extraction: drawbacks
• Necessary pupil dilatation can complicate centering of the keratoplasty	
• Most of the procedure is performed with open-sky surgery	
• Difficult extraction of the nucleus in hypotonic eyes	
• Difficult aspiration of the cortical mass	
• In the case of capsular rupture, vitreous loss may be problematic	
• In the case of choroidal or expulsive hemorrhage, the consequences can be devastating	

implantation) **(Figure 49.1)** in one surgical operation and the possibility of good visual recovery in a relatively short time. The drawbacks in triple procedure are shown in **Table 49.1**.

The following question has therefore emerged in recent years: *Why not perform phacoemulsification in triple procedures?*

We consider that this procedure would have certain advantages **(Table 49.2)** and perhaps, certain limitations rather than drawbacks.

TABLE 49.2	Triple procedure with phacoemulsification: advantages
• Most of the triple procedure is performed with closed-system surgery	
• Cortical aspiration is simpler	
• If the intraocular lens is implanted prior to the keratoplasty, the pupil may contract, thus facilitating centering of the keratoplasty	
• The zonule-capsular barrier, reinforced by implantation of the intraocular lens, maintains its ocular compartmentalization	
• Potential capsular rupture or choroidal hemorrhage is more controllable	

INDICATIONS

When considering a combined procedure (keratoplasty and cataract surgery) one has to evaluate not only the condition of the lens but also the state of the cornea and the degree of visual incapacity potentially justifying corneal and lens alteration.[5] When considering keratoplasty and based on its level of complexity, we must also evaluate the potential visual acuity of the affected eye.

CATARACT EVALUATION IN PATIENTS WITH CORNEAL OPACIFICATION

Having diagnosed the corneal problem, we must evaluate-interpret the degree of lens opacification in order to establish whether or not a simultaneous procedure is advisable.[6]

It is useful to evaluate the thickness of the affected cornea:

1. If opacification is superficial, we can consider either phototherapeutic excimer laser or superficial lamellar keratectomy. Phototherapeutic keratectomy can be useful if the opacification covers no more than the most superficial 140 μm of the cornea, although we must not forget that this technique can cause hyperopia, more pronounced the deeper and smaller in diameter the areas treated.[7]

2. Superficial keratectomy with microkeratome is useful if opacification of the anterior stroma only involves the anterior 180 μm of the cornea.[8] In none of these cases it is necessary to substitute eliminated anterior corneal tissue with donor tissue.

3. In cases where the corneal pathology lies in deeper anterior stromal layers, one can consider an anterior lamellar keratoplasty associated with phacoemulsification as an alternative to penetrating keratoplasty.

4. If almost all of the corneal thickness is opacified but the deepest membrane and endothelial-Descemet complex are normal, one can perform a deep anterior lamellar keratoplasty together with a phacoemulsification.[9,10]

CORNEAL EVALUATION IN PATIENTS WITH CATARACTS

The author occasionally has to consider the inverse situation: That of having to evaluate the state of the cornea in a patient with cataract, given that it is not unusual to come across cornea guttata, Fuchs' dystrophy or other corneal pathologies which tend to increase considerably in frequency and seriousness with age. When alterations in the corneal endothelium membrane exist, it could be useful to study the membrane in question with endothelial specular microscopy. Another examination which provides important information is ultrasound pachymetry **(Table 49.3)**.

However, practically speaking, the decision of whether to simply operate on the cataract or to perform a combined procedure (keratoplasty and cataract extraction) initially

TABLE 49.3	Corneal evaluation in patients with cataracts

- Endothelial specular microscopy
- Corneal edema
- Central corneal thickness by pachymetry
- Corneal topography

depends on two factors: (1) The corneal stromal edema; and (2) The central corneal pachymetry. If the pachymetric readings are higher than 640–650 μm and a stromal edema exists, a combined procedure is advisable. If there is no edema, and the reading is lower than 640 μm, an isolated phacoemulsification technique implies no great risk of endothelial decompensation, given that the latest cataract surgery advances and the appropriate use of viscoelastics has reduced the risk of corneal decompensation in pathologies like Fuchs' dystrophy.[11] However, we have to use a viscoelastic providing maximum endothelial protection in order to reduce this risk. In this respect, hyaluronate sodium and chondroitin sulphate seem to provide maximum intraoperative endothelial protection, causing a lower post-surgical loss of endothelial cells.[12,13]

Corneal topography may well be extremely useful when evaluating corneal status in these situations. This procedure helps to establish whether corneal opacity exists on the anterior surface of the cornea **(Figure 49.2)**, in which case it would become obvious, or inside the stroma (*vg* interstitial keratitis), where the topography would suffer no alteration. This differentiation is of capital importance and one must not forget that the anterior corneal surface is responsible for greater refractive power of the eye and that its alteration strongly compromises visual acuity. On the contrary, a relatively dense stromal scar may not cause obvious impairment to the visual function. Endeavoring to adapt a contact lens with a view to reducing irregular astigmatisms can be useful in evaluating potential visual acuity and can even improve the sight.

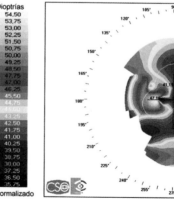

FIGURE 49.2: Corneal topography demonstrating anterior corneal surface damage

WHEN TO OPERATE?

Surgery must be considered when the corneal opacity and cataract are sufficiently dense to justify the visual limitations indicated by the patient and when optical and medical alternatives are not sufficient to recover the sight or to satisfy the patient's needs. On the other hand, recourse should be taken to non-surgical treatment when the visual function, esthetics and discomfort or pain can be improved and eased by other methods.

One must occasionally consider surgery when pain or ugliness justifies the decision without waiting for the recovery of sight; this said, it will probably not be necessary to perform a triple procedure in these cases, given that a keratoplasty may well be sufficient.

COMBINED OR TWO-STAGE PROCEDURE?

Having taken the decision to remove the cataract and perform a keratoplasty, we must ask ourselves whether to do so in two separate stages or in one single procedure.

COMBINED PROCEDURES

The advantages of performing cataract surgery and a keratoplasty in one single operation, as part of a combined procedure, are:

- A single operation
- The use of a standard, well-known technique
- Lower financial cost
- Less risk for the corneal endothelium than performing cataract surgery at a second time following penetrating keratoplasty;[14,15] this said, certain authors[16] find no particular difference in endothelial readings among patients on whom a combined procedure was performed and those on whom a second phacoemulsification was performed following keratoplasty, probably due to advances in phacoemulsification technology and the rational use of new viscoelastics
- Not having to repeat cataract surgery, a procedure which has almost become standard post-keratoplasty[17] due to the cataractogenic nature of corneal transplant surgery, in general, and to the use of steroids at the postoperative stage, in particular
- Evidence that posterior capsular opacification occurs less frequently (9.8% vs. 36.2%) and at a later stage (45.6 months vs. 24.3 months) with combined procedures than with isolated cataract extraction.[18]
- The higher tendency for the cataract to progress in patients previously treated with keratoplasty

The advantages of extracapsular surgical cataract extraction are obvious given the knowledge that intracapsular lens surgery is recognized as one of the risk factors behind the development of corneal failure in combined procedures. The risk of intracapsular extraction could be

the result of the vitreous/corneal endothelium contact arising with this technique due to the non-existence of anatomical barriers.[19] The differences between conventional extracapsular surgery and phacoemulsification are not as yet well defined.

TWO-STAGE PROCEDURE

Among the advantages of performing keratoplasty and cataract surgery in two stages, as independent procedures, we could underline:

- Improved refractive predictability when the cataract surgery is performed following keratoplasty, given the possibility of obtaining true keratometric readings. Numerous articles have been published in the past, indicating the results obtained with the triple procedure; these studies describe refractive errors varying between -14.7 diopters to +8.0 diopters, with the percentage of patients showing a final refraction of ± 2.0 diopters standing at between 26% and 68%[16]
- Technically speaking, independent keratoplasty is safer due to the fact that it can be carried out with the patient in miosis; hence the pupil becomes a useful reference for centring the keratoplasty
- Sequential cataract surgery, although complicated by the keratoplasty interface and occasionally by the presence of suturing, may be simpler, given that the performing of an open-sky capsulorhexis or cortical aspiration, as corresponding to a combined procedure, is more complex.

IOL CALCULATION

One of the greatest drawbacks of the combined procedure, an advantage therefore of the two-stage technique (keratoplasty followed by cataract surgery), is the difficulty of correctly calculating the power of the lens to be implanted during a triple procedure of cataract extraction, intraocular lens implantation and keratoplasty. One of the reasons for residual refractive error following triple procedures is not having preoperative knowledge of the keratometric reading resulting from the keratoplasty. Calculating the power of the lens to be implanted seems to be more predictable if we consider the refractive results obtained on carrying out the procedures separately, with up to 95% of patients showing readings of ± 2.0 diopters.[20]

Whatever the case, when performing two-stage surgery one must wait for a minimum of three months between the keratoplasty and cataract extraction for the keratometric readings to offer minimum reliability for lens calculation. Even so, the central corneal curvature will not be totally stable, until the corneal sutures have been removed (a year after the keratoplasty). And even then, calculating the power of the lens can bring more postoperative refractive surprises than using the postoperative K, generally more curved than the physiological preoperative version, especially if one uses donor grafts of a larger diameter than the recipient beds; using this K can cause defects in the ELP (Effective Lens Position) calculation if based on the SRK/T formula.[21] Given the above, in the case of keratoplasty followed by cataract surgery, one uses the double K method recommended for cataract surgery following corneal refractive surgery,[22] using the K of the contralateral eye, if it is normal, in the first part of the formula to calculate the ELP and the true keratometry following the keratoplasty in the second part of the formula serving to calculate the lens power for a specific keratometry and axial length. If the contralateral eye is not normal, we recommend that a normal average keratometry (43–44 diopters) be used in the first part of the formula serving to calculate the ELP.

WHAT TECHNIQUE SHOULD WE USE?

We have selected some of the above-mentioned alternatives based on our observations regarding the grade of corneal opacification and its depth (Table 49.4):

- The appropriate alternative in the case of superficial opacification (0-140 µm) is phototherapeutic keratectomy. One drawback of this option is that it has to be performed with an excimer laser, not always available in the same operating theater, meaning that the patient has to be moved. It can be performed at the same time as or prior to phacoemulsification. We must remember that this process will modify the corneal curvature, a factor which could condition the intraocular lens power calculation; if performed previously, this change can be considered in the biometric calculation; however, if performed simultaneously, one will not know the correct keratometry, a factor conditioning the refractive result.

- If opacification is somewhat deeper (0–180 µm), a free superficial keratectomy with microkeratome and no corneal substitution could be the solution in certain cases.[8] Here we would be faced with the same limitation as indicated above when calculating the intraocular lens. This said, free superficial keratectomy can be performed in the operating theater itself. Although true that the corneal surface following operation becomes irregular and can complicate the visualization of intraocular structures, the effect is not as great as corneal opacification; in this case, the given optical aids can be useful, the best of which is application of viscoelastic to the cornea.

- If the corneal pathology is located in deeper anterior stromal layers (0–300 µm), one can consider an anterior lamellar keratoplasty associated with phacoemulsification as an alternative to the penetrating keratoplasty. Here we would start by performing a free-running anterior keratectomy at the desired depth, followed by a phacoemulsification and finally transplant of the anterior corneal tissue.

- The chosen technique for deep opacities (0–500 µm) is anterior lamellar keratoplasty.[9] We first of all eliminate the anterior corneal stroma, performing a phacoemulsification after having applied viscoelastic to the deep corneal stroma to favor visualization, finally substituting the anterior corneal stroma at the end of the procedure.

- If the entire thickness of the cornea is compromised, complete trephination may be necessary. In this case, if one does not want to renounce phacoemulsification, one will have to use a transitory keratoprosthesis[23] or a transitory corneal graft[24] for substitution at a later date by the definitive cornea.

NINE OPTICAL AIDS FOR IMPROVING VISUALIZATION

The basic key for completion of the phacoemulsification on a cornea with obvious opacification is visualization of the anterior segment structures (Table 49.5).

The following procedures, listed from more to less simple, may be useful:[25]

1. Switching off the main lights in the operating theater.
2. Applying viscoelastics to the cornea which, once in place, magnify the anterior chamber structures, thus potentially facilitating the different phacoemulsification stages.
3. Using optic fiber, whether from outside of the eye or introducing it to the anterior chamber by paracentesis.
4. It is sometimes possible to focus the microscope beneath the cornea and obtain suitable visualization for proceeding with the phacoemulsification. Doing this can

TABLE 49.4	Phaco-keratoplasty: Selection of techniques
0–140 µm corneal opacity	Phototherapeutic keratectomy (PTK)
0–180 µm corneal opacity	Free superficial keratectomy
0–300 µm corneal opacity	Automated lamellar keratoplasty
0–500 µm corneal opacity	Deep anterior lamellar keratoplasty
Full thickness corneal opacity	Transitory keratoprosthesis or graft

TABLE 49.5	Optical and visual aids for phacoemulsification with corneal opacification

- Switching off the main lights in the operating theater
- Applying viscoelastics to the cornea
- Using optic fiber
- Focussing the microscope beneath the cornea for adequate visualization during phacoemulsification
- De-epithelializing in the case of epithelial edemas or irregular corneal epithelial surfaces
- Lamellar keratectomies of sufficient thickness to include corneal opacification
- Deep anterior lamellar keratoplasties in the case of corneal opacifications located in deep stromal layers
- Using trypan blue for capsular tincture
- Transitory corneal prosthesis

serve to modify the microscope angle of inclination and to move the ocular globe into different positions in the endeavor to find the areas of best visualization.

5. In the case of epithelial edemas or highly irregular corneal epithelial surfaces, it is useful to de-epithelialize the cornea before starting the procedure.

6. When the above measures are insufficient, performing lamellar keratoplasties of sufficient thickness to include the corneal opacity and smoothing the resulting surface with viscoelastic material facilitates lens visualization. This kind of keratectomy can be performed manually or automatically with a microkeratome. Using a microkeratome shortens surgical times.

7. If the above measures are insufficient, deep anterior lamellar keratoplasty will make it possible to overcome the visualization problems caused by deep corneal opacification.[9]

8. As a last option for dense corneal opacification when wishing to proceed with a phacoemulsification, one can perform a complete trephination, followed by a transitory corneal prosthesis, phacoemulsification, removal of the transitory prosthesis and transplant.

9. Another interesting option is to apply trypan blue for improved capsule visibility,[26] thus increasing contrast and potentially facilitating the capsulorhexis.

PHACOEMULSIFICATION AND PENETRATING KERATOPLASTY

The conventional combined procedure (cataract surgery and keratoplasty) consists of performing a corneal trephination, open-sky extracapsular lens extraction, intraocular lens implantation and suturing of the donor corneal button to the recipient bed. Nowadays, with the spreading of phacoemulsification as the generally preferred method for cataract extraction, another triple procedure has come to light: lens phacoemulsification, intraocular lens implantation and the performing of a keratoplasty as if one was dealing with a phakic eye. The only circumstance conditioning the performing of phaco-keratoplasty is the degree of corneal opacity and the only cases where this technique cannot be performed is where the cornea is sufficiently opaque, to prevent visualization of the anterior segment structures, as is the case with Schnyder's dystrophy.

INCISION

The author is of the opinion that making the incision in a clear cornea is not advisable when the phacoemulsification is to be associated with a keratoplasty. Although some people[27] do use this technique, the author believes that it can have a number of drawbacks: Proximity of the incision in the clear cornea to the donor-recipient interface means that mutual tractions threaten their watertightness once both have been sutured. In the author's opinion, making a frown-type incision in the superior sclera is the best option. Once

the conjunctiva has been dissected, one coagulates the scleral bed and marks a frown incision measuring 2.75–3.2 mm in width. The scleral incision is then tunnelled, performing an ancillary puncture (for right-handed surgeons) to the left of the frown, filling the anterior chamber via this puncture with viscoelastic liquid and proceeding to approach the anterior chamber through the sclera tunnel with a 2.75–3.2 mm scalpel. Here it is extremely important not to advance excessively on the cornea at the entrance to the anterior chamber, given that doing so could interfere with the borders of the corneal transplant **(Figure 49.3)**. It is precisely now, and at no other time, that one must apply viscoelastic to the cornea in the case of suspected visualization problems; before that, it it is not appropriate because it would complicate control of the entrance incision to the anterior chamber and later it may no longer be necessary and would oblige us to suspend the procedure, during the time it takes for the viscoelastic to spread over the corneal convexity.

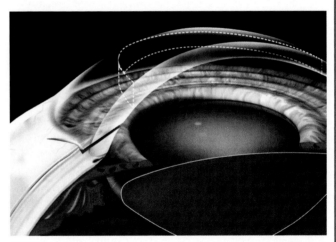

FIGURE 49.3: The entrance to the anterior chamber must not be too advanced given that it could damage the limits of the keratoplasty

CAPSULORHEXIS

Having filled the anterior chamber with viscoelastic, the next step is to perform the capsulorhexis. Here one must attempt to apply the options considered in the section on "Nine optical aids".Having started the capsulorhexis in the desired area with either a cystitome or forceps, it will be simpler to continue with forceps alone in the case of poor visibility. It is a good idea to control the anterior capsule, not by its line of progress, but by its radius **(Figure 49.4)**, an area in which visualization may be simpler given the formation of reflections at this level.

HYDRODISSECTION-HYDRODELAMINATION

This must be no different to the procedure employed in any other phacoemulsification process. Here the author would only point out that it must be sufficiently meticulous to ensure correct liberation of the crystalline lens nucleus without endangering capsular integrity, a risk which is

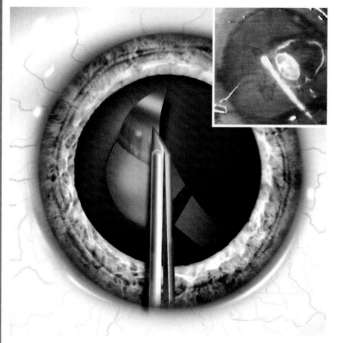

FIGURE 49.4: Controlling the capsulorhexis by visualizing its radius through a corneal opacification

greater in these cases due to deficient visualization of the different surgical steps.

NUCLEAR PHACOEMULSIFICATION

Nuclear phacoemulsification can be performed inside or outside of the capsular bag, as the surgeon prefers. The author is more familiar with phacoemulsification inside the bag, and performs it thus even in combined procedures. Other authors[27-33] suggest that the phacoemulsification be performed outside of the bag, in the anterior chamber, assuring that there is a lower risk of capsular rupture, a claim which may be true, while defending the fact that the greater loss of endothelial cells is of scant importance, given that the cornea is being transplanted immediately. However, one would say that not the whole cornea is transplanted; only the central button, and that a phacoemulsification in the anterior chamber may decrease endothelial density of the recipient cornea, even though one only conserves its rim. The author would add that being able to luxate the nucleus into the anterior chamber, either by hydrodissection or viscoexpression, requires having performed an extensive capsulorhexis.

ASPIRATION OF THE CORTEX

As far as parameters and strategies are concerned, irrigation-aspiration of the cortex is identical to that performed in other situations. The author uses an aspiration rate of 25 cc/min, vacuum of 500 mm Hg (linear mode) and bottle at 65–80 cm. On occasions, when visibility is exceedingly poor, one can use an aspiration rate of 18–20 cc/min, hence stressing safety over rapidity, while moving the globe towards areas in which the aspiration point is more visible.

INTRAOCULAR LENS IMPLANTATION

Having completed aspiration of the cortex, the author proceeds to fill the capsular bag with viscoelastic liquid and subsequently enlarge the scleral incision according to the lens to be implanted.

CLOSING THE SCLERAL INCISION

The situation described (frown incision when performing a phacokeratoplasty) is the only occasion on which the author goes about systematic suturing in a phacoemulsification with scleral incision; not in order to maintain watertightness of the globe during the keratoplasty, but to ensure that, once the donor button has been sutured, there is no traction on the anterior lip of the scleral incision. Although a traction of this kind could half-open the incision **(Figure 49.5)**, this is not the greatest concern, but rather the fact that it could provide poor support to the corneal rim of the bed receiving the keratoplasty at the phacoemulsification incision level. The author normally uses two radial sutures **(Figure 49.6)** or one horizontal Nylon 10/0 suture, subsequently burying the knot.

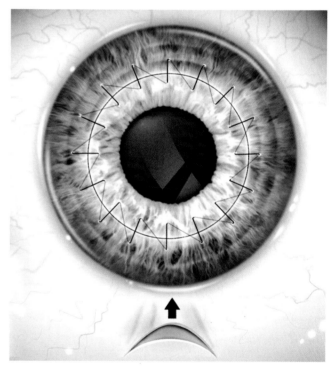

FIGURE 49.5: Closing the scleral incision. Traction on the keratoplasty suture of the frown incision if it does not suture

CORNEAL TREPHINATION

Before performing this operation, the author fills the anterior chamber with acetylcholine to achieve a good miosis, facilitating centring of the trephination. Before starting the corneal trephination, the author prepares the trephines and donor button at our surgery, storing the latter in viscoelastic liquid on an ancillary table. The technique is as follows: The author always trephines the donor button on its endothelial face (working with preserved corneal

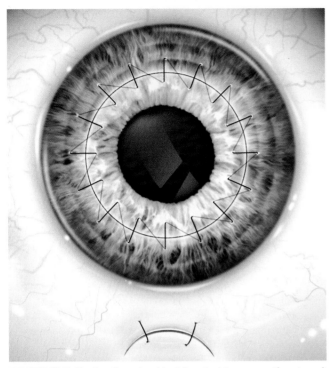

FIGURE 49.6: Closing the scleral incision. Incision correctly sutured

buttons) and similarly always does so with Hessburg-Barron trephines.

SUTURING THE KERATOPLASTY

The suturing of the graft is, together with the quality of the donor cornea, the main factor conditioning the final result of the operation. Correctly suturing the graft **(Figure 49.6)** to the host will determine its proper healing and can have a decisive influence on an ideal, or at least acceptable, refractive result permitting visual rehabilitation of the eye.

PHACOEMULSIFICATION AND LAMELLAR TECHNIQUES

The introduction in recent years of lamellar techniques means that we can use their surgical principles either to facilitate phacoemulsification and simultaneously perform a penetrating keratoplasty or to replace these with other lamellar keratoplasty techniques.

COMPLETE THICKNESS CORNEAL OPACITY

In this situation, if one wishes to perform a phacoemulsification, one has to take recourse to complete trephination of the cornea, its substitution with a transitory keratoprosthesis **(Figures 49.7A to D)**, the performing of phacoemulsification and replacement of the transitory prosthesis with the donor cornea. The choice of the author transitory prosthesis is Edkardt, the diameter of which obliges to perform trephinations of 7 mm.

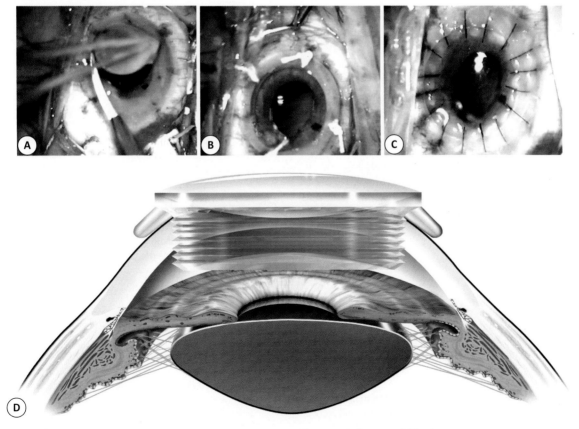

FIGURES 49.7A TO D: Keratoprosthesis and phacoemulsification

CONCLUSION

Despite varying opinions, the author believes that phacoemulsification as a cataract extraction technique within a triple procedure can offer certain advantages. In addition to the security offered by working in a closed system, in the author's experience it is obvious that extraction of the nucleus and of the cortex, despite poor corneal transparency, is much simpler than when working open-sky. The amount of time of ocular exposition without a corneal button is also shorter and complications of a capsular rupture or expulsive hemorrhage nature, if they occur, have less consequence.

KEY POINTS

- When considering a combined procedure (keratoplasty and cataract surgery) one has to evaluate not only the condition of the lens but also the state of the cornea and the degree of visual incapacity potentially justifying corneal and lens alteration.
- The decision of whether to simply operate on the cataract or to perform a combined procedure (keratoplasty and cataract extraction) initially depends on two factors: (1) The corneal stromal edema; and (2) The central corneal pachymetry.
- One of the greatest drawbacks of the combined procedure, an advantage therefore of the two-stage technique (keratoplasty followed by cataract surgery), is the difficulty of correctly calculating the power of the lens to be implanted during a triple procedure of cataract extraction, intraocular lens implantation and keratoplasty.
- The conventional combined procedure (cataract surgery and keratoplasty) consists of performing a corneal trephination, open-sky extracapsular lens extraction, intraocular lens implantation and suturing of the donor corneal button to the recipient bed.
- With the spreading of phacoemulsification as the generally preferred method for cataract extraction, another triple procedure has come to light: Lens phacoemulsification, intraocular lens implantation and the performing of a keratoplasty as if one was dealing with a phakic eye.

REFERENCES

1. Malbran ES, Malbran E, Buonsanti J, et al. Closed-system phacoemulsification and posterior chamber implant combined with penetrating keratoplasty. Ophthalmic Surg. 1993;24: 403-6.
2. Baca SL, Epstein RJ. Closed chamber capsulorhexis for cataract extraction combined with penetrating keratoplasty. J Cataract Refract Surg. 1998;24:581-4.
3. Caporossi A, Traversi C, Simi C, et al. Closed-system and open-sky capsulorhexis for combined cataract extraction and corneal transplantation. J Cataract Refract Surg. 2001;27:990-3.
4. Chu TG, Green RL. Suprachoroidal hemorrhage. Surv Ophthalmol. 1999;43:471-86.
5. Agency for Health Care Policy and Research. Cataract in adults: Management of Functional Impairment. Rockville: MD: US DHHS; AHCPR Publ No. 93-0542; 1993.
6. American Academy of Ophthalmology. Comprehensive Adult Eye Evaluation. Preferred Practice Pattern. San Francisco; 1992.
7. Dogru M, Katakami C, Yamanaka A. Refractive changes after excimer laser phototherapeutic keratectomy. J Cataract Refract Surg. 2001;27:686-92.
8. Pérez-Santonja JJ, Galal A, Muñoz G. Queratectomía lamelar superficial. In: Villarrubia A, Mendicute J, Pérez-Santonja JJ, et al (Eds). Queratoplastia lamelar: técnicas quirúrgicas. Madrid: Mac Line S.L, 2005. pp. 36-43.
9. Muraine MC, Collet A, Brasseur G. Deep lamellar keratoplasty combined with cataract surgery. Arch Ophthalmol. 2002;120: 812-5.
10. Alldredge CD, Alldredge OC Jr. Penetrating keratoplasty and cataract extraction. In: Krachmer JH, Mannis MJ, Holland EJ (Eds). Cornea, 3 vols. St. Louis: Mosby; 1997 II. pp. 1593-601.
11. Seitzman GD, Gottsch JD, Stark WJ. Cataract surgery in patients with Fuchs's corneal dystrophy: expanding recommendations for cataract surgery without simultaneous keratoplasty. Ophthalmology. 2005;112:441-6.
12. Craig MT, Olson RJ, Mamalis N. Air bubble endothelial damage during phacoemulsification in human eye bank eyes: the protective effects of Healon and Viscoat. J Cataract Refract Surg. 1990;16:597-602.
13. Koch DD, Liu JF, Glasser DB, et al. A comparison of corneal endothelial changes after use of Healon or Viscoat during phacoemulsification. Am J Ophthalmol. 1993;115:188-201.
14. Zacks CM, Abbott RL, Fine M. Long-term changes in corneal endothelium after keratoplasty. A follow-up study. Cornea. 1990;9:92-7.
15. Binder PS. Intraocular lens implantation after penetrating keratoplasty. Refract Corneal Surg. 1989;5:224-30.
16. Shimmura S, Ohashi Y, Shiroma H, et al. Corneal Opacity and cataract:triple procedure versus secondary approach. Cornea. 2003;22:234-8.
17. Martin TP, Reed JW, Legault C, et al. Cataract formation and cataract extraction after penetrating keratoplasty. Ophthalmology. 1994;101:113-9.
18. Dangel ME, Kirkham SM, Phipps MJ. Posterior capsule opacification in extracapsular cataract extraction and the triple procedure: a comparative study. Ophthalmic Surg. 1994;25: 82-7.
19. Bersudsky V, Rehany U, Rumelt S. Risk factors for failure of simultaneous penetrating keratoplasty and cataract extraction. J Cataract Refract Surg. 2004;30: 1940-7.
20. Geggel HS. Intraocular lens implantation after penetrating keratoplasty: improved unaided visual acuity, astigmatism, and safety in patients with combined corneal disease and cataract. Ophthalmology. 1990; 97:1470-7.
21. Nardi M, Giudice V, Marabotti A, et al. Temporary graft for closed-system cataract surgery during corneal triple procedures. J Cataract Refract Surg. 2001;27:1172-5.
22. Aramberri J. Intraocular lens power calculation after corneal refractive surgery: double-K method. J Cataract Refract Surg. 2003;29:2063-8.
23. Menapace R, Skorpik C, Grasl M. Modified triple procedure using a temporary keratoprosthesis for closed system, small-incision cataract surgery. J Cataract Refract Surg. 1990;16: 230-4.

24. Nardi M, Giudice V, Marabotti A, et al. Temporary graft for closed-system cataract surgery during corneal triple procedures. J Cataract Refract Surg. 2001;27:1172-5.

25. Mendicute J. Facoemulsificación y queratoplastia penetrante. In: Mendicute J, Cadarso L, Lorente R, et al (Eds). Facoemulsificación. Madrid: CF Comunicación; 1999. pp. 325-38.

26. Bhartiya P, Sharma N, Ray M, et al. Trypan blue assisted phacoemulsification in corneal opacities. Br J Ophthalmology. 2002;86:857-9.

27. Malbrán ES. Facoemulsificación, lente intraocular y queratoplastia. An Inst Barraquer 1996;25:599-604.

28. Lesiewska-Junk H, Kaluzny J, Malukiewicz-Wisniewska G. Long-term evaluation of endothelial cell loss after phacoemulsification. Eur J Ophthalmol. 2002;12:30-3.

29. Millá E, Vergés C, Ciprés MC. Corneal endothelium evaluation after phacoemulsification with continuous anterior chamber infusion. Cornea. 2005;24:78-282.

30. Melles GRJ, Eggink FAGJ, Lander F, et al. A surgical technique for posterior lamellar keratoplasty. Cornea 1998; 17: 618-26.

31. Melles GRJ, Lander F, van Dooren BTH, et al. Preliminary clinical results of posterior lamellar keratoplasty through a sclerocorneal pocket incision. Ophthalmology 2000;107:1850-7.

32. Melles GRJ, Rietveld FJR, Beekhuis WH, et al. A technique to visualize corneal incision and lamellar dissection depth during surgery. Cornea. 1999;18:80-6.

33. Mendicute J. Queratoplastia y cirugía de la catarata. In: Mendicute J, Aramberri J, Cadarso L, et al. (Eds). Biometría, Fórmulas y Manejo de la Sorpresa Refractiva. Madrid: Mac Line S.L; 2000:197-210.

CHAPTER 50

Conversion from Phaco to ECCE (Manual Non-phaco Techniques)

Soosan Jacob, Dhivya Ashok Kumar, Amar Agarwal

INTRODUCTION

Of all the surgeries in ophthalmology, cataract surgery is one of the most popular and successful. The speed at which advances are taking place in this field often leaves one emerging out of one learning curve only to plunge down another! So, one often wonders what the advantages of phaco are? With its added advantage of surgery under topical anesthesia, smaller incisions and no sutures, clearer uncorrected vision, phacoemulsification has become the preferred method of cataract extraction.

So, the pertinent question that arises now is "Is ECCE (extracapsular cataract extraction) dead or still alive?" In other words, is phaco preferable in all cases for all surgeons? Point is should one learn manual non-phaco techniques like the manual small incision cataract surgery techniques.

BRUNESCENT AND BLACK CATARACTS

In a black cataract **(Figure 50.1)** the use of excessive ultrasound energy, prolonged surgical time, increased stress on the bag-zonular complex and greater endothelial damage may lead to a dismal first postoperative day picture which often takes time to recover and sometimes does not. This is as compared to manual small incision cataract surgery (SICS) or an ECCE which generally gives very good anatomical results even in brown cataracts. Cracking and chopping both are difficult in these brown cataracts and are often incomplete. Repeated unsuccessful attempts at

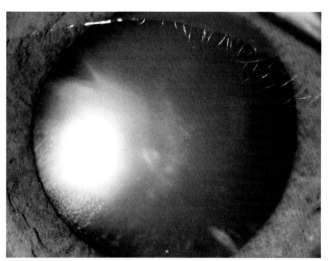

FIGURE 50.1: Black cataract

chopping in the bag could cause stress on the bag-zonular complex and may result in the disastrous complication of nucleus drop.

MORGAGNIAN CATARACTS

These are hypermature cataracts with weak zonules. The mobile, lax anterior capsule makes rhexis a challenge. The hyperdense, shrunken nucleus is also very mobile, thus increasing the chances of endothelial damage. The lack of a protective epinuclear and cortical shell increases the risk of a posterior capsule rupture and nucleus drop during phacoemulsification. Weak zonules could also result in a zonular dialysis.

SEVERE PSEUDOEXFOLIATION

This is associated with preoperative challenges such as a poorly dilating pupil, posterior synechiae, shallow anterior chamber, hard cataracts, weak zonules, phacodonesis or subluxated cataracts, all of which can increase the risks of phacoemulsification.

ZONULAR DIALYSIS OR WEAKNESS

With phaco, excessive traction on the capsule during rhexis can enlarge the zonulodialysis as can nucleus rotation, chopping and cracking maneuvers. Difficult surgery results in capsular or zonular tears and vitreous loss and this is a situation where surgical experience becomes a crucial factor. Performing an ECCE in such eyes, though also associated with a greater risk of intraoperative complications is still safer than phacoemulsification in novice/inexperienced hands.

EYES WITH SHALLOW ANTERIOR CHAMBERS

Shallow AC makes intraocular maneuvering difficult and increases the risk of endothelial touch as well as increases phaco energy related endothelial damage. Increased surge and increased risk of Descemet's detachment also exists.

SMALL PUPIL WITH HARD CATARACT

Though small pupils can be overcome with pupil expanders, it can still be a challenge, especially if also associated with a black cataract. The pupil can get more damaged by the phaco tip.

PHACOLYTIC GLAUCOMA

Corneal edema, hampering visualization, and weak zonules make the option of phaco nonviable.

BAD ENDOTHELIAL COUNT

In eyes with cornea guttata or dystrophies, phacoemulsi-fication may tip the scales of an already borderline endothelium, especially if associated with a hard nucleus or shallow anterior chamber, resulting in pseudophakic bullous keratopathy.

CONVERSION FROM PHACO

A die hard phaco surgeon may also need to be familiar with converting to an ECCE, **(Figures 50.2 to 50.4)** especially in case of complications such as a lengthening phaco time, high phaco energy levels, zonular dialysis, posterior capsular rent (PCR) or vitreous loss.

Extracapsular cataract extraction can be done using a can-opener or an envelope capsulotomy, the latter being preferable as three-fourth of the capsule is left intact until after *intraocular lens* (IOL) implantation, thus providing possible sulcus support in case of a posterior capsular rent. Application of controlled pressure-counter pressure allows safe and easy delivery of the nucleus. Applying two sutures prior to cortex aspiration gives a virtually closed chamber increasing the safety of the procedure.

Manual small incision cataract surgery (SICS) combines many of the advantages of ECCE as well as phaco. It is good for tackling tough cases such as brown cataracts while at the same time is sutureless and induces less astigmatism.

CONCLUSION

With an experienced surgeon, phacoemulsification may be

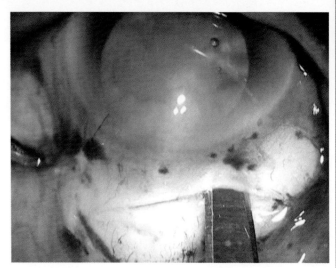

FIGURE 50.3: Conversion to manual non-phaco technique, i.e. small incision cataract surgery (SICS). Note that the temporal clear corneal incision is sutured. The conjunctiva is cut, cautery done and a scleral tunnel incision made

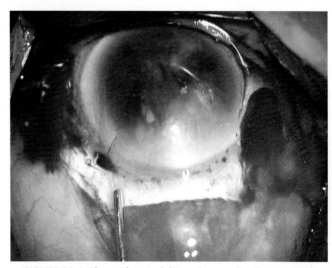

FIGURE 50.4: The nucleus is delivered manually. Then cortical aspiration done and the IOL of surgeon's choice implanted

possible in all cataract types but it is important to remember that the chances of complications with phaco are higher in the hands of someone who does not regularly perform such surgeries. Also, there are often instances when it is advisable to enlarge the phaco incision and convert it to an ECCE. Hence, ECCE and manual SICS or non-phaco manual techniques of cataract surgery are a very safe and useful alternative means of cataract surgery. They should therefore be a pre-requisite in every cataract surgeon's armamentarium. Yet, both ECCE and phaco have their own limitations. The ideal answer would be a technique that combines the best of both worlds and more, with the femtosecond laser coming into its own, femtosecond cataract surgery would evolve to combine the precision, predictability and safety of lasers with surgeon programmability and this may indeed prove to be the Holy Grail for all cataract surgeons. But up until then, the authors believe that ECCE is still alive.

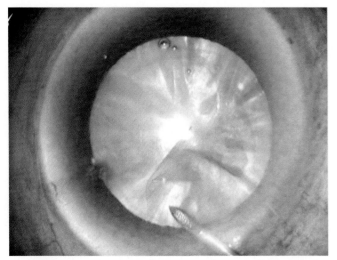

FIGURE 50.2: Rhexis running away in a hard brown cataract

CHAPTER 51

Cataract Surgery and Implantation of Intraocular Lenses in Severe Hyperopia

Roberto Bellucci

INTRODUCTION

Severe hyperopia can be defined as an optical defect above +4D, that is often associated with an axial length below 22 mm although short eyes are not always hyperopic. Out of 23239 eyes of the widest published series, 1107 (4.76%) had axial length below 5th percentile and were considered highly hyperopic.[1] These eyes have special anatomical features relevant for cataract surgery. As nuclear cataract often induces a reduction of the optical defect in an early phase, these eyes approach surgery later than emmetropic or myopic eyes. In addition, a high percentage of hyperopic eyes develop closed angle glaucoma, with prevalence of onset later in life because of the growth of the crystalline lens. Many of these eyes are administered prolonged miotic therapy, which causes severe miosis and formation of pupil membrane and of posterior synechiae.

Highly hyperopic eyes are associated with greater intraoperative and postoperative problems than non-hyperopic eyes, and severely hyperopic and microphthalmic eyes worry the surgeon most.[2-3] The recent techniques of cataract emulsification through a sub-2 mm incision under topical anesthesia have greatly improved the clinical outcome of these eyes. A whole series of maneuvers has been developed to reduce the complications even further.

At present, phacoemulsification can be performed in the severely hyperopic eye with almost the same safety level as in the normal eye. This has led many surgeons to perform lensectomy and intraocular lens implantation for refractive purposes, and especially after the wide availability of multifocal intraocular lenses,[4,5] However, the difficulties in the precise calculation of the power of the implant may limit refractive success. Short eyes do not fit in with statistical formulas despite all the modifications suggested, and even theoretical formulas are based on estimations of optical relations and therefore often they are not precise.[6] Moreover, high power intraocular lenses are rarely available in powers that exceed 30 diopters, and more than one lens may be necessary to emmetropize a severely hyperopic eye, originating a condition named polypseudophakia.

SURGICAL ANATOMY OF SEVERELY HYPEROPIC EYES

The understanding of the surgical anatomy of severely hyperopic eyes guides the surgical methods, explains the possible complications and is of great help in their prevention. From a general point of view, hyperopic eyes can be divided into two categories: those with small anterior segment and those with a normal anterior segment.[7]

Most hyperopic eyes have anterior segment that is proportional to the axial length, that means of small size. These eyes have reduced axial length, often lower than 22 mm; the size of the crystalline lens is more or less normal and tends to push the iris forward, reducing the depth of the anterior chamber. The corneal diameter can be small or normal. The iris is frequently dark and thick, the chamber angle is narrow (0-2 according to Shaffer). These eyes may develop acute glaucoma which sometimes can happen early in life.

Often these eyes underwent cataract extraction after a long history of closed angle glaucoma, of miotic therapy, of Nd:YAG laser iridotomy, and presented at surgery with narrow pupils that could not be dilated pharmacologically. Today Micro Incision Cataract Surgery (MICS) is of great help in controlling difficulties and surgery can be planned earlier. Corneal endothelial cell count is often reduced, and threatened by the reduced space available in the anterior chamber and by the thickness of the cataractous lens. The zonule is normally strong, excluding microphthalmic eyes where it is frequently weak. The sclera is thick and even the choroid is thickened and ready to dilate even further during surgery. The vitreous generally has normal consistency. Choroidal dilation and vitreous hydration are the basis of the posterior pressure that frequently complicates cataract surgery in these eyes.[3]

Sometimes severely hyperopic or microphthalmic eyes have normal anterior segment, not in proportion with the axial length. The depth of the anterior chamber appears to be normal, the chamber angle is wide and there is no risk of angle closure. In this case, severe hyperopia is only a refractive disturbance that compels the patient to use spectacles from a very young age.

These eyes present at surgery after many years of spectacles, but rather early in life because of the desire to eliminate or to reduce spectacles dependency. The zonule may be weak, and there may be a subluxation of the lens. The posterior segment is typical of hyperopic eyes with an increase in scleral and choroidal thickness, and maintained vitreous consistency. One eye we observed measured 16.4 mm axial length, and 7.6 mm from the corneal apex to the posterior lens pole. Vitreous chamber was 8.8 mm long. These features made the exact calculation of the implant power a difficult procedure.[6]

The two types of hyperopic eyes probably have geographical distribution depending on the characters of the population examined. **Table 51.1** reports two examples of personal observation. In a study published some years ago involving 93 hyperopic eyes, Holladay reports a prevalence of 83% of eyes with a normal anterior segment, with the remaining 17% having a small anterior segment.[7] Brannan reported a reduced anterior segment with microcornea and ACD of 2.41 mm in an eye measuring 26.6 mm. The fellow eye of this patient measured 21.5 mm yet had the same anterior segment.[8] Therefore, short eyes with normal anterior segment and little or no risk for angle-closure glaucoma are probably more frequent than usually perceived.

TABLE 51.1 Comparison of two short eyes with different anatomy				
	Small anterior segment		Normal anterior segment	
	Value	%	Value	%
Refraction (D)	+5.5		+11	
Axial length (mm)	21.0	100%	20.2	100%
Anterior chamber depth (mm)	1.9	9%	3.3	16.3%
Lens thickness (mm)	4.2	20%	4.2	20.8%
Vitreous length (mm)	14.9	71%	12.7	62.9%

PHACOEMULSIFICATION IN SEVERE HYPEROPIC EYES

Cataract surgery in a severely hyperopic eye will face greater intra- and postoperative complications. In these eyes I believe MICS is mandatory for a variety of reasons, including superior visibility due to the small instruments, increased chamber stability during all phases of the procedure, reduced incision size allowing better control of astigmatism in small corneas.

EYES WITH SHALLOW ANTERIOR CHAMBER

In these eyes, cataract surgery will also solve the closed-angle glaucoma,[9,10] with good results even years after surgery, and for this reason many patients are now offered surgery even if their lenses are still transparent.[11] At surgery, every attempt should be made to check intraocular pressure, and to reduce it to normal levels. The quick infusion of 10 cc/kg b.w. of 20% mannitol, administered 2–4 hours before surgery, can be of great help. **Table 51.2** reports our current preoperative schedule.

FIRST MANEUVERS

The aperture of the eye bulb with increased intraocular pressure may jeopardize the safety of the entire operation.

TABLE 51.2 Preoperative treatment of the hyperopic eye with narrow chamber angle
- Stop miotic therapy 48 hours prior to surgery - Add oral acetazolamide - Add topical non-miotic hypotensives - Administer 20% mannitol, 10 ml/kg body weight i.v. 2-4 hours before surgery - Avoid excessive administration of phenylephrine to overcome miosis

The eye should be decompressed gradually to give the choroidal vessels the time to adapt to the new pressure. The sudden drop in pressure may induce dilation of the choroidal vascular bed, rupture of choroidal vessels, and choroidal hemorrhage. Expulsive hemorrhages are virtually impossible with MICS, still sometimes choroidal hemorrhages can be observed.[3] Local anesthesia is the worst in these eyes, as it increases pressure against the eyeball. Topical anesthesia is preferred and in general is the best because blood pressure can also be controlled.

Endothelial cell count may be very low in severely hyperopic eyes, and therefore surgery must be particularly delicate. An adhesive viscoelastic substance should be injected several times into the anterior chamber during phacoemulsification, maintaining spaces and providing better protection of the corneal endothelium.

Particularly when the anterior chamber is less than 2 mm deep, clear cornea 2 mm incisions should be preferred to avoid iris damage or prolapse. The anterior chamber can then be deepened by high viscosity viscoelastic substance, that will allow room for the coaxial capsulorhexis forceps.

SMALL PUPIL

The reduced pupil diameter often observed in severely hyperopic eyes with shallow anterior chamber depends on the prolonged miotic therapy. Fibrosis of the pupil edge is often associated with the formation of a pale or pigmented ring. Sometimes a true pupillary membrane can be observed. Miosis cannot be solved with drugs, and frequently requires high viscosity viscoelastics, mechanical pupil enlargement by removal of fibrotic tissue, sphinctero-tomies, stretching (**Figure 51.1**), and positioning of rings or iris retractors (**Figure 51.2**). Following the cataract operation, many pupils dilated in this way return to a round shape. Capsulorhexis is rarely difficult with small pupil, and escape is an exceptional event because of the centripetal action on the pupil edge. With small pupils, MICS is mandatory (**Figure 51.3**). With hard nuclei, we use the "stop and chop" phacoemulsification technique to divide the nucleus into two parts and to avoid zonular rupture.

POSTERIOR PRESSURE

Excessive pressure in the vitreous chamber during cataract surgery is common in eyes affected by closed-angle glaucoma. Posterior pressure begins to rise shortly after the beginning of surgery, and may be evident towards the final

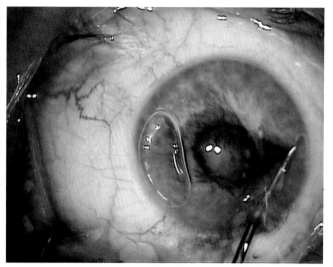

FIGURE 51.1: Pupil stretching after removal of papillary fibrotic ring due to prolonged miotic therapy

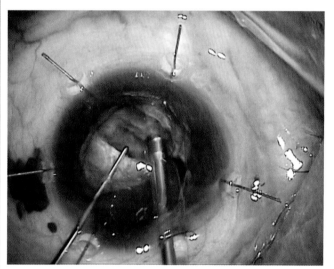

FIGURE 51.2: Iris retractors have been used in this microphthalmic eye

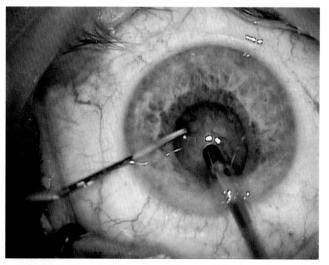

FIGURE 51.3: Micro Incision Cataract Surgery (MICS) employs smaller instruments and is particularly helpful in small eyes with small pupils

phase of irrigation and aspiration. The surgeon should never be afraid to interrupt the operation for a couple of hours or even to postpone it for a full day if the posterior pressure proves to be excessive.

The main causes of posterior pressure are choroidal dilation because of high blood pressure, and vitreous hydration because of BSS passing through the zonula into the vitreous cavity.[12] Better control of blood pressure, and better phaco fluidics not requiring high-pressure infusion can frequently avoid this complication.

Zonular weakness is rarely observed in these eyes but it may be a serious complication inducing anterior chamber oscillation during the early phases, and possibly posterior pressure later on.

LENS IMPLANTATION

The intraocular lens for severe hyperopia should be as thin as possible. Therefore, manufacturers produce high power IOLs that are either smaller than normal or made of high refractive index material. MICS lenses should be preferred, as they do not require incision enlargement **(Figure 51.4)**.

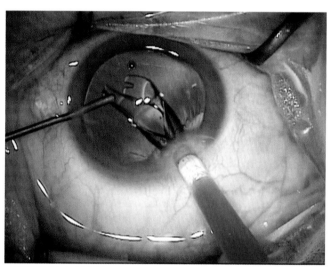

FIGURE 51.4: MICS lenses can be implanted into shallow anterior chambers through sub-2 mm incisions

COMPLICATIONS

Intraoperative complications of phacoemulsification in severely hyperopic eyes with shallow anterior chamber are the same as of normal cataract surgery, but they happen more frequently. Rupture of the posterior capsule can be favored by miosis in eyes where the lens is hard and the capsule is fragile, and it is managed in the same way as in normal cataract surgery. Incorrect IOL implant can also happen because of miosis, requiring iris pulling for visualization and correction. Posterior vitreous pressure can develop for a variety of reasons **(Table 51.3)**, but choroidal hemorrhage is extremely rare **(Figure 51.5)**.

Postoperatively, intraocular pressure can rise because of viscoelastic remnants inside the eye. Though it has been

TABLE 51.3	Increased vitreous pressure during phacoemulsification in severely hyperopic eyes
Risk factors	**Possible effects**
Peri/retrobulbar anesthesia	Increase of the intraorbitary pressure
Sympathomimetics	Increase of blood pressure with dilation of choroidal vessels
Pressure drop within the AC	Dilatation of choroidal vessels
Excessive irrigation	Vitreous hydration through the zonula

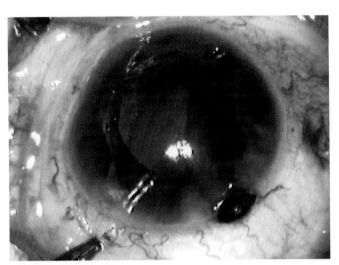

FIGURE 51.5: A choroidal hemorrage developed in this microphthalmic eye, requiring scleral puncture. The capsular bag is intact and received two MICS lenses three months later with good result

demonstrated that transitory increases in intraocular pressure does not cause any further damage to the visual field of these eyes,[13] any pressure increase should be corrected by paracentesis at the slit lamp.

Ciliary block or malignant glaucoma is a rare complication of eye surgery, but it is more frequent in hyperopic eyes. It involves the misdirection of aqueous humor towards the vitreous chamber instead of towards the posterior chamber.[14] Medical treatment consists of cycloplegic mydriatic eyedrops, while the surgical solution consists of capsulotomy with Nd:YAG laser through an iridectomy if present, or of posterior vitrectomy in more refractory cases.

Eyes with Normal Anterior Segment

When the anterior segment is normal, there are fewer surgical problems with respect to the previous case, and they are very similar to the complications of routine cataract surgery. Zonular relaxation is the only element that should be thoroughly considered. It can be identified through the enormous increase in the depth of the anterior chamber during phacoemulsification, with surgical difficulties due to the very posterior position of the capsular bag.

It is advisable to lower the infusion bottle, consequently lowering phaco aspiration to avoid chamber collapse. With MICS, a machine with perfect control of aspiration fluidics must be employed.

CALCULATION OF THE IMPLANT POWER

Besides being the basis of power calculation, the biometrical measurements will confirm whether the anterior segment of the hyperopic eye under investigation is normal or shorter than normal. Laser interference is the preferred method for measuring the axial length of highly hyperopic eyes, and recent machines will perform well even with many posterior polar cataracts. Ultrasound measurement of axial length can be easily obtained using focalized probes, as the return echo is increased in short eyes. Sometimes miosis complicates the measurement, particularly if the patient is not cooperative. However, the standard procedure is not very precise due to the considerable thickness of the crystalline lens, and the speed of the ultrasound inside the lens should be varied. Immersion biometry that avoids corneal flattening is of advantage.[15] Anterior chamber depth and lens thickness should be measured carefully, as the final position of the intraocular lens, and therefore its effective power, will depend on these anatomical structures.

The statistical formulas for the calculation of the power of intraocular lenses should not be used in severely hyperopic eyes because they underestimate severe ametropias. Moreover, they cannot consider the specific anatomical and biometrical characters of single eyes. Optical formulas are preferred, but despite all precautions the calculation of the power of the implant can still be inaccurate, originating residual ametropias that will require further correction.

CLEAR LENSECTOMY FOR REFRACTIVE PURPOSES

Patients affected by severe hyperopia have bad near and distant vision and always require spectacles. Visual discomfort increases as the patient ages because of presbyopia. Moreover, these patients tolerate contact lenses much less than their myopic counterparts. In practice, they cannot even manage the insertion of contact lenses without using spectacles.

The problems are increased by the aesthetic and functional limitations of thick spectacle lenses. These lenses are often very heavy, they leave residual aberration, and are expensive.

These problems promoted the extension of clear lens extraction to hyperopic eyes.[15-19] Severely hyperopic eyes take more advantage from refractive surgery than severely myopic eyes, but with fewer surgical options available. It is unlikely that corneal surgery can correct more than

| TABLE 51.4 | Studies on clear lens exchange in severely hyperopic eyes |

Author	Year	Technique	Eyes	Preop SphEq Min	Preop SphEq Max	Postop UCVA Media	Postop UCVA Min	Postop SphEq Min	Postop SphEq Max	Complications
Lyle[15]	1994	Phaco	6	+4.2	+7.9	NR	20/40	-0.75	+0.87	
Siganos[16]	1995	ECCE	17	+6.7	+13.7	20/25	20/30	-0.37	+0.50	Endoth cell loss 11%
Lyle[17]	1997	Phaco	20	+2.4	+7.6	20/35	20/60*	-2.25	+1.88	
Kolahdouz[18]	1999	Phaco	18	+4.5	+9.6	20/40	20/50	-2.50	+1.37	Malignant glaucoma 10%
Vicary[19]	1999	Phaco	58	+3.0	+11.6	20/28	20/50	NR	NR	

NR: Not reported   *Ambliopia

4-5 D even with the best laser and Lasik techniques; phakic intraocular lenses are not suitable for eyes with small anterior segment. In addition, hyperopic eyes may benefit from the positive effects of lensectomy against closed angle glaucoma, and are less subject to retinal detachment than myopic eyes because of the different anatomy (**Table 51.4**).

MULTIFOCAL INTRAOCULAR LENSES

Multifocal intraocular lenses are increasingly popular for hyperopic eyes, especially after clear lens extraction. Several papers report very good results in terms of refractive correction and patient satisfaction, obtained with almost every type of multifocal intraocular lens.[20-22] However, Lasik had to be performed in a percentage of eyes to obtain emmetropia, and early posterior capsulotomy has been required by patients for visual disturbances from posterior capsule wrinkling.[22,23] Patients with low preoperative refractive error complained about several visual disturbances, but patients with severe hyperopia did not.[24]

POLYPSEUDOPHAKIA

Many severely hyperopic eyes subjected to cataract operation require the implantation of very high power intraocular lenses. While hyperopic eyes with small anterior segment normally require lenses around +30 D, those with normal anterior segment frequently require lenses above +40 diopters, and sometimes above +50 D.

Table 51.5 reports the findings of a personal observation, and **Figure 51.6** shows the primary implantation of two MICS lenses in the same eye.

Such a high dioptric power can theoretically be obtained with intraocular lenses produced to size by the industry, but the thickness of the lens creates problems of refraction that are difficult to overcome.[25] Moreover, the implantation of 'custom built' lenses is not practical due to production time. The problem has been solved by implanting two intraocular lenses, a condition named polypseudophakia after Gayton.[26,27] Over years, polypseudophakia has become as a routine technique for achieving emmetropia in severely hyperopic eyes[28] and as a means to correct for pseudophakic refractive errors.[29] The refractive results proved to be good, with acceptable complication profile.

| TABLE 51.5 | Refractive outcome of a microphthalmic eye with normal anterior segment (see Figures 51.2 and 51.6) |

Hyperopia	+15	D
Axial length	16.8	mm
Anterior chamber depth	3.3	mm
Lens thickness	4.2	mm
Vitreous chamber depth	9.3	mm
Mean keratometry reading	43	D
Mean corneal diameter	10.5	mm
Implanted power	+50	D
Pseudophakic refraction	+2	D

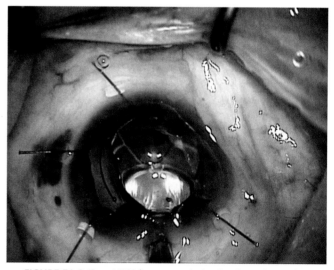

FIGURE 51.6: Two MICS lenses are being implanted into this microphthalmic eye

When the two lenses come into contact at the apex, the resulting optic system should be considered as a single lens, according to the suggestions from physical optics. The resulting power is the sum of the powers of the two lenses. It still has not been clarified whether it is better to split the dioptric power into two halves, or to implant lenses of different power.[27,30] The contact area between two foldable lenses is a small circle, with extension depending on the type of intraocular lens and on the dioptric power. The contact zone may be responsible for modest visual reduction and for some of the multifocal phenomena sometimes observed in polypseudophakia.[31]

Many severely hyperopic eyes retain some hyperopic refractive error in the pseudophakia. These eyes can be refocused by a secondary implant in the capsular bag or more often in the ciliary sulcus.

The refractive results of polypseudophakia are very good, with 53% of eyes within 0.5 D of emmetropia, and 82% within 1 D as reported by Gills.[32] However, there are also complications. A whitish viscoelastic material may persist between the two lenses which can reduce the postoperative visual acuity. Elschnig's pearls may proliferate between the two lenses again reducing visual acuity and increasing hyperopia[33] For this reason the implantation of two acrylic lenses in a single capsular bag is no longer recommended,[31] as it is not recommended to implant IOLs of different materials when the optics come in touch, because of possible opacification (**Figure 51.7**).

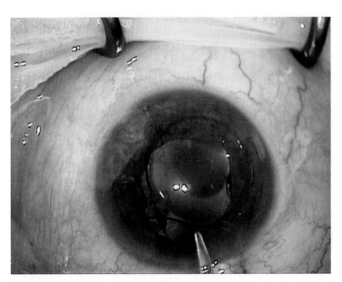

FIGURE 51.7: This hydrophilic lens in the capsular bag developed opacity in the area of contact with a piggyback hydrophobic lens secondarily implanted in the ciliary sulcus to correct for residual refractive error

CONCLUSION

The cataract operation in the severely hyperopic patient is now much safer thanks to phacoemulsification. These eyes should be operated quite precociously, in order to avoid the possibility of closed angle glaucoma in eyes with small anterior segment, and to improve vision in eyes with normal anterior segment.

The difficulties associated with the anatomical conditions of these eyes have been solved by MICS, a technique especially useful in these small eyes, and by a variety of devices and instruments to overcome specific problems. Power calculation challenges have been almost won by modern biometry and power calculation formulas.

Multifocal implants can reduce or cancel the need for spectacles. Thin MICS lenses can be implanted through sub-2 mm incisions, and more than one may be implanted in the case of excessive power requirement. In conclusion, modern cataract surgery can offer a valid option to these highly hyperopic eyes not only affected by cataracts, but also operated for refractive purposes.

REFERENCES

1. Hoffman PC, Hutz WW. Analysis of biometry and prevalence data for corneal astigmatism in 23239 eyes. J Cataract Refract Surg 2010;36:1479-85.
2. Jünemann A, Küchle M, Händel A, Naumann GO.[Cataract surgery in nanophthalmic eyes with an axial length of less than 20.5 mm]. Klin Monbl Augenheilkd 1998;212:13-22.
3. Yuzbasioglu E, Artunay O, Agachan A, Bilen H. Phacoemulsification in patients with nanophthalmos. Can J Ophthalmol 2009;44:534-39.
4. Pop M, Payette Y. Refractive lens exchange versus iris-claw Artisan phakic intraocular lens for hyperopia. J Refract Surg 2004;20:20-24.
5. Alfonso JF, Fernández-Vega L, Ortí S, Montés-Micó R. Refractive lens exchange with the Acri.Twin asymmetric diffractive bifocal intraocular lens system. Eur J Ophthalmol 2010;20:509-16.
6. Terzi E, Wang L, Kohnen T. Accuracy of modern intraocular lens power calculation formulas in refractive lens exchange for high myopia and high hyperopia. J Cataract Refract Surg 2009; 35:1181-89.
7. Holladay JR. Achieving emmetropia in extremely short eyes. American Academy Ophthalmology Meeting, Chicago, 1996.
8. Brannan SO, Kyle G. Bilateral microcornea and unilateral macrophthalmia resulting in incorrect intraocular lens selection. J Cataract Refract Surg 1999;25:1016-18.
9. Vizzeri G, Weinreb RN. Cataract surgery and glaucoma. Curr Opin Ophthalmol 2010;21:20-24.
10. Lee SJ, Lee CK, Kim WS. Long-term therapeutic efficacy of phacoemulsification with intraocular lens implantation in patients with phacomorphic glaucoma. J Cataract Refract Surg 2010;36:783-89.
11. Bhattacharjee H, Bhattacharjee K, Medhi J, DasGupta S. Clear lens extraction and intraocular lens implantation in a case of microspherophakia with secondary angle closure glaucoma. Indian J Ophthalmol 2010;58:67-70.
12. Bellucci R. Vitreous hydration: often a hidden complication of cataract surgery. Cataract Refract Surg Today Europe, 2006;1(2):50-52.
13. Krupin T, Feitl ME, Bishop KI. Postoperative intraocular pressure rise in open-angle glaucoma patients after cataract or combined cataract-filtration surgery. Ophthalmology 1989;96: 579-84.
14. Gunning FP, Greve EL. Lens extraction for uncontrolled angle-closure glaucoma: long-term follow-up. J Cataract Refract Surg 1998;24:1347-56.
15. Siganos DS, Siganos CS, Pallikaris IG. Clear lens extraction and intraocular lens implantation in normally sighted hyperopic eyes. J Refract Corneal Surg 1994;10:117-21.
16. Siganos DS, Pallikaris IG, Siganos CS. Clear lensectomy and intraocular lens implantation in normally sighted highly hyperopic eyes. Three-year follow-up. Eur J Implant Refract Surg 1995;7:128-33.

17. Lyle WA, Jin GJ. Clear lens extraction to correct hyperopia. J Cataract Refract Surg 1997;23:1051-56.

18. Kolahdouz-Isfahani AH, Rostamian K, Wallace D, Salz JJ. Clear lens extraction with intraocular lens implantation for hyperopia. J Refract Surg 1999;15:316-23.

19. Vicary D, Sun XY, Montgomery P. Refractive lensectomy to correct ametropia. J Cataract Refract Surg 1999; 25: 943-48.

20. Buznego C, Trattler WB. Presbyopia-correcting intraocular lenses. Curr Opin Ophthalmol 2009;20:13-18.

21. Cezón Prieto J, Bautista MJ. Visual outcomes after implantation of a refractive multifocal intraocular lens with a +3.00 D addition. J Cataract Refract Surg 2010;36:1508-16.

22. Fujimoto K, Honda K, Wada YR, Tanaka M, Irie T. Four-year experience with a silicone refractive multifocal intraocular lens. J Cataract Refract Surg 2010; 36: 1330-35.

23. Gauthier L, Lafuma A, Laurendeau C, Berdeaux G. Neodymium:YAG laser rates after bilateral implantation of hydrophobic or hydrophilic multifocal intraocular lenses: twenty-four month retrospective comparative study. J Cataract Refract Surg 2010;36:1195-1200.

24. Leccisotti A. Secondary procedures after presbyopic lens exchange. J Cataract Refract Surg 2004;30:1461-65.

25. Accou M, Hennekes R. Implantation of posterior chamber lenses of more than 30 dptr. Bull Soc Belge Ophthalmol 1996; 261: 121-24.

26. Gayton JL, Sanders VN. Implanting two posterior chamber intraocular lenses in a case of microphthalmos. J Cataract Refract Surg 1993;19:776-77.

27. Shugar JK, Lewis C, Lee A. Implantation of multiple foldable acrylic posterior chamber lenses in the capsular bag for high hyperopia. J Cataract Refract Surg 1996; 22 (Suppl 2):1368-72.

28. Holladay JT, Gills JP, Leidlein J, Cherchio M. Achieving emmetropia in extremely short eyes with two piggyback posterior chamber intraocular lenses. Ophthalmology 1996; 103: 1118-23.

29. Habot-Wilner Z, Sachs D, Cahane M, Alhalel A, Desatnik H, Schwalb E, Barequet IS. Refractive results with secondary piggyback implantation to correct pseudophakic refractive errors. J Cataract Refract Surg 2005;31: 2101-03.

30. Perrone DM. Modified intraocular lens power formula in polypseudophakia. J Cataract Refract Surg 1996;22:1392-93.

31. Findl O, Menapace R, Rainer G, Georgopoulos M. Contact zone of piggyback acrylic intraocular lenses. J Cataract Refract Surg 1999;25:860-2.

32. Gills JP, Cerchio M. Phacoemulsification in highly hyperopic cataract patients. In: Lu LW, Fine IH (Eds): Phacoemulsification in Difficult and Challenging Cases. Thieme, New York, 1999;21-31.

33. Gayton JL, Apple DJ, Peng Q, Visessook N, Sanders V, et al. Interlenticular opacification: clinicopathological correlation of a complication of posterior chamber piggyback intraocular lenses. J Cataract Refract Surg 2000; 26: 330-36.

CHAPTER 52

Cataract Surgery in the Patient with Uveitis

Enrique Chipont, Jorge L Alio

INTRODUCTION

Cataract development is a very common occurrence in any form of anterior and intermediate uveitis, because of: (i) the frequent relapses and chronic intraocular inflammation, and (ii) the chronic use of corticosteroid therapy. The reported incidence of cataract in uveitic patients varies between series but it approaches 50% in juvenile rheumatoid arthritis[1] and other forms of posterior uveitis,[2] and upto 75% in chronic anterior uveitis.[3]

The indications for proceeding with cataract surgery are more demanding in eyes with uveitis. Also complications of this surgery are higher in these patients than in no uveitic patients. Uncontrolled inflammation, hypotony, phthisis bulbi, among others are important challenges to the postoperative period in uveitic patients.[4] The time of surgery has to be justified on eyes with slightly decrease in visual acuity, but in functional vision that is not in danger of visual loss, but on the other hand we cannot delay the surgery so long that treatable problems worsen progressively the status of the eye.

There are some facts concerning these cataracts that make the therapeutical or surgical approach different from those associated with senior population: (i) cataracts associated with uveitis develop at an early age, affecting children and young adults, (ii) a higher incidence of subcapsular cataracts leads to glare disability and near vision difficulties, (iii) preoperative anti-inflammatory regimens must be carefully planned for each individual patient which differs from the routine surgical protocol, and (iv) postoperative follow-up should ensure the control of inflammation and monitor the higher incidence of complications including posterior capsule opacification, glaucoma, iritis recurrences, macular edema.

The improvement in surgical techniques and pre-and postoperative control of inflammation, thanks to new and safer small incision surgeries and the usage of corticosteroids pre- and postoperatively have led to better results of surgery in patients with uveitis. This has increased the tendency to operate these eyes earlier and earlier to prevent more important complications.

Surgery should be performed when the inflammation of the eyes is quiet. However, in some patients, it is impossible to clear every cell from the anterior chamber or vitreous. Furthermore, in patients with dense cataracts and primarily vitreoretinal inflammation, it is impossible to assess the activity of the disease behind the cataract.

CLINICAL EXAMINATION

SYMPTOMS

Complaints in those patients associated to the development of cataract will be in function of the age, type of uveitis and mostly the type of cataract. Decrease in vision is the most important symptom of the development of cataract in patients with uveitis. Glare, and sometimes halo can be referred to by the patient as the first complaint. Glare can be associated with subcapsular posterior cataract, anterior Tyndall, intermediate uveitis or glaucoma that must be ruled out in such patients.

SLIT LAMP EXAMINATION

In human studies of postsurgical inflammation the primary clinical variable examined to assess is the degree of postoperative intraocular inflammation. The presence of cells and flare in the anterior chamber is mandatory measured with the laser flare cell meter, fluorophotometry, or an inflammation severity score (USS). Ocular discomfort, bulbar conjunctival hyperthymia, ciliary flush, corneal edema, an even anterior vitreous reaction.

With development of the fluorophotometer and the laser flare cell meter, however, the task has been simplified, allowing the blood-aqueous barrier function to be used as a physiological, clinical parameter. The laser flare meter has been especially useful because it is noninvasive and easy to perform.

SURGICAL INDICATIONS

Two are the main indications for cataract surgery in patients with uveitis: (i) visually significant cataract if prospects for substantial improvement in visual acuity are good, and (ii) cataract that impairs fundus assessment in a patient with suspected fundus pathology.

VISUALLY SIGNIFICANT CATARACT

Cataract is not a reversible disease, so a detected decrease in visual acuity due to cataract precludes a subsequent decrease in few years. Techniques to estimate postoperative visual acuity can be performed in patients where standard acuity scales are not sufficient and the health of the macula is unclear. Potential acuity meter (PAM) and laser interferometry are the most reliable techniques in these patients.

Glare

Sometimes a 20/20 visual acuity is present in a patient with uveitis but still the patient complains of blurred vision. Explanation of the potential risks and benefits must be carefully done including the fact that cataract is not reversible and that those symptoms will augment with time.

Improvement of Posterior Pole Visualization

Those situations associated with visualization of the posterior pole either to assess the evolution of a given disease (posterior uveitis, vasculitis, macular edema) or the response to a treatment (systemic steroids or immunosuppressant) can be affected by the presence of a dense cataract or even a wide posterior subcapsular cataract.

PREOPERATIVE MANAGEMENT

The control of inflammation prior to cataract surgery in patients with a history of uveitis is critical. Total control of active inflammation for at least 3 months must be attempted. This goal is sometimes difficult to achieve, but with a stepladder approach to therapy a complete control of inflammation in most patients is possible. The single most important sign of inflammation is the presence or absence of inflammatory cells in the anterior chamber or vitreous. Aqueous flare in anterior chronic uveitis simply denotes vascular incompetence of the iris and ciliary body, a consequence of vascular damage from recurrent uveitis. Therefore, flare should not generally be used as a guidepost for inflammatory quiescence. The presence of inflammatory cells in the vitreous may be extremely difficult to discern through an advanced cataract. The presence of vitreous cells does not necessarily signify active disease because inflammatory cells clear more slowly than in the anterior chamber. Vitreous inflammation did not appear to be significantly associated with the presence of cataract development in patients with Vogt-Koyanagi-Harada (VKH) syndrome as reported by Moorthy et al.[5]

Our approach includes patients who will be divided into two groups: complicated cases and uncomplicated cases following the guidelines of the intraocular inflammation society (IOIS).[6]

Complicated patients will be those in which systemic or periocular therapy is necessary to maintain uveitis in a quiescent state or those in which surgery itself is expected to be difficult for the surgeon.

Uncomplicated patients will be those in which the uveitis is controlled with topical steroids and an operative routine is anticipated.

The therapeutic approach begins one week before surgery. Each subject will be given a topical corticosteroid (prednisolone acetate 1% or dexamethasone alcohol 0.5%) one drop four times daily. All subjects classified as "complicated" cases also receive 1 mg/kg/day of oral prednisone.

SURGERY: PHACOEMULSIFICATION

Intracapsular surgery is reserved for the situations in which an important phaco-induced component is revealed in prior contralateral surgery. If a chronic macular edema arises, a combined procedure anterior and posterior approach should be performed. Most surgeons opt for conventional pars plana vitrectomy techniques.[7]

Cataract surgery is sometimes complicated by the presence of iris atrophy, sclerosis of the pupillary sphincter, cyclitic membrane, posterior sinechiae, anterior capsular sclerosis, and possible hemorrhage from the iris and angle neovascularization; as a result a precise and delicate surgery is mandatory.

Phacoemulsification allows a small wound, causes minimal trauma and may therefore minimize postoperative inflammation. Young patients and patients with high doses of corticosteroids are at an advantage with this technique. General anesthesia is not necessary (though many patients are young and their treatment with general anesthesia is compulsory), and locoregional anesthesia by retrobulbar or peribulbar block are preferred. Topical anesthesia is not contraindicated but we do not use it in these cases.[8]

Clear corneal or scleral tunnel incision can be performed. Clear corneal incision has some advantages over scleral tunnels such as the absence of postoperative hyphemas, filtering blebs and need for cautery among others. This is our favored approach if no lens or a foldable lens is implanted, and if the implantation of a rigid polymethylmethacrylate (PMMA) lens is planned a limbal approach with a short scleral tunnel is performed. Viscoelastic substances are routinely used to release adhesions and aid mydriasis. Combinations of hyaluronic acid and chondroitin sulfate (Viscoat R) are preferred, and high viscosity viscoelastics can be used (Healon GVR, Amvisc plus R). Many patients with uveitis have sclerosis of the dilator muscle of the pupil or intense posterior synechiae, and under viscoelastic aid synechiolysis is performed with an iris spatula. If further mydriasis is desired we use four De Juan hooks placed at each quadrant through four small corneal incisions. Continuous circular capsulotomy (capsulorhexis) is always performed, even in intumescent cataracts, and if this is not possible a can-opener capsulotomy is opted for, but phacoemulsification is performed with caution.

The phacoemulsification procedure is accomplished by the most suitable technique for each case, with chop techniques if hardness of the nucleus is high. In general the nucleus is soft in young patients and phacoemulsification can be performed without any complications. Intensive cortical cleaning is mandatory to eliminate one of the sources of postoperative inflammatory reaction and the posterior surface of the anterior capsule must be aspirated with a low vacuum to eliminate proliferative cells and to remove one of the sources of posterior and possibly anterior capsule opacification. Bimanual techniques give excellent results in anterior cortical cleaning. Our guidelines for phacoemulsification are listed in **Table 52.1**.

TABLE 52.1	Phaco parameters (abstract)	
Soft cataracts	Power	30% pulsed
	Vacuum	400 mm Hg
	Aspiration	20 cc/min
	Burst	30 ms
Hard cataracts	Power	100%
	Vacuum	65 mm Hg
	Aspiration	20 cc/min
	Burst	30 ms
Fragment removal	Power	65%
	Vacuum	400 mm Hg
	Aspiration	20 cc/min
	Burst	30 ms
Irrigation/Aspiration	Aspiration	30 cc/min
	Vacuum	400 mm Hg

Where there is extensive membrane formation in the vitreous especially in the anterior part, vitrectomy after posterior central capsulorhexis must be considered. If the vitreous cavity shows extensive fibrosis and exudate formation transscleral pars plana vitrectomy may be indicated.[9]

INTRAOCULAR LENSES

Until recently, the existence of chronic uveitis has been regarded by most surgeons as a relative contraindication to IOL implantation. For these reasons, sulcus or anterior chamber implantation has always been contraindicated and capsular bag placement has been controversial. On the other hand, several studies have suggested that inserting a posterior chamber lens into the capsular bag poses no additional threat to ocular morbidity in selective uveitis cases, providing proper perioperative treatment for inflammation is given.[10,11] An ambitious study is being carried out under the auspices of Intraocular Inflammation Society (IOIS) to determine which IOL if any has the best behavior after implantation in uveitis patients.

Surface-modified IOLs such as the heparin coated models have been introduced. The heparin surface-modified IOL is created by inducing electrostatic absorption of heparin onto the surface of a PMMA IOL. Heparin-coated IOLs are recommended for patients with uveitis as they decrease the number and severity of deposits on the surface of the IOL.[12]

Limited information is available regarding small incision phacoemulsification and foldable IOL implantation in patients with chronic uveitis. Several controlled studies comparing flexible IOL implantation through a 3.2 mm incision and conventional PMMA IOL implantation through 5.5 mm or larger incisions have been reported. Postoperative inflammation is significantly less with smaller incisions.

Polymethylmethacrylate (PMMA) has been the most commonly used IOL material. It has proved to be inert and stable and numerous designs are manufactured by many companies.[13] New materials like silicone and hydrogel have been rapidly accepted for intraocular implantation, partly as a result of the worldwide popularity of phacoemulsification. The interest in these materials is based on their mechanical properties, which allow them to be folded and inserted through a small incision. New technology applied to PMMA lenses has enabled the development of a new generation of acrylic foldable lenses for small incision surgery.[14]

Silicone lenses have displayed greater inflammatory reaction in nonuveitic patients when compared to other IOL materials (PMMA, Heparin-modified, hydrogel).[14] After phacoemulsification procedures a number of complications have been described such as intense inflammatory reactions in the anterior chamber, total closure of the capsulorhexis and an increase in posterior capsule opacification when compared with PMMA implants.[15] We do not recommend the use of this material in patients whose blood-aqueous barrier is compromised. Nevertheless few reports of the use of silicone IOLs in patients with uveitis have been published. A 13-mm silicone IOL with a 6 mm optic was implanted through a 3.2 mm incision in a woman with sarcoidosis uveitis, and this case revealed perioperative tolerance to the silicone implant and rapid visual rehabilitation compared with the fellow eye which received a rigid PMMA lens.

The issues surrounding IOL placement in uveitic eyes after cataract extraction remains a key concern in management of the uveitic patient. Many features unique to a uveitic eye must be considered, including different types of uveitis and their diagnoses, preoperative inflammation and treatment, postoperative inflammation and specific complications. With newer techniques and modern posterior chamber lenses, IOLs are being implanted with fewer complications. These IOLs are well tolerated in selected patients, especially when the lens is placed in the capsular bag. Many questions remain unanswered regarding the uveitic eye in conjunction with IOL biocompatibility and inflammation. Valuable information can be gained through more experience with IOL use in these eyes.

Due the heterogeneity and the scarce number of patients multicentric studies are needed to determine which, if any, IOL material is better tolerated in a uveitic patient by evaluating postoperative responses in the operative eye. This will be accomplished by descriptively comparing the postoperative outcome of these eyes when implanted with IOLs made of various materials. Outcomes will be determined by measuring visual acuities and postoperative parameters such as posterior capsule opacification, inflammatory responses and endothelial cell counts.

COMBINED SURGERIES

GLAUCOMA

Glaucoma associated with uveitis is one of the most serious complications of intraocular inflammation. It occurs with various syndromes and it may be difficult to manage. Most patients respond poorly to surgery. It is of primary importance to determine the severity of the inflammation and if possible, the syndrome associated with it. Management includes treatment of the underlying inflammation and of glaucoma itself. Various mechanisms produce secondary glaucoma, and it is important to identify them to institute the appropriate therapy. Special considerations should be given to the management of acute or chronic intraocular inflammation and if it is certain that corticosteroids are not the cause of the elevated pressure. Pharmacologic intervention is the first step in the treatment of uveitic glaucoma. Corticosteroids, acetazolamide, beta-blockers, cycloplegics, etc.

In general the results of the surgery for glaucoma in uveitic patients is not as good as it is for glaucoma in patients without uveitis. The following procedures can be performed: laser iridotomy, surgical iridectomy, trabeculodialysis, trabeculectomy, trabeculectomy with wound modulation therapy, *ab interno* laser sclerostomy, drainage implantation, cycloablation therapy.

Trabeculectomy with Wound Modulation Therapy

Actually mitomycin-C is replacing the use of 5-fluorouracil in preventing the wound healing after trabeculectomy.[16] The use of antimetabolites in association with trabeculectomy has been used for at least 10 years. Good surgical results have been reported for secondary glaucomas such as traumatic, aphakic, and pseudophakic glaucomas with the use of mitomycin C. Some problems are associated with the use of these medications. The highest success rate of filtering surgery with modulation of wound healing is associated with an elevated risk for hypotony, bleb leaks, and late bleb related endophthalmitis.[17] We perform this technique by placing a hemostat 0.02 mg/ml concentration of mitomycin C covered by the scleral flap during two minutes and without washing the remnants before suturing.

Drainage Implantation

This surgical strategy seems to be promising when facing a progressive secondary glaucoma with uveitis. The most commonly used device is the Molteno implant.[18] What makes this uniquely suited for the benefit of inflammatory glaucoma is the simple fact that the artificial material of the tube is incapable of scaring. The surface area of this plate allows for the elaboration of a fibrotic bleb across from which there is absorption of the accumulated aqueous. These devices are reserved for the intractable glaucoma patients with uveitis who have failed to improve with other medical procedures and if intercurrent or recurrent inflammation is believed to be the reason for a standard filter drainage procedure.

CATARACT REMOVAL AND VITRECTOMY

Combined phacoemulsification and pars plana vitrectomy technique has displayed many advantages over other techniques.[19,20] A small incision (even 3.00 mm) guarantees minimal corneal distortion and manipulation and these incisions are water-tight so they allow perfect closure during the vitrectomy portion of the operation. Lens density is not a main problem for phacoemulsification and allows the posterior capsule to remain intact, enabling endocapsular fixation of a posterior chamber lens. Delaying the IOL implantation until completion of vitrectomy, if required, allows fast visual rehabilitation and functional unaided vision in patients who are considered poor candidates for aphakic contact lens wear. If a limbal approach to the cataract and posterior pars plana vitrectomy is intended, the scleral incisions for the vitrectomy should be made first. Fixed infusion method and upper sclerotomies occluded with scleral plugs. The advantage of this procedure lies in preserving part of the posterior capsule for the secondary implant of an IOL. We prefer this approach whenever possible, first performing phacoemulsification of the crystalline lens followed by pars plana vitrectomy. A capsulotomy or posterior capsulorhexis must be performed on completion of the vitrectomy due to the fast opacification occurring and because it allows the decompartmentalization of the eye, facilitating the access of anti-inflammatory drugs in the postoperative stage.

POSTOPERATIVE TREATMENT

A strategy for blocking postoperative inflammation, thereby, avoiding potential ocular complications, is desirable. Topical steroids have become the standard care during the immediate postoperative period to reduce the morbidity associated with ocular inflammation, to prevent structural damage to the eye, and to reduce patient's discomfort.[21] In contemporary surgical practice, the ophthalmologist usually prescribes prednisolone or dexamethasone four times daily beginning one day after surgery, then tappering the dosage over the following four to six weeks. Acetate or alcohol vehicles are the most adequate due to their superior ocular penetration.

Although topical steroids are currently the most widely used anti-inflammatory agents after cataract extraction, their potential side effects limit their clinical effectiveness in some settings. This is particularly true for steroids that have a predilection for elevating intraocular pressure (IOP). Thus, anti-inflammatory agents that control postoperative inflammation with little effect on IOP would be a useful adjunct to the surgeons therapeutic armamentarium. A current strategy underlying the development of new steroidal compounds for ocular use is therefore, to identify drugs that exhibit marked anti-inflammatory activity while decreasing the propensity to raise IOP or induce other side effects.

In emergency cases, no strict guidelines are available, when a previous uveitis is present a severe postsurgical exacerbation of pre-existing inflammation should be expected. Depending on the severity of the case one week prior to surgery topical or systemic corticosteroids should be administered. At the time of surgery a subconjunctival corticosteroid should be injected periocular far from any ocular wounds. During the postoperative period, both topical and systemic corticosteroids may be tapered based on the severity of ocular inflammation. In the most severe cases moderate to high doses of oral prednisone from 1 to 1.5 mg/kg/day, and intensive once per hour topical corticosteroid drops should be given prior to and tapered after surgery. In cases of steroid-induced glaucoma the management may be much more difficult. In these cases temporary immunosuppressive therapy may need to be substituted to control inflammation in the early post-operative period. These guidelines may be applied for all intraocular procedures in uveitis eyes.

Several recent studies have assessed the effectiveness of nonsteroidal anti-inflammatory drug (NSAID) to treat ocular inflammation. Most NSAIDs used today act by inhibiting the enzyme cyclo-oxygenase and thereby decreasing the formation of prostaglandins, which play a major role in ocular inflammation by producing and maintaining the rupture of the blood-aqueous barrier. Diclofenac drops were shown to reduce inflammation after argon laser trabeculoplasty,[22] and after cataract surgery.[23] The role of these drugs is then controversial in the post-operative control of inflammation even in uncomplicated senile cataracts. We cannot offer these drugs as an alternative to corticosteroids or even as an adjunct to treatment in uveitis patients with cataract.

FOLLOW-UP

Generally a low inflammatory reaction is observed after IOL implantation in patients with chronic anterior uveitis if preoperative and postoperative anti-inflammatory measures are undertaken. Complications associated with these patients in the follow-up are related to:

Posterior Capsule Opacification

It has been described that the frequency of this complication in some series is as high as 50% of cases.[24]

Membranes

The appearance of fibrous membranes mostly in pars planitis patients have been described.[25] These membranes are dense enough to resist Nd:YAG laser rupture with high levels of energy. The tendency to reform is known and they are associated with displacements of the lens and retinal detachment.

Decreased Visual Acuity

The major causes of decreased visual acuity in these patients are cystic macular edema,[4] epiretinal membrane,[26] and glaucomatous optic nerve damage.[5] Nevertheless a proper visual acuity can be achieved in the majority of patients in

the most important series of patients published.[6,2] Visual acuities better than 20/40 can be achieved in 20 to 75% of patients.[6,22]

Even low-grade chronic inflammation can result in permanent damage to the optic nerve, retina, anterior chamber angle and other structures that may preclude our efforts for a visual rehabilitation after cataract surgery. Early surgical intervention prior to the development of permanent structural damage from inflammation or corticosteroid therapy may be the option for the future. Better surgical approaches and the choice of the ideal lens for each patient is the goal for the present and the future in the surgical management of cataract in patients with uveitis.

SUMMARY

Cataract in patients with uveitis is a frequent event that must be managed by surgical intervention. The surgical approach must be always individualized attending to the symptoms referred to by the patient, especially visual acuity, the etiology of uveitis, the treatment necessary to maintain a quiescent state, and the expected difficulties of surgery. Preoperative and postoperative control of the inflammation is mandatory and none of these patients should be enrolled in a standard surgical approach for senile cataracts.

REFERENCES

1. Kanski JJ, Shun Shin GA. Systemic uveitis syndromes in childhood: an analysis of 340 cases. Ophthalmology 1984;91: 1247-52.
2. Tabbara KF, Chavis PS. Cataract extraction in patients with chronic posterior uveitis. Int Ophthalmol Clin 1995;35:121-31.
3. Ram J, Jain S, Pandav SS. Postoperative complications of intraocular lens implantation in patients with Fuch's hetero-chromic cyclitis. J Cataract Refract Surg 1995;21: 548-1.
4. Kaplan I IJ, Foster CS, Fong LP, et al. Cataract surgery and intraocular lens implantation in patients with uveitis. Ophthalmology 1989;96: 287-8.
5. Moorthy RS, Rajeev B, Smith RE, et al. Incidence and management of cataract in Vogt-Koyanagi-Harada syndrome. Am J Ophthalmol 1994;118:197-204.
6. Alió JL, Chipont E. Multicentrical IOIS study on surgery of cataract in the uveitic patient. First combined International Symposium on Ocular Immunology and Inflammation. Amsterdam June 1998 (Personal communication).
7. Hooper PL, Rao N. Cataract extraction in uveitis patients. Surv Ophthalmol 1990;35:120-45.
8. Alió JL, Ben Ezra D, Chipont E. Cataract in patients with uveitis. Symposium on Cataract IOL and Refractive Surgery, Seattle 1999 (Personal communication).
9. Alió JL, Chipont E. Inflamación en Cirugía de la catarata. Inflamaciones Culares EDIKAMED (Ed): Barcelona 1995; 407-28.
10. Alió JL, Chipont E, Sayans JA. Flare-cell meter measurement of inflammation after uneventful cataract surgery with intraocular lens implantation. J Cataract Refract Surg 1997;23: 935-9.
11. Lowenstein A, Bracha R, Lazar I. Intraocular lens implantation in an eye with Behcet's uveitis. J Cataract Refr Surg 1991;17: 95-7.

12. Percival SPB, Pai V. Heparin-modified lenses for eyes at risk for breakdown of the blood-aqueous barrier during cataract surgery. J Cataract Refrc Surg 1993;19: 760-5.

13. Drews RC. Lens implantation lessons learned from the first million. Trans Ophthalmol Soc UK 1982;102: 505-9.

14. Alió JL, Sayans J, Chipont E. Laser flare-cell measurement of inflammation after uneventful extracapsular cataract extraction and intraocular lens implantation. J Cataract Refract Surg 1996;22: 775-9.

15. Martinez JJ, Artola A, Chipont. Total anterior capsule closure after silicone intraocular lens implantation. J Cataract Refract Surg 1996;22: 269-71.

16. Palmer SS. Mitomycin as an adjunct chemotherapy with trabeculectomy. Ophthalmology 1991;98: 317-21.

17. Wolnetr B, Liebmann JM. Late bleb related endophthalmitis after trabeculectomy with adjunctive 5 Fluorouracil. Ophthalmology 1991;98: 1053-60.

18. Hill RA, Nguyen QH. Trabeculectomy and Molteno implantation for glaucomas associated with uveitis. Ophthalmology 1993;93: 903-8.

19. Koening SB, Han DP, Msfieler WF. Combined phacoemulsification and pars plana vitrectomy. Arch Ophthalmol 1990;108: 362-64.

20. MacKool RJ. Pars plana vitrectomy and posterior chamber intraocular lens implantation in diabetic patients. Ophthalmology 1989;96: 1679-80.

21. Jaanus SD. Anti-inflammatory drugs. In Bartlett JD, Jaanus SD (Eds): Clinical Ocular Pharmacology. Boston: Butterworth Publishers; 1989. pp. 163-97.

22. Herbort CP, Mermoud A. Antiinflammatory effect of Diclofenac drops after argon laser trabeculoplasty. Arch Ophthalmol 1993;111: 481-3.

23. Othenin P, Borruat X. Association declofenac-dexamethasone dans le traitement de linflammation postoperatorie. Klin Monatsbl Augenheilkd 1992;200: 362-6.

24. Akova YA, Foster CS. Cataract surgery in patients with sarcoidosis-associated uveitis. Ophthalmology 1994;101: 473-9.

25. Tessler HH, Faber MD. Intraocular lens implantation versus no implantation in patients with chronic iridocyclitis and pars planitis. Ophthalmology 1993;100: 1026-9.

26. Kaufman AH, Foster CS. Cataract extraction in patients with pars planitis. Ophthalmology 1993;100: 1210-7.

Complications

CHAPTER 53

Posterior Capsular Rupture

Dhivya Ashok Kumar, Amar Agarwal

INTRODUCTION

Any breach in the continuity of the posterior capsule is defined as a posterior capsule tear. Intrasurgical posterior capsule tears are common and can occur during any stage of cataract surgery.[1-3] The incidence of posterior capsule complications is related to the type of cataract and conditions of the eye. It increases with the grade of difficulty of the case, and furthermore is influenced by the surgeon's level of experience. Timely recognition and a planned management, depending upon the stage of surgery during which the posterior capsule tear has occurred, is required to ensure an optimal visual outcome.

COMMON RISK FACTORS FOR POSTERIOR CAPSULAR RUPTURE (PCR)

- Intraoperative factors causing variation in anterior chamber depth
- Type of cataract
- Extended rhexis.

INTRAOPERATIVE FACTORS CAUSING VARIATION IN ANTERIOR CHAMBER DEPTH

Intraoperative shallow anterior chamber could be due to various reasons. It may be a tight lid speculum, tight drapes or pull from the collecting bag. In all the above cases, one needs to remove the precipitating factors (to remove the speculum pressure and the tight drapes and collecting bags). Variation in the amount of space in the anterior and posterior chambers may result from changes in the intraocular pressure (IOP) due to an alteration in the equilibrium between inflow and outflow of fluid. Diminished inflow may be secondary to insufficient bottle height, tube occlusion or compression, bottle emptying, too tight incisions compressing the irrigation sleeve or the surgeon moving the phaco tip out of the incision, making the irrigation holes come out of the incision. Excessive outflow may be caused by too high vacuum/flow parameters or too large incisions with leakage. Another cause is the postocclusion surge. Use of air pump or gas forced infusion solves most of these problems of intraoperative shallow anterior chamber.[1]

TYPE OF CATARACT

A higher incidence of posterior capsule tear with vitreous loss is associated with cataract with pseudoexfoliation,

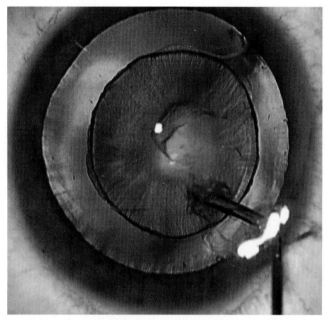

FIGURE 53.1: Hydrodelineation being performed in a posterior polar cataract

diabetes mellitus and trauma. Missing the diagnosis in a posterior polar cataract (**Figure 53.1**) can be catastrophic to the surgeon and the patient. It is frequently associated with a weakened or deficient posterior capsule. Posterior lenticonus, cataracts with persistent primary hyperplastic vitreous, cataracts following vitreoretinal surgery and morgagnian cataracts are some of the other types. In any intraoperative diagnosis of posterior polar cataract, it is to avoid hydrodissection with balanced salt solution (BSS). Hydrodissection may cause hydraulic perforation at the weakened area of the capsule, hence only a careful controlled hydrodelineation is preferred. One can also make multiple pockets of viscoelastic injection around the nucleus. If a capsular tear does occur, a closed system should be maintained by injecting viscoelastic before withdrawing the phaco tip. This helps to tamponade the vitreous backwards where a capsular dehiscence is present.

EXTENDED RHEXIS

Extension of anterior capsule can occur as a complication in MICS also. During capsulorhexis, anterior capsular tears can cause posterior capsule tear by extending to the periphery. In a new method of managing this situation, a nick is made from the opposite side of the rhexis using a cystitome or vannas and the capsulorhexis is completed. The viscoelastic in the anterior chamber (AC) is then expressed out to make the globe hypotonous, following which a gentle hydrodissection is done at 90° from the tear, while pressing the posterior lip of the incision to prevent any rise in intraocular pressure (IOP). No attempt is made to press on the center of the nucleus to complete the fluid wave. The fluid is usually sufficient to prolapse one pole of the nucleus out of the capsular bag; else it is removed by embedding the phacoemulsification probe, making sure not to exert any downward pressure and then gently pulling the nucleus anteriorly. The whole nucleus is brought out into the AC and no nuclear division techniques are tried in the bag. The entire nucleus is prolapsed into the anterior chamber and emulsified.

STEPS FOR MANAGEMENT OF PCR

Surgeon should be aware of the signs **(Table 53.1)** of posterior capsular tear. Posterior capsule tears can occur during any stage of phacoemulsification surgery. They occurred most frequently during the stage of nuclear emulsification, as reported by Mulhern et al[4](49%) and Osher et al[5] and during irrigation–aspiration, as reported by Gimbel et al.[6]

TABLE 53.1 Signs of posterior capsular rupture
• Sudden deepening of the chamber, with momentary expansion of the pupil
• Sudden, transitory appearance of a clear red reflex peripherally
• Apparent inability to rotate a previously mobile nucleus
• Excessive lateral mobility or displacement of the nucleus
• Excessive tipping of one pole of the nucleus
• Partial descent of the nucleus into the anterior vitreous space
• 'Pupil snap sign' – sudden marked pupil constriction after hydro-dissection

Three possible situations can happen in a posterior capsule rent namely:[7]
- Posterior capsule tear with hyaloid face intact and nuclear material present
- Posterior capsule tear with hyaloid face ruptured without luxation of nuclear material into vitreous
- Posterior capsule tear with hyaloid face ruptured and luxation of nuclear material into vitreous.

Immediate precautions are to be taken not to do further hydrate the vitreous and not to increase the size of the PCR. The conventional management consists of prevention of mixture of cortical matter with vitreous, dry aspiration and anterior vitrectomy, if required. In addition, during phacoemulsification, low flow rate, high vacuum and low ultrasound are advocated if a posterior capsule tear occurs.

REDUCE THE PARAMETERS

Lowering aspiration flow rate and decreasing the vacuum will control surge and will allow the bottle to be lowered,

diminishing turbulence inside the eye. If the nucleus is soft, only a small residual amount remains, and there is no vitreous prolapse, the procedure may be continued. If vitreous is already present, special care must be taken for preventing additional vitreous prolapse into the anterior chamber or to the wound. Small residual nucleus or cortex can be emulsified by bringing it out of the capsular bag and can be emulsified in the anterior chamber with viscoelastic underneath the corneal endothelium. In case of a small PCR and minimal residual nucleus **(Figure 53.2)**, a dispersive viscoelastic is injected to plug the posterior capsule tear. Subsequently, the nuclear material is moved into the anterior chamber with a spatula and emulsified. The recommended parameters are low bottle height (20–40 cm above the patient's head), low flow rate (10–15 cc/ min), high vacuum (120–200 mm Hg) and low ultrasound (20–40%).

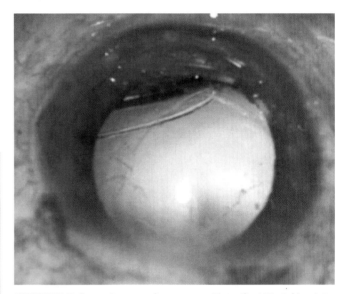

FIGURE 53.2: Posterior capsular rupture. Note the IOL sinking into the vitreous cavity. The white reflex indicates nuclear fragments also in the vitreous cavity. This patient was managed by vitrectomy, FAVIT (removal of the nuclear fragments) and the IOL repositioned in the sulcus

DRY CORTICAL ASPIRATION

If there is only a small amount or no vitreous prolapse in the presence of a small capsular rent, a dry cortical aspiration with 23 G cannula can be performed.

VISCOEXPRESSION

It is a method of removal of the residual nucleus by injecting viscoelastic underneath the nucleus to support it and the nucleus is expressed along with the viscoelastic.

CONVERSION TO EXTRACAPSULAR CATARACT EXTRACTION (ECCE)

If there is sizeable amount of residual nucleus, it is advisable to convert to a large incision ECCE to minimize the possibility of a dropped nucleus.

ANTERIOR BIMANUAL VITRECTOMY

Bimanual vitrectomy (**Figure 53.3**) is done in eyes with vitreous prolapse. Use 23 G irrigating cannula via side port after extending the side port incision. The irrigation bottle is positioned at the appropriate height to maintain the anterior chamber during vitrectomy. Vitrectomy should be performed with cutting rate (500–800 cuts per minute), an aspiration flow rate of 20 cc/min and a vacuum of 150–200 mm Hg.

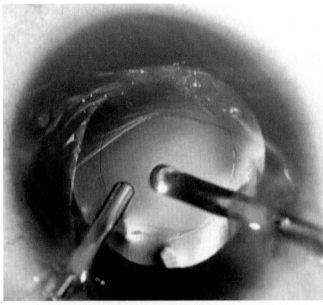

FIGURE 53.3: Bimanual vitrectomy is being performed in a posterior capsular tear with vitreous prolapse

ANTERIOR CHAMBER CLEARED OF VITREOUS

Vitrectomy is continued in the anterior chamber and the pupillary plane. A rod can be introduced into the anterior chamber to check the presence of any vitreous traction and the same should be released. Complete removal of the vitreous from the anterior chamber can be confirmed if one sees a circular, mobile pupil (**Figures 53.4A and B**) and

complete air bubble in the anterior chamber. The usage of the fiber of an endoilluminator, dimming the room lights and microscope lights, may be useful in cases of doubt, in order to identify vitreous strands. Another useful measure is the use of purified triamcinolone acetate suspension (Kenalog) to identify the vitreous described by Peyman.[8] Kenalog particles remain trapped on and within the vitreous gel, making it clearly visible.[9]

SUTURE THE WOUND

In cases with vitreous loss with PCR, it is recommended to suture the corneal wound as a prophylaxis to prevent infection. One should remove any residual vitreous in the incision site in the main and side port with vitrector or manually with Vannas scissors. If necessary, one needs to insert a rod via the side port and pass it over the surface of the iris, to release them.

IOL IMPLANTATION

Depending upon the state of the capsular bag and rhexis, IOL is implanted (**Table 53.2**).

TABLE 53.2	IOL implantation in PCR

- Insertion and rotation of IOL should always be away from the area of capsule tear
- The long axis of the IOL should cross the meridian of the posterior capsule tear
- Eyes with (< 6 mm) PCR with no vitreous loss, IOL can be placed in the capsular bag
- In the presence of a posterior capsule tear(>6 mm) with adequate anterior capsule rim, an IOL can be placed in the sulcus
- In deficient capsules, Glued IOL is a promising technique without complications of sutured scleral fixated or anterior chamber IOL

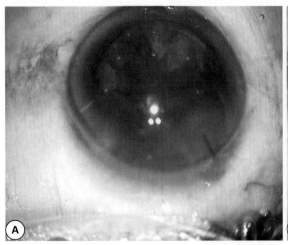

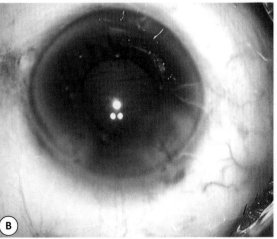

FIGURES 53.4A AND B: Clinical photographs showing the change in the anterior chamber after complete removal of the vitreous from the anterior chamber. (A) Before vitrectomy, (B) After vitrectomy

IN THE BAG

In the presence of a posterior capsule tear with good capsular bag, the IOL can be placed in the bag. Small PCR with no vitreous loss and good capsular bag, foldable IOL can be placed.

IN THE SULCUS

If the rent is large, if the capsular rim is available, then the IOL can be placed in the sulcus. The rigid IOL can be placed in the sulcus in large PCR over the residual anterior capsular rim with Mc Person forceps holding the optic. The "chopstick technique" is another method of placing IOL in sulcus. In this new chopstick forceps namely, 'Agarwal-Katena forceps' **(Figures 53.5A and B)** is used for IOL implantation. This chopstick technique refers to the IOL being held between two flangs of the forceps. The advantage is the smooth placement of the IOL in the sulcus without excess manipulation. Moreover, the IOL implantation is more controlled **(Figures 53.6A to D)** with the forceps as compared to other methods. Small PCR with

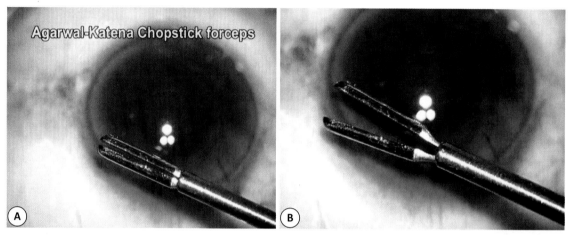

FIGURES 53.5A AND B: (A) Photograph of an 'Agarwal- Katena' forceps. (B) Reverse opening shown (Katena, USA)

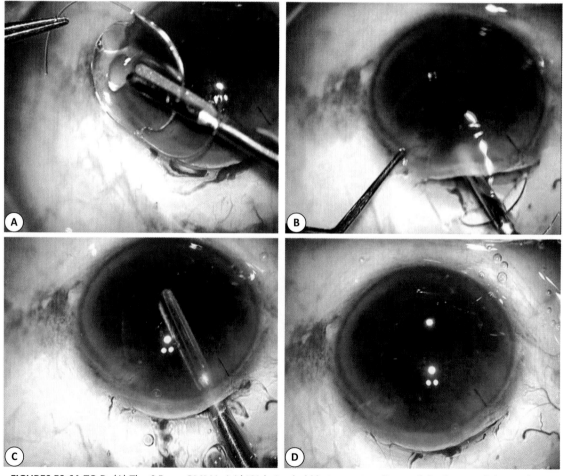

FIGURES 53.6A TO D: (A) The 6.5 mm PMMA rigid IOL being held between two flangs of the forceps. (B) IOL is being introduced through the limbal incision. (C) IOL is positioned in the sulcus. (D) IOL is well centered

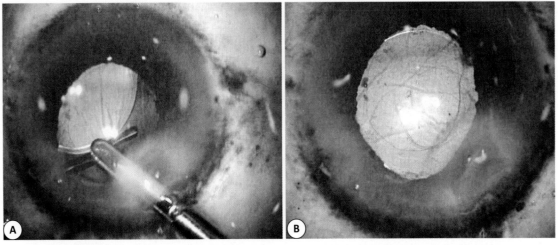

FIGURES 53.7A AND B: (A) Foldable IOL is placed with 'Agarwal-Katena' forceps into the sulcus, (B) IOL well centered on the capsular rim

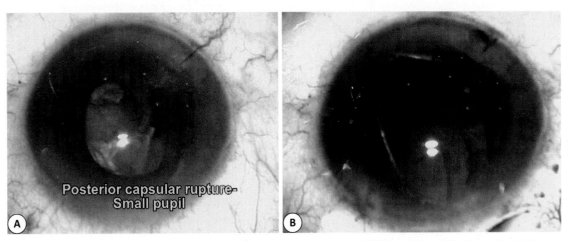

Posterior capsular rupture–
Small pupil

FIGURES 53.8A AND B: (A) Intraoperative miosis with posterior capsular tear. (B) Agarwal's modification of the Malyugin ring iris expansion: A 6-0 polyglactic vicryl suture passed in the leading scroll of the ring and injected. The end of the suture stays at the main port incision

no vitreous loss and good capsular bag, foldable IOL can be placed (**Figures 53.7A and B**). In eyes with intraoperative miosis with PCR, IOL can be implanted with the pupil expansion with "Agarwal's modified Malyugin ring" method (**Figures 53.8A and B**). In this method,[10] a 6-0 polyglactic suture is placed in the leading scroll of the Malyugin ring and injected into the pupillary plane (**Figures 53.9A and B**). The end of the suture stays at the main port incision. Once in place, the ring produced a stable mydriasis of about 6.0 mm. Hereby, IOL can be implanted easily in the sulcus with visualization and this prevents the inadvertent dropping of the iris expander into the vitreous during intraoperative manipulation.

DEFICIENT POSTERIOR CAPSULE

Now recently Glued IOL[11-13] is easily performed in such cases with deficient posterior capsules. Scleral fixated posterior chamber lenses and anterior chamber IOLs[14,15] can also be implanted when the posterior capsule tear is large.

SQUELAE AFTER POSTERIOR CAPSULAR RUPTURE

Vitreous Traction

Incomplete vitrectomy can produce dynamic traction on the retina leading to retinal breaks.

Retinal Detachment

Undetected long standing vitreous traction progresses to retinal break and detachment.

Macular Edema

Manipulation of vitreous will increase not only the traction transmitted to the retina but also the inflammation in the posterior segment and the risk of macular edema.

Vitritis

Over-enthusiastic use of viscoelastic into the vitreous can lead to sterile inflammation. Dropped minimal residual cortex can also present with postoperative vitritis.

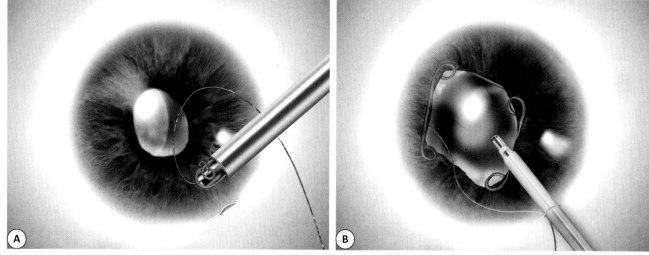

FIGURES 53.9A AND B: Illustration depicting the Agarwal modification of the Malyugin ring for cases with small pupil with a posterior capsular rupture. (A) 6/0 suture tied to the ring. (B) Malyugin ring in place in the pupil. The suture can be pulled at if the ring begins to fall into the vitreous

IOL RELATED COMPLICATIONS

Improperly placed IOL in the sulcus can lead to lens induced astigmatism and tilt.

CONCLUSION

The occurrence of a posterior capsule tear during cataract surgery is one of the most serious complications. It is important for a surgeon to diagnose the occurrence of a posterior capsule tear at an early stage, to avoid further enlargement of the tear and associated vitreous complications. The primary goal of all the maneuvers is to remove the remaining nucleus, epinucleus, and as much as cortex possible without causing vitreoretinal traction.

REFERENCES

1. Agarwal A. Phaco nightmares. Conquering Cataract Catastrophes. USA: Slack Inc; 2006.
2. Agarwal S, Agarwal A, Agarwal A. Phacoemulsification. 3rd edition. Delhi: Jaypee Brothers; 2004.
3. Fishkind WJ. Facing Down the 5 Most Common Cataract Complications. Review of Ophthalmology: 2001.
4. Mulhern M, Kelly G, Barry P. Effects of posterior capsular disruption on the outcome of phacoemulsification surgery. Br J Ophthalmol. 1995;79:1133–7.
5. Osher RH, Cionni RJ. The torn posterior capsule: its intraoperative behaviour, surgical management and long term consequences. J Cataract Refract Surg. 1990;16(4):490–4.
6. Gimbel HV. Posterior capsular tears during phacoemulsi-fication—causes, prevention and management. Eur J Refract Surg. 1990;2:63–9.
7. Vajpayee RB, Sharma N, Dada T, et al. Management of posterior capsule tears. Surv Ophthal. 2001;45:473-88.
8. Peyman GA, Cheema R, Conway MD, et al. Triamcinolone acetonide as an aid to visualization of the vitreous and the posterior hyaloid during pars plana vitrectomy. Retina. 2000;20:554-5.
9. Burk SE, Da Mata AP, Snyder ME, et al. Visualizing vitreous using Kenalog suspension. J Cataract Refract Surg. 2003;29:645-51.
10. Agarwal A, Malyugin B, Kumar DA, et al. Modified Malyugin ring iris expansion technique in small-pupil cataract surgery with posterior capsule defect. J Cataract Refract Surg. 2008;34(5):724-6.
11. Agarwal A, Kumar DA, Jacob S, et al. Fibrin glue–assisted sutureless posterior chamber intraocular lens implantation in eyes with deficient posterior capsules. J Cataract Refract Surg. 2008;34:1433–8.
12. Agarwal A, Kumar DA, Prakash G, et al. Fibrin glue–assisted sutureless posterior chamber intraocular lens implantation in eyes with deficient posterior capsules. [Reply to letter]. J Cataract Refract Surg. 2009;35:795-6.
13. Prakash G, Kumar DA, Jacob S, et al. Anterior segment optical coherence tomography–aided diagnosis and primary posterior chamber intraocular lens implantation with fibrin glue in traumatic phacocele with scleral perforation. J Cataract Refract Surg. 2009;35(4):782-4.
14. Bleckmann H, Kaczmarek U. Functional results of posterior chamber lens implantation with scleral fixation. J Cataract Refract Surg. 1994;20(3):321–6.
15. Numa A, Nakamura J, Takashima M, et al. Long-term corneal endothelial changes after intraocular lens implantation. Anterior vs posterior chamber lenses. Jpn J Ophthalmol. 1993;37(1): 78–87.

CHAPTER 54

Posterior Capsule Rupture and Vitreous Loss

Brian Little

INTRODUCTION

There has been a steady improvement in the safety of cataract surgery since the inception of phacoemulsification, so that now the risk of sight-threatening complications is reassuringly low and generally accepted to be in the order of 1 in 1000. However, there remains a small but persistent incidence of serious complications,[1-4] which can be measured using the validated proxy of posterior capsule rupture (PCR) and vitreous loss (VL) that run at approximately 2% of procedures.

PREVENTING VITREOUS LOSS

The importance of intraoperative complications lies in their potential seriousness, but their potential seriousness is usually determined not by their occurrence *per se*, but by the way in which they are managed. Therefore, the operating surgeon has principal responsibility for the incidence, the immediate impact and ultimately the final outcome of any complication. In order to achieve the best possible result the surgeon has to adopt a calm, strategic, methodical and careful approach. If this principle is followed then the final result can be just as good as if the complication had never happened, and this is the ideal outcome for everyone.

RISK FACTORS FOR VITREOUS LOSS

Fortunately one is now in a position to be able to quantify and take into account the various surgeon and patient factors that predict the relative risk of vitreous loss. This information is available from the data provided by large-scale prospective studies, such as the cataract national dataset from the UK (over 55,500 cases).

We can now recognize and quantify specific preoperative risk factors so that we are able to a degree, to bring them under some control. Factors such as advanced cataract, elderly patient, long and short axial length, small pupil, zonular weakness, poor visibility, etc. can be anticipated before surgery and planned for appropriately.

Of course the intraoperative risk factors for vitreous loss are less easy to anticipate but they come into play at every stage of the procedure from capsulorhexis through to final intracameral injection of an antibiotic or miotic at the end of surgery.

RISK FACTORS DURING CAPSULORHEXIS

Problems during capsulorhexis that increase the risk of vitreous loss include a small rhexis (broad shelf of anterior capsule vulnerable to tearing by the phaco tip or second instrument, increased risk of capsular block and posterior capsule (PC) tear during hydrodissection) and discontinuity of the edge such as an unrecognized notch or a radialized tear-out.

RISK FACTORS DURING HYDRODISSECTION

During hydrodissection itself there is a risk of posterior capsule tear from over-distending the bag due to capsular block or due to failure to ballotte the nucleus backwards when fluid is sequestered behind the nucleus, in front of the posterior capsule.

RISK FACTORS DURING PHACO

Early on during phaco, it is quite easy to phaco the edge of the rhexis whence it is likely to tear out into the zonules and possibly beyond resulting in a wrap-around tear. The risk of dropped nucleus or nuclear fragment is therefore high in this situation.

Successful removal of the nucleus is possible but difficult and hazardous in the presence of a radial anterior capsule tear (**Figure 54.1**). Meticulous care has to be taken during IOL implantation if it is decided to place it within the bag and, in particular, rapid removal of OVD at the end can

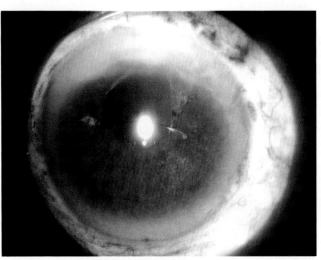

FIGURE 54.1: Dislocated endocapsular ring
(*Courtesy:* Dr Agarwal's Eye Hospital, India)

result in sudden decompression and chamber collapse that precipitates a wrap-around extension of the tear into the posterior capsule.

Pushing the phaco tip unnecessarily into the peripheral nucleus is seen early as well as later in the learning curve. In general, this should be avoided because of the high risk of damaging the peripheral capsule.

If the posterior capsule is torn early during nuclear fragmentation then the lens will no longer rotate freely in the bag. This is a specific and important sign that needs to be heeded, as the nucleus is very likely to drop if surgery is continued.

Inadequate hydrodissection performed earlier will come back to bite the surgeon towards the end of nucleus removal because he will now have to deal with a large bowl of epinucleus that remains stuck to the capsule. If this is pursued using the phaco tip then there is a high likelihood of aspirating and popping the peripheral posterior capsule.

The most common time to tear the posterior capsule during phaco is actually whilst removing the final nuclear fragment. At this point, postocclusion surge readily collapses the empty capsular bag, drawing the unsupported and floppy posterior capsule onto the phaco tip. Judicious use of a second instrument may help to keep the capsule away but lowering the vacuum for the final fragment also helps and using pulsed, burst or torsional phaco keeps the fragment impaled on the tip and thereby minimize vacuum break and postocclusion surge. Additionally, many surgeons now prefer in fact to withdraw the second instrument altogether during removal of the final fragment since its presence in the sideport tends to be accompanied by significant incisional leakage, leading to chamber instability. So, paradoxically, one could argue that a second instrument is needed in the first place in order to help with the problem that it causes by being there. In other words, the presence of the second instrument causes chamber instability so the second instrument is needed to hold back the posterior capsule that flops forward only because of the chamber instability that the second instrument has caused through incisional leakage.

It is worth remembering that the posterior capsule can be torn towards the end of phaco without necessarily breaking the anterior hyaloid face. If this is the case, then a free straight-edged flap of capsule is visible. It is critical not to panic at this point by withdrawing the irrigation, as this is all that is holding back the vitreous face. An ophthalmic viscosurgical device - balanced salt solution (OVD-BSS) exchange will keep the flap tamponaded and allow the surgeon to safely convert it into a primary posterior capsulorhexis.

If the irrigation is withdrawn in a panic then the vitreous will burst through the capsular defect as the chamber collapses.

Overall the most common stage of surgery for vitreous loss is during Irrigation-Aspiration (IA) when the capsular bag is empty and unsupported. Good visibility of the

aspiration port throughout IA is an important safety factor. It should be kept facing forwards at all times and not tilted sideways, which is often tempting when trying to reach less accessible sub-incisional cortex.

It is to beware that the edge on some aspiration ports, particularly of disposable cannulae, are sometimes sharp and unpolished, whilst those that are chamfered and polished are far less likely to tear the capsule once it has been aspirated.

There are a few factors during IOL implantation (**Figure 54.2**) that are worth mentioning as they represent an increased risk of vitreous loss. The first is to make sure that the capsular bag is fully inflated before attempting to implant the lens. An under-inflated bag is more likely to be snagged and dragged by the implant resulting in a capsular or zonular tear if the surgeon persists with the implantation.

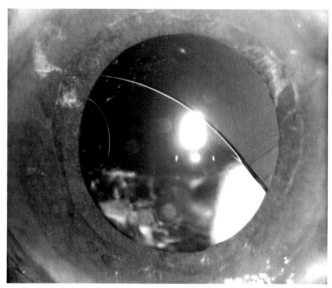

FIGURE 54.2: Dislocated PC IOL (*Courtesy:* Dr Agarwal's Eye Hospital, India)

Care also needs to be taken not to use excessive force when trying initially to push the implant through the incision. This is particularly likely if forceps are being used, instead of an injector, when the wound needs to be enlarged (symmetrically funnelled) to accommodate the bulk of the implant plus forceps. If excessive force is used, then the OVD is likely to be expressed from the eye and the implant delivered explosively through the wound, which is more likely to cause PC rupture and vitreous loss.

Finally there is a small but finite risk of shooting any cannula that is used for intracameral antibiotic or miotic through the posterior capsule at the end of an otherwise uneventful operation. This risk can be effectively zeroed by always using a Luer-Lock syringe whenever injecting any fluid into the eye.

So in summary, it is easy to forget that although the incidence of vitreous loss is low, its consequences are still potentially disastrous. In the presence of vitreous loss, there is a higher risk of endophthalmitis, cystoid macular edema, suprachoroidal hemorrhage, glaucoma and retinal detachment. In fact, the risk of retinal detachment following cataract surgery goes up by about 15-fold if the surgery is complicated by vitreous loss.

All these risk factors for vitreous loss can be largely quantified, anticipated and prevented by careful and strategic surgery. On detailed analysis the prevention of complications requires a balanced mixture of Anticipation, Attitude (avoiding denial and being self-disciplined), Adaptability (dealing calmly with the unexpected), Aptitude (innate or acquired competence) and Acquired Skill (that comes with experience and learning) in the operating surgeon. With the right fusion of these skills, something that nearly every motivated surgeon is capable of, the performance of an anterior vitrectomy or any other surgical procedure is likely to proceed to a successful outcome. With this background in mind, the practical details of carrying out anterior vitrectomy will now be discussed.

ANTERIOR VITRECTOMY AND TRIAMCINOLONE

Most trainees have never really been taught how to properly perform an anterior vitrectomy; to understand the instruments, how they work, to know the appropriate machine settings, how to use the instruments and the techniques for performing the vitrectomy **(Figure 54.3)**. These are critically important in order to obtain the best possible outcome; so that the final result following anterior vitrectomy is as good as if it had never happened.

There is a clear strategy for dealing with vitreous loss that can be summarized as follows:
• Do not panic
• Do not deny it
• Do not pull it
• Visualize it
• Remove it
• Follow it up

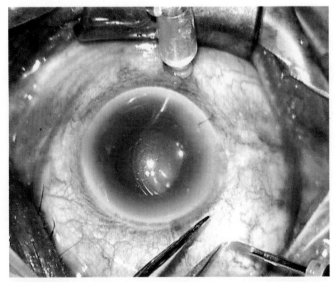

FIGURE 54.3: 23 G sutureless vitrectomy using trocar and cannula in a dislocated IOL (*Courtesy:* Dr Agarwal's Eye Hospital, India)

If one suspects that vitreous loss has occurred one should try to stay calm, which can be difficult, but one can definitely learn to override the immediate brainstem reflex, which is to withdraw the instruments from the eye. One should leave the irrigating instrument in the eye (whether phaco or I/A) with the irrigation still running, in order to keep the vitreous tamponaded whilst one performs a BSS/OVD exchange that will fill the chamber with viscoelastic. One does this by inserting the OVD cannula through the sideport and starts to inject the viscoelastic while turning off the irrigation. It is to leave the irrigating instrument in the eye in order to occlude the wound whilst the chamber fills with OVD. As it fills one can safely remove the irrigating instrument without the risk of chamber collapse and vitreous prolapse.

The first thing one can then assess is whether or not the vitreous face has indeed been ruptured or whether all one has is in fact a PC tear with an intact anterior hyaloid face. PC tears usually occur at the end of phaco with removal of the final fragment or most commonly during I/A. In either case, usually, there are fortunately no longer any nuclear fragments around. If this is the case, then the bag should be inflated with OVD and the PC tear then circularized, using rhexis forceps, into a primary posterior capsulorhexis when a lens can then be safely inserted into the bag as planned.

If there is obvious vitreous loss then one must strongly resist the immediate temptation to deny that it has happened. It can be almost irresistible to just continue as if everything was proceeding as normal. However, this is plainly dangerous and will work against a good outcome. If there is vitreous around in the anterior chamber then one should not be using a non-cutting instrument in the eye, which very much includes the phaco probe. Ultrasound does not cut vitreous. If one continues with phaco then vitreous will inevitably be aspirated into the tip and traction will thereby be transmitted to the vitreous base. Vitreous base traction is highly likely to pull a retinal tear, leading to retinal detachment. One should bear in mind that the retinal pigment epithelium (RPE) pump, holding the sensory retina to the underlying RPE, exerts a pressure of only 0.27 mm Hg. The exact same principles apply to using I/A in the eye when there is vitreous around. So one should simply refuse to submit to the temptation to pretend that nothing has happened; one should have the honesty and humility to admit that there is a problem and then sort it out. Pretending otherwise will cause greater problems and will result in a worse outcome.

One of the most significant innovations in the safe surgical management of vitreous gel has without doubt been the intraoperative use of triamcinolone acetonide to visualize invisible vitreous, pioneered by Scott Burk in 2003. Adoption of this technique has been slow but steady and has increased more recently, since licensed preservative-free preparations have become commercially available. Initially, the product used was triamcinolone acetonide (Kenalog, Bristol Myers Sqibb) 40 mg/ml for which intracameral use is off-label **(Figures 54.4 to 54.8)**. Other licensed products now available include Triesence from Alcon and Trivaris from Allergan. There are a number of other preparations available from different manufacturers, depending in which country one practices.

In principle, a suspension of 40 mg/ml (Trivaris is 80 mg/ml) is diluted between three and ten times with BSS and injected directly into the anterior chamber. It adheres to vitreous and visualizes otherwise invisible gel. A process accurately likened to "Cloaking the Ghost". The excess suspension is washed out of the chamber and then the stained gel vitrectomized. There is simply no other way of ensuring a complete and meticulous removal of all gel with total confidence. It is this complete removal which is so critical to preventing most of the complications associated with vitreous loss which nearly all relate to the persistence of residual vitreous gel in the anterior segment and incarcerated in the wounds (e.g. vitreous wick, endophthalmitis, VR traction, CMO, glaucoma and peaked pupil).

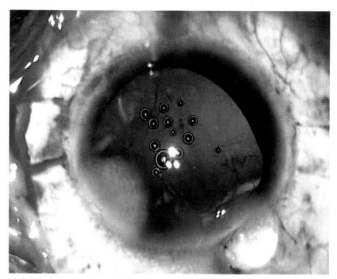

FIGURE 54.6: Vitreous loss (*Courtesy:* Dr Agarwal's Eye Hospital, India)

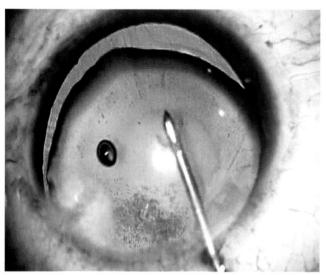

FIGURE 54.4: 8 Subluxated cataract with Posterior capsular rupture (*Courtesy:* Dr Agarwal's Eye Hospital, India)

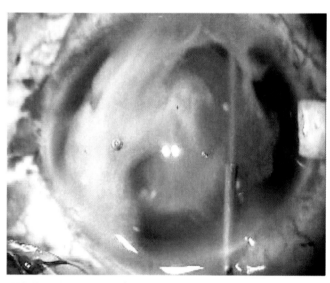

FIGURE 54.7: Triamcinolone injection (*Courtesy:* Dr Agarwal's Eye Hospital, India)

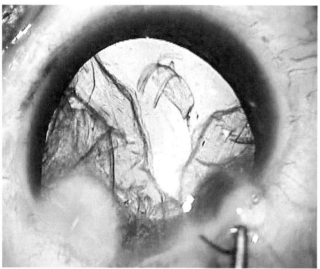

FIGURE 54.5: Subluxated cataract case has a posterior capsular rupture (*Courtesy:* Dr Agarwal's Eye Hospital, India)

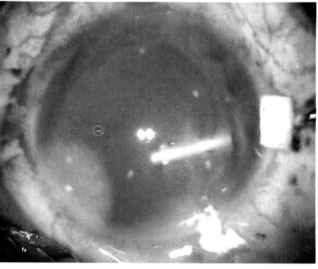

FIGURE 54.8: Vitrectomy done to clear the triamcinolone (*Courtesy:* Dr Agarwal's Eye Hospital, India)

The details of the technique and instrumentation that enables high quality anterior vitrectomy are straightforward but important to clearly understand. The key principles are to use separate disposable infusion and cutter (avoiding the older coaxial instruments) via an anterior approach (use corneal sideports; a pars plana approach has greater risks without demonstrable benefit) and to minimize pulling on the gel high cut rate (as high as the machine will allow) with low vacuum (100–150 mm Hg) minimizes vitreous traction. A low bottle height discourages turbulence and a tendency to additionally hydrate the gel and promote further anterior prolapse, but this has to be balanced against preventing collapse of the eye. In practice, a bottle height of around 30 cm usually works fine. One can use an AC maintainer instead of a separate infusion cannula although it is to beware that one tends to get higher flow rates for a given bottle height through this short, open-ended and relatively larger bored alternative.

The term "core vitrectomy" is the desired end-point and represents the generally referenced gold standard to which one is encouraged to aspire. It sounds precise and convincing theory. However in practice it is a very soft-edged concept that is impossible to define specifically. In general one is referring to the "central" gel, which is around one-third of the volume, whilst leaving the vitreous base and posterior gel alone, as this is not safely accessible using these instruments. In practice, a core vitrectomy is whatever it takes to remove all residual gel from the anterior chamber.

During vitrectomy, the cutter tip and aspiration port should always be visible to the surgeon and the temptation to pass it peripherally under the pupil should be resisted. This is unnecessary and potentially dangerous. One should keep the infusion cannula anterior to the iris pointing it across the chamber and not posteriorly. One moves the cutter around only small amounts within the pupil aperture using a gentle and smooth motion to avoid traction (it is to recall the RPE pump pressure of 0.27 mm Hg). One may want to turn up the vacuum to around 200 mm Hg as one makes progress but any higher is usually unnecessary and causes greater gel traction in between cuts.

If there is vitreous incarcerated in the main incision or sideport then one needs to remove it from within, using the cutter via the other sideport. Attempting to remove it through the main incision itself is impossible and will only encourage additional outflow and gel prolapse.

If there are still lens fragments present when the vitreous initially prolapses then, after using triamcinolone, the safest way of removing them is to perform a "dry" vitrectomy without any BSS infusion. This removes any entangled gel

from around the fragments, so that they can be floated out, enlarging the incision as needed. Performing phaco on these fragments is still a high-risk maneuver as gel traction is almost unavoidable. Any volume removed by the cutter is replaced using viscoelastic delivered simultaneously through a second sideport. This supports the fragments and prevents scleral collapse. Once the fragments are out, then irrigation can be used to complete the vitrectomy.

At whatever stage the anterior vitrectomy is performed, it is important to be careful not to damage the capsulorhexis, which in most cases will still be intact. One will be able to use the rhexis to optic capture the implant to secure it centrally in the correct anatomical plane. This only works with suitable three piece IOLs, not single piece acrylics whose haptics are too bulky. These thick haptics angulate forwards (or backwards) if the IOL is in front of (or behind) the anterior capsule when the optic is captured, and cause iris chaffing, etc.

Finally, these patients need an early postoperative peripheral retinal examination preferably with scleral indentation, in order to exclude any anterior breaks.

SUMMARY

In summary, vitreous loss is serious. It is to accept that it has happened, to stay calm and to decide on a surgical strategy. One needs to respect the vitreous base by using high cut-rate and low vacuum with gentle movement of the instruments. The gel needs to be cut and one should not pull it. One has to visualize the vitreous with triamcinolone to ensure meticulous and complete removal of all gel from the anterior chamber. It is to avoid collapsing the eye, especially during dry vitrectomy.

By adhering to these clear and simple principles for managing vitreous loss, one will be able to achieve a final result that really is as good as if it had never happened.

REFERENCES

1. Lois N, Wong D. Pseudophakic retinal detachment. Surv Ophthalmol 2003;48(5):467-87.
2. The Cataract National Dataset electronic multi-centre audit of 55,567 operations: variation in posterior capsule rupture rates between surgeons.
3. Johnston RL, Taylor H, Smith R, et al. Eye (Lond). 2010;24(5): 888-93.
4. The Cataract National Dataset electronic multi"centre audit of 55,567 operations: updating benchmark standards of care in the United Kingdom and internationally.Eye (Lond). 2009;23(1):38–49.

CHAPTER 55

Intraocular Lens (IOL) as a Scaffold to Prevent Nucleus Drop

Dhivya Ashok Kumar, Amar Agarwal

INTRODUCTION

Posterior capsular rupture (PCR) is one of the common complications during phacoemulsification.[1-3] PCR with vitreous prolapse and the nucleus still in the capsular bag is an impending situation for nucleus drop. As a preventive step it is usual for the cataract surgeon to extend the corneal incision and deliver the nucleus.[4-6] Lens glide or Viscoat assisted levitation has also been done to remove the nuclear fragments.[8] Another method is to emulsify the nucleus in the anterior chamber with low flow rate and vacuum. In this technique, we have used the foldable intraocular lens (IOL) as a scaffold for preventing the nucleus drop without extending the incision.

SURGICAL TECHNIQUE

When there is a posterior capsule rupture with the nucleus in the bag, an anterior chamber (AC) maintainer is introduced (Figure 55.1). Anterior vitrectomy is done with the vitrectomy cutter to remove the vitreous prolapsed in the anterior chamber. While doing this an Agarwal globe stabilization road (Katena, USA), pushes the fragment away from the PCR thus preventing the nucleus from falling down. A foldable IOL is then injected via the existing corneal wound and is moved below the nucleus. The leading haptic of the IOL is positioned in the sulcus and the trailing haptic is placed just out of the incision (Figure 55.2). The

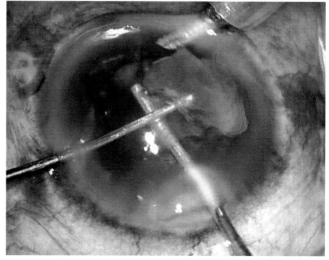

FIGURE 55.2: Vitrectomy

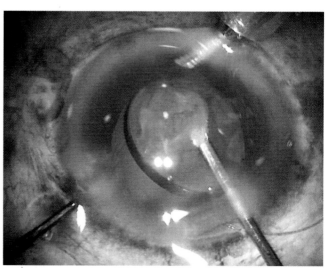

FIGURE 55.3: IOL as a scaffold

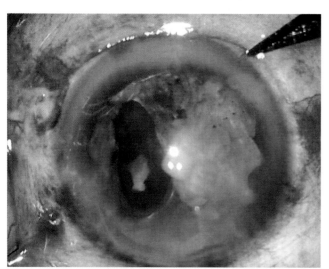

FIGURE 55.1: Posterior capsular rupture during phacoemulsification of the nucleus

nucleus fragment is then removed with the vitrectomy cutter or a phaco probe depending on the density of the nucleus (Figure 55.3). Once the whole nucleus is removed, the retained cortex is then cleaned with the vitrectomy cutter with gentle aspiration (Figure 55.4). The other haptic of the IOL is then positioned in the ciliary sulcus (Figures 55.5 and 55.6) and the AC maintainer is removed.

It is easier to manipulate the IOL by placing one haptic above the iris. The non-dominant hand adjusts the other optic haptic junction so that the IOL is well centered while emulsifying the nucleus (Figures 55.7 to 55.12).

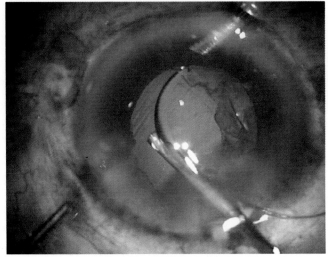

FIGURE 55.4: Cortical removal

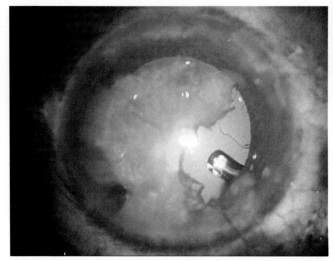

FIGURE 55.7: Nucleus in AC

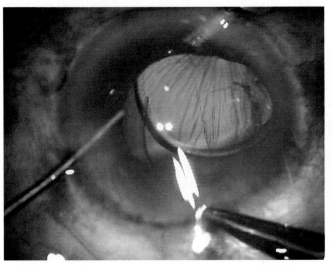

FIGURE 55.5: Foldable IOL positioned in the ciliary sulcus

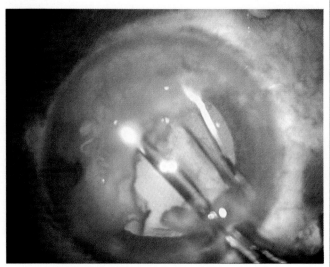

FIGURE 55.8: IOL injected with haptic above the iris

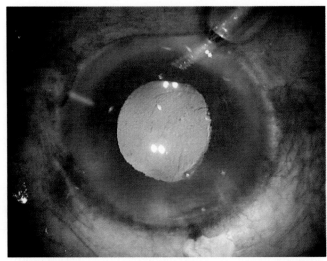

FIGURE 55.6: IOL well centered at the end of the procedure

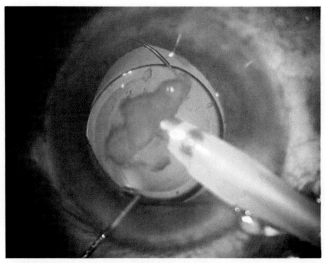

FIGURE 55.9: IOL acts as a scaffold. Note the nondominant hand using a dialer to help center the IOL

POSTERIOR CAPSULE RUPTURE AND VITREOUS LOSS

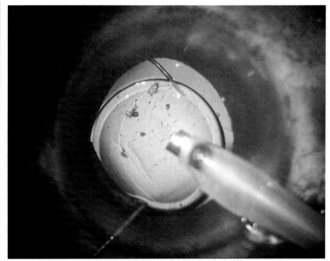

FIGURE 55.10: Nucleus emulsified

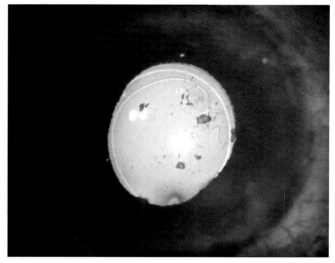

FIGURE 55.12: PC IOL in sulcus

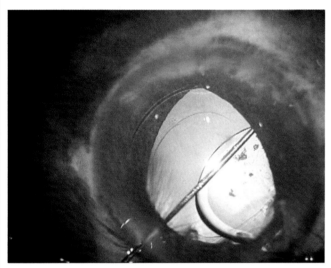

FIGURE 55.11: Haptic placed in sulcus

DISCUSSION

Posterior capsular rupture (PCR) is known to occur at any stage of phacoemulsification.[3] When it happens with the nucleus still left to emulsify, excess manipulation can cause extension of the PCR. The aim of any method at this stage is to prevent the nucleus fragment from dropping into the vitreous. The chances of nucleus drop increases with increasing size of the PCR and vitreous loss. Though a small fragment which descends into the vitreous is left for observation; large nucleus fragments always require surgical removal.[9,10] Nucleus drop can induce vitritis and macular edema thereby affecting the best corrected vision.[10] Moreover a second surgery for retrieving the dropped nucleus again can cause additional trauma to the eye. Hence, it is seldom better to prevent the complication from happening by proper management of the PCR.

Though there have been techniques performed to prevent nucleus fragment from descending into the vitreous after intraoperative PCR, this IOL scaffolding method has not been reported earlier. Conversion of phacoemulsification to extracapsular cataract extraction (ECCE)[4,5] is done when a large nucleus is still left. Some surgeons prefer to use the lens glide to deliver the nucleus. In both the conditions, corneal wound extension is required and this can increase the risk of postoperative suture induced astigmatism. Another way is the nucleus removal by phaco sandwich method,[6] where a vectis and a spatula are used. However, the incision in a phaco sandwich is sclerocorneal and requires extension. In eyes with nucleus displaced in the anterior vitreous, Viscoat posterior assisted levitation[7] is done followed by nucleus emulsification with phacoprobe above a trimmed sheet's glide[8] after wound extension. In the IOL scaffold technique, the wound remains clear corneal and there is no wound extension. The foldable IOL acts as the vitreous barrier and works like an artificial posterior capsule. Since one haptic is kept at the incision site the IOL position can be readily adjusted if the nucleus rotates in the anterior chamber and the chances of IOL drop is also not there as the haptic is controlled from the incision site. In all the three eyes we did not encounter vitritis or endophthalmitis. There was no loss of best corrected vision in any of the eyes.

When compared to an open wound (after extension), PCR during phacoemulsification is associated with a relatively low incidence of vitreous loss because the self-sealing small clear corneal wound provides control of ocular integrity. This maintains the anterior chamber and intraocular pressure, discouraging forward movement of the vitreous, which would occur in the presence of an "open globe" as in ECCE.

SUMMARY

Avoiding PCR is the goal of every cataract surgeon. If a tear occurs, management techniques and skills are required for preventing further complications. Early recognition of posterior capsular rupture combined with prevention of collapse of the anterior chamber may prevent extension of the tear, forward movement of the vitreous, and displacement of the lens posteriorly. Here in this technique, the anterior chamber is maintained by slow infusion, forward movement of the vitreous is prevented by the IOL scaffold and the nucleus fragment drop is stopped by the IOL which acts as a physical barrier. Thus, we favor this new IOL scaffolding technique in PCRs with non-emulsified moderate to soft nucleus during phacoemulsi-fication. However, in cases of hard cataract conversion to ECCE is ideal.

REFERENCES

1. Vejarano LF, Tello A. Posterior capsular rupture. In Amar Agarwal: Phaco Nightmares; Conquering cataract catastrophes; Slack Inc, USA 2006;253-64.
2. Vajpayee RB, Sharma N, Dada T, Gupta V, Kumar A, Dada VK. Management of posterior capsule tears. Surv Ophthalmol 2001;45(6):473-88.
3. Gimbel HV, Sun R, Ferensowicz M, Anderson Penno E, Kamal A. Intraoperative management of posterior capsule tears in phacoemulsification and intraocular lens implantation. Ophthalmology. 2001;108(12):2186-9; discussion 2190-2.
4. Dada T, Sharma N, Vajpayee RB, Dada VK. Conversion from phacoemulsification to extracapsular cataract extraction: incidence, risk factors, and visual outcome. J Cataract Refract Surg. 1998;24(11):1521-4.
5. Prasad S, Kamath GG. Converting from phacoemulsification to ECCE. J Cataract Refract Surg. 1999;25(4):462-3.
6. Thatte S, Raju VK. Phacosandwich technique. J Cataract Refract Surg. 1999;25(8):1039-40.
7. Chang DF, Packard RB. Posterior assisted levitation for nucleus retrieval using Viscoat after posterior capsule rupture. J Cataract Refract Surg. 2003;29(10):1860-5.
8. Michelson MA. Use of a Sheets' glide as a pseudo-posterior capsule in phacoemulsification complicated by posterior capsule rupture. Eur J Implant Refract Surg. 1993;5:70–72.
9. Hansson LJ, Larsson J.Vitrectomy for retained lens fragments in the vitreous after phacoemulsification. J Cataract Refract Surg. 2002;28(6):1007-11.
10. Monshizadeh R, Samiy N, Haimovici R. Management of retained intravitreal lens fragments after cataract surgery. Surv Ophthalmol. 1999;43(5):397-404.

CHAPTER 56

Management of Dropped Nucleus and IOLs

Kaladevi Satish, Dhivya Ashok Kumar, Amar Agarwal

INTRODUCTION

Management of intraoperative nucleus drop[1-3] in cataract surgery has always been a nightmare for anterior segment surgeons. Moreover postoperative dislocated or luxated IOL remain an infrequent but significant problem of complicated cataract surgery.[3,4] Hence the cataract surgeons should be equipped to manage these complications safely with available instruments. In this chapter, we have reviewed the literature and discussed the techniques used for managing these situations.

DROPPED NUCLEUS

Large posterior capsular tear or zonular dialysis[3] can cause the intraoperative nucleus drop. Similar to any surgical technique, complications can be encountered in the learning curve in microincision cataract surgery (MICS) phacoemulsification. Phaco surgeon should be more cautious in continuing the procedure to prevent excess manipulation in the vitreous.[1,2] This will prevent the unnecessary traction on the vitreous. Thus, the cataract surgeon must refrain from the temptation of passing a sharp instrument or lens loop into the mid or posterior vitreous cavity to engage the sinking lens fragments, or passing forceful irrigation fluid into the vitreous cavity to float the lens fragments. Surgeons who are equipped with retinal set up can convert the procedure to posterior vitrectomy; otherwise the patient has to be referred to a vitreoretinal surgeon.

INDICATIONS FOR SURGERY

OBSERVATION

Selected cases in which the displaced lens material is small (less than 5–10% of lens volume) or in which there is little or no intraocular inflammation and intraocular pressure (IOP) is easily controlled with topical medications.[5]

SURGICAL INTERVENTION

Nucleus segments greater than one-fourth of the total should be removed by vitrectomy because of the risk for chronic inflammation and secondary glaucoma.[6]

SURGICAL TECHNIQUES

STANDARD PARS PLANA VITRECTOMY

The standard three-port pars plana vitrectomy (PPV) approach is the most frequently employed method for the removal of posteriorly dislocated lens fragments in a safe and effective manner.[1] Initial step is the infusion cannula fixation port made in the inferotemporal quadrant. A 4–6 mm sized infusion tip with or without chandelier illumination is used. After passing a 6–0 polyglactil suture around the sclerotomy, the infusion cannula is positioned. Infusion cannula is connected to 500 ml bottle of balanced salt solution inserted through the sclerotomy. Fluid flow is started only after visualization of the tip of infusion cannula in the vitreous cavity. Two sclerotomies are then made in the superonasal and superotemporal quadrant in the pars plana. Conventional PPV is performed with 20 gauge vitrectomy probe and endoilluminator passed through the sclerotomy ports under visualization. In the end of all PPV, scleral depression is performed to confirm the absence of any peripheral retinal breaks.

PARS PLANA VITRECTOMY WITH PHACOFRAGMATOME

The first step involves the insertion of a posterior infusion cannula at the inferotemporal pars plana as explained above. Core vitrectomy is completed to carefully remove all of the vitreous fibers surrounding the posterior lens fragments before proceeding with phacofragmentation.[7] Otherwise there can be occlusion of the phaco tip by formed vitreous elements during the phacofragmentation process and traction on the retina. At the start of the pars plana phacoemulsification process, each lens fragment is first engaged at the phaco tip with the machine set at the aspiration mode and then brought to the mid-vitreous cavity for emulsification. During the emulsification of the lens fragments, the ultrasonic power is kept at a low or moderate setting in order to decrease the tendency of blowing the fragments from the phaco tip and repeatedly dropping them on the retina. The removal of dropped nucleus by phacofragmentation[8,9] eliminates the need for a large cornealscleral incision for nucleus removal. The disadvantages are the probability of causing a tissue burn at the sclerotomy site, difficulty of keeping the nuclear material stable at the tip, damage to the macula from ultrasonic power, and aspiration of vitreous fibrils that could not be removed adequately by PPV.

PARS PLANA VITRECTOMY WITH PHACOFRAGMATOME WITH PFCL

Pars plana vitrectomy with nucleus removal can be combined with perfluorocarbon liquid (PFCL). This is a

TABLE 56.1 Properties of perfluorocarbon liquids

Characteristic	Perfluoro-N-Octane	Perfluoro-tributylamine	Perfluoro-decaline	Perfluoro-phenanthrene
Chemical formula	C_3F_{18}	$C_{12}F_{27}N$	$C_{10}F_{18}$	$C_{14}F_{24}$
Molecular weight	438	671	462	624
Specific gravity	1.76	1.89	1.94	2.03
Refractive index	1.27	1.29	1.31	1.33
Surface tension (Dyne/cm at 25°C)	14	16	16	16
Viscosity (Centistokes- 25°C)	0.8	2.6	2.7	8.03
Vapor pressure (mm Hg at 37°C)	50	1.14	13.5	< 1

high density **(Table 56.1)**, low viscosity liquid with inert nature used for dislodging the nucleus.[10-13] Perfluorocarbon liquid is infused into the eye through the same pars plana sclerotomy. This serves as a cushion for protecting the underlying retina from the bouncing lens fragments during the process of lens emulsification. In hazy media due to corneal edema or opacity or vitritis, this is preferred. Limited amount of PFCL should be injected, since excessive perfluorocarbon liquid with a convex meniscus tends to displace the lens fragments away from the central visual axis and toward the peripheral fundus and the vitreous base. After the nucleus floats up, the phacofragmatome can be used to remove it. Residual PFCL should be removed at the end of the surgery followed by complete retinal examination to rule out any retinal breaks or hemorrhage.

FALLEN NUCLEUS FROM THE VITREOUS

Fallen nucleus from the vitreous (FAVIT) technique is a technique described by Agarwal et al.[1] FAVIT is an acronym for a technique to remove **FA**llen nucleus from the **VIT**reous **(Figure 56.1A)**. In this technique, a chandelier illumination system coupled to the infusion cannula to achieve visualization of the posterior segment is introduced in the inferotemporal port and an endoilluminator is inserted through a second port. The 20 gauge vitrectomy probe is used in a third port; all ports are through the pars plana; to achieve complete vitreous removal. Complete core pars plana vitrectomy is done and is performed till the nucleus is released of all tractions in the vitreous and starts moving

freely. Then the vitrectomy probe is replaced with the sleeveless phaco probe with a 700 micron phaco needle **(Figure 56.1B)**. Suction-only mode is used on the phaco probe to lift the lens off the retina and hold it while it is repositioned into the anterior chamber, where phaco or an enlarged limbal incision is used to remove the lens **(Figure 56.1C)**. If the nucleus is hard, one should extend the incision so that endothelial damage is prevented. Scleral depression is performed to identify and remove any residual lens material trapped in the vitreous base and to confirm the absence of any peripheral retinal breaks. This technique can be easily done without any special instrumentation.

POSTERIOR ASSISTED LEVITATION

Posterior assisted levitation (PAL) introduced by Kelman et al[1,14] in which a cyclodialysis spatula is passed through a pars plana stab incision to push the nucleus up into the anterior chamber from below. Then Packard[15] modified the technique using a Viscoat cannula, inserting it through a pars plana stab incision located 3.5 mm behind the limbus. Viscoat is first slowly injected downward well behind the nuclear piece to provide supplemental support. The nucleus is then elevated into the anterior chamber through a combination of additional Viscoat injection and manipulation of the cannula tip.

FAVIT WITH 20 GAUGE SUTURELESS VITRECTOMY

Three partial thickness scleral flaps **(Figures 56.2A to D)** are made. First flap (F1) is made in the inferotemporal quadrant. Next two flaps F2, F3 are made in the superior

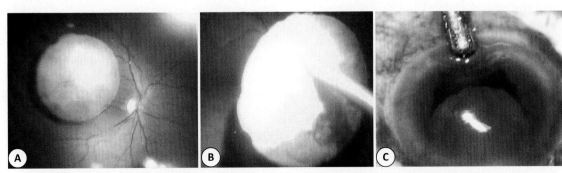

FIGURES 56.1A TO C: (A) Intraoperative photograph of a hard nucleus dropped on the retina, (B) 700 micron phaco needle is used to hold the nucleus, (C) Nucleus is brought through the limbal route

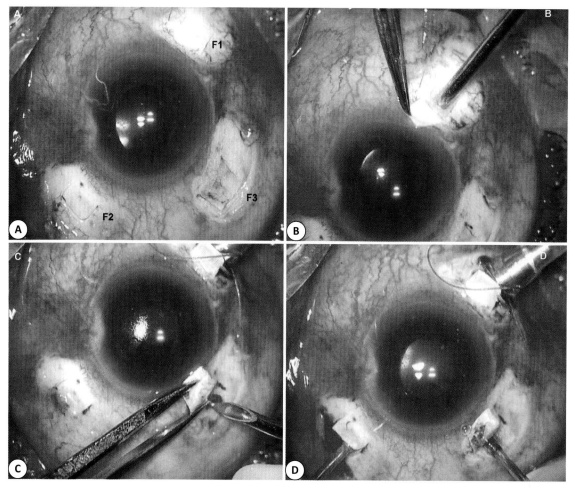

FIGURES 56.2A TO D: (A) Intraoperative photograph showing the three partial thickness scleral flaps (F1, F2, F3) made for 20 gauge sutureless vitrectomy, (B) Sclerotomy made for infusion cannula, (C) Pars plana sclerotomy made for vitrectomy probe, (D) Pars plana vitrectomy performed with 20 gauge instruments

nasal and superior temporal quadrant about 2 mm from the limbus. A straight sclerotomy is made under the scleral flap F1 about 3.5 mm from the limbus. A polyglactil 6–0 suture is placed and a 4 mm infusion cannula connected to 500 ml bottle of balanced salt solution is inserted through the sclerotomy. Two straight sclerotomies with a 20 gauge needle are made under the existing scleral flaps (F1, F2). Pars plana vitrectomy is completed with 20 gauge vitrectomy instruments (vitrectomy probe and endoilluminator). FAVIT is completed as explained above. At the end of the procedure, polyglactil suture and the infusion cannula are removed and the scleral flaps (F1, F2, F3) are sealed **(Figures 56.3A to D)** with the tissue glue (Tisseel, Baxter). Conjunctiva is also apposed at the peritomy sites with the glue.

ASSISTED TECHNIQUES

Staining of the vitreous material[9] with triamcinolone acetonide during vitrectomy and phacofragmentation surgery for luxated nuclei helped in total removal of the vitreous body, thus preventing the aspiration of peripheral vitreous fibrils by the phaco tip, which might induce retinal

detachment intraoperatively or postoperatively. Other methods are endoscopy assisted and cryoextraction procedures for nucleus removal.[1]

DROPPED INTRAOCULAR LENS

Intraoperative or postoperative IOL drop into the vitreous is infrequent but important sight-threatening complication. Several advances in microsurgical techniques have led to highly safe and effective cataract surgery. Despite such advances, dislocation of an IOL due to capsular rupture or zonular dehiscence remains. The key to the prevention of poor visual outcome for this complication is its proper management. Many highly effective surgical methods have been developed to manage a dislocated IOL.

PARS PLANA VITRECTOMY WITH IOL REMOVAL WITH PERFLUOROCARBON

Perfluorocarbon liquids have been used for the surgical treatment of various vitreoretinal disorders. Due to their heavier-than-water properties **(Table 56.1)**, and their ease of intraocular injection and removal, perfluorocarbon

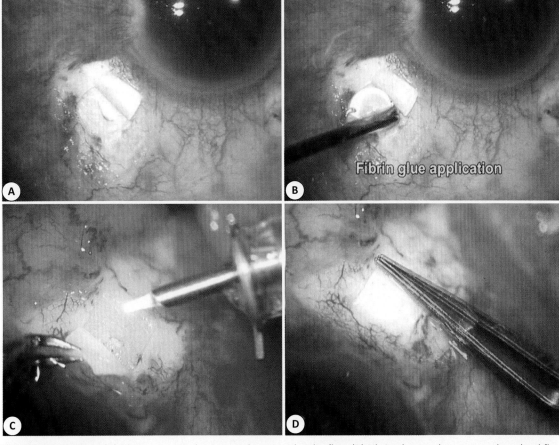

FIGURES 56.3A TO D: (A) 20 gauge pars plana wound seen under the flap, (B) Fibrin glue used to appose the scleral flaps, (C) Infusion cannula with Chandelier illumination removed, (D) Scleral flap opposed to the bed with fibrin glue

liquids are highly effective. After complete vitrectomy and freeing of the vitreous around the lens fragment, PFCL is injected over the optic nerve. The high specific gravity of the PFCL floats the IOL off the retinal surface into the midvitreous space **(Figures 56.4A and B)**, where it can be safely picked with the intravitreal forceps. Due to their unique physical properties, perfluorocarbon liquids are well suited for floating dropped IOL, in order to insulate the underlying retina from damage. At the same time, the anterior displacement of the dislocated IOL by the

perfluorocarbon liquids facilitates its removal or repositioning. With intravitreal forceps IOL is held with intravitreal forceps and brought out through the limbal route.

PARS PLANA VITRECTOMY WITH IOL REMOVAL WITHOUT PERFLUOROCARBON

In this method, pars plana vitrectomy should be done first followed by IOL removal with intravitreal forceps under direct visualization of the IOL. The IOL is released from

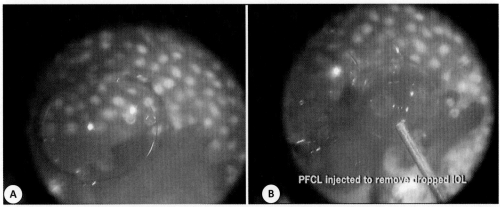

FIGURES 56.4A AND B: (A) Intraoperative picture showing dislocated IOL, (B) Perfluorocarbon liquid is injected to dislodge the IOL

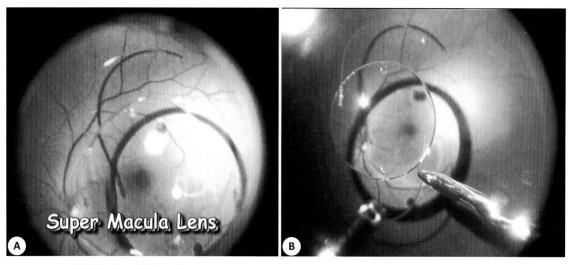

FIGURES 56.5A AND B: (A) Fundus view as seen through super macula lens, (B) Dislocated IOL removed under super macula using intravitreal forceps

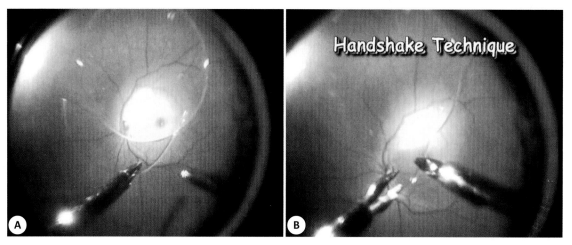

FIGURES 56.6A AND B: "Handshake" technique demonstrated. (A) IOL haptic is held with the left hand intravitreal forceps, (B) IOL haptic is transferred to the other hand to another intravitreal forceps

all the vitreous traction. The under wide angle view the IOL is picked with the intravitreal forceps and retrieved through the limbal incision. Thus in this method, PFCL is not used. The risk of injury to the retina or vasculature exits during manipulation. However, this can be overcome by using super macula lens viewing system **(Figures 56.5A and B)** which gives greater magnification and stereopsis. "Handshake technique" is the method in which the IOL is transferred from one hand to other hand with the intravitreal forceps **(Figures 56.6A and B)**.

REPOSITIONING THE DISLOCATED IOL

Localized peritomy and wet cautery of the sclera at 3, 9 and 7 o' clock was performed. Two partial thickness limbal based scleral flaps F1, F2, 2.5 mm × 3 mm were created exactly 180 degrees diagonally apart and 1 mm from the limbus. A third scleral flap **(Figures 56.7A and B)** F3 was made about 2 mm from the limbus. A pars plana sclerotomy about 3 mm from the limbus was made with a 20 gauge needle under the scleral flap F3. A polyglactil 6–0 suture was placed and a

4 mm infusion cannula connected to 500 ml bottle of balanced salt solution was inserted through the sclerotomy. Infusion cannula with a halogen light source (Chandelier illumination) can also be used. Two straight sclerotomies with a 20 gauge needle were made about 1 mm from the limbus under the existing scleral flaps (F1, F2). Accurus® 400 VS (Alcon Laboratories, Inc., Fort Worth, TX) vitrectomy system was used for posterior vitrectomy. Posterior vitreous detachment was induced mechanically using suction of the 20 gauge vitrectomy probe. A thorough vitrectomy to free all the IOL attachments was done with 20 gauge vitrectomy probe and endoilluminator. When the vitreous tractions were released, a diamond coated 20 gauge intravitreal forceps (Grieshaber, Alcon, Fort Worth, TX) was used to hold the haptic tip. The IOL was gently lifted up to bring it at the level of the sclerotomy sites. The intravitreal forceps (holding the haptic) was then withdrawn from the sclerotomy site (F1), externalizing the haptic in the process. With the assistant holding the tip of the externalized haptic, the other haptic was pulled **(Figure 56.7C and D)** through the other sclerotomy (F2)

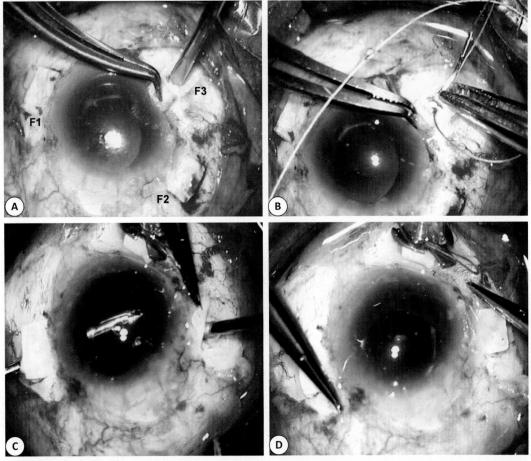

FIGURES 56.7A TO D: Three scleral flaps made (F1, F2, F3). (A) The scleral flaps F1, F2 are about 1 mm from the limbus and F3 is 2 mm from the limbus, (B) Pars plana sclerotomy made and infusion cannula attached with 6–0 polyglactil suture at 3 mm from the limbus, (C) Vitrectomy done through the pars plicata and IOL haptic externalized with an intravitreal forceps, (D) Both the haptics externalized through the pars plicata port and tucked into the scleral tunnel

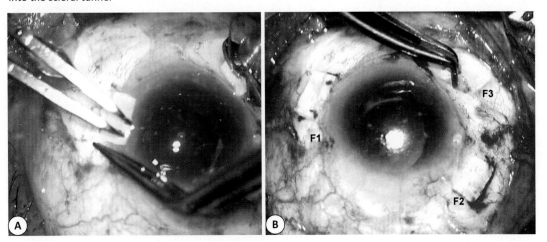

FIGURES 56.8A AND B: Scleral flaps being closed with fibrin glue after tucking; (A) the haptics (F1, F2) and after the removal; (B) of the infusion cannula (F3)

using intravitreal forceps. The tips of the haptic were then tucked through an intralamellar scleral tunnel made with a 26 gauge needle at the point of externalization **(Figure 56.8A)**. Scleral flaps (F1, F2) were closed with fibrin glue (Tisseel, Baxter). Polyglactil suture and the infusion cannula were removed and the third scleral flap (F3) **(Figure 56.8B)** was also sealed with the glue. Conjunctiva was also apposed at the peritomy sites with the tissue glue. Ultrasound biomicroscopy with 50 MHz frequency and 50 μ resolution **(Figures 56.9A and B)** showed no vitreous traction or uveal incarceration in pars plicata ports in the postoperative period. The anterior segment Visante™ OCT (Carl Zeiss Meditec, Dublin, California, USA) can be used to scan across the pars plicata region **(Figures 56.10A and B)**.

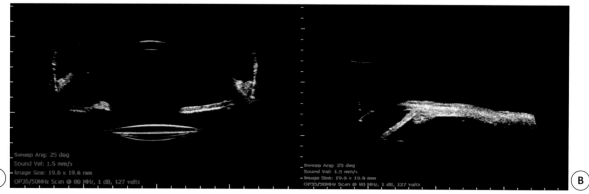

FIGURES 56.9A AND B: Ultrasound biomicroscopy image showing good glued IOL centration (A) and pars plicata port site with no vitreous traction or incarceration (B)

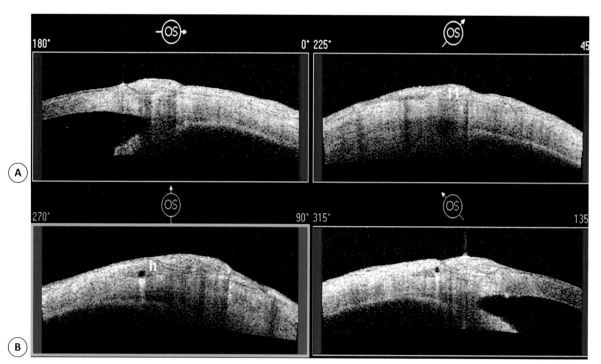

FIGURES 56.10A AND B: High resolution anterior segment OCT images of scleral flaps (F1) taken along 360 degrees. End on view of the haptic (h) at the site of externalization is seen

COMPLICATIONS AND PREVENTION

The worst strategy for recovering a descending nucleus is to try to chase and spear the nucleus with the phaco tip. The best strategy is avoiding nuclear material in the posterior segment, so when in front of an impending dropped nucleus it is necessary to take every measure to maintain it in the anterior segment. A good option is to levitate it into the pupillary plane or anterior chamber for extraction through a standard ECCE incision.

Attempting to emulsify or aspirate it may snag vitreous into the tip, potentially leading to retinal tears or detachment. Similarly in case of dislocated IOL, proper vitreoretinal set up is required to do three port vitrectomy. Untreated dropped nucleus or IOLs can lead to vitritis, macular edema, vitreous membranes, retinal traction and on long-term loss of best corrected vision. Gilliland et al[16] has shown that removal of retained lens fragments allows rapid visual restoration, enhances resolution of uveitis, and improves control of glaucoma. Precautions should be taken while implanting IOL in posterior capsular tear. If the support is not adequate one can go for Glued IOL[17,18] or anterior chamber IOL. Double IOL **(Figure 56.11)** can also be managed with the pars plana vitrectomy. Complications like broken optic or haptic **(Figure 56.12)** can occur during removal of the dislocated IOL when it is held with the forceps. Hence, it is better not to give excess pressure over the haptics. Broken IOL or haptic can hit the retina and may lead to retinal tear, macular edema or vitreous hemorrhage. However, proper execution of the surgical skill in the appropriate time will prevent these complications.

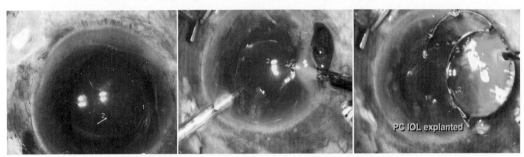

FIGURE 56.11: Intraoperative image showing the removal of a dislocated IOL (IOL 2) in an already existing PC IOL (IOL1)

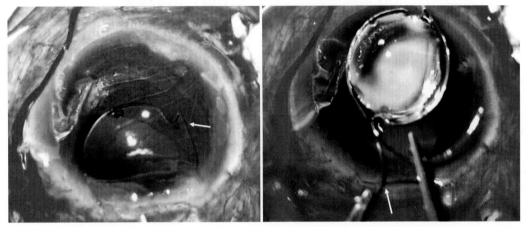

FIGURE 56.12: Haptic broken (shown in arrows) during intraoperative manipulation

CONCLUSION

Thus vitreoretinal surgery offers a variety of effective techniques for the safe removal of posteriorly dislocated lens fragments and IOLs. Besides the standard 3-port pars plana vitrectomy with phacoemulsification, FAVIT, 20 gauge sutureless vitrectomy and Glued IOL are expedient alternatives for the cataract surgeon. This helps promptly to remove the lens fragments or reposition the IOLs with minimal additional setup during the primary surgery.

REFERENCES

1. Amar Agarwal. Phaco Nightmares. Conquering cataract catastrophes. Slack Inc., USA; 2006.
2. Sunita Agarwal, Athiya Agarwal, Amar Agarwal. Phacoemulsification –Two volume set. Third Edition. Jaypee Brothers: Delhi; 2004.
3. Vajpayee RB, Sharma N, Dada T, et al. Management of posterior capsule tears. Surv Ophthal. 2001;45:473-88.
4. Chan CK, Agarwal A, Agarwal S, et al. Management of dislocated intraocular implants. In: Nagpal PN, Fine IH (Eds). Ophthalmology Clinics of North America, Posterior Segment Complications of Cataract Surgery. Philadelphia: WB Saunders; 2001; p. 681.
5. Monshizadeh R, Samiy N, Haimovici R. Management of retained intravitreal lens fragments after cataract surgery. Surv Ophthalmol. 1999;43(5):397-404.
6. Blodi BA, Flynn HW Jr, Blodi CF, et al. Retained nuclei after cataract surgery. Ophthalmology. 1992;99:41-4.
7. Chan CK. Managing dislocated lens fragments. In: Amar Agarwal. Phaco Nightmares; Conquering cataract catastrophes; Slack Inc., USA; 2006.
8. Kim JE, Flynn HW Jr, Smiddy WE, et al. Retained lens fragments after phacoemulsification. Ophthalmology 1994;101: 1827-32.
9. Kaynak S, Celik L, Kocak N, et al. Staining of vitreous with triamcinolone acetonide in retained lens surgery with phaco-fragmentation. J Cataract Refract Surg. 2006;32(1):56-9.
10. Chang S. Perfluorocarbon liquids in vitreo-retinal surgery. International Ophthalmology Clinics-New approaches to vitreo-retinal surgery. 1992;32(2):153.
11. Liu K, Peyman GA, Chen M, et al. Use of high density vitreous substitute in the removal of posteriorly dislocated lenses or intraocular lenses. Ophthalmic Surg. 1991;22:503.
12. Charles S. Posterior dislocation of lens material during cataract surgery. In: Agarwal S, Agarwal A, Sachdev MS, et al (Eds). Phacoemulsification, Laser Cataract Surgery, and Foldable IOLs. 2nd Edition. New Delhi: Jaypee Brothers Medical Publishers Ltd; 2000. p 517.
13. Topping TM. Management of dislocated lens fragments during phacoemulsification, and, retained intravitreal lens fragments after cataract surgery [Discussion]. Ophthalmology 1992; 99:1268.
14. Kelman C. New PAL method may save difficult cataract cases. Ophthalmology Times. 1994;19:51.
15. Packard R. Technique prevents nucleus drop through capsular tear. Ocular Surgery News. 2001;19:14.
16. Gilliland GD, Hutton WL, Fuller DG. Retained intravitreal lens fragments after cataract surgery. Ophthalmology. 1992;99(8): 1263-7.
17. Agarwal A, Kumar DA, Jacob S, et al. Fibrin glue–assisted sutureless posterior chamber intraocular lens implantation in eyes with deficient posterior capsules. J Cataract Refract Surg. 2008;34:1433-8.
18. Prakash G, Kumar DA, Jacob S, et al. Anterior segment optical coherence tomography-aided diagnosis and primary posterior chamber intraocular lens implantation with fibrin glue in traumatic phacocele with scleral perforation. J Cataract Refract Surg. 2009;35:782-4.

CHAPTER 57

Posterior Dislocation of Lens Material During Cataract Surgery

Steve Charles

SURGICAL PSYCHODYNAMICS

Cataract surgery has been one of the most frequently performed surgical procedures worldwide for over a century. While inexperience is known to cause a higher complication rate, high volumes and phenomenal success rates can also lead to complacency and judgement errors when complications do occur. Busy schedules, observers, and videography may contribute to faulty decision making when the capsule ruptures. High success rates, outpatient surgery, no stitch, no patch, emmetropia, and topical anesthesia elevate patient expectations unrealistically furthering the problem.

EARLY RECOGNITION AND MANAGEMENT OF DEFECTS IN THE LENS CAPSULE

Optical systems that enhance the red-reflex and the clear corneas achievable with modern cataract surgery assist in early recognition of capsular defects. The surgeon must admit that the defect has occurred rather than rationalize because of the psychological factors described above. When a capsular defect is recognized, the first action should be to construct a barrier between the posterior capsule and the anterior vitreous cortex. Colvard has proposed a plastic barrier that can be deployed in this space, but none are available at this time. High viscosity viscoelastics injected into the defect can serve as a temporary barrier enabling removal of remaining lens material. Many surgeons focus exclusively on prevention or management of posterior dislocation of lens material rather than the more serious matter of reducing vitreoretinal traction and subsequent retinal detachment. Any maneuver designed to prevent posterior dislocation that increases vitreoretinal traction should not be used. Kelman has described use of a needle through the pars plana to prevent lens material from falling posteriorly. This method ignores the pressure that must be placed on the eye to place the needle and the anterior movement of the vitreous that occurs without a barrier. The next section discusses management of vitreous that prolapses through the capsular defect. This discussion intentionally precedes the discussion of the management of lens material because retinal detachment prevention is the most important issue.

VITREOUS LOSS

Use of the phacoemulsifier to remove vitreous is a dangerous step that should never be undertaken. Phaco probes liquefy hyaluronic acid but do not cut collagen fibers. Use of a large bore needle to aspirate "liquid" vitreous should be avoided because of the obligate vitreoretinal traction it creates. The theoretical "pockets" of liquid vitreous are more difficult to locate than the fountain of youth.

Cellulose sponge vitrectomy as reported by Kasner has been an obsolete and dangerous method for two decades in spite of the important role it played at one time. A cellulose sponge causes significant traction on the retina as the sponge is lifted to transect the adherent vitreous. Removal of all vitreous by a vitreous cutter causes virtually no inflammation, while marked inflammation is the rule after sponge vitrectomy. Mechanical damage to the iris caused by contact with the sponge as it swells and is lifted appears to be the cause of this inflammation. The author had also observed cellulose material on the anterior vitreous cortex after sponge vitrectomy had been performed. One can speculate that this retained material causes inflammation in addition to that caused by iris trauma. Testing for vitreous can be accomplished by injecting air into the anterior chamber via the sideport incision and looking for fragmentation of the bubble. Alternatively, a single drop of sterile fluorescein from a newly opened ampoule can be used to stain the vitreous.

Vitrectomy with a high quality vitreous cutter is the preferred method of managing vitreous that presents in the anterior chamber. Alcon builds high quality cutters for use with their phaco systems such as Legacy. These cutters should be operated at the highest possible cutting frequency and very low vacuum. Posterior vitreous surgeons use vacuum settings rather than flow for better control over vitreoretinal traction. The anterior segment machines frequently utilize peristaltic pumps, which cannot be directly controlled for vacuum. The best procedure is to use very low flow rate and vacuum settings to reduce traction on the retina. The cutter should be advanced or held stationary during vitrectomy, never retracted. ***Pulling the cutter back while vacuum is applied dramatically increases vitreoretinal traction.*** Sideport infusion is preferable to "dry" vitrectomy, because it prevents hypotony and therefore reduces the chance of choroidal hemorrhage. Air can be used instead of infusion fluid to keep the vitreous from hydrating. The air helps to delineate the surface of the vitreous and keep it confined by surface tension. Sweeping the wound for vitreous is dangerous because of the vitreoretinal traction it causes.

DISLOCATED LENS MATERIAL

Phacoemulsifiers, lens loops, and saline fluid streams should never be utilized in an attempt to extract lens material from the vitreous cavity **(Figures 57.1A to C).**

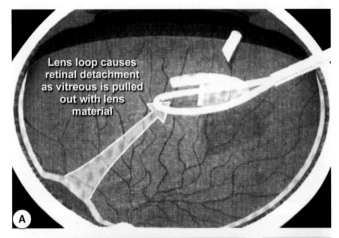

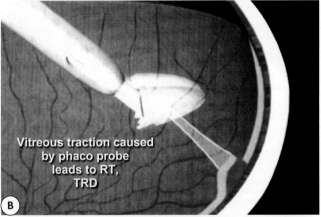

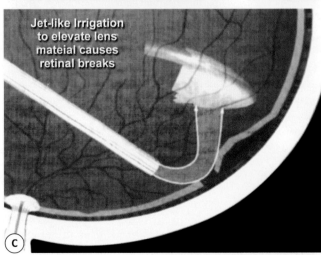

FIGURES 57.1A TO C: Dislocated lens material: What not to do?

If lens material falls posteriorly, there is a natural tendency for the surgeon to chase it with the phaco probe. The phaco probe gives the appearance of vitreous emulsification, but does not sever the collagen fibers. The surgeon must consciously stop, relax, and plan before performing any further maneuvers. The best plan is usually to let the material fall posteriorly and focus on vitreous clean-up and IOL implantation. Lens loops can put significant traction on the retina and cause retinal breaks and detachments. Saline injected under pressure was used by Foulds and later Machemer to create experimental retinal detachments. There is significant risk of retinal breaks if saline is used in an attempt to move the lens material anteriorly.

If the pupil is large, the cornea clear, and the surgeon and available staff are optimum for posterior vitrectomy, immediate intervention may be undertaken. In most instances, it is preferable to perform posterior vitrectomy and removal of lens material at a second procedure **(Figure 57.2).** This procedure should be performed when the cornea is clear, the wound is sealed, and the pupil well dilated. The timing can be from several days to weeks later. If there is a moderate amount of cortex, no inflammation, no glaucoma, and no lens-corneal touch, vitrectomy may not be necessary.

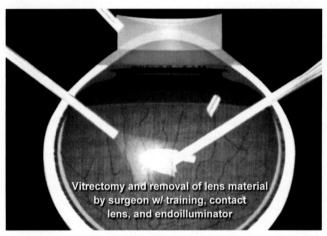

FIGURE 57.2: Dislocated lens material: What to do?

Posterior vitrectomy requires the surgeon specifically trained in posterior techniques and a sophisticated vitrectomy system. A suture supported infusion cannula placed through the pars plana is essential. A hand-held, planoconcave fundus contact lens (Machemer) is easier and faster to use than a sewed-on contact lens. Wide-angle visualization systems increase cost, complexity, and the learning curve although they provide an excellent view. A fiberoptic endoilluminator is essential for all cases. Light reflexes from the cornea prevent the surgeon from having an optimal view if coaxial illumination is used. Iris retractors increase inflammation, cost and may cause a distorted pupil after surgery.

All vitreous should be removed before aspirating any dislocated lens material **(Figures 57.3A and B).** *Many*

POSTERIOR DISLOCATION OF LENS MATERIAL DURING CATARACT SURGERY

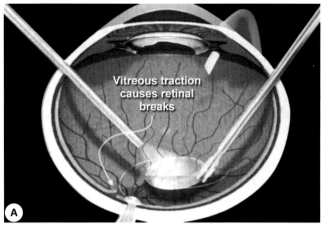

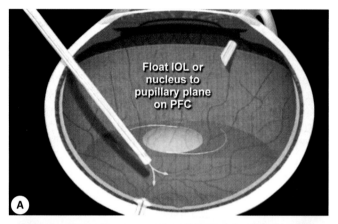

FIGURES 57.3A AND B: Dislocated lens: Precautions

stabilizing the retina during dissection of epiretinal membranes **(Figures 57.4 and 57.5)**. PFC liquids can also be used to float the lens material away from the retina allowing aspiration-fragmentation to be performed anteriorly. This method increases cost and requires subsequent procedures to remove residual PFC liquids. The PFC liquid method is safe, but unnecessary unless there is extremely dense nuclear sclerosis that should not have been managed with phaco in the first place.

surgeons function under the false concept that lens material can damage the retina if it falls posteriorly. Inappropriate techniques, not the lens, damage the retina. It is dangerous and unnecessary to leave a layer of vitreous under the lens material until it is removed. Some cortex may be removed with the vitreous cutter, but nuclear material requires the phacofragmenter. Fragmenters are 20-gauge like vitreous cutters eliminating the need for the larger wounds required for phacoemulsifier probes. The Alcon titanium fragmenter utilizes the same drive electronics and piezo driver as the Legacy phaco probe and is able to handle the majority of nuclear sclerosis cases.

After removal of the vitreous, the fragmenter is introduced with the endoilluminator in the other sclerotomy. The fragmenter is moved to the surface of the lens material and suction applied with the linear (proportional) suction. The lens material is moved away from the retina and then the footpedal is used to activate sonification. The fragmenter power is adjusted until sufficient sculpting without bouncing is accomplished.If the fragmenter drills into the lens, the endoilluminator is used to push the fragment off the tip. Alternatively, the endoilluminator can be used to crush and divide the fragment that is speared on the fragmenter tip. This process is continued until all lens fragments are removed.

Perfluorocarbon (PFC) liquids (Chang) were introduced to vitreoretinal surgery for unfolding giant breaks and

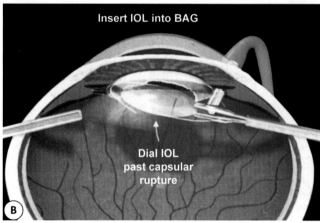

FIGURES 57.4A AND B: Removal of dislocated IOL with perfluorocarbon liquids

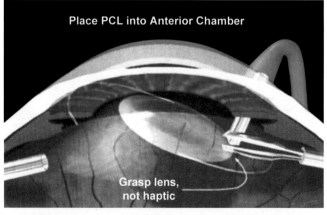

FIGURE 57.5: Removal of dislocated IOL with perfluorocarbon liquids

INTRAOCULAR LENS IMPLANTATION

Some retinal surgeons are opposed to lens implantation in cases of posterior dislocation of lens material. The author recommends lens implantation unless there is insufficient capsular support and low corneal endothelial cell counts or significant glaucoma. If the capsule can support an IOL, it can be placed in the bag with the haptics rotated away from the capsular defect. If the posterior capsule will not support an IOL, the IOL can be implanted in the ciliary sulcus anterior to the stronger anterior lens capsule.

If the capsule is not sufficient to support the IOL, an anterior chamber lens can be used. Anterior chamber lenses are contraindicated if there are low endothelial cell counts or open angle glaucoma. Judgement is required to set the level of cell counts and severity of glaucoma that represent contraindications.

SUMMARY

It is essential for the cataract surgeon to mentally rehearse a plan for capsular rupture, vitreous in the anterior chamber, and posterior dislocation of lens material. Simulation of rare complications is similar to that used in flight simulator-based pilot training. Constant attention to prevention of vitreoretinal traction and retinal detachment rather than an obsession with prevention of posterior dislocation of lens material is crucial. Sophisticated mechanical vitrectomy rather than cellulose sponge vitrectomy must become the standard.

CHAPTER 58

The Malpositioned Intraocular Implant

Clement K Chan, Amar Agarwal

INTRODUCTION

Numerous advances in microsurgical techniques have led to highly safe and effective cataract surgery. Two of the current trends in the evolution of modern cataract techniques include increasingly smaller surgical incisions associated with phacoemulsification (e.g. 1.4 mm incisions as in Phakonit with rollable IOL implantation),[1] as well as the movement from retrobulbar and peribulbar anesthesia to topical anesthesia, and even "no anesthesia" techniques.[2] Despite such advances, the malpositioning or dislocation of an intraocular lens (IOL) due to capsular rupture or zonular dehiscence remains an infrequent but important sight-threatening complication for contemporary cataract surgery. The key to the prevention of poor visual outcome for this complication is its proper management. Many highly effective surgical methods have been developed to manage a dislocated IOL. They include manipulating the IOL with perfluorocarbon liquids, scleral loop fixation, using a snare, employing 25 gauge IOL forceps, temporary haptic externalization, as well as managing the one-piece plate IOL and two simultaneous intraocular implants.[3-13]

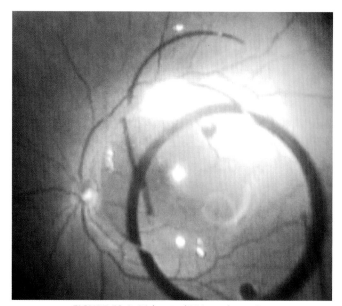

FIGURE 58.1: Dislocated IOL on the retina

MANAGEMENT OF A MALPOSITIONED IOL

Disturbing visual symptoms such as diplopia, metamorphopsia, and hazy images are associated with a dislocated IOL **(Figure 58.1)**. If not properly managed, a malpositioned IOL may also induce sight-threatening ocular complications, including persistent cystoid macular edema, intraocular hemorrhage, retinal breaks, and retinal detachment. Contemporaneous with advances in phakonit microsurgical techniques for treating cataracts, a number of highly effective surgical methods have been developed for managing a dislocated IOL.

CHANDELIER ILLUMINATION

Visualization is done using a Chandelier illumination in which xenon light is attached to the infusion cannula. This gives excellent illumination and one can perform a proper bimanual vitrectomy as an endoilluminator is not necessary for the surgeon to hold in the hand **(Figure 58.2)**. An inverter has to be used if one is using a wide field lens. The supermacula lens helps give better steropsis so that one

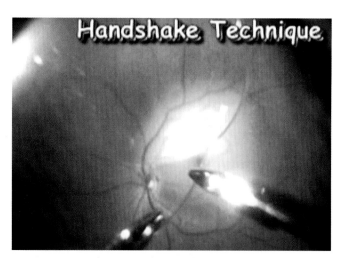

FIGURE 58.2: IOL lying over the macula. Notice the wide field view of the retina. This is because of the wide field contact lens being used and the Chandelier illumination which is seen in the upper left hand corner. Using two forceps one can hold the IOL comfortably and can bring it anteriorly

will not have any difficulty in holding the IOL with a diamond tipped forceps. When one is using the Chandelier illumination system one hand can hold the IOL with the forceps and the other hand can hold a vitrectomy probe to cut the adhesions of the vitreous thus doing a bimanual vitrectomy, one can also use two forceps to hold the lens thus performing a handshake technique **(Figure 58.2)**.

Characteristic	Perfluoro-N-octane	Perfluoro-tributylamine	Perfluoro-decaline	Perfluoro-phenanthrene
Chemical Formula	C_3F_{18}	$C_{12}F_{27}N$	$C_{10}F_{18}$	$C_{14}F_{24}$
Molecular Weight	438	671	462	624
Specific Gravity	1.76	1.89	1.94	2.03
Refractive index	1.27	1.29	1.31	1.33
Surface Tension (Dyne/cm at 25°C)	14	16	16	16
Viscosity (Centistokes- 25°C)	0.8	2.6	2.7	8.03
Vapor pressure(mm Hg at 37°C)	50	1.14	13.5	<1

TABLE 58.1 Properties of perfluorocarbon liquids

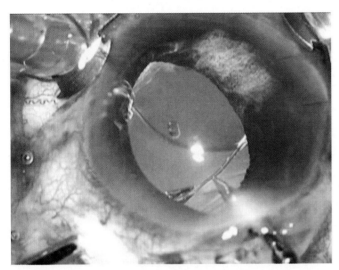

FIGURE 58.3: IOL brought out anteriorly through the limbal route. Notice in the upper right and left corners infusion cannulas fixed. One is for infusion and the other for the Chandelier illumination. One can also have the same infusion cannula with the Chandelier illumination

The lens is then brought out anteriorly and removed through the limbal route (**Figure 58.3**).

Other techniques include IOL manipulation with perfluorocarbon liquids, scleral loop fixation, use of a snare, employing 25 gauge IOL forceps, temporary haptic externalization, as well as managing the single plate implant and two simultaneous intraocular implants. The primary aim of such methods is to reposition the dislocated IOL close to the original site of the crystalline lens in an expeditious manner whenever possible, and with minimal morbidity, enhancing the chance of good visual outcome.

PERFLUOROCARBON LIQUIDS

Chang popularized the use of perfluorocarbon liquids for the surgical treatment of various vitreoretinal disorders.[3] Due to their heavier-than-water properties, and their ease of intraocular injection and removal,[14-17] perfluorocarbon liquids are highly effective for flattening detached retina, tamponading retinal tears, limiting intraocular hemorrhage, as well as floating dropped crystalline lens fragments and a dislocated IOL.[18-25]

TYPES OF PERFLUOROCARBON LIQUIDS

Four types of perfluorocarbon liquids are frequently employed for intraocular surgery. They include the following:
1. Perfluoro-N-Octane
2. Perfluoro-Tributylamine
3. Perfluoro-Decaline
4. Perfluoro-Phenanthrene.

Their physical properties are outlined in **Table 58.1.**

IOL MANIPULATION WITH PERFLUORO-CARBON LIQUIDS

Due to their unique physical properties, perfluorocarbon liquids are well suited for floating dropped lens fragments and dislocated IOL, in order to insulate the underlying retina from damages. At the same time, the anterior displacement of the dislocated IOL by the perfluorocarbon liquids facilitates its removal or repositioning.[18-27]

ANTERIOR CHAMBER INTRAOCULAR LENS (ACIOL)

Dislocation of the ACIOL into the vitreous cavity is relatively infrequent in comparison to the posterior chamber intraocular lens (PCIOL). However, the ACIOL may dislocate during trauma, particularly in the presence of a large sector iridectomy. A subluxated or posteriorly dislocated ACIOL may be simply repositioned into the anterior chamber.[28,29] If the dislocated ACIOL is attached to formed vitreous or is sitting deep in the posterior vitreous cavity, an initial partial vitrectomy to eliminate the vitreoretinal traction is preferred before the repositioning or removal of the ACIOL.[29] If there is any substantial anterior segment injury associated with the dislocation (e.g. marked iridodialysis, large hyphema, excessive angle damage, etc.), it is best to remove the dislocated ACIOL through a limbal incision.

OPENED EYE OR EXTERNAL APPROACH

This approach involves modifications of various suturing techniques for inserting an external primary or secondary PCIOL; sometimes in association with aphakic penetrating keratoplasty, or with an IOL exchange, in the absence of appropriate capsular or zonular support.[40-50] The suture material can be easily tied to the externally located IOL before its re-insertion. A relatively large limbal incision is required for the externalization and the subsequent re-insertion of the entire dislocated PCIOL.

CLOSED EYE OR INTERNAL APPROACH—PARS PLANA TECHNIQUES

This approach avoids the making of a large surgical incision that may induce undesirable astigmatism or tissue injury. The integrity of the globe is maintained, and the fluctuation of the intraocular pressure is minimized throughout the case. However, many internal techniques require the passage of sharp instruments or needles into the eye, which sometimes can be associated with the risk of an injury to the intraocular structures. Relatively intricate intraocular maneuvers may also be involved. In recent years, a number of internal techniques for the repositioning of the PCIOL with a pars plana approach have become increasingly popular.[4-11,25,26,51,52]

SCLERAL LOOP FIXATION

In 1991, Maguire and Blumenkranz, et al. described the preparation of a 9–0 or 10–0 polypropylene suture loop by making a simple knot or a series of twists on the suture with a pair of microforceps.[4] The same microforceps are used to grasp the suture adjacent to the suture loop for insertion through an anterior sclerotomy corresponding to the location of the ciliary sulcus, after a partial pars plana vitrectomy to eliminate the vitreoretinal traction. The inserted suture loop is then used to engage one of the dislocated haptics for anchoring at the anterior sclerotomy. The same maneuver is repeated for the opposite haptic.

THE GRIESHABER SNARE

Grieshaber first manufactured a snare designed by Packo in the early 1990s. It consists of a 20 gauge tube and a handle with a movable spring-loaded finger slide for adjusting the size of a protruding polypropylene loop. The distal portion of the tube with the polypropylene loop is inserted through an anterior sclerotomy for engaging a dislocated haptic in the vitreous cavity. Once the looped haptic is pulled up against the anterior sclerotomy, the external portion of the polypropylene loop is cut free and guided through a 30 gauge needle for anchoring by the

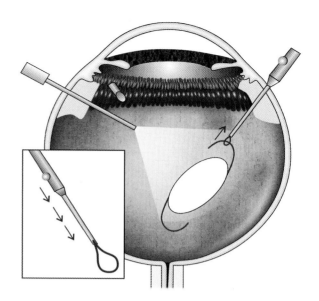

FIGURE 58.4: The Grieshaber snare consists of a 20 G tube and handle with a movable spring-loaded finger slide for adjusting the amount of a protruding polypropylene suture loop. The suture loop is inserted posteriorly to engage a dislocated haptic. The external portion of the suture loop is then cut free and guided through a 30 gauge needle for anchoring at the sclera, after the engaged haptic is pulled up against the anterior sclerotomy

anterior sclerotomy **(Figure 58.4)**. Little et al reported the successful transscleral fixation of the dislocated PCIOL with the snare method in a series of cases in 1993.[5]

THE 25 GAUGE IOL FORCEPS

In 1994, Chang introduced the 25 gauge IOL forceps.[6] His passive-action forceps have smooth platforms at the distal end for grasping tissue or holding a suture, and a small groove at the proximal end for gripping a haptic.[6] After a partial vitrectomy, a sharp 25 gauge, 5/8 inch needle is inserted through a scleral groove at 0.8 mm posterior to the corneoscleral limbus, to create a tract for the 25 gauge forceps. The forceps holding a slip knot (lasso) on a 10–0 polypropylene suture is then inserted through the grooved scleral incision into the eye for engaging an IOL haptic. After looping the haptic, the forceps are released from the suture and are used to regrasp the end of the haptic; thus preventing the suture from slipping off the haptic. After tightening the slip knot, the IOL is repositioned in the ciliary sulcus by anchoring the needle of the 10–0 polypropylene suture within the scleral groove **(Figure 58.5)**. The same maneuver may be repeated for the opposite haptic, if necessary. The scleral groove is closed with an interrupted 10–0 nylon suture.

TEMPORARY HAPTIC EXTERNALIZATION

Chan first described this method in 1992.[7] Its main features involve temporary haptic externalization for suture placement after a pars plana vitrectomy, followed by re-

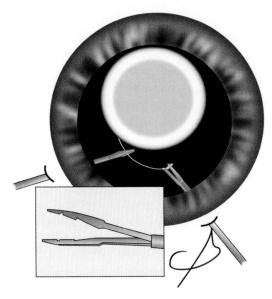

FIGURE 58.5: These 25 gauge Chang passive-action IOL forceps have smooth distal platforms for grasping tissues or sutures, and a proximal groove for gripping a haptic. A slip knot is inserted through a paralimbal scleral groove incision to engage the haptic of the IOL. The forceps are then used to re-grasp the distal end of the haptic to prevent the slippage of the suture loop. After tightening the slip knot, the needle of the 10–0 polypropylene suture is anchored within the scleral groove for the implant fixation in the ciliary sulcus

internalization of the haptics tied with 9–0 or 10–0 polypropylene sutures for secured anchoring by the anterior sclerotomies.[7] The details of this technique include the following:[7,8]

- A 3-port pars plana vitrectomy is performed for the removal of the anterior and central vitreous adjacent to the dislocated IOL, in order to prevent any vitreoretinal traction during the process of manipulating the IOL.
- Two diametrically opposed limbal-based partial thickness triangular scleral flaps are prepared along the

horizontal meridians at 3 and 9'o clock. Anterior sclerotomies within the beds under the scleral flaps are made at 1–1.5 mm from the limbus **(Figure 58.6A)**. As an alternative to the scleral flaps, the anterior sclerotomies may be made within scleral grooves at 1–1.5 mm from the horizontal limbus.

- A fiberoptic light pipe is inserted through one of the posterior sclerotomies, while a pair of fine non-angled positive action forceps (e.g. Grieshaber 612.8) is inserted through the anterior sclerotomy of the opposing quadrant to engage one haptic of the dislocated IOL for temporary externalization **(Figure 58.6B)**. A double-armed 9–0 (Ethicon TG 160-8 plus, Somerville NJ) or 10–0 polypropylene suture (Ethicon CS 160-6 Somerville NJ) is tied around the externalized haptic to make a secured knot. The same process is repeated for the other haptic after the surgeon switches the instruments to his opposite hands.
- The externalized haptics with the tied sutures are re-internalized through the corresponding anterior sclerotomies with the same forceps **(Figure 58.6C)**. The surgeon anchors the internalized haptics securely in the ciliary sulcus by taking scleral bites with the external suture needles on the lips of the anterior sclerotomies. By adjusting the tension of the opposing sutures while tying the polypropylene suture knots by the anterior sclerotomies, the optic is centered behind the pupil, and the haptics are anchored in the ciliary sulcus.

Several important features of this technique include:[7,8]

1. The horizontal meridians are chosen for the location of the anterior sclerotomies for easier manipulation of the forceps, haptics and sutures during the repositioning process.
2. The locations of the anterior sclerotomies determine the final position of the IOL. Previous anatomic studies have

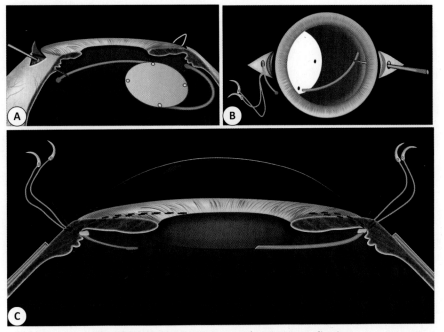

FIGURES 58.6A TO C: Temporary haptic externalization

reported the ciliary sulcus to be between 0.46–0.8 mm from the limbus.[53] Thus the distance of 1–1.5 mm from the limbus places the anterior sclerotomies close to the external surface of the ciliary sulcus. Making the anterior sclerotomies at less than 1 mm from the limbus increases the risk of injuring the anterior chamber angle or the iris root.

3. The following steps are taken to ease the passage of the haptics through the anterior sclerotomies and reduce the chance of haptic breakage: (a) The anterior sclerotomies should have adequate size. If necessary, they may be widened before haptic re-internalization. (b) Fine non-angled positive action intraocular forceps are used for the haptic manipulation to give the surgeon the maximal "feel" and "control". Excessive pinching of the haptics is avoided during the passage of the haptics.

Several measures may also be taken to prevent the decentering and tilting of the IOL:

a. The anterior sclerotomies are made at 180° from each other.

b. The sutures are tied at equal distance from the ends of both haptics.

c. A four-point-fixation option: to enhance more stability, two separate polypropylene sutures can be tied on each haptic, and the associated needles are anchored on the two "corners" of each anterior sclerotomy. This allows a stable configuration of four-point fixation of the IOL.

This repositioning technique combines the best features of the external and the internal approaches, while avoiding any intricate and cumbersome intraocular manipulations. With the easy placement of the anchoring sutures in an "opened" environment and the maintenance of the integrity of the globe in a "closed" environment, this technique allows a precise and secured fixation of the dislocated IOL in the ciliary sulcus on a consistent basis.[7-9]

ONE-PIECE SILICONE PLATE IOL

There is a lack of fibrous adhesion between the lens capsule and the one-piece silicone IOL with plate haptics even years after its insertion into the capsular bag.[54-56] The "slippery" surface of the one-piece silicone plate implant makes it relatively mobile, even years after its placement. The silicone plate implant is fixated in the capsular bag by capsular contraction.[54-56] After its implantation, there is fibrotic fusion of the anterior and posterior capsules as well as capsular purse-stringing due to anterior capsular contraction.[54-56] These effects induce the posterior bowing of the silicone plate implant against the posterior capsule, resulting in the posterior capsular tightening and stretching.[54-56] Thus any dehiscence of the capsular bag outside of the capsulorhexis allows the release of the "built-up" tension, and the expulsion of the implant through the dehiscence.[10,11,54-56] Frequently, further capsular contraction after a posterior YAG capsulotomy may then vault the

one-piece silicone plate implant through the opening into the vitreous cavity, in a delayed fashion.[10,11,54-56]

Previous reports have advocated the repositioning of the dislocated silicone plate implant anterior to the capsular remnants or in the ciliary sulcus.[10,11] Schneiderman and Johnson described the technique of picking the slippery silicone plate implant off the retinal surface with a lighted pick.[10,11] The surgeon extends the tip of the pick under the edge of the silicone plate implant to gently elevate it off the retinal surface. The elevated edge is then grasped with the intraocular forceps for the repositioning or removal of the implant. Alternatively, the plate implant may be brought anteriorly by hooking the lighted pick through one of its positioning holes, and then grasped with forceps at the anterior or mid-vitreous cavity **(Figure 58.7)**. Another method is to aspirate the plate implant with a soft-tip cannula. As discussed above, perfluorocarbon liquids may also be used to float the dislocated plate implant. The one-piece silicone plate implant is designed for insertion into the capsular bag. Thus repositioning the silicone plate implant anterior to the capsular remnants or in the ciliary sulcus tends to be unstable, particularly without the support of sutures. None of the suturing methods (including the temporary haptic externalization technique described) work well for the one-piece silicone IOL with plate haptics. The temporary externalization of the bulky plate haptics of the silicone plate implant is awkward, and the suture placement through its "floppy" surface tends to result in the "cheese-wiring" of the implant. Frequently, the best approach for managing the dislocated one-piece silicone plate implant is its removal.

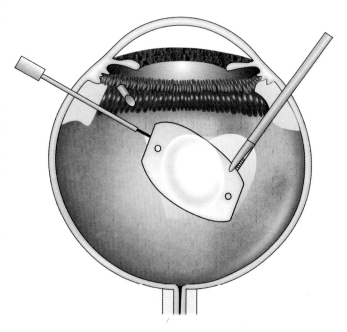

FIGURE 58.7: The slippery plate implant may be lifted on its edge or hooked through a positioning hole with a lighted pick, and then grasped with intraocular forceps for its repositioning or removal

MANAGING EYES WITH TWO INTRAOCULAR IMPLANTS

The presence of two intraocular implants complicates the surgical management. This usually occurs when the cataract surgeon inserts a second implant (usually an ACIOL) without removing the posteriorly dislocated implant. If a dislocated implant is made out of relatively soft and inert material (e.g. one-piece silicone implant with plate haptics), it may not cause a retinal injury. In that situation, surgical intervention may be avoided, although intraocular movements of the loose implant may create a visual disturbance. Mobile dislocated implants with hard surfaces and sharp edges may induce an intraocular injury, and therefore should be removed. The association of vitreous hemorrhage, glaucoma, uveitis, retinal breaks, or a retinal detachment with the dislocated implant also requires surgical intervention. The presence of the second intraocular implant eliminates the option of repositioning the dislocated implant, and it also interferes with the removal of the dislocated implant. A number of techniques have been described in the removal of the dislocated implant in the presence of a second implant. The dislocated implant may be treated as an intraocular foreign body, and removed through a pars plana incision with standard vitreoretinal techniques, as reported by Williams et al.[12] The dislocated implant may also be removed through a limbal incision with or without the simultaneous removal of the second implant.[13] Wong recently described a technique of temporarily suspending the dislocated implant at the anterior vitreous cavity by passing a 6–0 nylon suture through one of the IOL positioning holes; followed by gently tilting up the edge of the second implant to allow the delivery of the dislocated implant out of the eye through a limbal incision.[13] Another option is the removal of the second implant followed by the repositioning of the dislocated implant. This option may be chosen if there is marked anterior segment pathology associated with a second anterior chamber implant (marked iridodialysis or hyphema, progressive corneal edema, etc.), and the dislocated posterior chamber implant can be safely fixated in the ciliary sulcus. The final option is the removal of both implants, particularly when the presence of any implant may aggravate a serious ocular condition; such as poorly controlled glaucoma, or an advanced retinal detachment with severe proliferative vitreoretinopathy. Whether the removal of one or both implants is through a limbal or pars plana opening, a relatively large incision is required, and complex maneuvers are necessary. This increases the chance of ocular morbidities. Thus, the placement of a second implant should be avoided in the setting of a posteriorly dislocated implant.

SUMMARY

Capsular rupture or zonular dehiscence during cataract surgery predisposes subsequent malpositioning or dislocation of an IOL. If the surgeon decides to insert a PCIOL after the loss of capsular or zonular integrity, he should consider a large-diameter (6.0 or 6.5 mm) IOL, in order to decrease the chance of IOL malpositioning or dislocation. Placing the PCIOL in the ciliary sulcus or inserting an ACIOL may also diminish subsequent complications. The management of a malpositioned or dislocated intraocular implant is best accomplished via modern pars plana technology. The basic principles of management include initial anterior and posterior vitrectomy to eliminate any vitreous traction, followed by the use of various intraocular microforceps and small sutures to engage the dislocated IOL for its removal or repositioning. Due to their heavier-than-water properties, perfluorocarbon liquids are particularly valuable supplementary agents for manipulating the dislocated IOL in conjunction with various methods of IOL management. A dislocated ACIOL may be removed or repositioned. The repositioning of a dislocated PCIOL in the ciliary sulcus with modern vitreoretinal techniques provides the optimal environment for visual recovery. The PCIOL repositioning techniques may be broadly divided into the external and the internal approaches. The former involves modifications of suturing techniques for a primary or secondary implant in the absence of appropriate capsular or zonular support, while the latter is best accomplished with pars plana technology. Some of the recent vitreoretinal methods of PCIOL repositioning gaining wide acceptance include scleral loop fixation,[24] the snare approach,[27] the use of perfluorocarbon,[30,32,33] employing the 25 gauge implant forceps,[35] and temporary haptic externalization.[36] The temporary haptic externalization method combines the best features of the external and the internal approaches, avoids difficult intraocular maneuvers, and allows consistent IOL fixation in the ciliary sulcus. Unique features are associated with one-piece silicone plate implants. The capsular contraction after a posterior YAG capsulotomy often leads to a delayed posterior dislocation of the plate implant. Special techniques can be used to pick up the slippery plate implant from the retinal surface for its removal or repositioning. The plate implant repositioned anterior to capsular remnants or in the ciliary sulcus may be unstable, and it is often best to remove the dislocated plate implant. The placement of a second implant in the presence of a dislocated implant is ill advised, as it complicates subsequent surgical management. Surgical options include the removal of the dislocated implant through a pars plana or a limbal incision with special techniques, the repositioning of the dislocated implant after removing the second implant, or the removal of both implants. Surgical maneuvers in the setting of double implants are associated with increased morbidities and complications.

REFERENCES

1. Agarwal A, Agarwal S, Agarwal A. Phakonit: Lens removal through a 0.9 mm incision. In: Agarwal A. Phacoemulsification, Laser Cataract Surgery and Foldable IOLs. 1st Edition. Jaypee Brothers Medical Publishers, New Delhi; 1998.

2. Agarwal A, Agarwal A, Agarwal S. No anesthesia cataract surgery. In: Agarwal A. Phacoemulsification, Laser Cataract Surgery and Foldable IOLs. 2nd Edition. Jaypee Brothers Medical Publishers, New Delhi; 2000.

3. Chang S. Perfluorocarbon liquids in vitreo-retinal surgery. International Ophthalmology Clinics-New approaches to vitreo-retinal surgery. Spring. 92:153-63.

4. Maguire AM, Blumenkranz MS, Ward TG, et al. Scleral loop fixation for posteriorly dislocated intraocular lenses. Operative technique and long-term results. Arch Ophthalmol. 1991; 109:1754-8.

5. Little BC, Rosen PH, Orr G, et al. Trans-scleral fixation of dislocated posterior chamber intraocular lenses using a 9-0 microsurgical polypropylene snare. Eye. 1993;7:740-3.

6. Chang S, Coll GE. Surgical techniques for repositioning a dislocated intraocular lens, repair of iridodialysis, and secondary intraocular lens implantation using innovative 25 gauge forceps. Am J Ophthalmol. 1995;119:165-74.

7. Chan CK. An improved technique for management of dislocated posterior chamber implants. Ophthalmol. 1992;99:51-7.

8. Chan CK, Agarwal A, Agarwal S, et al. Management of dislocated intraocular implants. In: P.N. Nagpal, I. H. Fine. (Eds). Ophthalmology Clinics of North America, Posterior Segment Complications of Cataract Surgery. W. B. Saunders: Philadelphia; 2001. pp. 681-93.

9. Thach AB, Dugel PU, Sipperley JO, et al. Outcome of sulcus fixation of dislocated PCIOL's using temporary externalization of the haptics. AAO Annual Meeting. New Orleans: Louisiana; 1998.

10. Schneiderman TE, Johnson MW, Smiddy WE, et al. Surgical management of posteriorly dislocated silicone plate haptic intraocular lenses. Am J Ophthalmol. 1997;123:629-35.

11. Johnson MW, Schneiderman TE. Surgical management of posteriorly dislocated silicone plate intraocular lenses. Curr Opin Ophthalmol. 1998;9:11-5.

12. Williams DF, Del Piero EJ, Ferrone PJ, et al. Management of complications in eyes containing two intraocular lenses. Ophthalmol. 1998;105:2017-22.

13. Wong KL, Grabow HB. Simplified technique to remove posteriorly dislocated lens implants. Arch Ophthalmol. 2001; 119:273-4.

14. Lakshminarayanan K, Venkataraman M. Physics. KCS Desikan & Co: Madras; 1992.

15. Leopold LB, Davis KS. Life Science Library Matter. Time Life International BV: USA; 1974.

16. Lapp RE. Life Science Library Matter. Time Life International BV: USA; 1974.

17. Subramanyam N, Lal B. A Text-book of BSc Physics. S Chand & Company Ltd: Delhi; 1985.

18. Glaser BM, Carter JB, Kuppermann BD, et al. Perfluoro-octane in the treatment of giant retinal tears with proliferative vitreo-retinopathy. International Ophthalmology Clinics - New approaches to vitreo-retinal surgery. Vol.32,No.2. Spring. 92;1-14.

19. Nabih M, Peyman GA, Clark Jr LC, et al. Experimental evaluation of perfluorophenanthrene as a high specific gravity vitreous substitute: A preliminary report. Ophthalmic Surgery. 1989;20:286-93.

20. Blinder KJ, Peyman GA, Paris CL, et al. Vitreon, a new perfluorocarbon. Br J Ophthalmology. 1991;75:240-4.

21. Shapiro MJ, Resnick KI, Kim SH, et al. Management of the dislocated crystalline lens with a perfluorocarbon liquid. Am J Ophthalmol. 1991;112:401-5.

22. Liu K, Peyman GA, Chen M, et al. Use of high density vitreous substitute in the removal of posteriorly dislocated lenses or intraocular lenses. Ophthalmic Surg. 1991;22:503-7.

23. Lewis H. Blumenkranz MS, Chang S. Treatment of dislocated crystalline lens and retinal detachment with perfluorocarbon liquids. Retina. 1992;12:299-304.

24. Rowson NJ, Bacon AS, Rosen PH. Perfluorocarbon heavy liquids in the management of posterior dislocation of the lens nucleus during phakoemulsification. Br J Ophthalmol. 1992;176(3):169-70.

25. Greve MD, Peyman GA, Mehta NJ, et al. Use of perfluoro-perhydrophenanthrene in the management of posteriorly dislocated crystalline and intraocular lenses. Ophthalmic Surg. 1993;24(9):593-7.

26. Lewis H, Sanchez G. The use of perfluorocarbon liquids in the repositioning of posteriorly dislocated intraocular lenses. Ophthalmol. 1993;100:1055-9.

27. Elizalde J. Combined use of perfluorocarbon liquids and viscoelastics for safer surgical approach to posterior lens luxation [poster]. The Vitreous Society 17th Annual Meeting. 1999; Rome Italy.

28. Flynn HW Jr. Pars plana vitrectomy in the management of subluxated and posteriorly dislocated intraocular lenses. Graefes Arch Clin Exp Ophthalmol. 1987;225:169-72.

29. Flynn HW Jr. Buus D, Culbertson WW. Management of subluxated and posteriorly dislocated intraocular lenses using pars plana vitrectomy instrumentation. J Cataract Refract Surg. 1990;16:51-6.

30. Jacobi KW, Krey H. Surgical management of intraocular lens dislocation into the vitreous: case report. J Am Intraocul Implant Soc. 1983;9:58-9.

31. Mittra RA, Connor TB, Han DP, et al. Removal of dislocated intraocular lenses using pars plana vitrectomy with placement of an open-loop, flexible anterior chamber lens. Ophthalmol. 1998;105:1011-4.

32. McCannel MA. A retrievable suture idea for anterior uveal problems. Ophthalmic Surg. 1976;7(2):98-103.

33. Stark WJ, Bruner WE. Management of posteriorly dislocated intraocular lenses. Ophthalmic Surg. 1980;11:495-7.

34. Sternberg P Jr, Michels RG. Treatment of dislocated posterior chamber intraocular lenses. Arch Ophthalmol. 1986;104:1391-3.

35. Girard LJ. Pars plana phacoprosthesis (aphakic intraocular implant): a preliminary report. Ophthalmic Surg. 1981;12:19-22.

36. Girard LJ, Nino N, Wesson M, et al. Scleral fixation of a subluxated posterior chamber intraocular lens. J Cataract Refract Surg. 1988;14:326-7.

37. Smiddy WE. Dislocated posterior chamber intraocular lens. A new technique of management. Arch Ophthalmol. 1989;107:1678-80.

38. Campo RV, Chung KD, Oyakawa RT. Pars plana vitrectomy in the management of dislocated posterior chamber lenses. Am J Ophthalmol. 1989;108:529-34.

39. Anand R, Bowman RW. Simplified technique for suturing dislocated posterior chamber intraocular lens to the ciliary sulcus [letter]. Arch Ophthalmol. 1990;108:1205-6

40. Stark WJ, Goodman G, Goodman D, et al. Posterior chamber intraocular lens implantation in the absence of posterior capsular support. Ophthalmic Surg. 1988;19:240-3.

41. Hu BV, Shin DH, Gibbs KA, et al. Implantation of posterior chamber lens in the absence of posterior capsular and zonular support. Arch Ophthalmol. 1988;106:416-20.

42. Shin DH, Hu BV, Hong YJ, et al. Posterior chamber lens implantation in the absence of posterior capsular support [letter]. Ophthalmic Surg. 1988;19:606-7.

43. Dahan E. Implantation in the posterior chamber without capsular support. J Cataract Refract Surg. 1989;15:339-42.

44. Pannu JS. A new suturing technique for ciliary sulcus fixation in the absence of posterior capsule. Ophthalmic Surg 1988; 19: 751-4.

45. Spigelman AV, Lindstrom RL, Nichols BD, et al. Implantation of a posterior chamber lens without capsular support during penetrating keratoplasty or as a secondary lens implant. Ophthalmic Surg. 1988;19:396-8.

46. Drews RC. Posterior chamber lens implantation during keratoplasty without posterior lens capsule support. Cornea. 1987;6:38-40.

47. Wong SK, Stark WJ, Gottsch SD, et al. Use of posterior chamber lenses in pseudophakic bullous keratopathy. Arch Ophthalmol. 1987;105:856-8.

48. Waring GO III, Stulting RD, Street D. Penetrating keratoplasty for pseudophakic corneal edema with exchange of intraocular lenses. Arch Ophthalmol. 1987;105:58-62.

49. Shin DH. Implantation of a posterior chamber lens without capsular support during penetrating keratoplasty or as a secondary lens [letter]. Ophthalmic Surg. 1988;19: 755-6.

50. Lindstrom RL, Harris WS, Lyle WA. Secondary and exchange posterior chamber lens implantation. J Am Intraocul Implant Soc 1982;8:353-6.

51. Bloom SM, Wyszynski RE, Brucker AJ. Scleral fixation suture for dislocated posterior chamber intraocular lens. Ophthalmic Surg 1990;21:851-4.

52. Friedberg MA, Pilkerton AR. A new technique for repositioning and fixating a dislocated intraocular lens. Arch Ophthalmol. 1992;110:413-5.

53. Duffey RJ, Holland EJ, Agapitos PJ, et al. Anatomic study of transsclerally sutured intraocular lens implantation. Am J Ophthalmol. 1989;108:300-9.

54. Milauskas AT. Posterior capsule opacification after silicone lens implantation and its management. J Cataract Refract Surg. 1987;13:644-8.

55. Milauskas AT. Capsular bag fixation of one-piece silicone lenses. J Cataract Refract Surg. 1990;16:583-6.

56. Joo CK, Shin JA, Kim JH. Capsular opening contraction after continuous curvilinear capsulorrhexis and intraocular lens implantation. J Cataract Refract Surg. 1996;22:585-90.

CHAPTER 59

Evaluation of IOL Tilt with Anterior Segment Optical Coherence Tomography

Dhivya Ashok Kumar, Amar Agarwal

INTRODUCTION

The accurate positioning of an intraocular lens (IOL) in the capsular bag is vital in preventing postoperative IOL tilt and astigmatism. IOL tilt is one of the components of malposition which invariably leads to pseudophakic astigmatism, loss of best corrected vision and change in wavefront aberrations.[1-3] Ultrasound biomicroscopy (UBM), Schiempflug images and anterior segment optical coherence tomography has been used in IOL position evaluation.[3-6] The author has utilized anterior segment optical coherence tomography (OCT) for estimation of tilt in IOLs implanted within the capsular bag after uneventful phacoemulsification and its correlation with the refractive outcome.

CASES

Hundred and twenty three eyes of 92 patients who had uneventful phacoemulsification with posterior capsule (PC) IOL in the capsular bag were included in this observational case series. Informed consent was obtained from all patients. The inclusion criteria were eyes with "in the bag" fixated IOL after uneventful phacoemulsification and the exclusion criteria were complicated cataract surgeries with posterior capsular rent or post neodymium-doped yttrium aluminium garnet (Nd YAG) capsulotomy. The pupils were dilated to 6 mm with 0.5% tropicamide and images were taken in mesopic illumination. The headrest and chinrest of the OCT was adjusted to guarantee a perpendicular position of the patient's head for each examination. Cross-sectional imaging of the IOL was done with visante anterior segment OCT (Carl Zeiss Meditec, Dublin, California, USA). Anterior segment single scan mode was used. Images were taken in four axes, namely 180°-0°, 225°-45°, 315°-135° and 270°-90°.

The images were then analyzed with the caliper tools in the software of AS OCT for iris vault (D1, D2- Distance in mm between the iris margin and the anterior surface of IOL) (**Figure 59.1**). Using MatLab version 7.1, the anterior segment single scan images were analyzed. A line (L) passing through the limbus on either side of the image was marked as the reference line (**Figure 59.2**). The horizontal axis of the IOL was determined by the following method. The image from OCT was converted to binary for subsequent extraction of edge coordinates. The selected

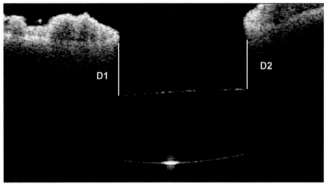

FIGURE 59.1: IOL position seen with corneal high resolution OCT image. D1, D2: distance in mm from iris margin to IOL edge

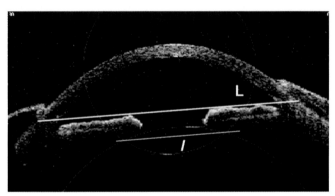

FIGURE 59.2: Anterior segment OCT analysis of IOL position. X1, X2, X3, X4,Y1,Y2,Y3,Y4 co-ordinates. L-slope of limbus, *l*- slope of IOL

points on the anterior and posterior arc edges of IOL were taken. The mathematical representation to fit the anterior and posterior arc of IOL was derived from the equation of the circles passing through the given points (**Figure 59.2**). The intersection points of the two circles were joined to form the horizontal axis of IOL. This was executed in all the four quadrants (180°-0°, 225°-45°, 315°-135° and 270°-90°) in all the eyes. The slopes were calculated for both the straight lines (L, *l*)."

When the reference line along the limbus and the IOL optic were parallel, the optic was considered as not tilted. The angle (θ) in degrees between the two lines (L& *l*) was determined. Slope ratio was obtained by dividing slope of IOL by slope of limbus. Corneal topography was obtained from Orbscan (Bausch & Lomb). All patients underwent refraction and retinoscopy. Best corrected spectacle vision (BCVA) was determined with Snellen's distant vision charts.

DISCUSSION

Optical coherence tomography (OCT) is a noninvasive, high-resolution imaging method that provides cross sectional tomography of the ocular structures *in vivo*. It has many promising clinical applications in cataract and refractive surgery, as well as in glaucoma diagnosis and anterior segment tumor imaging.[7-10] Here the author has described the application of IOL tilt examination with the aid of AS OCT. Intraocular lens (IOL) malposition is one of the indications for the removal, exchange or repositioning of a posterior chamber IOL. Even though there have been reports on examination of an IOL with OCT, there are no reports on the IOL tilt analysis.[6,11,12] The high speed OCT with 1310 nm wavelength used in the author's study has an axial resolution of 18 microns and transverse resolution of 60 microns. It has a scan speed of about 8 frames/sec. With the anterior segment scan, 16 × 6 mm image was obtained and corneal vertex, limbus and the IOL were visualized. The high resolution corneal scan gives a high resolution, cross sectional, quantitative imaging of the IOL position. Ultrasound biomicroscopy (UBM) has been used to examine the intraocular position of the IOL haptics after phacoemulsification, ECCE, and transscleral or iris fixation of posterior chamber lenses.[4,6]

The main advantage of the OCT over the UBM is the noninvasiveness (noncontact), high resolution and less time consumption. Hence, this can be performed in the early postoperative period and in traumatized corneas. Schiempflug images taken from Pentacam have also been used for tilt analysis. Purkinje reflections, photographic documentation and anterior segment analysis system were the other methods used for evaluation of IOL position.[13-15]

Akkin et al has studied the IOL tilt in the bag fixated IOLs and reported a mean 1.13 degrees tilt after in the bag fixation after continuous curvilinear capsulorhexis (CCC) technique.[16] The study by Mutlu et al. showed that if the IOLs were placed properly in the capsular bag after continuous circular capsulorhexis, foldable acrylic IOLs with polymethylmethacrylate (PMMA) haptics were superior in terms of tilt and decentration.[17] All the author's patients had CCC and there was no significant difference in the IOL tilt among the groups. The mean angle between IOL and limbus was 1.49.° Although slope ratio was falling in wide range, there was no significant difference in IOL position noted between them. This shows that a normal capsule fixated IOL has an angle between the limbus and if it extends beyond the range the tilt can be significant. It was observed that the capsule (both anterior and posterior) is usually stuck to the IOL. It is difficult to delineate the capsular bag unless it is freely mobile behind or forms a thin layer. Eyes with posterior capsular opacity or pigment dispersion on the IOL can produce an artifact on the IOL reflection. Prominent IOL reflection can be seen in these eyes with thick posterior capsular opacification or multiple pigment dispersion on the optic. The aim of the study was to identify the ability of the anterior segment OCT to detect IOL position in "in the bag" IOLs following an uneventful phacoemulsification. The same has been shown by deriving the slopes of the limbus and IOL. The author has taken the limbus as the anatomical reference line as it can be delineated easily in the image and is easy for any observer. This can be done in eyes in the immediate postoperative period and in eyes with poor corneal clarity due to edema. The limitation is that pupillary dilatation is required for evaluation. In the author's study it was noted that 180-0° axis was the most suitable axis for good visualization of an IOL. However, 360° IOL position was possible in 22.7% of the eyes. As compared to other studies, the author did not obtain any significant difference in tilt depending on the IOL types.[16,17] Nevertheless, this high speed anterior segment OCT can be used in analysis of tilt and position in eyes with sulcus fixated glued IOLs and sutured scleral fixated IOLs as well. One might require a prospective observational case study with the anterior segment OCT in malpositioned IOLs in a large population in the near future.

REFERENCES

1. Takei K, Hommura S, Okajima H. Optimum form of posterior chamber intraocular lenses to minimize aberrational astigmatism. Jpn J Ophthalmol. 1995;39(4):390-401.
2. Taketani F, Matuura T, Yukawa E, et al. Influence of intraocular lens tilt and decentration on wavefront aberrations. J Cataract Refract Surg. 2004;30(10):2158–62.
3. Oshika T, Sugita G, Miyata K, et al. Influence of tilt and decentration of scleral-sutured intraocular lens on ocular higher-order wavefront aberration. BJO. 2007;91(2):185-8.
4. Loya N, Lichter H, Barash D, et al. Posterior chamber intraocular lens implantation after capsular tear: ultrasound biomicroscopy evaluation. J Cataract Refract Surg 2001; 27(9):1423-7.
5. Hayashi K, Hayashi H. Comparison of the stability of 1-piece and 3-piece acrylic intraocular lenses in the lens capsule. J Cataract Refract Surg. 2005;31(2):337-42.
6. Detry-Morel ML, Van Acker E, Pourjavan S, et al. .Anterior segment imaging using optical coherence tomography and ultrasound biomicroscopy in secondary pigmentary glaucoma associated with in-the-bag intraocular lens. J Cataract Refract Surg. 2006;32(11):1866-9.
7. Li Y, Shekhar R, Huang D. Corneal pachymetry mapping with high-speed optical coherence tomography. Ophthalmology. 2006;113(5):792–9.
8. Tang M, Li Y, Avila M, et al. Measuring total cornealpower before and after laser in situ keratomileusis with high-speed optical coherence tomography. J Cataract Refract Surg. 2006;32(11):1843–50.
9. Memarzadeh F, Li Y, Chopra V, et al. Anterior segment optical coherence tomography for imaging the anterior chamber after laser peripheral iridotomy. Am J Ophthalmol. 2007;143(5):877-9.
10. Bakri SJ, Singh AD, Lowder CY, et al. Imaging of iris lesions with high-speed optical coherence tomography. Ophthalmic Surg Lasers Imaging. 2007;38(1):27–34.
11. Wolffsohn JS, Davies LN. Advances in anterior segment imaging. Curr Opin Ophthalmol. 2007;18(1):32-8.

12. Garcia JP Jr, Rosen RB. Anterior segment imaging: optical coherence tomography versus ultrasound biomicroscopy. Ophthalmic Surg Lasers Imaging. 2008;39(6):476-84.

13. Mester U, Sauer T, Kaymak H. Decentration and tilt of a single-piece aspheric intraocular lens compared with the lens position in young phakic eyes. J Cataract Refract Surg. 2009;35(3):485- 90.

14. Schaeffel F. Binocular lens tilt and decentration measurements in healthy subjects with phakic eyes. Invest Ophthalmol Vis Sci. 2008;49(5):2216–22.

15. Sasaki K, Sakamoto Y, Shibata T, et al. The multi-purpose camera: a new anterior eye segment analysis system. Ophthalmic Res. 1990;22 Suppl 1:3-8.

16. Cezmi A, Serdar AO, Jale M. Tilt and decentration of bag-fixated intraocular lenses: A comparative study between capsulorhexis and envelope techniques. Doc Ophhalmol. 1994;87(3):199-209.

17. Mutlu FM, Bilge AH, Altinsoy HI,et al. The role of capsulotomy and intraocular lens type on tilt and decentration of polymethylmethacrylate and foldable acrylic lenses. Ophthalmologica. 1998;212(6):359-63.

CHAPTER 60

Expulsive Hemorrhage

Soosan Jacob, Amar Agarwal

INTRODUCTION

Expulsive hemorrhage is one of the most devastating complications for both the surgeon and the patient. Unlike other complications, the surgeon is generally caught totally unaware and unprepared. It can occur during any kind of intraocular surgery right from phacoemulsification to vitreoretinal surgeries, but certain surgeries are more predisposed to developing an expulsive hemorrhage and these include intracapsular cataract extraction, open sky procedures such as penetrating keratoplasty, etc. It is also more commonly seen in elderly patients with generalized arteriosclerosis, hypertension, etc. Patients with history of expulsive hemorrhage are at higher risk of developing an expulsive in the other eye as well. Local ocular conditions predisposing to an expulsive hemorrhage include glaucoma, increased intraocular pressure (IOP), low scleral rigidity, high myopia, etc. Other intraoperative factors that can be important include sudden rise in blood pressure, a positive Valsalva maneuver such as coughing, straining, squeezing of the lids by the patient, a tight lid speculum causing pressure on the globe, vitreous loss, etc. during surgery. It has an incidence of about 0.05–0.4%. About 50% of expulsive hemorrhages occur within the first few days of surgery. An expulsive hemorrhage may be self-limiting and confined to only one or two quadrants. On the other hand, it may lead to an expulsive bleeding with extrusion of intraocular contents, which is more likely if the eye is also open at the same time.

EXPULSIVE HEMORRHAGE

Sudden hypotony caused by opening the globe leads to lowering of the intraocular pressure to atmospheric levels. This leaves the intraocular vascular bed unsupported, leading to a rupture of one of the ciliary vessels. This leads to a suprachoroidal bleed which lifts up the retina and choroid leading in turn to stretching and rupture of progressively more of the posterior ciliary vessels. The process can cascade eventually resulting in extrusion of all intraocular contents. Bleeding generally starts from one of the short posterior ciliary arteries. The vessels are especially prone to rupture if they are also necrotic secondary to glaucoma or arteriosclerosis. Events might also begin with a serous choroidal detachment which leads to a sudden stretching of the ciliary vessels leading to their rupture.

It is recognized intraoperatively as a shallowing of the anterior chamber, spontaneous expulsion of the lens or intraocular lens (IOL), progressive vitreous loss, wound gape, a dark, expanding choroidal mass along with hemorrhage through the wound and finally the appearance of retina and choroid in the wound (**Figures 60.1 and 60.2**). With a closed globe or in eyes with self sealing incisions such as phacoemulsification, an expulsive hemorrhage is recognized as shallowing of the chamber and progressive firmness of the globe.

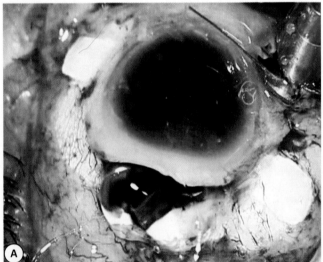

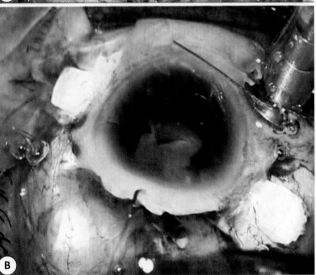

FIGURES 60.1A AND B: Expulsive hemorrhage: (A) Early stage of an expulsive hemorrhage with vitreous prolapse and wound gape, (B) Late stage of the same case with extrusion of intraocular contents including retina

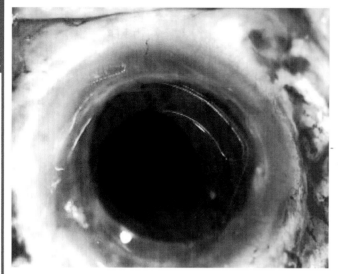

FIGURE 60.2: A dark, expanding choroidal mass is seen, signifying impending expulsive hemorrhage. Prompt action may save the eye in this case

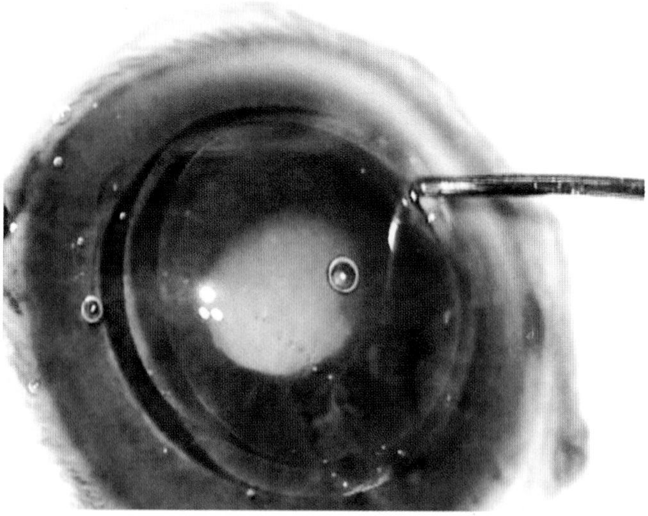

FIGURE 60.3: The donor cornea with a top hat shaped cut created by the IntraLase is seen. A similar cut is also made on the recipient cornea. The donor thus fits into the recipient bed like a jig-saw puzzle

PREVENTION

Patients at high risk need maximal ocular hypotension preoperatively with acetazolamide, liquid glycerol and intravenous mannitol. The blood pressure should be lowered in hypertensives and adrenaline should be avoided during surgery. A good block with application of Super Pinky ball for decreasing the intraocular as well as intraorbital pressure is invaluable. A facial block may also be given to avoid lid squeezing by the patient. Surgery should be done with the head end elevated to avoid venous congestion.

Preplaced sutures in extracapsular cataract surgery helps in rapid closure of the wound. Slow decompression of the anterior chamber, especially in eyes with glaucoma or in eyes with low scleral rigidity is important. Penetrating keratoplasty is associated with a higher risk of intraoperative hemorrhage because of the longer open sky time. The donor graft must always be prepared and kept ready before removing the recipient button and should be sutured rapidly in place. IntraLase Enabled Keratoplasty (IEK) can be performed to obtain shaped cuts in both the donor and recipient buttons which fit together like jig-saw puzzles **(Figure 60.3)**. With IEK, application of just the four cardinal sutures results in an air tight chamber rapidly **(Figure 60.4)**. It is advisable to not cut the host button fully but leave it attached by a hinge in cases of eyes requiring a longer open sky time because of the need of associated pupilloplasty or cataract extraction. This allows rapid closure of the globe in case of a sudden eventuality. In penetrating keratoplasty with secondary IOL planned, as compared to a sutured scleral fixated IOL, the glued IOL decreases open sky time by allowing rapid exteriorization of haptics following which the graft can be sutured in place **(Figures 60.5A and B)**. The haptics are then tucked intrasclerally after the globe is formed well. An anterior chamber

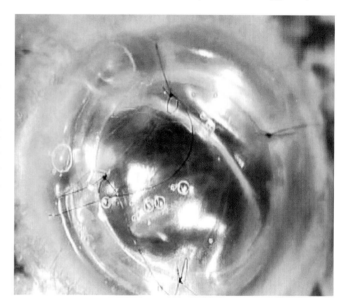

FIGURE 60.4: Placement of just the four cardinal sutures allows creation of an air-tight chamber in IntraLase enabled shaped keratoplasties such as top-hat, mushroom or zig-zag keratoplasty

IOL might not be preferred in this case because of the decreased IOL to endothelium distance.

MANAGEMENT

If the surgeon is faced with an expulsive hemorrhage, the first priority is to stem the intraocular hemorrhage as quickly as possible. This can be done by rapid suturing or even more quickly by applying the finger over the wound to plug it **(Figures 60.6A and B)**. This was first published by Osher senior the father of Robert Osher. At the same time, posterior sclerotomies are made to allow external drainage of the blood and to avoid lifting of the choroid and retina by the expanding supra-choroidal hemorrhage. This combination may prove effective in halting the hemorrhage and allowing the blood to drain externally.

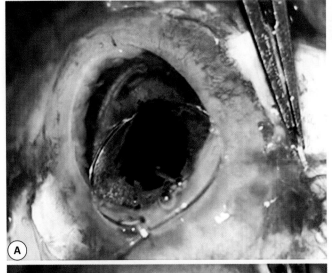

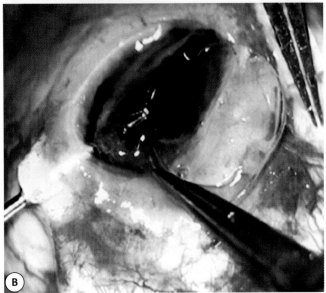

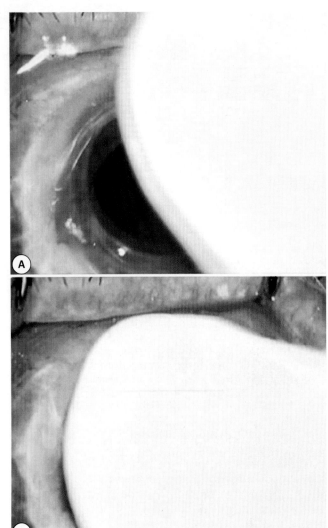

FIGURES 60.5A AND B: A combined PK with glued IOL is seen: (A) One haptic of the IOL has been exteriorized under a scleral flap using a 23 gauge end-gripping MST forceps, (B) The trailing haptic is then grasped with the forceps and similarly exteriorized. Both haptics are then tucked intrasclerally

FIGURES 60.6A AND B: (A) An impending expulsive hemorrhage is seen, (B) Applying finger pressure to close the open globe is very effective in stopping the expulsive hemorrhage along with making posterior sclerotomies

CONCLUSION

An expulsive hemorrhage usually strikes at a time when the surgeon is both unwary and unprepared. The final prognosis depends on the time of hemorrhage, the size of the vessel involved and speedy therapy. Rapid recognition and institution of appropriate measures can help save an otherwise unsalvageable eye.

CHAPTER 61

Postoperative Inflammation after Cataract Extraction by Phacoemulsification

AT Gasch, Chi-Chao Chan

INTRODUCTION

Postoperative inflammation after cataract extraction by phacoemulsification has many causes (**Table 61.1**). The causes can be categorized as infectious or noninfectious (sterile), both of which will be discussed below. It is of utmost importance to rapidly differentiate the former from the latter because prompt treatment with specific anti-microbial therapy can have a major impact on the visual outcome of infectious postoperative inflammation.[1]

TABLE 61.1 Some causes of postoperative inflammation after cataract extraction by phacoemulsification

Infectious
- Acute
    - Gram positive bacteria = primary cause
      (especially *Staphylococcus epidermidis* and *aureus*)
- Chronic
    - *Propionibacterium acnes* = primary cause
      Fungi = rare cause

Noninfectious (Sterile)
- Surgical trauma
- Surgical complications
  Exacerbation of preexisting uveitis
- Lens-induced uveitis
- Residual lens epithelial cells
- Intraocular lens-related factors
    i. Surface contaminants
    ii. Design and finish
    iii. Material
    iv. Placement
- Miotic agents
- Intraocular solutions
- Residual contaminants on sterilized instruments
    i. Denatured viscoelastic material
    ii. Heat-stable endotoxin
- Particulate contaminants
- Toxic anterior segment syndrome

INFECTIOUS POSTOPERATIVE INFLAMMATION/ENDOPHTHALMITIS

Infectious endophthalmitis can be classified as acute or chronic. The organisms most commonly associated with these two classifications differ. Thus, this categorization assists in determining etiology, treatment, and prognosis.

Overall, despite prompt, appropriate treatment, visual acuity outcome is worse than 20/400 in 27 to 61% of the cases of infectious endophthalmitis after cataract surgery.[1-5] Favorable outcome has been associated with good visual acuity and a red reflex at initial presentation, absence of retinal detachment, negative cultures, less virulent organisms, and prompt therapy.[6]

ACUTE POSTOPERATIVE ENDOPHTHALMITIS

Acute bacterial endophthalmitis occurs most frequently after intraocular surgery[1-2,4-5,7-8] and is a surgical emergency.[9] Fortunately, the incidence after cataract surgery is less than 0.5%.[10-11] Wound closure problems[9] and posterior capsule rupture[12] are facilitating factors, presumably because they aid the spread of infection. Administration of subconjunctival antibiotics at the conclusion of surgery does not necessarily prevent postoperative endophthalmitis—even that due to organisms sensitive to the antibiotics used.[3]

Usually a single organism is responsible. Gram-positive organisms are the most common cause (56 to 90% of culture isolates), particularly *Staphylococcus epidermidis* and *S. aureus* (30 to 50% and 10 to 30% of gram-positive culture isolates respectively). Less commonly, gram-negative organisms are responsible (7 to 29% of culture isolates), especially *Proteus* and *Pseudomonas aeruginosa* (30 to 40% and 20% of gram-negative culture isolates respectively).[3-5,7,13]

Potential sources of infection include inadequately prepped lids and conjunctivae, airborne contaminants, operating room personnel, and contaminated instruments, solutions or intraocular lenses (IOLs).[10,14]

Onset of most aerobic bacterial infections occurs 3 to 7 days after surgery and progression usually is rapid. Classically, there is sudden onset of increasing eye pain and decreasing vision with lid edema, conjunctival hyperemia, chemosis, severe anterior uveitis with fibrin and a hypopyon in the anterior chamber, vitritis, and a reduced red reflex.[6,9] However, the classic findings of pain and hypopyon are not necessarily present particularly when *S. epidermidis* is responsible.[15] Retinal periphlebitis may be an early sign.[16] Corneal opacification may occur in severe cases.[6]

The diagnosis should be suspected whenever there is more ocular inflammation than would be expected after the procedure performed.[6] In some cases, ultrasound is useful diagnostically. Thickening of the retinochoroid layer and echoes in the anterior and/or posterior vitreous are consistent with the diagnosis.[17] A definitive diagnosis is made by culture of an organism from aqueous and/or vitreous specimens—not conjunctival specimens, which may be falsely negative or positive for an unrelated organism.[6] Vitreous cultures are more likely to yield growth than aqueous cultures, even after anterior segment surgery.[18] However, both aqueous and vitreous cultures should be obtained because culture of the aqueous may be positive when that of the vitreous is negative.[1,3] About 55 to 75% of cultures from patients with the clinical diagnosis of infectious endophthalmitis any positive.[1,3,5-7,8] Nevertheless, any patient suspected of having infectious endophthalmitis clinically should be treated as such until there is improvement on until further clinical findings indicate another diagnosis.[9]

Aqueous and vitreous specimens are cultured on blood (at 25 and 37°C), chocolate, and Sabouraud agar, thioglycolate broth, and an anaerobic medium. In addition, if fungus is suspected, evaluation of fresh vitreous with Cellufluor of Calcofluor white is done (see below). Usually smears are examined by microscopy with Gram's and Giemsa stains. However, Gram staining has limited utility in directing therapy because in about one-third of cases, it is inconsistent with culture results or falsely negative.[5]

Organism recovery from direct injection of vitreous specimens into blood culture bottles correlates highly with that from membrane filter techniques. This simplified culture technique could be useful in settings with limited microbiologic laboratory support.[19]

After obtaining specimens for culture and microscopic examination, medical therapy should be given promptly and later revised if indicated by culture results. For suspected bacterial cases, gram-positive and gram-negative organisms must be covered. Suggested therapy for acute bacterial endophthalmitis is as follows.

Intravitreal injection of: (i) vancomycin (1.0 mg in 0.1 ml) or clindamycin (1 mg in 0.1-0.2 ml), (ii) amikacin (0.4 mg in 0.1 ml) or gentamicin (0.1 0.4 mg in 0.1 ml), and (iii) ±dexamethasone (0.4 mg; of particular benefit with severe inflammation). Intravitreal injections are given at the time of vitrectomy and repeated only if organisms persist on culture of smear or if clinical deterioration occurs.

Subconjunctival injection of: (i) vancomycin (25-50 mg) or clindamycin (40 mg), and (iii) gentamicin (20 mg). May be repeated daily if bacteria are isolated.

Topical fortified antibiotics: (i) cefazolin (50 mg/ml) q 1 hour, (ii) gentamicin or tobramycin (15 mg/ml) q 1 hour, alternating every 1/2 hour, (iii) prednisolone acetate 1% 6 times/day, and (iv) cycloplegic (e.g. atropine 1%) 3–4 times/day.

Systemic (i) vancomycin or cefazolin, and (ii) gentamicin for 5 to 7 days with surveillance for toxicity (at 72 hours systemic aminoglycoside treatment is discontinued if there is microbial sensitivity to the other systemic antibiotic being used).[6,20]

Amikacin is substituted for gentamicin subconjunctivally, topically, and systemically only if there is bacterial resistance to gentamicin on culture or clinical deterioration.[6] Steroids are contraindicated when fungus is suspected, which is unusual in acute-onset postoperative endophthalmitis.[20] Antibiotics and steroids are withheld until after vitrectomy (if done) unless there will be a prolonged delay before surgery.[20]

Although vitrectomy often is done to diagnose and treat endophthalmitis, only the endophthalmitis vitrectomy study (EVS) has examined the results after cataract extraction (and secondary IOL implantation), Outcome measures in the EVS were visual acuity and media clarity. For eyes with better than light-perception visual acuity at presentation, outcome measurements were equal between the immediate pars plana vitrectomy group and the vitreous biopsy/tap group. However, for eyes with light-perception-only at presentation, the vitrectomy group had significantly better outcomes.[21]

Vitrectomy offers the potential advantages of clearing the ocular media, removing potentially toxic bacterial products, reducing the load of organisms, eliminating vitreous scaffold, and facilitating intravitreal drug administration and circulation. However, there are potential disadvantages, including delay of medical therapy, and creation of retinal holes or detachments or choroidal hemorrhage.[6]

The IOL usually is retained except in cases of infection with filamentous fungi, which adhere tenaciously to IOLs. Treatment of fungal endophthalmitis is discussed below.[3]

CHRONIC POSTOPERATIVE ENDOPHTHALMITIS

Although most cases of postsurgical infectious endophthalmitis present acutely and progress rapidly, some cases are chronic and indolent.[9] The latter may have a delayed onset.[9] Partially treated acute bacterial endophthalmitis can manifest as persistent, low-grade inflammation.[20] However, unlike the usual organisms causing acute endophthalmitis, those implicated in chronic, indolent endophthalmitis usually grow slowly and are difficult to culture.[9] The most common cause of chronic postoperative endophthalmitis is *Propionibacterium acnes*, but *P. granulosum, Achromobacter, Staphylococcus epidermidis, Corynebacterium,*[6] *Streptococcus viridans, Rhodococcus erythropodes, R. luteus,*[22] *Pseudomonas,*[23] and fungi[6] have also been implicated. Common symptoms include insidiously decreasing vision with increasing eye pain. Common signs are reduced visual acuity, progressive conjunctival injection, anterior chamber cells and flare, and vitreous cells and haze. A hypopyon and/or clumps of inflammatory byproducts in the anterior chamber, on the iris, or along the pupillary border are also common. However, the typical signs and symptoms of *P. acnes* endophthalmitis differ somewhat.[20]

Propionibacterium acnes Usually, *P. acnes* endophthalmitis occurs 2 months to 2 years after cataract surgery.[9]

Typically, it manifests as a recurrent, granulomatous, low-grade anterior uveitis. Sometime a hypopyon is present conjunctival injection and pain usually are minimal.[20] A white plaque comprised of bacteria may be evident between the IOL and posterior capsule or on the IOL haptics. It is visualized best when the pupil is dilated.[6]

Topical corticosteroids may transiently suppress the inflammation early in the course of the disease.[9] The clinical course may resemble lens-induced uveitis.[24,25]

Diagnosis is made by culture of the organism from aqueous and/or vitreous, which must be maintained for 14 days because of the slow growth of the organism. Many microbiology laboratories discard cultures after 3 to 4 days unless instructed not to do so.[9]

Optimal therapy is unknown. Recommended initial treatment is vitrectomy with posterior capsulectomy, intravitreal vancomycin, and systemic cephalosporin.[6] However, because lens material may sequester bacterial growth,[26] incomplete removal of the material may result in recurrences of *P. acnes* endophthalmitis. Recommended treatment for recurrences is removal of the IOL and residual lens capsule, and repeat intravitreal vancomycin[6]—and possibly IOL reimplantation. With complete capsule removal, IOL exchange during active *P. acnes* endophthalmitis has not been associated with recurrent or persistent endophthalmitis.[27]

Visual prognosis is good even when treatment is delayed.[9]

Fungi Fungal endophthalmitis is rare. Studies suggest that it accounts for 8 to 13% of culture-positive isolates[3,18] and less than 1% of postoperative endophthalmitis cases (calculated from the incidence of positive culture results).[6] Risk factors include intravenous drug use (which particularly increases risk for *Candida* and *Aspergillus*) and immunosuppression.[9] *Candida* predominates.[3,18]

Fungal endophthalmitis is rare within one week of surgery, and may not become symptomatic until weeks to months after surgery. Typical complaints are blurred vision, pain, and eye redness, all of which progress insidiously. Initially, often there is low-grade anterior uveitis and/or vitritis. With time vitreous "fluff balls" (particularly with *Candida* and *Aspergillus*), yellow-white chorioretinal lesions, and panuveitis may occur. In contrast, *Torulopsis candida* endophthalmitis has been reported to simulate *P. acnes* endophthalmitis.[27] Corticosteroids, which should be avoided, can transiently ameliorate signs and symptoms early in the disease course.[9]

The diagnosis should be suspected when postoperative inflammation occurs weeks to months after surgery. diagnosis can be facilitated with Cellufluor or Calcofluor white staining of vitreous sample and by passing vitreous specimen through a millipore filter (to concentrate the fungus) and culturing the filter.[9]

Until fungus is identified in a smear of culture, suspected fungal endophthalmitis is treated as acute postoperative endophthalmitis but without steroids and with intravitreal amphotericin B (5-10 μg) injection at the time of vitrectomy (if done initially).[20] Once fungus is identified, intravitreal and systemic antifungal therapy with vitrectomy and IOL removal are advocated.[9] IOL removal is recommended because filamentous fungi tend to adhere tenaciously to IOLs.[6] However, some cases of *Candida* endophthalmitis have been managed successfully without IOL removal.[29] Amphotericin B is injected intravitreally (if not done initially) and repeated once if indicated. If there is no response, miconazole is injected intravitreally.[9] Systemically, some recommend ketoconazole as primary therapy instead of amphoteracin B, which has been used traditionally (initially 0.25-0.3 mg/kg/day in test doses of 1 mg, gradually increasing to 0.75-1.0 mg/kg/day IV in divided doses),[20] because ketoconazole is associated with fewer side effects.[30] Oral flucytosine (37.5 mg/kg po q 6 hrs) can be useful for nonresistant *Candida* infections.[9,20] In addition, infections involving the cornea may require topical (natamycin q 1hr) and subconjunctival (miconazole 10 mg in 1.0 ml) antifungal treatment.[9,20]

No treatment and delayed treatment usually results in blindness.[9] Studies suggest that 33 of 75% of treated eyes attain visual acuity of 20/400 or better.[6]

NONINFECTIOUS (STERILE) POSTOPERATIVE INFLAMMATION/ ENDOPHTHALMITIS

Noninfectious postoperative inflammation can mimic infectious endophthalmitis, which always requires immediate cultures and antimicrobial therapy if suspected.[9] There are many causes. Roles of the following factors will be discussed below—trauma from the surgical procedure, surgical complications, exacerbation of preexisting uveitis, lens-induced uveitis, residual lens epithelial cells, IOL-related factors (surface contaminants, design and finish, material, placement), miotic agents, intraocular solutions, residual contaminants on sterilized instruments (denatured viscoelastic material, heat-stable endotoxin), and particulate contaminants. Often the cause of noninfectious postoperative inflammation is unclear, as in "toxin anterior segment syndrome", which is also discussed below. Nevertheless, it is important to try to define the etiology not only to determine appropriate treatment to prevent ocular sequelae of inflammation, but also to prevent recurrence.

One study indicated that the following factors (in order from most to least important) are associated with a significant probability of developing increased postoperative inflammation after extracapsular cataract extraction (ECCE): (i) history of uveitis, (ii) pseudoexfoliation syndrome, (iii) inability to obtain adequate mydriasis at the start of surgery, (iv) IOL implantation problems, and (v) pigment effusion during surgery.[29] Another study suggested that: (i) a history of ocular disease, (ii) glaucoma, (iii) previous ocular surgery, and (iv) prolonged surgery are significant risk factors for fibrinoid reaction after ECCE with posterior chamber IOL implantation. Systemic disease, age, gender, operative method, and surgeon were not associated with increased risk of this outcome.[30] In contrast, several other studies have indicated that diabetes mellitus is associated with an increased risk of a fibrinoid reaction after cataract extraction.[31-33] The above findings for a history of uveitis, pseudoexfoliation syndrome, and glaucoma have been corroborated.[31,33-36] Although the above associations pertained to ECCE, there is evidence that at least some also apply to phacoemulsification, though perhaps to a lesser degree because phacoemulsification, particularly with a clear corneal, self-sealing incision, is associated with a lower risk of fibrinous reaction than ECCE.[37]

INFLAMMATION DUE TO SURGICAL TRAUMA

ROUTINE POSTOPERATIVE INFLAMMATION

Low-grade intraocular inflammation is common after cataract extraction due to tissue manipulation.[9] It appears to be mediated by prostaglandins[38] and can be diminished with prostaglandin inhibitors, including topical 0.1% diclofenac sodium,[39-42] 0.03% flurbiprofen,[43-44] and 0.5% ketorolac.[45-47] These three topical agents appear to be as effective as 0.1% dexamethasone phosphate in diminishing routine inflammation after phacoemulsification,[42,44,46] and 0.1% diclofenac may be as effective as 1% prednisolone acetate in this regard.[40] Furthermore, pretreatment with topical 0.1% diclofenac sodium before cataract surgery may reduce the amount of initial postoperative inflammation.[48]

Noncompliance taking anti-inflammatory medications, inadequate shaking of steroid drops, and tapering of anti-inflammatory medications that is too abrupt can cause persistent postoperative inflammation.[20]

SYMPATHETIC OPHTHALMIA

Sympathetic ophthalmia is a potential cause of inflammation after any intraocular procedure, including laser treatment. However, unlike other causes of postoperative inflammation discussed in this chapter, it is always bilateral. Onset is usually 2 to 8 weeks after ocular trauma with a range of about 10 days to 50 years. Typical symptoms are bilateral eye pain, photophobia, and decreased vision. Often near acuity is affected before distance acuity. Initially, there may be loss of accommodation and/or mild anterior or posterior uveitis in the uninjured eye. Classically, there is progression to severe, bilateral, granulomatous panuveitis with small hypopigmented lesions at the level of the retinal pigment epithelium— Dalen-Fuchs nodules and thickening of the uveal tract. Nodular iris infiltrates, peripheral anterior synechiae, iris neovascularization, pupil occlusion or seclusion, exudative retinal detachment, and papillitis may occur.[20]

The initial treatment usually is steroids with a cycloplegic agent (e.g. scopolamine 0.25% tid). Topical prednisolone

acetate 1% (q 1-2 hrs.), subconjunctival dexamethasone (4-5 mg, 2-3X/week), and systemic prednisolone (60-80 mg, po,q day with an antacid or H_2 blocker) used concomitantly have been recommended. If steroids are ineffective or contraindicated, an immunosuppressant agent is often used.[20]

INFLAMMATION DUE TO SURGICAL COMPLICATIONS

Iris or vitreous incarceration in the wound can result in chronic postoperative inflammation.[20] In addition, retinal detachment may produce a low-grade anterior chamber reaction.[20] Furthermore, epithelial downgrowth or ingrowth should also be considered in the differential diagnosis of persistent postoperative inflammation. Epithelial down/ingrowth involves growth of corneal epithelium or fibrous tissue into the eye through a corneal wound. The tissue may spread across the posterior corneal surface and/or the anterior chamber angle into the iris, which may appear flattened. Large cells in the anterior chamber and elevated intraocular pressure (IOP) may be present. Medium-power argon laser application to iris covered by the membrane immediately produces white spots and can confirm the diagnosis.[20]

EXACERBATION OF PRE-EXISTING UVEITIS

Cataract extraction may precipitate a flare of pre-existing uveitis, particularly in young patients and those with sarcoidosis or diabetes. Such a flare may be associated with fibrin, which may be so dense that it mimics vitreous bands. It may also mimic infectious endophthalmitis. However, in contrast, severe pain and hypopyon are rare.[9]

Flares of pre-existing uveitis usually occur 3 to 7 days after surgery in patients who receive sub-conjunctival corticosteroids at the conclusion of surgery and earlier in patients who do not.[9]

The following guidelines can help to minimize intraocular inflammation after cataract extraction in uveitis patients.
- Postponement of surgery until inflammation has been quiescent for 3 months
- If the patient is not receiving systemic corticosteroids, initiation of corticosteroid therapy (usually at 1 mg/kg/day) the day before or the day of surgery
- Administration of intravenous corticosteroid (e.g. 50-100 mg methylprednisolone) at the conclusion of surgery
- Injection of subconjunctival corticosteroid at the end of surgery.[9]

LENS-INDUCED UVEITIS

Phacoanaphylactic (phacoantigenic) uveitis is a granulomatous inflammation that is thought to be an autoimmune reaction to lens proteins exposed after surgical, traumatic, or spontaneous disruption of the lens capsule. The term "phacoanaphylactic: is a misnomer because the reaction is not an anaphylactoid (type I) hypersensitivity reaction. Although it is distinguished from phacogenic (phacotoxic) uveitis, which is nongranulomatous, both entities may represent varying degrees of severity of the same immunologic process, which has been termed "lens-induced uveitis".[9]

Phacoanaphylactic uveitis has not been reported after intracapsular cataract extraction (ICCE), but it has been reported after both ECCE[24,49] and phacoemulsification.[49] Onset is usually 1 to 14 days after disruption of the lens capsule.[24,49]

Typical symptoms are pain, redness, photophobia, and decreased vision. Examination shows more anterior chamber inflammatory signs than is usual after surgery—more cells and flare, sometimes a hypopyon and/or "mutton-fat" keratic precipitates.[22] A hyphema may also be present. Eyelid edema, chemosis, posterior synechiae, elevated intraocular pressure, and vitritis may be present. Thus, the inflammation can be severe.[20]

Marked intraocular inflammation and hypopyon has been reported as an initial manifestation of retained lens fragments after phacoemulsification.[51-52] Histologic findings are consistent with a striking inflammatory response to retained lens material. Ultrasonography can be useful in establishing the diagnosis.[51] Usually the course is indolent with waxing and waning inflammation, which initially may respond to steroid treatment.[24,49] Thus, clinically phacoanaphylactic uveitis may be indistinguishable from chronic infectious endophthalmitis, such as that due to *P. acnes*. If infectious endophthalmitis cannot be ruled out, cultures should be obtained and antimicrobial agents started.[20]

It is important to bear in mind that concomitant infectious endophthalmitis and phacoanaphylactic uveitis may occur and have been reported after phacoemulsification. Recommended treatment for such cases is removal of retained lens fragments and intraocular injection of antibiotics.[52]

Mild cases of phacoanaphylactic uveitis alone may be treated with topical steroids and periocular steroid injections. Severe cases may require systemic steroids and surgical removal of residual lens and capsule material after the inflammation has subsided. If lens material is mixed with vitreous, a vitrectomy may be indicated. Removal of all lens and capsule usually is curative. All cases need to be monitored for elevation of IOP.[20]

RESIDUAL LENS EPITHELIAL CELLS

There is evidence that residual lens epithelial cells may participate in postoperative inflammation, including fibrin reaction, after phacoemulsification. It has been proposed that they do so by breaking down the blood-aqueous barrier as they proliferate.[53]

INFLAMMATION RELATED TO INTRAOCULAR LENSES

IOL sterilizing agents,[54-56] surface contaminants,[57-58] design,[59-62] finishing,[63] and placement[64-66] all have been implicated as causes inflammation after cataract extraction. *The materials constituting IOLs do not appear to play a role in inducing inflammation.*

STERILIZING AGENTS

Around 1980, sterile early postoperative hypopyons were reported after cataract extraction with IOL implantation. This syndrome was called "toxic lens syndrome".[67-68] However, this term is a misnomer because in at least some cases the inflammation was not caused by the IOL itself, but, rather, by lens sterilization techniques and polishing compounds.[56]

Early IOL sterilization methods employed quaternary ammonium compounds (e.g. cetrimide),[56] ultraviolet irradiation,[69] and sodium hydroxide ("wet pack" sterilization),[70] all of which have been abandoned. Quaternary ammonium compounds caused sterile hypopyon and fibrinoid anterior chamber inflammation.[56] Ultraviolet radiation was implicated in damaging the IOL material polymethylmethacrylate (PMMA).[69] Although used extensively until the late 1970s, wet pack, sodium hydroxide sterilization was banned by the US Food and Drug Administration (FDA) after it was associated with two major outbreaks of postoperative infections due to contamination of the sodium hydroxide-neutralizing solution by *Paecilomyces lilacinus* fungus[71] and *Pseudomonas aeruginosa*.[72]

Subsequently, "dry pack" sterilization with ethylene oxide gas was developed. Initially, it was associated with increased anterior segment inflammation.[54-56] However, improvement of the technique with proper aeration of IOLs has eliminated this problem. Presently, anterior segment inflammation from IOL sterilization is very rare. Nevertheless it may occur.

SURFACE CONTAMINANTS

Residual polishing compounds on IOL surfaces have been associated with hypopyon.[57] Surface films and gross particulate contaminants have also been found on IOL surfaces.[58] Improved manufacturing techniques and quality control have virtually eliminated the problem of IOL surface contaminants. However, it may happen.

DESIGN AND FINISH

Early anterior chamber IOLs are infamous for causing anterior segment inflammation after cataract surgery. Both the closed-loop design[52-60] and poor finishing with resultant sharp optic edges and gaping where the haptic was stuck to the optic[63] contributed to the problem.

Although initially attributed to warped IOL footplates,[73] the first cases of uveitis-glaucoma-hyphema (UGH) syndrome, actually were due to sharp, irregular IOL edges.[59] After the syndrome initially was reported in 1977,[73] vitreous hemorrhage (UGH plus syndrome), corneal decompensation, and cystoid macular edema (CME) were noted in some cases.

The incidence of anterior segment inflammation associated with anterior chamber IOLs has diminished significantly due to several factors—the adoption of an open design with broad haptics, improved finishing techniques, and better quality control.[59] Because of the lower complication rates of anterior chamber IOLs currently available, use of these lenses has been advocated for secondary or exchange lens implantation or as an alternative to aphakic spectacles in developing countries.[75]

MATERIALS

There is no evidence in the literature that IOL polymers, including PMMA, polypropylene, silicone, and hydrogel, directly cause postoperative inflammation. Polypropylene haptics have exhibited superficial degradation, particularly in areas of direct contact with uvea for more than two years.[76] However, there is no evidence that this phenomenon causes inflammation. Furthermore, capsular bag fixation of posterior chamber IOLs, which is generally preferred, minimizes IOL-uveal contact. Similarly, nylon haptics exhibited surface degradation, most prominent in areas of uveal contact.[76-77] Consequently, nylon hapatics were abandoned, despite no evidence of causing inflammation. Surface degradation of PMMA has not been reported.

In pseudoexfoliation syndrome, compared with regular PMMA IOLs heparin surface modified PMMA IOLs have been associated with a lower incidence of fibrinoid reaction, IOL pigment and cell deposits, and posterior synechiae between the iris and implant or lens capsule.[78]

PLACEMENT

IOL placement in the capsular bag is associated with less inflammation than uncomplicated fixation in the sulcus.[66] Furthermore, sulcus fixation has been associated with the following problems.

- Contact between the posterior iris and a nonaggulated sulcus-fixated IOL has caused intermittent episodes of decreased vision with white and/or red blood cells in the anterior chamber. This phenomenon has been called the "intermittent visual white-out syndrome".[65]
- Microhyphemas with iris transillumination defects[79] and some cases of pigmentary glaucoma[80-81] have also been attributed to chafing of the iris by a posterior chamber IOL.
- Erosion of a posterior chamber IOL loop into the ciliary sulcus with occlusion of the major arterial circle of the iris has caused anterior segment ischemia and severe anterior uveitis.[64]

MIOTIC AGENTS

The miotic agents acetylcholine (Miochol) and carbachol (Miostat) are often used at the conclusion of cataract surgery to constrict the pupil. Carbachol may promote more prolonged aqueous-iris barrier breakdown and more inflammation than acetylcholine.[82,83] However, the clinical significance is unclear.

INTRAOCULAR SOLUTIONS

Inappropriate pH, osmolality, or composition of intraocular irrigation solutions and viscoelastic agents could cause inflammation. Severe anterior segment inflammation after cataract extraction has been attributed to an increase in pH of the balanced salt solution (BSS) used during surgery.

RESIDUAL CONTAMINANTS ON STERILIZED INSTRUMENTS

DENATURED VISCOELASTIC MATERIAL

Acute anterior uveitis with keratopathy has been attributed to anterior chamber injection of residual denatured viscoelastic material in sterilized, reusable cannulas.[84,85] However, in cats, neither heat-denatured nor untreated sodium hyaluronate had this effect. Rather, anterior segment inflammation was induced by preservatives and chemical contaminants mixed with sodium hyaluronate.[86] Use of disposable cannulas could alleviate problems due to residua in reusable cannulas.

HEAT-STABLE ENDOTOXIN

Both enhanced anterior segment inflammation on the first postoperative day and sterile hypopyon in the immediate postoperative period after uncomplicated cataract surgery, have been attributed to heat-stable endotoxin that remained on instruments after cleaning and sterilization. The sources of the endotoxin were contaminated ultrasound cleaning baths[87-88] and liquid detergent used to clean the instruments.[87]

PARTICULATE CONTAMINANTS

Talc from surgical gloves was postulated as a cause of inflammation after cataract surgery in a patient who had anterior uveitis and deposits on the IOL surface.[90]

In addition, rubber stopper "coring" has been pushed into ocular irrigating solution during insertion of the plastic spike for the infusion line.[91] Although a potential cause of problems inducing inflammation, none has been reported.

POSTOPERATIVE INFLAMMATION AFTER CATARACT EXTRACT BY PHACOEMULSIFICATION

TOXIC ANTERIOR SEGMENT SYNDROME (TASS)

Three unrelated cases of acute, sterile, anterior segment inflammation with diffuse corneal endothelial damage and edema, a fixed and dilated pupil, iris atrophy, and secondary glaucoma have been reported after uncomplicated cataract extraction with posterior chamber IOL placement. Onset was on the first postoperative day. Introduction of an unidentified toxic insult into the anterior chamber at the time of surgery was the postulated cause.[92]

REFERENCES

1. Bohigian GM, Olk RJ. Factors associated with a poor visual result in endophthalmitis. Am J Ophthalmol. 1986;101: 332-34.

2. Diamond JG. Intraocular management of endophthalmitis. Arch Ophthalmol. 1981;99: 96-99.

3. Driebe WT Jr, Mandelbaum S, Forster RK, et al. Pseudophakic endophthalmitis—diagnosis and management. Ophthalmology. 1986;93: 442-48.

4. Puliafito CA, Baker AS, Haaf J, et al. Infectious endophthalmitis. Ophthalmology. 1982;89: 921-29.

5. Rowsey JJ, Newsom DL, Sexton DJ, et al. Endothalmitis—current approaches. Ophthalmology. 1982;89: 1055-55.

6. D'Amico DJ, Noorily SW. Postoperative endophthalmitis. In Albert DM, Jakobiec FA, (Eds): Principles and Practices of Ophthalmology: Clinical Practice Philadelphia: WB Saunders. 1994;2(102).

7. Forster RK, Abbott RL, Gelender H. Management of infectious endophthalmitis. Ophthalmology. 1980;87: 313-19.

8. Nelsen PT, Marcus DA, Bovino JA. Retinal detachment following endophthalmitis. Ophthalmology. 1985;92: 1112-17.

9. Nussenblatt RB, Whitcup SM, Palestine AG. Uveitis: Fundamentals and Clinical Practice (2nd ed). St. Louis: Mosby. 1996;256-61.

10. Allen HF, Mangiarcaine AB. Bacterial endophthalmitis after cataract extraction: II—incidence in 36,000 consecutive operations with special reference to preoperative topical antibiotics. Arch Ophthalmol. 1974;91: 3-7.

11. Koul S. Philpson A, Philipson BT. Incidence of endophthalmitis in Sweden. Acta Ophthalmol. 1989;67: 499-503.

12. Beyer TL, Vogler G, Sharma D, et al. Protective barrier effect of the posterior lens capsule in exogenous bacterial endophthalmitis—an experimental primate study. Invest Ophthalmol Vis Sci. 1984;25: 108-12.

13. Olson JC, Flynn HW, Forster RK, et al. Results in the treatment of postoperative endophthalmitis. Ophthalmology. 1983;90: 692-99.

14. Sherwood DR, Rich WJ, Jacob JS, et al. Bacterial contamination of intraocular and extraocular fluids during extracapsular cataract extraction. Eye. 1989;3:308-12.

15. Deutsch TA, Goldberg MF. Painless endophthalmitis after cataract surgery. Ophthalmic Surg. 1984;15: 837-40.

16. Packer AJ, Weingeist TA, Abrams GW: Retinal periphlebitis as an early sign of bacterial endophthalmitis. Am J Ophthalmol. 1983;96: 66-71.

17. Chan Im, Jalkh AE, Trempe CL, et al. Ultrasonography findings in endophthalmitis. Ann Ophthalmol. 1984;16:778-84.

18. Forster RK, Zachary IG, cottingham AJ, et al. Further observation on the diagnosis, cause, and treatment of endophthalmitis. Am J Ophthalmol. 1976;81: 52-56.

19. Joondeph B, Flynn HW, Miller DM, et al. A new culture method for infectious endophthalmitis. Arch Ophthalmol. 1989;107: 1334-37.

20. Friedberg MA, Rapuano CJ. Wills Eye Hospital Office and Emergency Room Diagnosis and Treatment of Eye Disease. Philadelphia: JB Lippincott. 1990;353: 58.

21. Endophthalmitis Vitrectomy Study Group. Results of the endophthalmitis vitrectomy study—a randomized trial of immediate vitrectomy and intravenous antibiotics for treatment of postoperative bacterial endophthalmitis. Arch Ophthalmol. 1995;113:479-96.

22. Wenkel H, Rummelt V, Knorr H, et al. Chronic postoperative endophthalmitis following cataract extraction and intraocular lens implantation—report on nine patients. Ger J Ophthalmol. 1993;2: 419-25.

23. Fong DS, Pesavento RD: Pseudomonas endophthalmitis presenting as subacute inflammation. Arch Ophthalmol. 1995;113: 265.

24. Apple DJ, Mamalis N, Steinmetz RL, et al. Phacoanaphylactic endophthalmitis associated with extracapsular cataract extraction and posterior chamber lens. Arch Ophthalmol. 1984;102: 1528-32.

25. McMahon MS, Weiss JS, Riedel KG, et al. Clinically unsuspected phacoanaphylaxis after extracapsular cataract extraction with intraocular lens. Br J Ophthalmol. 1985;69: 836-40.

26. Cheung MK, Martin DG, Nussenblatt RB, Chan C-C. Clinical pathologic findings of Propionibacterium acnes endophthalmitis. Ocul Immunol Inflam. 1995;4: 69-73.

27. Winward KE, Pflugfelder SC, Flynn HW Jr, et al. Postoperative Propionibacterium endophthalmitis—treatment strategies and long-term results. Ophthalmology. 1993;100: 447-51.

28. Rao HA, Nerenberg AV, Forster DJ. Torulopsis candida (Candida famata) simultating Propionibacterium acnes syndrome. Arch Ophthalmol. 1991;109: 1718-21.

29. Drolsum L, Davanger M, Haaskjold E. Risk factors for an inflammatory response after extracapsular cataract extraction and posterior chamber IOL. Acta Ophthalmol. 1994;72: 21-26.

30. Rossa V, Sundmacher R, Willers R. Risk factors for fibrinoid reaction after posterior chamber lens implantation—a retrospective study. Klin Monatsbl Augenheilkd 1992;200:101-04.

31. Baltatzis S, Georgopoulos G, Theodossiadis P. Fibrin reaction after extracapsular cataract extraction—a statistical evaluation. Eur J Ophthalmol. 1993;3: 95-97.

32. Krupsky S, Zalish M, Oliver M, et al. Anterior segment complications in diabetic patients following extracapsular cataract extraction and posterior chamber intraocular lens implantation. Ophthalmic Surg. 1991;22: 526-30.

33. Siskova E, Cernak A, Pont'uchova E, et al. Fibrin reaction after implantation of posterior chamber intraocular lenses. Cesk Oftalmol. 1994;50: 361-66.

34. Zetterstom C, Olivestedt G, Lundvall A. Exfoliation syndrome and extracapsular cataract extraction with implantation of posterior chamber lens. Acta Ophthalmol. 1992;70: 85-90.

35. Walinder PE, Olivius EO, Nordell SI, et al. Fibrinoid reaction after extracapsular cataract extraction and relationship to exfoliation syndrome. J Cataract Refract Surg. 1989;15: 526-30.

36. Geerards AJ, Langerhorst CT. Pupillary membrane after cataract extraction with posterior chamber lens in glaucoma patients. Doc Ophthalmol. 1990;5: 233-37.

37. Muller-Jensen K, Rorig M, Hagele J, et al. Effect of cataract technique and duration of surgery on fibrin reaction after IOL implantation. Ophthalmologe. 1977;94: 38-40.

38. Huang K, Peyman GA, McGetrick J, et al. Indomethacin inhibition of prostaglandin mediated inflammation following intraocular surgery. Invest Ophthalmol Vis Sci. 1977;16: 1760-62.

39. Brennan KM, Brown RM, Roberts CW. A comparison of topical non-steroidal antiinflammatory drugs to steroids for control of post cataract inflammation. Insight. 1993;18: 8-9.

40. Roberts CW, Brennan KM. A comparison of topical diclofenac with prednisolone for postcataract inflammation. Arch Ophthalmol. 1995;113: 725-27.

41. Brown RM, Roberts CW. preoperative and postoperative use of nonsteroidal antiinflammatory drugs in cataract surgery. Insight. 1996;21: 13-16.

42. Othenin-Girard P, Tritten JJ, Pittet N, et al. Dexamethasone versus diclofenac sodium eyedrops to treat inflammation after cataract surgery. J Cataract Refract Surg. 1994;20: 9-12.

43. Blaydes JE Jr, Kelley EP, Walt JG, et al. Flurbiprofen 03% for the control of inflammation following cataract extraction by phacoemulsification. J Cataract Refract Surg. 1993;19: 481-87.

44. Drews RC. Management of postoperative inflammation—dexamethasone versus flurbiprofen, a quantitative study using the new flare cell meter. Ophthalmic Surg. 1990;21: 560-62.

45. Flach AJ, Graham J, Kruger LP, et al. Quantitative assessment of postsurgical breakdown of the blood-aqueous barrier following administration of 0.5% ketorolac tromethamine solution—a double-masked, paired comparison with vehicle-placebo solution study. Arch Ophthalmol. 1988;106: 344-47.

46. Flach, AJ, Kraff MC, Sanders DR, et al. The quantitative effect of .5% ketorolac tromethamine solution and 0.1% dexamethasone sodium phosphate solution on postsurgical blood-aqueous barrier. Arch Ophthalmol 1988;106: 480-83.

47. Flach AJ, Lavelle CJ, Olander KW, et al. The effect of ketorolac tromethamine solution 0.5% in reducing post-operative inflammation after cataract extraction and intraocular lens implantation. Ophthalmology 1988;95: 1279-84.

48. Roberts CW. Pretreatment with topical diclofenac sodium to decrease postoperative inflammation. Ophthalmology 1996; 103: 636-39.

49. Marak GE. Phacoanphylactic endophthalmitis. Surv Ophthalmol. 1992;36: 325-39.

50. Smith, RE, Weiner P. Unusual presentation of phacoanaphy-laxis following phacoemulsification. Ophthalmic Surg. 1976;7: 65-68.

51. Irvine WD, Flynn HW. Jr, Murrey TG, et al. Retained lens fragments after phacoemulsification manifesting as marked intraocular inflammation with hypopyon. Am J Ophthalmol. 1992;114: 610-14.

52. Kim JE, Flynn HW. Jr, Rubsamen PE, et al. Endophthalmitis in patients with retained lens fragments after phacoemulsi-fication. Ophthalmology. 1996;103: 75-78.

53. Nishi O, Nishi K. Disruption of the blood-aqueous barrier by residual lens epithelial cells after intraocular lens implantation. Ophthalmic Surg. 1992;23: 325-29.

54. Boyaner D, Soloman LD. Ocular reaction to the use of wet-pack versus dry-pack intraocular lenses. J Am Intraocul Implant Soc. 1980;6: 252-54.

55. Stark WJ, Rosenbaum P, Maumenee AE, et al. Postoperative inflammatory reactions to intraocular lenses sterilized with ethleneoxide. Ophthalmology. 1980;87: 385-89.

56. Worst JGF. A retrospective review on the sterilization of intraocular lenses and the incidence of sterile hypopyon. J Am Intraocul Implant Soc. 1980;6: 10-12.

57. Meltzer DW. Sterile hypopyon following intraocular lens surgery. Arch Ophthalmol. 1980;98: 100-04.

58. Ratner BD. Analysis of surface contaminants on intraocular lenses. Arch Ophthalmol. 1983;101: 1434-38.

59. Apple DJ, Brems RN, Park RB, et al. Anterior chamber lenses: I—complications and pathology and a review of designs. J Cataract Refract Surg. 1987;13: 157-74.

60. Apple DJ, Olson RJ. Closed-loop anterior chamber intraocular lenses: Arch Ophthalmol 1987;105: 19-20.

61. Jsenberg RA, Apple DJ, Reidy JJ, et al. Histopathologic and scanning electron microscopic study of one type of intraocular lens. Arch Ophthalmol. 1986;104: 683-86.

62. Reidy JJ, Apple DJ, Googe JM, et al. An analysis of semi-flexible, closed-loop anterior chamber intraocular lenses. J Am Intraocul Implant Soc. 1985;11: 344-52.

63. Mamalis N, Apple DJ, Brady SE, et al. Pathologic and scanning electron microscopic evaluation of the 91Z intraocular lens. J Am Intraocul Implant Soc. 1984;10: 191-99.

64. Apple DJ, Craythorn JM, Olson RJ, et al. Anterior segment complications and neovascular glaucoma following implantation of a posterior chamber intraocular lens. Ophthalmology. 1984;91: 403-19.

65. Lieppman ME. Intermittent visual "white-out"—a new intraocular lens complication. Ophthalmology. 1982;89: 109-12.

66. Martin RG, Sanders DR, Souchek, et al. Effect of posterior chamber intraocular lens design and surgical placement on postoperative outcome. J Cataract Refract Surg. 1992;18: 333-41.

67. Alpar JJ. Toxic lens syndrome. J Ocul Ther Surg. 1982;1: 306-08.

68. Shepherd DD. The "toxic lens" syndrome. Contact Intraocul Lens Med J. 1980;6: 158-61.

69. Binkhorst CD, Flu PP. Sterilization of intraocular acrylic lens prostheses with ultraviolet rays. Br J Ophthalmol. 1956;40: 655-68.

70. Ridley F. Safety requirements for acrylic implants. Br J Ophthalmol. 1957;41: 359-67.

71. Pettit TH, Olson RJ, Foos RY, et al. Fungal endophthalmitis following intraocular lens implantation—a surgical epidemic. Arch Ophthalmol. 1980;98: 1025-39.

72. Gerding DN, Poley BJ, Hall WH, et al. Treatment of Pseudomonas endophthalmitis associated with prosthetic intraocular lens implant. Am J Ophthalmol. 1979;88: 902-08.

73. Ellingson FT. Complications with the Choyce Mark VIII anterior chamber lens implant (uveitis-glaucoma-hyphema). J Am Intraocul Implant Soc. 1977;3: 199-201.

74. Hagan JC III. A comparative study of the 91Z and other anterior chamber intraocular lenses. J Am Intraocul Implant Soc. 1984;10: 324-80.

75. Auffarth GU, Wesendahl TA, Brown SJ, et al. Are there acceptable anterior chamber intraocular lenses for clinical use in the 1990's? An analysis of 4104 explanted anterior chamber intraocular lenses. Ophthalmology. 1995;101: 1913-22.

76. Apple DJ, Mamalis N, Brady SC, et al. Biocompatibility of implant materials—a review and scanning electron microscopic study. J Am Intraocul Implant Soc. 1984;10: 53-66.

77. Drews RC, Smith ME, Okun N. Scanning electron microscopy of intraocular lenses. Ophthalmology. 1978;85: 415-24.

78. Zetterstrom C, Lundvall A, Olivestedt G. Exfoliation syndrome and heparin surface modified intraocular lenses. Acta Ophthalmol. 1992;70: 91-95.

79. Johnson SH, Kratz RP, Olson PF. Iris transillumination defects and microhyphema syndrome. J Am Intraocul Implant Soc. 1984;10: 425-28.

80. Masket S. Pseudophakic posterior iris chafing syndrome. J Cataract Refract Surg. 1986;12: 252-56.

81. Samples JR, Van Buskirk EM. Pigmentary glaucoma associated with posterior chamber intraocular lenses. Am J Ophthalmol. 1985;100: 385-88.

82. Roberts CW. Intraocular miotics and postoperative inflam-mation. J Cataract Refract Surg. 1993;19: 731-34.

83. Yee RW, Edelhouser HF. Comparison of intraocular acetylcholine and carbachol. J Cataract Refract Surg 1986;12: 18-22.

84. Kim JH. Intraocular inflammation of denatured viscoelastic substance in cases of cataract extraction and lens implantation. J Cataract Refract Surg. 1987;13: 537-42.

85. Sutphin JE, Papadimus TJ. Post-cataract extraction corneal edema—epidemiological intervention and control. Invest Ophthalmol Vis Sci. 1989;30(Suppl): 165.

86. Ohguro N, Matsuda N, Kinoshita S. The effects of denatured sodium hyaluronate on the corneal endothelium in cats. Am J Ophthalmol. 1991;112: 424-30.

87. Kreisler KR, Martin SS, Young CS, et al. Postoperative inflammation following cataract extraction caused by bacterial contamination of the cleaning bath detergent. J Cataract Refract Surg. 1992;18: 106-10.

88. Richburg FA, Reidy JJ, Apple Dj, et al. Sterile hypopyon secondary to ultrasonic cleaning solution. J Cataract Refract Surg. 1986;12: 248-51.

89. Googe JM, Mamalis M, Apple Dj, et al. BSS warning. J Am Intraocul Implant Soc. 1984;10: 202.

90. Bene C, Kranias G: Possible intraocular lens contamination by surgical glove powder. Ophthalmic Surg. 1986;17: 290-91.

91. Ullman S, Clevenger CE, Parker GR. Coring-a potential source of intraocular contamination. J Cataract Refract Surgery. 1990;16: 338.

92. Monson MC, Mamalis N, Olson RJ: Toxic anterior segment inflammation following cataract surgery. J Cataract Refract Surg. 1992;18: 184-90.

CHAPTER 62

Toxic Anterior Segment Syndrome

Nick Mamalis, Stanley Fuller

INTRODUCTION

Toxic anterior segment syndrome (TASS) is a sterile, inflammatory, postoperative syndrome that can occur as a significant complication of anterior segment surgery, especially cataract surgery. TASS may occur sporadically in individual patients, or may occur in "outbreaks" or clusters, involving several patients who undergo cataract or anterior segment surgery at a particular surgical center. Cases of a severe form of anterior segment inflammation following cataract surgery have been reported since the 1980s and were originally referred to as sterile postoperative endophthalmitis. This term did not accurately describe the condition, as it was limited to only the anterior segment, thus the term "toxic anterior segment syndrome" was giving to the condition by Monson et al in 1992.[1] An episode of TASS can have long-term sequelae, therefore it is imperative for an ophthalmologist to be able to recognize the symptoms and treat it appropriately. An understanding of the many causes of TASS and the methods used to prevent this condition is of great benefit to a surgeon's patients. Even greater benefit can come from the establishment of protocols and guidelines that can be followed by all operating room personnel to further ensure that TASS is prevented from occurring in the first place.

CLINICAL PRESENTATION OF TASS

TASS is first presented anywhere from 12–48 hours postoperatively, although typically within 24 hours. It is always Gram stain and culture negative, and is characterized by clinical symptoms of significant blurred vision, and often an irritated and injected eye. On exam, patients will have diffuse, "limbus-to-limbus" corneal edema secondary to widespread corneal endothelial cell damage, which is distinct from the focal edema that is often noted following difficult cataract surgery (**Figure 62.1**). In the majority of cases, patients will also present with inflammatory cells and fibrin in the anterior chamber, secondary to a breakdown in the blood-aqueous barrier, often causing a hypopyon, as the cells settle inferiorly in the anterior chamber (**Figure 62.2**).[2,3]

Additional signs associated with acute TASS presentation include difficult to manage glaucoma from trabecular meshwork damage and pupil irregularities and permanent iris dilation from damage to the iris. The iris in these cases will usually be thin and allow transillumination on exam.

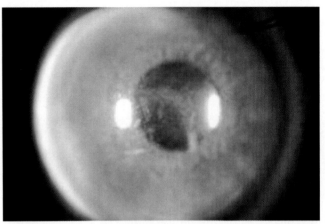

FIGURE 62.1: Diffuse corneal edema with Descemet's membrane folds

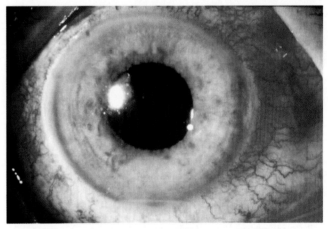

FIGURE 62.2: Anterior segment inflammation with hypopyon

While most cases present within the time frame of 12–48 hours, there is a variant of TASS that can present with delayed onset, however this variant is rarely seen. It should also be noted that cases with more localized corneal endothelial damage have been termed toxic endothelial cell destruction syndrome.[4]

DIFFERENTIAL DIAGNOSIS

There are several causes of anterior segment inflammation following cataract surgery, including surgical trauma, retained lens material, bacteria, sterile toxic substances and more uncommon causes such as previous uveitis. In making a diagnosis of TASS, it is important to distinguish acute TASS from an infectious etiology such as postoperative endophthalmitis, as they share the common complaints of postoperative blurry vision, eye redness, anterior segment inflammation, and pain in some cases. It is beneficial to note the time of onset of the patient's symptoms, which is 12–48 hours in TASS, versus a more delayed, 2–7 day onset of symptoms in infectious endophthalmitis. In fact, more recent reports show a trend towards an even more delayed onset of infectious endophthalmitis.[5] Most organisms will not cause infectious endophthalmitis symptoms in the first 24 hours; however, it is recognized that highly virulent strains are more likely to present sooner than more benign strains and could possibly present within the window of time in which one would expect to see TASS.

There are other signs that can be used to further assist the ophthalmologist in making the diagnosis of TASS versus infectious endophthalmitis. One sign particular to TASS is involvement of the anterior chamber only with rare spillover into the vitreous, whereas infectious endophthalmitis has prominent vitreous involvement. As TASS is sterile by definition, Gram stains and cultures will be negative. While most patients with endophthalmitis have pain, most with TASS do not unless the inflammation is severe. In addition, the diffuse corneal edema characteristic of TASS is not usually seen in infectious endophthalmitis. Similarly, iris and pupil changes are relatively uncommon acutely in infectious endophthalmitis. A final differentiating factor is that TASS improves with intense corticosteroid treatment, which may not help the clinician in initial diagnosis, but can serve as a marker of the correctness of the diagnosis once the treatment regimen has begun. To summarize, TASS is characterized by relatively immediate onset of symptoms, anterior chamber involvement only, diffuse corneal edema, pupil/iris changes, and lack of pain unless the symptoms are severe.

The true incidence of TASS has been difficult to accurately determine. Although surgical centers with TASS outbreaks are motivated to report their cases and get help identifying the cause, if the number of cases is small or the patients have mild cases that are easily treatable, it is suspected that TASS cases may not be reported in all instances. Although not indicating incidence, to give an idea of the frequency of occurrence in surgical centers with TASS cases reported, a recent study of the TASS cases reported to the TASS task force through the ASCRS showed that of the 68 centers experiencing TASS cases, there were 909 cases of TASS reported in 50,114 cataract surgeries performed concurrently at the reporting centers.[6]

ETIOLOGY OF TASS

The causes of TASS are many and varied, and although rare, represent a growing problem for intraocular surgeons. When an outbreak occurs, it can be difficult for a surgeon and surgical center to isolate and identify the etiology, but an understanding of the known causes of TASS can be a helpful starting point and can provide a framework to guide the investigational efforts and prevention of future outbreaks.

In general, TASS is caused by any substance, excluding infectious agents, which enters or is inserted into the anterior chamber of the eye either during or immediately after surgery, causing damage through toxicity to the intraocular tissues and an inflammatory response. Some of the etiologic agents include intraocular solutions used during surgery, intraocular anesthetics and antibiotics, contaminating residues of denatured ophthalmic visco-surgical devices, bacterial endotoxins, and remnants of materials used to clean and sterilize ophthalmic instruments. It should be understood that with the constant advent of new chemicals, medications, materials, products and equipment used in and around intraocular surgery, there is an ever expanding list of possible etiologies of TASS, adding greater complexity to the already difficult task of preventing outbreaks and identifying a source during an outbreak.

SOLUTIONS, INJECTABLES AND MEDICATIONS

The intraocular tissues, particularly the corneal endothelium, are exquisitely sensitive to toxic insult, and thus the surgeon has to be highly cognizant of what is put inside and on the eye during surgery. Something as common and widely used as BSS can be the source of a TASS outbreak, if contaminated or improperly manufactured. In a 2005 outbreak of TASS in the United States, surgeons began to notice clusters of patients with acute postoperative inflammation and negative anterior chamber and vitreous cultures that responded to intense topical corticosteroid treatments. A total of 112 cases were reported, and an investigation revealed that the vast majority of cases involved a particular brand of BSS. The BSS in question was tested and some lots were found to contain endotoxin levels above the allowable limit of 0.5 endotoxin units per milliliter (EU/mL). The BSS brand was pulled from the market and the outbreak was terminated.[7]

Medications or solutions, such as epinephrine or antibiotics, are frequently added to BSS for surgery and must also be considered as a potential source in an outbreak of TASS. If the concentration of the added medication is inadvertently increased, or if the additive includes stabilizing agents or preservatives, such as benzalkonium chloride, tissue damage can result and TASS ensue. Common stabilizing agents that are added to epinephrine include bisulfites and metasulfites, both of which have been found to be toxic to the corneal endothelium and other cells in the anterior segment of the eye.[8] Also to consider with BSS is the pH, osmolarity, and ionic composition of the solution, which if abnormal can damage intraocular tissue and lead to TASS.[9-12]

Ophthalmic viscoelastic devices (OVDs) are a potential source of TASS, with the patient at risk, if too much is left behind in the anterior chamber, or if it is allowed to dry on the surgical instruments (especially reusable cannulas or handpieces) and subsequently gains access to the anterior chamber during surgery in a following patient. In addition, dried OVD denatures when undergoing high temperature sterilization, and in its denatured form it is more likely to cause TASS if particles or debris of OVD are irrigated into the anterior chamber.[13] It has also been theorized that residual OVD may help retain enzymes and detergents used in cleaning the instruments, thus becoming the carrier of such agents into the anterior chamber during surgery.[2] A study of the centers with TASS outbreaks reported to the American Society of Cataract and Refractive Surgeons (ASCRS) over a two year period from 2007 to 2009 found that 89% of the centers reporting TASS were not following the recommended guidelines for flushing and cleaning the phaco and I/A handpieces.[6] The recommendations to prevent the transferring of dried OVD include keeping the handpieces moist, or in sterile water, until they are flushed with at least 120 cc of fluid per port. The final flush through the port should be with sterile distilled or deionized water. To ensure adequate removal of all agents that could potentially cause TASS, it is recommended that each handpiece should be flushed after each patient, as previously described.[14,15]

Topical drops and intraocular anesthetics are a potential source of TASS, primarily through the common use of preservatives or stabilizing agents that are toxic to the corneal endothelium. If the topical drops gain access to the anterior chamber following surgery (such as through a leaking or improperly constructed wound), they can cause tissue damage. A commonly used preservative that is highly toxic to corneal endothelium and found in several topical medications is benzalkonium chloride (BAK). While generally safe to the corneal endothelium when used topically in appropriate doses, it seems that too often it is inadvertently irrigated into the anterior chamber during surgery, causing endothelial damage and new TASS cases. Any medication that contains BAK should not be used in the anterior segment of the eye or be allowed to gain access to the anterior chamber.[16-18] Another common preservative to avoid is methylparaben, which is often used in lidocaine solutions. One percent methylparaben-free (MPF) lidocaine is available and can be used as an intraocular anesthetic without causing endothelial toxicity. In addition to damage from preservatives, intracameral anesthetics at higher concentration (such as lidocaine 2.0% or higher) can lead to endothelial tissue damage and have been known to cause corneal thickening and opacification.[17]

The use of intraocular antibiotics in the irrigating solution during surgery or injected intracamerally at the conclusion of surgery has been discussed for many years as a means of preventing infectious endophthalmitis. More recently, concerns over the possible toxicity of vancomycin and gentamicin, the fear over vancomycin resistant organisms, and the lack of pharmacologic efficacy has resulted in their falling out of regular use. Cefuroxime however, when used in proper concentration of 1 mg/0.1 cc, has been shown in recent studies to be nontoxic and efficacious in the prevention of infectious endophthalmitis.[19] At the time of this printing, cefuroxime is used throughout Europe in this manner, but is not approved in the United States for intracameral injections. Should intracameral antibiotics of any kind be used, care should be taken to ensure proper and accurate dilution to prevent possible anterior segment inflammation due to an excessive concentration. In addition, TASS-like syndromes have occurred when antibiotics or ointments placed on the eye at the end of surgery have gained access to the anterior chamber through poorly constructed wounds that are not water tight. In these cases, the anterior chamber or intraocular lens were found to have a filmy or oily-like substance consistent with a topical corticosteroid-antibiotic put on the patients' eyes after surgery.[20] There is some thought that postsurgical tight pressure patching may influence the ingress of ointment into the anterior chamber in the setting of an incompetent wound.

In cases of delayed onset, TASS which have been known to present as far out as 21 days postoperatively, the etiology is most commonly associated with the intraocular lens. Elements of the lens that are thought to be involved include the finish and design, polishing compounds, cleaning agents and sterilizing techniques used by the lens manufacturer.[21]

OPHTHALMIC INSTRUMENT CLEANING AND STERILIZATION

A critical factor in preventing the occurrence of TASS is the appropriate cleaning and sterilization of ophthalmic instruments. Due to constraints on time and personnel at many surgical centers, there may be a tendency to short-cut the recommendations for appropriate cleaning and sterilization, putting the patients at increased risk. Ultrasound and irrigation/aspiration handpieces that are not properly flushed can allow for the build-up of residual OVD and cortex, which during subsequent surgeries can be injected or irrigated into the anterior chamber and cause inflammation leading to TASS. In addition, the reuse of small bore instruments, such as cannulas, which are not properly flushed in between cases, increases the risk of the surgery resulting in a case of TASS. Due to the difficulty in cleaning and sterilizing reusable cannulas, it is recommended that when possible, disposable cannulas be used. After the proper cleaning and flushing of the instruments, if they are wiped with or stored on towels, the towels should be lint free.[3,14]

In addition to a lack of appropriate flushing leading to TASS, the use of enzymes and detergents for cleaning ophthalmic instruments is an important factor in the etiology of TASS. When instruments are cleaned with these agents, residues can accumulate on the inner surface, especially if there is retained OVD or biomaterial present, which can lead to their gaining access to the anterior chamber during subsequent surgeries. These agents have been shown to be toxic to corneal endothelium in both humans and animal models. It should be noted that enzymes and detergents are not completely inactivated by the high temperature of autoclaving, thus again pointing out the importance of adequate flushing to cleanse these instruments.[4,22]

Another potential source of TASS is the use of water baths or ultrasound baths to clean ophthalmic instruments. It has been shown that these baths can become contaminated with gram-negative bacteria that produce heat-stable endotoxin, particularly baths that are not changed regularly or cleaned appropriately.[23] Even the water in autoclave reservoirs can become contaminated with bacterial endotoxin if not changed regularly. The bacteria can be killed by the heat of autoclaving, but the endotoxin remains viable and attaches to the instruments. The endotoxin can be very difficult to remove from the instruments, requiring rinsing and wiping with alcohol or acetone. The use of the contaminated instruments can lead to corneal toxicity if the endotoxin is injected into the eye. While these baths are useful in removing gross biomaterial from the instruments, as would be found in general surgery, the lack of significant biomaterial on ophthalmic instruments that have been appropriately flushed and the risk of gram-negative endotoxin contamination has lead to the recommendation that ultrasound baths are not be used unless strict protocols are followed to prevent contamination.[23]

An additional factor in TASS cases that should be considered is the level of impurities in the water used to clean the instruments. High levels of heavy metal condensates, sulfate condensates, and impurities in the water supplying an autoclave machine can lead to a build up of residue that can eventually contaminate the autoclave steam. An outbreak of TASS has been reported in which the autoclave steam sterilizer was not appropriately maintained, allowing for heavy metals to be deposited on the instruments. The condition of the instruments themselves should also be analyzed, as areas of chrome breakdown can lead to exposed brass metal and allow for a toxic residue of copper and zinc deposits to accumulate and subsequently be flushed into the eye during surgery.[24]

A helpful and informative guide to the proper cleaning and sterilizing of instruments was prepared as a special report in February of 2007 by an Ad Hoc task force, sponsored by the ASCRS and the American Society of Ophthalmic Registered Nurses (ASORN). The goal of the report was to provide generic, evidence-based recommendations on the cleaning and sterilizing of all surgical instruments to help prevent single facility outbreaks of TASS related to contaminated or degraded instruments.[14]

TREATMENT

Once an infectious etiology has been ruled out and the diagnosis established, treatment for TASS should begin immediately. Topical steroids are the primary medications used, with topical prednisolone acetate 1% drops being the mainstay. The drops are administered every 1 to 2 hours in an attempt to suppress the inflammatory response to the toxic insult and thus limit the damage to sensitive intraocular structures. If the response is not adequate, some surgeons recommend adding oral prednisone, topical nonsteroidal anti-inflammatory drops, and/or hypertonic drops. The use of periocular steroids can be considered and is used by some surgeons. If the surgeon is able to detect any residual material within the eye, such as ointment or cortex, the material should be evacuated rapidly. This can prevent a chronic inflammation and delayed onset (smoldering) TASS. There is no evidence that routine anterior chamber washout upon an initial diagnosis of TASS is beneficial unless there is obvious residual material in the anterior segment.[2,3]

Close follow-up, including slit-lamp exam several hours after initiating treatment and daily for several days, is imperative in ensuring adequate response to treatment and expected resolution. Intraocular pressure (IOP) should be measured as part of each exam. Early in the course of treatment the IOP is often low, but with increased aqueous production as the eye begins to recover and the susceptibility of the trabecular meshwork to significant damage, a rapid increase in IOP can be seen. Once the cornea begins to clear and inflammation subsides, a gonioscopic exam to evaluate the anterior chamber angle and trabecular meshwork should be performed. Specular or confocal microscopy can also be performed at this point to establish the extent of corneal endothelial cell damage. The presence of peripheral anterior synechiae may indicate that trabecular meshwork has been damaged enough to cause chronic, long-term complications.[2,3]

PROGNOSIS

The prognosis and outcome of patients with TASS depends on the degree of insult to the intraocular tissue, which correlates with the amount and type of substance involved and the duration of the exposure. The corneal endothelium has been shown to be highly sensitive to toxic agents, and was shown by Edelhauser et al to undergo an acute breakdown of endothelial junctions and loss of the barrier function. The toxic load results in the death of many endothelial cells and if the remaining endothelial cells cannot migrate and spread to cover the damaged area, permanent corneal edema can result. Mild cases that are treated early tend to have the inflammation resolve rapidly with topical steroid drops and the corneal edema resolve over a period of days to weeks, with little to no long-term sequelae. Moderate cases can see the corneal edema last from weeks to months, with the possibility of mild residual edema and/or increased IOP. Severe cases or cases that have a delayed onset of treatment can see significant chronic corneal edema, glaucoma from trabecular meshwork damage that can be resistant to medical management, transient or permanent cystoid macular edema from anterior segment inflammation, or iris damage that leads to a permanently fixed, dilated pupil. These patients may require multiple surgical interventions such as corneal transplants and glaucoma valves or setons. Long-term follow-up is recommended to evaluate for potential problems with corneal edema and glaucoma, as well as sequelae of anterior segment inflammation.[2,3]

OUTBREAK ANALYSIS

Should an outbreak of TASS occur, it is recommended that a team be established to search for possible causes. All medications, fluids, solutions, and injectables that are part of the surgery should be analyzed for appropriate pH, concentration, dosage, and the presence of preservatives and stabilizing agents. Staff that handles, prepares, and dispenses such items should be included in the investigational team, and should actively ensure that all items are prepared accurately and handled appropriately. Thorough flushing of handpieces and cannulas should be ensured, using at least 120 cc of water with the last flush being with sterile deionized/distilled water. Surgical centers also should evaluate across the board the protocols and policies involved with cleaning and sterilizing instruments, with special consideration given to the use of enzymes, detergents, and ultrasound baths in the cleaning and sterilization process. If an autoclave instrument is used as part of the sterilization process, proper cleaning, maintenance, and a clean water supply should be ensured. All aspects and details of cataract surgery at a TASS outbreak site must be analyzed with the understanding that the cause could be from any of the above categories as well as a previously unanticipated source.

In addition to the above measures, any center or physician from around the world can contact the TASS task force, established in conjunction with the Intermountain Ocular Research Center at the University of Utah, the ASCRS, and members of industry. Through the ASCRS website (www.ascrs.org), surgical centers or physicians can report cases and receive help in sorting through the complex task of finding the etiology of the outbreak. Questionnaires have been developed by the TASS task force to aid the surgical center in its evaluation of the products used during surgery as well as the instrument cleaning and sterilization. Ophthalmology research fellows are available to provide analysis of TASS outbreaks and subsequent recommendations on the prevention of future occurrences, and TASS Task Force nurses are available to provide onsite analysis within the United States.

CONCLUSION

TASS, although rare, can be a significant problem for a surgeon and surgical center and can lead to significant long-term sequelae for the affected patients. The causes of TASS are many and prevention of TASS is the key. Protocols should be established and followed to ensure that each solution, medication, or ointment that is injected, irrigated, or has access to the anterior chamber is at its proper dosage, without contaminants and harmful preservatives or additives. The surgeon and surgical staff should be aware of and follow appropriate protocols for cleaning, processing, and sterilization of instruments to help prevent outbreaks. All involved personnel must stay vigilant in the prevention of TASS, and should an outbreak occur, it is the surgeon's responsibility to alert the surgical team and center that a case has occurred so that a detailed investigation can take place to determine the possible etiology. Outbreaks can be reported and resources are available to help in sorting through the complex task of finding the causative agent.

REFERENCES

1. Monson MC, Mamalis N, Olson RJ. Toxic anterior segment inflammation following cataract surgery. J Cataract Refract Surg. 1992;18:184-9.
2. Mamalis N. Toxic anterior segment syndrome. AAO Focal Points. 2009;10:1-13.
3. Mamalis N, Edelhauser HF, Dawson DG, et al. Toxic anterior segment syndrome. J Cataract and Refract Surg. 2006;32: 324-33.
4. Breebaart AC, Nuyts RMMA, Pels E, et al. Toxic endothelial cell destruction of the cornea after routine extracapsular cataract surgery. Arch Ophthalmology. 1990;108:1121-5.
5. Moshirfar M, Feiz V, Vitale AT, et al. Endophthalmitis after Uncomplicated Cataract Surgery with the Use of Fourth-Generation Fluoroquinolones. A Retrospective Observational Case Series. Ophthalmology. 2007;114 (4):686-91.
6. Peck CM, Brubaker J, Clouser S, et al. Toxic anterior segment syndrome: common causes. J Cataract and Refract Surg. 2010;36:1073-80.
7. Kutty PK, Forster TS, Wood-Koob C, et al. Multistate outbreak of toxic anterior segment syndrome, J Cataract and Refract Surg. 2005;34:585-90.
8. Hull DS, Chemotti MT, Edelhauser HF, et al. Effect of epinephrine on the corneal endothelium. Am J Ophthalmol. 1975;79:245-50.
9. Edelhauser HF, Van Horn DL, Schultz RO, et al. Comparative toxicity of intraocular irrigating solutions on the corneal endothelium. Am J Ophthalmol. 1976;81:473-81.
10. Carter LM, Duncan G, Rennie GK. Effects of detergents on the ionic balance and permeability of isolated bovine cornea. Exp Eye Res. 1973;17:409-16.
11. Gonnering R, Edelhauser HF, Van Horn DL, et al. The pH tolerance of rabbit and human corneal endothelium. Invest Ophthalmol Vis Sci. 1979;18:373-90.
12. Edelhauser HF, Hanneken AM, Pederson HJ, et al. Osmotic tolerance of rabbit and human corneal endothelium. Arch Ophthalmol. 1981;99:1281-7.
13. Kim JH. Intraocular inflammation of denatured viscoelastic substance in cases of cataract extraction and lens implantation. J Cataract Refract Surg. 1987;13:537-42.
14. American Society of Cataract and Refractive Surgery and the American Society of Ophthalmic Registered Nurses. Recommended practices for cleaning and sterilizing intraocular surgical instruments. J Cataract Refract Surg. 2007;33:1095-100.
15. AORN. Recommended practices for sterilization in the perioperative setting. In: Association of Operating Room Nurses. Standards, Recommended Practices & Guidelines. AORN; 2007. pp. 673-87.

16. Liu H, Routley I, Teichmann K. Toxic endothelial cell destruction from intraocular benzalkonium chloride. J Cataract Refract Surg. 2001;27:1746-50.

17. Parikh CH, Edelhauser HF. Ocular surgical pharmacology: corneal endothelial safety and toxicity. Curr Opin Ophthalmol. 2003;14:178-85.

18. Britton B, Hervey R, Kasten K, et al. Intraocular irritation evaluation of benzalkonium chloride in rabbits. Ophthalmic Surg. 1976;7(3):46-55.

19. ESCRS Endophthalmitis Study Group. Prophylaxis of postoperative endophthalmitis following cataract surgery: results of the ESCRS multicenter study and identification of risk factors. J Cataract Refract Surg. 2007;33:978-88.

20. Werner L, Sher JH, Taylor JR, et al. Toxic anterior segment syndrome and possible association with ointment in the anterior chamber following cataract surgery. J Cataract Refract Surg. 2006;32:227-35.

21. Jehan FS, Mamalis N, Spencer TS, et al. Postoperative sterile endophthalmitis (TASS) associated with the MemoryLens. J Cataract Refract Surg. 2000;26:1773-7.

22. Parikh C, Sippy BD, Martin DF, et al. Effects of enzymatic sterilization detergents on the corneal endothelium. Arch Ophthalmol. 2002;120:165-72.

23. Kriesler KR, Martin SS, Young CW, et al. Postoperative inflammation following cataract extraction caused by bacterial contamination of the cleaning bath detergent. J Cataract and Refract Surg. 1992;18:106-10.

24. Hellinger WC, Hasan SC, Bacalis LP, et al. Outbreak of toxic anterior segment syndrome following cataract surgery associated with impurities of autoclave steam moisture. Infect Control Hosp Epidem. 2006;27:294-8.

CHAPTER 63

Pseudophakic Cystoid Macular Edema

Carlos F Fernandez, J Fernando Arevalo

INTRODUCTION

Cystoid macular edema (CME) following cataract surgery was initially reported by Irvine in 1953 and is known as the Irvine-Gass syndrome.[1,2] CME is one of the most common causes of unexpected decreased visual acuity after ophthalmic surgery. Despite recent advances in cataract surgery technique and instrumentation, pseudophakic cystoid macular edema (PCME) occurs most frequently after cataract surgery even after uncomplicated surgery **(Figures 63.1A and B)**.[3] CME exhibits dilation of normal retinal capillaries around the fovea, with consequent fluid leakage and microcystoid formation. It is the pooling of fluorescein in these microcystoid spaces that produces the typical petaloid appearance. CME is often accompanied by disruption of the blood-retinal barrier or blood-aqueous barrier, and in fact, it is suggested clinically that the condition is not limited to the macula, but spreads so as to become diffuse in the eye.

Although no definitive treatment regimen exists, the long-term goal of treatment is to reduce clinical macular edema and improve visual acuity.

The objective of this chapter is to review the most important aspects of the histology, pathogenesis, natural history, differential diagnosis, clinical presentation, prevention and management of PCME.

HISTOLOGY

Cystoid macular edema consists of a localized expansion of the retinal intracellular and/or extracellular space in the macular area. This predilection to the macular region is probably associated with the loose binding of inner connecting fibers in Henle's layer, allowing accumulation of fluid leaking from perifoveal capillaries. The absence of Müller cells in the foveal region is also a contributing factor. Radially orientated cystoid spaces consisting of ophthalmoscopically clear fluid are often clinically detectable in the macular area. The cysts are characterized by an altered light reflex with a decreased central reflex and a thin, highly reflective edge. Histological studies show the cysts to be areas of retina in which the cells have been displaced **(Figure 63.2)**.[4] Recently Antcliff et al[5] monitored the hydraulic conductivity of the human retina following progressive ablation of retinal layers performed with the aid of an excimer laser. They concluded that the inner and outer plexiform layers constitute high resistance barriers to fluid flow through the retina, which accounts for the characteristic distribution of CME seen in histological specimens and with optical coherence tomography (OCT). In CME associated with cataract extraction, the cysts were most prominent in the inner nuclear layer and less prominent in the outer plexiform layer.

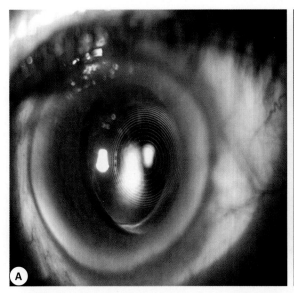 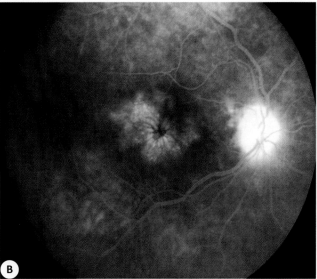

FIGURES 63.1A AND B: (A) Anterior segment after uneventful cataract surgery showing a multifocal intraocular lens in the posterior chamber; (B) Fluorescein angiography shows pseudophakic cystoid macular edema

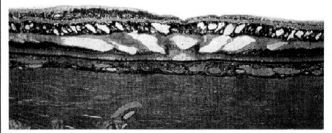

FIGURE 63.2: Histology of pseudophakic cystoid macular edema showing cystic spaces in the outer plexiform layer (Reprinted with permission from Folberg R. Retina: Cystoid Macular Edema. In: Pathology of the eye (CDROM). Folberg R (Ed). Mosby-Year Book: St Louis; 1996).

PATHOGENESIS

Several theories exist regarding the pathogenesis of CME,[6,7] and the rationale for its treatment is dictated by the pathogenetic theory. The theories involve changes in the perifoveal retina where the vascular permeability of the retinal capillaries is altered, leading to leakage of plasma into the central retina, which causes it to thicken because of excess interstitial fluid. The excess interstitial fluid is likely to disrupt ion fluxes, and the thickening of the macula results in stretching and distortion of the neurons. There is reversible reduction in visual acuity, but over time the perturbed neurons die, which results in permanent visual loss.[8]

The macular region by virtue of its anatomic structure is the site of predilection for the accumulation of interstitial fluid. Here the long neural receptor cell axons radiating outward from the foveal area form the outer plexiform layer of Henle, which acts much like a sponge in that it is capable of interstitial accumulation of large quantities of fluid exuding from the neighboring capillaries. As this fluid dissects into the nerve fiber layer, it displaces the nerve fibers to form large lakes of intercellular fluid. Larger lakes develop centrally as a result of the longer nerve fiber layers present centrally in Henle's fiber layer.

Fluorescein angiograms often show that the capillaries in the macular region (and disc) are preferentially affected. They show obvious dye leakage while capillaries in other parts of the retina do not. There is thus something about these capillaries, or their relation to the vitreous, which makes them preferentially susceptible. The explanation for this preferential increased permeability of the macular capillaries is unknown.

All treatment schemes have been related to theoretical factors believed to be associated with its pathogenesis. These include hypotony, hyaluronidase in the local anesthetic, topical adrenergic compounds, phototoxicity induced by the coaxial illumination of the operating microscope, vitreomacular traction, inflammation of macular capillaries potentiated or produced by mediators such as prostaglandins and the specificities of the cataract technique.

DIRECT VITREOUS TRACTION

Autopsy studies show that the incidence of posterior vitreous detachment in patients in the senile cataract age range (60–80 years of age) is not as high as clinical observations have led us to believe. Instead, large syneresis cavities are often mistaken clinically for posterior vitreous detachment. Foos[9] found the incidence of total posterior vitreous detachment in phakic subjects to be only 17% in the seventh decade, 51% in the eighth decade and 55% in the ninth decade, whereas in all aphakic subjects over the age of 45, it was approximately 75%. Therefore, lens extraction would seem to produce posterior vitreous detachment in roughly 50% of the patients, an incidence comparable to that reported for transient cystoid macular edema following lens extraction. However, the theory of direct vitreous traction on the macula is no longer generally accepted.

INFLAMMATION

It is now generally believed that inflammation is the cause of cystoid macular edema after cataract extraction. Surgical trauma to the iris/ciliary body or lens epithelial cells induces synthesis of prostaglandins (PGs) in the aqueous humor. This substance then causes a disruption of the blood-aqueous barrier, which results in the accumulation of not only PGs but also other inflammatory mediators such as endotoxin, immune complex, and cytokines in the aqueous humor. Inflammatory mediators that have accumulated in the aqueous humor diffuse to the vitreous and reach the retina, where they cause a disruption of the blood-retinal barrier. Thus, these mediators stimulate capillaries of the retina and the nerve head, and in a regular postoperative process serum leaks from the blood vessels and pools in the retinal tissue **(Figure 63.3)**. When the serum reaches a certain level, the condition can be identified clinically as CME by fluorescein angiography.

The key in this hypothesis is that the disruptions of the blood-aqueous barrier and the blood-retinal barrier are truly parallel, i.e. if the disruption in the blood-aqueous barrier is large, then the disruption in the blood-retinal barrier is also large; if the disruption in the blood-aqueous barrier is small, then so is that in the blood-retinal barrier.

Histologically, inflammatory cells have been found in the retina and ciliary body. The increased vascular permeability which forms the basis for the fluorescein leakage is most easily explained as the effect of inflammation. Clinically, it appears that a vasoactive stimulus from inflammatory debris in the vitreous is probably more important in producing the retinal vascular leakage than direct inflammation of the retinal vessels.

Most research on the formative mechanism of CME has been done on the role of prostaglandins following cataract

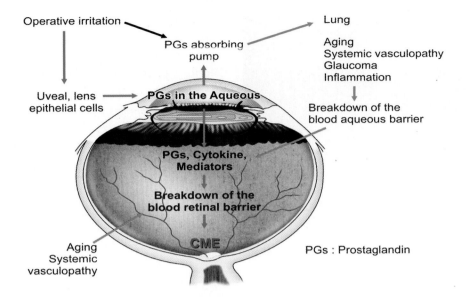

FIGURE 63.3: Inflammatory hypothesis on the pathogenesis of pseudophakic cystoid macular edema. (Modified with permission from Miyake K, Ibaraki N. Prostaglandins and cystoid macular edema. Surv Ophthalmol. 2002;47 Suppl 1:S203-18)

surgery. Prostaglandins, which are metabolic products of arachidonic acid, are the most studied of the chemical transmitters contributing to general edema in systemic tissues, including eye tissue. The synthesis of prostaglandins is known to cause irritative reactions after ocular or surgical traumas.

Products of the arachidonic acid cascade are not the only chemical transmitters related to postoperative and other inflammations. Complement, platelet-activating factor (PAF), lysosomal enzymes, cytokines, nitric oxide, and endothelin have also been implicated in inflammatory conditions such as postoperative inflammation. Markedly increased levels of interleukin in the aqueous humor of patients who underwent cataract surgery can be seen, and these increases closely paralleled to clinical symptoms. It has also been shown that cytokines correlate to induce cyclo-oxygenase-2. Moreover, it has been suggested that platelet-activating factor forms the inflammatory condition through various interactions with interleukin and prostaglandins. It has also been reported that endothelin-1 induces the arachidonic acid cascade.

In addition to the above-mentioned cytokines related to inflammation, vascular endothelial growth factor (VEGF) and insulin-like growth factor-1 (IGF- 1) have also been suggested to cause disruption of the blood-retinal barrier and contribute to the onset of macular edema, including CME.

Vascular endothelial growth factor is a cause of the breakdown of the blood-retinal barrier. Moreover, VEGF also acts in coordination with PGs, nitric oxide, and PAF. This indicates that VEGF is also a mediator in the inflammatory macular edema.[10]

LIGHT TOXICITY

High levels of light delivered to the eye during cataract surgery have been documented by various investigators. By extracting the lens, a natural barrier to light penetration is removed. An intact posterior capsule provides no shield to the passage of the ultraviolet light. Light, particularly the blue end of the visible spectrum and ultraviolet wavelengths, can cause permanent nonthermal damage to primate blue cones. On the basis of this circumstantial evidence, it has been suggested that light toxicity from the operating microscope could cause CME.[11]

SYSTEMIC FACTORS

Systemic diseases may be important in the development of CME. The presence of hypertension, diabetes mellitus, and ocular inflammatory diseases has been suggested to be contributory to the development of CME.[12]

Cystoid macular edema is one of the leading causes of poor postoperative visual acuity after cataract surgery in uveitis patients **(Figure 63.4).** Foster et al[13] in a retrospective study of uveitis patients undergoing extracapsular cataract extraction and posterior chamber intraocular lens implantation, reported 46% incidence of postoperative macular edema, but in all cases improved or resolved with corticosteroid therapy. It has been suggested that the risk of macular edema is greater in uveitis patients with severe postoperative uveitis and preoperative anterior uveitis.

Cataract surgery in diabetic patients may result in a dramatic acceleration of pre-existing diabetic macular edema leading to poor functional visual outcome **(Figures 63.5A to C).** This can be prevented provided the severity

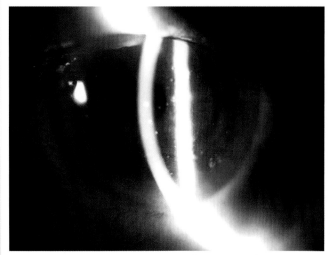

FIGURE 63.4: Anterior segment after uneventful cataract surgery showing posterior keratic precipitates in a uveitis patient

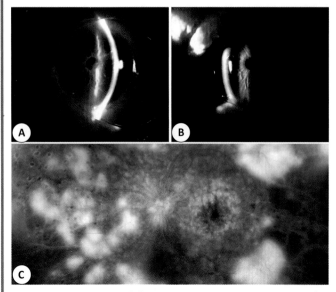

FIGURES 63.5A TO C: (A) Anterior segment after uneventful phacoemulsification cataract surgery showing anterior chamber fibrin in a patient with diabetes; (B) Anterior segment post treatment with tissue plasminogen activator (tPA) in the anterior chamber showing disappearance of the fibrin; (C) Fluorescein angiography after cataract surgery showing macular edema and proliferative diabetic retinopathy

of the retinopathy is recognized preoperatively and treated appropriately with prompt laser photocoagulation either before surgery, if there is adequate fundal view, or shortly afterward.

NATURAL HISTORY

Approximately 20% of the patients who undergo uncomplicated phacoemulsification or extracapsular extraction develop angiographically proven CME. However, a clinically significant decrease in visual acuity is seen only in about 1% of these eyes. If cataract extraction is complicated by posterior capsule rupture and vitreous loss,

severe iris trauma or vitreous traction at the wound, there is a significantly higher incidence (up to 20%) of clinically apparent CME, which is unrelated to the presence of anterior chamber-intraocular lens. Clinically significant CME usually occurs within 3–12 weeks postoperatively, but in some instances its onset may be delayed for months or many years after surgery. Spontaneous resolution of the CME with subsequent visual improvement may occur within 3–12 months in 80% of the patients. Chronic CME is defined as a persistent decline in visual acuity for more than six months. The longer the CME persists, the less likely the CME will resolve spontaneously. These chronic changes, including the presence of photoreceptor/retinal pigment epithelium changes or lamellar holes, may result in poor visual acuity even after the CME resolves.

Interestingly, complicated cataract extraction is associated with an increased risk for clinically significant CME. Cystoid macular edema is more often seen in association with some complications of cataract surgery, such as disruption of the anterior vitreous hyaloid (**Figure 63.6**), vitreous loss (**Figures 63.7A to C),** retention of lens cortex (**Figure 63.8**), vitreous strands to the wound (**Figures 63.9A and B**), dislocated intraocular lens (IOL) (**Figure 63.10**), inadequate wound closure and chronic inflammation.[14]

DIFFERENTIAL DIAGNOSIS

There are a variety of ocular and systemic diseases that can mimic pseudophakic CME, the differential diagnosis can be extensive. Branch retinal vein occlusion or diabetic macular edema can be responsible for the macular edema. Inflammatory diseases can be responsible for macular edema because of the release of inflammatory mediators. Retained lens material may act as a potential source for the release of inflammatory mediators, leading to the development of postoperative CME. Epiretinal membrane formation, vitreomacular traction syndrome are another

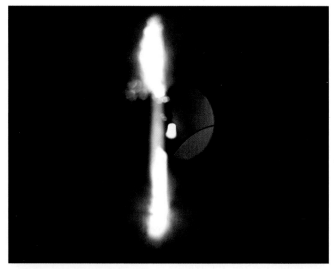

FIGURE 63.6: Anterior segment showing absent posterior capsule with anterior hyaloid rupture and luxation of the intraocular lens

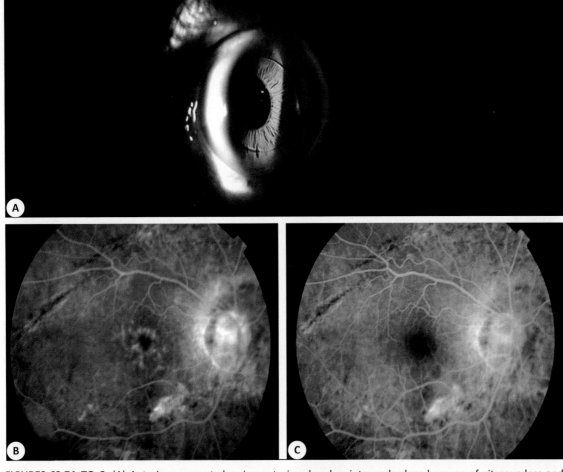

FIGURES 63.7A TO C: (A) Anterior segment showing anterior chamber intraocular lens because of vitreous loss and posterior capsule rupture; (B) Fluorescein angiograpy showing pseudophakic cystoid macular edema; (C) Fluorescein angiography showing the resolution of the cystoid macular edema after intravitreal bevacizumab

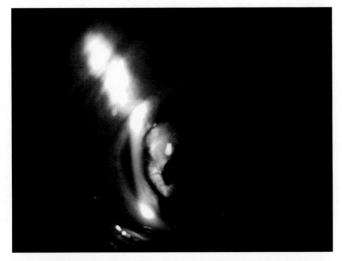

FIGURE 63.8: Anterior segment showing retention of lens cortex in the posterior chamber

important causes of mechanical thickening. Finally, the topical use of epinephrine in aphakic patients, prostaglandin analogues and the use of high doses of nicotinic acid for the treatment of hypercholesterolemia can produce cystoid macular edema.

CLINICAL PRESENTATION

Pseudophakic CME should be suspected when a patient without underlying risk factors complains of decreased vision or metamorphopsia following cataract extraction. Clinically, intraretinal edema contained in cyst-like spaces in a honeycomb pattern around the fovea can be seen. A yellow spot in the deep retina replace the normal foveal reflex. Small intraretinal hemorrhages may be present sometimes within the cystoid spaces. The cystoid spaces may coalesce into a central larger space in chronic edema and a lamellar hole can develop. Diagnosis is based on the clinical findings and characteristic appearance on fundus fluorescein angiography and OCT.

Angiographic CME is defined as cystoid macular edema that is not clinically noted by the physician or patient and is only detectable with fluorescein angiography. The angiogram is characteristic. Early phases of fluorescein angiography demonstrate dye leakage from the parafoveal retinal capillaries, and later phases of the angiogram demonstrate the petaloid pattern of leakage into the parafoveal intraretinal spaces along with optic disc hyperfluorescence **(Figure 63.11)**.

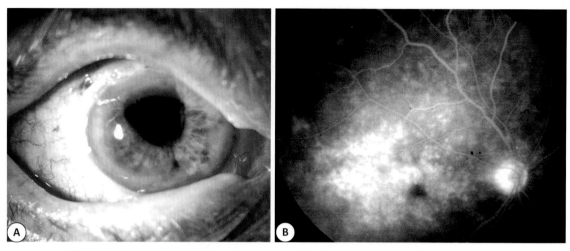

FIGURES 63.9A AND B: (A) Anterior segment showing vitreous strands to the wound; (B) Fluorescein angiography showing cystoid macular edema

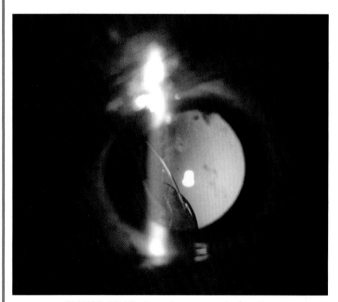

FIGURE 63.10: Anterior segment showing dislocated intraocular lens

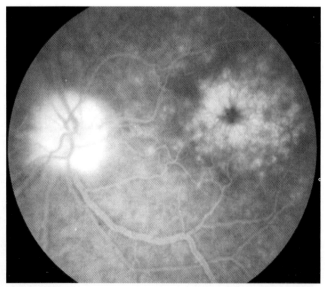

FIGURE 63.11: Fluorescein angiography showing the classic petaloid appearance in a patient with pseudophakic cystoid macular edema

OCT is a sensitive noninvasive tool that can clearly demonstrate these cystoid spaces as well as calculate central macular thickness and total macular volume. Spectral-domain OCT (SD-OCT), can be used to describe the ultrastructural changes, it can show an increased thickness of the fovea and presence of large cystoid spaces in the outer plexiform layer with stretching of the Müller cell processes. OCT can also show increased thickness of the outer nuclear layer. Photoreceptor layer [as represented by inner segment-outer segment line (IS-OS line)] can be intact and the continuity of the external limiting membrane (ELM) can be maintained **(Figure 63.12)**.

HIGH-RISK CHARACTERISTICS FOR CYSTOID MACULAR EDEMA

A variety of medical and ocular maladies may predispose patients to the development of pseudophakic cystoid macular edema. Between these conditions are epiretinal membrane, a history of vein occlusion, diabetes mellitus, hypertension, preoperative use of prostaglandin analogues, previous ocular surgery and complicated cataract extraction. Prophylactic therapy with topical nonsteroidal anti-inflammatory drugs (NSAIDs) should be utilized to reduce the risk of developing pseudophakic cystoid macular edema.[15]

PREVENTION

There have been several trials evaluating the effect of prophylactic NSAIDs and they show that the prophylactic use of NSAIDs reduces the incidence of pseudophakic cystoid macular edema. The efficacy of prophylactic nonsteroidal anti-inflammatory therapy is greatest when started at least three days preoperatively and continued postoperatively for several weeks. Yabas et al[16] reported that topical indomethacin for three days preoperatively followed

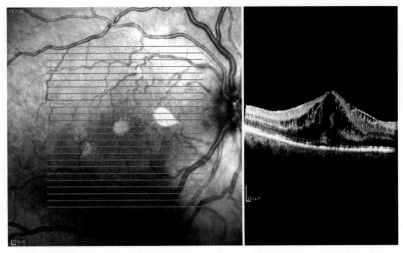

FIGURE 63.12: Spectral-domain optical coherence tomography (SD-OCT), can be used to describe the ultrastructural changes, it can show an increased thickness of the fovea and presence of large cystoid spaces in the outer plexiform layer with stretching of the Müller cell processes. In cystoid macular edema associated with cataract extraction, the cysts are most prominent in the inner nuclear layer and less prominent in the outer plexiform layer (*Courtesy:* Lihteh Wu, MD)

by combination therapy, postoperative combination therapy only, or corticosteroid only, the incidence of angiographic pseudophakic cystoid macular edema was reduced from 32.8% (corticosteroid only) to 15% (postoperative combination) to 0% (preoperative and postoperative NSAIDs).

Another study reported a reduction in pseudophakic cystoid macular edema from 12% (corticosteroid postoperatively only) to 0% with two days of preoperative diclofenac sodium (Voltaren) and combination diclofenac/corticosteroid postoperatively.[17] Recently, a randomized prospective trial comparing three days of preoperative ketorolac and combination therapy to corticosteroid alone reported that, the corticosteroid group had a 2.4% incidence of pseudophakic cystoid macular compared to 0% in the combination group.[18]

Wolf et al reported that the addition of nepafenac sodium (Nevanac) to a postoperative corticosteroid therapy reduced pseudophakic cystoid macular edema rates from 2.1% to 0%.[19] However, the exact timing and duration of preoperative and postoperative treatment, and the identification of patients who would benefit most, remain as yet undetermined.

TREATMENT OPTIONS

The primary goal of postsurgical CME treatment is to improve visual acuity by decreasing the amount of macular edema once it has formed. Effective and rational treatment rests on the understanding of the pathophysiology of the disease process itself.

NONSTEROIDAL ANTI-INFLAMMATORY AGENTS

Nonsteroidal anti-inflammatory drugs are cyclo-oxygenase inhibitors that work by preventing the synthesis of prostaglandins. As NSAIDs have no effect on preformed or existing prostaglandin levels, treatment before surgical trauma is essential. Topical ketorolac tromethamine (Acular) demonstrates a sustained beneficial effect on the visual acuity of treated patients with pseudophakic CME.

Flach et al[20] demonstrated that 8 of 13 patients treated with ketorolac had improved Snellen visual acuity of two or more lines in contrast to 1 of 13 patients treated with placebo after two months of therapy. Visual acuity deteriorated when ketorolac tromethamine therapy was stopped and the visual acuity was reversed when ketorolac tromethamine therapy was reinstated for one month.

Newer generation NSAIDs, such as bromfenac sodium (Xibrom) and nepafenac, have modifications to their chemical structure, increasing their ocular penetration and theoretical potency.[21] Waterbury et al found that the relative potency of COX-2 inhibition is 18 times greater for bromfenac than ketorolac.[22] Other study revealed that aqueous humor concentrations of nepafenac is significantly greater than that of either bromfenac or ketorolac.[23] However, it is not known whether these differences in penetration and potency translate into improved clinical outcomes.

NONSTEROIDAL ANTI-INFLAMMATORY DRUGS AND CORTICOSTEROIDS

Several studies have shown the beneficial effect of topical NSAIDs in the prophylaxis and treatment of postoperative CME. Heier et al[24] described a trial that showed that the treatment of acute, visually significant pseudophakic CME with combination corticosteroid and NSAID therapy resulted in greater gains of visual acuity, faster recovery, and greater likelihood of improvement in contrast sensitivity than monotherapy. Combination therapy of topical

CORTICOSTEROID INJECTIONS

Corticosteroids work inhibiting the release of arachidonic acid from cell membrane phospholipids, thereby preventing the formation of both leukotrienes and prostaglandins. Debate continues regarding the most efficacious route of administration (sub-Tenon's versus intravitreal), optimal dosage (4 mg versus greater), and patient safety (risks of ocular hypertension, retinal detachment, vitreous hemorrhage and endophthalmitis).

Some studies have demonstrated the usefulness of an intravitreal (IVT) injection of triamcinolone acetate in the reduction of pseudophakic cystoid macular edema (**Figures 63.13A and B**). However, no randomized clinical trials exist evaluating these modes of treatment, and published results appear contradictory. Koutsandrea et al found that intravitreal triamcinolone for persistent pseudophakic cystoid macular edema resulted in improved visual acuity, decreased macular thickness and increased multifocal electroretinogram values.[25] However, Boscia et al[26] reported that the use of 4 mg of IVTA in chronic refractory pseudophakic cystoid macular edema resulted in anatomic and functional improvement after one month. However, the beneficial effect was temporary as visual acuity and macular thickness returned to preinjection levels despite multiple treatments. Another study reported that patients maintained an improvement in acuity and decreased macular thickness following a single dose of 4 mg IVTA for refractory pseudophakic cystoid macular edema.[27]

CARBONIC ANHYDRASE INHIBITION

Acetazolamide increases subretinal fluid transport and has been shown to remove foveal cystoid edema in disorders such as retinitis pigmentosa, aphakia and macular epiretinal membrane formation. No patients with primary retinal vascular disorders such as central retinal vein occlusion or branch retinal vein occlusion, however, benefited from such treatment. There are few case reports correlating the resolution of PCME with use of oral acetazolamide, but to date, no clinical trials have been performed. Use of acetazolamide is complicated by many potential adverse effects, including bone marrow depression, paresthesias, aplastic anemia, gastrointestinal distress and psychological disturbances.

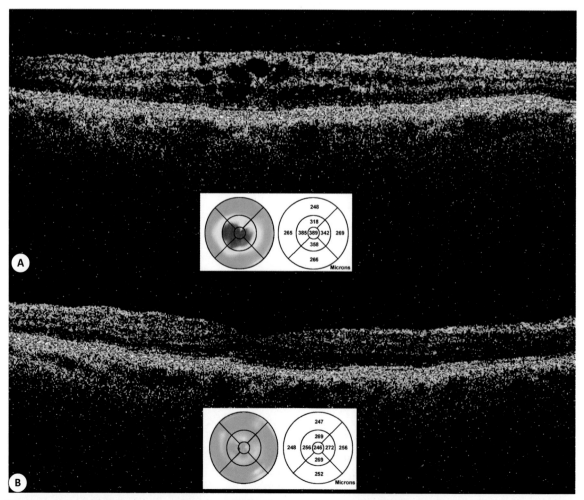

FIGURES 63.13A AND B: (A) Time domain optical coherence tomography (OCT) showing cystoid macular edema. (B) OCT after treatment with intravitreal triamcinolone acetonide with resolution of the cystoid macular edema

ANTIVASCULAR ENDOTHELIAL GROWTH FACTOR AGENTS

Surgical trauma leads to postoperative inflammation which can lead to pseudophakic cystoid macular edema through an increase in the production of vasopermeable factors such as vascular endothelial growth factor. Vascular endothelial growth factor (VEGF) has been associated with breakdown of the blood-retinal barrier, and contributes to the onset of macular edema. Vascular endothelial growth factor has been demonstrated to increase retinal vessel permeability by increasing the phosphorylation of tight junction proteins. Recent studies showed elevated levels of VEGF and interleukin-6 in ocular fluids of patients with macular edema.[28]

Bevacizumab (Avastin; Genentech, Inc., San Francisco, CA) is a complete full-length humanized antibody that binds to all subtypes of VEGF-A and is used successfully in tumor therapy as a systemic drug. Recent studies have demonstrated the usefulness of an intravitreal (IVT) injection of bevacizumab in the reduction of refractory pseudophakic cystoid macular edema. The mechanism for bevacizumab induced reduction of CME may be associated with a downregulation of many cytokines and VEGF combined with conformational changes in the tight junctions of retinal vascular endothelial cell and decrease of vascular permeability.[28]

Recently, the Pan-American Collaborative Retina Study Group (PACORES) published a retrospective study of consecutive eyes with pseudophakic CME treated with primary IVT bevacizumab as initial therapy and demonstrated both anatomic and functional significant improvement at six months. Twenty eyes (71.4%) demonstrated improvement of best-corrected visual acuity (BCVA) [Two Early Treatment Diabetic Retinopathy Study (ETDRS) lines], and no eye experienced worsening of BCVA.[29] and another study by Barone et al reported that all eyes in their series had a statistically significant improvement in vision.[30] However, Spitzer et al reported that intravitreal bevacizumab did not improve visual acuity in patients with PCME.[31]

The PACORES group reported another study of 36 eyes of 31 patients with refractory pseudophakic cystoid macular edema after cataract surgery treated with 1.25 or 2.5 mg of intravitreal bevacizumab. Patients were followed up for 12 months following which 72.2% of the eyes were observed to show anatomical and functional improvement. In addition, these results suggest a reduced risk of VA loss in eyes with CME treated with IVT bevacizumab (100% of eyes). Twenty-six (72.2 %) eyes received reinjections at a mean of 15 weeks. This strongly suggests that VEGF is a stimulus for retinal thickening, which is a conclusion supported by the added improvement in foveal thickness that is achieved with additional injections of bevacizumab. The anatomic and visual benefit of IVT bevacizumab was found to maintain itself over 12 months.[32] Statistically significant differences in duration or anatomic or functional effectiveness were not found between the 2 doses of bevacizumab evaluated. In addition, the difference between the previous primary study[29] and the current study[32] (refractory group) does not seem to be significant with regard to BCVA and OCT measurements.

In the future, this new therapeutic method may be established as alternative treatment for refractory CME after cataract surgery. Safety concerns were not detected in these studies. The results were very promising and suggest the need for further investigation.

VITRECTOMY

Pars plana vitrectomy with membrane peeling may be considered in cases of PCME with a mechanical component as identified either on clinical exam or by OCT, or in cases of chronic refractory edema unresponsive to medical therapy. In a small series, surgical intervention resulted in a greater than three line improvement in BCVA in most patients, and resolution of PCME in all cases.[33] There are also case reports in the literature indicating visual improvement following vitrectomy and peeling of the internal limiting membrane.[34] As mentioned earlier, pars plana vitrectomy should be considered in cases of retained lens fragments, IOL malposition or *Propionibacterium acnes* infection.

ND:YAG VITREOLYSIS

Pseudophakic CME with vitreous incarceration in the corneoscleral wound responds more slowly than without vitreous incarceration. There are several reports where the Nd:YAG vitreolysis is effective in the resolution of pseudophakic CME in selected patients with vitreous incarceration.[35,36] Because of the natural history of pseudophakic CME to spontaneously improve, the lack of controls with previous studies, and the confounding treatment of patients with corticosteroids, however, the precise benefit of this treatment cannot be stated with certainty until a randomized, controlled, prospective clinical study is performed.

FUTURE DIRECTIONS

As mentioned earlier, corticosteroids work at the beginning of the inflammatory cascade. Posurdex (Allergan, Irvine, CA, USA) is a biodegradable sustained dexamethasone delivery system that is implanted into the vitreous cavity. Its polymer matrix gradually transforms into lactic and glycolic acid, which are in turn broken down into water and carbon dioxide. In a phase II study, 54% of patients suffering from PCME and uveitis-associated CME showed an improvement of at least 10 letters of acuity at post-implant day 90, as compared to only 14% showing a similar result in the observation group (Allergan Phase II study data).

Recently, the FDA approved Triesence (Alcon Labs., Fort Worth, TX, USA), triamcinolone acetonide for intravitreal injection during surgery. This drug may be used off-label in the treatment algorithm of recalcitrant PCME.

SUMMARY

In summary, it is important to understand the varied pathogenesis, risk factors and proper management of PCME. It is now generally believed that inflammation is the cause of cystoid macular edema after cataract extraction. Surgical trauma to the iris/ciliary body or lens epithelial cells induces synthesis of PGs in the aqueous humor. This substance then causes a disruption of the blood-aqueous barrier, which results in the accumulation of not only PGs but also other inflammatory mediators such as endotoxin, immune complex, and cytokines in the aqueous humor. Inflammatory mediators that have accumulated in the aqueous humor diffuse to the vitreous and reach the retina, where they cause a disruption of the blood-retinal barrier. Thus, these mediators stimulate capillaries of the retina and the nerve head, and in a regular postoperative process serum leaks from the blood vessels and pools in the retinal tissue. When the serum reaches a certain level, the condition can be identified clinically as CME by fluorescein angiography.

In addition, surgical trauma leads to postoperative inflammation which can lead to PCME through an increase in the production of vasopermeable factors such as vascular endothelial growth factor. Vascular endothelial growth factor has been associated with breakdown of the blood-retinal barrier, and contributes to the onset of macular edema. Vascular endothelial growth factor has been demonstrated to increase retinal vessel permeability by increasing the phosphorylation of tight junction proteins. Recent studies showed elevated levels of VEGF and interleukin-6 in ocular fluids of patients with macular edema.

OCT is a sensitive noninvasive tool that can clearly demonstrate these cystoid spaces as well as calculate central macular thickness and total macular volume. Spectral-domain OCT, can be used to describe the ultrastructural changes, it can show an increased thickness of the fovea and presence of large cystoid spaces in the outer plexiform layer with stretching of the Müller cell processes. OCT also can show increased thickness of the outer nuclear layer.

Current management includes non-steroidal anti-inflammatory agents, NSAIDs plus corticosteroids, corticosteroid injections, carbonic anhydrase inhibition, anti-VEGF agents, vitrectomy, and Nd:YAG vitreolysis. New technology has and will revolutionize the diagnosis, prognosis and treatment of this condition.

REFERENCES

1. Irvine SR. A newly defined vitreous syndrome following cataract surgery. Am J Ophthalmol. 1953;36:599-619.
2. Gass JD, Norton EW. Follow-up study of cystoid macular edema following cataract extraction. Trans Am Acad Ophthalmol Otolaryngol. 1969;73:665-82.
3. Wright PL, Wilkinson CP, Balyeat HD, et al. Angiographic cystoid macular edema after posterior chamber lens implantation. Arch Ophthalmol. 1988;106:740-4.
4. Tso MO. Pathology of cystoid macular edema. Ophthalmology. 1982;89:902-15.
5. Antcliff RJ, Hussain AA, Marshall J. Hydraulic conductivity of fixed retinal tissue after sequential excimer laser ablation: barriers limiting fluid distribution and implications for cystoid macular edema. Arch Ophthalmol. 2001;119:539-44.
6. Flach AJ. The incidence, pathogenesis and treatment of cystoid macular edema following cataract surgery. Trans Am Ophthalmol Soc. 1998;96:557-634.
7. Stark WJ Jr, Maumenee AE, Fagadau W, et al. Cystoid macular edema in pseudophakia. Surv Ophthalmol. 1984;28(suppl): 442-51.
8. Nguyen QD, Tatlipinar S, Shah SM, et al. Vascular endothelial growth factor is a critical stimulus for diabetic macular edema. Am J Ophthalmol. 2006;142:961-9.
9. Foos RY. Posterior vitreous detachment. Trans Am Acad Ophthalmol Otolaryngol. 1972;76:480.
10. Miyake K, Ibaraki N. Prostaglandins and cystoid macular edema. Surv Ophthalmol. 2002;Suppl 1:S203-18.
11. Yannuzzi LA. A perspective on the treatment of aphakic cystoid macular edema. Surv Ophthalmol. 1984;28 Suppl:540-53.
12. Jampol LM, Sanders DR, Kraff MC. Prophylaxis and therapy of aphakic cystoid macular edema. Surv Ophthalmol. 1984;28 Suppl:535-9.
13. Foster RE, Lowder CY, Meisler DM, et al. Extracapsular cataract extraction and posterior chamber intraocular lens implantation in uveitis patients. Ophthalmology. 1992;99:1234-41.
14. Spaide RF, Yannuzzi LA, Sisco LJ. Chronic cystoid macular edema and predictors of visual acuity. Ophthalmic Surg. 1993;24:262.
15. Henderson BA, Kim JY, Ament CS, et al. Clinical pseudophakic cystoid macular edema. Risk factors for development and duration after treatment. J Cataract Refract Surg. 2007; 33:1550-8.
16. Yavas GF, Oztürk F, Küsbeci T. Preoperative topical indomethacin to prevent pseudophakic cystoid macular edema. J Cataract Refract Surg. 2007;33:804-7.
17. McColgin AZ, Raizman MB. Efficacy of topical Voltaren in reducing the incidence of postoperative cystoid macular edema. Invest Ophthmol Vis Sci. 1999;40:S289.
18. Wittpenn JR, Silverstein S, Heier J, et al. A randomized, masked comparison of topical ketorolac 0.4 percent plus steroid vs steroid alone in low-risk cataract surgery patients. Am J Ophthalmol. 2008;146:554-60.
19. Wolf EJ, Braunstein A, Shih C, et al. Incidence of visually significant pseudophakic macular edema after uneventful phacoemulsification in patients treated with nepafenac. J Cataract Refract Surg. 2007;33:1546-9.
20. Flach AJ, Stegman RC, Graham J, et al. Prophylaxis of aphakic cystoid macular edema without corticosteroids. A paired-comparison, placebo-controlled double-masked study. Ophthalmology. 1990;97:1253-8.
21. Walsh DA, Moran HW, Shamblee DA, et al. Antiinflammatory agents 3. Synthesis and pharmacological evaluation of 2-amino-3-benzoylphenylacetic acid and analogues. J Medicinal Chem. 1984;27:1379-88.
22. Waterbury LD, Silliman D, Jolas T. Comparison of cyclo-oxygenase inhibitory activity and ocular anti-inflammatory effects of ketorolac tromethamine and bromfenac sodium. Curr Med Res Opin. 2006;22:1133-40.

23. Walters TR, Raizman M, Ernest P, et al. In vivo pharmacokinetics and in vitro pharmacodynamics of nepafenac, amfenac, ketorolac, and bromfenac. J Cataract Refract Surg. 2007; 33; 1539-45.

24. Heier JS, Topping TM, Baumann W, et al. Ketorolac versus prednisolone versus combination therapy in the treatment of acute pseudophakic cystoid macular edema. Ophthalmology. 2000;107:2034-8.

25. Koutsandrea C, Moschos MM, Brouzas D, et al. Intraocular triamcinolone acetonide for pseudophakic cystoid macular edema: Optical coherence tomography and multifocal electroretinography study. Retina. 2007;27:159-64.

26. Boscia F, Furino C, Dammacco R, et al. Intravitreal triamcinolone acetonide in refractory pseudophakic cystoid macular edema: Functional and anatomic results. Eur J Ophthalmol. 2005;15:89-95.

27. Karacorlu M, Ozdemir H, Karacorlu S. Intravitreal triamcinolone acetonide for the treatment of chronic pseudophakic cystoid macular oedema. Acta Ophthalmol Scand. 2003;81: 648-52.

28. Noma H, Minamoto A, Funatsu H, et al. Intravitreal levels of vascular endothelial growth factor and interleukin-6 are correlated with macular edema in branch retinal vein occlusion. Graefes Arch Clin Exp Ophthalmol. 2006;244:309-15.

29. Arevalo JF, Garcia-Amaris RA, Roca JA, et al. Primary intravitreal bevacizumab for the management of pseudophakic cystoid macular edema: Pilot study of the Pan-American Collaborative Retina Study Group. J Cataract Refract Surg. 2007;33:2098-2105.

30. Barone A, Russo V, Prascina F, et al. Short-term safety and efficacy of Intravitreal Bevacizumab for Pseudophakic Cystoid Macular Edema. Retina. 2009;29:33-7.

31. Spitzer MS, Ziemssen F, Yoeruek E, et al. Efficacy of intravitreal bevacizumab in treating postoperative pseudophakic cystoid macular edema. J Cataract Refract Surg. 2008;34: 70-5.

32. Arevalo JF, Maia M, Garcia-Amaris RA, et al. Pan-American Collaborative Retina Study Group. Intravitreal bevacizumab for refractory pseudophakic cystoid macular edema: the Pan-American Collaborative Retina Study Group results. Ophthalmology. 2009;116:1481-7.

33. Pendergast SD, Margherio RR, Williams GA, et al. Vitrectomy for chronic pseudophakic cystoid macular edema. Am J Ophthalmol. 1999;128:317-23.

34. Peyman GA, Canakis C, Livir-Rallatos C, et al. The effect of internal limiting membrane peeling on chronic recalcitrant pseudophakic cystoid macular edema: A report of two cases. Am J Ophthalmol. 2002;133:571-2.

35. Steinert RF, Puliafito CA. The Nd:YAG laser in ophthalmology: principles and clinical applications of photodisruption. Philadelphia: WB Saunders; 1985; 115-23.

36. Steinert RF, Wasson PJ. Neodmium:YAG laser anterior vitreolysis for Irvine-Gass cystoid macular edema. J Cataract Refract Surg. 1989;15:304-6.

CHAPTER 64

Postoperative Endophthalmitis

Clement K Chan

INCIDENCE AND PRESENTATION

The literature reported the incidence of endophthalmitis to range from approximately 0.1 to 0.5%.[1-7] It is estimated that about 1000 cases of endophthalmitis developed after eye surgery in the United States each year.[4,8-12] Although most cases of postoperative endophthalmitis are associated with cataract surgery, any eye surgery has the potential for inducing endophthalmitis (e.g. strabismus surgery, transscleral fixation of an implant, penetrating keratoplasty and refractive surgery, etc.).[6,8,10] The most common presentation of acute postoperative endophthalmitis includes severe vision loss associated with marked ocular pain and headaches within 2 to 5 days after surgery. However, the Endophthalmitis vitrectomy study (EVS) showed that 25% of the cases that developed endophthalmitis in that study lacked pain.[9] The typical ocular findings include a red and painful eye, usually involving lid and corneal edema, chemosis and conjunctival injection and discharge, as well as intraocular infiltrates, i.e. hypopyon and vitreous infiltrates **(Figures 64.1A and B)**.[8] However, the EVS showed that 14% of the cases in that study lacked a hypopyon. In addition, the characteristic clinical signs may be absent or masked due to the application of postoperative antibiotic and corticosteroid drops or an organism with low virulence.[3,9,13,14] Untreated endophthalmitis or poor responses to its treatment usually leads to severe ocular tissue damages involving the optic nerve and the retina. It may also predispose the affected eye to subsequent retinal breaks and detachment.[8,15] The end result can be severe vision loss.

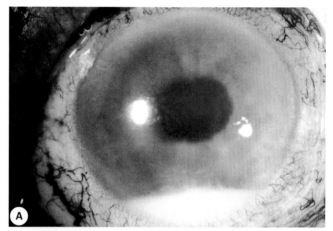

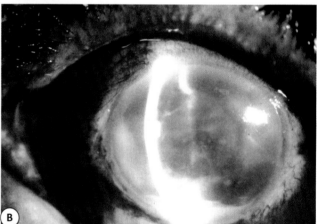

FIGURES 64.1A AND B: Typical examples of acute postoperative endophthalmitis associated with cataract surgery shows the following clinical findings: (A and B) Conjunctival injection, hypopyon and vitreous infiltrates (*Courtesy*: Flynn Jr HW, MD)

CAUSATIVE ORGANISMS

ACUTE-ONSET CASES

Gram-positive and coagulase-negative *Staphylococcus* is the most frequent microbial isolate associated with acute postoperative endophthalmitis.[3,13,14,16-18] In fact, EVS showed that 70% of the culture-positive endophthalmitis was due to coagulase-negative *staphylococcus*.[10,19,20] Other gram-positive organisms reported by EVS included *Staphylococcus aureus* (9.9%), *Streptococcus* species (9.0%), *Enterococcus* species (2.2%), *miscellaneous gram-positive* species (3.1%), *Propionibacterium* species (0.6%), *Corynebacterium* species (1.2%), *Bacillus* species (0.6%) and *Diphtheroid* (0.6%).[2,9,17] In addition, EVS,[9,17] reported only 5.9% of the cases to be related to gram-

negative organisms: *Proteus mirabilis* (1.9%), *Pseudomonas* species (1.2%), *Morganella morganii* (0.6%), *Citrobacter diversus* (0.6%), *Serratia marcescens* (0.3%), *Enterobacter* species (0.6%) and F*lavobacterium* species (0.3%). The underestimation of gram-negative infection by the EVS cannot be ruled out, since eyes with severe corneal opacities precluding a vitrectomy were excluded from that study.[2,9,17] Other unusual gram-positive bacilli such as *Listeria monocytogenes*,[21,22] and gram-negative bacilli such as *Haemophilis influenzae*,[23] *Actinobacillus* species,[24] *Escherichia coli*,[25] *Pseudomonas* species,[26,27] *Serratia marcescens*[28] and *Mycobacterium tuberculosis*[29,30] are found with increasing frequency in endogenous cases, but rarely encountered in postoperative cases.

TABLE 64.1	Microbial spectra of endophthalmitis (in percentages)	
Organism	**Acute Postoperative*** (N=323)	**Bleb-related§** (N=30)
Coagulase-negative	70%	
Staphylococcus	9.9%	6.7%
Streptococcus	9.0%	56.7%
Bacillus species	0.6%	0%
Pseudomonas	1.5%	6.7%
Hemophilus	0%	23.3%
Other Gram-	4.3%	3.3%
Fungi	0%	3.3%
Others	5.3%	0%
mixed flora	‡ 9.3%	0%

* Data from EVS.[58]

§ Data from Mandelbaum et al[87]

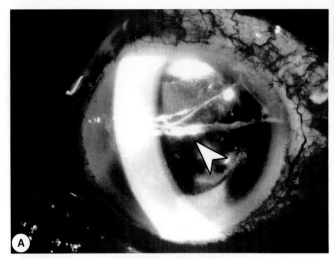

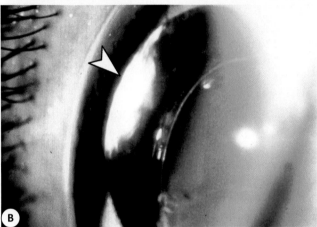

FIGURES 64.2A AND B: The distinctive features of delayed-onset postoperative Propionibacterium acne consist of low-grade iridocyclitis and vitreous infiltrates, as well as (A) Beaded fibrin strands in the anterior chamber (arrow head), and (B) Prominent whitish plaque on residual capsular remnants, (arrow head) (*Courtesy:* Flynn HW Jr, MD, Miami, Florida)

Table 64.1 presents the typical spectrum of causative organisms associated with acute postsurgical endophthalmitis.[17,31]

DELAYED-ONSET CASES

Certain cases of postoperative endophthalmitis may have a delayed onset. The most common bacterium responsible for delayed-onset and low-grade infection is P*ropionibacterium acnes (P. acnes).*[32-38] *Staphylococcus epidermidis* and *Achromobacter* species may also induce late-onset endophthalmitis on an occasional basis.[33,39] Meisler et al first identified *Propionibacterium acnes* to be the causative agent of delayed-onset endophthalmitis in 1986, usually from 2 to 6 months after surgery.[36] This opportunistic gram-positive, pleomorpic anaerobic bacillus is ubiquitous in nature, and a frequent component of the ocular and periocular bacterial flora.[35,40] Its typical clinical presentation includes large white granulomatous or nongranulomatous keratic precipitates, beaded fibrin strands **(Figure 64.2A)**, hypopyon, vitritis, intraretinal hemorrhage and infiltrates and a whitish lenticular capsular plaque **(Figure 64.2B)**.[32-38] The last feature is considered a hallmark sign for *P. acnes* endophthalmitis.[35,40] The sequestered *P. acnes* organisms can be identified from biopsied capsular remnants with the typical whitish plaque.[34-38] *P. acnes* responsible for chronic infection may be quite resistant to treatment, frequently requiring extensive topical and intraocular antibiotic treatment, repeated vitrectomy, and even explantation of the intraocular implant and capsular remnants for its eradication.[32,33,35,36,40,41] It has been reported that *P. acnes* isolated from cases of acute-onset endophthalmitis may behave differently than *P. acnes* associated with the delayed-onset cases, since it can be easily eradicated with treatment in the former situation in contrast to the latter situation.[40] It is possible that the sequestration of *P. acnes* in the operated eye on a chronic basis allows it to develop increased resistance to eradication or that *P. acnes* in the chronic cases constitutes a different strain of *P. acnes*.

Fungal endophthalmitis is another example of delayed-onset infection after surgery.[3,42] Fox et al reported 16% of delayed-onset cases to be due to *Candida parapsilosis*.[3,33] Other causative fungal organisms include *Curvularia* species, *Penicillium* species and *Volutella* specie*s*, etc.[3,43,44] In 1980, Pettit et al reported 13 cases involving intraocular lenses contaminated with *Acremonium* species, *Aspergillus* species, *Blastomycetes* and *Paecilomyces lilacinus*.[3,45,46] Mild ocular discomfort accompanied by a low-grade iridocyclitis, and a smoldering course of anterior chamber and vitreous inflammation starting two weeks or later after surgery, most pronounced at the iris-pupillary margin, are typical clinical features of fungal endophthalmitis **(Figure 64.3)**.[3,44] Eventually, clumps of exudates may appear in the anterior chamber, vitreous cavity, and on the retinal surface (fluff balls). Advanced cases may show marked corneal edema, chemosis and conjunctival injection, as well as hypopyon. Besides *Propionibacterium acnes* and fungal organisms, other organisms reported to be associated with a delayed-onset infection include the *Corynebacterium* species, *Achromobacter* species, *Actinomyces* species and *Norcardia asteroids*.[3,33,39,47-50]

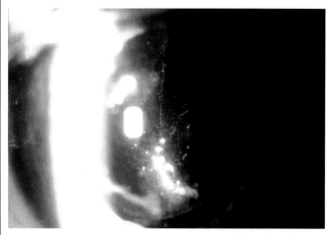

FIGURE 64.3: Low-grade iridocyclitis and mild vitreous infiltrates with a delayed onset are characteristics of postoperative fungal endophthalmitis found in this patient with postoperative fungal endophthalmitis (*Candida parapsilosis*) (*Courtesy:* Flynn HW Jr, MD, Miami, Florida)

BLEB-ASSOCIATED CASES

Bleb-associated ocular infection constitutes another distinct category of postoperative ocular infection. The first type involves a less serious and localized form of bleb-related infection and has been given a term of blebitis,[51,52] including the conjunctival bleb and the surrounding structures but without vitreous involvement. The second category of bleb-related endophthalmitis is one of the most fulminant forms of ocular infection.[31,51,53-55] Photopsia, conjunctival injection and discharge associated with an opaque filtering bleb, variable aqueous reactions including Seidel-positive results on the filtering bleb, are typical findings of blebitis.[51,52] In general, blebitis has a favorable prognosis following intense topical broad-spectrum antibiotic and anti-inflammatory treatment with or without intraocular treatment. In contrast, bleb-related endophthalmitis is usually associated with a poor prognosis.[3,19,31,52] The latter condition usually presents with acute ocular pain and redness associated with an infected bleb leading to rapid and severe vision loss, months to years after the original filtering surgery **(Figures 64.4A and B)**. The surface of the infected bleb may appear to be falsely intact in spite of a positive Seidel test.[31,52] A rapid progression of anterior chamber and vitreous infiltrates is typical. The increased usage of anti-metabolites (i.e. Mitomycin-C and 5-fluoro-uracil) tends to create thin conjunctival blebs vulnerable for postoperative bleb-related infection.[53-55] However, Mandelbaum reported bleb-related endophthalmitis for thick-walled blebs as well.[31] Multiple reports also showed a much higher risk of bleb-related endophthalmitis for inferiorly than superiorly-located blebs (9.4% versus 3%).[53-55] Male gender and age below 60 are other risk factors for bleb-related endophthalmitis for unknown reasons.

Perhaps the increased exposure of inferiorly located blebs and greater physical activities of males and younger patients

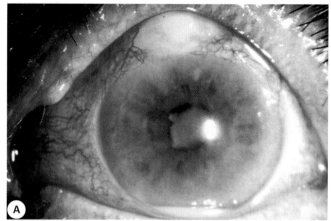

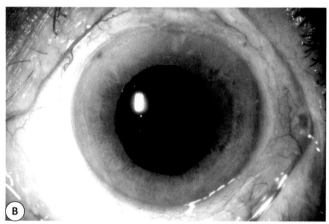

FIGURES 64.4A AND B: (A) Bleb-related endophthalmitis was diagnosed for this eye with a sudden onset of ocular pain associated with a purulent conjunctival bleb, marked conjunctival injection, a miotic pupil and marked vitreous infiltrates, and severe vision loss (hand motions) months after the initial glaucoma-filtering surgery. (B) Performance of a pars plana vitrectomy and intravitreal antibiotic injections after the mechanical dilation of the pupils with iris hooks resulted in the visual recovery of 20/40 (*Courtesy:* Flynn HW Jr, MD, Miami, Florida)

leading to repeated disturbance of the blebs may account for the increased risk. Thus, the ophthalmic surgeon should pay close attention to the correction of any lid and lacrimal drainage abnormalities, blepharitis, distichiasis, and deficiency of tear function, prior to a glaucoma drainage procedure. Most cases of bleb-related endophthalmitis tend to be late-onset.[54] However, some cases may have an acute onset (within 6 weeks after surgery). Apparently, the causative organisms associated with the late-onset cases are vastly different than those responsible for the acute-onset cases.[14,18,52] For late-onset endophthalmitis, streptococcal species (*S. pneumoniae*, *S. faecalis*, *S. Viridans*, and beta hemolytic *streptococcus*) and gram-negative organisms are the most common microbial isolates.[14,18,52] In Mandelbaum's study, *Streptococcus* species were isolated in 57% of cases, *Hemophilus influenzae* in *23% of cases*, *Staphylococcus aureus* in two cases, *Pseudomonas aeruginosa* in two cases, *Morazella nonliquefaciens* in one case and *Fusarium* species in one case.[31] In contrast, coagulase-negative *Staphylococcus* is the most common organism associated with the acute type of bleb-related endophthalmitis, similar to the situation for acute endophthalmitis after cataract surgery.[31,52] Such a difference in the causative organisms can be explained by the predominance of coagulase-negative *Staphylococcus* in the natural ocular flora of the acute cases, and the more time-consuming penetration through the conjunctival barrier by the more virulent streptococcal and gram-negative organisms in the late cases. The potent toxins released by the virulent streptococcal and gram-negative species are responsible for generally poor vision outcome for cases of bleb-related endophthalmitis despite its prompt treatment.[52,56]

STERILE ENDOPHTHALMITIS

Severe noninfectious intraocular inflammation may develop after surgery for certain eyes. Most such cases are free of ocular pain, which is an important sign for most cases of infectious endophthalmitis. As mentioned above, however, the EVS showed that 25% of the cases with infectious endophthalmitis may manifest no pain.[4,17] The sterile inflammation usually starts in the first 24 to 36 hours following surgery, somewhat earlier than most of the infectious cases.[57] The clinical findings are also milder than the infectious cases. Conjunctival injection and chemosis may be mild or absent. Anterior chamber reaction may vary from mild to severe. Thus, there may be variable flare and cells, fibrin deposits and hypopyon. The mild to moderate vitreous infiltrates associated with a sterile case may still allow a residual red reflex from the fundus, in contrast to a severe case of infectious endophthalmitis.[57] Typically, the noninfectious inflammation responds rapidly to steroidal and nonsteroidal medical treatment, without any need for antimicrobial therapy. A high index of suspicion for a missed infection or alternative etiology is needed, in case of a lack of favorable response to anti-inflammatory therapy after 36 to 48 hours. Persistent sterile inflammation may lead to substantial cystoid macular edema and central visual deficit.

Factors reported to increase the risk for sterile endophthalmitis may include prior history of uveitis, difficult surgical course, pseudoexfoliation syndrome, brown irides, inadequate mydriasis at the start of the surgery, intraoperative excessive pigment release and difficulties with intraocular lens implantation during surgery.[57-59] Irvine et al also reported multiple eyes that developed hypopyon associated with retained lens fragments after extracapsular cataract surgery or phacoemulsification.[60] Others also reported mechanical irritation of the iris due to intraocular lenses, residual monomers on the PMMA lenses, and inadvertent intraocular entry of topical anesthetic agents or nylon suture material inducing excessive postoperative inflammation.[57,61] Until proven otherwise, any case of excessive inflammation after surgery must be treated as an infectious case, considering the devastating consequences of infectious endophthalmitis if not managed properly and promptly.[57]

CLINICAL EVALUATION AND DIAGNOSTIC STUDIES

A careful eye examination is required prior to the treatment of the endophthalmitis. The clinician must search for factors predisposing to the endophthalmitis that may be rectified, i.e. iris or vitreous prolapse, wound leak or dehiscence, flat anterior chamber, corneal or suture abscess, bleb defects and eroding scleral suture associated with a sutured posterior chamber implant, etc.[8,10] In addition, the clinician must differentiate other conditions that mimic infectious endophthalmitis, i.e. sterile endophthalmitis, corneal ulcer associated with excessive intraocular inflammation and phacotoxic or phacoanaphylactic reactions, etc. At the same time, he or she must search for concurrent complications that may respond to surgical corrections, including vitreous hemorrhage, retinal breaks or detachment, choroidal detachment, retained lens fragments and intraocular foreign bodies, etc. Besides slit-lamp biomicroscopy and indirect ophthalmoscopy, B-scan ultrasonography can be a useful diagnostic tool for the evaluation of such cases.

Although empirical antibiotic therapy utilizing a series of topical and intravitreal antimicrobial agents with a broad spectrum of coverage in a "shot-gun" approach is the currently recommended method for treating infectious endophthalmitis, a careful microbiological work-up is indicated during the course of management of the endophthalmitis for sound reasons.[3,4,17] The EVS reported that 99.4% of infectious cases were appropriately treated with the initial empirical antimicrobial therapy. Only 7.4% of cases with a baseline visual acuity of hand motions or better, and 19.1% of cases with a baseline visual acuity of light perception required additional therapy after the initial empirical therapy in the EVS.[2,9,51] Nevertheless, a thorough work-up provides the following advantages for the treating clinician:[8] 1) Differentiation of infectious versus sterile endophthalmitis, 2) Specific tailoring of the antimicrobial treatment according to the identity and susceptibility of the organism for optimal outcome as a part of the currently accepted practice pattern and medicolegal requirements, and 3) Creation of sufficient space for delivery of intraocular antimicrobial agents after the vitreous tap. A delay in the specimen collection (particularly after the onset of antimicrobial therapy) may lower the yield of culture-positive results. Previously, Maylath and Leopold showed a higher yield of positive culture results with a vitreous than an aqueous tap.[62] Subsequent clinical studies confirmed their observation of the greater importance of vitreous over aqueous cultures.[3,4,9,19,20, 63] Forster et al reported 35% of those with positive culture results showed positive growth from the vitreous but not the aqueous specimens.[3,19] The EVS reported 54.9% confirmed growth from undiluted vitreous specimens alone, and 22.5% confirmed growth from aqueous specimens alone.[4,63] Only 13% of the EVS eyes required both vitreous and aqueous specimens for confirmed growth.[4,63] EVS showed the rare occurrence of a positive aqueous culture in the presence of a negative vitreous culture in only 4.2% of cases. Thus, the EVS showed positive culture results from a specimen of any one source alone: aqueous, undiluted vitreous or cassette fluid. It also showed a high positive predictive value associated with a positive gram stain (95–97% positive culture results), but a low negative predictive value associated with a negative gram stain (23–67% negative culture results).[4,63]

The standard methods of collecting the aqueous and vitreous specimens may involve a needle tap, a mechanical vitrectomy, or both. The needle tap method consists of the use of a 30, 27 or 25-gauge needle for the collection of 0.1 to 0.25 ml of aqueous specimen, and a 27, 25 or larger-gauge needle for the collection of 0.1 to 0.3 ml of more viscous vitreous specimen. A vitrectomy employs a 20, 23 or 25-gauge probe with cutting and aspiration functions for collecting up to 0.5 ml of undiluted vitreous specimen through a one, two or three-port approach (**Figure 64.5A**). Donahue et al reported greater culture yield by concentrating the specimen obtained from a vitrectomy cassette alone in comparison to a needle or limited vitreous biopsy alone (74% versus 43%).[64] For concentration of diluted specimens, either the suction-filtered method or the centrifuged method may yield the optimal outcome (**Figures 64.5B and C**).[3,4,8,16] The former involves passing a diluted specimen in an upper sterile chamber through a membrane filter with 0.45-micron pores into a lower chamber connected to suction. Using sterile forceps and scissors or knives, the membrane filter containing the concentrated specimen is then cut into small pieces for direct inoculation on solid or liquid media for culturing (**Figure 64.5B**).[3,4,8,16] Smears may also be prepared from the concentrated specimen. The centrifuged method involves the transfer of the diluted specimen into a sterile centrifuge tube for high-speed centrifuging.

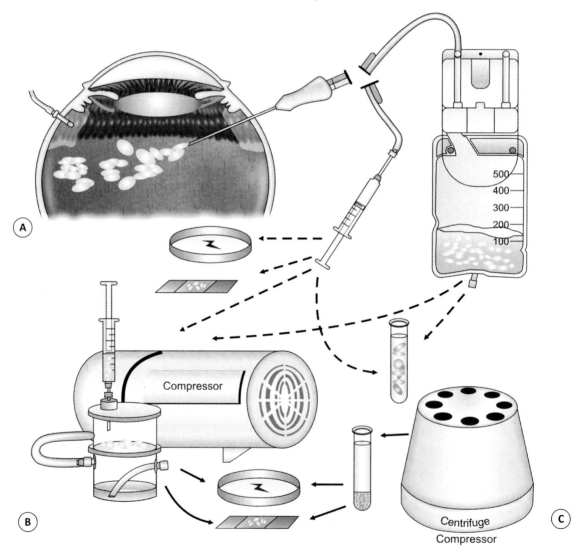

FIGURES 64.5A TO C: (A) The smear preparation and inoculation of culture media can be achieved without further processing for undiluted aqueous and vitreous specimens. A diluted specimen collected in a syringe or vitrectomy cassette needs concentration first via either; (B) The vacuum method by passing the diluted fluid in a sterile upper chamber through a 0.45-micron membrane filter into a lower sterile chamber; or (C) The centrifuge method by high-speed centrifuge in a sterile tube. The cut pieces of the membrane filter containing the concentrated EVS specimen or the sediments from the centrifuged tube are then applied on smears for staining and inoculated in culture media for culturing

The sediments obtained from the centrifuged tube are then processed for microbiological stains and cultures **(Figure 64.5C)**.[8]

The most recent advances in diagnostic tools for microbiological work-up for endophthalmitis involve immunologic and molecular genetic technologies that may enhance the speed and specificity of identifying the organisms.[57,65] For instance, Hykin et al employed DNA polymerase chain reaction to amplify small amounts of DNA for the diagnosis of delayed postoperative endophthalmitis related to *P. Acnes*.[65]

Undiluted specimens and concentrates of diluted specimens must be promptly inoculated onto fresh enriched media, such as blood agar and chocolate agar for aerobic organisms, as well as liquid thioglycollate or other media for anaerobic organisms (e.g. chopped meat or egg meat medium and brain heart infusion, etc.).[3,8,57] Immediate incubation of the above-inoculated media at 35°C (body temperature) allows bacterial isolation. In addition, blood and chocolate agar should be incubated in a 3 to 5% carbon dioxide atmosphere, while the anaerobic cultures should be kept in an anaerobic environment. Specimens with suspected fungal organisms are inoculated onto Sabouraud agar, brain heart infusion agar or blood agar. The inoculated medium is then maintained at a temperature of 25° to 30° C (room temperature) for fungal isolation. A few drops of the specimen are applied on slides for Gram or Giemsa staining, and an immediate search for bacterial and certain fungal organisms is then carried out. A wet mount or KOH smear, and a Grocott's methenamine silver stain is sometimes prepared for identification of fungal organisms.[3,8,9,17,19,66]

Recently, a new culture method involving the direct inoculation of blood culture bottles at the time of the vitreous biopsy was reported to be a reliable means of increasing culture-positive rates.[67] Although most aerobic organisms will grow within 24 to 48 hours, all aerobic cultures should be held for seven or more days to allow the isolation of certain slow-growing organisms. Anaerobic cultures are typical slow-growers and should be kept for a minimum of 14 days. Fungal and Actinomyces cultures should be maintained for 4 to 6 weeks, while mycobacterial cultures should be incubated at 35° C in a 5 to 10% carbon dioxide atmosphere for six weeks. A laboratory "confirmed" positive culture is defined as growth of the same microbe on two or more media, semiconfluent growth on one or more solid media, or growth on one medium supported by a positive Gram stain. Growth in only one liquid medium or scant growth in one solid medium is considered as "equivocal".[3,9,17,66]

PROPHYLACTIC THERAPY

Paying close attention to sterile techniques during surgery and prophylactic antimicrobial treatment constitutes the key measures for preventing postoperative endophthalmitis. The goal is to lower the concentration of bacterial flora within the operative field. Appropriate sterile prepping and draping, and the retraction of the eyelids and lashes with a sterile lid speculum are crucial steps in achieving this goal.[57] The application of topical povidone-iodine solution before or during surgery has been shown to be the most effective means of preventing postoperative endophthalmitis.[68-70] The commercially available 5% povidone-iodine solution (Alcon Laboratories Inc., Forth Worth, Texas) specifically manufactured for ophthalmic application is the most commonly used povidone-iodone solution for eye surgery. Tornambe and Hilton advocated the off-labeled use of the higher-strength 10% povidone-iodine solution instead, based on anecdotal evidence of enhanced efficacy in preventing an infection, in comparison to the 5% solution (Personal communication, Tornambe et al). However, the more potent 10% solution has greater potential for inducing ocular toxic reactions, such as punctuate keratopathy and corneal abrasion. A previous prospective study has shown the administration of 5% povidone-iodine solution to reduce the conjunctival bacterial load and lower the incidence of culture-positive endophthalmitis.[70] In addition, the same group of investigators also found that the administration of preoperative topical antibiotic beginning at three days before surgery besides applying povidone-iodine at the start of surgery further reduced the bacterial flora on the conjunctiva.[68,71] Currently, antibiotics with a broad-spectrum coverage (i.e. 3rd or 4th-generation quinolones) are most commonly used before and after surgery. Multiple retrospective studies and surveys have also substantiated the efficacy of povidone-iodine in decreasing the risk of postoperative infection and culture-positive endophthalmitis.[57,69,72] However, multiple uncontrolled variables might have confounded the results of these retrospective studies and surveys, lowering the reliability of their conclusions.

The value of topical, subconjunctival and intracameral antibiotic therapy, as well as the intraoperative use of antibiotics in the irrigating fluid as prophylaxis against postoperative endophthalmitis has not been proven with controlled prospective studies, and lacks consensus.[57,72,73] Critics against prophylactic antibiotic therapy point out that the inconsistent concentration of the antibiotics in irrigating solutions, and the transient contact of the antibiotics in the irrigating solutions to the bacteria, may lower their effectiveness in prophylaxis.[57] The prior controversial practice of utilizing aminoglycosides (i.e. gentamicin or tobramycin) in the irrigating solutions has largely been abandoned due to the lack of efficacy of such antibiotics against most cases of postoperative endophthalmitis related to gram-positive organisms. Frequent usage of various forms of prophylactic antibiotics may also increase the risk of antibiotic resistance.[57,74] Recently, Mamalis et al pointed out the theoretical advantage of direct intracameral injection of an antibiotic into the capsular bag at the conclusion of surgery in preventing postoperative infections.[57] They suggested that such a targeted approach may provide greater precision and duration of the antibiotic for prophylaxis against an infection, and lower the risk of ocular toxicity related to the antibiotic.

Similar to the high supportive evidence of prophylactic povidone-iodine before surgery, Apt et al have shown the superior efficacy of topical 5% povidone-iodine solution, in comparison to broad-spectrum topical antibiotics at the conclusion of surgery in reducing the number of colony-forming bacterial flora, for the first 24 hours after surgery in a well-conducted prospective study.[75] Despite such a report, the most common practice against infection after ophthalmic surgery remains to be the application of a broad-spectrum antibiotic (e.g. 3rd or 4th generation fluoroquinolone) with efficacy against most gram-positive and gram-negative organisms instead of a povidone-iodine solution.[7] To reduce the development of antibiotic resistance, the application of postoperative antibiotics should be limited to 7 to 10 days, and the cessation of therapy should be abrupt instead of a tapered fashion.[57,76]

TREATMENT OF ENDOPHTHALMITIS

Although previous studies have shown the lack of efficacy of topical and subconjunctival antimicrobials, once a sufficient quantity of organisms is inoculated into the eye, consistent application of postoperative antimicrobials remains to be an essential part of effective treatment for postoperative endophthalmitis, particularly in the case of a corneal ulcer, suture or wound abscess and bleb infection associated with the endophthalmitis.[1,3,4,8] Otherwise, topical and subconjunctival therapy constitutes only adjunctive treatment for postoperative endophthalmitis. The standard regimen of topical antibiotic therapy includes the frequent application of broad-spectrum antibiotics effective against both gram-positive and gram-negative organisms, and the repeated administration of anti-inflammatory corticosteroid and cycloplegic medications. Corticosteroid drops are usually avoided for fungal endophthalmitis. The use of customized topical fortified antimicrobial therapy for treating postoperative endophthalmitis is a common but controversial practice (e.g. 45 to 50 mg per ml of vancomycin, 50 mg per ml of cefazolin, cefamandole or ceftazidime, 50 mg per ml of ampicillin, 50 mg per ml of clindamycin, 1% solution of methicillin, 8 to 15 mg per ml of tobramycin, 10 to 20 mg per ml of gentamicin or amikacin, 0.15 to 0.5% of amphotericin B or 10 mg per ml of miconazole, etc.)[4,8,9] Their superiority over the regular doses of commercially-available antimicrobials remains to be unproven. Another frequent but controversial practice is the administration of supplemental subconjunctival antimicrobial injections (e.g. 25 mg of vancomycin, 100 to 125 mg of cefazolin or ceftazidime, 75 mg of cefamandole, 100 mg of ampicillin or methicillin, 20–40 mg of gentamicin, tobramycin or amikacin, 30 mg of clindamycin, or 5 mg of miconazole).[3,4,9] The synergistic effects of subconjunctival and topical antimicrobial therapy with intravitreal anti-microbial therapy are unproven.

INTRAVITREAL ANTIMICROBIALS

Intravitreal antimicrobial therapy constitutes the mainstay of treatment for postoperative endophthalmitis. The prompt administration of properly prepared intravitreal antibiotics with effective coverage against a broad-spectrum of gram-positive and gram-negative organisms on an empirical basis is crucial for the success for treating these cases.[3,4,94] This "shot-gun" approach is required due to the potentially rapid and devastating ocular damages by the infectious agents, preventing the luxury of waiting until the availability of the culture and antimicrobial susceptibility results before instituting therapy. The ideal condition for preparing intravitreal antimicrobials involves specially trained personnel working under a hood that provides a laminar airflow for enhancing an aseptic environment.[8] Appropriately prepared and administered intravitreal antimicrobials with the proper dosages have been shown to be highly safe and effective.[3,9,12,18,19,77-80] Currently, vancomycin has superseded first-generation cephalosporins and gentamicin as the primary drug of choice for intravitreal therapy due to the susceptibility of most gram-positive organisms to vancomycin and their increasing resistance to the other antibiotics, including coagulase-negative and positive *Staphylococcus* and *Streptococcus* species, etc.[3,4,8,17,81,82] In the EVS, 100% of the gram-positive organisms were susceptible to vancomycin treatment.[3,8,17] Another advantage of vancomycin is its relatively low retinal toxicity over a wide range.[82] For appropriate coverage of gram-negative organisms, aminoglycosides have been shown to be the drugs of choice for intravitreal administration.[17] Recently, amikacin has superseded gentamicin and tobramycin as the preferred aminoglycoside for gram-negative coverage, due to its lower toxic potential in comparison to other aminoglycosides, as shown by D'Amico et al, and others.[8,83-86,19,21,26,30,94] In addition, amikacin has been shown to provide a synergistic effect with vancomycin against certain organisms (e.g. various *Streptococcus*, *Enterococcus* and *Staphylococcus* species).[87-89] In contrast to beta-lactams (i.e. cephalosporins), aminoglycosides demonstrate "concentration-dependent killing" (i.e. increasing concentration raises bactericidal effect), and are less susceptible to the "inoculum effect" (reduced antimicrobial activity with high microbial concentrations).[87] One major disadvantage of aminoglycosides is their relatively high toxic potential over a narrow range. Recent studies have shown that ceftazidime, a third-generation cephalosporin, provides approximately equivalent coverage for most gram-negative organisms but with a greater safety profile, in comparison to aminoglycosides.[79,90-93] Certain gram-negative organisms (i.e. *H. influenza*) are also more susceptible to ceftazidime than aminoglycosides.[3] Therefore, some favor ceftazidime over aminoglycosides for gram-negative coverage. The EVS confirmed similar antimicrobial coverage for amikacin and ceftazidime. In the EVS, all tested gram-negative organisms except two were susceptible to amikacin and ceftazidime (89.5%).[17] One *Pseudomonas* species and one *Flavobacterium* species were resistant to both amikacin and ceftazidime.[17]

Currently, the typical empirical antibiotic regimens for intravitreal injections include the following:[3,4,9]

1. Vancomycin (1.0 mg in 0.1 ml) and ceftazidime (2.25 mg in 0.1 ml); or
2. Vancomycin (1.0 mg in 0.1 ml) and amikacin (100 to 400 micrograms in 0.1 ml) for beta-lactam sensitive patients.

For postoperative fungal endophthalmitis, amphotericin B (5 to 10 micrograms per 0.1 ml) is the drug of choice for intravitreal injections.[3,94] Because of its potential toxicity, the dosage of amphotericin B needs to be precise.[94] It should also be shielded from light due to its tendency to degrade with light exposure. The alternative is miconazole (25 micrograms per 0.1 ml).[3] Supplemental therapy with subconjunctival miconazole (10 mg in 1 ml), and the concurrent intake of oral flucytosine (150 mg/ kg/ day in four divided doses) may provide a synergistic effect with amphotericin B against the fungus.[44,95]

Recent studies advocated the use of oral fluconazole for certain fungal endophthalmitis, due to its favorable ocular penetration as well as safety and efficacy profiles.[3,60,96] The usual adult dose of oral fluconazole, ketoconazole or itraconazole is 200 to 400 mg per day for two to four weeks. Fluconazole is also available in an intravenous solution (2 mg per ml).[97] Fluconazole is better tolerated than ketoconazole and itraconazole due to less associated systemic side effects (nausea, vomiting, diarrhea, abdominal pain and headache, etc).[97]

Most recently, intravitreal voriconazole, a new-generation triazole (100 micrograms per 0.1 ml), has been found to possess high safety and efficacy profiles for treating postoperative and endogenous fungal endophthalmitis.[98-101] Besides intravitreal injections, this medication may also be given by topical, oral and intravenous routes.[102-104]

Table 64.2 outlines detailed information on the preparation and dosages of various antimicrobial drugs for intravitreal injections.[3,8,95,105]

SYSTEMIC ANTIBIOTICS AND CORTICOSTEROID THERAPY

The EVS determined the lack of additional benefits provided by systemic antibiotics besides intravitreal antibiotics in treating postoperative endophthalmitis.[9,106] However, some have criticized the limitation of systemic antibiotics to ceftazidime or ciprofloxacin and amikacin in the EVS, since the use of vancomycin or clindamycin might have yielded a different conclusion due to the higher susceptibility of most gram-positive organisms to the latter two medications.[8,106] Despite this controversy, the current recommendation is to reserve systemic antibiotics as primary therapy for endogenous endophthalmitis, and supplemental therapy for bleb-related and traumatic endophthalmitis.[31,52,54,106] Regarding ciprofloxacin, a fluoroquinolone, it was detected to reach intraocular therapeutic levels against a wide variety of gram-positive

and gram-negative bacteria. It is therefore a good alternative to Ceftazidime for a broad-spectrum coverage for patients with penicillin allergy or beta-lactam sensitivity.[9,17] Its oral route of administration (750 mg every 12 hours) is also convenient for many patients. Unfortunately, it is generally ineffective against the *Streptococcus* species, despite its strong activity against most staphylococci and gram-negative organisms.[62] Certain *Pseudomonas* species are also relatively resistant to it.[62] For the majority of postoperative endophthalmitis, intravitreal injections instead of systemic administration remain to be the primary antimicrobial therapy.[9,107] For persistent cases of postoperative endophthalmitis (e.g. bleb-related infection), intravenous vancomycin has great potential for effective supplemental coverage to intravitreal antibiotic injection and vitrectomy for most gram-positive organisms, whereas intravenous ceftazidime is highly effective against most gram-negative organisms.[93]

Regarding intravitreal corticosteroid therapy, there is a lack of consensus.[4,108] Theoretical benefits of corticosteroid therapy include counter-activity against macrophage and neutrophil migration, stabilization of lysosomal membranes and decreased degranulation of inflammatory cells (neutrophils, mast cells, macrophages and basophils), and reduction in prostaglandin synthesis and capillary permeability due to inhibition of phospholipase A2.[108] However, its harmful effects include potential reduction in the killing power of inflammatory cells, changes in the bioavailability and doses of the intravitreal antibiotics, potentiation of the infection in the absence of appropriate antibiotic therapy, risk of retinal toxicity due to medication errors, and inability to counteract bacterial toxin-induced damages.[108] There are multiple experimental and clinical studies for and against corticosteroid therapy for postoperative endophthalmitis. For instance, experimental studies have reported the reduction of histological and clinical severity of the infection within 24 hours after administration of corticosteroid therapy, and clinical studies have also shown the lack of worsening infection or visual outcome associated with corticosteroid therapy.[91,109-115] However, the negative effects of corticosteroid therapy for endophthalmitis have been reported by multiple investigators, including decreased bacteriocidal effects of ciprofloxacin in combination with intraocular dexamethasone, increased corneal and retinal toxicity after dexamethasone injections for *S. aureus* infection, and the inability of corticosteroid to reduce the retinal damages induced by *E. faecalis* infection.[4,56,108,114,116,117] Kwak and D'Amico reported potential toxic reactions of intravitreal dosages of dexamethasone above 500 microns,[118] and Hida et al published retinal toxicity profiles associated with intraocular injections of a series of commercially-available corticosteroids.[119] Yoshizumi reported potential toxic effects related to repeated intraocular injections of dexamethasone in

| TABLE 64.2 | Protocol for intravitreal antibiotic preparation |

Vancomycin Hydrochloride: 1 mg in 0.1 ml
1. Add 10 ml of diluent to 500 mg powder in vial, resulting in 50 mg/ml concentration.
2. Insert 2 ml (100 mg) or reconstituted drug into 10 ml sterile empty vial, and add 8 ml of diluent, resulting in a final solution of 10 mg/ml.*

Ceftazidime Hydrochloride: 2.25 mg in 0.1 ml
1. Add 10 ml of diluent to 500 mg powder in vial to result in 50 mg/ml concentration.
2. Insert 1 ml (50 mg) of reconstituted drug into a 10 ml sterile empty vial, and mix with 1.2 ml of diluent, for a final solution of 22.5 mg/ml. *

Cefazolin sodium: 2.25 mg in 0.1 ml
1. Add 2 ml of diluent to 500-mg powder in vial to result in concentration of 225 mg/ml.
2. Insert 1 ml (22.5 mg) of reconstituted drug into a 10-ml sterile empty vial, and mix with additional 9 ml of diluent, for a final solution of 22.5 mg/ ml. *

Amikacin sulfate: 0.2 to 0.4 mg in 0.1 ml
1. Original vial contains 500 mg in 2 ml (250 mg/ml) solution.
2. Add 0.8 ml (200 mg) solution into a 10-ml sterile empty vial, and mix with additional 9.2 ml of diluent, to achieve a concentration of 200 mg in 10 ml (20mg/ml).
3. Withdraw 0.2 ml (4 mg) and mix with 0.8 ml of diluent in a second sterile empty vial to achieve final solution of 0.4 mg/ml *; or withdraw 0.1ml (2mg) and mix with 0.9ml of diluent to achieve a final solution of 0.2 mg/ml.*

Gentamicin sulfate: 0.1 to 0.2 mg in 0.1 ml
1. Original vial contains 80 mg in 2 ml (40 mg/ml) solution.
2. Add 0.1 ml (4 mg) solution into a 10-ml sterile empty vial, and mix with 3.9 ml of diluent to achieve a solution of 4 mg in 4 ml or 1 mg/1 ml *; or add 0.2 ml (8 mg) solution into a 10-ml sterile empty vial, and mix with 3.9 ml of diluent to achieve a solution of 8 mg in 4 ml or 2 mg/1 ml *

Clindamycin phosphate: 1 mg in 0.1 ml
1. Original vial contains a 600 mg in 4 ml solution (150 mg/1 ml)
2. Add 0.2 ml (30 mg) solution into a 10-ml sterile empty vial and mix with 2.8 ml of diluent to achieve a solution of 30 mg in 3 ml or 10 mg/ml.*

Chloramphenicol sodium succinate : 2 mg in 0.1 ml
1. Original vial contains 1000 mg powder.
2. Add 10 ml of diluent to reconstitute 1000 mg powder for a concentration of 100 mg /ml.
3. Withdraw 1 ml of reconstituted drug (100 mg) and mix with 4 ml of diluent in a 10-ml sterile empty vial to achieve a final solution of 20 mg/1ml.*

Amphotericin B: 0.005 mg in 0.1 ml
1. Original vial contains 50 mg powder.
2. Add 10 ml of diluent to reconstitute the 50 mg powder into a concentration of 5 mg/ml.
3. Add 0.1 ml (0.5 mg)of reconstituted solution into a 10-ml sterile empty vial, and mix with 9.9 ml of diluent to achieve a final solution of 0.05 mg/ 1ml. *

Miconazole: 0.025 mg in 0.1 ml
1. Original ampule contains 20 ml of 10 mg/ml solution.
2. Remove glass particles and impurities by passing solution into a 5 μm filter needle.
3. Add 0.25 ml (2.5 mg) of filtered solution into a 10-ml sterile empty vial, and mix with 9.75 ml of diluent to achieve a final solution of 2.5 mg in 10 ml or 0.25 mg/1ml.*

Recommendation: For optimal results, the drug dilution and preparation should be performed by trained personnel in the controlled environment of a hospital pharmacy.[3,105] Nonbacteriostatic sterile water is used as diluent for Vancomycin and Amphotericin B. For all others, nonbacteriostatic sterile water or 0.9 % sodium chloride solution is used as diluent.[3,105] For all medications, the volume from the final solution for intravitreal injection is 0.1 ml drawn into a tuberculin syringe and delivered with a 27-or 30-gauge needle at the pars plana.[3,105]

combination with commonly used antibiotics.[115,120] Such toxic reactions may be due to the enhanced elimination of vancomycin associated with less virulent organisms, but prolongation of its half-life by certain virulent organisms (e.g. *Pneumococcus*) after intravitreal dexamethasone administration.[4,121,122] In a retrospective study, Shah et al showed that those patients with endophthalmitis receiving both antibiotics and corticosteroid injections were 3.5 times less likely to achieve a 3-line visual acuity gain, in comparison to those receiving antibiotic injections alone.[123] Given the controversy, intravitreal corticosteroid injections should be used with caution for treatment of postoperative endophthalmitis. The typical dosage of intravitreal dexamethasone is 360 to 400 micrograms per 0.1 ml.[3,4,8,110,118] In the case of fungal endophthalmitis, corticosteroid therapy should either be avoided altogether or applied cautiously under the coverage of antifungal medications.[8,124,125] Hasany et al reported that corticosteroid administration may weaken the host defenses and increase the rate of growth and pathogenicity of saprophytic fungi.[125] However, Coats and Peyman reported that intravitreal corticosteroid injections did not interfere with fungal killing (*C. albicans*) in the treatment of exogenous fungal endophthalmitis in their animal study.[124] Besides intravitreal injections, other routes of corticosteroid therapy may involve subconjunctival injections (4 to 12 mg of dexamethasone, or 40 to 80 mg of triamcinolone or depomedrol) and systemic therapy (1 mg per kg per day for five days followed by rapid tapering).[4,9,108]

VITRECTOMY FOR TREATING ENDOPHTHALMITIS

Prior to the EVS, multiple studies suggested superior outcome with vitrectomy and intravitreal antibiotic injections, in comparison to intravitreal antibiotic injections alone for treating these cases.[3,8,9,12,117,126-128] There are multiple theoretical advantages associated with a vitrectomy for endophthalmitis. For instance, it allows rapid elimination of sequestered infectious infiltrates and vitreous opacities, reduction in inflammatory mediators, relief of vitreoretinal traction, more room for intravitreal injections and enhanced diffusion of medications.[3,9] However, most of the reports advocating vitrectomy involved retrospective and un-controlled studies with multiple confounding variables.[8,19,126,127-129] Early vitrectomy remains to be vital for enhancing the successful treatment of postoperative endophthalmitis associated with chronic *P. acnes* and bleb-related infections.[31,33,35-37,40,41,106,127] The EVS was conducted to determine the value of vitrectomy for postoperative endophthalmitis.[130]

ENDOPHTHALMITIS VITRECTOMY STUDY

The EVS was a carefully designed multicenter controlled prospective clinical trial sponsored by the National Eye Institute.[2,9,130] Its definitive conclusions were reported in 1995.[2,9] The main conclusion of EVS was that for those eyes undergoing cataract extraction with an intraocular implant that developed postoperative endophthalmitis, vitreous tap and intravitreal antibiotic injections alone (TAP) yielded equivalent outcome in comparison to those eyes treated with immediate vitrectomy and intravitreal antibiotic injections (VIT), (66% versus 62% with final visual acuity [VA] of 20/40 or better), as long as the baseline VA was hand motions or better.[9] However, EVS determined that for those infected eyes with a baseline VA of light perception only, the VIT group fared better than the TAP group.[9] In this latter category, a three-fold increase in the rate of achieving a VA of 20/40 or better was found in the VIT group in comparison to the TAP group (33% versus 11%). There was also a two-fold increase in the rate of achieving a VA of 20/100 and a 50% reduction in the rate of severe vision loss (VA < 5/200) in the VIT group in comparison to the TAP group (56% versus 30%, and 20% versus 47%, respectively) for these eyes with a baseline VA of worse than hand motions.[9] For the EVS,

the designation of achieving a VA of hand motions required the patient to correctly identify four of five presentations of hand movements shown at two feet (60 centimeters) away with a light source emanating from behind the patient and directed towards the examiner's hand. Therefore, if the patient could only recognize hand motions at less than two feet, the VA would be considered as light perception only, and a vitrectomy with antibiotic injections would be recommended.[4,9] Furthermore, the EVS reported the lack of additional benefit in the use of systemic antibiotics with respect to the final visual outcome or media clarity.[9] In evaluating the microbial spectrum isolated in their study, EVS showed 70% of the organisms to be coagulase-negative *Staphylococcus*, 24.2% to be other gram-positive species, and only 5.9% to be gram-negative species.[17] Following subsequent subgroup analysis in 2001, the EVS reported a trend of more frequent achievement of a VA of 20/40 or better for diabetic patients with acute postoperative endophthalmitis in the VIT group over the TAP group (57% versus 40%), even if their baseline VA was hand motions or better.[131] However, this difference did not reach statistical significance, possibly due to insufficient numbers.

The EVS also showed comparable positive culture results for the TAP eyes associated with only a needle paracentesis, versus the TAP eyes associated with mechanized vitreous biopsy, and the vitrectomy eyes (68.6% versus 66.1% and 73.5%).[4,63] Similar retinal detachment rates were detected for the mechanized vitreous biopsy eyes and the needle tap eyes (8% versus 11%) in the EVS, although absolute rates of difference of 10% or less could not be ruled out.[4,132] The overall rate of 8.3% of retinal detachment in the EVS was less than the rates of 10 to 16% reported in previous studies.[15,133] The frequency of a retinal detachment was higher for eyes with more virulent organisms (e.g. gram negative), poor presenting VA, open posterior capsule, and requirement for additional procedure in the early course of the study.[132] Eyes without a retinal detachment had better final visual outcome than those with one (55% of final VA of 20/40 or better for the former versus 27% for the latter).[132] Eight percent of VIT eyes and 13% of TAP eyes required additional procedures within one week of study entry (14% for complications of the initial procedure and 86% for worsening ocular inflammation or infection). Eyes requiring additional procedures had more severe disease than those that did not, with only 15% of the former versus 57% of the latter achieving a VA of 20/40 or better.[63]

Another intriguing finding of the EVS was that there was a statistically higher rate of gram-positive and coagulase-negative isolates for those eyes with a posterior chamber intraocular lenses (IOL) than those with an anterior chamber IOL (51.8% versus 34%).[17] The reason for this difference is unknown. One plausible explanation is the differential adherence of *Staphylococcus epidermidis* to various IOL materials. This difference held even when the eyes were subdivided into those with primary cataract extraction (51.9% for PCIOL versus 37.9% for ACIOL), and secondary IOL implantation (40% for PCIOL versus 27.8% for ACIOL). In contrast, there was less than half the rate of infection with gram-positive and coagulase-negative micrococci (21.7% versus 48%), as well as greater than twice the rate of infection (30.4% versus 14.6%) with other gram-positive organisms (i.e. *Staphylococcus aureus*, *Streptococcus* and *Enterococcus* species), when comparing the secondary IOL implantation group with the primary cataract extraction group in the EVS.[17] The reason for this difference is unclear, but could be related to the confounding variable of a much higher percentage of ACIOL inserted for secondary implantation eyes than the primary cataract surgery eyes (78% versus 7%). However, this difference held even when the IOL type was considered. Of particular interest is the fact that the microbiological spectrum was not influenced by vitreous loss, anterior vitrectomy and posterior capsulotomy made during surgery.[17]

Some have emphasized the limited application of the conclusions of the EVS to only eyes undergoing cataract extraction with implant insertion. They point out that for eyes with chronic or delayed-onset endophthalmitis after surgery (e.g. *P. acnes* infection) and those associated with bleb-related endophthalmitis, a vitrectomy besides antibiotic injections is frequently required for an optimal outcome.[31,33,35-37,40,106,127] Furthermore, they question the validity of its conclusion on the lack of additional benefit with systemic antibiotics, due to the limitation of the systemic antibiotics to only ceftazidime or ciprofloxacin and amikacin in the EVS (See previous section on systemic antibiotics for detailed discussion).[8,106] In the EVS, eyes treated with systemic antibiotics had a lower rate of a retinal detachment (5%) than those not treated with them (11%).[132] The significance of this difference is unclear.

VITRECTOMY TECHNIQUES

Pars plana vitrectomy for postoperative endophthalmitis may utilize a 2 or 3-port 20-guage, 23-gauge, or 25-gauge technique. In addition, single-port 23-gauge vitrectors are now available for simple vitreous biopsy in the office setting [i.e. Josephberg 1-port vitrectomy biopsy cutter (Beton Dickinson, Inc) Intrector (Insight Instruments Inc, Stuart, Florida)].

If possible, utilizing a long infusion cannula (i.e. 6 mm) during a vitrectomy lowers the risk of inadvertent subretinal and choroidal infusion for pseudophakic eyes with postoperative endophthalmitis, given the multiple predisposing factors of such eyes for surgical complications (e.g. limited intraocular tissue visibility, increased choroidal congestion and frequent hypotony, etc).[8] To further avoid such surgical complications, the surgeon must ensure that the tip of the infusion cannula is well within the vitreous cavity before turning on the infusion fluid. For a case with very cloudy media, the surgeon may confirm the proper position of the infusion cannula's tip by gently rubbing the

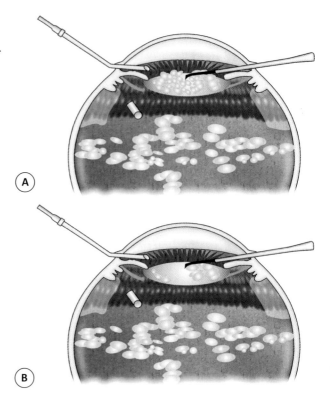

FIGURES 64.6A AND B: Clearance of anterior chamber before vitrectomy: (A) Anterior chamber wash-out is utilized to eliminate cloudy fibrin deposits and hyphema to allow appropriate visualization for the surgeon before a vitrectomy can be performed; (B) The surgeon may employ a microsurgical pick or hook inserted through the limbus to scrape off the cloudy material from the surfaces of the IOL and iris for removal with a vitrectomy probe. Separate infusion via a cannula connected to a separate infusion line is usually needed through a second limbal incision to prevent the collapse of the anterior chamber during this portion of the procedure. Upon achievement of appropriate clarity of the anterior chamber, the proper location of the posterior infusion cannula is then ascertained by visualizing its tip before turning on the posterior infusion line

tip of a microvitreoretinal blade inserted through one of the superior sclerotomies against the tip of the infusion cannula. Frequently, a separate anterior chamber wash-out through the limbus is required to eliminate cloudy fibrin deposits or hyphema from the anterior chamber first, before attaining sufficient clarity in the anterior portion of the eye for a pars plana vitrectomy.[8] Various microsurgical hooks and picks may be inserted through the limbus to scrape off infiltrates in the anterior chamber and fibrin membranes layered on the surfaces of the implant and the iris before removing them with a vitrectomy probe from the anterior chamber (**Figures 64.6A and B**). A separate infusion line may be required through the limbus for the anterior chamber wash-out to prevent chamber collapse. When performing a core vitrectomy, care must be taken to engage in only gentle intraocular movements and avoid vigorous surgical maneuvers that may induce vitreoretinal traction, such as aggressive epiretinal membrane removal and fibrin clean- up. Despite the intentional avoidance of their direct removal during the vitrectomy, the posterior epiretinal fibrin deposits and hemorrhage tend to slowly dissolve following the injections of intravitreal antimicrobial and anti-inflammatory medications after surgery. Keeping the intraocular instruments well within the anterior and central vitreous cavity and staying away from the fragile infected retina during surgery, will reduce the chance of retinal complications. The vitreous specimen for microbial investigation is either collected into a syringe connected to the aspiration line of the vitrectomy probe or into a cassette of the vitrectomy machine for subsequent processing **(Figures 64.6A and B)**.[4] Finally, the eye is made sufficiently soft to allow room for injections of medications and the sclerotomies are closed tightly to avoid leakage, before the injection of intravitreal drugs at the end of the surgery.

POSTOPERATIVE CARE

Although the patient usually reports decreased ocular pain and headaches, the ocular media may still be quite cloudy during the first 24 hours following intravitreal anti-microbial injections and even after a vitrectomy, often due to temporary layering of the residual fibrin infiltrates on the intraocular implant and corneal surfaces during their anterior migration.[4,8] Progressive clinical improvement usually occurs by 48 to 60 hours after treatment. During the postoperative course, intense topical broad-spectrum antibiotics, cycloplegic and corticosteroid medications are applied. Frequently, additional intravitreal antimicrobial injections are necessary after 48 to 72 hours.

Instead of a "shot-gun" approach similar to the initial therapy, the choice of the repeat antimicrobial injection may be tailored based on the antimicrobial susceptibility of the cultured organism.[3,4] In the case of a gram-positive organism, vancomycin injection may be repeated.[3,9,17] In the case of a gram-negative organism, amikacin or ceftazidime injection may be repeated.[3,9,17] The latter is particularly appropriate for the *Hemophilus* species.[3] A repeat vitrectomy may be needed for recalcitrant cases, such as certain cases of chronic or delayed-onset endophthalmitis. For instance, repeat surgery may be needed for removal of capsular remnants or implant associated with sequestered organisms for certain cases of *P. acnes*.[33,35-37,40] The EVS reported that 8 % of VIT eyes and 13 % of TAP eyes required additional procedures within seven days after the initial therapy.[4,134]

VISUAL OUTCOME

The visual outcome after prompt and appropriate treatment of postoperative endophthalmitis associated with cataract surgery is generally more favorable than other types of endophthalmitis. Primarily due to the predominance of coagulase-negative *Staphylococcus* with relatively low virulence, the EVS showed that 53% of patients achieved a VA of 20/40 or better, 74% achieved a VA of 20/100 or better, and only 15% developed a VA of worse than 5/200 (5% with LP at final visit), 46 at 9 to 12 months after

treatment. Such favorable results are consistent with other studies on postoperative endophthalmitis associated with cataract surgery.[3,14,124,135] The EVS confirmed that the visual prognosis was strongly associated with the identity of the infecting organism and gram-stain results (VA of 20/100 or better for 84% of eyes with gram-positive and coagulase-negative micrococci, 50% eyes with *Staphylococcus aureus*, 30% of eyes with streptococci, 14% eyes with enterococci and 56% of eyes with gram-negative organisms).[2] However, the EVS and other studies also showed that the presenting VA was a more reliable indicator than microbiologic factors in predicting the final visual outcome, confirming the importance of prompt therapeutic intervention.[2,135] The visual outcome for delayed-onset endophthalmitis caused by the *Propionibacterium* species is also relatively favorable but can be variable.[32-38,40] Studies of small series of *P. acnes* endophthalmitis reported the final VA to range from 20/20 to 20/400.[32-38,40] Bleb-related endophthalmitis is associated with a poor visual outcome as a result of the high virulence of the organisms (mostly *Streptococcus* species and gram-negative organisms) and the frequent delay in the correct diagnosis. Mandelbaum et al reported that only 24% of their series of bleb-related endophthalmitis achieved useful vision, 19% achieved a VA of 20/400 or better and 37% developed no light perception.[31] Another study on streptococcal endophthalmitis showed that 31% of eyes achieved a VA of 20/400 or better, the best results associated with enterococci (54% with 20/400 or better for *Streptococcus faecalis*), and the worst results associated with beta-hemolytic streptococci (all less than 20/400).[136]

Recently, Horio et al proposed the use of flash electroretinography (ERG) to objectively quantify the severity of endophthalmitis, since it is not inhibited by media opacity.[137] Their recommendation was based on the report of reduced b-wave amplitudes of the scotopic electroretinogram within 2 to 3 days after inoculation of highly virulent organisms into animal eyes.[27,137-139] They reported that those eyes with a b-wave to a-wave ratio of less than 1.0 and early onset of endophthalmitis (less than one week) were associated with more virulent organisms (e.g. *Pseudomonas aeruginosa* and *Enterococcus faecalis*) and worse visual results (no light perception to 20/200). Thus, flash ERG can predict the visual prognosis of eyes with postoperative endophthalmitis, and also be utilized as an objective clinical tool besides the presenting VA to determine the need for vitreous tap and anti-microbial injections alone versus an immediate vitrectomy with antimicrobial injections.[137]

CONCLUSION

For the majority of postoperative endophthalmitis following cataract surgery, relatively favorable visual outcome can be achieved with prompt and appropriate therapy, due to the predominance of coagulase-negative *Staphylococcus* and other low-virulent gram-positive organisms responsible for the infection. The EVS clearly showed that for those eyes diagnosed with postoperative endophthalmitis after cataract surgery and a presenting VA of hand motions or better, simple vitreous tap and antimicrobial injections alone in the office setting fares as well as immediate vitrectomy and antimicrobial injections. Those eyes with chronic or delayed-onset postoperative endophthalmitis (e.g. *P. acnes* and fungal infections) may develop variable visual outcome. For bleb-related endophthalmitis, the highly virulent organisms usually induce poor visual outcome. The empirical intravitreal injections of specially prepared anti-microbials with specific concentrations and a wide-spectrum of antimicrobial coverage in a "shot-gun" approach constitute the first-line therapy for postoperative endophthalmitis. Repeat injections of more selective antimicrobial after obtaining culture and antimicrobial susceptibility results may follow. Vitrectomy remains a first-line therapy for certain cases of postoperative endophthalmitis with poor presenting vision, resistant cases and bleb-related cases. The two key factors with the greatest influence on the final visual outcome for postoperative endophthalmitis are the identity of the organism and the duration of the infection. Despite substantial advances in treating postoperative endophthalmitis in the modern era allowing the eradication of the infection for almost all cases after proper treatment, achieving favorable visual outcome across the entire spectrum of responsible organisms remains to be an elusive goal. Therapeutic breakthrough in preventing severe tissue damages due to highly potent toxins from virulent organisms is needed, before major improvement in the vision outcome for treating these cases can be expected. Until then, postoperative endophthalmitis remains a condition with the potential for inducing devastating ocular consequences.

REFERENCES

1. Christy NE, Lall P. Postoperative endophthalmitis following cataract surgery. Arch Ophthalmol. 1973;90:361-6.
2. Endophthalmitis Vitrectomy Study Group. Microbiologic factors and visual outcome in the Endophthalmitis Vitrectomy Study. Am J Ophthalmol. 1996;122:830-46.
3. Forster RK. Endophthalmitis. In: Tasman W, Jaeger EA (Eds). Duane's Clinical Ophthalmology, Vol 4, chapter 24, Philadelphia: Lippincott-Raven; 1996. pp. 1-29.
4. Han DP. Acute-onset postoperative endophthalmitis: current recommendations. In syllabus: Subspecialty Day-Retina, Management of posterior segment complications of anterior segment surgery; 1998.
5. Kattan HM, Flynn HW Jr, Pflugfelder S, et al. Nosocomial endophthalmitis survey. Ophthalmology. 1991;98:227-38.
6. Leveille AS, McMullan FD, Cavanagh HD. Endophthalmitis following penetrating keratoplasty. Ophthalmology. 1983;90:38-9.
7. Starr MB. Prophylactic antibiotics for ophthalmic surgery. Surv Ophthalmol. 1983;27:353-73.
8. Chan CK, Lin SG. Current concepts in managing infectious endophthalmitis: a comprehensive review. In: Agarwal S, Agarwal A, Agarwal A (Eds). Phako, Phakonit, And Laser Phako, A Quest For The Best. Section VII. Complications, 1st edn, Chapter 47. Slack Incorporated and Highlights of Ophthalmology; 2002. pp. 505-34.
9. Endophthalmitis Vitrectomy Study Group. Results of the Endophthalmitis Vitrectomy Study. A randomized trial of immediate vitrectomy and intravenous antibiotics for the treatment of postoperative bacterial endophthalmitis. Arch Ophthalmol. 1995;113:1479-96.
10. Heilskov T, Joondeph BC, Olsen KR, et al. Case report: Late endophthalmitis after transscleral fixation of a posterior chamber intraocular lens. Arch Ophthalmol. 1989;107:1427.
11. Javitt JC, Vitale S, Canner JK, et al. National outcomes of cataract extraction. Arch Ophthalmol. 1991;109:1085-9.
12. Rowsey JJ, Newsom DL, Sexton DJ, et al. Endophthalmitis, Current approaches. Ophthalmology. 1982;89:1055-66.
13. Bode DD, Gelender H, Forster RK. A retrospective review of endophthalmitis due to coagulase-negative staphylococci. Br J Ophthalmol. 1985;69:915-9.
14. Ormerod LD, Ho DD, Becker LE, et al. Endophthalmitis caused by the coagulase-negative staphylococci: 1. Disease spectrum and outcome. Ophthalmology. 1993;100:715-23.
15. Nelson PT, Marcus DA, Bovino JA. Retinal detachment following endophthalmitis. Ophthalmology. 1985;92:1112-7.
16. Forster RK. Symposium: Postoperative endophthalmitis: Etiology and diagnosis of bacterial postoperative endophthalmitis. Ophthalmology. 1978;85:320-6.
17. Han DP, Wisniewski SR, Wilson LA, et al. Spectrum and susceptibilities of microbiologic isolates in the Endophthalmitis Vitrectomy Study. Am J Ophthalmol. 1996;112:1-17.
18. Puliafito CA, Baker AS, Haaf J, et al. Infectious endophthalmitis. Ophthalmology. 1982;89:921-9.
19. Forster RK, Abbott RL, Gelender H. Management of infectious endophthalmitis. Ophthalmology. 1980;87:313-9.
20. Forster RK, Zachary IG, Cottingham AJ Jr, et al. Further observations on the diagnosis, cause, and treatment of endophthalmitis. Am J Ophthalmol. 1976;81:52-6.
21. Abbott RL, Forster RK, Rebell G. Listeria monocytogenes endophthalmitis with a black hypopyon. Am J Ophthalmol. 1978;86:715-9.
22. Ballan PH, Loffredo FR, Painter B. Listeria endophthalmitis. Arch Ophthalmol. 1979;97:101-2.
23. Boomla K, Quilliam RP. Haemophilis influenzae endophthalmitis. Br Med J. 1981;282:989-90.
24. Lass JH, Varley MP, Frank KE, et al. Actinobacillus actinomycetemcomitans endophthalmitis with subacute endocarditis. Ann Ophthalmol. 1984;16:54-61.
25. Cohen P, Kirshner J, Whiting G. Bilateral endogenous Escherichia coli endophthalmitis. Arch Intern Med. 1980;140: 1088-9.
26. Cowan CL Jr, Saeed T, Stevens J, et al. Successful management of Pseudomonas endogenous endophthalmitis. Ann Ophthalmol. 1983;15:559-61.
27. Hatano H, Sasaki T, Tanaka N. Pseudomonas endophthalmitis in rabbits: intravitreal inoculation of two Pseudomonas strains. Acta Soc Ophthalmol. 1988;92:1758-64.
28. Gammon JA, Schwab I, Joseph P. Gentamicin-resistant Serratia marcescens endophthalmitis. Arch Ophthalmol. 1980;98: 1221-3.
29. Darrel RW. Acute tuberculous panophthalmitis. Arch Ophthalmol. 1967;78:51-4.
30. Dvorak-Theobald G. Acute tuberculous endophthalmitis. Am J Ophthalmol. 1958;45:403-7.

31. Mandelbaum S, Forster RK, Gelender H, et al. Late onset endophthalmitis associated with filtering blebs. Ophthalmology. 1985;92:964-72.

32. Brady SE, Cohen EJ, Fischer DH. Diagnosis and treatment of chronic postoperative bacterial endophthalmitis. Ophthalmic Surg. 1988;19:580-4.

33. Fox GM, Joondeph BC, Flynn HW Jr, et al. Delayed-onset pseudophakic endophthalmitis. Am J Ophthalmol. 1991;111: 163-73.

34. Jaffe GJ, Whitcher JP, Biswell R, et al. Propionibacterium acnes endophthalmitis seven months after extracapsular cataract extraction and intraocular lens implantation. Ophthalmic Surg. 1986;17:791-3.

35. Meisler DM, Mandelbaum S. Propionibacterium-associated endophthalmitis after extracapsular cataract extraction. Review of reported cases. Ophthalmology. 1989;96:54-61.

36. Meisler DM, Palestine AG, Vastine DW, et al. Chronic Propionibacterium endophthalmitis after cataract extraction and intraocular lens implantation. Am J Ophthalmol. 1986;102: 733-9.

37. Meisler DM, Zakov ZN, Bruner WE, et al. Endophthalmitis associated with sequestered intraocular Propionibacterium acnes [letter]. Am J Ophthalmol. 1987;104:428-9.

38. Roussel TJ, Culbertson WW, Jaffe NS. Chronic postoperative endophthalmitis associated with Propionibacterium acnes. Arch Ophthalmol. 1987;105:1199-201.

39. Ficker L, Meredith TA, Wilson LA ,et al. Chronic bacterial endophthalmitis. Am J Ophthalmol. 1987;103:745-8.

40. Zambrano W, Flynn HW Jr, Pflugfelder SC, et al. Management options for Propionibacterium acnes endophthalmitis. Ophthalmology. 1989;96:1100-5.

41. Winward KE, Pflugfelder SC, Flynn HW Jr, et al. Postoperative Propionibacterium endophthalmitis. Ophthalmology. 1993; 100:447-51.

42. Stern WH, Tamura E, Jacobs RA, et al. Epidemic post-surgical Candida parapsilosis endophthalmitis. Ophthalmology. 1985;92:1701-9.

43. Theodore FH. Symposium: Postoperative endophthalmitis; Etiology and diagnosis of fungal postoperative endophthalmitis. Ophthalmology. 1978;85:327-40.

44. Wilson FM, Wilson II FM. Postoperative uveitis. In: Tasman W, Jaeger EA (Eds). Duane's Clinical Ophthalmology, Vol 4, chapter 55, Philadelphia: Lippincott-Raven; 1996. pp. 1-18.

45. Aziz AA, Bullock JD, Mcguire TW, et al. Aspergillus endophthalmitis: a clinical and experimental study. Trans Am Ophthalmol Soc. 1992;90:317-42, discussion 342-6.

46. Pettit TH, Olson RJ, Foos RY, et al. Fungal endophthalmitis following intraocular lens implantation. Arch Ophthalmol. 1980;98:1025-39.

47. Jampol LM, Strauch BS, Albert DM. Intraocular nocardiosis. Am J Ophthalmol. 1973;76:568-73.

48. Roussel TJ, Olson ER, Rice T, et al. Chronic postoperative endophthalmitis associated with Actinomyces species. Arch Ophthalmol. 1991;109;60-2.

49. Sher NA, Hill CW, Eifrig DE. Bilateral intraocular Nocardia asteroides infection. Arch Ophthalmol. 1977;95:1415-8.

50. Zimmerman PL, Mamalis N, Alder JB, et al. Chronic Nocardia asteroides endophthalmitis after extracapsular cataract extraction. Arch Ophthalmol. 1993;111:837-40.

51. Brown RH, Yang LH, Walker SD, et al. Treatment of bleb infection after glaucoma surgery. Arch Ophthalmol. 1994; 112:57-61.

52. Ciulla TA, Beck AD, Topping TM, et al. Blebitis, early endophthalmitis, and late endophthalmitis after glaucoma-filtering surgery. Ophthalmology. 1997;104:986-95.

53. Higginbotham EJ, Stevens RK, Musch D, et al. Bleb-related endophthalmitis after trabeculectomy with mitomycin C. Ophthalmology. 1996;103:650-6.

54. Parrish R, Minckler D. Late endophthalmitis-Filtering surgery time bomb? [editorial]. Ophthalmology. 1996;103:1167-8.

55. Wolner B, Liebermann JM, Sassan JW, et al. Late bleb-related endophthalmitis after trabeculectomy with adjunctive 5-fluorouracil. Ophthalmology. 1991;98:1053-60.

56. Jett BD, Jensen HG, Atkuri RV, et al. Evaluation of therapeutic measures for treating endophthalmitis caused by isogenic toxin producing and toxin-nonproducing Enterococcus faecalis strains. Invest Ophthalmol Vis Sci. 1995;36:9-15.

57. Mamalis N, Nagpal M, Nagpal K, et al. Endophthalmitis following cataract surgery, Posterior segment complications of cataract surgery. Ophthalmol Clinics No Amer. 2001;14: 661-74.

58. Corbett MC, Hingorani M, Boulton JE, et al. Factors predisposing to postoperative intraocular inflammation. Eur J Ophthalmol. 1995;5:40-7.

59. Drolsum L, Davanger K, Haaskjold E. Risk factors for an inflammatory response after extracapsular cataract extraction and posterior chamber IOL. Acta Ophthalmol (Copenh). 1994;72:21-6.

60. Oncel M, Ercikan C. Penetration of oral fluconazole into the vitreous in humans. Invest Ophthalmol Vis Sci. 1992;33:747.

61. Sullivan LJ, Su C, Snibson G, et al. Sterile ocular inflammatory reactions to monofilament suture material. Aust N Z J Ophthalmol. 1994;22:175-81.

62. Baum J. Antibiotics use in ophthalmology. In: Tasman W, Jaeger EA (eds). Duane's Clinical Ophthalmology, Vol 4, chapter 24. Philadelphia: Lippincott-Raven; 1996. pp. 1-26.

63. Barza M, Pavan PR, Doft BH, et al. Evaluation of microbiological diagnostic techniques in postoperative endophthalmitis in the Endophthalmitis Vitrectomy Study. Arch Ophthalmol. 1997;115:1142-50.

64. Donahue SP, Kowalski RP, Jewar BH, et al. Vitreous cultures in suspected endophthalmitis: biopsy or vitrectomy? Ophthalmology. 1993;100:452-5.

65. Hykin PG, Tobal K, McIntyre G, et al. The diagnosis of delayed post-operative endophthalmitis by polymerase chain reaction of bacterial DNA in vitreous samples. J Med Microbiol. 1994;40:408-15.

66. Brinser JH, Weiss A. Laboratory diagnosis in ocular disease. In: Tasman W, Jaeger EA (Eds). Duane's clinical Ophthalmology, Vol 4, chapter 1. Philadelphia: Lippincott-Raven; 1996. pp. 1-14.

67. Joondeph BC, Flynn HW Jr, Miller D, et al. A new culture method for infectious endophthalmitis. Arch Ophthalmol. 1989;107:1334-7.

68. Apt L, Isenberg S, Yoshimori R, et al. Chemical preparation of the eye in ophthalmic surgery III. Effect of povidone-iodine on the conjunctiva. Arch Ophthalmol. 1984;102:728-9.

69. Bohigan GM. A study of the incidence of culture-positive endophthalmitis after cataract surgery in an ambulatory care center. Ophthalmic Surg Lasers. 1999;30:295-8.

70. Speaker MG, Menikoff JA. Prophylaxis of endophthalmitis with topical povidone-iodine. Ophthalmology. 1991;98:1769-75.

71. Isenberg SJ, Apt L, Yoshimori R, et al. Chemical preparation of the eye in ophthalmic surgery. IV. Comparison of povidone-iodine on the conjunctiva with a prophylactic antibiotic. Arch Ophthalmol. 1985;103:1340-2.

72. Schmitz S, Dick HB, Krummenauer F, et al. Endophthalmitis in cataract surgery: results of a German survey. Ophthalmology. 1999;106:1869-77.

73. Masket S. Preventing, diagnosing, and treating endophthalmitis (Guest editorial). J Cataract Refract Surg. 1998;24:725-6.

74. Speaker MG. How to head off endophthalmitis. Rev Ophthalmol. 2000;7:74-9.

75. Apt L, Isenberg SJ, Yoshimori R, et al. The effect of povidone-iodine solution applied at the conclusion of ophthalmic surgery. Am J Ophthalmol. 1998;119:701-5.

76. Donnenfeld ED, Perry HD. Cataract surgery. Five ways to prevent endophthalmitis. Review Ophthalmol. 1995;3:67-72.

77. Forster RK. Experimental postoperative endophthalmitis. Trans Am Ophthalmol Soc. 1992;90:505-59.

78. May DR, Ericson ES, Peyman GA, et al. Intraocular injection of gentamicin: single injection therapy of experimental bacterial endophthalmitis. Arch Ophthalmol. 1974;91:487-9.

79. Meredith TA. Antimicrobial pharmacokinetics in endophthalmitis treatment: studies of ceftazidime. Trans Am Ophthalmol Soc. 1993;91:653-99.

80. Stern GA. Factors affecting the efficacy of antibiotics in the treatment of experimental postoperative endophthalmitis. Trans Am Ophthalmol Soc. 1993;91:775-844.

81. Davis JL, Koidou-Tsiligianni A, Pflugfelder SC, et al. Coagulase-negative staphylococcal endophthalmitis. Ophthalmology. 1988;95:1404-10.

82. Pflugfelder SC, Hernandez E. Fliesler SJ, et al. Intravitreal vancomycin: retinal toxicity, clearance, and interaction with gentamicin. Arch Ophthalmol. 1987;105:831-7.

83. Campochiaro PA, Conway BP. Aminoglycoside toxicity: a survey of retinal specialists. Arch Ophthalmol. 1991;109:946-50.

84. Conway BP, Campochiaro PA. Macular infarction after endophthalmitis treated with vitrectomy and intravitreal gentamicin. Arch Ophthalmol. 1986;104:367-71.

85. D'Amico DJ, Caspers-Velu L, Libert J, et al. Comparative toxicity of intravitreal aminoglycoside antibiotics. Am J Ophthalmol. 1985;100:264-75.

86. McDonald HR, Schatz H, Allen AW, et al. Retinal toxicity secondary to intraocular gentamicin injection. Ophthalmology. 1986;93:871-7.

87. Doft BH, Barza M. Ceftazidime or amikacin: choice of intravitreal antimicrobials in the treatment of postoperative endophthalmitis. Arch Ophthalmol. 1994;112:17-8.

88. Watanakunakorn C, Bakie C. Synergism of vancomycin-gentamicin and vancomycin-streptomycin against enterococci. Antimicrob Agents Chemother. 1973;4:120-4.

89. Watanakunakorn C, Tisone JC. Synergism between vancomycin and gentamicin or tobramycin for methicillin-susceptible and methicillin-resistant Staphylococcus aureus strains. Antimicrob Agents Chemother. 1982;22:903-5.

90. Campochiaro PA, Green WR. Toxicity of intravitreous ceftazidime in primate retina. Arch Ophthalmol. 1992;110:1625-9.

91. Irvine WD, Flynn HW Jr, Miller D, et al. Endophthalmitis caused by gram-negative organisms. Arch Ophthalmol. 1992;110:1450-4.

92. Lim JI, Campochiaro PA. Successful treatment of gram-negative endophthalmitis with intravitreous ceftazidime. Arch Ophthalmol. 1992;110:1686.

93. The Medical Letter on Drugs and Therapeutics: the choice of antimicrobial drugs. New Rochelle, New York, Medical Letter; 1986. pp. 33-40.

94. Axelrod AJ, Peyman GA, Apple DJ. Toxicity of intravitreal injection of amphotericin B. Am J Ophthalmol. 1973;76:678-83.

95. Bohigan GM. Intravitreal antibiotic preparation, pp. 64-7. Antifungal agents. pp.158-63. In: External diseases of the eye, Fort Worth: Alcon Laboratories; 1980.

96. O'Day DM, Foulds G, William TE, et al. Ocular uptake of fluconazole following oral administration. Arch Ophthalmol. 1990;108:1006-8.

97. Jones DB. Diagnosis and management of fungal keratitis. In: Tasman W, Jaeger EA (Eds). Duane's Clinical Ophthalmology, Vol 4, chapter 21. Philadelphia, Lippincott-Raven; 1996. pp. 1-19.

98. Gao H, Pennesi ME, Shah K, et al. Intravitreal voriconazole: an electroretinographic and histopathologic study. Arch Ophthalmol. 2005;123:130.

99. Kernt M, Neubauer AS, De Kaspar HM, et al. Intravitreal voriconazole: in vitro safety-profile for fungal endophthalmitis. Retina. 2009;29:362-70.

100. Lin RC, Sanduja N, Hariprasad SM. Successful treatment of postoperative fungal endophthalmitis using intravitreal and intra-cameral voriconazole. J Ocul Pharmacol Ther. 2008;24:245-8.

101. Sen P, Gopal L, Sen PR. Intravitreal voriconazole: in vitro safety-profile for fungal endophthalmitis. Retina. 2009;29:362-70.

102. Hariprasad SM, Mieler WF, Holz ER, et al. Determination of vitreous, aqueous, and plasma concentration of orally administered voriconazole in humans. Arch Ophthalmol. 2004;22:42-7.

103. Nehemy MB, Vasconcelos-Santos DV, Torqueti-Costa L, et al. Chronic endophthalmitis due to verticillium species after cataract surgery treated (or managed) with pars plana vitrectomy and oral and intravitreal voriconazole. Retina. 2006;26:225-7.

104. Vemulakonda GA, Hariprasad SM, Mieler WF, et al. Aqueous and vitreous concentrations following topical administration of 1% voriconazole in humans. Arch Ophthalmol. 2008;126:18-22.

105. Jeglum EL, Rosenberg SB, Benson WE. Preparation of intravitreal drug doses. Ophthalmic Surg. 1981;12:355-9.

106. Sternberg P Jr, Martin DF. Management of endophthalmitis in the post-Endophthalmitis Vitrectomy Study era [editorial]. Arch Ophthalmol. 2001;119:754-5.

107. Baum J, Peyman GA, Barza M. Intravitreal administration of antibiotics in the treatment of bacterial endophthalmitis. III: Consensus. Surv Ophthalmol. 1982;26:204-6.

108. Han DP. Corticosteroids in the management of postoperative endophthalmitis. In Syllabus: Subspecialty Day-Retina 2000: Management of posterior segment disease, Drugs and Bugs. Dallas; 2000. pp. 229-34.

109. Baum JL, Barza M, Lugar J, et al. The effect of corticosteroids in the treatment of experimental bacterial endophthalmitis. Am J Ophthalmol. 1975;80:513-5.

110. Das T, Jalali S, Gothwal VK, et al. Intravitreal dexamethasone in exogenous bacterial endophthalmitis: results of a prospective randomised study. Br J Ophthalmol. 1999;83:1050-5.

111. Graham RO, Peyman GA. Intravitreal injection of dexamethasone. Treatment of experimentally induced endophthalmitis. Arch Ophthalmol. 1974;92:149-54.

112. Mao LK, Flynn HW Jr, Miller D, et al. Endophthalmitis caused by Staphylococcus aureus. Am J Ophthalmol. 1993;116:584-9.

113. Maxwell DP, Brent BD, Diamond JG, et al. Effects of intravitreal dexamethasone on ocular histopathology in a rabbit model of endophthalmitis. Ophthalmology. 1991;98:1370-5.

114. Meredith TA, Aguilar E, Drews C, et al. Intraocular dexamethasone produces a harmful effect on treatment of experimental Staphylococcus aureus endophthalmitis. Trans Am Ophthalmol Soc. 1996;94:241-52.

115. Yoshizumi MO, Lee GC, Equi RA, et al. Timing of dexamethasone treatment in experimental Staphylococcus aureus endophthalmitis. Retina. 1998;18:130-5.

116. Kim IT, Chung KH, Koo BS. Efficacy of ciprofloxacin and dexamethasone in experimental Pseudomonas endophthalmitis. Korean J Ophthalmol. 1996;10:8-17.

117. Meredith TA, Aguilar HE, Miller MJ, et al. Comparative treatment of experimental Staphylococcus epidermidis endophthalmitis. Arch Ophthalmol. 1990;108:857-60.

118. Kwak HW, D'Amico DJ. Evaluation of the retinal toxicity and pharmacokinetics of dexamethasone after intravitreal injection. Arch Ophthalmol. 1992;110:259-66.

119. Hida T, Chandler D, Arena JE, et al. Experimental and clinical observations of the intraocular toxicity of commercial corticosteroid preparations. Am J Ophthalmol. 1986;101;190-95.

120. Yoshizumi MO, Bhavsar AR, Dessouki A, et al. Safety of repeated intravitreous injections of antibiotics and dexamethasone. Retina. 1999;19:437-41.

121. Park SS, Vallar RV, Hong CH, et al. Intravitreal dexamethasone effect on intravitreal vancomycin elimination in endophthalmitis. Arch Ophthalmol. 1999;117:1058-62.

122. Smith MA, Sorenson JA, Smith C, et al. Effects of intravitreal dexamethasone on concentration of intravitreal vancomycin in experimental methicillin-resistant Staphylococcus epidermides endophthalmitis. Antimicrob Agents Chemother. 1991;35:1298-302.

123. Shah GK, Stein JD, Sharma S, et al. Visual outcomes following the use of intravitreal steroids in the treatment of postoperative endophthalmitis. Ophthalmology. 2000;107:486-9.

124. Coats MI, Peyman GA. Intravitreal corticosteroids in the treatment of exogenous fungal endophthalmitis. Retina. 1992;12:46-51.

125. Hasany SM, Basu PK, Kazden JJ. Production of corneal ulcer by opportunistic and saprophytic fungi. Can J Ophthalmol. 1973;8:119-31.

126. Cottingham AJ, Forster RK. Vitrectomy in endophthalmitis: results of study using vitrectomy, intraocular antibiotics, or a combination of both. arch Ophthalmol. 1976;94:2078-81.

127. Peyman GA, Raichand M, Bennett TO, et al. Management of endophthalmitis with pars plana vitrectomy. Br J Ophthalmol. 1980;64:472-5.

128. Talley AR, D'Amico DJ, Talamo JH, et al. The role of vitrectomy in the treatment of postoperative bacterial endophthalmitis: an experimental study. Arch Ophthalmol. 1987;105:1699-702.

129. Diamond JG. Intraocular management of endophthalmitis. A systematic approach. Arch Ophthalmol. 1981;99:96-9.

130. Doft BH. The Endophthalmitis Vitrectomy Study. Arch Ophthalmol. 1991; 109:487-9.

131. Doft BH, Wisniewski SR, Kelsey SF, et al. Diabetes and postoperative endophthalmitis in the Endophthalmitis Vitrectomy Study. Arch Ophthalmol. 2001;119:650-6.

132. Doft BM, Kelsey SF, Wisniewski SR, for the Endophthalmitis Vitrectomy Study Group. Retinal detachment in the Endophthalmitis Vitrectomy Study. Arch Ophthalmol. 2000;118:1661-5.

133. Olson JC, Flynn HW Jr, Forster RK, et al. Results in the treatment of postoperative endophthalmitis. Ophthalmology. 1983;90:692-9.

134. Doft BH, Kelsey SF, Wisniewski SR, the EVS Study Group. Additional procedures after the initial vitrectomy or tap-biopsy in the endophthalmitis vitrectomy study. Ophthalmology. 1998;105:707-16.

135. Bohigan GM, Olk RJ. Factors associated with a poor visual result in endophthalmitis. Am J Ophthalmol. 1986;101:332-4.

136. Mao LK, Flynn HW Jr, Miller D, et al. Endophthalmitis caused by streptococcal species. Arch Ophthalmol. 1992;110:798-801.

137. Horio N, Terasaki H, Yamamoto E, Miyake Y. Electroretinogram in the diagnosis of Endophthalmitis after intraocular lens implantation. Am J Ophthalmol. 2001;132:258-9.

138. Kim IT, Park SK, Lim JH. Inflammatory response in experimental Staphylococcus and Pseudomonas endophthalmitis. Ophthalmologica. 1999;213:305-10.

139. Stevens SX, Jensen HG, Jett BD, et al. A hemolysin-encoding plasmid contributes to bacterial virulence in experimental Enterococcus faecalis endophthalmitis. Invest Ophthalmol Vis Sci. 1992;33:1650-6.

CHAPTER 65

Delayed Postoperative IOL Opacification

Suresh K Pandey, Liliana Werner, Andrea M Izak, David J Apple

INTRODUCTION

It has been over 50 years since Harold Ridley's first implant and the cataract-intraocular lense (IOL) procedure has reached an extraordinarily high level of quality and performance. Still complications like IOL opacification do occur **(Figure 65.1)**.

DELAYED OPACIFICATION OF POLYMETHYLMETHACRYLATE (PMMA) IOL OPTIC BIOMATERIAL: "SNOWFLAKE" OR CRYSTALLINE OPACIFICATION

Over the past 50 years PMMA has been rightly considered a safe, tried and true material for IOL manufacturing with good and high quality control. PMMA biomaterial was used as an optic biomaterial in Sir Harold Ridley's original IOL, manufactured by Rayner Intraocular lenses Ltd, London, UK, and first implanted in 1949-1950.[1] Although surgeons in the industrialized world and in selected areas in the developing world have largely transitioned to foldable IOL biomaterials, PMMA does remain in widespread use in many regions. Biomaterial studies on PMMA IOL optics were rarely required. Until now, any untoward complications such as PMMA-optic material alteration/breakdown have not been seen with this material and its fabrication.

However, the author has recently reported gradual but progressive late postoperative alteration/destruction of PMMA optic biomaterial causing significant decrease in visual acuity, sometimes to a severity that requires IOL explantation **(Figure 65.2)**. The first clinical case of the type that the author observed was a documentation of photographs sent by David Davis, MD, of Hayward, CA, in 1993. He noted "crystalline" formations in 7 IOPTEX Research (Azuza, CA) 3-piece PMMA IOLs. Over the past four years, 25 cases including nine explanted IOLs were submitted to Center for Research on Ocular Therapeutics and Biodevices **(Figure 65.2)**.[2,3]

All of the explanted IOLs were 3-piece posterior chamber (PC)-IOLs with rigid PMMA optical components and blue polypropylene or extruded PMMA haptics. These had been implanted in the early 1980s to early 1990s in most cases and the clinical symptoms appeared late postoperatively, 8–15 years after the implantation. The clinical, gross, light and electron microscopic profiles of all the cases showed almost identical findings, differing only in the degree of intensity of the "snowflake" lesions that in turn reflected the severity and probably the duration of the opacification. In the early stages of many of the cases, the lesions were first noted clinically by a routine slit-lamp examination, in the absence of visual disturbances. Most examiners described the white-brown opacities within the IOL optics as "crystalline deposits" **(Figure 65.3)**. They appeared to progress gradually in most cases. Clinically, the slowly progressive opacities of the IOL optics usually start as scattered white-brown spots within the substance of the IOL optic. These usually do not have an impact on the patients' veterans administration (VA). They gradually increase in intensity and number, eventually reaching a point where the VA loss necessitates removal or exchange

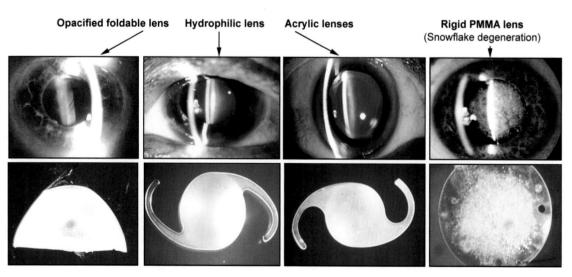

Opacified foldable lens **Hydrophilic lens** **Acrylic lenses** **Rigid PMMA lens**
(Snowflake degeneration)

FIGURE 65.1: Opacification of rigid and foldable lenses

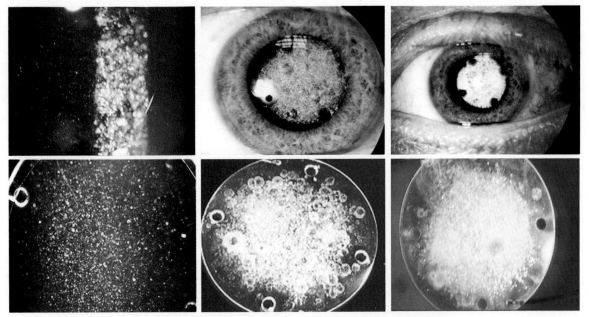

FIGURE 65.2: "Snowflake" opacification of PMMA IOLs

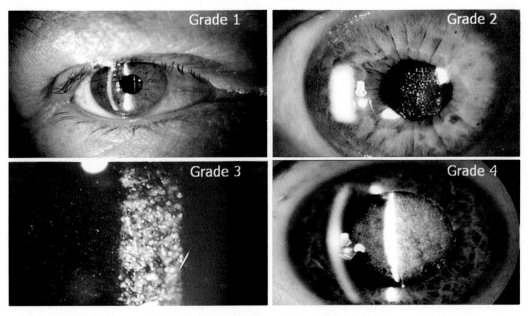

FIGURE 65.3:. Classification of "Snowflake" lesion*

of the IOL. In addition to visual loss, the symptoms included decrease in contrast sensitivity and various visual disturbances and aberrations, including glare. **Figure 65.3** presents the classification of snowflake lesions as proposed by Apple et al.[2,3]

CLINICOPATHOLOGICAL STUDY OF EXPLANTED LENSES

The opacities of the IOL optics may start as scattered white-brown spots within the substance of the IOL optic and remain stable or slowly progressive. Some may gradually increase in intensity and numbers, eventually reaching a point where a visual acuity loss may necessitate removal or exchange of the IOL. Besides visual loss, there were

other symptoms such as decrease in contrast sensitivity as well as various visual disturbances and aberrations, including glare. In early stages there was usually no effect on Snellen visual acuity but a gradual decrease of visual acuity was noted in the late stage of the process. Associated systemic disorders were not described. Metabolic imbalances have not been implicated as pathogenetic factors. Because the lesions invariably appeared years later in a very late postoperative period, there is almost certainly no direct connection between the opacities and substances used intraoperatively. In the examinations, the author performed to identify the nature of the deposits, including Energy dispersive spectroscopy (EDS). The authors did not document any exogenous chemicals apart from elements present in PMMA itself (carbon, oxygen).

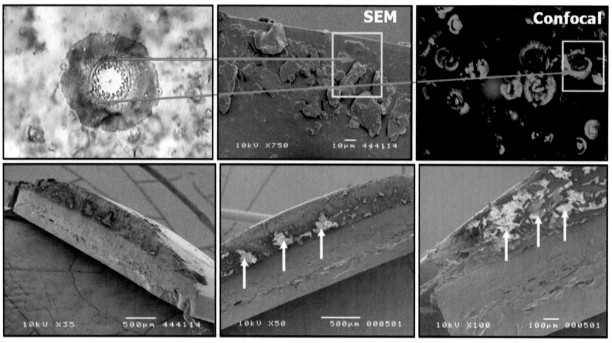

FIGURE 65.4: "Snowflake" lesions of PMMA IOL: microscopic, ultrastructural appearance

High power three-dimensional light microscopy (**Figure 65.4**, top left) and SEM (**Figure 65.4** top middle) of the surfaces of bisected IOL optics were the most informative examinations with regard to determining the structure of the opacifications. The term "snowflake" applies best to the clinical and low power microscopic appearance of each lesion (**Figure 65.4**, top left). High power examination revealed that the lesions are spherical or stellate, the shape depending on the contour of the surrounding pseudocapsule (**Figure 65.4**). The interior of the sphere does not appear to contain fluid.

To date, there have not been any clinicopathologic reports on this complication nor any hypotheses regarding its pathogenesis. The author suggests that manufacturing variations in some lenses fabricated in the 1980s and early 1990s may be responsible. It is possible that the late change in the PMMA material process is facilitated by long-term ultraviolet (UV, solar) exposure. This is supported by two pathologic observations. First, many opacities have been indeed clustered in the central zone of the optic, extending to mid-peripheral portion but often leaving the distal peripheral rim free of the opacities. This observation would support the hypothesis that the slow and sometimes progressive lesion formation noted here might relate to the fact that the IOL's central optic is exposed to ultraviolet radiation over an extended period, whereas the peripheral optic may be protected by the iris. Furthermore, the opacities are present most commonly and intensely within the anterior one-third of the optics substance (**Figure 65.4,** bottom). Since the anterior strata of the optic are the first to encounter the ultraviolet light, this might explain why the opacities are seen more frequently in this zone.

Since it is plausible that the lesions may be ultraviolet-induced, and it is highly unlikely that nonporous PMMA allows an entrance of aqueous into the optic substance, the author postulates that the lesions are "dry" and that the PMMA disruption might be related to a specific manufacturing problem that eaves the optic susceptible to damage.

- PMMA is manufactured by polymerization of the methylmethacrylate (MMA) monomer. This manufacturing process utilizes many different polymerization techniques and various components, such as UV absorbers and initiators. Therefore, various impurity profiles are possible. An initiator substance starts such process. A frequently used initiator is azo-bis-isobutyryl nitrile (AIBN).[4-6] It is possible that UV radiation is a contributing factor, however, the exact pathogenesis can as of now only be hypothesized. Potential causes of a snowflake lesion include:
- Insufficient post-annealing of the cured PMMA polymer
- Excessive thermal energy during the curing process leaving voids in the polymer matrix
- Nonhomogeneous dispersement of the UV chromophore and/or thermal initiator into the polymer chain
- Poor filtration of the pre-cured monomeric components (MMA, UV blocker, thermal initiator).

Another possible pathogenic factor could be an inadvertent use of excessive initiator substance during the polymerization process that may facilitate the formation of the snowflake lesions. The N=N bond of the AIBN initiator may be disrupted by gradual UV exposure with a release of nitrogen gas (N_2). Such gas formation can be caused by either heat or UV light exposure. Indeed the normal polymerization process for PMMA synthesis consists in part of a heat-induced N_2 formation as a byproduct. During normal polymerization, the N_2 escapes from the mixture. However, with a poor manufacturing process, e.g. using excessive initiator more than the fractional amount required unwanted initiator may be entrapped in the PMMA substance. Slow release of gaseous N_2 within the PMMA substance trigged by long-term UV exposure would explain the formation of the cavitations within the "snowflake" lesions. The outer "pseudocapsule" might consist of PMMA, whereas the central space contains the N_2 gas admixed with convoluted material also possibly consisting of degenerated PMMA. There is nothing in the molecular structure of the PMMA that in and of itself could be compressed to form such an expansile material that might create the round circular cavitations of the snowflake lesions.

These hypothetical mechanisms have the potential to form microheterogeneity within the PMMA polymer that, over time and potentially with exposure to UV radiation, could result in a lesion within the polymer. Additional experimentation is necessary to determine if any of these proposed mechanisms for the formation of a "snowflake" lesion are realized.

Awareness of this delayed complication may be warranted in developing countries, where PMMA IOLs are still used in the majority of cases. Virtually all IOLs manufactured today appear to be satisfactory. However, one should always be aware that some early IOLs from American manufacturers, including some described in this report, have been delivered to the developing world over the years, sometimes implanted without regard to expiration dates on the packaging. It would be very unfortunate to see this complication showing up in underprivileged areas where patients have almost no recourse to treat visual loss/ blindness of this type.

The emergence of this complication could have represented a true disaster, except for the fact that many of the patients implanted with these IOLs are now deceased. However, there is probably still sufficient number of patients living with varying stages of this complication. This necessitates that today's ophthalmologists to be aware of, to diagnose, and to know when not to explant and/or exchange these lenses. It is important to know the nature of this syndrome in order to spare by now elderly patients and their doctors unwarranted anxiety about the cause of his or her visual problems/loss and also to obviate request for unwarranted diagnostic testing.

OPACIFICATION OF FOLDABLE HYDROPHILIC ACRYLIC LENSES

INTRODUCTION

Small incision cataract surgery with implantation of foldable lenses has evolved significantly over the past two decades. Presently, available foldable intraocular lens (IOL) biomaterials include silicone, hydrophobic acrylic and recently introduced hydrophilic acrylic or hydrogel materials. Foldable hydrophilic acrylic intraocular lenses

(IOLs), also known as hydrogel lenses are not yet available in the United States but have been marketed by several firms for several years in international markets. Most of the currently available hydrophilic acrylic lenses are manufactured from different copolymers acrylic with water contents ranging from 18 to 28%, and an incorporated UV absorber.[6,7] They are packaged in a vial containing distilled water or balanced salt solutions (BSS), thus being already implanted in the hydrated state and in their final dimensions. Hydration renders these lenses flexible, enabling the surgeons to fold and insert/inject them through small incisions. Many surgeons have adopted the use of hydrophilic acrylic IOLs because of their easier-handling properties and biocompatibility.[8,9] Although hydrophilic surfaces have been shown to lower the inflammatory cytological response to the IOL,[9] some currently available hydrophilic acrylic IOL designs have been associated to reports on late postoperative opacification caused by calcium precipitation.[10-35] Postoperative opacification of the foldable hydrophilic acrylic lens designs is a major concern among surgeons and manufacturers. The majority of cases are reported from Asia, Australia, Canada, Europe, Latin America and South Africa.

In the later section of the chapter on IOL opacification, the author describes the analyses performed in the laboratory on hydrophilic acrylic lenses of three major designs during past three years (**Figure 65.5**). They were all explanted because of whitish discoloration of the optic component or of the whole lens, related to different forms and degrees of dystrophic calcification. (Werner L, Apple DJ, Pandey SK. Late postoperative opacification of hydrophilic intraocular lens designs; presented at the ASCRS Symposium on Cataract, IOL and Refractive Surgery, Best Paper of the Session, San Diego, CA, April 28, 2001; Pandey SK, Werner L, Apple D, Kaskaloglu MM, Izak AM, Cionni RJ). Intraocular lens opacification, second prize in the category Intraocular Lenses at the ASCRS/ Alcon Annual Video Festival, Congress of the American Society of Cataract and Refractive Surgeons, Philadelphia, PA, USA.

Figure 65.6 illustrates the first group of explanted hydrophilic acrylic lenses analyzed because whitish discoloration was represented by the Bausch and Lomb Surgical (Rochester, NY). Hydroview[TM] IOL.

Figure 65.7 represents the second group of the SC60B-OUV[TM] lens, which is another hydrophilic IOL to be recently associated with clinically significant postoperative optic opacification. The manufacturer and distributor of this design is Medical Developmental Research (MDR Inc, Clearwater, FL). The clinical characteristics of these lenses were different from the previously described "granularity" covering the optical surfaces of the Hydroview™ design. The clinical appearance of the SC60B-OUV[TM] lenses was that of a clouding similar to a "nuclear cataract".

Figure 65.8 represents the explanted Aqua-Sense™ lenses, manufactured by Ophthalmic Innovations

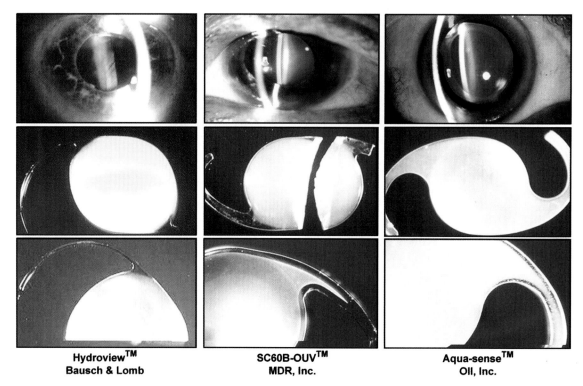

Hydroview™
Bausch & Lomb

SC60B-OUV™
MDR, Inc.

Aqua-sense™
OII, Inc.

FIGURE 65.5: Hydrophilic acrylic lens designs presented with delayed postoperative opacification

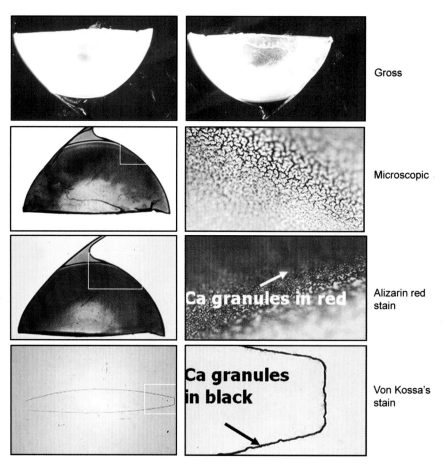

Gross

Microscopic

Alizarin red stain

Von Kossa's stain

FIGURE 65.6: Hydroview™ IOL: microscopic and histochemical evaluation

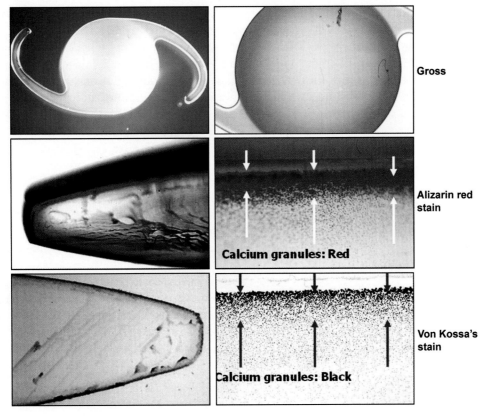

FIGURE 65.7: SC60B-OUV™ IOL: microscopic and histochemical evaluation

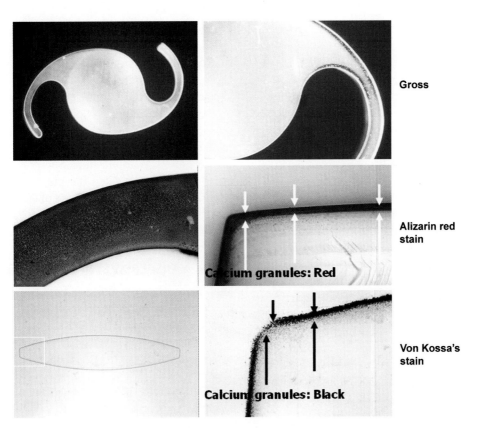

FIGURE 65.8: AQUA-SENSE™ IOL: microscopic and histochemical evaluation

International, Inc, (OII), Ontario, CA, USA.[34,35] The clinical appearance of the Aqua-Sense™ lenses was also that of a clouding similar to a "nuclear cataract". As with the two above-mentioned designs, neodymium-doped yttrium aluminium garnet (Nd: YAG) laser was performed in some cases in an attempt to "clean" the optical surfaces, without success.

CLINICOPATHOLOGICAL ANALYSES

The explanted hydrogel IOLs were submitted by several ophthalmic surgeons from various countries (Australia, China, Sweden, Egypt, Germany, South Africa, Turkey, UK and others) for pathological analysis. Gross (macroscopic) analysis of the explanted IOLs was performed and gross pictures were taken using a camera (Nikon N905 AF, Nikon Corporation, Tokyo, Japan) fitted to an operating microscope (Leica/Wild MZ-8 Zoom Stereomicroscope, Vashaw Scientific, Inc, Norcross, GA, USA). The unstained lenses were then microscopically evaluated and photographed under a light microscope (Olympus, Optical Co. Ltd., Japan). They were rinsed in distilled water, immersed in a 1% alizarin red solution (a special stain for calcium) for 2 minutes, rinsed again in distilled water and re-examined under the light microscope.[35-38]

The author then performed full thickness sections through the optic of the explanted lenses. Some of the resultant cylindrical blocks were directly stained with 1% alizarin red. Calcium salts stain in dark brown with this technique.[35-38] Some lenses in each group were air-dried at room temperature for seven days, sputter-coated with aluminum and examined under a JEOL JSM 5410LV scanning electron microscope (SEM) equipped with a Kevex X-ray detector with light element capabilities for Energy dispersive X-ray analyses (EDS). Incisional biopsies of conjunctiva and iris were also obtained from one patient during removal and exchange of a Hydroview™ IOL.[18] This was done in order to rule out the presence of dystrophic calcification in those tissues.

Figures 65.6 to 65.8 summarized the gross, microscopic and histochemical findings in three different types of opacified explanted foldable hydrophilic lenses manufactured by the Bausch and Lomb, Medical Developmental Research (MDR) and OII Inc, respectively. **Figure 65.6** illustrates the deposits on the surfaces of the Hydroview™, IOLs stained positive with alizarin red in all cases (**Figure 65.6**). Sagittal histological sections through the optic of this lens design stained using von Kossa's method showed a continuous layer of dark brown, irregular granules on the anterior and posterior optical surfaces, and the edges of the lenses (**Figure 65.6**). Histochemical evaluations of the conjunctival and iris biopsies obtained from one of the patients were negative.

Alizarin red staining of the surfaces of the SC60B-OUV™ lenses was in general negative. Analysis of the cut sections (sagittal view) of the lens optics revealed multiple granules of variable sizes in a region beneath the external

anterior and posterior surfaces of the IOLs. The granules were distributed in a line parallel to the anterior and posterior curvatures of the optics. They stained positive with alizarin red (**Figure 65.7**). Sagittal histological sections stained with the von Kossa method also confirmed the presence of multiple dark brown/black granules mostly concentrated in a region immediately beneath the anterior and posterior optical surfaces (**Figure 65.7**).

Staining with alizarin red revealed spots of granular deposits on the external surfaces of the Aqua-Sense™ lenses (**Figure 65.8**). In some cases, a fine granularity was covering the lenses' external surfaces. Analysis of cut sections (sagittal view) of the lens optic revealed multiple granules of variable sizes in a region beneath the external anterior and posterior surfaces of the IOLs. As with the previous lens design, the granules were distributed in a line parallel to the anterior and posterior curvatures of the optics and they stained positive with alizarin red and the von Kossa method (**Figure 65.8**).

SCANNING ELECTRON MICROSCOPY (SEM)

Figure 65.9 summarized the ultrastructural findings in three different types of opacified explanted foldable hydrophilic lenses manufactured by the Bausch and Lomb, MDR and OII Inc, respectively. The aspect of the three lens designs observed under light microscopy was confirmed by SEM. Analyses of the anterior optical surfaces of some Hydroview™ lenses revealed granular deposits composed of multiple spherical-ovoid globules, scattered in some areas, and confluent in others (**Figure 65.9**). SEM analysis of cut sections (sagittal view) of the optic of some SC60B-OUV™ lenses confirmed that the region immediately subjacent to the IOLs' outer surfaces as well as the central area of the optical cut sections were free of deposits. This also revealed the presence of the granules in the intermediate region beneath the anterior and posterior surfaces (**Figure 65.9**). With the Aqua-Sense™ lenses, SEM of the anterior surface revealed the presence of small granular deposits (**Figure 65.9**). Analyses of cut sections of this lens design demonstrated features similar to those described with the SC60B-OUV™ lens (**Figure 65.9**).

ENERGY DISPERSIVE X-RAY SPECTROSCOPY (EDS)

With the three lenses designs, EDS performed precisely on the deposits revealed the presence of calcium and phosphate peaks (**Figure 65.9**). The EDS was also performed on areas free of deposits to serve as controls, showing only peaks of carbon and oxygen (**Figure 65.9**).

LATE POSTOPERATIVE OPACIFICATION OF CIBA VISION MEMORY® LENS

The author recently reported clinical, pathologic, histochemical, ultrastructural, and spectroscopic analyses of memory lens intraocular lenses (IOLs) explanted from patients who had visual disturbances caused by postope-

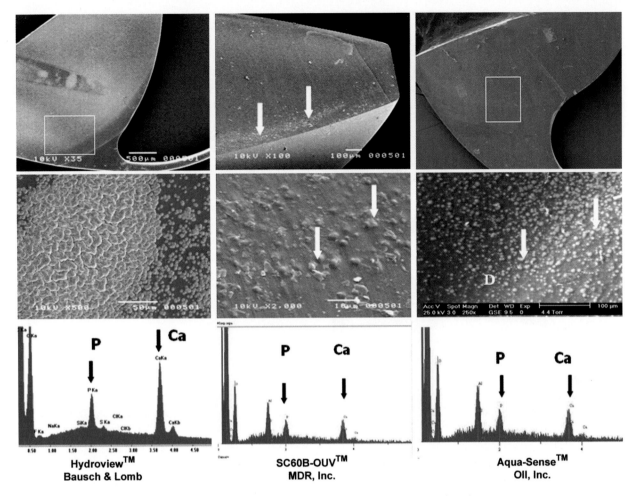

FIGURE 65.9: Opacified hydrogel lenses: ultrastructural evaluation

rative opacification of the lens optic (Neuhann I, Werner L, Pandey SK, et al. Opacification of the Memory Lens, presented at the ASCRS Symposium on Cataract, IOL, and Refractive Surgery, San Diego, CA, May 2004, USA). A total of 106 hydrophilic acrylic IOLs of the same design explanted from 106 different patients **(Figures 65.10 and 65.11)**. All patients had decreased visual acuity at presentation approximately 2 years after cataract surgery, associated with a whitish fine granularity on the optical surfaces of the IOLs. The explanted IOLs were submitted to the John A Moran Eye Center and were examined under light microscopy, histochemically, and with scanning electron microscopy (SEM) equipped with an EDS with light element capabilities **(Figures 65.10 and 65.11)**. The IOLs were examined for distribution, structure, and composition of the deposits causing opacification of their optic components. The average interval between lens implantation and opacification was 25.8 ± 11.9 months. The most frequently associated medical and ophthalmic conditions were diabetes and glaucoma. However, some patients did not have any pre-existing medical or ophthalmic conditions. Most of the IOLs had been implanted in 1999 and 2000. Microscopic analyses revealed the presence of multiple fine, granular deposits of variable sizes on the anterior and posterior optic surfaces, especially on the

anterior surface **(Figures 65.10 and 65.11)**. The deposits stained positive for calcium. The EDS confirmed the presence of calcium and phosphate within the deposits. In conclusion, late postoperative opacification due to surface deposit formation in a series of 106 Memory Lens® IOLs. The deposits were probably caused by an altered surface energy, which under certain circumstances, allowed adsorption of proteins with the deposition of calcium on top of the protein film. Further studies should be undertaken to evaluate the possible interactions of biomaterials with their surroundings, as well as their stability in biological systems over time, as theoretically no material might be spared from the complication of calcification.

OPACIFICATION OF THE SILICONE LENSES

Recently, some cases of silicone intraocular lens (IOL) opacification (SI-40NB, AMO Inc.) were reported **(Figures 65.12 and 65.13)**. The opacification was observed on the first postoperative day in all cases, who had phacoemulsification between April and June 2003. The appearance of the silicone IOLs ranged from milky gray to a yellow hue and affected the entire optical component homogeneously **(Figures 65.12A to D)**. The patients did not complain about their vision, and visual acuity was only slightly affected; three of the four patients had a best

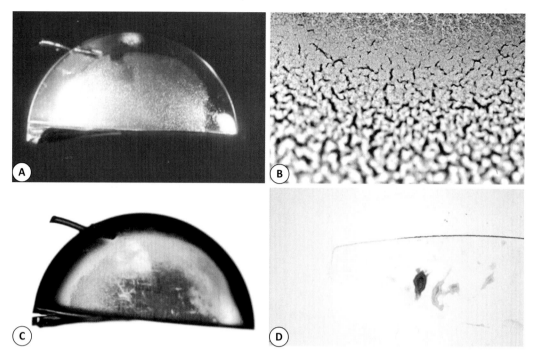

FIGURES 65.10A TO D: Opacification of memory IOL: gross and histochemical evaluation

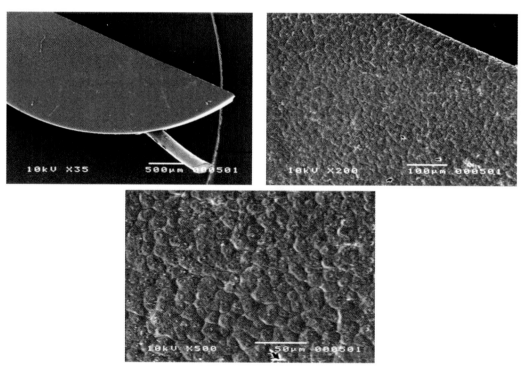

FIGURE 65.11: Opacification of memory IOL: ultrastructural evaluation

corrected visual acuity of 20/30, and no anterior chamber reaction was observed. Contrast sensitivity was reduced in all cases.

The author recently became aware of cases in which IOLs, analyzed elsewhere became cloudy *in vivo*, apparently after exposure to aerosol fumigants prior to implantation **(Figure 65.13).** One explanted lens was sent for chemical analysis by gas chromatography/ mass spectrometry. The key finding was the presence of a chemical in the cloudy lens that was not present in a control lens. The chemical was not used in the IOL manufacturing process but was, however, the primary nonaqueous component in a disinfectant solution used in the operating theater at the site that submitted the lens for evaluation. Laboratory studies were subsequently conducted on clear IOLs by exposing them to gaseous diffusion from a disinfectant solution. These lenses became cloudy upon immersion in water. This supports the hypothesis that

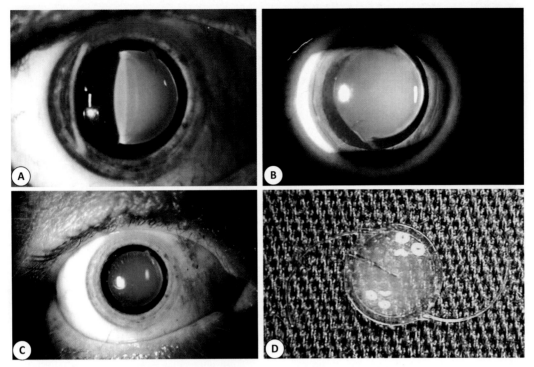

FIGURES 65.12A TO D: Opacification of silicone (AMO SI40) IOL

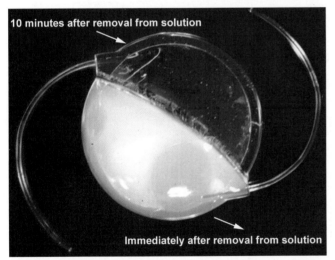

10 minutes after removal from solution

Immediately after removal from solution

FIGURE 65.13: Opacification of AMO SI40 IOLs: gross evaluation

environmental conditions are capable of producing unexpected changes in IOLs during storage and that this may impact how the lenses behave when exposed to the aqueous environment of the eye. Most IOLs are enclosed in semipermeable packages to allow sterilization by ethylene oxide gas. This may also unexpectedly allow other aerosolized chemicals to seep into the unopened package and come into contact with the lens inside. Storage facilities and operating theaters that are sprayed with aerosolized disinfectants, insecticides, cleaning solutions or other volatile chemicals may be inadvertently introducing chemicals through the package and onto the lenses. As a general precautionary measure, all IOLs should be stored in a clean, dry environment, at room temperature, and be protected from potentially harmful fumigant sprays.

PREVENTION AND TREATMENT

The opacification described in the author's reports have an entirely different appearance than classic posterior capsule opacification or anterior lens epithelial cell proliferation.

Excessive Nd:YAG laser treatment, in an attempt to clean the optical surfaces of the lenses may jeopardize implantation of a new lens in the capsular bag after explantation of the opacified lens. The adherence of the deposits to the optical surfaces of the lenses seems to be extremely strong and Nd: YAG laser treatment was proven to be ineffective in the cleaning of the lenses' surfaces. The cause of this condition seems to be multifactorial, and until the pathogenic mechanism is not fully clarified, explantation and exchange of the IOL is the only available treatment.

Surgeons usually face two important challenges during explantation of these opacified lenses. Firstly, fibrosis along the capsulorhexis edge and secondly the capsular adhesions around the lens haptics. A few radial incisions may be helpful to increase the rhexis diameter and to remove the capsular flap. It is very important to well viscodissect the lens from the capsular bag, in order to liberate any adherence to this structure. The lens is removed after being folded inside the eye bisected or intact through a larger incision. The status of the capsular bag should then be carefully inspected, which will influence the decision about the site for fixation of the new lens. Methods for the prevention of this condition are also not completely defined to date. Long-term clinical studies will determine the efficacy of modifications performed on IOL polymers and packaging for prevention of lens calcification.

SUMMARY

Each hydrophilic acrylic IOL design available in the market is manufactured from a different copolymer acrylic. To the best of our knowledge, the calcification problem described in this text cannot be generalized to all of the lenses in this category. The incidence of IOL explantation because of calcification remains low, much less than 1% in each of the three groups described here. The mechanism is not fully understood, but it does not seem to be directly related to substances used during the surgery as it occurred in the late postoperative period. Also, the substances used during the surgery were not the same in all cases. The majority of the patients involved had an associated systemic disease; therefore, the possibility of a patient-related factor, such as a metabolic imbalance cannot be ruled out.

A lot of history, component history, process changes, surgical setting and techniques, environmental factors, pre-existing patients' conditions and packaging have been examined. It is now important to carefully follow clinical outcomes of these lens designs, in order to assure that this phenomenon will disappear, following the changes in polymer source or packaging.

ACKNOWLEDGMENT

The authors would like to thank all the ophthalmic surgeons around the world for submitting the explanted rigid PMMA and hydrogel intraocular lenses for pathological analysis at the David J Apple, MD, Laboratory for Ophthalmic Devices Research, Moran Eye Center, Salt Lake City, Utah, USA.

KEY POINTS

- The opacities of the IOL optics may start as scattered white-brown spots within the substance of the IOL optic and remain stable or slowly progressive. Some may gradually increase in intensity and numbers, eventually reaching a point where a visual acuity loss may necessitate removal or exchange of the IOL.
- In addition to visual loss, the reported symptoms included decrease in contrast sensitivity and various visual disturbances and aberrations, including glare.
- Surgeons usually face two important challenges during explantation of these opacified lenses. Firstly, fibrosis along the capsulorhexis edge and secondly the capsular adhesions around the lens haptics.
- The IOL can be removed after being folded inside the eye, bisected or intact through a larger incision.
- Methods for the prevention of this condition are also not completely defined to date.

REFERENCES

1. Ridley NHL. Artificial intraocular lenses after cataract extraction. St Thomas Hospital Reports. 1951;7:12-4.

2. Apple DJ, Peng Q, Arthur SN, et al. Snowflake degeneration of polymethyl methacrylate (PMMA) posterior chamber intraocular lens optic material: a newly described clinical condition caused by an unexpected late opacification of PMMA. Ophthalmology. 2002;109(9):1666-75.

3. Peng Q, Apple DJ, Arthur SA, et al. "Snowflake" opacification of poly(methyl methacrylate) intraocular lens optic biomaterial: a newly described syndrome. Int Ophthalmol Clin. 2001; 41(3):91-107.

4. Park JB. Biomaterials: an introduction. New York: Plenum Press; 1979. pp. 88-91.

5. Sugaya H. Sakai Y. Polymethylmethacrylate: from polymer to dialyzer. Contrib Nephrol. 1999;125:1-8.

6. Christ FR, Buchen SY, Deacon J, et al. Biomaterials used for intraocular lenses. In: Wise DL, et al (Eds). Encyclopedic Handbook of Biomaterials and Bioengineering. New York: Marcel Dekker Inc; 1995. p. 1277.

7. Chehade M, Elder MJ. Intraocular lens materials and styles: a review. Aust N Z J Ophthalmol. 1997;25(4):255-63.

8. Schauersberger J, Kruger A, Abela C, et al. Course of postoperative inflammation after implantation of 4 types of foldable intraocular lenses. J Cataract Refract Surg. 1999; 25(8): 1116-20.

9. Hollick EJ, Spalton DJ, Ursell PG. Surface cytologic features on intraocular lenses: can increased biocompatibility have disadvantages? Arch Ophthalmol. 1999;117(7):872-8.

10. Chang BYP, Davey KG, Gupta M, et al. Late clouding of an acrylic intraocular lens following routine phacoemulsification. Eye(Lond). 1999;13(Pt 6):807-8.

11. Murray RI. Two cases of late opacification of the hydroview hydrogel intraocular lens. J Catract Refract Surg. 2000;26(9): 1272-3.

12. Fernando GT, Crayford BB. Visually significant calcification of hydrogel intraocular lenses necessitating explantation. Clin Experiment Ophthalmol. 2000;28(4):280-6.

13. Apple DJ, Werner L, Escobar-Gomez M, et al. Deposits on the optical surfaces of Hydroview™ intraocular lenses. J Cataract Refract Surg. 2000;26(6):796-7.

14. Werner L, Apple DJ, Escobar-Gomez M, et al. Postoperative deposition of calcium on the surfaces of a hydrogel intraocular lens. Ophthalmology. 2000;107(12):2179-85.

15. Izak AM, Werner L, Pandey SK, et al. Calcification on the surface of the Bausch & Lomb Hydroview™ intraocular lens. Int Ophthalmol Clin. 2001;41(3):63-77.

16. Apple DJ, Werner L, Pandey SK. Newly recognized complications of posterior chamber intraocular lenses. Arch Ophthalmol. 2001;119(4):581-2.

17. Pandey SK, Werner L, Apple DJ, et al. Hydrophilic acrylic intraocular lens optic and haptics opacification in a diabetic patient: Bilateral case report and clinicopathological correlation. Ophthalmology. 2002;109(11):2042-51.

18. Pandey SK, Werner L, Apple DJ, et al. Calcium precipitation on the optical surfaces of a foldable intraocular lens: a clinicopathological correlation. Arch Ophthalmol. 2002;120(3): 391-3.

19. Yu AK, Shek TW. Hydroxyapatite formation on implanted hydrogel intraocular lenses. Arch Ophthalmol. 2001;119(4): 611-4.

20. Yu AK, Kwan KY, Chan DH, et al. Clinical features of 46 eyes with calcified hydrogel intraocular lenses. J Cataract Refract Surg. 2001;27(10):1596-606.

21. Groh JMM, Schlotzer-Schrehardt U, Rummelt C, et al. Postoperative Kunstlinsen-Eintrubungen bei 12 Hydrogel-Intraokularlinsen (Hydroview). Klin Monatsbl Augenheilkd. 2001; 218:645-8.

22. Shek TW, Wong A, Yau B, et al. Opacification of artificial intraocular lens: an electron microscopic study. Ultrastruct Pathol. 2001;25(4):281-3.

23. Buchen SY, Cunanan CM, Gwon A, et al. Assessing intraocular lens calcification in an animal model. J Cataract Refract Surg. 2001; 27(9):1473-84.

24. Frohn A, Dick B, Augustin AJ, et al. Late opacification of the foldable hydrophilic acrylic lens SC60B-OUV. Ophthalmology. 2001;108(11):1999-2004.

25. Mamalis N. Hydrophilic acrylic intraocular lenses. J Cataract Refract Surg. 2001;27:1339-40.

26. Werner L, Apple DJ, Kaskaloglu M, et al. Dense Opacification of the optical component of a hydrophilic intraocular lens: a clinicopathological analysis of 9 explanted lenses. J Cataract Refract Surg. 2001;27(9):1485-92.

27. Macky TA, Trivedi RH, Werner L, et al. Degeneration of UV absorber material and calcium deposits within the optic of a hydrophilic IOL lens. Int Ophthalmol Clin. 2001;41(3):79-90.

28. Apple DJ, Werner L, Pandey SK. Opalescence of hydrophilic acrylic lenses. Eye. 2001;15:97-8.

29. Izak AM, Werner L, Pandey SK, et al Opacification of modern foldable hydrogel intraocular lens designs. Eye. 2003.

30. Sharma TK, Chawdhary S. The opalescence of hydrogel intraocular lens. Eye(Lond). 2001;15(Pt 1):97-8.

31. Sharma A, Ram J, Gupta A. Late clouding of an acrylic intraocular lens following routine phacoemulsification. Eye. (Lond) 2001;15(Pt 3):362.

32. Woodruff SA, Khan J, Dhingra N, et al. Late clouding of an acrylic intraocular lens following routine phacoemulsification. Eye (Lond). 2001;15(Pt 3):361-2.

33. Pavlovic S, Magdowski G, Brueckel B,et al. Ultrastructural analysis of opacities seen in a hydrophilic acrylic intraocular lens. Eye (Lond). 2001;15(Pt 5):657-9.

34. Werner L, Apple DJ, Izak AM. Discoloration/opacification of modern foldable hydrogel intraocular lens designs. In: Buratto L, Zanini R, Apple DJ, Werner L (Eds). Phacoemulsification, Principles and Techniques. Thorofare NJ: Slack Inc; 2002; 659-70.

35. Werner L, Izak AM, Apple DJ, et al. Complete calcification of a hydrogel lens design: case reports and clinicopathological correlation. Am J Ophthalmol, 2003.

36. McGee-Russell SM. Histochemical methods for calcium. J Histochem Cytochem. 1958;6(1):22-42.

37. Carr LB, Rambo ON, Feichtmeir TV. A method of demonstrating calcium in tissue sections using chloranilic acid. J Histochem Cytochem. 1961;9:415-7.

38. Pizzolato P. Histochemical recognition of calcium oxalate. J Histochem Cytochem. 1964;12:333-6.

39. Jensen MK, Crandall AS, Mamalis N, et al. Crystallization on intraocular lens surfaces associated with the use of Healon GV. Arch Ophthalmol. 1994;112(8):1037-42.

40. Olson RJ. New cases of crystalline deposits on intraocular lenses not related to any specific viscoelastic. Arch Ophthalmol. 1995;113(10):1229.

41. Olson RJ, Caldwell KD, Crandall AS, et al. Intraoperative crystallization on the intraocular lens surface. Am J Ophthalmol. 1998;126(2):177-84.

42. Amon M, Menapace R. Cellular invasion on hydrogel and poly(methyl methacrylate) implants: An in vivo study. J Cataract Refract Surg. 1991;17(6):774-9.

43. Amon M, Menapace R. In vivo observation of surface precipitates of 200 consecutive hydrogel intraocular lenses. Ophthalmologica. 1992;204(1):13-8.

44. Bucher PJM, Buchi ER, Daicker BC. Dystrophic calcification of an implanted hydroxyethylmethacrylate intraocular lens. Arch Ophthalmol. 1995;113(11):1431-5.

45. Ullman S, Lichtenstein SB, Heerlein K. Corneal opacities secondary to Viscoat®. J Cataract Refract Surg. 1986;12(5): 489-92.

46. Binder PS, Deg JK, Kohl FS. Calcific band keratopathy after intraocular chondroitin sulfate. Arch Ophthalmol. 1987; 105(9):1243-7.

47. Jensen OA. Ocular calcifications in primary hyperparathyroidism. Histochemical and ultrastructural study of a case. Comparison with ocular calcifications in idiopathic hypercalcemia of infancy and in renal failure. Acta Ophthalmol (Copenh). 1975;53(2):173-86.

48. Pandey SK, Thakur J, Werner L, et al. Classification, clinical applications and complications of ophthalmic viscosurgical devices: an update. In: Garg A, Pandey SK (Eds). Textbook of Ocular Therapeutics. New Delhi, India: Jaypee Brothers; 2002. pp. 392-407.

49. Gasset AR, Lobo L, Houde W. Permanent wear of soft contact lenses in aphakic eyes. Am J Ophthalmol. 1977;83(1):115-20.

50. Winder AF, Ruben M, Sheraidah GA. Tear calcium levels and contact lens wear. Br J Ophthalmol. 1977;61(8):539-43.

51. Levy B. Calcium deposits on glyceryl methyl methacrylate and hydroxyethyl methacrylate contact lenses. Am J Optomet Physiol Opt. 1984;61(9):605-7.

52. Bowers RWJ, Tighe BJ. Studies in the ocular compatibility of hydrogels: a review of the clinical manifestations of spoilation. Biomaterial. 1987;8(2):83-8.

53. Bowers RWJ, Tighe BJ. Studies of the ocular compatibility of hydrogels: white spot deposits: chemical composition and geological arrangement of components. Biomaterial. 1987;8(3):172-6.

54. Tripathi RC, Tripathi BJ, Silverman RA, et al. Contact lens deposits and spoilage: identification and management. Int Ophthalmol Clin. 1991;3(2):91-120.

55. Dhaliwal DK, Mamamlis N, Olson RJ, et al. Visual significance of glistenings seen in the AcrySof intraocular lens. J Cataract Refract Surg. 1996;22(4):452-7.

56. Omar O, Pirayesh A, Mamalis N, et al. In vitro analysis of AcrySof intraocular lens glistenings in AcryPak and Wagon Wheel Packaging. J Cataract Refract Surg. 1998;24(1):107-13.

57. Anderson C, Koch DD, Green G, et al. Alcon AcrySof™ acrylic intraocular lens. In: Martin RG, Gills JP, Sanders DR, (Eds). Foldable Intraocular Lenses. Thorofare, NJ: Slack; 1993.pp. 161-77.

58. Milauskas AT. Silicone intraocular lens implant discoloration in humans. Arch Ophthalmol. 1991;109(7):913-5.

59. Watt RH. Discoloration of a silicone intraocular lens 6 weeks after surgery. Arch Ophthalmol. 1991;109(11):1494-5.

60. Koch DD, Heit Le. Discoloration of silicone intraocular lenses. Arch Ophthalmol. 1992;110(3):319-20.

Explanting a Posterior Chamber Intraocular Lens

Thomas A Oetting

INTRODUCTION

Occasionally, an intraocular lens (IOL) must be removed. The IOL may have simply been of the wrong power or not tolerated due to glare or dysphotopsia. The IOL may have opacified with time; or most commonly, the IOL may have become unstable or subluxed due to progressive zonular laxity.[1] Removing an IOL can be difficult, especially if it has been in place for several years. The first step to explant an IOL is to free the IOL from its capsular adhesions. Then the IOL when free, is pulled from the eye using the smallest wound which allows safe removal.

INDICATIONS FOR IOL EXPLANTATION

Dr Nick Mamalis and his colleagues at the University of Utah, in great service to ophthalmology, have periodically collected surveys of explanted IOLs to allow analysis of this procedure and its indications.[1] In his latest survey, the indications for IOL explantation depend on the type of IOL (**Table 66.1**) but in general, IOL explantation is most commonly performed for a dislocated or decentered IOL. The strategy for and the issues surrounding explantation differ depending on the reason for explantation.

TABLE 66.1	IOL explantation by IOL type (From Mamalis 2007[1])	
IOL type	**Primary explantation indication**	**Percent of IOLs explanted**
Single piece acrylic	Dislocation/decentration	24%
Multifocal acrylic	Visual aberration	23%
3-piece silicon	Visual aberration	20%
3-piece acrylic	Incorrect IOL power	19%
Single piece silicon	Dislocation/decentration	6%

INCORRECT POWER IOL

In many ways, the simplest indication for IOL explantation comes when the wrong power of IOL is placed. It may be difficult to explain to the patient when an error has been made by the surgical team which resulted in placing the wrong power of IOL; but the actual surgery is relatively easy. The surgery is straightforward as the surgeon typically detects that the wrong IOL power was placed early in the postoperative period. As such, the capsular bag is not

excessively adherent to the IOL which allows one to easily free the IOL from the capsule which is often the most difficult part of the explantation procedure.

Jin, Crandall, and Jones prepared a nice series of cases where the wrong power of IOL was placed. They showed that the most common reason for placing the wrong power of IOL was incorrect estimation of the corneal power, followed by incorrect axial eye length (AEL), followed by simply placing the incorrect IOL.[2] The time from original surgery to the exchange varied from 1 day to 14 months with an average of 2.6 months.[2] Following exchange in their series, 95% of patients had a best corrected visual acuity of better than 20/40.[2] Another option in patients with the wrong power IOL is to use refractive corneal surgery rather than lens exchange.[3]

VISUAL ABERRATION

Visual aberrations such as glare disturbances, halos, and dysphotopsia are a common indication for IOL explantation, especially with multifocal IOLs.[1] Unlike the situation where the wrong power IOL is placed, the decision to remove the IOL with visual aberrations is often delayed as the surgeon waits for symptoms to resolve.[4] As a result, removing these lenses can be difficult as the capsule may be adherent to the optic and more importantly to the haptics. In addition, it can be difficult to determine if the symptoms are related to the IOL, the wound or the posterior capsule.

Davison reported on a large series of acrylic IOLs and described the positive and negative dysphotopsia with these popular square edge optic high refractive index IOLs.[5] However, these visual aberrations have been associated with most all of the IOLs in use now including even the rounded 3-piece silicon IOLs.[1] Vámosi reported on several cases of negative dysphotopsia and noted that in three cases that required lens exchange, the one-third with replacement of the IOL into the bag had continued symptoms whereas the two-thirds where the replacement lens was placed in the sulcus has cessation of symptoms.[6]

Multifocal IOLs explantation is especially associated with visual aberrations. Galor reported on a series of 10 dissatisfied patients that had 12 IOL exchange procedures removing presbyopic IOLs, most of which were multifocal.[7] Eight of ten patients were satisfied following the procedure, but two continued to report symptoms that included blurred vision, decreased contrast sensitivity and glare or halos.[7]

INAPPROPRIATE IOL IN THE SULCUS

The perfect IOL for sulcus placement has a large optic (6 mm or greater), large thin haptics (13 mm or greater) and smooth anterior optic surface to lessen iris irritation. In addition, avoiding silicon may be of some benefit if the patient is at risk for the future placement of silicon oil or an air fluid exchange during pars plana vitrectomy, as the silicon lenses can cloud with these procedures.

Unfortunately, not all IOLs placed in the sulcus are suited for sulcus placement. The popularity of single piece acrylic (SPA) IOLs has led some to place SPA IOLs in the sulcus either inadvertently or when presented with an intraocular complication such as a posterior capsular tear. Dr David Chang and the cataract clinical committee of the American society of cataract and refractive surgery (ASCRS) reported on a series of patients with poorly placed SPA IOLs.[8] In this series, at least one of the SPA haptics was in the sulcus. These thick square edged haptics in the sulcus led to a variety of problems including chronic uveitis, glaucoma and hemorrhage.

The surgical strategy for eliminating the problems associated with SPA IOLs in the sulcus involves removing the thick SPA haptic from the sulcus, by either repositioning the IOL such that both haptics are in the capsular bag or by removing the SPA IOL and exchanging for a large 3-piece IOL better suited for the sulcus. In several cases in Chang's series of misplaced SPA IOLs, one haptic was in the bag and one was in the sulcus. In this situation, Ophthalmic viscoelastic devices (OVD) should be used to separate the haptic from the bag to allow explantation of the SPA.[8] Masket has described the technique of simply cutting off and removing only the offending sulcus based haptic when the remaining portions of the SPA IOL are firmly in the bag.[9] In some cases, one may be able to reform the capsular bag with OVD and position the sulcus haptic into its proper location in the bag.[10]

DISLOCATION/DECENTRATION IOL

The most common reason for IOL explantation is decentration or dislocation.[1] Decentration is when the IOL is in the proper plane, but not centered. Decentration, especially when it occurs early in the postoperative period, is often caused by inadvertent placement of one haptic in the sulcus and one in the bag. Occasionally, decentration can be caused by a damaged haptic, but this is less common especially with the commonly used SPA IOLs. Decentration of IOLs with both haptics placed in the sulcus is more common when the IOL haptics are too short for sulcus placement (less than 12.5 mm). Dislocation of IOLs where the IOL may also be too posterior or loose (pseudophaco-donesis) is typically caused by areas of weakened zonules which can occur even years after implantation.

Rather than explanting a decentered IOL, often the best strategy is to secure or reposition the existing IOL (**Table 66.2**). Sometimes the IOL can simply be repositioned and secured using the existing remnant of the capsule. More often the decentered IOL is freed from capsular remnants and sutured to the iris or sclera or glued to the sclera as described by Agarwal.[11] If it is possible to secure the existing IOL, this is usually the best approach, as it minimizes the trauma to the eye that comes with an exchange of the IOL.

When the iris will constrict and is not damaged, often the best strategy for a decentered IOL is to suture the IOL to the iris. Stark nicely described this technique using a McCannel suture to attach the peripheral iris to the 3-piece IOL haptic.[12] Chang described a modification of this procedure using a Siepser sliding knot for fixation of the iris to the haptics.[13] However, in order to suture the IOL to the iris, the IOL must be a 3-piece IOL and must be free in the sulcus. If the IOL is in the bag, it is difficult to suture in the bag and must be freed from the capsular bag prior to suturing to the iris.

One of the most difficult situations which the anterior segment surgeons face is present when the IOL is in the bag, but the bag itself is loose. This situation seems to be more common as one operates sooner on patients and as they live longer. This is especially noted in patients with pseudoexfoliation, uveitis, trauma or other conditions with weakened zonules. The surgeon has three choices in this situation:
1. Suture the IOL and the bag to the sclera
2. Remove the IOL from the bag and secure the IOL only to the sclera or iris
3. Or finally to explant the IOL.

The choice depends on the type of IOL, the amount of residual lens material in the capsular bag with the IOL and the age of the patient. In older patients with lots of residual lens material, it may make the most sense to suture the IOL to the sclera.[12] In younger patients with a SPA IOL, it may make more sense to simply remove the IOL and place an anterior chamber IOL through a 6.0 mm wound.

STRATEGIES TO FREE THE IOL FROM THE CAPSULE

The ease of IOL removal is mostly dependent on how long the IOL has been in the bag. IOLs which have been in the bag for a few weeks, such as when the wrong IOL is placed, are very easy to free from the bag. IOLs that have been in the bag for years, such as with opacified IOLs, can be very hard to remove. Removing an IOL with an intact posterior capsule is far easier than when the patient has had an yttrium aluminum garnet (YAG) posterior capsulotomy. When the IOL is in the sulcus, it is typically not adherent to the capsule and can easily be removed.

The first step to free the IOL from the bag is to somehow get a dissection plane started between the IOL and the capsule. The author likes to use a viscous and dispersive OVD (e.g. Viscoat) especially when the posterior capsule is not intact. With IOLs that have been in place for a while (e.g. more than a year) the author suggests using a 27-gauge needle attached to the viscoat syringe and to use the sharp end of the needle to get under the capsule and then inject

TABLE 66.2 IOL decentration

IOL Location	Typical cause of decentration	Explantation strategy	Secure existing IOL strategy
Both haptics in secure capsular bag	Capsular phimosis Damaged haptic Both haptics are not really in bag	Free IOL from capsule and remove IOL	Free IOL from capsule and suture to iris
Both haptics in loose capsular bag(dislocation)	Zonular weakness	Remove capsule and IOL through large incision Free IOL from capsule and remove IOL	Suture IOL/capsule to sclera Free IOL from capsule suture to iris Free IOL from capsule Suture/glue to sclera
3-piece IOL One haptic in bag one in sulcus	Not placed properly	Free optic and one haptic from capsule and remove IOL	Free optic and haptic from bag and leave in sulcus
SPA IOL One haptic in bag one in sulcus	Not placed properly	Free optic and one haptic from capsule and remove IOL	Separate capsule and place both haptics in bag
3-piece IOL Both haptics in sulcus	IOL too small Zonular weakness	IOL is usually free	Suture IOL to iris Glue IOL to sclera (Agarwal technique) Suture IOL to sclera
SPA Both haptics in sulcus	Not placed properly	IOL is usually free	Separate capsule and place both haptics in bag

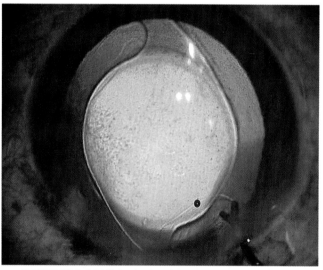

FIGURE 66.1: PC IOL in the bag (*Courtesy:* Dr Agarwal's Eye Hospital, India)

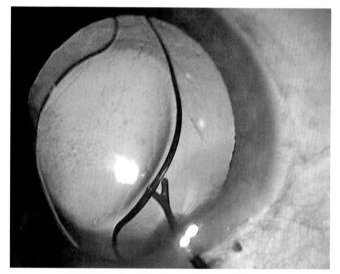

FIGURE 66.2: PC IOL brought out of the bag (*Courtesy:* Dr Agarwal's Eye Hospital, India)

the OVD to start the dissection (**Figure 66.1**). Sometimes the author will use the microforceps (such as the MST Duet microforceps) to lift the capsule to allow a cannula to get access under the anterior chamber which allows vigorous viscodissection (**Figure 66.2**). The author also likes to use a flat hydrodissection cannula attached to the OVD syringe for viscodissection, as the flat surface of the cannula makes it easier to get between the capsule and the IOL yet still allows for vigorous flow of the OVD.

When freeing the IOL, most of the attention should be directed to freeing up the haptics with the viscodissection. If the posterior capsule is intact, the OVD will often track around the optic which makes freeing the optic of its posterior

attachments fairly easily. However, freeing the haptics can often be very difficult. One should use generous OVD dissection to separate the anterior and posterior capsule in the area of the two haptics and carry the viscodissection as posterior as possible. When one thinks one has freed the capsular adhesions to the haptics, it is to try to spin the IOL clockwise to allow the haptics to work free of the capsule. Sometimes the haptics are just too stuck and must be cut to free the IOL (**Figure 66.3**). One can simply leave the cut haptic in the bag and remove the remainder of the IOL. Sometimes the cut haptics will come out more easily without the optic as one will have a better angle for removing it through the dissected portion of the capsular leaflets.

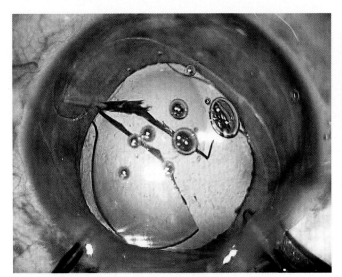

FIGURE 66.3: PC IOL cut so that it can then be explanted
(*Courtesy:* Dr Agarwal's Eye Hospital, India)

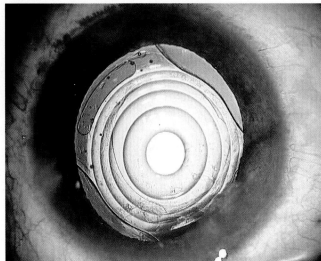

FIGURE 66.4: Multifocal IOL in the bag
(*Courtesy:* Dr Agarwal's Eye Hospital, India)

TABLE 66.3 Removing IOLs

IOL type	Removal technique	Example
AcrySof®SPA	Refold in anterior chamber Henderson technique Cut in anterior chamber	SN60WF SA60AT
AcrySof® Multifocal acrylic	Refold in anterior chamber Cut in anterior chamber	MA60AT
Other acrylic	Cut in anterior chamber	AR40
3-piece silicon	Cut in anterior chamber	SI30
Single piece silicon	Cut in anterior chamber	Plate haptic
PMMA	Enlarge wound to 6.0 mm	

STRATEGIES TO REMOVE THE IOL

The IOL can be removed through a small incision (refolding or cutting) or by extending the incision to the size of the optic (**Figures 66.1 to 66.3 and Table 66.3**).

The high index of refraction acrylic IOLs (e.g. MA60, SA60, IQ) can be refolded within the eye, either using the folding forceps or the Henderson technique. The standard refolding technique uses a paracentesis across from the main wound (3.5 mm) to introduce a spatula to place under the optic, while using an open IOL insertion forceps above the optic in the anterior chamber. While lifting with the spatula and coming down on top of the optic with the open insertion forceps, the IOL can be folded in the anterior chamber (**Figure 66.4**). Once folded, the IOL is simply removed through a 3.5 mm or so wound. It is important of course to place OVD above and below the IOL during the refolding process. Refolding the IOL only works well with thin acrylic IOLs like the single piece and multipiece Alcon AcrySof® IOLs and in the author's hands, is virtually impossible with thick acrylic IOLs like the AR40 and the slippery IOLs like the silicon 3-piece IOLs.

An interesting refolding technique comes from Henderson (Bonnie Henderson Ophthalmic Consultants of Boston) for folding high index of refraction (i.e. thin) acrylic SPA such as the Alcon SN60WF IQ. Dr Henderson's technique is to simply pull on an externalized haptic (with 0.12 or similar toothed forceps) through a 2.5–3.0 mm wound while pushing on the optic180 across from the wound (inside the eye) with a hook (e.g. Kuglen). For some reason, amazingly and almost magically, the IOL folds itself and pops out of the eye.[14]

There are several ways to cut an IOL to get the optic small enough to remove through a small incision (**Figures 66.4 to 66.8**). One classic technique is to only cut about two-thirds through the IOL and make what looks like a "Pac Man" and rotate the IOL out through the wound. Another technique is to simply cut the IOL completely in half or into thirds and bring out the pieces. The author likes to use the Osher mildly serrated cutter from Duckworth and Kent. One can usually keep the IOL from flopping around too much by holding the externalized haptic with this cutter. Sometimes the author will use a Duet micro forceps (MST) through a paracentesis to hold the IOL, while cutting it through the main incision to make sure the IOL tilting does not cause corneal damage (**Figure 66.5**). MST also makes an IOL cutting scissor than can be used though a paracentesis. If one is in a bind, one can even use Vanna scissors to cut most IOLs.

Polymethyl methacrylate (PMMA) IOLs are harder to cut than silicon or acrylic IOLs. In general for these PMMA IOLs such as AC IOLs and CZ70 sutured IOLs, the author would suggest making a short scleral tunnel and removing the IOL in one piece. As always, one wants to place a lot of OVD above and below the IOL while removing it. As one is already making a large incision to remove the IOL, placing an AC IOL will be easy in this situation.

EXPLANTING A POSTERIOR CHAMBER INTRAOCULAR LENS

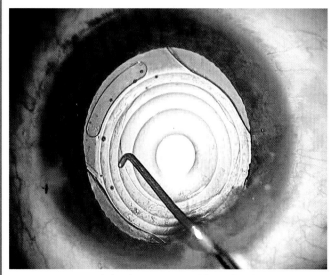

FIGURE 66.5: Multifocal IOL separated from the rhexis margins (*Courtesy:* Dr Agarwal's Eye Hospital, India)

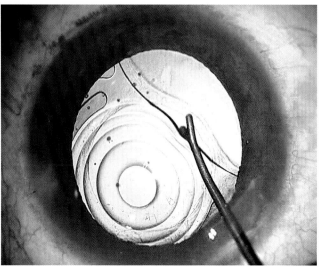

FIGURE 66.6: Multifocal IOL manipulated out of the bag (*Courtesy:* Dr Agarwal's Eye Hospital, India)

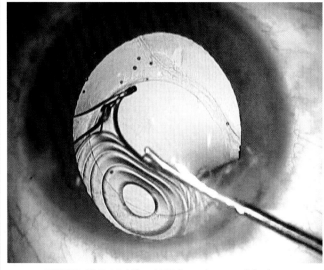

FIGURE 66.7: Multifocal IOL brought out of the bag (*Courtesy:* Dr Agarwal's Eye Hospital, India)

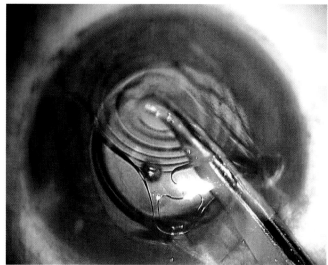

FIGURE 66.8: Another new IOL put in the bag. Then the multifocal IOL is cut. This way the new IOL prevents the scissor from damaging the posterior capsule (*Courtesy:* Dr Agarwal's Eye Hospital, India)

SUMMARY

IOL explantation techniques are important to master for anterior segment surgeons. The indications for IOL removal include implantation of the wrong power IOL, visual aberrations (e.g. halos, glare, and dysphotopsia) and most commonly decentration/dislocation. In general, if the existing IOL can be secured or repositioned that is preferable to IOL exchange. Explantation of the IOL from the capsular bag gets more difficult with time as the capsule becomes more adherent especially to the haptics. The IOL can be removed from the eye with a small incision by folding or cutting the IOL or simply can be removed through a large incision.

REFERENCES

1. Mamalis N, Brubaker J, Davis D, et al. Complications of foldable intraocular lenses requiring explantation or secondary intervention-2007 survey update. J Cataract Refract Surg. 2008;34(9):1584-91.
2. Jin GJ, Crandall AS, Jones JJ. Intraocular lens exchange due to incorrect lens power. Ophthalmology. 2007;114(3):417-24.
3. Jin GJ, Merkley KH, Crandall AS, et al. Laser in situ keratomileusis versus lens-based surgery for correcting residual refractive error after cataract surgery. J Cataract Refract Surg. 2008;34(4):562-9.
4. Osher RH. Negative dysphotopsia: long-term study and possible explanation for transient symptoms. J Cataract Refract Surg. 2008;34(10):1699-707.
5. Davison JA. Positive and negative dysphotopsia in patients with acrylic intraocular lenses. J Cataract Refract Surg. 2000;26(9):1346-55.
6. Vámosi P, Csákány B, Németh J. Intraocular lens exchange in patients with negative dysphotopsia symptoms. J Cataract Refract Surg. 2010;36(3):371-2.
7. Galor A, Gonzalez M, Goldman D, et al. Intraocular lens exchange surgery in dissatisfied patients with refractive intraocular lenses. J Cataract Refract Surg. 2009;35(10):1706-10.

8. Chang DF, Masket S, Miller KM, et al. ASCRS Cataract Clinical Committee. Complications of sulcus placement of single-piece acrylic intraocular lenses: Recommendations for backup IOL implantation following posterior capsule rupture. J Cataract Refract Surg. 2009;35(8):1445-58.

9. Masket S. Personal Communication, 2009.

10. Oetting TA. (2010). Pseudoamaurosis. [online] Available from http://www.facebook.com/cataract.surgery?v=app_2392950137&ref=ts#!/video/video.php?v=227256076140, [Accessed on 6/22/2010].

11. Kumar DA, Agarwal A, Prakash G, et al. Glued posterior chamber IOL in eyes with deficient capsular support: a retrospective analysis of 1-year postoperative outcomes. Eye (Lond). 2010;24(7):1143-8.

12. Stutzman RD, Stark WJ. Surgical technique for suture fixation of an acrylic intraocular lens in the absence of capsule support. J Cataract Refract Surg. 2003;29(9):1658-62.

13. Chang DF. Siepser slipknot for McCannel iris-suture fixation of subluxated intraocular lenses. J Cataract Refract Surg. 2004;30(6):1170-6.

14. Oetting TA. (2010). Remove IOL ala Henderson", [online] Available from http://www.facebook.com/cataract.surgery?v=app_2392950137&ref=ts#!/video/video.php?v=264444166140. [Accessed 6/22/2010].

CHAPTER 67

Posterior Capsular Opacification

Suresh K Pandey, Liliana Werner, David J Apple, Andrea M Izak

INTRODUCTION

Posterior capsular opacification (PCO, secondary cataract, after cataract) is a nagging complication of cataract-intraocular lens (IOL) surgery since the beginning of extracapsular cataract extraction (ECCE) and IOL implantation. PCO needs to be eliminated since deleterious sequelae of this complication occur and Neodymium: Yttrium Aluminum Garnet (Nd:YAG) laser treatment now constitutes a major and unnecessary financial burden on the health care system. A successful expansion of ECCE-IOL surgery in the developing world depends on eradication of PCO, since patient follow-up is difficult and access to the Nd:YAG laser is not widely available. Advances in the surgical techniques, IOL designs/biomaterials have been instrumental in gradual, and unnoticed decrease in the incidence of the PCO. The author strongly believes that the overall incidence of PCO and hence the incidence of Nd:YAG laser posterior capsulotomy is now rapidly decreasing from rates as high as 50% in the 1980s-early 1990s to less than 10% in the developed World. The author's two decades of active research and information derived from other experimental and clinical studies from several other centers have revealed that the tools, surgical procedures, skills and appropriate IOLs designs are now available to significantly reduce this complication.

BACKGROUND

Opacification of the posterior capsule caused by post-operative proliferation of cells in the capsular bag remains the most frequent complication of cataract-intraocular lens surgery.[1,2] In addition to classic posterior capsular opacification (PCO, secondary cataract, after cataract), postoperative lens epithelial cell (LEC) proliferation is also involved in the pathogenesis of anterior capsular opacification/fibrosis (ACO) and interlenticular opacification (ILO).[3-6] Secondary cataract (PCO) has been recognized since the origin of extracapsular cataract surgery (ECCE) and was noted by Sir Harold Ridley in his first IOL implantations.[7,8] It was particularly common and severe in the early days of IOL surgery (in late 1970s and early 1980s) when the importance of cortical cleanup was less appreciated. Through the 1980s and early 1990s, the incidence of PCO ranged between 25–50%.[9] PCO is a major problem in pediatric cataract surgery where the incidence approached 100%.[10-12]

One of the crowning achievements of modern cataract surgery has been a gradual, almost unnoticed decrease in the incidence of this complication. The author's data at present show that with modern techniques and IOLs, the expected rate of PCO and the need for subsequent Neodymium: Yttrium Aluminum Garnet (Nd:YAG) laser posterior capsulotomy rate is decreasing to single digit (less than 10%).[13,14]

REASONS TO ERADICATE POSTERIOR CAPSULAR OPACIFICATION

Although cataract is the most common cause of blindness in the world, after-cataract (PCO or secondary cataract) is an extremely common cause as well. Jan GF Worst has stated—"the most meaningful development in intraocular implant research in the next five years will be effective prevention of secondary cataract formation (International Intraocular Implant Club Report, Vol. 1, No. 2, January 1999)". Eradication of PCO following ECCE has major medical and financial implications:

- Nd:YAG laser secondary posterior capsulotomy, can be associated with significant complications. Potential problems include IOL optic damage/pitting, postoperative intraocular pressure elevation, cystoid macular edema, retinal detachment and IOL subluxation.[15-18]
- Dense PCO and secondary membrane formation is particularly common following pediatric IOL implantation.[10-12] A delay in diagnosis can cause irreparable amblyopia.
- PCO represents a significant cost to the US health care system. Nd:YAG laser treatments of almost one million patients per year have cost up to $250 million annually.[9]
- A posterior capsulotomy can increase the risk of posterior segment complications in high myopes and patients with uveitis, glaucoma and diabetic retinopathy.
- PCO of even a mild degree can decrease near acuity through a multifocal IOL, and may interfere with the function of refractive/accommodating IOL designs.
- A significant incidence of PCO means that cataract surgery, alone, may not restore lasting sight to the 25 million people worldwide who are blind from cataract.[19]
- Finally, a successful expansion of ECCE-IOL surgery in the developing world depends on eradication or at least diminishing of PCO, since patient follow-up is difficult and access to the Nd:YAG laser is not widely available.[19]

ETIOPATHOGENESIS

In the normal crystalline lens, the lens epithelial cells (LECs) are confined to the anterior surface at the equatorial region and the equatorial lens bow. This single row of cuboidal cells can be divided into two different biological zones (**Figure 67.1**):

- The anterior-central zone (corresponding to the zone of the anterior lens capsule) consists of a monolayer of flat cuboidal, epithelial cells with minimal mitotic activity. In response to a variety of stimuli, the anterior epithelial cells ("A" cells) proliferate and undergo fibrous metaplasia. This has been called "pseudofibrous metaplasia" by Font and Brownstein.[20]
- The second zone is important in the pathogenesis of "pearl" formation. This layer is a continuation of anterior lens cells around the equator, forming the equatorial lens bow ("E" cells). Unlike within the A-cell layer, cell mitosis division and multiplication are quite active in this region. New lens fibers are continuously produced in this zone throughout life.

In addition to classic PCO, postoperative LEC proliferation is also involved in the pathogenesis of other entities, such as anterior capsular opacification/fibrosis (ACO)[3,4] and interlenticular opacification(ILO); a more recently described complication related to piggyback IOLs.[5,6] Thus, there are three distinct anatomic locations within the capsular bag where clinically significant opacification may occur postoperatively (**Figure 67.1**). Ophthalmic researchers are now developing surgical techniques/devices not only to eliminate PCO, but also to eliminate capsular bag opacification, secondary to proliferation of LECs.

Although both types of cells (from the anterior central zone and from the equatorial lens bow) have the potential to produce visually significant opacification, most cases of classic PCO are caused by proliferation of the equatorial cells. The term posterior capsular opacification implies that the capsule opacifies. Rather, an opaque membrane develops over the capsule as retained cells proliferate and migrate onto the posterior capsular surface.

The opacification usually takes one of two morphologic forms. One form consists of capsular pearls, which can consist of clusters of swollen, opacified epithelial "pearls" or clusters of posteriorly migrated equatorial epithelial (E) cells (bladder or Wedl cells). It is probable that both LEC types can also contribute to the fibrous form of opacification. Anterior epithelial (A) cells are probably important in the pathogenesis of fibrosis PCO, since the primary type of response of these cells is to undergo fibrous metaplasia. Although the preferred type of growth of the equatorial epithelial (E) cells is in the direction of bloated, swollen, bullous-like bladder (Wedl) cells, these also may contribute to formation of the fibrous form of PCO by undergoing a fibrous metaplasia. This is a particularly common occurrence in cataracts in developing world settings where cataract surgery has been delayed for many years, and where posterior subcapsular cataracts have turned into fibrous plaques.[21]

Capsulorhexis contraction (capsular phimosis) is an important complication related to extreme fibrous proliferation of the anterior capsule.[2-4] Capsular phimosis can be avoided by not making the capsulorhexis too small. In general, a diameter less than 5.0 mm is undesirable.

In contrast to the lesions of the anterior (A cells) capsule that cause phenomena related to fibrosis, the E cells of the equatorial lens bow tend to form cells that differentiate toward pearls (bladder cells) and cortex. Equatorial cells (E-cells) are also responsible for formation of a Soemmering's ring. The Soemmering's ring, a dumb-bell or donut shaped lesion that often forms following any type of rupture of the anterior capsule, was first described in connection with ocular trauma. The pathogenetic basis of a Soemmering's ring is rupture of the anterior lens capsule with extrusion of nuclear and some central lens material. The extruded cortical remnants then transform into Elschnig pearls. It is not widely appreciated that a Soemmering's ring forms virtually every time that any form of ECCE is done, whether manual, automated or with phacoemulsification. This material is derived from proliferation of the epithelial cells (E-cells) of the equatorial lens bow. The author has noted that these cells have the capability to proliferate and migrate posteriorly across the visual axis, thereby opacifying the posterior capsule. Because the Soemmering's ring is a direct precursor to PCO, surgeons should strive to prevent its formation.

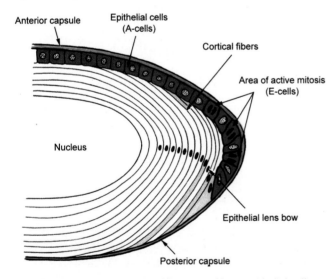

FIGURE 67.1: Postoperative proliferation of lens epithelial cells can also lead to postoperative opacification of capsular bag secondary to development of anterior capsular opacification/fibrosis (ACO) and interlenticular opacifcation (ILO)

Schematic illustration of the microscopic anatomy of the lens and the capsular bag, showing the "A" cells of the anterior epithelium and the "E" cells, the important germinal epithelial cells of the equatorial lens bow. The primary cells of origin for posterior capsular opacification (PCO) are the mitotic germinal cells of the epithelial lens bow. These cells normally migrate centrally from the lens equator and contribute to formation of the nucleus or epinucleus throughout life. In pathologic states, they tend to migrate posteriorly to form such lesions as a posterior subcapsular cataract, as well as postoperative PCO following ECCE

Cells types other than lens epithelial cells may be involved in PCO. As ECCE is always associated with some breakdown of the blood-aqueous barrier, inflammatory cells, erythrocytes and many other inflammatory mediators may be released into the aqueous humor. The severity of this inflammatory response may be exacerbated by the IOL. This foreign body elicits a three-stage immune response that involves many different cell types, including polymorphonuclear leukocytes, giant cells and fibroblasts. Collagen deposition onto the IOL and onto the capsule may cause opacities and fine wrinkles to form in the posterior capsule. In most cases, however, this inflammatory response is clinically insignificant. Iris melanocytes also have been shown to adhere to and migrate over the anterior surface of the posterior capsule.

LENS EPITHELIAL CELLS PROLIFERATION: ROLE OF GROWTH FACTORS

Cataract surgery causes major changes in the ocular environment. Not only because of breakdown of the blood aqueous barrier, as mentioned above, but also through the release/activation of endogenous cytokines and growth factors from endogenous sources during wound healing. Aqueous and vitreous humors are rich in growth and regulatory factors and there is now abundant evidence that differences in the distribution of such factors between aqueous and vitreous compartments determine normal lens polarity and growth patterns; that is, factors in the vitreous environment promote the differentiation of fiber cells whereas the aqueous factors promote epithelial differentiation and growth.[22]

The lens itself expresses members of major growth factor families and a variety of growth factor receptors and molecules involved in a range of signaling pathways.[23] Studies over the last couple of decades have mostly concentrated on identifying the factor(s) that controls the differentiation of lens epithelial cells into fibers and there is now compelling evidence that members of the fibroblast growth factors (FGF) growth factor family are required for induction of this process.[22] Recent studies have also indicated that the Wnt growth factor family plays a key role in promoting the differentiation of the epithelial sheet.[24] However, in relation to PCO, the most interesting studies have been on the transforming growth factor-beta (TGF-β) family.[25]

TGF-β is abundant in the lens, and the surrounding ocular media.[26] The effects of TGF-β on lens cells were initially studied in rats using epithelial explants and whole lens cultures. TGF-β induces lens epithelial cells to commit to a differentiation pathway that is distinct from that seen in the normal lens. In cultured lenses, TGF-β induces the formation of subcapsular opacities.[27] These correspond to plaques of spindle-shaped cells that contain α-smooth muscle actin and desmin and accumulations of extracellular matrix that include collagen types I and III, fibronectin and tenascin.[28] TGF-β also induces localized wrinkling of the capsule in epithelial explants and cultured lenses.[27,29] Similarly, overexpression of TGF-β in transgenic mice also results in the development of anterior subcapsular fibrotic plaques that grow progressively with age.[28,30] These studies clearly show that TGF-β disrupts the normal lens epithelial architecture and induces an epithelial-mesenchymal transition that is a central feature of the fibrotic growth that results in opacification and disturbed vision.

Similar patterns of aberrant growth and differentiation are found in subcapsular cataracts in humans. Following eye trauma, surgery, or associated with other disorders (e.g. atopic dermatitis and retinitis pigmentosa), anterior subcapsular cataracts (ASC) can arise.[31] These exhibit similar fibrotic changes to that described for PCO. In this form of cataract in humans, it also appears that members of the TGF-β family initiate the epithelial mesenchymal transition that is a central feature of this condition. In addition, it appears that an initial TGF-β insult induces connective tissue growth factor, TGF-β-inducible gene-H3 and other autocrine signaling pathways, including endogenous TGF-β signaling, that promotes the progressive fibrosis that leads to cataract.[25,32,33]

As TGF-β is expressed by lens cells and the ocular media have abundant supplies, TGF-β bioavailability must be tightly regulated, otherwise all lenses would develop cataract. It appears that there may be multiple levels of TGF-β regulation. For example, it is well known that TGF-β is generally produced in a latent form that requires conversion to the mature (active) form. In addition, the ocular media, particularly vitreous, normally contain molecule(s) that inhibit active TGF-β and block its cataract-inducing effects.[32] The sensitivity of lens cells to TGF-β may also be modulated by many factors. For example, studies with rats have shown that estrogen can protect the lens from TGF-β-induced cataract.[35] This is consistent with epidemiological studies that report female hormones may help prevent or slow the development of some forms of cataract.[36]

In summary, during cataract surgery many growth factors are upregulated and/or activated in the lens and the ocular media. Not only does this disturb the normal distribution and activity of factors in the aqueous and vitreous compartments that are critical for determining normal growth patterns, but additional events such as activation of latent stores of TGF-β in the ocular media result in the induction of aberrant growth and differentiation in the lens. Clearly procedures that reduce the trauma of cataract surgery will be beneficial, as this will minimize disruption of the growth factor composition in and around the lens. A better understanding of lens cell biology also opens up possibilities of introducing molecules that will effectively kill residual lens cells. In addition, blockers of TGF-β could be included in irrigation solutions during surgery, and as coatings of IOLs, to ensure that any residual lens cells do not undergo epithelial mesenchymal transition, but rather maintain a normal epithelial phenotype.

CLINICAL MANIFESTATIONS AND TREATMENT

The interval between surgery and PCO varies widely, ranging anywhere from three months to four years after the surgery. Although the causes of PCO are multifactorial, as reported in several studies,[9,37,38] there is an inverse correlation with age. Young age is a significant risk factor for PCO, and its occurrence is a virtual certainty in pediatric patients.[10-12]

Visual symptoms do not always correlate to the observed amount of PCO. Some patients with significant PCO on slit-lamp examination are relatively asymptomatic while others have significant symptoms with mild apparent haze, which is reversed by capsulotomy.[39]

Visually significant PCO usually managed by creating an opening within the opaque capsule using the Nd:YAG laser. A surgical posterior capsulotomy may be indicated in children for dense PCO associated with secondary membrane formation. The technical details, parameters, preoperative and postoperative treatments, complications and recommendations for surgical and Nd:YAG laser posterior capsulotomy are discussed in literature[15-18] and not covered in this chapter. In brief, indications for Nd:YAG laser capsulotomy include: presence of a thickened capsule leading to functional impairment of vision and the need to evaluate and treat posterior segment pathology. However, caution should be exercised if there is any signs suggestive of intraocular inflammation, raised intraocular pressure, macular edema and a predisposition to retinal detachment (e.g. high myopia). As mentioned before Nd:YAG laser posterior capsulotomy may be rarely associated with complications such as transient rise in intraocular pressure, enhanced risk of retinal detachment, which is particularly marked in axial myopia, cystoid macular edema, IOL subluxation, lens optic damage/pitting, exacerbation of local endophthalmitis and vitreous prolapse into the anterior chamber and anterior hyaloid disruption.

SURGICAL AND IMPLANT RELATED FACTORS FOR PREVENTION OF POSTERIOR CAPSULAR OPACIFICATION

Based upon the author's twenty years research experience on evaluation of 17,500 IOL related specimens (7523 human eyes obtained postmortem; 6127 eyes implanted with rigid lenses and 1396 eyes implanted with foldable lenses) using Miyake-Apple technique, and published studies from the author's Center and other Centers,[1,9,13,14,19,40-45] it is possible to review the principles of PCO prevention. These measures can be divided into two categories. One strategy is to minimize the number of retained/regenerated cells and cortex (including the Soemmering's ring) through cortical cleanup. The second strategy is to prevent the remaining cells from migrating posteriorly. The edge of the IOL optic is critical in the formation of such a physical barrier.

The author has identified three surgery-related factors and three IOL-related factors that are particularly important in the prevention of PCO (**Table 67.1**).[40-45]

Surgery-Related Factors to Reduce PCO

Hydrodissection-Enhanced Cortical Cleanup: A very important and underrated surgical step is hydrodissection. Dr I Howard Fine perfected and popularized this technique and coined the term cortical cleaving hydrodissection.[46] Until fairly recently, many surgeons had a rather fatalistic attitude regarding removal of lens cortex and cells during ECCE either manual or automated or with phacoemulsification. A common opinion was that removing all or even most equatorial cells from the bag is impossible. PCO was therefore considered an inevitable complication. This conclusion arose, in part, because PCO occurred in up to 50% of cases.

The necessary tenting up of the anterior capsule during subcapsular (or cortical cleaving) hydrodissection is best achieved by using a cannula with a bend at the tip, allowing a flow of fluid toward the capsule to efficiently separate capsule from cortex (**Figures 67.2A to C**). By freeing and rotating the lens nucleus, hydrodissection facilitates lens nucleus and cortex removal without zonular-capsular rupture.[47] The author now knows from autopsy and experimental studies that thorough cortical and cellular cleanup from the capsular bag can be accomplished in most cases.[42] Use of hydrodissection during cataract surgery allowed more efficient removal of cortex and LECs (which in turn reduces PCO), when compared to control eyes where hydrodissection was not utilized (**see Figure 67.5**).[42] A successfully performed cortical cleaving hydrodissection provides an easy way to remove the entire lens cortex as well as nucleus. Occasionally, this can even occur without the need for cortical aspiration with a separate irrigation/aspiration instrument.

Surgeons use balanced salt solution (Alcon Inc., Fort Worth, TX, USA) while performing cortical cleaving hydrodissection. Recent experimental animal studies from the author's center have shown that use of preservative-free lidocaine 1% during hydrodissection may diminish the amount of live LECs by facilitating cortical cleanup, by loosening the desmosomal area of cell-cell adhesion with decreased cellular adherence or by a direct toxic effect.[48] Corneal endothelial toxicity continues to be a major concern of using hypo-osmolar agents (to loosen the cell-cell adhesion) during hydrodissection or any step of cataract surgery, in absence of a sealed capsular bag. However, it is now possible to irrigate the entire capsular bag using an injection-molded silicone disposable innovative device known as PerfectCapsule™ (Milvella Pty. Ltd., Sydney, Australia). Sealed capsule irrigation (SCI) isolates the internal lens capsule, and facilitates removal of residual cortical material as well as lens epithelial cells, and thus prevents/delays capsular bag opacification.[49,50] The SCI technique is pioneered by one of the authors (AJM), and discussed in details in later part of this chapter.

TABLE 67.1 Factors that significantly influence the formation of PCO. Three factors are related to the type and quality of surgery and three are related to IOL biomaterial/design

3 Surgery-related factors (capsular surgery)	3 IOL-related factors (Ideal IOL)
1. Hydrodissection-enhanced cortical clean-up	1. Biocompatible IOL to reduce stimulation of cellular proliferation
2. In-the-bag fixation	2. Maximal IOL optic—posterior capsule contact with angulated haptics, "adhesive" biomaterial to create a "shrink wrap" of the capsule
3. Small capsulorhexis with anterior capsular edge on the IOL surface to sequester the capsular bag (shrink wrap the capsule around the IOL optic).	3. IOL optic geometry a square, truncated edge for 360 degrees.

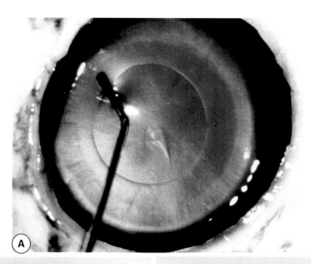

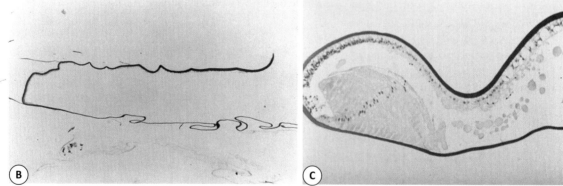

FIGURES 67 2A TO C: In the author's laboratory studies on human eyes obtained postmortem, the author was pleasantly surprised that with copious hydrodissection and meticulous cortical cleanup, most cortex and most if not all lens epithelial cells from the equator (E cells) could be removed, when compared to eyes without hydrodissection

A. Gross photograph of experimental surgery on a human cadaver eye from anterior (surgeon's) view showing the technique of subcapsular hydrodissection (cortical cleaving hydrodissection). It is to note that the 27-gauge bent cannula is immediately under the edge of the capsulorhexis

B. Photomicrograph of the lens capsular bag of one of the eye that underwent experimental cataract surgery associated with copious hydrodissection. It is to note the excellent removal of lens material and E cells a very clear capsular bag (Periodic acid-Schiff stain, original magnification 750x)

C. Photomicrograph of a sagittal view of a crystalline lens without hydrodissection in human cadaver eyes. One needs to note residual cortical material and equatorial lens epithelial cells (Periodic acid-Schiff stain, original magnification 250x)

In-the-Bag (Capsular) IOL Fixation: The hallmark of modern cataract surgery is the achievement of consistent and secure in-the-bag (capsular) fixation (**see Table 67.1**). The most obvious advantage of in-the-bag fixation is the accomplishment of good optic centration and sequestration of the IOL from adjacent uveal tissues. Numerous other advantages have been described elsewhere.[51,52] However, it is not often appreciated that this is also extremely important in reducing the amount of PCO.

One desired goal of in-the-bag fixation is enhancing the IOL optic barrier effect, which is functional and maximal when the lens optic is fully in-the-bag with direct contact with the posterior capsule. In case one or both haptics are not placed in the bag, a potential space is created, allowing an avenue for cells to grow posteriorly toward the visual axis. The reader may recall the barrier ridge IOL design devised by Kenneth Hoffer in the 1980s, which did not function sufficiently at the time.[9] The reason was not a problem with the concept or the IOLs themselves, but rather that only about 30% of posterior chamber IOLs were implanted inside the bag at the time.

With non-phaco ECCE in-the-bag fixation of IOLs occurs about 60% of the time. One explanation is that many cases combined rigid design IOLs with can-opener anterior capsulotomies. Secure and permanent in-the-bag fixation only occurred in approximately 60% of cases.[40] However, when considering modern foldable lens implantation, the number rapidly rises to over 90%. It is not the foldable IOL itself or even the small incision in and of itself that provides this positive result, but rather the fact that successful foldable IOL insertion generally requires meticulous surgery, with the necessity of performing a continuous curvilinear capsulorhexis (CCC) and secures implantation of both IOL loops in the bag.[40]

Capsulorhexis Edge on IOL Surface: A less obvious, but significant addition to precise in-the-bag fixation, is creating a CCC diameter slightly smaller than that of the IOL optic. For example, if the IOL optic were 6.0 mm, the capsulorhexis diameter would ideally be slightly smaller, perhaps 5.0–5.5 mm. This places the cut anterior capsule edge on the anterior surface of the optic, providing a tight fit (analogous to a "shrink wrap") and helping to sequester the optic in the capsular bag from the surrounding aqueous humor (**see Table 67.1**). This mechanism may support protecting the milieu within the capsule from at least some potentially deleterious factors within the aqueous, especially some macromolecules and some inflammatory mediators. The concept of capsular sequestration based on the CCC size and shape is subtle, but more and more surgeons appear to be applying this principle and seeing its advantages.

However, a recent study by Vasavada and Raj[53] suggested that with certain IOLs biomaterial such as 3-Piece AcrySof IOL, the relationship of the anterior capsule and the IOL does not seem to be a factor that relates to the development of central PCO. In a prospective, randomized, controlled trial, these authors evaluated the relationship of the anterior capsule and the AcrySof MA30BA IOL and its impact on the development of central PCO in 202 patients with senile cataracts. Patients were randomized prospectively to receive one of the three possibilities of anterior capsule and IOL optic relationship:

- Group 1: Total anterior capsule cover (360°) of the optic;
- Group 2: No anterior capsule cover (360°) of the optic;
- Group 3: Partial anterior capsule cover (<360°) of the optic.

After surgery, slit-lamp video photography was performed every six months for three years. The posterior capsule was divided into three zones: peripheral, central 3 mm and midperipheral (the space between the peripheral and the central zones). At three years, the rate of central PCO was 6.4% in group 1, 7.1% in group 2 and 5.9% in group 3 (p = 0.9). Midperipheral PCO was present in 24.2% in group 1, 16% in group 2 and 20.6% in group 3 (p = 0.9). Peripheral PCO was seen in 100% of patients in all groups. The Nd:YAG posterior capsulotomy rate was 0% in all groups. The authors concluded that there was no significant difference in the incidence of development of central PCO among the three groups.

Implant-Related Factors to Reduce PCO

In addition to the three above-mentioned surgery-related factors the author will describe briefly the three IOL-related factors, which in the author's opinion play an important role in the eradication of PCO.

IOL Biocompatibility: Lens material biocompatibility (**see Table 67.1**) is an often-misunderstood term. It can be defined by many criteria, e.g. the ability to inhibit stimulation of epithelial cellular proliferation. The less the cell proliferates, the lower the chance is for secondary cataract formation. In the author's large series of post-mortem human eyes, the Alcon AcrySof® IOLs presented with minimal to absent Soemmering's ring formation, PCO and ACO (**Figures 67.3A and B**).[1-4,13,14,41,51] In addition, the amount of cell proliferation is greatly influenced by surgical factors, such as copious cortical cleanup. Furthermore, the time factor also plays a role, such as the duration of the implant in the eye. Additional long-term studies are required to assess the overall role of "biocompatibility" in the pathogenesis of PCO.

Maximal IOL Optic-Posterior Capsule Contact: Other contributing factors in reducing PCO are posterior angulation of the IOL haptic and posterior convexity of the optic (**see Table 67.1**). This is due to the creation of a "shrink wrap", a tight fit of the posterior capsule against the back of the IOL optic. The relative "stickiness" of the IOL optic biomaterial probably helps producing an adhesion between the capsule and IOL optic. There is preliminary evidence that the hydrophobic acrylic IOL biomaterial provides enhanced capsular adhesion, or "bioadhesion".[54-56]

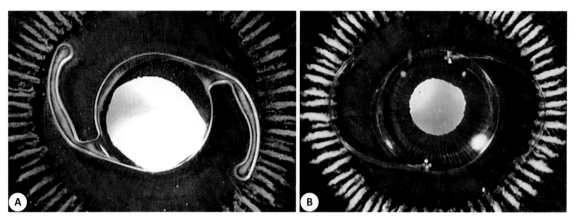

FIGURES 67.3A AND B: Among nine different types of rigid and foldable lens designs studies in psudeophakic human eyes, hydrophobic acrylic IOLs had the lowest PCO formation and therefore the Nd:YAG laser posterior capsulotomy rates. The lowest PCO score was confirmed by gross and histological evaluation

A. Human eye obtained postmortem, Miyake-Apple posterior photographic technique of a single-piece hydrophobic acrylic optic/haptics (Alcon AcrySof®) PC-IOL showing a symmetric fixation and excellent centration. The surgical technique was excellent and there is virtually no retained/regenerative material (Soemmering's ring). This obviously represents good cortical cleanup, and also suggests good biocompatibility with minimal proliferation

B. A 3-piece acrylic optic/PMMA haptics (Alcon AcrySof®) showing a good example of excellent cortical cleanup, and also suggesting good biocompatibility, with minimal cellular proliferation

RJ Linnola, proposed the sandwich theory for explanation of less PCO with hydrophobic IOL biomaterial.[54-56] According to this theory if the IOL is made of a bioactive material it would allow a single lens epithelial cell layer to bond both to the IOL and the posterior capsule at the same time. This would produce a sandwich pattern including the IOL, the cell monolayer and the posterior capsule. The sealed sandwich structure would prevent further epithelial ingrowth. The degree of bioactivity of the IOL could explain the basic difference in the incidence of PCO and capsulotomy rates with different IOL materials.

The sandwich theory was tested in pseudophakic autopsy eyes implanted with PMMA, silicone, soft hydrophobic acrylate or hydrogel IOLs. Histological sections were prepared from the capsular bag and immunohistochemical analyses were performed for fibronectin, vitronectin, laminin and collagen type IV. Results of this study suggested that soft hydrophobic acrylate IOLs had significantly more adhesion of fibronectin to their surfaces than PMMA or silicone IOLs. Also, more vitronectin was attached to hydrophobic acrylate IOLs than to the other IOL materials. Silicone IOLs had more collagen type IV adhesion in comparison to the other IOL materials studied. In histologic sections a sandwich-like structure (anterior or posterior capsule-fibronectin-one cell layer-fibronectin-IOL surface) was seen significantly more often in eyes with hydrophobic acrylate IOLs than in PMMA, silicone or hydrogel IOL eyes. These studies support the sandwich theory for PCO after cataract surgery with IOLs. The results suggest that fibronectin may be the major extracellular protein responsible for the attachment of hydrophobic acrylic IOLs to the capsular bag. This may represent a true bioactive bond between the IOL and the LECs, and between the IOL and the capsular bag. This may explain the reason for clinical observations of less PCO and lower capsulotomy rates with

the soft hydrophobic acrylate material of AcrySof® IOLs compared to the other IOL materials studied.

Barrier Effect of the IOL Optic: The IOL optic barrier effect **(Table 67.1),** plays an important role as a second line of defense against PCO, especially in cases where retained cortex and cells remain following ECCE. The concept of the barrier effect goes back to the original Ridley lens.[8] If accurately implanted in the capsular bag, it provided an excellent barrier effect, with almost complete filling of the capsular bag and contact of the posterior IOL optic to the posterior capsule ("no space, no cells"). A lens with one or both haptics "out-of-the-bag" has much less of a chance to produce a barrier effect. Indeed, the IOL optic's barrier function has been one of the main reasons that PC-IOLs implanted after ECCE throughout the decades did not produce an unacceptably high incidence of florid PCO.

A subtle difference between classic optics with a round tapered edge and optics with a square truncated edge became evident recently **(see Table 67.1).** The effect of a square-edge optic design as a barrier was first discussed by Nishi et al[57,58] in articles related to PCO. In a clinico-pathological study, the author's laboratory was the first to confirm this phenomenon in human eyes **(Figures 67.4A and B).**[32,33] The author reported results of a large histopathological analysis covering the IOL barrier effect, with special reference to the efficacy of the truncated edge **(Figures 67.4A and B).** A truncated, square-edged optic rim appears to cause a complete blockade of cells at the optic edge, preventing epithelial ingrowth over the posterior capsule.[60-67] The enhanced barrier effect of this particular edge geometry provides another supplemental factor, in addition to the five above-mentioned factors, that has significantly diminished the overall incidence of clinical PCO.

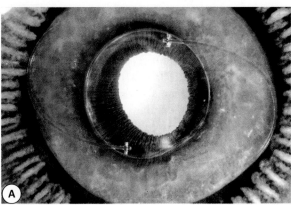
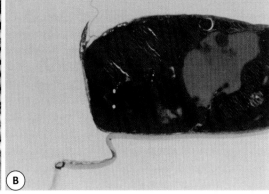

FIGURES 67.4A AND B: Even when a significant Soemmering's ring remains in the eye, a square truncated edge such as what exists on the AcrySof® IOL provides a second line of defense against cortical in growth. Other IOLs with square or truncated optic edges include the Ciba Mentor MemoryLens™, the Staar Surgical/Bausch and Lomb Surgical elastimide-polyimide silicone design, the Pfizer CeeOn Edge™ 911 silicone IOL, Advanced Medical Optics Sensar OptiEdge™ and plate haptic IOLs

A. Gross photograph from behind (Miyake-Apple posterior photographic technique) of a human eye obtained postmortem containing an AcrySof® IOL. Some cortical remnants (a Soemmering's ring) remain peripherally but the optical zone remains totally cell-free, with no encroachment of cells past the edge of the IOL optic

B. Photomicrograph of an eye in which an Alcon AcrySof® IOL was implanted. Cleanup was not complete and a Soemmering's ring resulted. However, the Soemmering's ring remnants (red) were blocked by the square optic edge, leaving the posterior capsule cell-free (Masson's trichrome stain, original magnification 100x.)

The authors past studies,[13,14] demonstrated that the original, three-piece MA60 AcrySof® (Alcon Inc., Fort Worth, TX) IOL successfully combined these three IOL-related factors **(see Table 67.1, Figures 67.3 and 67.4)** in a way that produced a major PCO advantage. Other manufacturers have begun to incorporate these PCO preventing features, such as a sharp or squared-posterior edge. The Cee-On 911™ silicone IOL (Pfizer Inc., New York, NY) was the first silicone IOL to feature a squared edge. The Sensar™ hydrophobic acrylic (Advanced Medical Optics Inc., Santa Ana, CA) and Clariflex™ silicone (Advanced Medical Optics Inc, Santa Ana, CA) IOLs now feature a sharp posterior edge, combined with a rounded anterior edge. Modification in the Centerflex® one-piece hydrpophilic IOL design (Rayner Inc., Hove East Sussex, UK) has been incorporated to prevent cellular ingrowth at the broad optic-haptic junction. The modified profile provides a square edge (barrier, ridge, wall) for 360 degrees around the lens optic (enhanced square edge), eliminating the potential defect **(Figure 67.5)**. This further minimizes the ingrowth of migrating LECs toward the visual axis.

A major disadvantage of the truncated edge is the production of clinical visual aberrations, such as glare, halos and crescents.[68] Subtle changes in manufacturing are now helping alleviate glare and other optical complications.

PHARMACOLOGICAL PREVENTION OF POSTERIOR CAPSULAR OPACIFICATION

Intraocular application of pharmacologic agents has also been investigated by several authors as a means to prevent PCO.[71-76] The idea was to selectively destroy the LECs and avoid toxic side effects on other intraocular tissues, such

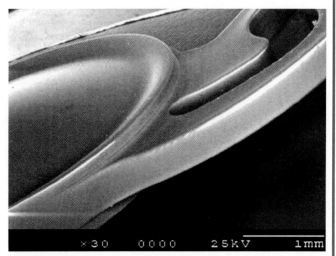

FIGURE 67.5: Scanning electron photograph obtained at the level of the optic-haptic junction of the Rayner Centerflex™ one-piece hydrpophilic IOL. This profile provides a square edge (barrier, ridge, wall) for 360 degrees around the lens optic, eliminating the potential defect. The round tapered edge of classic one-piece IOL design at the optic edge that subtends the optic-haptic junction represents a theoretical "Achilles' heel" in which when ingrowing cells may bypass the desired barrier

as the sensitive corneal endothelium. Pharmacologic agents being investigated include cancer chemotherapeutic drugs (e.g. antimetabolites such as methotraxate, mitomycin, daunomycin, 5-FU, colchicine and daunorubicin), anti-inflammatory substances, hypo-osmolar drugs and immunological agents.

The author designed an intracapsular ring to prevent capsular bag contraction and also to inhibit LECs proliferation and metaplasia by sustained release of 5-FU.[77-79] The effects of the intracapsular ring on the prevention of

PCO was prospectively studied by analyzing postmortem ocular specimens macroscopically using Miyake-Apple technique[81,82] and histologically. The author also evaluated the toxic effects of 5-FU (Fluorouracil) on the corneal endothelium, capsular bag and retina of rabbits. Results of this study suggested that implantation of intracapsular ring may prevent central PCO after cataract surgery by mechanically blocking migration of lens epithelial cells towards the central visual axis. The potential pharmacological effect of 5-FU for PCO prevention was not demonstrated in this experimental study.[77]

Toxicity to corneal endothelium and other ocular structure remains one of the major concern for using cancer chemotherapeutic drugs, anti-inflammatory substances, hypo-osmolar drugs and immunological agents, when intralenticular compartment is in direct contact with anterior chamber. However, with the development of a SCI device, it is now possible to precisely deliver the pharmacological/hypo-osmolar agents to the lens epithelial cells within the capsular bag, while minimizing the potential for collateral ocular damage.[49,50]

Sealed capsule irrigation (SCI) device may allow the isolated safe delivery of pharmacologic agents into the capsular bag following cataract surgery (**Figures 67.6A to D**).[49,50] Developed by one of the co-author (AJM), SCI is a form of Sealed Irrigation System applied to the internal eye, and may be applied elsewhere to the body. In the eye, the technique of capsular bag irrigation may be used with pharmacologic agents to target LECs, eliminate PCO and help maintain capsular bag transparency. The author considers that SCI should meet the following requirements:

- It should be minimally invasive, be easy to use, fit through a small incision,
- Be relatively inexpensive, provide a repeatable seal with the lens capsule, and be not add significantly to the duration of routine cataract surgery.

The intact human lens capsule is functionally a separate compartment within the eye. Once breached, the intralenticular compartment becomes continuous with the anterior chamber and the rest of the eye. However, since intact capsulorhexis is now routinely performed, the author devised a technique to reseal the capsular bag following lens removal. By resealing the capsular bag, the author recompartmentalizes the lens and allows for the selective irrigation of the internal contents of the capsular bag.

The SCI device called Perfect Capsule™ (Milvella Pty. Ltd., Sydney, Australia), which is made from biomedical

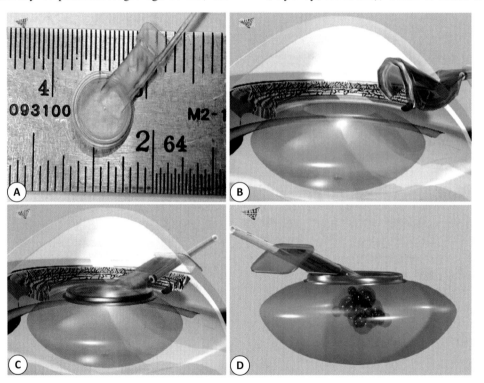

FIGURES 67.6A TO D: Schematic diagrams illustrating the concept of Sealed Capsule Irrigating Device (PerfectCapsule,™ Milvella Pty. Ltd., Sydney, Australia). This device is designed to hold the capsular bag by means of a toroidal suction ring connected to a locking suction syringe. An irrigation/aspiration port allows fluids to be injected through the device into the empty capsule, significantly reducing the concentration of irrigation fluid able to contact other ocular structures and thus perform sealed capsule irrigation

A. Sealed capsule irrigation device viewed from the top. It consists of a round plate that seals against the capsule and an extension arm that passes outside the wound to provide to the internal lens capsule
B. Sealed capsule irrigation device is folded and inserted through a 3 mm incision
C. Sealed capsule irrigation device is placed onto the capsular bag and vacuum-activated by a syringe
D. Internal irrigation of the capsular bag using sealed capsule irrigation device

grade soft silicone, allows the surgeon to reseal the capsular bag. The device consists of a rounded plate containing a suction ring, which abuts the anterior capsule, and an extension arm that passes through a phacoemulsification wound. This extension arm carries a vacuum channel which supplies vacuum to the suction ring, and a combined irrigation and aspiration channel. The irrigation and aspiration channels allow for communication between the sealed capsular bag and the external eye.

The author has performed initial testing on postmortem porcine lens capsules and demonstrated the effectiveness of sealed capsule irrigation.[49] The author has further refined the device to incorporate changes which would allow it to be used in small incision cataract surgery, and address the potential risk of pseudosuction, which would result in loss of sealing of the capsular bag. The author considered the properties of the adult capsule to be less elastic than the pediatric capsule, and less prone to pseudosuction. To prevent pseudosuction, the device was modified to contain a vacuum manifold within the suction ring that ensures no focal occlusion of the suction ring is possible at any point, and that the vacuum is evenly distributed to the entire

ring. This has been further developed using a cog-wheel design.

In performing product validation, 13 randomly chosen devices were subjected to testing on pig capsule. In all cases, the devices sealed the capsule using vacuum generated by a 20 ml lockable syringe, resulting in a maximal vacuum pressure of greater than 700 mm Hg on application, with no evidence of pseudosuction with less than 2.5% reduction in vacuum pressure over a 1 min period. One of these devices was then selected for repeat testing for a period of 10 min with less than 5% reduction in vacuum at 10 min.

The author is continuing to demonstrate that selective capsular bag irrigation can be performed in animals and humans. In a rabbit study,[50] the author assessed the ability to deliver a non-specific extremely toxic agent directly to the LECs post crystalline lens removal, and assessed the eyes histologically for evidence of collateral damage (**Figures 67.7 to 67.9**). A total of six New Zealand white rabbit eyes were selected. The eyes were divided into three groups of four eyes. All eyes underwent phacoaspiration of the crystalline lens via a 3.2 mm corneal incision. Group

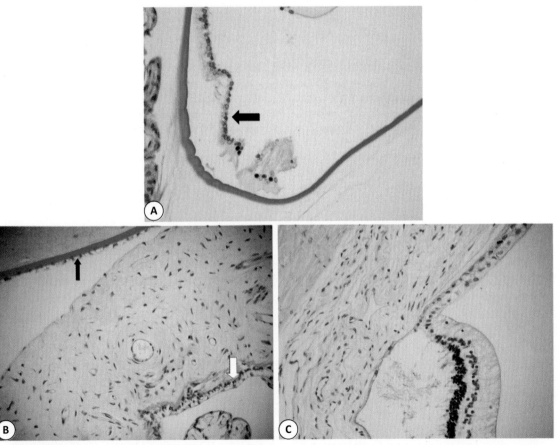

FIGURES 67.7A TO C: Histological findings of the rabbit eyes in Group 1 (phacoaspiration surgery without any treatment, Control Group)

A. Photomicrograph showing the capsular bag. It is to note the presence of residual viable LECs with in the capsular bag (Periodic acid-Schiff stain, original magnification 40x)

B. Photomicrograph showing healthy corneal endothelial cells and posterior iris epithelium (Periodic acid-Schiff stain, original magnification 40x).

C. Photomicrograph showing undamaged retinal tissue and epithelium. There is postmortem artefactual detachment at the ora serata (Periodic acid-Schiff stain, original magnification 40x).

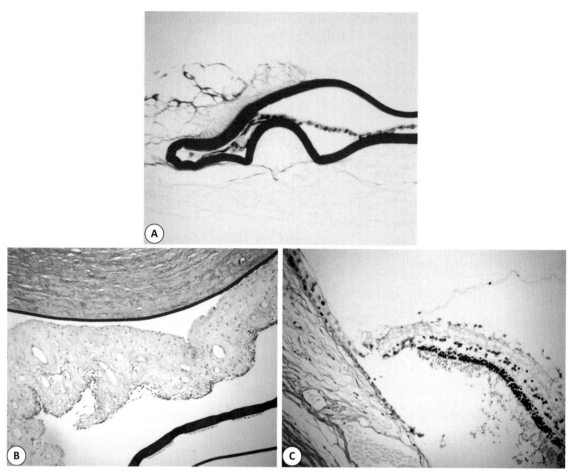

FIGURES 67.8A TO C: Histological findings of the rabbit eyes in Group 2 (phacoaspiration surgery and nonselective irrigation of the capsular bag with DWI and TTX-100 without SCI)

A. Photomicrograph showing the collapsed fornices of the capsular bag. One has to note the presence of viable LECs at the anterior and equatorial region of the capsular bag (Periodic acid-Schiff stain, original magnification 40x)

B. Photomicrograph showing almost total loss of corneal endothelial cells, with bare Descemet's membrane. There is a loss of integrity of posterior iris epithelium (Periodic acid-Schiff stain, original magnification 40x)

C. Photomicrograph of the peripheral retina showing significant disorganization of the retinal tissue and epithelium (Periodic acid-Schiff stain, original magnification 40x)

one eyes were used as control. In Group two eyes, the capsular bag was irrigated with 1% Triton X-100 and demineralized water for injection (DWI) for 5 min. In Group 3 eyes, the capsular bag was isolated from the anterior segment using the PerfectCapsule™. Immediately after the surgery, all (six) rabbits were humanly euthanised. The enucleated eyes were immediately fixed in 10% neutral buffered formalin and histological analysis was performed to assess the corneal endothelium, iris and retina. The capsular bag was also assessed and residual equatorial LECs were evaluated. There was no intraoperative complication in any eye. The capsular bag was sealed and inflated under SCI, PerfectCapsule™, in all treatment eyes in Group three. Histological evaluation revealed no evidence of any collateral damage in Group one (control, group) and Group three (with SCI) **(Figures 67.7 and 67.9)**. Significant histological damage to the cornea, iris and peripheral retina was noted in Group two eyes, which underwent irrigation with DWI and Triton X-100 (without SCI) **(Figures 67.8A to C).** Histological evaluation of capsular bag suggests

presence of LECs in Group one (control, group) and Group two (without SCI) **(Figures 67.7 and 67.8)**. In the presence of SCI, Triton X-100 caused almost complete destruction of LECs in the capsular bag **(Figures 67.9A to C)**. Result of this pilot study suggests that SCI allows selective delivery of toxic agents directly into the capsular bag preventing collateral damage to surrounding intraocular structures in a rabbit eye. The SCI device kept the capsular bag well inflated intraoperatively and therefore it may allow the isolated safe delivery of pharmacological agents into the capsular bag during cataract surgery.

The author has recently completed a one-year follow-up on a total of nine human eyes underwent cataract-IOL surgery using SCI with distilled water and silicone lenses (SI40NB, Clariflex®, Advanced Medical Optics, Santa Ana, CA, USA). A control group of nine eyes, underwent cataract surgery with implantation of silicone lenses, without SCI. All eyes in the treatment group, underwent internal irrigation of the capsular bag using 20cc of distilled water for 60–90 sec using the PerfectCapsule™.

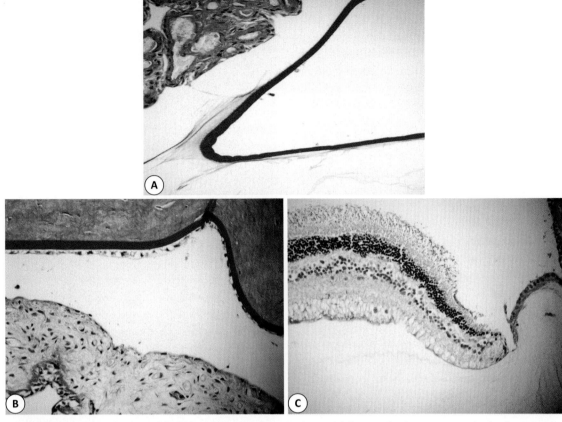

FIGURES 67.9A TO C: Histological findings of the rabbit eyes in Group 3 (phacoaspiration surgery and selective irrigation of the capsular bag with DWI & TTX-100 with SCI)

A. Photomicrograph showing the capsular bag. Note the absence of viable LECs within the capsular fornices. Some nuclear remnants are visible lying on the capsule (Periodic acid-Schiff stain, original magnification 40x)

B. Photomicrograph showing healthy corneal endothelial cells and posterior iris epithelium (Periodic acid-Schiff stain, original magnification 40x)

C. Photomicrograph showing undamaged peripheral retinal tissue and epithelium (Periodic acid-Schiff stain, original magnification 40x)

Fluorescein sodium (0.01%) or trypan blue (0.01%) was used to identify any leakage into the anterior chamber during the SCI procedure. Slit-lamp biomicroscopic examination was performed at 1 day, 1 week, 3, 6, and 12 months to evaluate anterior capsular opacification (ACO), capsular folds/wrinkling, capsular phimosis and posterior capsular opacification (PCO) (area/severity). Intraoperatively, there was no visible leakage of fluorescein sodium/ trypan blue dyes into the anterior chamber during SCI in all eyes in Group AA and AS, indicative of effective seal provided by the SCI device. Follow-up examination at six and 12 months demonstrated a significant reduction in ACO in all eyes, which had undergone SCI with distilled water treatment in comparison to control eyes. In addition, the degree of capsular phimosis was significantly reduced in treatment group, compared to control groups.

Using SCI technique, targeting of lens epithelial cells to prevent PCO can be safely conducted using precise delivery of known doses of pharmacologic agents, with much less fear of toxicity to surrounding intraocular structures. This method may be utilized to eliminate or modulate LEC activity after cataract surgery, which may lead to less postoperative inflammation and a theoretical reduction in the risk of postoperative cystoid macular edema, reduced anterior and posterior capsular opacification, and allow for definitive implantation of multifocal and accommodative lenses, so that the treatment of presbyopia may finally become a reality. Clinical studies will be needed to test efficacy of SCI during pediatric cataract surgery. Theoretically, SCI may be helpful to elimination of LECs and therefore avoid the PCO/ secondary membrane formation postoperatively. It may obviate the need for primary posterior capsulotomy with anterior vitrectomy intraoperatively.

MODULATION OF THE LENS EPITHELIAL CELLS

The human lens capsular bag provides a unique environment within the body for selective specific targeting of tissue. Within this environment, an ideal approach would be to target LEC's for modulation of cell function, rather than cell death. Concern remains over the viability of a denuded lens capsule within the human eyes. It is not known how long the denuded lens capsule will support a lens and stay clear; to date, this has not been achieved. Conventional Methods to destroy remaining LECs result in significant damage to surrounding structures.

The environment of the anterior chamber immediately following cataract surgery contains TGF-β. There is breakdown of blood aqueous barrier and the presence of inflammatory mediators. Clinically, this corresponds with proliferation of LEC's, commonly seen at growing onto the surface of hydrophobic acrylic lenses one month, reaching a peak at six weeks, then stabilizing. In culture medium, LEC's are noted to very rapidly grow over capsule over one week under conditions of accelerated growth, and a similar effect may occur in the human eye. Modulation of the LECs can be another option to prevent visually significant capsular bag opacification. The effect of lithium chloride (LiCl) on the morphology and behavior of lens epithelial cells is profound. In low density, NaCl (20 mm) treated cells display a loosely packed squamous profile with numerous pseudopodia. By contrast, LiCl (20 mm) treated cells form aggregated islands and remain tightly packed with an apical-basal polarized profile and rounded cobblestone appearance. LiCl abrogates cell spreading over a concentration range of 10–40 mm compared with NaCl controls.

LiCl has distinct and dichotomous roles in influencing the behavior of lens epithelial cells. LiCl is both a potent inhibitor of lens cell proliferation, migration and differentiation and, at similar concentrations; LiCl promotes cell adhesion and maintenance of epithelial characteristics, i.e. apical-basal polarity. LiCl also blocks the TGF-β-induced epithelial-to-mesenchymal transition (EMT). Evidence for the inhibition of GSK-3 by LiCl in lens cells was demonstrated by an increase in expression of active β-catenin (AβC). With LiCl, active β-catenin preferentially accumulates on membranes and does not move into the nucleus. However, under similar conditions, nuclear expression of AβC does occur with addition of a specific GSK-3 inhibitor. These results support the view that, while LiCl promotes stabilization of AβC, this does necessarily result in nuclear transactivation. The author's pilot study also implicates pathways other than Wnt/β-catenin in the LiCl response, these are: inhibition of proliferation and migration which coincides with abrogation of phospho-ERK expression, implying LiCl-induced modulation of the MAPK pathway; promotion of tight packing, polarized cells and increased expression of ZO-1 and MARCKS. MARCKS proteins bind and cross-link actin suggesting a role in stabilizing polarized cells. Therefore, LiCl promotes tight junction formation and membrane expression of AβC and ZO-1, through inhibition of GSK-3 and possibly activation of Protein Kinase C (PKC). Inhibition of GSK3 promotes stabilization of β-catenin, allowing canonical Wnt signaling. Formation of the Wnt/Frizzled/LRP complex activates β-catenin. In the nucleus, active β-catenin complexes with TCF and regulates gene expression. Active β-catenin also binds to E-cadherin and becomes localized at the cell membrane.

REMOVAL OF LENS EPITHELIAL CELLS USING Aqualase® LIQUEFACTION DEVICE

AquaLase® liquefaction device is a new advancement in lens removal technology which is a part of the newly introduced Infiniti™ Vision System (Alcon Inc., Fort Worth, Tx, USA).[82] The AquaLase® liquefaction hand piece proved to be effective to remove nuclear cataracts of up to grade two with reasonable efficiency, as of this writing, and this technology may have applications in polishing the capsule and removing lens equatorial cells, thus minimizing the postoperative cellular proliferation of the LECs, thereby minimizing or eliminating the risk of capsular bag fibrosis (ACO/PCO).

The AquaLase® tip is composed of a soft polymer and has soft, rounded edges. This design makes the instrument more capsule-friendly than metal ultrasound tips. The AquaLase® hand piece propels small pulses of balanced saline solution (BSS®) warmed to 57°C to liquefy lens material just inside the aspiration port of the tip. The BSS pulses are delivered at a maximum rate of 50 Hz, and the surgeon controls the magnitude of the pulses with the Infiniti™ foot pedal.

SUMMARY AND CONCLUSION

The tools, surgical procedures, skills and appropriate IOLs are now available to eradicate PCO. Continued motivation to apply the six factors noted in this article, the efficacy of which have been further suggested in a recent study,[54] will help diminish this final major complication of cataract-IOL surgery exactly 50 years after Sir Ridley's first encounter with this complication. A major reduction of Nd:YAG laser capsulotomy rates towards single digits is now possible because of application of aforementioned surgical factors and factors related to modern lens designs/biomaterials at least in the industrialized world. This will obviously be of great benefit to patients in achieving improved long-term results and avoidance of Nd:YAG laser capsulotomy complications. Eradication of the Nd:YAG laser procedure will help control what has been the one of the most expensive costs to the health care system. To date, one cannot precisely determine the relative proportion or contribution of IOL design vs. surgical techniques to the decrease of Nd:YAG laser rates observed here. However, this could be possible with continuing analysis including annual updates and increasing numbers of pseudophakic autopsy eyes.

In summary, the author has ascertained various factors that help bring about the very positive conclusion that surgeons now have the sufficient tools and appropriate IOLs to help reduce the incidence of PCO. The recent advent of SCI is a significant step to eliminate PCO and to maintain long-term capsular bag clarity that is necessary for success of accommodative/refractive lenses. The SCI will also be helpful for maintaining the long-term clear visual axis in pediatric cataract-IOL surgery. However, further experimental studies and multicentric clinical trials are necessary to test its efficacy.

KEY POINTS

- In addition to classic posterior capsular opacification (PCO, secondary cataract, after cataract), postoperative lens epithelial cell (LEC) proliferation is also involved in the pathogenesis of anterior capsular opacification/fibrosis (ACO) and interlenticular opacification (ILO).
- Nd:YAG laser secondary posterior capsulotomy, can be associated with significant complications. Potential problems include IOL optic damage/pitting, postoperative intraocular pressure elevation, cystoid macular edema, retinal detachment and IOL subluxation.
- Although both types of cells (from the anterior central zone and from the equatorial lens bow) have the potential to produce visually significant opacification, most cases of classic PCO are caused by proliferation of the equatorial cells. The term posterior capsular opacification implies that the capsule opacifies. Rather, an opaque membrane develops over the capsule as retained cells proliferate and migrate onto the posterior capsular surface.
- One strategy to reduce posterior capsular opacification is to minimize the number of retained/regenerated cells and cortex (including the Soemmering's ring) through cortical cleanup. The second strategy is to prevent the remaining cells from migrating posteriorly. The edge of the IOL optic is critical in the formation of such a physical barrier.
- Sealed capsule irrigation (SCI) device may allow the isolated safe delivery of pharmacologic agents into the capsular bag following cataract surgery.

REFERENCES

1. Apple DJ. Influence of intraocular lens material and design on postoperative intracapsular cellular reactivity. Trans Am Ophthalmol Soc. 2000;98:257-83.
2. Werner L, Apple DJ, Pandey SK. Postoperative proliferation of anterior and equatorial lens epithelial cells: A comparison between various foldable IOL designs. In: Buratto L, Osher R, Masket S (Eds). Cataract Surgery In Complicated Cases. Thorofare NJ: Slack Inc; 2000.pp 399-417.
3. Werner L, Pandey SK, Escobar-Gomez M, et al. Anterior capsular opacification: A histopathological study comparing different IOL styles. Ophthalmology. 2000;107(3):463-7.
4. Werner L, Pandey SK, Apple DJ, et al. Anterior capsular opacification: Correlation of pathological findings with clinical sequelae. Ophthalmology. 2001;108(9):1675-81.
5. Gayton JL, Apple DJ, Peng Q, et al. Interlenticular opacification: Clinicopathological correlation of a complication of posterior chamber piggyback intraocular lenses. J Cataract Refract Surg. 2000;26(3):330-6.
6. Werner L, Apple DJ, Pandey SK, et al. Analysis of elements of interlenticular opacification. Am J Ophthalmol. 2002; 133(3):320-6.
7. Ridley H. The origin and objectives of intraocular lenticular implants. Trans Am Acad Ophthalmol Otolaryngol. 1976; 81(1):65-6.
8. Ridley H. Long-term results of acrylic lens surgery. Proc R Soc Med. 1970;63(3):309-10.
9. Apple DJ, Solomon KD, Tetz MR, et al. Posterior capsular opacification. Surv Ophthalmol. 1992;37(2):73-116.
10. Pandey SK, Wilson ME, Trivedi RH, et al. Pediatric cataract surgery and intraocular lens implantation: Current techniques, complications and management. Int Ophthalmol Clin. 2001;41(3):175-96.
11. Pandey SK, Ram J, Werner L, et al. Visual results and postoperative complications of capsular bag versus sulcus fixation of posterior chamber intraocular lenses for traumatic cataract in children. J Cataract Refract Surg. 1999;25(12):1576-84.
12. Pandey SK, Wilson ME, Werner L, et al. Childhood cataract surgical technique, complications and management. In: Garg A, Pandey SK (Eds). Textbook of Ocular Therapeutics. New Delhi, India: Jaypee Brothers Medical Publishers; 2002. pp. 457-86.
13. Apple DJ, Peng Q, Visessook N, et al. Eradication of posterior capsular opacification. Documentation of a marked decrease in Nd:YAG laser posterior capsulotomy rates noted in an analysis of 5416 pseudophakic human eyes obtained postmortem. Ophthalmology. 2001;108(3):505-18.
14. Apple DJ, Peng Q, Visessook N, et al. Surgical prevention of posterior capsular opacification. Part I. Progress in eliminating this complication of cataract surgery. J Cataract Refract Surg. 2000;26(2):180-7.
15. Holweger RR, Marefat B. Intraocular pressure change after Neodymium:YAG capsulotomy. J Cataract Refract Surg. 1997;23(1):115-21.
16. Hu CY, Woung LC, Wang MC. Change in the area of laser posterior capsulotomy: 3 months follow-up. J Cataract Refract Surg. 2001;27(4):537-42.
17. Richter CU, Steinert RF. Neodymium: Yttrium Aluminium Garnet laser posterior capsulotomy. In: Steinert RF (Ed). Cataract Surgery: Techniques, Complications and Management. Philadelphia, PA: WB Saunders Company; 1995. pp 378-8.
18. Koch D, Liu J, Gill P, et al. Axial myopia increases the risk of retinal complications after Neodymium-YAG laser posterior capsulotomy. Arch Ophthalmol. 1989;107(7):986-90.
19. Apple DJ, Ram J, Foster A, et al. Elimination of cataract blindness: A global perspective entering the new millennium. Surv Ophthalmol. 2000;45 (Suppl 1):S70-99.
20. Font RL, Brownstein S. A light and electron microscopic study of anterior subcapsular cataracts. Am J Ophthalmol. 1974;78(6):972-84.
21. Peng Q, Hennig A, Vasavada AR, et al. Posterior capsular plaque: A common feature of cataract surgery in the developing world. Am J Ophthalmol. 1998;125(5):621-6.
22. McAvoy JW, Chamberlain CG. Growth factors in the eye. Prog Growth Factor Res. 1990;2(1):29-43.
23. Lang RA, McAvoy JW. Growth Factors In Lens Development. In: Lovicu FJ, Robinson ML (Eds). Development of the Ocular Lens. New York: Cambridge University Press; 2004.
24. Stump RJ, Ang S, Chen Y, et al. A role for Wnt/beta-catenin signaling in lens epithelial differentiation. Dev Biol. 2003; 259(1):48-61.
25. Wormstone IM. Posterior capsular opacification: A cell biological perspective. Exp Eye Res. 2002;74(3):337-47.
26. Gordon-Thomson C, deIongh RU, Hales AM, et al. Differential cataractogenic potency of TGF--beta1, -beta2, and -beta3 and their expression in the postnatal rat eye. Invest Ophthalmol. Vis Sci. 1998;39:1399-409.

27. Hales AM, Chamberlain CG, McAvoy JW. Cataract induction in lenses cultured with transforming growth factor-beta. Invest Ophthalmol Vis Sci. 1995;36(8):1709-13.

28. Lovicu FJ, Schulz MW, Hales AM, et al. TGF-beta induces morphological and molecular changes similar to human anterior subcapsular cataract. Br J Ophthalmol. 2002;86(2):220-6.

29. Liu J, Hales AM, Chamberlain CG, et al. Induction of cataract-like changes in rat lens epithelial explants by transforming growth factor beta. Invest Ophthalmol Vis Sci. 1994;35(2):388-401.

30. Srinivasan Y, Lovicu FJ, Overbeek PA. Lens-specific expression of transforming growth factor beta1 in transgenic mice causes anterior subcapsular cataracts. J Clin Invest. 1998;101(3):625-34.

31. Sasaki K, Kojima M, Nakaizumi H, et al. Early lens changes seen in patients with atopic dermatitis applying image analysis processing of Scheimpflug and specular microscopic images. Ophthalmologica. 1998;212(2):88-94.

32. Lee EH, Seomun Y, Hwang KH, et al. Overexpression of the transforming growth factor-beta-inducible gene betaig-h3 in anterior polar cataracts. Invest Ophthalmol Vis Sci. 2000;41(7):1840-5.

33. Saika S, Miyamoto T, Ishida I, et al. TGF-β-Smad signalling in postoperative human lens epithelial cells. Br J Ophthalmol. 2002;86(12):1428-33.

34. Schulz MW, Chamberlain CG, McAvoy JW. Inhibition of TGF-β-induced cataractous changes in lens explants by ocular media and 2-macroblobulin. Invest Ophthalmol Vis Sci. 1996;37:1509-19.

35. Hales AM, Chamberlain CG, Murphy CR, et al. Estrogen protects lenses against cataract induced by TGF-β. J Exp Med. 1997;185(2):273-80.

36. Younan C, Mitchell P, Cumming RG, et al. Hormone replacement therapy, reproductive factors, and the incidence of cataract and cataract surgery: The Blue Mountains Eye Study. Am J Epidemiol. 2002;155(11):997-1006.

37. Ram J, Kaushik S, Brar GS, et al. Neodymium:YAG capsulotomy rates following phacoemulsification with implantation of PMMA, silicone, and Acrylic intraocular lenses. Ophthalmic Surg Lasers. 2001;32:375-82.

38. Schaumberg DA, Dana MR, Christen WG, et al. A systematic overview of the incidence of posterior capsular opacification. Ophthalmology. 1998;105(7):1213-21.

39. Cheng CY, Yen MY, Chen SJ, et al. Visual acuity and contrast sensitivity in different types of posterior capsular opacification. J Cataract Refract Surg. 2001;27(7):1055-60.

40. Ram J, Apple DJ, Peng Q, et al. Update on fixation of rigid and foldable posterior chamber intraocular lenses. Part II. Choosing the correct haptic fixation and intraocular lens design to help eradicate posterior capsular opacification. Ophthalmology. 1999;106(5):891-900.

41. Apple DJ, Auffarth GU, Peng Q, et al. Foldable intraocular lenses. In: Evolution, Clinicopathologic Correlations, Complications. Thorofare, NJ: Slack Inc; 2000. pp.157-215.

42. Peng Q, Apple DJ, Visessook N, et al. Surgical prevention of posterior capsular opacification. Part II. Enhancement of cortical clean up by focusing on hydrodissection. J Cataract Refract Surg. 2000;26(2):188-97.

43. Peng Q, Visessook N, Apple DJ, et al. Surgical prevention of posterior capsular opacification. Part III. Intraocular lens optic barrier effect as a second line of defense. J Cataract Refract Surg. 2000;26(2):198-213.

44. Vargas LG, Peng Q, Apple DJ, et al. Evaluation of 3 modern single-piece foldable intraocular lenses: clinicopathological study of posterior capsular opacification in a rabbit model. J Cataract Refract Surg. 2002;28(7):1241-50.

45. Vargas LG, Izak AM, Apple DJ, et al. Single Piece AcrySof Implantation of a single-piece, hydrophilic, acrylic, minus-power foldable posterior chamber intraocular lens in a rabbit model: clinicopathologic study of posterior capsular opacification. J Cataract Refract Surg. 2003;29:1613-20.

46. Fine IH. Cortical cleaving hydrodissection. J Cataract Refract Surg. 1992;18(5):508-12.

47. Vasavada AR, Singh R, Apple DJ, et al. Efficacy of hydrodissection step in the phacoemulsification for age related senile cataract. J Cataract Refract Surg. 2002;28:1623-8.

48. Vargas LG, Escobar-Gomez M, Apple DJ, et al. Pharmacologic prevention of posterior capsular opacification: in vitro effects of preservative-free lidocaine 1% on lens epithelial cells. J Cataract Refract Surg. 2003;29(8):1585-92.

49. Maloof AJ, Neilson G, Milverton EJ, et al. Selective and specific targeting of lens epithelial cells during cataract surgery using sealed-capsule irrigation. J Cataract Refract Surg. 2003;29(8):1566-8.

50. Maloof AJ, Pandey SK, Neilson G, et al. Selective death of lens epithelial cells using demineralised water and triton X-100 with PerfectCapsule™ sealed capsule irrigation: A histological study in rabbit eyes. Arch Ophthalmol. 2005;123(10):1378-84.

51. Ram J, Apple DJ, Peng Q, et al. Update on fixation of rigid and foldable posterior chamber intraocular lenses. Part I: Elimination of fixation-induced decentration to achieve precise optical correction and visual rehabilitation. Ophthalmology. 1999;106(5):883-90.

52. Apple DJ, Reidy JJ, Googe JM, et al. A comparison of ciliary sulcus and capsular bag fixation of posterior chamber intraocular lenses. J Am Intraocul Implant Soc. 1985;11(1):44-63.

53. Vasavada AR, Raj SM. Anterior capsule relationship of the AcrySof intraocular lens optic and posterior capsular opacification: A prospective randomized clinical trial. Ophthalmology. 2004;111(5):886-94.

54. Linnola RJ. Sandwich theory: Bioactivity-based explanation for posterior capsular opacification. J Cataract Refract Surg. 1997;23(10):1539-42.

55. Linnola RJ, Werner L, Pandey SK, et al. Adhesion of fibronectin, vitronectin, laminin and collagen type IV to intraocular lens materials in human autopsy eyes. Part I: histological sections. J Cataract Refract Surg. 2000;26(12):1792-806.

56. Linnola RJ, Werner L, Pandey SK, et al. Adhesion of fibronectin, vitronectin, laminin and collagen type IV to intraocular lens materials in human autopsy eyes. Part II: explanted IOLs. J Cataract Refract Surg. 2000;26(12):1807-18.

57. Nishi O, Nishi K, Akura J, et al. Effect of round-edged acrylic intraocular lenses on preventing posterior capsular opacification. J Cataract Refract Surg. 2001;27(4):608-13.

58. Nishi O, Nishi K, Menapace R, et al. Capsular bending ring to prevent posterior capsular opacification: 2 years follow-up. J Cataract Refract Surg. 2001;27(9):1359-65.

59. Kruger AJ, Schauersberger J, Abela C, et al. Two year results: Sharp versus rounded optic edges on silicone lenses. J Cataract Refract Surg. 2000;26(4):566-70.

60. Kucuksumer Y, Bayraktar S, Sahin S, et al. Posterior capsular opacification 3 years after implantation of an AcrySof and a MemoryLens in fellow eyes. J Cataract Refract Surg. 2000;26(8):1176-82.

61. Meacock WR, Spalton DJ, Boyce JF, et al. Effect of optic size on posterior capsular opacification: 5.5 mm versus 6.0 mm AcrySof intraocular lenses. J Cataract Refract Surg. 2001;27(8):1194-8.

62. Nishi O. Posterior capsular opacification. Part 1: Experimental investigations. J Cataract Refract Surg. 1999;25(1):106-17.

63. Nishi O, Nishi K. Effect of the optic size of a single-piece acrylic intraocular lens on posterior capsular opacification. J Cataract Refract Surg. 2003;29(2):348-53.

64. Hollick EJ, Spalton DJ, Ursell PG, et al. Posterior capsular opacification with hydrogel, polymethylmethacrylate, and silicone intraocular lenses: Two-year results of a randomized prospective trial. Am J Ophthalmol. 2000;129(5):577-84.

65. Buehl W, Findl O, Menapace R, et al. Effect of an acrylic intraocular lens with a sharp posterior optic edge on posterior capsular opacification. J Cataract Refract Surg. 2002;28(7): 1105-11.

66. Aasuri MK, Shah U, Veenashree MP, et al. Performance of a truncated-edged silicone foldable intraocular lens in Indian eyes. J Cataract Refract Surg. 2002;28(7):1135-40.

67. Auffarth GU, Golescu A, Becker KA, et al. Quantification of posterior capsular opacification with round and sharp edge intraocular lenses. Ophthalmology. 2003;110(4):772-80.

68. Masket S. Truncated edge design, dysphotopsia, and inhibition of posterior capsular opacification. J Cataract Refract Surg. 2000;26(1):145-7.

69. Ram J, Pandey SK, Apple DJ, et al. Effect of in-the-bag intraocular lens fixation on the prevention of posterior capsular opacification. J Cataract Refract Surg. 2001;27(7):1039-46.

70. Ravalico G, Tognetto D, Palomba M, et al. Capsulorhexis size and posterior capsular opacification. J Cataract Refract Surg. 1996;22(1):98-103.

71. Chung HS, Lim SJ, Kim HB. Effect of mitomycin-C on posterior capsular opacification in rabbit eyes. J Cataract Refract Surg. 2000;26(10):1537-42.

72. Power WJ, Neylan D, Collum LM. Daunorubicin as an inhibitor of human lens epithelial cell proliferation in culture. J Cataract Refract Surg. 1994;20(3):287-90.

73. Rakic JM, Galand A, Vrensen GF. Lens epithelial cell proliferation in human posterior capsular opacification. Exp Eye Res. 2000;71(5):489-94.

74. Rootman J, Tisdall J, Gudauskas G, et al. Intraocular penetration of subconjunctivally administered ^{14}C-fluorouracil in rabbits. Arch Ophthalmol. 1979;97(12):2375-8.

75. Legler UF, Apple DJ, Assia EI, et al. Inhibition of posterior capsular opacification: The effect of colchicine in a sustained drug delivery system. J Cataract Refract Surg. 1993;19(4):462-70.

76. Tetz MR, Ries MW, Lucas C, et al. Inhibition of posterior capsular opacification by an intraocular–lens–bound sustained drug delivery system: An experimental animal study and literature review. J Cataract Refract Surg 1996;22(8):1070-8.

77. Pandey SK, Cochener B, Apple DJ, et al. Intracapsular ring sustained 5-fluorouracil delivery system for prevention of posterior capsular opacification in rabbits: A histological study. J Cataract Refract Surg. 2002;28(1):139-48.

78. Cochener B, Bougaran R, Pandey SK, et al. Non-biodegradable drug-sustained capsular ring for prevention of secondary cataract. Part I: *In vitro* evaluation. J Fr Ophthalmol. 2003; 26(3):223-31.

79. Cochener B, Pandey SK, Apple DJ, et al. Nonbiodegradable drug-sustained capsular ring for prevention of secondary cataract. Part II: *In vivo* evaluation. J Fr Ophthalmol. 2003; 26(3):439-52.

80. Miyake K, Miyake C. Intraoperative posterior chamber lens haptic fixation in the human cadaver eye. Ophthalmic Surg. 1985;16(4):230-6.

81. Apple DJ, Lim ES, Morgan RC, et al. Preparation and study of human eyes obtained postmortem with the Miyake posterior photographic technique. Ophthalmology. 1990;97(6):810-6.

82. Mackool RJ, Brint SF. AquaLase: A new technology for cataract extraction. Curr Opin Ophthalmol. 2004;15(1):40-3.

IOL Implantation in Eyes without a Capsule

CHAPTER 68

Sutured Scleral Fixated IOL

Amar Agarwal, Soosan Jacob

INTRODUCTION

There are many conditions where an IOL needs to be implanted in the absence of adequate capsular support. These include a posterior capsular rent with inadequate sulcus support, large zonulodialysis or large subluxations of the lens or IOL and primary aphakias for secondary IOL fixation. Secondary IOL fixation can be done in the form of anterior chamber IOLs, iris sutured IOLs, sutured scleral fixated IOL or glued IOL.

SURGICAL TECHNIQUE

Sutured scleral fixated IOL needs a special IOL with eyelets on both the haptics through which the suture is tied. The sutured scleral fixated IOL is fixated to the sclera using 9-0 or 10-0 prolene. The suturing of the IOL can be done via an ab interno or an ab externo approach, though the latter is generally preferred. For both the techniques, partial lamellar rectangular or triangular scleral flaps are made **(Figure 68.1)**. These should be adequately thick enough to cover the suture knots so as to avoid knot exposure. They are made 180 degrees apart in the horizontal meridian. Adequate anterior vitrectomy should be done to avoid vitreous traction during the procedure.

Ab INTERNO SUTURED SCLERAL FIXATED IOL

Here, the needles are passed from the inside of the eye outwards. Two needles are passed on either side to emerge out from under the scleral flap. The IOL is tied to the other end of the two sutures. The IOL is then inserted behind the pupil. Both sutures are tied down and the IOL is thus suspended from the scleral wall. The scleral flaps are sutured over the scleral knot.

Ab EXTERNO SUTURED SCLERAL FIXATED IOL

Here the needle is passed from outside to inside the eye. A long, straight needle on a 9-0 prolene suture is used. It is passed through the bed of the scleral flap to pierce the sclera and enter the eye. At the same time, a 26 gauge needle is inserted from the opposite side from under the opposite scleral flap. The straight needle is directed into the 26 gauge needle so as to dock into it **(Figure 68.2)**. The 26 gauge needle is then withdrawn back out. This brings the straight needle out through the opposite scleral flap with the suture passing through the eye **(Figure 68.3)**. The suture is then hooked through a corneoscleral section and pulled out from the eye to form a loop **(Figure 68.4)**. This loop is then cut to get two free suture ends each of which pass outwards from under the scleral flap. Each of these cut ends of the suture are tied to the eyelets on the scleral fixated IOL **(Figure 68.5)**. The scleral fixated IOL is then inserted into

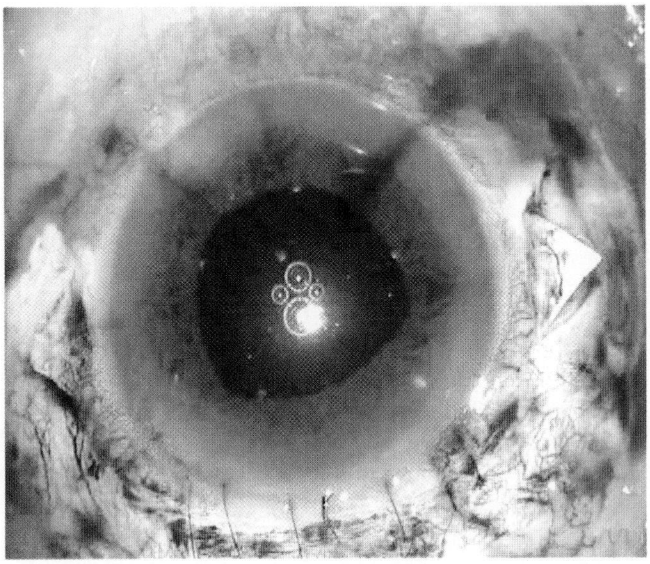

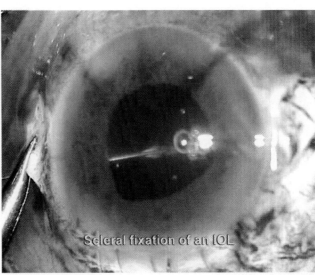

FIGURE 68.1: Two partial lamellar scleral flaps are created 180° apart from each other

FIGURE 68.2: A straight needle is passed from one side and docked into a 26 gauge needle passed in from the other side

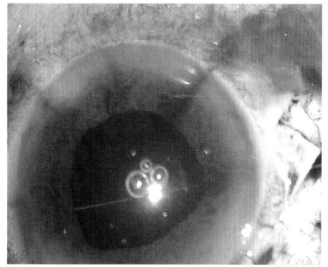

FIGURE 68.3: The suture is seen passing in from one side and out onto the other side

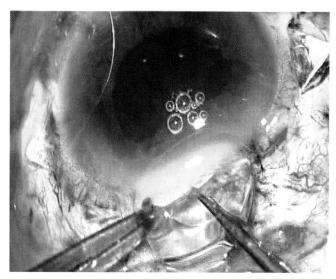

FIGURE 68.6: The IOL is inserted into the eye

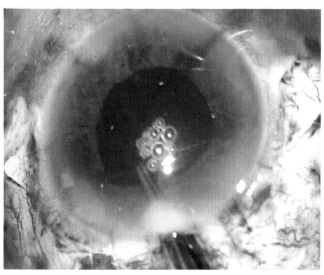

FIGURE 68.4: The suture is pulled out as a loop from the corneo-scleral section

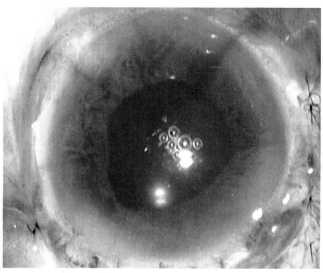

FIGURE 68.7: The IOL as seen at the end of the surgery

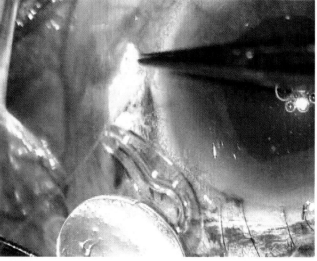

FIGURE 68.5: The loop is cut and both cut ends are tied onto the eyelets of a scleral fixated IOL

the eye behind the pupil (**Figure 68.6**). Pulling apart both the sutures emerging on the surface of the eye brings the IOL into position. The sutures are then tied down under the scleral flaps making sure the IOL is centered in the eye. The scleral flaps are sutured over the scleral knot (**Figure 68.7**).

COMPLICATIONS

Complications can arise as the needle is passed within the eye especially in the ab interno technique. Improper passage of the needle can result in retinal detachment. Sutures may degrade, erode and the knot may give way. This can be especially problematic in pediatric eyes where the IOL needs to remain well centered for decades together. The tension on the individual sutures decides the centering of the IOL as well as the degree of pseudophakodonesis. If one of the sutures is tied tighter than the other, it can result in a decentered IOL and consequent diplopia, edge glare effects, etc. Loose suturing can give rise to excessive intra-ocular mobility of the IOL which can result in pseudo-phakodonesis. Too much anteriorly sutured IOL can result in the lens rubbing on the iris which can result in pigment dispersion and uveitis-glaucoma hyphema syndrome.

DISCUSSION

Scleral fixation of IOLs can be done with either suture or by trans-sclerally fixating the IOL into a scleral tunnel such as in the glued IOL technique. The sutured scleral fixated IOL requires a special IOL. This requires the surgeon to have at hand a large inventory of these lenses in the event of having a posterior capsular rent with inadequate sulcus support. Also, 9–0 and 10–0 prolene sutures can degrade over time resulting in late IOL subluxation. The knots can

get exposed or eroded which can also result in late IOL subluxation. These problems are avoided with a glued IOL as no special IOL is required for this. Any nonfoldable IOL or three-piece foldable IOL can be fixed using the glued technique. As it is the haptics that are fixated trans-sclerally, all suture related problems are avoided. It is also more stable and posterior segment complications that are associated with endophthalmodonesis secondary to pseudophakodonesis would therefore be less with the glued IOL.

SUMMARY

Scleral fixated IOL may be used as a technique for secondary IOL fixation in eyes with insufficient capsular support either as a primary or as a secondary procedure.

CHAPTER 69

Iris Suture Fixation of Intraocular Lenses

Roger F Steinert

Iris fixation of an intraocular lens (IOL) for stabilization of a subluxating IOL or for secondary IOL implantation is an attractive option in many cases. The advantages of iris fixation compared to trans-scleral fixation are as follows:

1. Absence of conjunctival surgery.
2. The ability to perform the suturing through the small side-port incisions and, if the lens needs to be inserted, the insertion of a foldable IOL through small incisions.
3. Absence of any external sutures that can later erode to the surface and be the source for foreign body irritation and a track for organisms to enter the eye, causing endophthalmitis.
4. The apparent lower rate of late postoperative suture breakage and dislocation of the implant compared to trans-scleral suture fixation.

Concerns about iris sutured IOLs mainly relate to the potential for inflammation. Certainly, pupil fixation of the old design IOLs such as the Sputnik and the Worst Medallion proved that the iris sphincter is a source of inflammatory reaction when materials chronically irritate the sphincter. However, the peripheral iris does not appear to have this potential for chronic inflammation, at least when the implant is secure and not moving against the uveal tissue.

PRINCIPLES

Peripheral iris suture fixation requires that the patient has adequate iris tissue for suture fixation, of course, and successful outcomes depend upon attention to several surgical principles. If those principles are observed, an excellent functional and cosmetically acceptable outcome can be achieved reliably.

PRINCIPLE 1

Peripheral Short Suture Bites

In order to attain a round pupil that is reasonably mobile postoperatively, the peripheral suture bites must be in the far periphery and be as short as possible. Observing these two requirements avoids a fixed pupil that is oval, with a so-called "cat's eye" shape.

PRINCIPLE 2

Suture from the Concave Side of the Haptic

It is technically easier to obtain short and peripheral suture bites when approaching the haptic from the concave rather than convex side. In some cases the orbital anatomy will not allow the surgeon to pass the needle into the eye and suture the haptic from the concave side for both haptics, but this principle should be observed whenever possible. **Figure 69.1** shows a sequence of operative photos illustrating short peripheral suture bites when the needle is passed from the concave side. There is difficulty in having a peripheral suture bite when the haptic is approached from the convex side.

PRINCIPLE 3

Use a Three-Piece IOL

The IOL must be a three-piece design with flexible polymethyl methacrylate (PMMA) haptics. One-piece hydrophobic acrylic lenses have bulky and sharp-edged haptics that have the potential of causing iris chafe and chronic inflammation when the IOL haptic is tightly opposed to the backside of the iris. In addition, the tight suture can "cheese wire" through the soft haptic material resulting in a later dislocation of the IOL. Current hydrophilic acrylic IOLs do not have haptic shapes that permit peripheral iris sutures, and the soft material would also be expected to be vulnerable to cheese-wiring of the suture through the material.

PRINCIPLE 4

Use a Dense Cohesive Viscoadaptive Device to Visualize the Haptic

In order to successfully iris fixate the implant, the surgeon needs to be able to visualize the haptics during surgery. The fundamental technique begins with capturing the optic anteriorly through the pupil, with the haptics posterior to the iris. In order to know the precise location of the haptic and minimize the length of the suture bite, the iris must drape itself over the haptic. In that manner, the surgeon can visualize the location of the haptic reliably. Iris draping over the haptic is facilitated by two maneuvers. The first step is to employ a moderately dense cohesive ophthalmic viscoadaptive device (OVD) (the author's personal preference is Healon GV, Abbott Medical Optics, Santa Ana, CA, USA). The OVD is injected over the iris in the area of the haptic. The OVD will keep the iris in the posterior position when the haptic then is lifted anteriorly with the second maneuver, which is to elevate the optic with a second instrument. Options for elevating the optic include the use of a cyclodialysis spatula or a forcep which can grasp and hold the optic reliably, or the OVD cannula itself. When the optic is lifted in the anterior direction the OVD then drapes the iris over the haptic. Because of the cohesive nature and higher density of the preferred OVD, the haptic will remain visible for several minutes before settling back down, giving the surgeon time enough to pass the suture around the haptic.

PRINCIPLE 5

Tying the Suture

The surgeon must be familiar and comfortable with several alternate methods of suture tying in the setting of small incisions. The easiest method is illustrated in **Figures 69.1 to 69.3**. A long needle (Ethicon CTC-6L or equivalent, Ethicon Corporation, Somerville, NJ, USA) punctures ab externo through the peripheral cornea, passes in and out of the iris under the haptic, and then exits the peripheral cornea through another puncture ab interno. Following that, a side-port incision is made directly over the location of the suture where it is passed under the haptic. Both ends of the suture are drawn out through the side-port incision, utilizing a hook, and tied externally, taking great care to make sure that the suture is tied tightly and secured with at least four throws of the knot. The challenge with this technique is to make sure that the knot is tight, as the knot is actually being tied externally, which requires that the haptic suturing be very close to the side-port incision and be able to be drawn up to the side port (**Figure 69.4**).

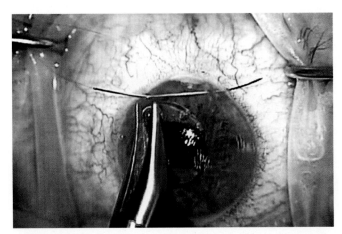

FIGURE 69.1: Method of suturing the haptic from the concave side. After puncturing the cornea in the periphery, the tip of the needle passes through the iris. The tip of the needle is lifted anteriorly so that the needle can then exit from behind the iris with only a small amount of iris within the bite of the suture. The tip of the needle is then driven *ab interno* through the peripheral cornea, grasped, and removed from the eye*

---

* Note: When the haptic is approached from the convex side, because the haptic is curving away from the entry point of the needle, the surgeon finds it difficult to keep the suture around the far periphery of the iris. A mid-peripheral iris suture typically results.

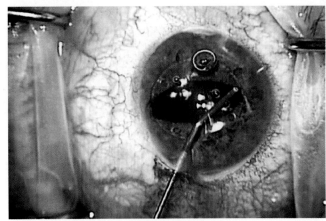

FIGURE 69.2: A high concentration cohesive ophthalmic viscoelastic device (OVD) is employed to disclose the precise location of the haptic that is under the iris. Before injecting the OVD, there is no indentation of the iris by the posteriorly located haptic. This is especially true with thicker, more darkly pigmented iris tissue. The OVD is injected over the iris in the periphery. The OVD cannula is repositioned under the optic and lifts the optic anteriorly. The iris then drapes over the haptic, allowing accurate placement of the suture bite around the haptic

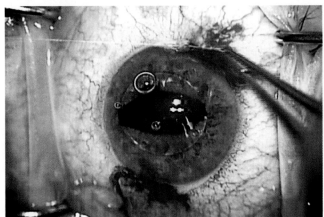

FIGURE 69.3: The easiest method of tying the suture is by creating a short side port incision directly over the location of the haptic suture. One at a time, each of the suture ends is hooked by an instrument such as a Lester hook. With the needle cut off, the suture is drawn out through the side port incision. The surgeon must hold onto the other end of the suture to avoid inadvertent pulling out the wrong end due to the friction. The suture is then tied externally but tightly with four throws of square knots. A short side port and a peripheral iris suture are important to allow the suture to be tight and secure around the haptic. The suture is then cut short and the knot falls back into the anterior chamber

If there is any distance between the haptic and the side-port, an inadequately tight knot will result. The alternative, therefore, is to use the Siepser slip-knot technique. The slip knot is a versatile method first described by Dr Steven Siepser. This technique allows the knot to be advanced anywhere within the eye without putting any tension on the area being sutured. This is helpful in repair of iris defects and other intraocular suturing situations, and, in the case suturing an IOL, assures the surgeon that the knot will be tight. This technique does take more time, however, and practice with large materials such as a string prior to going into surgery will help the surgeon feel more secure about the methodology. This technique is discussed and illustrated in detail in Snyder ME, Steinert RF, Khng C, Burk SE. "Iris Repair" in Steinert RF (Ed). Cataract Surgery, 3rd edn London: Saunders Elsevier; 2009. pp. 370-1 and Figure 31.1.

After completion of the suturing of both haptics, the optic is reposited behind the pupil, as shown in **Figure 69.4**.

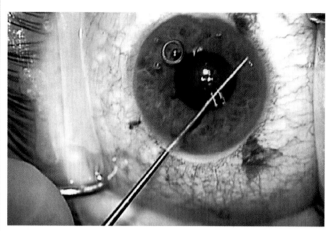

FIGURE 69.4: After completion of suturing both haptics, the optic is reposited posterior to the pupil, beginning by pressing on one side of the optic followed by the other side of the optic. If the pupil is not fully round, the peripheral iris is stroked gently with the Lester hook towards the center of the eye. If the suture bites are short and peripheral, it will result in a round pupil with a centered IOL

PRINCIPLE 6

Insertion of a New IOL without Capsular Support

When the peripheral iris suture fixation is employed to repair a subluxating IOL whose type and condition allow it to be retained, then positioning the haptics posterior to the iris and temporarily capturing the optic in the pupil is straightforward. If a new IOL must be inserted and there is adequate posterior capsule in the periphery, reasonable care in the insertion of the new IOL so that the haptics pass between the iris and the residual capsule will also give the surgeon a stable situation to begin the repair.

When the posterior capsule is inadequate or completely absent, however, insertion of the IOL into the correct position for suturing can be daunting. The potential for the IOL to fall posteriorly into the vitreous cavity is substantial. If the IOL is folded in a "moustache" fashion, both haptics can be inserted posteriorly through the pupil and then, as the folding forceps starts to release the optic and the taco folded optic starts to open, the surgeon supports the optic with a cyclodialysis spatula to prevent it from falling posteriorly through the pupil.

A less risky and more reliable technique is to control the optic at all times with a forceps firmly grasping the optic at all times. In this manner, each haptic can be maneuvered through the pupil, then lifting the optic anteriorly and capturing the optic in the miotic pupil.

A moderately small pupil of about 3–4 mm diameter is important for secure pupillary capture of a 6 mm IOL optic during the suturing. A much smaller pupil makes insertion of the haptics challenging. Preoperative pupillary dilation should be avoided. A retrobulbar injection of anesthetic will result in moderate pupillary dilation, which is easily reversed with intraoperative miotic agents.

If the pupil is large and cannot be constricted adequately for secure optic fixation, then the safest technique is to insert only one haptic behind the iris initially, suture that haptic, and then insert the second haptic behind the iris. The surgeon must secure and stabilize the optic in order to insert the second haptic without excessive traction on the first sutured haptic and the suture itself, risking hemorrhage and tearing the iris. The optic is firmly grasped with one forcep while manipulating the second haptic with either a hook such as Lester or Kuglen hook or a microforceps in order to bend the haptic gently and manipulate the haptic through the pupil.

CONCLUSION

Peripheral iris suture fixation of an IOL is a valuable technique for complex cataract surgery and repair of subluxating IOLs. In many cases it is the procedure of choice for secondary posterior chamber IOL implants in the absence of support from the capsular bag. Mastering the technique will enrich any surgeon's surgical repertoire.

CHAPTER 70

Sutureless Posterior Chamber IOL Fixation with Intrascleral Haptic Fixation

Gabor B Scharioth

INTRODUCTION

In eyes with insufficient or no capsular support, IOL implantation and fixation techniques are still controversial. Many reports in the literature confirm that the IOL can be implanted in the anterior chamber or fixated to the iris and, alternatively, a posterior chamber IOL can be fixated in the ciliary sulcus using transscleral suturing or glueing.[1-22] We recently developed a sutureless technique for sulcus fixation of a posterior chamber IOL using permanent incarceration of the haptics in a scleral tunnel parallel to the limbus. This method combines the control of a closed-eye system with the postoperative axial stability of the posterior chamber IOL **(Figure 70.1)**.[23]

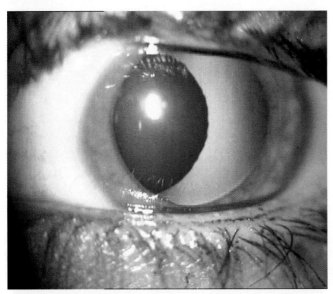

FIGURE 70.1: Preoperative situation in a patient with subluxated crystalline lens in Marfan´s syndrome

SURGICAL TECHNIQUE

After peritomy, the eye is stabilized either by 25-gauge pars plana infusion or with an anterior chamber maintainer. We try to prevent any diathermy of episcleral vessels to reduce the risk for scleral atrophy. Two straight sclerotomies ab externo are prepared with a sharp, 23- or 24-gauge cannula located 1.5–2.0 mm postlimbal and exactly 180° from each other **(Figures 70.2 to 70.6)**.

The cannulas are then used to create a limbus-parallel tunnel at approximately 50 percent scleral thickness,

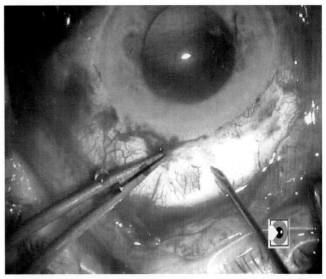

FIGURE 70.2: Preparing the ciliary sulcus sclerotomy 1.5 mm postlimbal

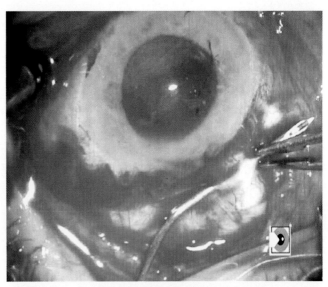

FIGURE 70.3: Preparing the limbus-parallel intrascleral tunnel with a 24-gauge cannula, note that 25 gauge pars plana infusion is used for stabilization of the eye

starting from the ciliary sulcus sclerotomies and ending with externalization of the cannula after 2 or 3 mm. Alternatively, a 23 gauge MVR blade could be used. A standard three-piece IOL with a haptic design fitting to the diameter of the ciliary sulcus is implanted with an injector, and the tailing haptic is fixated in the corneal incision. The leading

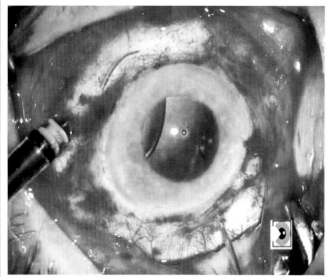

FIGURE 70.4: Inferior temporary externalized haptic, tip of trailing haptic grasped with 25 gauge endgripping forceps

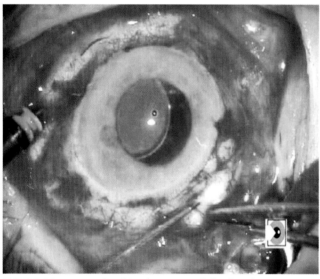

FIGURE 70.5: Intrascleral implantation of the first haptic using a special designed 25 gauge endgripping forceps (DORC, Netherlands)

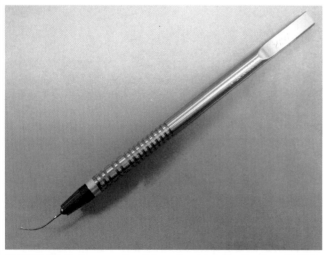

FIGURE 70.6: Forceps for intrascleral haptic fixation (DORC, Netherlands), curved end for easier haptic insertion, special designed end gripping tip for reduced trauma to IOL haptic

haptic is then grasped at its tip with an end-gripping 25-gauge forceps, pulled through the sclerotomy, and left externalized. With a special 25-gauge forceps (DORC, Netherlands), the haptic is then introduced into the intrascleral tunnel. The same maneuvers are performed with the trailing haptic. The ends of the haptic are left in the tunnel to prevent foreign body sensation and erosion of the conjuctiva and to reduce the risk for inflammation. The sclerotomies are checked for leakage. If necessary, they are sutured with 8 x 0 Vicryl. Conjunctiva is closed with adsorbable suture (**Figures 70.7 to 70.9**).

We have used this technique in more then 100 eyes over the past four years. Our standard IOLs are the Sensar AR40e (Abbott Medical Optics, Inc., Santa Ana, California) and the AcrySof (Alcon Laboratories, Inc, Fort Worth, Texas); however, we have also used multifocal IOLs, such as the ReZoom and Tecnis Multifocal (Abbott Medical Optics, Inc.).

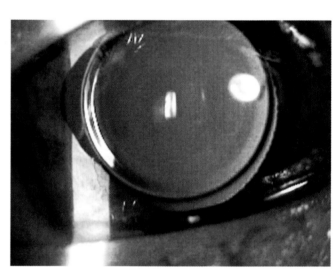

FIGURE 70.7: Postoperative situation after sutureless intrascleral fixation of a multifocal IOL (ReZoom, AMO, USA) in a Marfan´s case with luxated crystalline lens

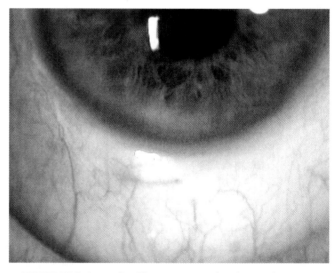

FIGURE 70.8: Intrascleral haptic 24 months after implantation

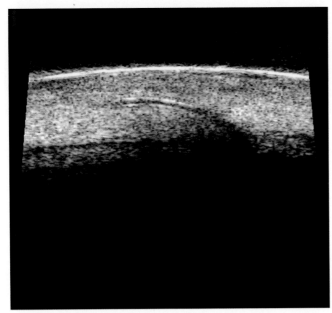

FIGURE 70.9: UBM image of intrascleral haptic. Please note that there is no sign of inflammation or leakage

DISCUSSION

Management of secondary implantation or refixation of dislocated posterior chamber IOLs with scleral tunnel fixation of the haptic is less technically demanding because it stabilizes the IOL in the posterior chamber without the need for difficult suturing procedures. This technique also enables the surgeon to easily recenter the IOL. Posterior chamber IOL torsion and decentration can be minimized by accurate placement of the haptics in the scleral tunnel above the ciliary sulcus. To avoid torsion, the haptic design of the implanted three-piece IOL should be at least as the diameter of the ciliary sulcus. Incarcerating a longer part of the haptic stabilizes the axial position of the IOL, which should decrease the incidence of tilt.[24]

Intraoperative IOL centration is possible due to adjustments made to the final intrascleral position of the haptics. The technique is appropriate for fixation of standard three-piece posterior chamber IOLs. However, it should not be used to fixate newer single-piece acrylic or silicone IOLs.

The potential complications of using sutures for transscleral fixation of posterior chamber IOLs include suture erosion, suture knot exposure, and recurrent dislocation caused by a broken suture.[25,26] All are preventable with the sutureless technique. Some techniques for scleral fixation of secondary IOLs, located within a scleral pocket, require two suture passes through the sclera for each haptic. This creates twice as many potential adverse bleeding events and endophthalmitis ports as our non-suturing technique.

Intrascleral fixation is an established technique in retinal surgery (i.e. silicone in buckling procedures) as well as refractive surgery. Because of the overall diameter of the IOLs, the author does not exert higher forces on the sclera. Scleral tunnels are well known in cataract surgery procedures, and scleromalacia should not be expected unless the patient has pre-existing inflammation, such as scleritis, episcleritis, rheumatoid arthritis, or herpes zoster ophthalmicus.[27-29] Because the tips of the haptics are buried, conjunctival erosion should not occur. The risk for chronic inflammation or recurrent bleeding is potentially lower than with any other sulcus-fixated IOL because there is no contact with the ciliary body.

Recently four European centers reported in their interim results of this technique.[30] Very low complication rate was observed and after four weeks postoperative period no complication has been occurred. This indicates a very good long term stability for lenses with intrascleral haptic fixation.

Power calculation of intraocular lens is same or 0.5 diopter less then for intracapsular implantation. In case of postoperative emmetropia Bioptics with excimer refractive surface treatment can be used for "fine tunning" of refraction. In this case using a suction ring for flap creation should be avoided.

Pearls of intrascleral PCIOL haptic fixation are as follows:
- No contraindication
- Standardized technique
- Standard PCIOL with no extra storage, easy logistic, routine biometry
- Excellent centration
- Sutureless
- Sclerafixation
- Minimal uveal contact
- Independent from iris changes
- Also for special IOL like multifocal and toric
- In combination with refractive surgery (Bioptics).

CONCLUSION

A modified technique can be performed for any procedure that requires trans-scleral fixation. This includes implantation of secondary IOLs, repairing dislocated IOLs,[19,31-33] and use of adjunctive surgical devices, such as the Ahmed capsular tension segment and Cionni capsular tension ring (both manufactured by Morcher GmbH, Germany). This technique simplifies scleral fixation of dislocated posterior chamber IOLs and allows successful repositioning of dislocated and subluxated posterior chamber IOLs. It also minimizes intraoperative maneuvers and could thus reduce the risk for intraoperative trauma. Furthermore, this technique can be performed with standard three-piece posterior chamber IOLs without the need for special haptic architecture or preparation. Additionally, there is no need to store or order special IOLs for rare indications as it is independent from iris changes.

REFERENCES

1. Anand R, Bowman RW. Simplified technique for suturing dislocated posterior chamber intraocular lens to the ciliary sulcus. Arch Ophthalmol. 1990;108:1205-6.

2. Azar DT, Wiley WF. Double-knot trans-scleral suture fixation technique for displaced intraocular lenses. Am J Ophthalmol. 1999;128:644-6.

3. Bloom SM, Wyszynski RE, Brucker AJ. Scleral fixation suture for dislocated posterior chamber intraocular lens. Ophthalmic Surg. 1990;21:851-4.

4. Chan CK. An improved technique for management of dislocated posterior chamber implants. Ophthalmology. 1992;99:51-7.

5. Chang S. Perfluorocarbon liquids in vitreoretinal surgery. Int Ophthalmol Clin. 1992;32(2):153-63.

6. Chang S, Coll GE. Surgical techniques for repositioning a dislocated intraocular lens, repair of iridodialysis, and secondary intraocular lens implantation using innovative 25-gauge forceps. Am J Ophthalmol. 1995;119:165-74.

7. Fanous MM, Friedman SM. Ciliary sulcus fixation of a dislocated posterior chamber intraocular lens using liquid perfluorophenanthrene. Ophthalmic Surg. 1992;23:551-2.

8. Friedberg MA, Pilkerton AR. A new technique for repositioning and fixating a dislocated intraocular lens. Arch Ophthalmol. 1992;110:413-5.

9. Kokame GT, Yamamoto I, Mandel H. Scleral fixation of dislocated posterior chamber intraocular lenses; temporary haptic externalization through a clear corneal incision. J Cataract Refract Surg. 2004;30:1049-56.

10. Little BC, Rosen PH, Orr G, et al. Trans-scleral fixation of dislocated posterior chamber intraocular lenses using a 9/0 microsurgical polypropylene snare. Eye. 1993;7:740-3.

11. Maguire AM, Blumenkranz MS, Ward TG, et al. Scleral loop fixation for posteriorly dislocated intraocular lenses; operative technique and long-term results. Arch Ophthalmol. 1991; 109:1754-8.

12. Nabors G, Varley MP, Charles S. Ciliary sulcus suturing of a posterior chamber intraocular lens. Ophthalmic Surg. 1990;21:263-5.

13. Schneiderman TE, Johnson MW, Smiddy WE, et al. Surgical management of posteriorly dislocated silicone plate haptic intraocular lenses. Am J Ophthalmol. 1997;123:629-35.

14. Shin DH, Hu BV, Hong YJ, et al. Posterior chamber lens implantation in the absence of posterior capsular support. Ophthalmic Surg. 1988;19:606-7.

15. Smiddy WE. Dislocated posterior chamber intraocular lens; a new technique of management. Arch Ophthalmol. 1989;107:1678-80.

16. Smiddy WE, Flynn HW Jr. Needle-assisted scleral fixation suture technique for relocating posteriorly dislocated IOLs. Arch Ophthalmol. 1993;111:161-2.

17. Smiddy WE, Ibanez GV, Alfonso E, et al. Surgical management of dislocated intraocular lenses. J Cataract Refract Surg. 1995;21:64-9.

18. Thach AB, Dugel PU, Sipperley JO, et al. Outcome of sulcus fixation of dislocated posterior chamber intraocular lenses using temporary externalization of the haptics. Ophthalmology. 2000;107:480-484; discussion by WF Mieler, 2000;107:485.

19. Koh HJ, Kim CY, Lim SJ, et al. Scleral fixation technique using 2 corneal tunnels for a dislocated intraocular lens. J Cataract Refract Surg. 2000;26:1439-41.

20. Lewis JS. Ab externo sulcus fixation. Ophthalmic Surg. 1991;22:692-5.

21. Mohr A, Hengerer F, Eckardt C. Retropupillare Fixation der Irisklauenlinse bei Aphakie; Einjahresergebnisse einer neuen Implantationstechnik. [Retropupillary fixation of the iris claw lens in aphakia; 1 year outcome of a new implantation technique.] Ophthalmologe. 2002;99:580-3.

22. Agarwal A, Kumar DA, Jacob S, et al. Fibrin glue-assisted sutureless posterior chamber intraocular lens implantation in eyes with deficient posterior capsules. J Cataract Refract Surgery. 2008;34:1433-8.

23. Gabor SG, Pavlidis MM. Sutureless intrascleral posterior chamber intraocular lens fixation. J Cataract Refract Surg. 2007;33:1851-4.

24. Teichmann KD, Teichmann IAM. The torque and tilt gamble. J Cataract Refract Surg. 1997;23:413-8.

25. Por YM, Lavin MJ. Techniques of intraocular lens suspension in the absence of capsular/zonular support. Surv Ophthalmol. 2005;50:429-62.

26. Wagoner MD, Cox TA, Ariyasu RG, et al. Intraocular lens implantation in the absence of capsular support; a report by the American Academy of Ophthalmology. Ophthalmology. 2003;110:840-59.

27. Ahmed TY, Carrim ZI, Diaper CJM, et al. Spontaneous intraocular lens extrusion in a patient with scleromalacia secondary to herpes zoster ophthalmicus. J Cataract Refract Surg. 2007;33:925-6.

28. Mamalis N, Johnson MD, Haines JM, et al. Corneal-scleral melt in association with cataract surgery and intraocular lenses: A report of four cases. J Cataract Refract Surg. 1990;16:108-115.

29. Watson PG, Hayreh SS. Scleritis and episcleritis. Br J Ophthalmol. 1976;60:163-91.

30. Scharioth GB, Prasad S, Georgalas I, et al. Intermediate results of sutureless intrascleral posterior chamber intraocular lens fixation. J Cataract Refractive Surg. 2010;36(2):254-9.

31. Moreno-Montan̄eś J, Heras H, Ferna̕ndez-Hortelano A. Surgical treatment of a dislocated intraocular lens-capsular bag-capsular tension ring complex. J Cataract Refract Surg. 2005;31:270-3.

32. Gross JG, Kokame GT, Weinberg DV. In-the-bag intraocular Lens Dislocation; the Dislocated In-the-Bag Intraocular Lens Study. Am J Ophthalmol. 2004;137:630-5.

33. Jehan FS, Mamalis N, Crandall AS. Spontaneous late dislocation of intraocular lens within the capsular bag in pseudoexfoliation patients. Ophthalmology. 2001;108: 1727-31.

CHAPTER 71

Glued PC IOL Implantation with Intralamellar Scleral Tuck in Eyes with Deficient Capsule

Dhivya Ashok Kumar, Amar Agarwal

INTRODUCTION

Posterior capsular rent (PCR)[1,2] can occur in early learning curve in phacoemulsification. intraoperative dialysis or large PCR will prevent intraocular lens (IOL) implantation in the capsular bag. Implantation of IOL in the sulcus will be possible in adequate anterior capsular support. The first glued PC IOL implantation in an eye with a deficient capsule was done by the authors on 14th of December 2007. In eyes with inadequate anterior capsular rim and deficient posterior capsule, the new technique of IOL implantation is the fibrin glue assisted sutureless IOL implantation with scleral tuck.[3-7]

SURGICAL TECHNIQUE

Under peribulbar anesthesia, superior rectus is caught and clamped. Localized peritomy and wet cautery of the sclera at the desired site of exit of the IOL haptics is done. Infusion cannula or anterior chamber maintainer is inserted. If using an infusion cannula, one can use a 23 G sutureless trocar and cannula. Positioning of the infusion cannula should be preferably in inferonasal quadrant to prevent interference in creating the scleral flaps. Two partial thickness limbal based scleral flaps about 2.5 mm × 3 mm are created exactly 180 degrees diagonally apart (**Figures 71.1A and B**). This is followed by 23 G vitrectomy via pars plana or anterior route to remove all vitreous traction. Two straight sclerotomies with a 20G/22G needle are made about 1.0 mm from the limbus under the existing scleral flaps.

A clear corneal/scleral tunnel incision is then prepared for introducing the IOL. While the IOL is being introduced with the one hand of the surgeon using a McPherson forceps or injector (depending upon the type of IOL), an end gripping 23 G/25 G microrhexis forceps (Micro Surgical Technology, USA) is passed through the inferior sclerotomy with the other hand. One can use any end opening forceps like a micro rhexis forceps. The tip of the leading haptic is then grasped with the microrhexis forceps, pulled through the inferior sclerotomy following the curve of the haptic (**Figures 71.2A and B**) and is externalized under the inferior scleral flap. Similarly, the trailing haptic is also externalized through the superior sclerotomy under the scleral flap. The tips of the haptics are then tucked inside a scleral tunnel made with 26 G needle at the point of extension. Scleral flaps are closed with fibrin glue (**Figures 71.3A and B**). The anterior chamber maintainer or the infusion cannula is removed. Limbal wound is sutured with 10-0 monofilament nylon if it is a sclera tunnel incision or closed with glue (in corneal wound). Conjunctiva is also closed with the same fibrin glue (**Figures 71.4A to C**).

FIBRIN GLUE

The fibrin kit the author used is Reliseal (Reliance Life Sciences, India). Another widely used tissue glue namely Tisseel (Baxter) can also be used. The fibrinogen and thrombin are first reconstituted according to the manufacturer's instructions. The commercially available fibrin glue that is virus inactivated is checked for viral antigen and antibodies with polymerase chain reaction; hence the

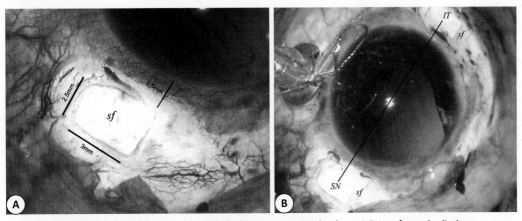

FIGURES 71.1A and B: Scleral flaps (*sf*) of 2.5 x 3 mm made about 1.5 mm from the limbus. Two flaps 180 degrees diagonally apart

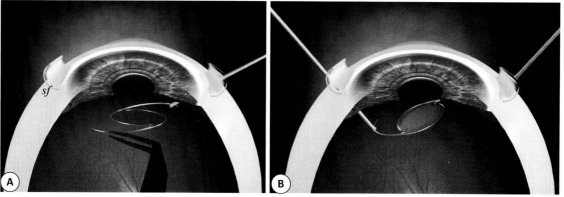

FIGURES 71.2A AND B: Image showing sclerotomy made with 22 G needle beneath the flaps
Haptics exteriorized by 25 G forceps beneath the scleral flaps (*sf*)

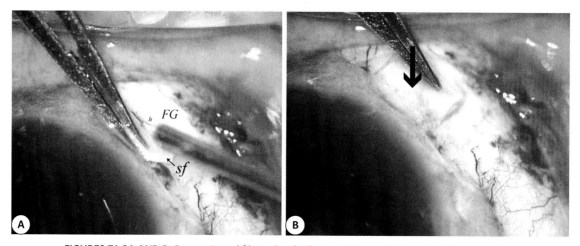

FIGURES 71.3A AND B: Reconstituted fibrin glue (FG) injected beneath the scleral flaps over the
haptics and scleral flaps (*sf*) closed

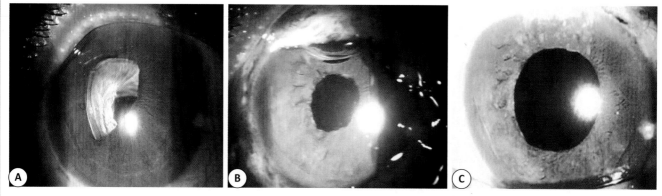

FIGURES 71.4A TO C: (A) Preoperative slit lamp image showing anterior subluxated IOL;
(B) Day one postoperative period; (C) Three months after surgery

chances of transmission of infection are very low. But with tissue derivatives, there is always a theoretical possibility of transmission of viral infections.

Reconstitution of Reliseal

It is available in a sealed pack, which contains freeze dried human fibrinogen (20 mg/0.5 ml), freeze dried human thrombin (250 IU/0.5 ml), aprotinin solution (1500 kiu in 0.5 ml), one ampoule of sterile water, four 21G needles, two 20 G blunt application needles and an applicator with two mixing chambers and one plunger guide. First, the aprotinin solution is taken in a 2 ml sterile syringe and mixed with the freeze dried fibrinogen and is then shaken by slow circular motion. The reconstituted vial is then placed in a preheated water bath of 37 degrees for not more than 10 minutes. Next, about 0.5 ml of water for injection is aspirated and injected into the vial of freeze dried thrombin followed by gentle agitation of the vial. Reconstitution is considered complete when no undissolved particles are visible. Both the reconstituted fibrinogen and the thrombin are loaded separately in two 2 ml sterile syringes and mounted on to the Reliseal applicator for use.

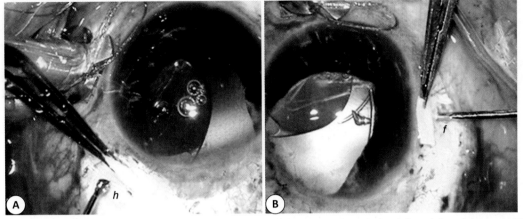

FIGURES 71.5A AND B: Haptics *(h)* exteriorized by 25G forceps *(f)* beneath the scleral flaps *(sf)* in dislocated IOL

Then, the reconstituted fibrin glue thus prepared is injected through the cannula of the double syringe delivery system under the superior and inferior scleral flaps. Local pressure is given over the flaps for about 10–20 seconds for the formation of fibrin polypeptides.

Special Situations

In case of those patients who had a luxated IOL, similar lamellar scleral flaps as described earlier are made and the luxated IOL haptic is then grasped with the 23/25 gauge rhexis forceps and externalized and glued under the scleral flaps **(Figures 71.5A and B)**.

Advantages

This fibrin glue assisted sutureless PCIOL implantation technique would be useful in a myriad of clinical situations where scleral fixated IOLs are indicated, such as luxated IOL, dislocated IOL, zonulopathy or secondary IOL implantation.

No special IOLs: It can be performed well with rigid PMMA IOL, 3 piece PC IOL or IOLs with modified PMMA haptics. One, therefore, does not need to have an entire inventory of special SFIOLs with eyelets, unlike in sutured SFIOLs. In dislocated posterior chamber PMMA IOL, the same IOL can be repositioned, thereby reducing the need for further manipulation. Furthermore, there is no need for newer haptic designs or special instruments other than the 25 gauge forceps.

No tilt: Since the overall diameter of the routine IOL is about 12–13 mm, with the haptic being placed in its normal curved configuration and without any traction, there is no distortion or change in shape of the IOL optic **(Figure 71.6)**. Externalization of the greater part of the haptics along its curvature stabilizes the axial positioning of the IOL and thereby prevents any IOL tilt.[8]

Less pseudophacodonesis: When the eye moves, it acquires kinetic energy from its muscles and attachments and the energy is dissipated to the internal fluids as it stops. Thus,

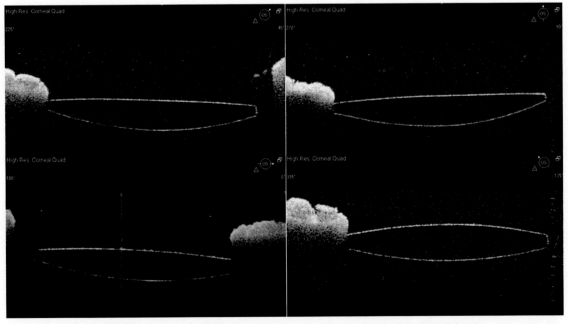

FIGURE 71.6: Anterior segment OCT showing 360 degrees good centration of the IOL

pseudophacodonesis is the result of oscillations of the fluids in the anterior and posterior segment of the eye. These oscillations, initiated by movement of the eye, result in shearing forces on the corneal endothelium as well as vitreous motion lead to permanent damage. Since the IOL haptic is stuck beneath the flap, it would prevent the further movement of the haptic and thereby reducing the pseudophacodonesis.[9]

Less UGH syndrome: The authors expect less incidence of UGH syndrome in fibrin glue assisted IOL implantation, as compared to sutured scleral fixated IOL. This is because; in the former, the IOL is well stabilized and stuck onto the scleral bed and thereby, has decreased intraocular mobility, whereas in the latter, there is increased possibility of IOL movement or persistent rub over the ciliary body.

No suture related complications: Visually significant complications due to late subluxation[10] which has been known to occur in sutured scleral fixated IOL may also be prevented as sutures are totally avoided in this technique. Another important advantage of this technique is the prevention of suture related complications,[11,12] like suture erosion, suture knot exposure or dislocation of IOL after suture disintegration or broken suture.

Rapidity and ease of surgery: All the time taken in SFIOL for passing suture into the IOL haptic eyelets, to ensure good centeration before tying down the knots, as well as time for suturing scleral flaps and closing conjunctiva are significantly reduced. The risk of retinal photic injury[13] which is known to occur in SFIOL would also be reduced in this technique due to the short surgical time. Fibrin glue takes less time [Reliseal (20 seconds)/Tisseel (3 seconds)] to act in the scleral bed and it helps in adhesion as well as hemostasis. The preparation time can also be reduced in elective procedures by preparing it prior to surgery as it remains stable up to four hours from the time of reconstitution. Fibrin glue has been shown to provide airtight closure and by the time the fibrin starts degrading, surgical adhesions would have already occurred in the scleral bed. This is well shown in the follow-up anterior segment OCT (**Figures 71.7A and B**) where postoperative perfect scleral flap adhesion is observed.

Stability of the IOL Haptic

As the flaps are manually created, the rough apposing surfaces of the flap and bed heal rapidly and firmly around the haptic, being helped by the fibrin glue early on. The major uncertainty here is the stability of the fibrin matrix *in vivo*. Numerous animal studies have shown that the fibrin glue is still present at 4–6 weeks. Because postoperative fibrosis starts early, the flaps become stuck secondary to fibrosis even prior to full degradation of the glue (**Figures 71.8A to D**). The ensuing fibrosis acts like a firm scaffold around the haptic which prevents movement along the long axis (**Figure 71.9A**). To further make the IOL rock stable, the author has started tucking the haptic tip into the scleral wall through a tunnel. This prevents all movement of the haptic along the transverse axis as well (**Figure 71.9B**). The stability of the lens first comes through the tucking of the haptics in the scleral pocket created. The tissue glue then gives it extra stability and also seals the flap down. Externalization of the greater part of the haptics along its curvature stabilizes the axial positioning of the IOL and thereby prevents any IOL tilt.

Steps of Surgery for a Glued IOL

It is to look at the various steps of surgery for a glued IOL (**Figures 71.10 to 71.38**). This shows the way that an injectable foldable IOL can be glued into an eye with no capsules.

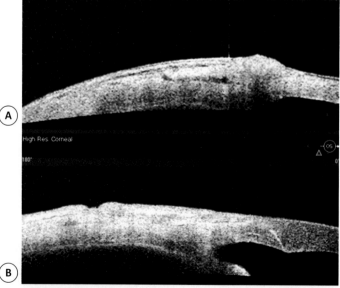

FIGURES 71.7A AND B: (A) Anterior segment OCT showing the scleral flap placement on day 1 and (B) Adhesion well maintained till six weeks

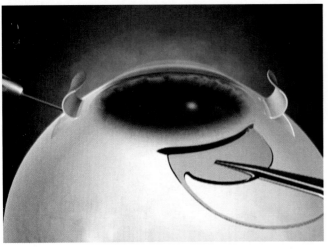

(A) IOL haptic grasped with a microsurgical technology MST forceps (USA)

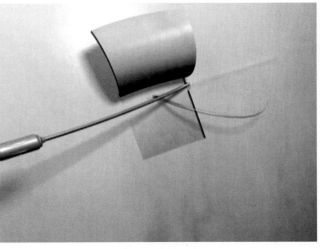

(B) 26-Gauge needle creates a scleral pocket at the edge of the flap

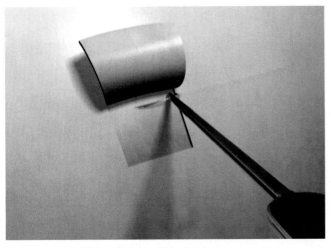

(C) IOL haptic tucked into the scleral pocket

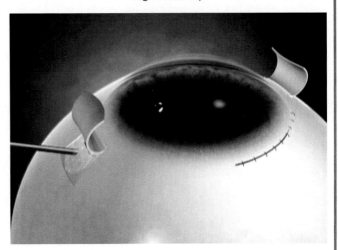

(D) Fibrin glue applied under the scleral flaps

FIGURES 71.8A TO D: Surgical technique of the glued IOL

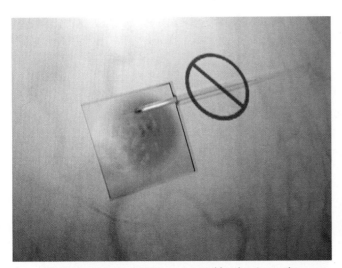

(A) Long axis movement is prevented by the tissue glue

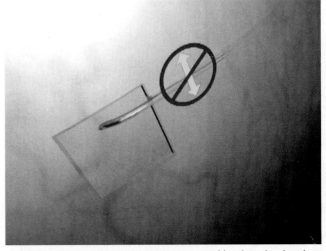

(B) Transverse axis movement is prevented by the scleral tuck

FIGURES 71.9A AND B: Stability of the IOL

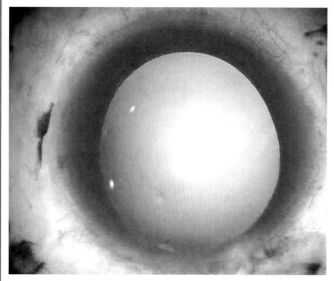

FIGURE 71.10: Aphakic case. No capsule seen

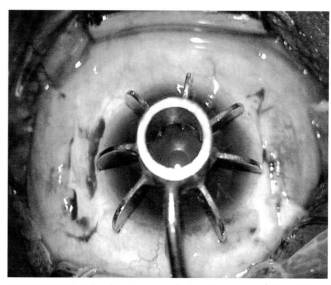

FIGURE 71.11: Scleral markers applied on the cornea. This will help to get marks created on the cornea 180 degrees apart to make sclera flaps

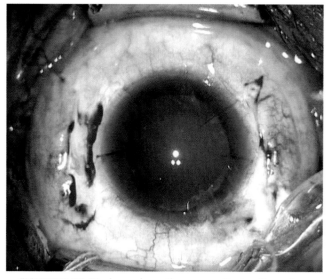

FIGURE 71.12: Marks made on the cornea. Conjunctiva cut on either side of the marks

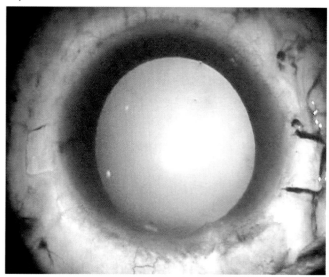

FIGURE 71.13: Scleral flaps made 180 degrees apart

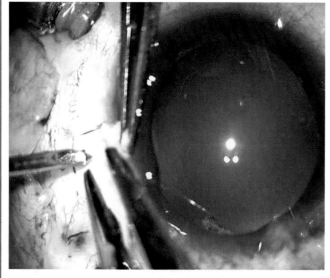

FIGURE 71.14: Sclerotomy made 1 mm from the limbus under the sclera flap using a 20 G needle

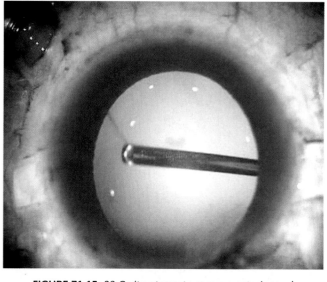

FIGURE 71.15: 23 G vitrectomy to remove anterior and midvitreous

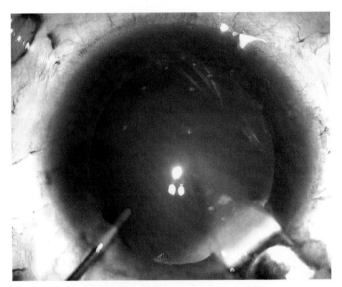

FIGURE 71.16: Clear corneal incision

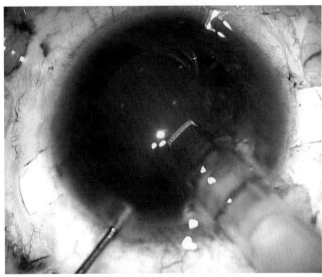

FIGURE 71.17: Foldable 3 piece IOL being injected slowly. It is to note that the cartridge is inside the eye. One should not do wound assisted as the injection might happen too fast. This can either break the IOL or push it so fast that it might go into the vitreous cavity

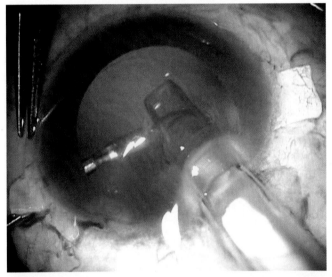

FIGURE 71.18: Foldable IOL injection continued with one hand. This injector has a pushing mechanism so one hand can be used. The other hand holds an end opening microrhexis forceps (23 G) and is passed through the sclerotomy under the sclera flap and is ready to grab the haptic

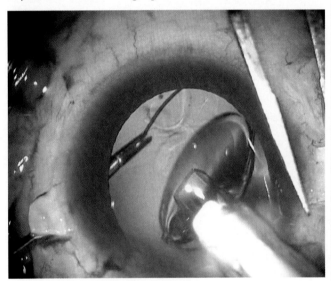

FIGURE 71.19: End opening forceps grabs the haptic tip

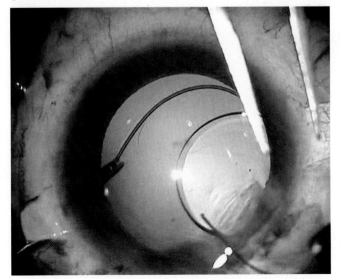

FIGURE 71.20: Forceps pulls the haptic while injection of the foldable IOL is continued

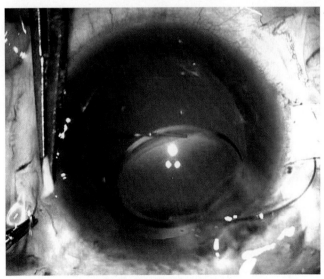

FIGURE 71.21: Haptic externalized

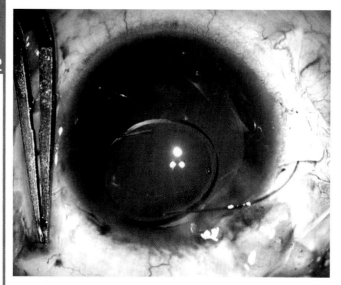

FIGURE 71.22: Assistant holds the haptic which is externalized

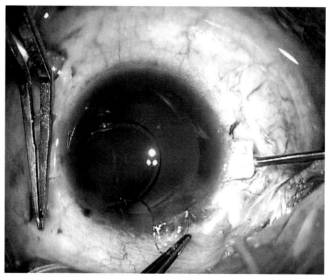

FIGURE 71.23: Trailing haptic is flexed into the anterior chamber. The other hand holds the end opening microrhexis forceps and is passed through the other sclerotomy under the sclera flap

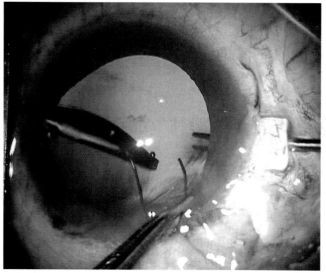

FIGURE 71.24: End opening forceps ready to grab the haptic tip

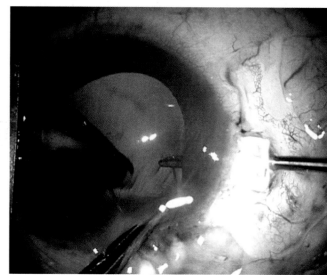

FIGURE 71.25: Haptic caught

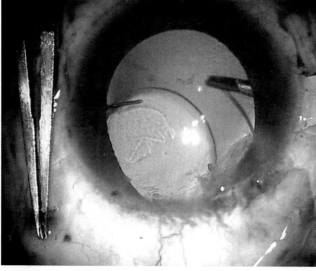

FIGURE 71.26: Haptic is gradually pulled towards the sclerotomy

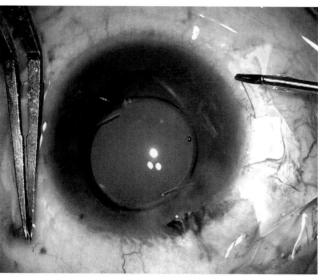

FIGURE 71.27: Haptic externalized

PHACOEMULSIFICATION

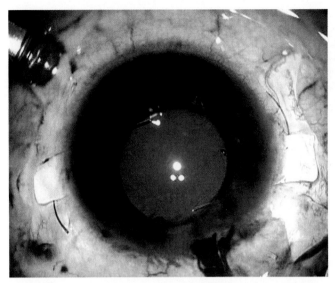

FIGURE 71.28: Both haptics externalized and can be seen lying under the sclera flaps

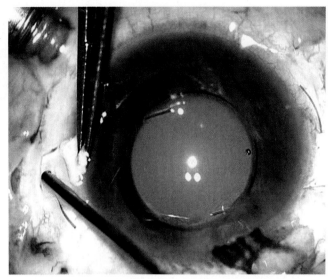

FIGURE 71.29: Vitrectomy done at the sclerotomy site

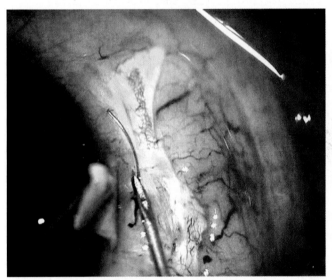

FIGURE 71.30: 26 G needle makes a sclera pocket at the edge of the flap where the haptic is seen

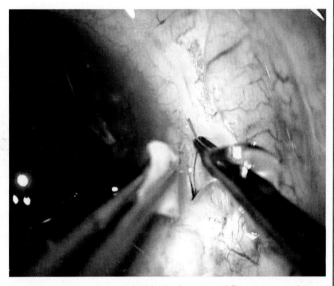

FIGURE 71.31: Forceps holds the haptic and flexes it to tuck it inside the scleral pocket

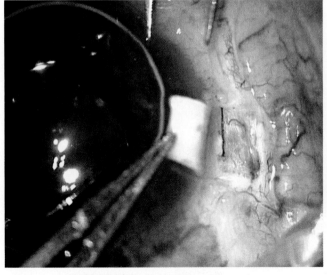

FIGURE 71.32: Haptic in the sclera pocket

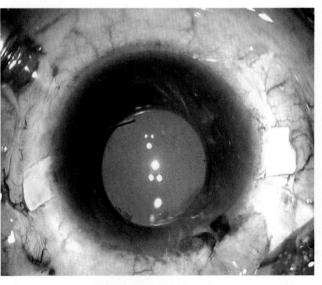

FIGURE 71.33: PC IOL stable

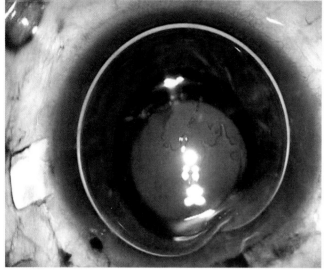

FIGURE 71.34: Infusion cut off and air fills the anterior chamber

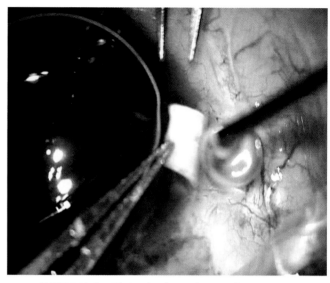

FIGURE 71.35: Fibrin glue (Tiessel, Baxter) application

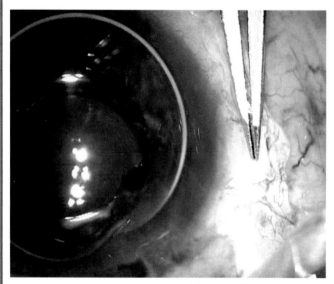

FIGURE 71.36: Scleral flap sealed

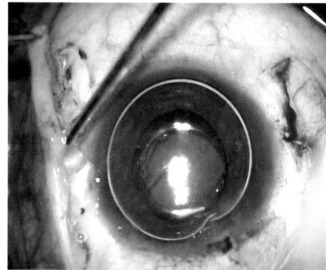

FIGURE 71.37: Fibrin glue applied on conjunctiva and clear corneal incison to seal them

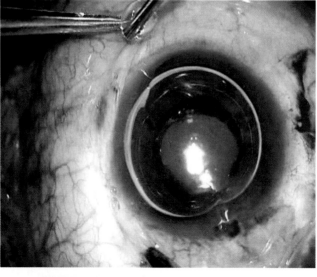

FIGURE 71.38: Immediate postoperation on table

REFERENCES

1. Vajpayee RB, Sharma N, Dada T, et al. Management of posterior capsule tears. Surv Ophthal. 2001;45:473-88.
2. Wu MC, Bhandari A. Managing the broken capsule. Curr Opin Ophthalmol. 2008;19:36-40.
3. Agarwal A, Kumar DA, Jacob S, et al. Fibrin glue-assisted sutureless posterior chamber intraocular lens implantation in eyes with deficient posterior capsules. J Cataract Refract Surg. 2008;34:1433-8.
4. Prakash G, Kumar DA, Jacob S, et al. Anterior segment optical coherence tomography-aided diagnosis and primary posterior chamber intraocular lens implantation with fibrin glue in traumatic phacocele with scleral perforation. J Cataract Refract Surg. 2009;35:782-4.
5. Prakash G, Jacob S, Kumar DA, et al. Femtosecond assisted keratoplasty with fibrin glue-assisted sutureless posterior chamber lens implantation: a new triple procedure. J Cataract Refract Surg. In press (manuscript no 08-919).
6. Agarwal A, Kumar DA, Prakash G, et al. Fibrin glue–assisted sutureless posterior chamber intraocular lens implantation in eyes with deficient posterior capsules [Reply to letter]. J Cataract Refract Surg. 2009;35:795-6.
7. Nair V, Kumar DA, Prakash G, et al. Bilateral spontaneous in-the-bag anterior subluxation of PC IOL managed with glued IOL technique: a case report. Eye Contact Lens. 2009;35(4):215-7.
8. Teichmann KD, Teichmann IAM. The torque and tilt gamble. J Cataract Refract Surg. 1997;23:413-8.
9. Jacobi KW, Jagger WS. Physical forces involved in pseudophacodonesis and iridodonesis. Albrecht Von Graefes Arch Klin Exp Ophthalmol. 1981;216:49-53.
10. Price MO, Price FW Jr, Werner L, et al. Late dislocation of scleral-sutured posterior chamber intraocular lenses. J Cataract Refract Surg. 2005;31(7):1320-6.
11. Solomon K, Gussler JR, Gussler C, et al. Incidence and management of complications of transsclerally sutured posterior chamber lenses. J Cataract Refract Surg. 1993;19:488-93.
12. Asadi R, Kheirkhah A. Long-term results of scleral fixation of posterior chamber intraocular lenses in children. Ophthalmology. 2008;115(1):67-72.
13. Lanzetta P, Menchini U, Virgili G, et al. Scleral fixated intraocular lenses: an angiographic study. Retina. 1998;18:515-20.

Miscellaneous

CHAPTER 72

Femtosecond Laser-Assisted Refractive Cataract Surgery

Glauco Reggiani Mello, Jonathan H Talamo, Ronald R Krueger

The main objective in the surgical management of cataracts has always been the treatment of a disease. Residual refractive errors, delayed recovery and even complications were accepted and even expected by both patients and physicians. While numerous advances in intraocular lens design have occurred since the time of Sir Harold Ridley, cataract surgical technology itself has not undergone fundamental changes since the introduction of phacoemulsification over 40 years ago. Following the development of intraocular lenses and small incision surgical technique, patients and doctors became less tolerant of imperfect or unexpected results. The drive within our profession to continually improve efficacy and safety is pushing to what will likely become the greatest paradigm shift in cataract surgery since the development of ultrasonic phacoemulsification: femtosecond laser-assisted refractive cataract surgery (FLARCS). Through automation of many of the most delicate and critical steps of the procedure, this technology has the potential to improve the results of both standard and premium cataract surgery.

Modern cataract surgery is fast becoming a refractive surgical procedure. Despite the excellent results obtained with the current technology, perfection is demanded by patients and surgeons alike. Femtosecond laser technology is expected to improve safety and uncorrected visual acuity (UCVA) results, due to a reduction in postoperative astigmatism, wound dehiscence, IOL decentration and potentially visually disabling complications such as capsular tears and vitreous loss. This technology is able to correct pre-existing and induced astigmatism with corneal incisions (using precisely created multiplanar clear corneal entry and limbal relaxing incisions of uniform depth and radius) and likely improve effective intraocular lens positioning through the use of fastidiously sized, centered and shaped anterior capsulorhexis incisions. In the years ahead, uncorrected visual acuity expectations and results after cataract surgery will likely rival those experienced after LASIK.

LIMITATIONS OF MANUAL CATARACT SURGERY

Modern cataract surgery is comprised of five principal surgical steps: incisions, capsulotomy, emulsification, IOL insertion (and centration) and astigmatism correction (toric IOL or limbal relaxing incisions). Each of these steps is currently performed by the surgeon's hand, and each is critical to the success and outcome of the procedure. Imperfect execution of these steps can lead to a less than desirable outcome and/or serious complications.

A clear corneal incision that leaks can allow entry of extraocular fluids into the anterior chamber, potentially leading to a severe endophthalmitis that can result in an enucleation.[1] A torn capsulotomy can lead to problems with IOL placement and centration, posterior capsular rupture and/or vitreous loss. An excessively small capsulotomy can increase the difficulty of lens extraction and likelihood of anterior capsular phimosis, which can decenter and tilt the IOL.[2] During lens emulsification, excessive ultrasound energy can cause a thermal incision burn[3] (increased chance of a leaking incision, astigmatism induction or tissue necrosis). The need to manually segment the lens nucleus is also a risk factor for posterior capsular rupture, particularly when the cataractous lens is very dense or compromised zonular integrity is present. A hand-made limbal relaxing incision can result in corneal perforation, flipped astigmatism axis, under correction or irregular astigmatism. Clinical data is not yet substantial enough to unequivocally demonstrate improved safety and efficacy of femtosecond laser cataract surgery over existing techniques. Complications unique to this technology, that have not yet been recognized, could arise, however, preliminary clinical experience suggests that routine use of femtosecond laser technology will likely decrease the overall rate of all of the above complications, resulting in safer and more precise cataract surgery.

FEMTOSECOND LASER TECHNOLOGY

The femtosecond laser was first introduced to the field of ophthalmology following the discovery that it could perform intrastromal only cuts (i.e no damage to the epithelium). Acting as a precise "laser blade", femtosecond lasers were successfully used to perform LASIK flaps, serving as a substitute for the microkeratome. Applications of the technology have expanded to other corneal procedures (i.e. corneal transplants, intrastromal corneal ring channels, astigmatic keratotomy/limbal relaxing incisions) proving to be major surgical refinements in ophthalmologic care. In addition to the expected changes in refractive, corneal and cataract surgery, future innovative

TABLE 72.1 Characteristics of lasers in ophthalmology

Laser	Wavelength	Effect
Excimer	193 nm	Photoablation
Argon	514–488 nm	Photocoagulation
Femtosecond	1053 nm	Photodisruption/Photodissection
Nd:Yag	1064 nm	Photodisruption
Carbon dioxide	10600 nm	Photothermal

Nd:YAG – Neodymium-doped yttrium aluminum garnet

procedures with the femtosecond laser can be expected in glaucoma,[4] vitreoretinal surgery[5] and in the preparation of keratolimbal[6] and possibly corneal endothelial grafts.

The currently available femtosecond laser devices use a near infrared laser with a wavelength of about 1053 nm. Unique, ultrashort duration laser pulses (10^{-15} seconds) cause significantly less damage in surrounding tissue and allows its use as a "laser blade" in a process called photodisruption or photodissection. The wavelength of the femtosecond laser is very similar to the one found in the Nd:YAG laser **(Table 72.1)**. However, the longer duration of the pulses in the latter (10^{-9} seconds) cause significant thermal damage in the surrounding tissue.[7] Varying the duration of the laser pulses and energy applied can generate different effects on the tissue **(Figure 72.1)**. The main technical specifications that play a role in the femtosecond laser are the following:

• Laser pulse repetition rate
• Spot size
• Pulse energy
• Pulse pattern

There is an inverse relation between the laser pulse duration and the energy required in each pulse to generate the optical breakdown.[8] Since there is nearly ten years experience with femtosecond laser technology for flap creation, ideal parameters to cut the cornea are now better understood. The earliest devices used for creating flaps operated with a low kilohertz repetition rate and needed a higher energy with

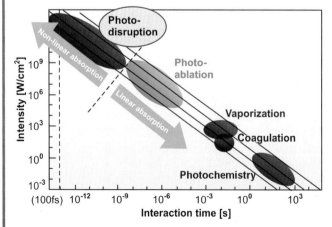

FIGURE 72.1: Effects of the relation between laser interaction time and energy intensity

larger spacing to achieve photodissection. Newer devices tend to increase repetition rate, which makes the procedure duration shorter, the spacing smaller and the energy lower, with the goal of reducing inflammation. The spot size and separation is also made smaller when using higher repetition rates, to produce smoother surface cuts without significantly increasing the time of the procedure.

In summary, the ideal device to cut the cornea and other avascular intraocular tissues (i.e. the lens) would include a high repetition rate, small spot size and low pulse energy. However, there is not yet data available regarding these technical specifications in the femtosecond laser cataract devices. The complexity in generating ideal femtosecond laser parameters for cataract surgery is greater, since the scope of laser-tissue interactions in one system must differ depending on location within the eye (cornea, anterior capsule and lens).

The potential geometry for cutting ocular tissues with femtosecond lasers is theoretically limitless. Vertical, horizontal, multiplanar and every imaginable geometrical pattern can be applied if appropriate software and hardware is utilized.

SYSTEMS AVAILABLE

Currently, three companies ("LensAR" – LensAR Inc., Winter Park, FL; "LenSx" - LenSx Lasers Inc., Aliso Viejo, CA; and "Optimedica" - OptiMedica Corporation, Santa Clara, CA) are developing femtosecond technology to make primary clear corneal incision, paracentesis, capsulotomy, lens fragmentation and limbal relaxing incisions. The first commercial systems are expected to become available in the 2011. The femtosecond laser devices for cataract surgery are more complex than the ones for flap creation. They require very precise imaging systems and a docking system that does not dramatically increase the intraocular pressure and preserves the anatomy of the cornea and intraocular structures.

IMAGING SYSTEMS

The imaging system is one of the most crucial parts in a femtosecond laser cataract surgery device. Displacement of the laser pulses by a fraction of a millimeter can cause a posterior capsular rupture and its further complications. The LenSx laser and the OptiMedica laser use real-time, high-resolution OCT. Further specifications regarding resolution and technical specifications have not yet been disclosed by the companies. The LensAR laser system uses a high-resolution 3D confocal structured illumination (CSI), a form of infrared-based scanning laser imaging. Regular OCT technologies usually have lower lateral resolution compared to axial (Visante has 18 µm axial and 60 µm lateral). In high-resolution commercially available OCT (axial resolution 5 µm, lateral 15 µm) it is not possible to get the entire image of the cornea in one picture, so combining pictures become necessary. LensAR's 3D CSI can achieve a

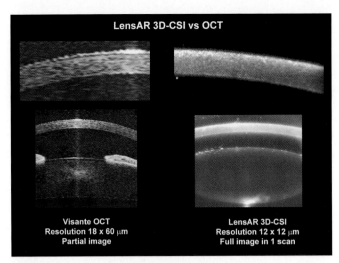

FIGURE 72.2: Visante (Carl Zeiss Meditec, Inc., Dublin,CA) in high-resolution mode (left) versus 3D-CSI (right) of the cornea, anterior chamber and crystalline lens. Image Courtesy from LensAR Inc., Winter Park, FL

resolution of approximately 12 μm (**Figure 72.2**) in any axis in one high-resolution image (it is not necessary to combine several images). A high contrast image is used with computer algorithms that can determine the grade of lens opacity based on light scattering. The computer then generates the plan of necessary laser pulse power and pattern needed for that specific nucleus density. Higher-grades cataracts have always been a challenge, and the full potential of each of the three technologies in those cases has yet to be proven.

DOCKING SYSTEM

There is no eyetracking system capable of the micron precision needed by the femtosecond technology, so fixating the eye with a docking system is required. The first devices for flap creation used a flat applanating glass, which allows good centration and is relatively easy to apply, however they produce high intraocular pressure and displace the intraocular structures. There are also devices that use a curved docking system, which allows less tissue deformation and lower intraocular pressure. The companies have not disclosed data regarding the docking systems of Optimedica and LenSx devices. The LensAR Laser system uses a different approach. The patient's interface is a no-touch, non-applanating suction fixation device (an automatically filled miniature water chamber). Since there is no touch in the cornea by a flat or curved device, the company claims that the corneal shape does not change, preserving the natural position of the ocular structures, with a beneficial effect on astigmatic outcomes. More data about the differences among the devices are expected after they become commercially available.

PROCEDURE

The femtosecond cataract surgery procedure can be performed in either a separate laser room outside the

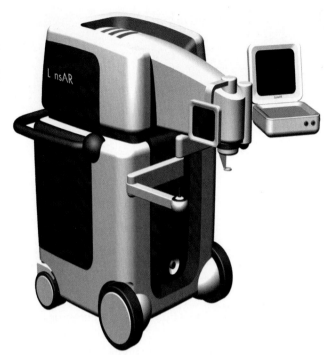

FIGURE 72.3: LensAR laser system. The device is a little larger than a phacoemulsification system and can function in a separate laser room or in the OR. Image Courtesy from LensAR Inc., Winter Park, FL

surgical theater or within the OR itself. These devices are a little larger than a regular phacoemulsification device (**Figure 72.3**). After anesthesia with topical drops or a block, the docking system is applied. The imaging system then recognizes the position of all the intraocular structures. After confirming the data for perfect placement of all the corneal incisions, capsulotomy and nucleus fragmentation in a monitor, the surgeon authorizes the procedure. After the laser pulses are applied and the suction is off, the device is removed and surgery completed in a sterile OR with aspiration of the nucleus and IOL insertion.

PRIMARY INCISION

The primary incision and the paracentesis shape, size and location can be customized. The cutting geometry profile is limitless and the ideal incision shape is yet to be determined. The precision and reproducibility with this technology to perform incisions is unprecedented. Further studies are needed to prove if there is indeed less incision leaking and consequently less endophthalmitis compared to manual incisions. **Figures 72.4 to 72.6** show possible different wound architectures and a comparison between intend and the achieved cut as seen in an OCT postoperatively (**Figure 72.7**).

CAPSULOTOMY

A reproducible, centered and precisely sized and shaped capsulotomy is one of the obvious advantages of using a femtosecond laser in cataract surgery. Initial studies show a high accuracy and very low standard deviation in laser-

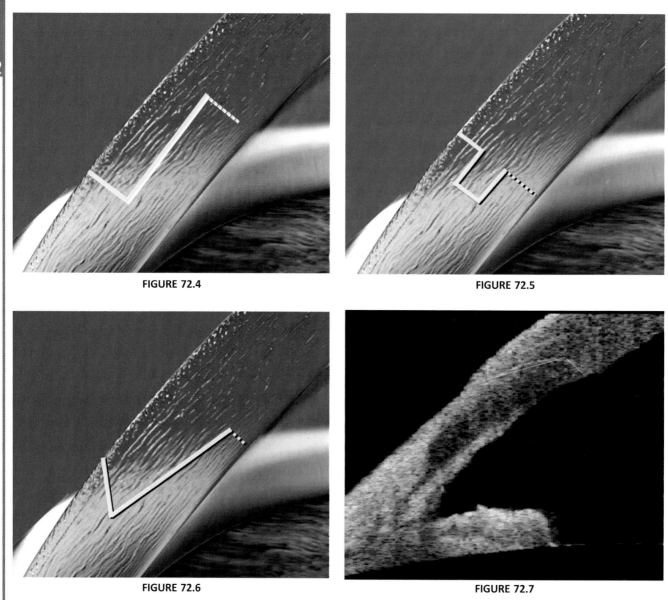

FIGURE 72.4

FIGURE 72.5

FIGURE 72.6

FIGURE 72.7

FIGURES 72.4 TO 72.7: Different incision shapes and sizes. The ideal pattern is not yet determined. An OCT image **(Figure 72.7)** showing the cut as it was programmed (*Courtesy:* OptiMedica Corporation, Santa Clara, CA)

performed capsulotomies (for an intended diameter capsulotomy of 5 mm, the average achieved was 5.88+/- 0.73 mm with the manual technique and 5.02+/-0.04 mm in the laser treated group),[9] with the same or better strength resistance compared to the manual technique.[9] A well-sized and centered capsulotomy **(Figure 72.8)** is crucial for IOL centration, which assumes great importance when accommodating and multifocal IOLs are implanted. The precision in achieving the desired capsulotomy size is much greater, and less variable than in manual techniques. A recent study (Slade SG et al., unpublished data) implanting the first 50 accommodating IOLs assisted by a femtosecond laser shows better IOL-capsule overlap and reduced variability in effective lens position, as well as less induced coma and astigmatism than found after manual capsulotomies. Besides the superior results in comparison to a successful manual capsulotomy, a poorly executed capsulorhexis can lead to posterior capsule rupture, increase

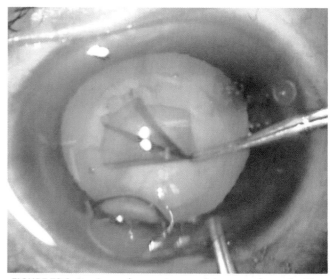

FIGURE 72.8: Precise and accurate capsulotomy performed with a femtosecond laser (*Courtesy:* LensAR Inc., Winter Park, FL)

the rate of capsular phimosis and reduce safety in the further steps of the surgery.

NUCLEUS FRAGMENTATION

The fragmentation of the nucleus is one of the most important steps in cataract surgery. Two main factors must be considered: energy applied to the endothelium and safety. The femtosecond laser causes very little damage in the surrounding tissue, extending to no more than 100 μm from the desired focus of the beam (very far from the endothelium, which is likely unaffected). However, the femtosecond laser is a cutting device that can only fracture and soften the lens to a point, with phaco energy still being needed to emulsify the nucleus in some cases (only irrigation and aspiration is possible in softer lenses). The reduction in ultrasound energy is greater in softer nuclei, but even in hard ones a decrease in total amount of energy used is observed.[9] Several different patterns (cubes, crosses, circles and many other shapes, **Figure 72.9)** of nucleus disassembly are being studied to determine which is most effective. The cube pattern has been shown to be one of easiest to aspirate with lower phaco energy **(Figures 72.10**

and 72.11) However, it is possible that different patterns and combinations would be optimal for different densities of nuclear sclerosis.

The safety concerns with femtosecond lasers are primarily related to displacement of the laser pulses, which can damage the posterior capsule. As such, it is important to program a safety zone, or "buffer" between the lens tissue targeted for photodisruption and the posterior capsule. The profiles of fragmentation are using a safe distance of about 300–500 μm from the capsule.

ASTIGMATIC CORRECTION

After the introduction of small incision cataract surgery and premium IOLs, residual astigmatism became problematic, as "left over" cylinder would often lead to a reduction in unaided postoperative visual acuity. Four main options are currently available for the treatment of astigmatism: excimer laser photoablation, manual limbal relaxing incisions, astigmatic keratotomy and toric IOLs.

In a cataract surgery patient, excimer photoablation of residual astigmatism necessitates a separate procedure.

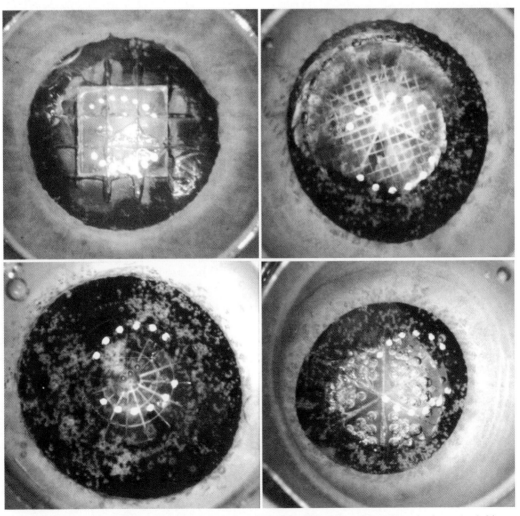

FIGURE 72.9: Four different profiles of laser pulses to fragment the nucleus. The cube (superior left) is the most used pattern (*Courtesy:* LensAR Inc., Winter Park, FL)

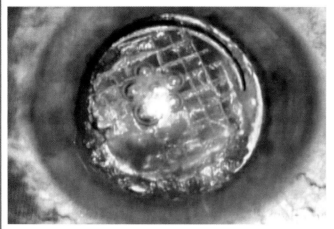

FIGURE 72.10: The cube pattern in a softer lens (*Courtesy:* LensAR Inc., Winter Park, FL)

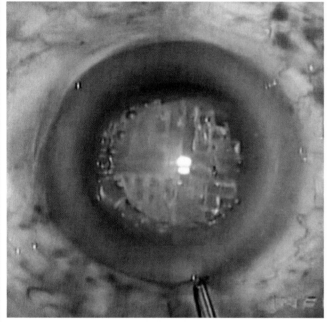

FIGURE 72.11: Nucleus fragmentation in a harder crystalline lens with the Optimedica system (*Courtesy:* OptiMedica Corporation, Santa Clara, CA)

Also, nonorthogonal astigmatism cannot be treated with astigmatic excimer laser photoablation, and topographic customization is not currently available in United States.

The rotational stability of toric IOLs has improved in the last decade, with current models showing excellent results. Thus, they are often the procedure of choice for correcting astigmatism in a cataract patient, and visual results are superior when compared to manual limbal relaxing incisions.[10] However, at the present time, the placement of a toric IOL is not possible when using a multifocal or accommodative implant.

Manual limbal relaxing incisions have been used successfully to correct low-grade astigmatism (less than 1.5 diopters) during cataract surgery.[11] However, one must be aware of the lack of length, depth and orientation precision during manual incision placement.

Astigmatic keratotomy (AK) has been widely performed during the radial keratotomy era, but because of resultant irregular astigmatism, instability and imprecision, it was essentially abandoned, except for high postkeratoplasty astigmatism.[12]

Initial studies of femtosecond laser- assisted astigmatism correction have begun with promising results.[13,14] In higher degrees of astigmatism (postkeratoplasty and high naturally occurring astigmatism), laser astigmatic keratotomy is effective, while among lower astigmatic eyes; limbal relaxing incisions seem best **(Figure 72.12)**. The results for high postkeratoplasty astigmatism shows greater accuracy and less complication compared to manual techniques.[15]

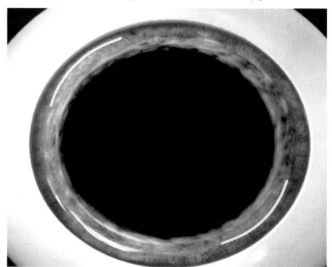

FIGURE 72.12: Limbal relaxing incisions can be customized in a micron precision (*Courtesy:* OptiMedica Corporation, Santa Clara, CA)

Besides the precision involved in a laser incision compared to manual limbal relaxing incisions, another great advantage of using femtosecond laser-assisted astigmatic incision compared to excimer laser photoablation in cataract patients is that there would be just one procedure. In addition, femtosecond lasers can create intrastromal only astigmatic incisions. Although these are expected to be less effective, they may prove to be safer and more stable because Bowman's layer remains intact; however, these benefits need to be proven through further clinical studies.

The precision of femtosecond laser technology for creation of corneal incisions remains a nascent technology, and still awaits the development of nomograms to allow routine and accurate correction of astigmatism. Also, precise imaging systems and flexible geometric cutting profiles will be required for a better placement of the incisions.[16] This technology is still evolving and advanced refinements are currently being developed in the newer generation femtosecond laser cataract surgery devices.

COMPLICATIONS, RISKS AND LIMITATIONS

Since the technology is new, there are no complications reported up to date. The major risks involved in the surgery are loss of suction during the procedure and displacement of the laser pulses. This can lead to posterior capsular rupture and, in an eye with increased pressure due to suction, potentially migration of nucleus fragments into the vitreous. Displaced laser pulses could also damage the iris, causing hemorrhage in the anterior segment, or damage the corneal endothelium. Irregular astigmatism could also occur with displaced limbal relaxing incisions.

Complex cataract cases, such as those with very opaque nuclei, corneal opacity or edema, conjunctival bleb due to previous filtration surgery and poor iris dilation are the contraindications for the procedure. The laser cannot penetrate well into an opaque cornea, which may lead to irregular cuts. Very hard nuclei can be challenging, because higher energy must be applied to obtain the fracture and, due to light scattering, energy delivery to the posterior part of the nucleus would not be ideal. Previous filtration blebs can prevent conjunctival docking and bleb rupture with extrusion of intraocular contents could result. However, the most common contraindication will be poor iris dilation. The risk of iris hemorrhage, imprecise or small capsulotomy, poor nucleus fragmentation and the need to surgically dilate the pupil (rings or hooks) will mandate the conversion to the conventional phacoemulsification when poor dilation is present.

ECONOMICS

Despite all the advantages of the femtosecond laser in cataract surgery, such as increased precision, reproducibility and safety, the major disadvantage at this time is the increased cost. Expenses may increase for both cost per case (i.e. cost of laser and related disposables) and increased surgical time, which, will in the short-term, reduce the number of cases that a surgeon or OR can perform on any given day. Economic considerations may initially limit access to these devices to large volume cataract surgery centers. Nevertheless, in the long run, as was true for phacoemulsification and all-laser LASIK surgery, improved results will ultimately drive the acceptance (or rejection) of Femtosecond laser cataract technology.

CONCLUSION AND FUTURE

The surgical precision offered by Femtosecond lasers promises a safer and more predictable cataract surgery, and could be responsible for the most important evolution since the transition to phacoemulsification. The first result shows a more reproducible and stronger capsulotomy, excellent incision architecture[17] (less leakage and less potential endophthalmitis), and less ultrasound energy used (less potential endothelial damage).[9]

The enhanced safety and predictability can improve outcomes, especially with premium IOLs, which depend on a regular, well-centered capsulotomy and minimum residual corneal astigmatism. These can lead to an expansion of the indications of refractive lens exchange and limbal relaxing incisions, bringing the revolution not only to cataract surgery but also in the refractive surgery area.

Future research with the Femtosecond laser technology will focus on enhancing the concept of these systems as precise intraocular cutting tools, determining the best nomograms for relaxing incisions, the best architecture for cataract incisions, capsulotomy and the ideal energy parameters for each of these steps and circumstances.

REFERENCES

1. Belazzougui R, Monod SD, Baudouin C, et al. Architectural analysis of clear corneal incisions using Visante OCT in acute postoperative endophthalmitis. Journal Français d'ophtalmologie. 2010;33(1):10-5.
2. Oner FH, Durak I, Soylev M, et al. Long-term results of various anterior capsulotomies and radial tears on intraocular lens centration. Ophthalmic Surgery and Lasers. 32(2):118-23.
3. Ernest P, Rhem M, McDermott M, et al. Phacoemulsification conditions resulting in thermal wound injury. Journal of Cataract and Refractive Surgery. 2001;27(11):1829-39.
4. Liu Y, Nakamura H, Witt TE, et al. Femtosecond laser photodisruption of porcine anterior chamber angle: an ex vivo study. Ophthalmic surgery, lasers & imaging. 2008;39(6):485-90.
5. Hild M, Krause M, Riemann I, et al. Femtosecond laser-assisted retinal imaging and ablation: experimental pilot study. Current eye research. 2008;33(4):351-63.
6. Choi SK, Kim JH, Lee D, et al. A New Surgical Technique: A Femtosecond Laser-Assisted Keratolimbal Allograft Procedure. Cornea. 2010;29(8):924-9.
7. Faktorovich E. Femtodynamics. First Edition. Thorofare, NJ - USA: Slack Incorporated; 2009.
8. Vogel A, Busch S, Jungnickel K, et al. Mechanisms of intraocular photodisruption with picosecond and nanosecond laser pulses. Lasers in Surgery and Medicine. 1994;15(1):32-43.
9. Nagy Z, Takacs A, Filkorn T, et al. Initial clinical evaluation of an intraocular femtosecond laser in cataract surgery. Journal of Refractive Surgery. 2009;25(12):1053-60.
10. Mendicute J, Irigoyen C, Ruiz M, et al. Toric intraocular lens versus opposite clear corneal incisions to correct astigmatism in eyes having cataract surgery. Journal of Cataract and Refractive Surgery. 2009;35(3):451-8.
11. Carvalho MJ, Suzuki SH, Freitas LL et al. Limbal relaxing incisions to correct corneal astigmatism during phacoemulsification. Journal of Refractive Surgery. 2007;23(5):499-504.
12. Poole TR, Ficker LA. Astigmatic keratotomy for post-keratoplasty astigmatism. Journal of Cataract and Refractive Surgery. 2006;32(7):1175-9.
13. Nubile M, Carpineto P, Lanzini M, et al. Femtosecond Laser Arcuate Keratotomy for the Correction of High Astigmatism after Keratoplasty. Ophthalmology. 2009;116(6):1083-92.
14. Abbey A, Ide T, Kymionis GD, et al. Femtosecond laser-assisted astigmatic keratotomy in naturally occurring high astigmatism. British Journal Ophthalmology. 2009;93:1566-9.
15. Kymionis GD, Yoo SH, Ide T, et al. Femtosecond-assisted astigmatic keratotomy for post-keratoplasty irregular astigmatism. Journal of Cataract and Refractive Surgery. 2009; 35(1):11-3.
16. Kumar NL, Kaiserman I, Shehadeh-Mashor R, et al. IntraLase-enabled astigmatic keratotomy for post-keratoplasty astigmatism: on-axis vector analysis. Ophthalmology. 2010;117(6):1228-35.e1.
17. Masket S, Sarayba M, Ignacio T, et al. Femtosecond laser-assisted cataract incisions: architectural stability and reproducibility. Journal of Cataract and Refractive Surgery. 2010;36(6):1048-9.

CHAPTER 73

Use of High-Definition 3D Visual Systems in Cataract Surgery

Robert J Weinstock

One of the most exciting and dynamic aspects of the practice of ophthalmology is the prospect to continually be exposed to new and improving technology. Whether it is diagnostic devices, surgical instruments or lasers, ophthalmic surgeons around the world are able to relentlessly improve the way they practice by incorporating novel devices into their armamentarium. Advancements in microscope technology have allowed surgeons to perform better and safer microscopic surgery throughout the years but recently there have been minimal changes. Three years ago, however, a high-definition 3D camera designed to attach to a surgical microscope via a binocular beam splitter was introduced to the ophthalmic and neurosurgical communities. This unique camera allows the surgeon to view the surgical field by looking at a 3D flat panel display, rather than through the oculars, in the same manner employed by endoscopic surgeons, with the notable exception that the view is three dimensional instead of two. TrueVision Systems, Inc. in Santa Barbara, California, has developed and continues to improve upon this novel 3D system.

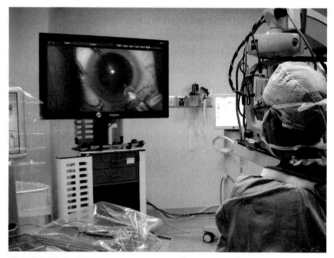

FIGURE 73.1: Cataract surgery is performed easily and comfortably by looking at the 3D display

THE TRUEVISION® 3D HD SYSTEM

This, as shown in **Figures 73.1 and 73.2**, consists of:
- A high-definition 3D camera which attaches to the surgical microscope
- A computer that processes the digital information and image fusion
- A high-definition 3D flat panel video monitor.

The whole system is designed to fit easily in a standard operating room. The latest design incorporates a mobile cart for the 3D flat panel and computer. The 3D camera easily attaches to a binocular beam splitter and does not hinder the surgeon from looking through the oculars if desired. There is a wireless keypad designed to be used by the operating room staff to enter text and manipulate a 3D mouse to control the software. For complete stereopsis and proper depth perception while using the 3D system, the surgeon must wear a pair of specially polarized 3D glasses. For improved contrast resolution and clarity it is helpful to turn off the overhead lights as well. The learning curve is surprisingly rapid when using the heads-up system. Usually, it takes only 2–3 days of experience with the system before a surgeon becomes fully comfortable operating by looking

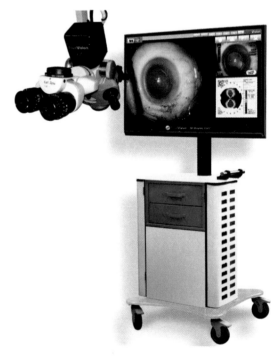

FIGURE 73.2: The 3D camera attaches to surgical microscopes that connect to an intelligent image processing unit in the 3D display cart

at the screen instead of through the microscope's oculars. Since there is a binocular beam splitter, the surgeon still has the opportunity to look through the oculars at any time and easily move back and forth between the two.

THE TRUEVISION® CATARACT AND REFRACTIVE TOOLSET SOFTWARE

TrueVision Systems has also been working on software, pending FDA approval, most notable is a cataract and refractive toolset designed to help guide the surgeon for certain delicate maneuvers during cataract surgery, such as capsulorhexis formation, limbal relaxing incision formation and toric IOL rotational positioning. The TrueVision® Cataract and Refractive Toolset software has a built in eye tracker which allows the use of computer graphics templates to show a surgeon where to perform certain surgical maneuvers. For example, the capsulorhexis software is designed to place a capsulorhexis template of a specific size over the image of the eye on the screen. The surgeon can then use this template to guide the shape and size of the

capsulorhexis **(Figure 73.3)**. This will become increasingly important as premium intraocular lens surgery becomes more commonplace.

Another application is the limbal relaxing incision (LRI) software, designed to take preoperative data and place templates of limbal relaxing incision arcs on the screen overlying the corneal limbus in the proper axis, orientation and length. The software incorporates surgeon tailored, built-in nomograms and pre-specified surgically induced astigmatism to calculate in real-time the optimal LRI arc shape. The built in tracking system keeps these templates in the proper position on the eye, while the surgeon uses the templates to make the necessary incisions **(Figure 73.4)**. Retrospective analysis of LRIs using these templates compared to standard techniques revealed improved results and less residual astigmatism when using the software.

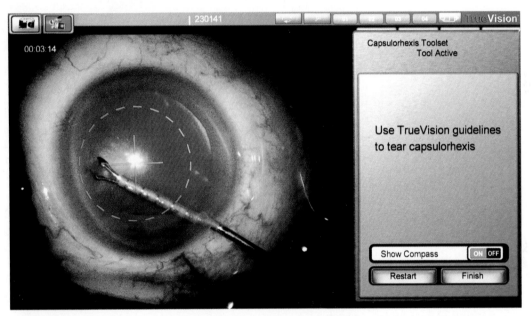

FIGURE 73.3: 3D capsulorhexis template on the 3D display is used to guide the surgical maneuver

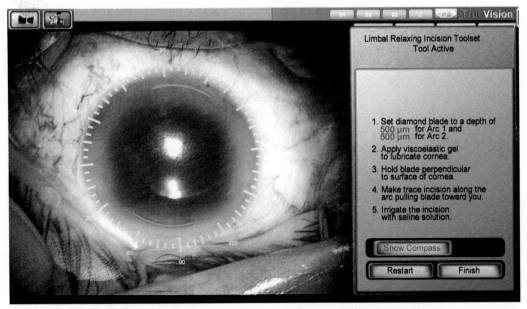

FIGURE 73.4: LRI template on the 3D display guides astigmatism correction

These are just the first of many software applications that the TrueVision 3D system will be able to provide to cataract surgeons and other microsurgery specialists. Software is presently being developed to provide the surgeon with auditory or visual clues, as to where an instrument is inside the eye. For instance, how deep a phaco tip is, and whether or not it is approaching a vital structure such as the endothelium or posterior capsule. In addition, the engineers at TrueVision are exploring different filters that can be applied to the digital image to help improve the view and highlight certain tissue structures which will guide and aid in the surgical removal of cataracts making it a safer procedure. Applications for retina surgery, glaucoma surgery and other specialties are also underway.

SITTING POSITION

One of the greatest benefits for the surgeon in using the TrueVision® system is the ability to sit back in a comfortable, natural position to operate. No longer is there a need to put the surgeon's stool too high or too low to accommodate the patient's bed or surgical microscope position. In addition, the surgeon is not required to lean forward and bend his neck to look through the oculars (**Figure 73.5**). Studies have shown that at least half of all microscopic surgeons suffer from chronic back and neck pain. One of the most significant benefits of this technology is the ability to reduce or eliminate that risk. Obviously, if a surgeon is sitting in a comfortable position, he or she is likely to perform better surgery with fewer complications. Technologically improved ergonomics may also work their way into the clinic where physicians will have the ability to look at a 3D screen on a desk instead of having to bend forward and look through the slit lamp.

TEACHING

A compeling advantage of the TrueVision® 3D system is the ability of all the personnel in the operating room (as well as visiting surgeons or residents in training) to be able to view the surgical field in 3D, in real-time, and have the same view that the surgeon does. The operating room staff is able to anticipate the needs of the surgeon because they are able to see exactly what the surgeon is doing. This can translate into quicker, more efficient surgery and less time spent waiting for the appropriate instrument. The staff is more in tune with the surgical procedure and is better able to anticipate the surgeon's needs. In addition, The author has experienced a tremendous advantage in teaching not only other surgeons, fellows and residents but also for ophthalmic personnel of all types. Engineers from implant manufacturing and phaco companies have found it extremely helpful to watch cataract surgery in 3D.

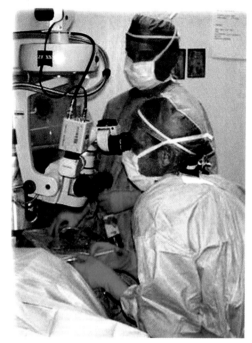

FIGURE 73.5: A Surgeon taking an awkward position in order to see through the oculars of a conventional microscope

They develop a much greater appreciation for the dynamics of the implants and instruments and how they behave inside the eye. Training surgeons by watching live 3D surgery is requisite for the future of ophthalmology.

Another valuable feature of the TrueVision® 3D camera and display system is the ability to not only view live 3D surgery on the screen but also to record the surgery in 3D for future legal and educational value. Over the past several years some surgeons have been recording interesting and unique cases in 3D and showing them (in 3D) at national meetings. Another interesting application is the ability to use the 3D format to provide patient education.

CONCLUSION

In conclusion, these are just a few of the many applications for 3D high definition operative displays. Ophthalmology is not the only specialty which will benefit from these early stages of the technology. Neurosurgeons and otolaryngology surgeons are also beginning to see the benefits of operating in a heads-up fashion where collaboration, ergonomics, visual display, computer graphics and digital overlays can tremendously improve the way surgery is performed. One has only experienced the very early benefits of these systems to date. Based on the continued trend towards minimally invasive surgery, digital integration, and software applications in the operating room, it seems clear that this technology will continue to make its way into the microscopic surgeon's hands.

CHAPTER 74

A New Sulcus Implanted Mirror Telescopic IOL for Age-related Macular Diseases and Other Macular Disorders: The LMI-SI (ORILENS©)

Soosan Jacob, Issac Lipshitz, Amar Agarwal

INTRODUCTION

With an aging population and with the increased longevity that modern medicine has made possible, there is an increasing population of cataract patients with other associated eye diseases such as AMD, diabetes, etc. thus presenting to the eye surgeon with a complex situation. The difficulties that comorbid pathologies induce are being experienced by surgeons all over the world. The prevalence of AMD in Asia has been found to be similar to that in Caucasian populations and has been variously reported as ranging from 1.4 to 12.7% for early AMD and 0.2 to 1.9% for late AMD. The presence of cortical cataract and prior cataract surgery are significantly associated with increased prevalence of AMD showing that these age related conditions often co-exist.

Dry AMD constitutes 85–90% of AMD patients and most of these patients have no medical treatment at all, other than vitamins and anti-oxidants. These patients can be treated only with optical means. Amongst the wet AMD, only 10-15% can be assisted by medical treatment and these go on to become the dry types, who then again need to be visually rehabilitated.

The important factor to realize here is that despite performing cataract surgery successfully in these patients, they do not benefit as much visually because of the co-existing retinal pathology. There is therefore, a significant difference between treating the disease pathology with medical management/ lasers/ cataract surgery and with being able to successfully rehabilitate the patient visually. Visual benefits from treatment are after all what actually affects the quality of life of the patient and what is meaningful to the patient.

LMI-SI (ORILENS©)

Cataract surgery *per se* is not a problem in eyes with AMD but lack of post-op visual improvement is definitely a cause of concern. One of us (Dr Isaac Lipshitz) designed the LMI-SI (OriLens©) which is a telescopic lens working on the principle of using mirrors to magnify the central image while the peripheral field remains normal. The LMI is designed so that it is positioned in the sulcus over a regular

bag implanted IOL. It is a telescopic IOL that is designed to magnify the image on the central retina. It looks like a regular PMMA IOL and is 5.00–6.00 mm in diameter (loop diameter is 13.50 mm), and it contains loops that have a similar configuration as a regular IOL. The only significant difference compared to a regular IOL is its central thickness. The LMI is thicker (central thickness of 1.25 mm, which is higher thickness than a normal IOL). The first worldwide implantation of this lens was done by one of us (Prof Amar Agarwal).

PREOPERATIVE EVALUATION

Preoperatively, as soon as a patient with AMD comes, a full medical eye examination including slit lamp for evaluation of the cornea, iris, anterior chamber, lens and vitreous are done. A thorough retinal examination is done including Fundus Fluorescein Angiography and Optical Coherence Tomography and the IOP is checked.

The distance and near visual acuity are checked in each eye separately using the ETDRS chart with best correction. The best corrected, distance and near visual acuity with x2.5 external telescope is again checked using the ETDRS chart. If a patient shows improvement with the external telescope, he/she is a good candidate for the LMI-SI (OriLens©). A cycloplegic refraction is also done. Specular microscopy is done for endothelial cell count. A-scan is done for anterior chamber depth and IOL calculations. Keratometric readings are taken with the keratometer or with corneal topography.

SURGERY FOR IMPLANTING THE LMI-SI (ORILENS©)

Intraoperatively, anesthesia is given according to the surgeon's preference. A corneal or limbal incision may be used and the size of the incision is made according to the surgical technique used. If the eye is phakic, a routine phaco or ECCE procedure is performed and the IOL (power calculated according to biometry) planned for the patient is inserted into the capsular bag. The incision is then enlarged to 5.00–5.50 mm. The anterior chamber is filled

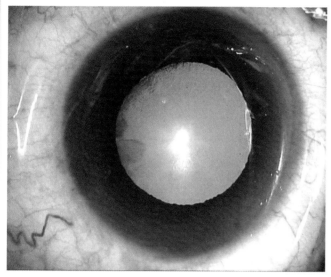

FIGURES 74.1A: Patient with cataract and AMD

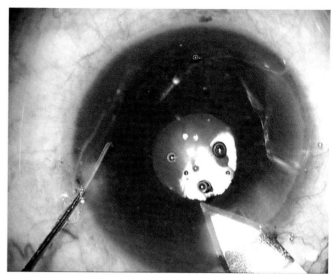

FIGURE 74.1B: A conventional foldable IOL in the bag after performing cataract surgery

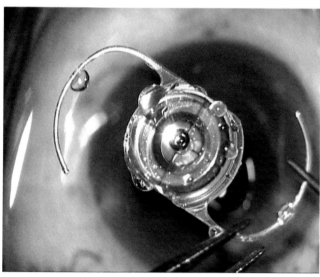

FIGURE 74.2: The LMI-SI (OriLens©) is seen

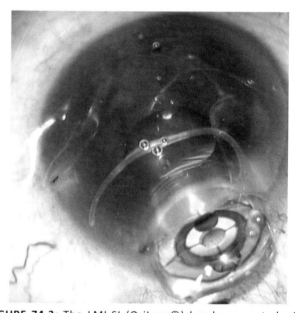

FIGURE 74.3: The LMI-SI (OriLens©) has been coated with viscoelastic and inserted through the clear corneal incision which has been extended just enough to allow implantation

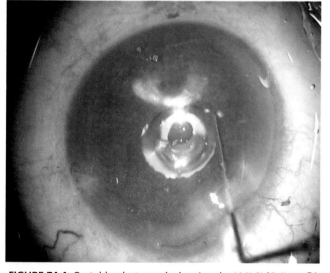

FIGURE 74.4: On table photograph showing the LMI-SI (OriLens©) well centered with a clear cornea

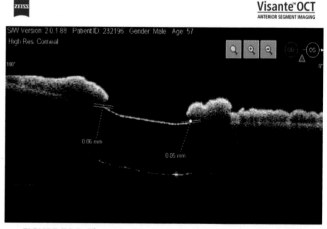

FIGURE 74.5: The anterior segment OCT showing the LMI-SI (OriLens©) in the sulcus above the bag implanted IOL

PHACOEMULSIFICATION

with viscoelastic and the implant is also coated with viscoelastic. It is then grasped by the loops or the base of the loop, taking care not to touch the lens optic itself. It is inserted into the sulcus as a piggy-back IOL with the posterior mirror (ring shaped) pointing towards the surgeon. It is confirmed that the pupil on the operated eye is central. In case of an eccentric pupil, a pupilloplasty may be needed. A peripheral iridectomy is then done surgically (Yag laser should not be used). All the viscoelastic is removed and the incision is sutured.

Postoperative care is similar to that of a regular cataract extraction except that a closer watch is kept for anterior synechiae and IOP spike. Post-op tests are carried out at days 1, 2, 7, 30, 3 months, 6 months and 12 months. The centration and position of the lens are checked for and the patient is refracted for distance and near uncorrected and best corrected visual acuity using ETDRS (each eye separately). Postoperative specular microscopy is done.

RESULTS

The initial outcomes are encouraging and a trial with larger number of patients recruited and a longer follow up is being planned. Proper patient recruitment is a key factor in ensuring good outcomes as in every other case. The inclusion criteria for our pilot trial of the LMI-SI (OriLens©) included patients with bilateral AMD (dry type, wet type, scar stage) or other similar macular lesions where the visual acuity ranged between 20/60 to 20/600 in each eye and improved for distance and/or near when tested with a X2.5 magnification using an external telescope. Presence of any other systemic or ocular diseases (other than cataract/ pseudophakia, AMD or another macular lesion) excluded them as also any other previous eye surgery other than cataract. Only those patients who were easy to communicate with, responsible and understood his/her condition, who knew the risks and potential benefits involved and who were highly motivated to read and improve visual capabilities were included. It was made sure that they understood that they would have to be available for follow up of one-year post-op. All the patients signed an informed consent. All other patients were excluded as also those patients where

the fellow eye suffers from medical problems, which would not enable the patient to use his peripheral vision, eg. those with glaucoma or retinitis pigmentosa.

ADVANTAGES OF THE LMI-SI

The advantages that the LMI-SI (OriLens©) offers as compared to other available intraocular telescopic devices are many. It can be implanted in both eyes and it is surgeon friendly. It is a simple and safe surgery and can be performed by any cataract surgeon. It does not lie close to the corneal endothelium and hence chances of damage to the corneal endothelium are very low. It also offers a quick recovery for the patients who do not need prolonged and complicated postoperative training sessions for visual rehabilitation. It preserves part of the peripheral vision while magnifying the central field. It is also complementary to all other retinal treatments (injections, lasers, etc.) and can also be used for other retinal diseases.

Another big advantage of this IOL is the fact that it is placed in the sulcus over another IOL. As we know, a large majority of AMD patients may have already undergone cataract surgery with IOL implantation before presenting to the treating doctor. In such a case, it is still possible to offer the patient the opportunity of visual rehabilitation without having to undergo a complicated procedure such as explantation of the existing IOL and reimplantation of another telescopic device. As the LMI-SI (OriLens©) can be easily placed in the sulcus, surgery is simple and it is also a-one-lens-fits-all situation as the previously placed IOL in the bag takes care of the refractive error of the patient. Hence the same LMI-SI (OriLens©) can be offered to all patients irrespective of the biometric calculation of IOL power.

FINANCIAL DISCLOSURES

Isaac Lipshitz has a financial interest in the LMI-SI (OriLens©). None of the other authors have any financial interests relevant to the products or procedures mentioned here.

Index

(The letter f after page number in the index denotes Figure and t denotes Table)